Diagnostic Immunohistochemistry

David J. Dabbs, MD
Professor of Pathology
University of Pittsburgh School of Medicine
Director of Anatomic Pathology
Magee-Women's Hospital
Pittsburgh, Pennsylvania

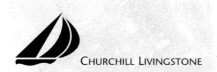

CHURCHILL LIVINGSTONE

An Imprint of Elsevier Science
New York   Edinburgh   London   Philadelphia

CHURCHILL LIVINGSTONE
An Imprint of Elsevier Science

The Curtis Center
Independence Square West
Philadelphia, Pennsylvania 19106

Library of Congress Cataloging-in-Publication Data

Dabbs, David J.
Diagnostic immunohistochemistry / David J. Dabbs

    p. : cm.

Includes bibliographical references and index.

ISBN 0–443–06566–7

1. Diagnostic immunohistochemistry.
   [DNLM: 1. Immunohistochemistry—methods.   2. Diagnostic Techniques
and Procedures.   3. Neoplasms—diagnosis.   QY 250 D111d 2002]   I.
Title.

RB46.6 .D33 2002

616.07'583—dc21   2001042148

Editor-in-Chief: Richard Zorab
Acquisitions Editor: Marc Strauss
Manuscript Editor: Jodi Kaye
Production Manager: Peter Faber
Illustration Specialist: Peg Shaw
Book Designer: Steven Stave
Illustrator: Esteban Cabrera

DIAGNOSTIC IMMUNOHISTOCHEMISTRY   ISBN 0–443–06566–7

Printed in China

Last digit is the print number: 9   8   7   6   5   4

To Kirstie Anne, the most amazing person that I have the pleasure to know.

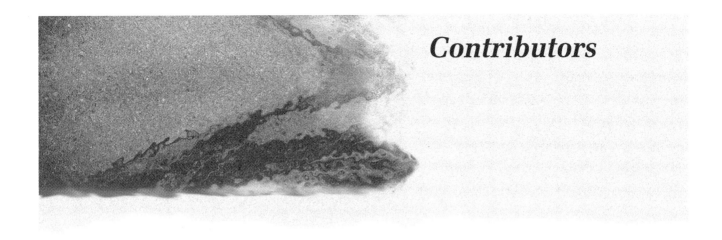

Contributors

Nancy J. Barr, MD
Keck School of Medicine, University of Southern
California, Los Angeles, California
*Techniques of Immunohistochemistry: Principles,
Pitfalls, and Standardization*

Deborah Belchis, MD
Assistant Professor of Pathology, Penn State
University College of Medicine, Hershey,
Pennsylvania
*Diagnostic Immunohistochemistry of Pediatric Small
Round Cell Tumors*

David G. Bostwick, MD, MBA
Clinical Professor of Pathology, University of
Virginia School of Medicine, Charlottesville,
Virginia; Medical Director, Bostwick
Laboratories, Richmond, Virginia
*Immunohistochemistry of the Prostate and Bladder,
Testis, and Renal Tumors*

Lisa A. Cerilli, MD
Assistant Professor of Pathology, University of
Virginia School of Medicine, Charlottesville,
Virginia
*Immunohistology of Soft Tissue and Osseous
Neoplasms*

David J. Dabbs, MD
Professor of Pathology, University of Pittsburgh
School of Medicine, Pittsburgh, Pennsylvania;
Director of Anatomic Pathology, Magee-Women's
Hospital, Pittsburgh, Pennsylvania
*Carcinomatous Differentiation and Metastatic
Carcinoma of Unknown Primary; Diagnostic
Immunohistochemistry of the Breast; Immunocytology*

Ronald A. DeLellis, MD
Professor of Pathology, Weill Medical College of
Cornell University; Vice Chairman for Anatomic
Pathology, New York Presbyterian Hospital, New
York, New York
*Diagnostic Immunohistochemistry of Endocrine
Tumors*

Eduardo J. Eyzaguirre, MD
Assistant Professor, Department of Pathology,
University of Texas Medical Branch at
Galveston; Surgical Pathologist, John Sealy
Hospital, Galveston, Texas
Immunohistochemistry of Infectious Diseases

Christopher D. Gocke, MD
Associate Professor, Department of Pathology,
University of Maryland, Baltimore, Maryland
Non-Hodgkin's Lymphoma

Neal S. Goldstein, MD
Staff Anatomic Pathologist, Department of
Anatomic Pathology, William Beaumont
Hospital, Royal Oak, Michigan
*Immunohistochemistry of the Gastrointestinal Tract,
Pancreas, Bile Ducts, Gallbladder, and Liver*

Samuel P. Hammar, MD
Clinical Professor of Environmental Sciences,
University of Washington School of Medicine,
Seattle, Washington; Pathologist and Director,
Diagnostic Specialties Laboratory, Harrison
Memorial Hospital, Bremerton, Washington
Lung and Pleural Neoplasms

Klaus F. Helm, MD
Associate Professor of Dermatology and Pathology,
Penn State Milton S. Hershey Medical Center,
Hershey, Pennsylvania
Immunohistochemistry of Skin Tumors

Christina Isacson, MD
Pathologist, Virginia Mason Medical Center,
Seattle, Washington
*Diagnostic Immunohistochemistry of the Female
Genital Tract*

Marshall E. Kadin, MD
Associate Professor of Pathology, Harvard Medical
School; Director of Hematopathology, Beth Israel
Deaconess Medical Center, Boston, Massachusetts
Hodgkin's Lymphoma

v

Paul E. McKeever, MD, PhD
Professor of Pathology, University of Michigan
  Medical School; Chief, Neuropathology Service,
  University of Michigan Medical Center, Ann
  Arbor, Michigan
Immunohistochemistry of the Nervous System

Junqi Qian, MD
Director of Molecular Diagnostics, Bostwick
  Laboratories, Richmond, Virginina
*Immunohistochemistry of the Prostate and Bladder,
Testis, and Renal Tumors*

Stephen S. Raab, MD
Associate Professor of Pathology and Laboratory
  Medicine, MCP Hahneman University, School of
  Medicine, Philadelphia, Pennsylvania; Director
  of Cytology and Outcomes Research, Allegheny
  General Hospital, Pittsburgh, Pennsylvania
Cost-Effectiveness of Immunohistochemistry

Dharamdas M. Ramnani, MD
Medical Director, Virginia Urology Center
  Laboratory, Richmond, Virginia
*Immunohistochemistry of the Prostate and Bladder,
Testis, and Renal Tumors*

Shan-Rong Shi, MD
Keck School of Medicine, University of Southern
  California, Los Angeles, California
*Techniques of Immunohistochemistry: Principles,
Pitfalls, and Standardization*

Sandra J. Shin, MD
Professor of Pathology, Weill Medical College of
  Cornell University; Attending Pathologist, New
  York Presbyterian Hospital, New York, New York
*Diagnostic Immunohistochemistry of Endocrine
Tumors*

Jan F. Silverman, MD
Professor and Chair, Department of Pathology and
  Laboratory Medicine, Allegheny General
  Hospital, Pittsburgh, Pennsylvania
*Immunohistochemistry of the Gastrointestinal Tract,
Pancreas, Bile Ducts, Gallbladder, and Liver*

Robert A. Soslow, MD
Associate Professor of Pathology, Weill Medical
  College of Cornell University; Associate
  Attending Pathologist, Memorial Sloan-Kettering
  Cancer Center, New York, New York
*Diagnostic Immunohistochemistry of the Female
Genital Tract*

Michael W. Stanley, MD
Chief, Department of Pathology, Hennepin County
  Medical Center, Minneapolis, Minnesota
*Head and Neck, Ear, Salivary Gland, Larynx, and
Trachea*

Clive R. Taylor, MD, PhD
Professor and Chair, Department of Pathology,
  Keck School of Medicine, University of Southern
  California, Los Angeles, California
*Techniques of Immunohistochemistry: Principles,
Pitfalls, and Standardization*

David H. Walker, MD
Professor and Chair, Department of Pathology;
  Director, World Health Organization
  Collaborating Center for Tropical Diseases,
  University of Texas Medical Branch at
  Galveston, Galveston, Texas
Immunohistochemistry of Infectious Diseases

Mark R. Wick, MD
Professor of Pathology and Clinical Dermatology,
  University of Virginia Medical Center; Staff
  Pathologist, University of Virginia Medical
  Center, Charlottesville, Virginia
*Immunohistology of Soft Tissue and Osseous
Neoplasms; Immunohistology of the Mediastinum;
Immunohistologic Features of Melanocytic Neoplasms*

Nancy Wu, MD
Keck School of Medicine, University of Southern
  California, Los Angeles, California
*Techniques of Immunohistochemistry: Principles,
Pitfalls, and Standardization*

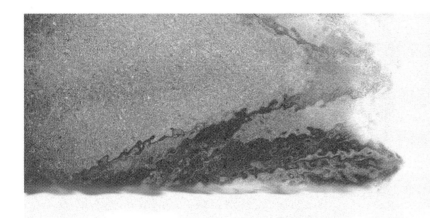

Foreword

Many are the "special" techniques that pathologists have used over the years to confirm, complement, and refine the information they were able to obtain with their "old faithful" armamentarium, that is, formalin fixation, paraffin embedding, and hematoxylin-eosin staining. These techniques have come and gone, their usual life cycle beginning with an initial period of unrestrained enthusiasm turning to a phase of disappointment, and finally leading to a more sober and realistic assessment. Many of these methods have left a permanent mark on the practice of the profession, even if often it was not as deep or wide-ranging as initially touted. These techniques include special stains, tissue culture, electron microscopy, immunohistochemistry, and, of late, molecular biology methods, such as in situ hybridization and polymerase chain reaction (PCR). Much was expected of the first three, and infinitely more is anticipated of the last, but it is fair to say that as of today no special technique has influenced the way that pathology is practiced as profoundly as immunohistochemistry, or has come even close to it. I don't think it would be an exaggeration to speak of a revolution, particularly in the field of tumor pathology. Those of us who have lived through it certainly feel that way. The newer generations of pathologists who order so glibly an HMB-45 or a factor VIII stain to identify melanocytes and vascular endothelial cells, respectively, do not seem to have much feeling for the efforts one had to make to achieve that identification only a few years ago. The virtues of the technique are so apparent and numerous as to make it as close to perfect as any biologic method carried out in human tissue obtained under routine (which means under less than ideal) conditions can be: It is compatible with standard fixation and embedding procedures; it can be performed retrospectively in material that has been archived for years; it is remarkably sensitive and specific; it can be applied to virtually any immunogenic molecule; and it can be evaluated against the morphologic backgrounds with which pathologists have long been familiar.

As with many other breakthroughs in medicine, immunohistochemistry started with a brilliant yet disarmingly simple idea: to have antibodies bind the specific antigens being sought and to make those antibodies visible by hooking them to a fluorescent compound. All subsequent modifications, such as the use of nonfluorescent chromogens, the amplification of the reaction, and the unmasking of antigens, merely represented technical improvements, although certainly not ones to be minimized. It is because of these technical advances that the technique spread beyond the research laboratories and is now applied so pervasively in pathology laboratories throughout the world. Of course, like any other biologic technique, it has its drawbacks. Antigens once believed to be specific for a given cell type have later been found to be expressed by other tissues; cross-reactions may occur between unrelated antigens; nonspecific absorption of the antibody may supervene; entrapped non-neoplastic cells reacting for a particular marker may be misinterpreted as part of the tumor and, most treacherously, antigen may diffuse out of a normal cell and find its way inside an adjacent tumor cell. Any of these pitfalls may lead to a misinterpretation of the reaction and a misdiagnosis; worse, it may lead to a final mistaken diagnosis after an initially correct interpretation of the hematoxylin-stained slides. A good defense against this danger is a thorough knowledge of these pitfalls and how to avoid them. An even more important safeguard is a solid background in basic anatomic pathology to be able to question the validity of any unexpected immunohistochemical result, whether positive or negative. There is nothing more dangerous (or expensive) than a neophyte in pathology making diagnoses on the basis of immunohistochemical "profiles" in disregard of the cytoarchitectural features of the lesions. Alas, this is true of any other "special" technique applied for diagnostic purposes to human tissue, molecular biology being the latest and most blatant example. However, when applied selectively and judiciously, immunohistochemistry is a notably powerful tool, in addition to being refreshingly cost-effective. As a matter of fact, pathologists can no longer afford to do without it, one of the reasons being that failure to make a diagnosis because of the omission of a key immunohistochemical reaction may be regarded as grounds for a malpractice action.

Any listing of the virtues of immunohistochemistry would be incomplete if it did not include the visual pleasure derived from the examination of this material. I am only half kidding when making this remark. There is undoubtedly an aesthetic component to the practice of histology, as masters of the technique such as Pio del Rio Hortega and Pierre Masson used to say. It is sad that these superb artists of morphology left the scene without having had the opportunity to marvel at the beauty of a well-done immunohistochemical preparation, but let's not be carried away. Instead, let's enjoy this excellent book, edited by one of the experts in the application of the technique and with a superb group of contributors—a book that summarizes in a lucid and comprehensive fashion the current knowledge in the field, in terms of both the technical aspects and the practical applications. In addition to the considerable authority of all of the contributors, this publication benefits from perfect timing. Although further progress in the area is surely forthcoming, enough information has accumulated and settled to give most of the statements made in this book a sense of credibility and permanency. Last, but not least, the publisher's felicitous decision to reproduce all the immunohistochemical illustrations in color adds considerably to the attractiveness of this treatise, which is likely to remain the standard reference in the field for years to come.

Juan Rosai, MD
Milan, Italy

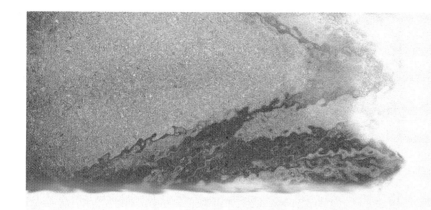

Preface

The challenge of creating *Diagnostic Immunohistochemistry* has been to bring some semblance of order to the vast body of knowledge of immunohistochemistry that has been published over the past decade. Diagnostic pathology will never be the same because of the profound contributions that immunohistochemistry has made to patient care. In reality, all of us in pathology are contributors to this continually growing body of knowledge, and herein lies the second challenge for this publication.

We realized that one of the potential pitfalls in creating *Diagnostic Immunohistochemistry* was to make sure that the base of knowledge in each chapter be relevant long after the ink has dried. The contributions of expert authors in each of their respective disciplines has helped to make this possible. Each chapter includes a base of time-tested knowledge and recent experience by an expert author.

The goal of this book is to provide a reference for pathologists who practice diagnostic surgical pathology and cytopathology. Each chapter is meant to be comprehensive in the diagnostic sense; this book was not meant to be encyclopedic of immunohistochemistry in general. The book is structured in the organ system approach to tumor pathology, and each chapter is capable of standing alone for the sake of reference convenience so that the user does not have to scour multiple places in the book to obtain useful diagnostic information. Inherent in this approach is redundancy of content, which not only is efficient for the user but also helps inculcate concepts that are useful, especially for the beginner.

David J. Dabbs, MD

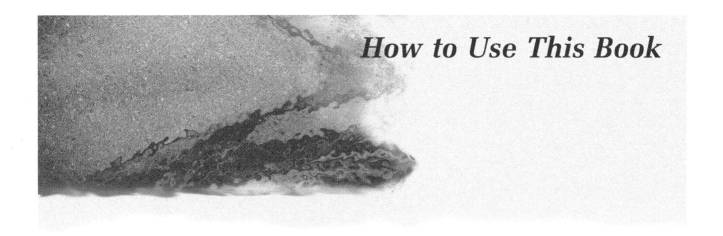

How to Use This Book

The first chapter includes data and modeling of the cost-effectiveness of the immunohistochemical test, and there are two chapters devoted to methods and techniques for surgical pathology and cytopathology. Immunohistochemical diagnosis of infectious diseases is dealt with in a separate chapter.

The remaining chapters deal primarily with tumor pathology using the organ system approach. Each chapter is organized to provide an introduction, the relevant antigens and antibodies and methods used in the study of that system, and a literature review of the subject matter. "Immuno-histograms" depicting immunostaining patterns of tumors, along with numerous tables, are structured for easy reference. Diagnostic algorithms for diagnosis are used where relevant, and many areas of the text are punctuated by summary "key diagnostic points," which may include diagnostic pitfalls. To maintain a constant terminology throughout the chapters, the following abbreviations in the text and tables are used: +, the result is always strongly, diffusely positive; +/−, most cases are strongly positive; −/+, most cases are negative; R, only rare cells may be positive; N, negative. The majority of the cited literature of immunohistochemical results and techniques is from the early 1990s on, a literature that includes techniques of antigen retrieval.

It is my hope that this text will be a starting point for the building and dissemination of knowledge in immunohistochemistry for the diagnostician.

David J. Dabbs, MD

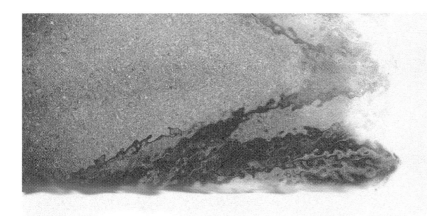

Contents

PART I

Introduction

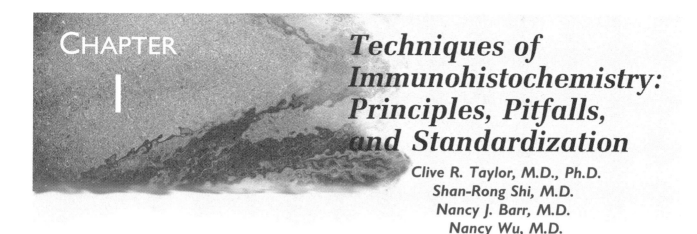

CHAPTER 1

Techniques of Immunohistochemistry: Principles, Pitfalls, and Standardization

Clive R. Taylor, M.D., Ph.D.
Shan-Rong Shi, M.D.
Nancy J. Barr, M.D.
Nancy Wu, M.D.

Immunohistochemistry (IHC), or immunocyto-chemistry, is a method for localizing specific antigens in tissues or cells based on antigen-antibody recognition; it seeks to exploit the specificity provided by the binding of an antibody with its antigen at a light microscopic level. IHC has a long history, extending more than half a century from 1940, when Coons developed an immunofluorescence technique to detect corresponding antigens in frozen tissue sections.[1] However, only since the early 1990s has the method found general application in surgical pathology.[2–4] A series of technical developments in IHC have created sensitive detection systems. Among them is the enzymatic label (horseradish peroxidase) developed by Avrameas and colleagues,[5, 6] which, in the presence of a suitable colorogenic substrate system, allowed visualization of the labeled antibody by orthodox light microscopy. One of the critical issues in the development of immunoperoxidase techniques was related to the need to achieve greater sensitivity, from the simplest one-step direct conjugate method to multiple-step detection techniques such as the peroxidase antiperoxidase (PAP), avidin-biotin conjugate (ABC) and biotin-streptavidin (B-SA) methods, together with amplification methods (such as tyramide), and the highly sensitive "polymer-based" labeling systems.[4, 7–19]

The development of the hybridoma technique[20] facilitated the development of IHC and the manufacture of abundant, highly specific monoclonal antibodies, many of which found early application in staining of tissues. Initial success in cryostat sections was eventually extended to routinely processed paraffin, celloidin, or other plastic-embedded tissue sections. Only when the IHC technique became applicable to routinely formalin-fixed, paraffin-embedded tissue sections did it usher in the "brown revolution."[21] The critical significance of rendering the IHC technique suitable for routine paraffin sections was illustrated by Taylor and colleagues, who in 1974 showed that it was possible to demonstrate at least some antigens in routinely processed tissue.[22] The collective appetites of path-ologists worldwide, once whetted by these initial studies, led to serious attempts to improve further the ability to perform IHC staining on formalin-paraffin sections.[22-27] Although great effort has been expended in the search for alternative fixatives (formalin substitutes) in order to preserve antigenicity without compromising preservation of morphologic features, no ideal fixatives have been found to date, as was pointed out by Larsson who said, "An ideal immunocytochemical fixative applicable to all antigens may never be found."[28] In addition, preservation of morphologic features is not always comparable with formalin fixation.

Enzyme digestion was introduced by Huang and colleagues[29] as a pretreatment to IHC staining to "unmask" some antigens that had been altered by formalin fixation. However, the enzyme digestion method, while widely applied, did not improve IHC staining of the majority of antigens, as reviewed by Leong and colleagues.[30] Another drawback of enzyme digestion was that it proved difficult to control the optimal "digestion" conditions for individual tissue sections when stained with different antibodies. These difficulties in standardization provided a powerful incentive for the development of a new technique, with the requirements that it should be more powerful, more widely applicable, and easier to use than enzyme digestion. In addition, it should enhance immunohistochemical staining of routinely formalin-fixed, paraffin-embedded tissue sections in a reproducible and reliable manner.

The antigen retrieval (AR) technique, based on a series of biochemical studies by Fraenkel-Conrat and coworkers,[31–33] was developed by Shi and associates in 1991.[34] In contrast to enzyme digestion, the AR technique is a simple method that involves heating routinely processed paraffin sections at high temperature (e.g., in a microwave oven) before IHC staining procedures. An alternative method that did not use heating was developed for celloidin-embedded tissues.[35–37] The intensity of IHC staining was increased dramatically after AR pretreatment, as demonstrated by the original articles and by more than 100 articles published subsequently.[38–42] Various modifications of the AR technique have been described, the majority of which use different buffer solutions as the AR solution in place of metal salt solutions, which may have a potentially toxic effect.[38, 39, 42–53] Worldwide application of AR-IHC in pathology has validated the feasibility of AR-IHC and expanded its use in molecular morphology, while raising some basic questions and practical issues for further study.[2, 3, 38, 39, 54–59]

This chapter focuses on IHC as applied to archival formalin-fixed, paraffin-embedded tissue sections for diagnostic pathologic study. In addition to basic principles and practical technical issues, the limitations and pitfalls of IHC are discussed, with the intention of providing "food for thought" in the further development of IHC, particularly for standardization and quantitative IHC.

BASIC PRINCIPLES OF IMMUNOHISTOCHEMISTRY

Pathologists have long recognized their fallibility, although they have not always publicized it.[2, 3, 24, 25] They have therefore sought more certain means of validating morphologic judgments. A variety of "special stains" were developed to facilitate cell recognition and diagnosis; most of these early stains were based on chemical reactions of cell and tissue components in frozen sections (histochemistry). In certain circumstances, these histochemical stains proved to be of critical value in specific cell identification. More often, they served merely to highlight or emphasize cellular or histologic features that supported a particular interpretation without providing truly specific confirmation. The ability to use a wide variety of truly specific special stains became available, at least in potential form, with the advent of the new field of IHC.

The aims of IHC are akin to those of histochemistry. Indeed, IHC builds on the foundations of histochemistry; it does not replace histochemistry but rather serves as a valuable adjunct that greatly extends the variety of tissue components that can be demonstrated specifically within tissue sections or other cell preparations. As emphasized by pioneers in this field of functional morphology, "the object of all staining is to recognize microchemically the existence and distribution of substances which we have been made aware of macrochemically."[60] The basic critical principle of IHC, as with any other special staining method, is a sharp localization of target components in the cell and tissue, based on a satisfactory signal-to-noise ratio. Amplifying the signal while reducing nonspecific background staining (noise) is the major strategy to achieve a satisfactory and practically useful result. After more than two decades, advances in IHC have provided a feasible approach to performing immunostaining on routinely processed tissues, such that

this method is now "routine" in surgical pathology laboratories (Appendix A).

Antibodies as Specific Staining Reagents

An antibody is a molecule that has the property of combining specifically with a second molecule, termed the *antigen*. Further, the production of antibody by an animal is induced specifically by the presence of antigen; this forms part of the basic immune response. Antigen-antibody recognition is based on the three-dimensional structure of protein (or other antigen), which is a critical issue in understanding the effectiveness of IHC (particularly after formalin-induced modification of protein conformation ["masking"]) as well as the mechanisms of AR, as described further on.

Antibodies are immunoglobulin molecules consisting of two basic units: a pair of light chains (either a kappa or a lambda pair) and a pair of heavy chains (gamma, alpha, mu, delta, or epsilon). An antigen may be any molecule that is sufficiently complex that it maintains a relatively rigid three-dimensional profile and is foreign to the animal into which it is introduced. Proteins and carbohydrates that are sufficiently complex to possess unique three-dimensional "charge-shape" profiles are good antigens; in fact, such molecules may bear more than one unique three-dimensional structure capable of inducing antibody formation (Fig. 1–1); each of these individual sites on a molecule may be termed an *antigenic determinant* (or *epitope)*, the determinant being the exact site on the molecule with which the antibody combines. The term *epitope* corresponds to a cluster of amino acid residues that binds specifically to the paratope of an antibody.[61] An epitope is a functional unit, not a fixed structural element of a protein and cannot be recognized independently of its paratope partner.[61] Antigenic determinants (epitopes) may be classified as continuous and discontinuous. The former are composed of a continuum of residues in a polypeptide chain, whereas the latter consist of residues from different parts of a poly-

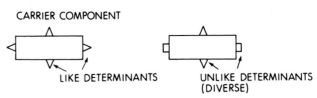

CARRIER COMPONENT

LIKE DETERMINANTS — UNLIKE DETERMINANTS (DIVERSE)

▧ *Figure 1–1.* Antigens and antigenic determinants. An antigenic molecule may be considered to consist of an immunologically "inert" carrier component and one or more antigenic determinants of like type *(left)* or diverse types *(right).* From Taylor RT, Cote RJ. Immunomicroscopy: A Diagnostic Tool for the Surgical Pathologist, 2nd ed. Philadelphia: WB Saunders, 1994, p 7.

peptide chain, brought together by the folding of the protein conformation.[62] This is an interesting issue that may reflect the variable influence of formalin fixation on antigenicity.

Any rigid part of an antibody molecule may serve as the antigenic determinant to induce an antibody. The fact that immunoglobulin molecules can serve both as antibodies, binding specifically to tissue antigens, and as antigens, providing antigenic determinants to which secondary antibodies may be attached, is exploited in IHC techniques (Fig. 1–2).

Evaluation of an antibody for use in IHC is based on two points: the sensitivity and the specificity of the antibody-antigen reaction for IHC. The development of the hybridoma technique[20] provided an almost limitless source of highly specific antibodies. Although monoclonal antibodies do not guarantee antigen specificity, since different antigens may share similar or cross-reactive epitopes, the "practical" specificity reflected by IHC is excellent for most monoclonal antibodies tested. In contrast, a "polyclonal antibody" is in fact an antiserum, which contains several different molecular species of antibody having varying affinities and even varying specificities against the different antigens or antigenic determinants used to immunize the animal. It is important to remember that "polyclonal antibodies" may also include varying amounts of antibody to a whole range of antigens, including bacteria and viruses, that the immunized animal encountered before its use as a source of antibody. As a result, polyclonal antibodies may give more nonspecific background staining in slides than the staining obtained using monoclonal antibodies. By the same token, however, the presence of a mixture of different antibodies may on occasion confer an advantage to the use of polyclonal antibodies in the staining of certain "hard to detect" antigens in fixed tissues, if monoclonal antibodies and AR fail to give satisfactory results. For these reasons, the use of highly purified antigen preparations to produce high-affinity conventional polyclonal antibodies (antisera), which are then subjected to multiple absorption procedures to maximize specificity, is of value for certain applications. However, it is important to emphasize that in the assessment of such antisera, immunodiffusion assays for specificity may fail to detect "trace" antibody specificities, which become apparent only when the antiserum is applied to tissue sections containing many different antigens. IHC performed on both fresh and archival tissue sections, or Western blotting techniques, is the preferred approach to the evaluation of specificity and sensitivity for such antibodies.

Comparison of sensitivity and specificity between polyclonal and monoclonal antibodies indicate that polyclonal antibody may be more sensitive but less specific than monoclonal antibody. The reason may be that polyclonal antibody (actually a composite of many antibodies) may recog-

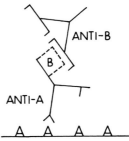

Figure 1–2. Antibodies as antigens. Anti-A antibody binds specifically to antigen A in the tissue section. Antigen B (B) is depicted as a second antigenic determinant that is part of the anti-A molecule; anti-B antibody, made in a second species, will bind to this determinant. Thus anti-B (the so-called secondary antibody) can be used to locate the site of binding of anti-A (the primary antibody) in a tissue section. From Taylor RT, Cote RJ. Immunomicroscopy: A Diagnostic Tool for the Surgical Pathologist, 2nd ed. Philadelphia: WB Saunders, 1994, p 9.

nize several different binding sites (epitopes) on a single protein (antigen), whereas a monoclonal antibody recognizes only a single type of epitope. Sophisticated amplification techniques, coupled with the use of the AR technique, have reduced the practical importance of this distinction.

Although the specificity of monoclonal antibody has been questioned regarding cross-reactivity with nontarget molecules,[63] most commercially available monoclonal antibodies are highly reliable for IHC, but again the ultimate specificity control should be the observation of the expected pattern of staining in control tissue sections, with the corresponding lack of unexpected or inexplicable staining reactions. Johnson[63] recommended simple methods to check the specificity of a particular antibody, that is, correlation of the staining result with the literature references for antigen distribution and comparing the staining of the test antibody with that of a second antibody known to bind to the same antigen but to a different epitope.

Blocking Nonspecific Background Staining

There are two aspects to the blocking of background staining of tissues: nonspecific antibody binding and the presence of endogenous enzymes. Nonspecific antibody binding is generally more of a problem with polyclonal antibody, because multiple "unwanted" antibodies may exist in antiserum. The greater the optimal working dilution, the smaller the problem. If necessary, it is advisable to preincubate the tissue section with normal serum from the same species of animal in order to occupy "unwanted" binding sites before incubation with the primary antibody. Another form of nonspecific binding may result from the fact that antibodies are highly charged molecules and may bind nonspecifically to tissue components bearing reciprocal charges (e.g., collagen). Such nonspecific binding may lead to localization of either the primary antibody or the labeled moiety (conjugate, PAP, and so on), producing false-positive staining of collagen and other tissue components of sufficient degree to obscure specific staining (Fig. 1–3*A*). Pre-incubation with normal serum may also reduce this kind of nonspecific binding. In theory, proteins in the normal serum occupy the charged sites within the tissue section, excluding (or at least reducing) nonspecific attachment of the specific primary antibody and other antibodies added subsequently. In practice, it is customary to use normal serum of the same species as the bridge antibody (in the PAP method) or the secondary antibody (in conjugate and ABC methods) because this normal serum neither interferes with nor participates in the immunologic reactions that occur as part of the immunostaining procedure.

Blocking endogenous enzyme activity is also important. The degree of susceptibility of an enzyme to denaturation and inactivation during fixation varies. Some, like peroxidase, are preserved in both paraffin and frozen sections; others, like alkaline phosphatase, are completely inactivated by routine fixation and paraffin-embedding procedures. Any residual activity of these endogenous enzymes must be abolished during immunostaining in order to avoid false-positive reactions when using the same or similar enzymes as labels. Peroxidase activity is present in a number of normal and neoplastic cells, including erythrocytes, neutrophils, eosinophils, and hepatocytes. When performing an immunohistochemical study in tissues rich in blood cells, such as bone marrow, it is recommended that a "peroxidase-blocking" step be used coupled with a "substrate control" (i.e., a sec-

tion treated only with the hydrogen peroxide-chromogen mixture to visualize the extent of endogenous peroxidase activity). Otherwise, alternative methods, such as the immunogold or glucose oxidase method, may be used to avoid the possibility of confusion with any endogenous enzyme activity.

To risk stating the obvious, it is essential that blocking of endogenous enzymatic activity be carried out before the addition of enzyme-labeled antibody or the PAP complexes, otherwise, the enzyme label is also inactivated by the blocking procedure, resulting in a false-negative result. Various approaches have been devised to inhibit peroxidase activity. Streefkerk[64] suggested incubating the sections with a mixture of methanol and H_2O_2 before the IHC procedure. Burns[65] increased the H_2O_2 concentration in stepwise fashion to about 10%, with the additional purpose of bleaching hematin. Weir and colleagues[66] succeeded in neutralizing endogenous peroxidase activity and obtained good preservation of immunoglobulin antigenicity by incubating sections with 0.075% hydrochloric acid in ethanol at room temperature for 15 minutes before immunostaining.

For general purposes, and in most situations, we have obtained satisfactory results with a 15-minute incubation in a methanol/H_2O_2 combination.

For those who encounter difficulty, or who wish to explore other approaches, a more detailed discussion follows. Some investigators[68, 69] believe that the methanol-H_2O_2 approach is too drastic and may cause some denaturation of antigen. Strauss[68, 69] advocated the use of phenylhydrazine, which appears to preserve the antigenicity of many molecules but suffers from the disadvantage that it does not completely inhibit the endogenous peroxidase activity of eosinophils. A combination of phenylhydrazine, nascent H_2O_2 freshly produced by a glu-

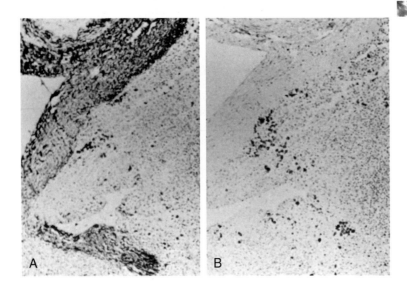

Figure 1–3. Example of the effectiveness of "blocking" nonspecific binding of primary and secondary antibodies. *A,* A section of spleen stained for IgG by the PAP method; scattered positive plasma cells *(black dots)* are seen, but there is heavy staining of collagen bands. *B,* The adjacent parallel section treated in an identical fashion except that normal serum from the same species as the linking antibody (in this case normal swine serum to match the swine antirabbit Ig-linking antibody) was added before the primary antibody. In this instance, the plasma cells are seen even more clearly because the heavy nonspecific staining of collagen is markedly diminished. Paraffin sections, DAB with hematoxylin counterstain. (×60) From Taylor RT, Cote RJ. Immunomicroscopy: A Diagnostic Tool for the Surgical Pathologist, 2nd ed. Philadelphia: WB Saunders, 1994, p 68.

cose oxidase-glucose mixture, and sodium azide inhibits endogenous peroxidase activity with little damage to surface antigens of lymphocytes.[70] A mixture Of H_2O_2 (0.3%) in 0.1% sodium azide was also found to be a simple and effective technique.[71] More recently, cyclopropanone hydrate was shown to inhibit endogenous peroxidase without adverse effects on antigenicity.[72] Robinson and Dawson,[73] in their study of gastrin, avoided antigenic denaturation by first developing the endogenous peroxidase with 4-chloro-1-naphthol (giving a blue-gray color); next they performed the immunohistologic staining procedure, developing the peroxidase label with diaminobenzidine (giving a contrasting brown reaction product). A similar approach was used by one of the authors in the initial reports describing the feasibility of demonstrating immunoglobulin antigens in paraffin sections; alpha-naphthol pyronine was used for endogenous peroxidase (pink), followed by diaminobenzidine (brown) for the horseradish peroxidase label.[22, 23]

Heyderman and Neville[74, 75] introduced a procedure in which sections are first incubated with 7.5% H_2O_2 in distilled water to inhibit the acid hematin and then in 2.28% periodic acid in distilled water to block endogenous peroxidase. Because the aldehyde groups formed during periodic acid treatment may lead to nonspecific staining phenomena, the sections should be incubated with 0.02% sodium borohydride[76] in distilled water before the addition of the antibodies. This method has given good immunostaining of carcinoembryonic antigen (CEA) and epithelial cell membrane antigens but may denature carbohydrate determinants (e.g., blood group antigens). It was shown in frozen sections of intestinal biopsy specimens from coeliac patients that a short incubation period (45 seconds) of the slides with a low concentration of periodic acid (0.28%) inhibits endogenous peroxidase activity effectively without loss of antigenicity of lymphocyte surface markers.[77] Comparing various inhibition procedures used for both frozen and paraffin sections, Hittmair and Schmid[78] reported that methanol-H_2O_2 is deleterious to certain sensitive antigens, including intermediate filament proteins.

Detection Systems

Antibody molecules cannot be seen with the light microscope or even with the electron microscope unless they are labeled or flagged by some method that permits their visualization. Essentially, detection systems attach certain labels or flags to primary or secondary antibodies in order to visualize the target antibody-antigen localization in the tissue sections. A variety of labels or flags have been used, including fluorescent compounds and active enzymes that can be visualized by virtue of their property of inducing the formation of a colored reaction product from a suitable substrate system. Such methods have worked well in light microscopy and can be adapted to electron microscopy if the products are rendered electron-dense by suitable treatment. Alternatively, labels that are visible directly by electron microscopy may be used, such as gold, ferritin, or virus particles.

Enhancement of sensitivity through amplification of signal is also an important goal of various detection systems, as described further on.

DIRECT CONJUGATE-LABELED ANTIBODY METHOD

The method of attaching a label by chemical means to an antibody and then directly applying this labeled conjugate to tissue sections (Fig. 1–4) has been used widely in immunohistology. In preparing a labeled antibody conjugate, the aim is to attach the maximal number of molecules of label to each individual antibody molecule. It is desirable to label 100% of antibody molecules and to render none of them immunologically inactive by the labeling process. Similarly, the labeling process must not inactivate the label (e.g., destroy the active site of the horseradish peroxidase enzyme). The final labeled reagent should not contain free molecules of label that might undergo nonspecific binding with the tissue section. Likewise, there should be no free molecules of unlabeled antibody and no molecules of antibody linked to inactivated label.

These are exacting requirements that are difficult to meet in the routine surgical pathology laboratory. However, conjugation methods have improved immensely since the early 1980s, and high-quality conjugates, including peroxidase, glucose oxidase, and alkaline phosphatase, are available from a number of commercial sources.

The direct conjugate procedure has the advantages of rapidity and ease of performance. With this procedure, the purity (i.e., monospecificity) of an antibody or antiserum (polyclonal antibody) is of critical importance. As noted previously, an antiserum contains a range of antibody molecules of differing specificity in addition to the antibody

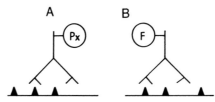

Figure 1–4. *A* and *B*, Direct conjugate method. The label, or flag, is attached directly to the antibody having specificity for the antigen under study. Px, peroxidase; F, fluorescein. From Taylor RT, Cote RJ. Immunomicroscopy: A Diagnostic Tool for the Surgical Pathologist, 2nd ed. Philadelphia: WB Saunders, 1994, p 10.

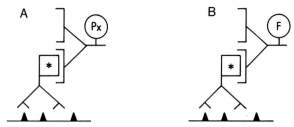

Figure 1–5. A and *B,* Indirect conjugate (sandwich) method. The primary antibody is unlabeled. The method uses a labelled secondary antibody, having specificity against the primary antibody. Boxed antigen determinant on primary antibody. Px, peroxidase label; F, fluorescein label. From Taylor RT, Cote RJ. Immunomicroscopy: A Diagnostic Tool for the Surgical Pathologist, 2nd ed. Philadelphia: WB Saunders, 1994, p 11.

having the desired specificity; all these antibodies are labeled during the conjugation procedure, and any or all may produce positive staining in tissue sections, leading to erroneous interpretation. The direct procedure is useful with monoclonal antibodies (see further on) that are truly monospecific, with the caveat that monoclonal antibodies prepared as an ascites (as opposed to in vitro culture) do contain contaminating murine immunoglobulins (antibody) of unknown specificity.

One practical disadvantage of the direct conjugate procedure is that to detect different antigens, it is necessary to conjugate the appropriate primary antibodies separately. Also, with regard to precious (scarce) antibodies, the direct conjugate procedure usually demands that the primary antibody be used at a relatively high concentration in comparison with indirect and unlabeled antibody methods.

INDIRECT, OR SANDWICH, PROCEDURE

The indirect, or sandwich, conjugate procedure (Fig. 1–5) is a relatively simple modification of the direct conjugate method. It has the following advantages:

1. Versatility is increased, in that a single conjugated antibody can be used with several different primary antibodies.
2. The conjugation process is applied only to the secondary antibody.
3. The primary antibody can often be used at a higher working dilution (than in the direct method) to achieve successful staining.
4. The secondary antibody, produced against immunoglobulin of the species from which the primary antibody is derived, is readily prepared with a high order of specificity and affinity; many commercial sources are available for conjugated secondary antibodies.
5. The method lends itself to additional specificity controls in that the primary specific antibody may be omitted, or another antibody of irrelevant specificity may be substituted, providing a

valuable assessment of the validity of any staining pattern observed.

All labeled antibody methods performed by the indirect procedure are strictly analogous in principle; the peroxidase and fluorescent indirect conjugate methods are illustrated in Figures 1–5*A and B,* respectively. The primary antibody that has specificity against the antigen in question (e.g., rabbit anti-A), is added to the section; the excess is washed off. The labeled secondary antibody, which has specificity against an antigenic determinant present on the primary rabbit antibody (e.g., swine antibody versus rabbit immunoglobulin), is then added; it serves to label the sites of tissue localization of the primary antibody, which, in turn, is bound to the antigen.

UNLABELED ANTIBODY METHODS

Enzyme Bridge Technique. The disadvantages of the chemical conjugation procedure may be entirely avoided by devising techniques whereby the labeled moiety is linked to the antigen solely by immunologic binding. To achieve this end, Mason and colleagues[79] developed a technique that has become known as the *enzyme bridge method* (Fig. 1–6). This method is little used today.

Peroxidase Antiperoxidase Method. The PAP method (Fig. 1–7) is a second unlabeled antibody procedure that also avoids the problems inherent in chemical conjugation. First employed by Sternberger and colleagues for the detection of antitreponemal antibodies,[80] the PAP system was reported to enjoy a sensitivity 100- to 1000-fold greater than that of comparable conjugate procedures. The principle of the PAP method is similar to that of the enzyme bridge method (see Fig. 1–6). The acronym *PAP* denotes the peroxidase anti-

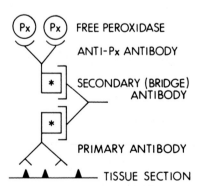

Figure 1–6. Enzyme bridge method. A second antibody is used to link (bridge) the primary antibody to an antiperoxidase antibody, which, in turn binds to free peroxidase. Boxed asterisk represents antigen determinant on primary and secondary antibodies. Px, peroxidase label. From Taylor RT, Cote RJ. Immunomicroscopy: A Diagnostic Tool for the Surgical Pathologist, 2nd ed. Philadelphia: WB Saunders, 1994, p 12.

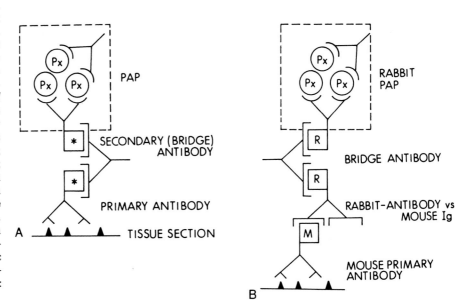

Figure 1-7. *A,* Peroxidase-antiperoxidase (PAP) method (three-stage). PAP reagent *(dashed lines)* is a preformed stable immune complex; it is linked to the primary antibody by a "bridging" antibody. *B,* PAP method (four-stage). PAP reagent *(dashed line)* is a preformed stable immune complex. Primary antibody in this example is murine (mouse Ig as in a monoclonal antibody [M]); this antibody is followed by a rabbit antimouse Ig (R), a bridge antibody (e.g., swine antirabbit Ig) and rabbit PAP. Px, peroxidase label. From Taylor RT, Cote RJ. Immunomicroscopy: A Diagnostic Tool for the Surgical Pathologist, 2nd ed. Philadelphia: WB Saunders, 1994, p 12.

peroxidase reagent that represents the third stage in this procedure.

The PAP reagent consists of antibody against horseradish peroxidase and horseradish peroxidase antigen in the form of a small, stable immune complex. Available evidence suggests that this immune complex typically consists of two antibody molecules and three horseradish peroxidase molecules in the configuration shown in Figure 1-7. The PAP reagent and the primary antibody must be from the same species (or from closely related species with common antigenic determinants), whereas the bridge antibody is derived from a second species and has specificity against the primary antibody (e.g., rabbit antisigma) and the immunoglobulin incorporated into the PAP complex (e.g., rabbit antiperoxidase). In the example depicted in Figure 1-7A, the primary antisigma antibody is made in rabbit; the bridge antibody is made in swine (i.e., it is a swine antibody against rabbit IgG), whereas the PAP reagent is made from rabbit antibody against horseradish peroxidase (rabbit antiperoxidase) complexed with horseradish peroxidase antigen. The bridge antibody serves as a "specific glue" to bind the PAP-labeled moiety to the primary antibody, which, in turn, is bound to the antigen under study. This method has become widely used in routinely processed paraffin sections because of its reputation for a high degree of sensitivity coupled with the specificity and stability of the reagents.

One limitation of the PAP method is that the antibody incorporated into the PAP reagent should be of the same species as the primary antibody. This requirement has caused difficulty for some thrifty investigators who have "mixed" reagents from different kits, only to find that a rabbit PAP from one kit will not link with a goat primary from another, even if so-called universal linking reagents (mixtures of two or more bridge antibodies) are used. In order to use mouse or goat antibodies with rabbit PAP, one may adopt a four-stage procedure (Fig. 1-7B), for example, mouse antisigma followed by a rabbit antibody against mouse immunoglobulin, a bridge reagent, and then the rabbit PAP.

PAP reagents prepared in goat, mouse, rat, and chimpanzee (cross-reactive with human immunoglobulin) are now available for use with goat, mouse, rat, and human primary antibodies, respectively.

BIOTIN-AVIDIN PROCEDURE

The biotin-avidin procedure (Fig. 1-8) exploits the high-affinity binding between biotin and avidin. Biotin can be linked chemically to the primary antibody (see Fig. 1-8A), producing a biotinylated conjugate that, when added to the tissue section, localizes to the sites of antigen within the section. Subsequently, avidin, chemically conjugated to horseradish peroxidase, is added; the avidin binds tightly to the biotinylated antibody, thus localizing the peroxidase moiety at the site of antigen in the tissue section. This method is rapid and has been used particularly in an indirect procedure (see Fig. 1-8B).

Two potential disadvantages exist. First, it has become apparent that different batches of biotin and different batches of avidin have differing affinities for one other, and this drastically affects the sensitivity and reproducibility of the procedure in different laboratories. Second, some tissues contain significant amounts of endogenous biotin that may

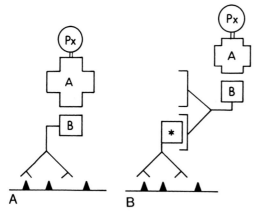

Figure 1–8. *A,* Direct biotin-avidin method. The primary antibody is linked to biotin (B); an avidin-peroxidase-conjugate (A-Px) is then added. *B,* Indirect biotin-avidin method. Used for monoclonal antibodies, the primary antibody is not conjugated; its localization is detected by a biotinylated secondary antibody. Boxed asterisk represents antigen determinant on primary antibody. Px, peroxidase label; A, avidin; B, biotin. From Taylor RT, Cote RJ. Immunomicroscopy: A Diagnostic Tool for the Surgical Pathologist, 2nd ed. Philadelphia: WB Saunders, 1994, p 13.

bind the avidin-peroxidase complex directly, thus producing nonspecific (false-positive) staining. This can be combated by suitable blocking techniques, as described further on.

AVIDIN-BIOTIN CONJUGATE PROCEDURE

Hsu and colleagues[13, 14] developed a further modification of the biotin-avidin system that greatly enhanced its sensitivity. The method can be used either as a direct or an indirect technique. In the indirect technique (Fig. 1–9), the primary antibody is added, followed by a biotinylated secondary antibody and next by preformed complexes of avidin and biotin horseradish peroxidase conjugate. This complex serves to localize several molecules of horseradish peroxidase at the site of the antigen. The time it takes to perform the ABC conjugate procedure compares favorably with that of the PAP method. Binding to endogenous biotin remains a problem.

BIOTIN-STREPTAVIDIN SYSTEMS

The B-SA method overcomes several of the problems associated with the ABC systems by substituting streptavidin for avidin and directly conjugating the streptavidin to the enzyme molecule. Streptavidin, a tetrameric 60-kd avidin analog isolated from the bacterium *Streptomyces avidinii,* is capable of binding biotin with a very high affinity. Theoretically, this affinity is approximately 10 times higher than that of most antibodies for their antigens and provides very specific detection and amplification

of the antigen-antibody binding event. The use of streptavidin is preferred to avidin for several reasons:

1. Streptavidin contains no carbohydrates, which can bind nonspecifically to lectin-like substances found in normal tissue from kidney, liver, brain, and mast cells.
2. The isoelectric point of streptavidin is close to neutrality, whereas avidin has an isoelectric point of 10; thus streptavidin conjugates do not exhibit the nonspecific electrostatic binding characteristic of avidin conjugates, which are positively charged under physiologic conditions.
3. Because the enzyme is directly conjugated to streptavidin in the B-SA system, it is a highly stable reagent that can be diluted and stored for long periods in a ready to use form.

With the B-SA systems (BioGenex, Shandon-Lipshaw, Immunon, DAKO), the secondary and labeling reagents can be modified to maximize the amounts of biotin and enzyme label present, providing substantial increases in sensitivity. The improved sensitivity can allow increased dilution of expensive primary antibodies. Either peroxidase or alkaline phosphatase may be used as the enzyme label.

POLYVALENT SYSTEMS

Many commercial suppliers now offer "polyvalent detection systems" (BioGenex, Shandon-Lipshaw, Immunon, DAKO). These systems provide a secondary reagent that is a "cocktail" of antibodies raised against immunoglobulins from different species. This allows one secondary reagent to be used for both polyclonal and monoclonal antibodies.

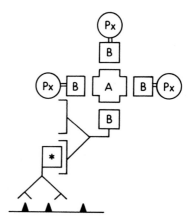

Figure 1–9. Avidin-biotin-conjugate (ABC) method. A biotinylated secondary antibody serves to link the primary antibody to a large preformed complex of avidin, biotin, and peroxidase. Boxed asterisk represents antigen determinant on primary antibody. A, avidin; B, biotin; Px, peroxidase label. From Taylor RT, Cote RJ. Immunomicroscopy: A Diagnostic Tool for the Surgical Pathologist, 2nd ed. Philadelphia: WB Saunders, 1994, p 14.

ALKALINE PHOSPHATASE ANTI–ALKALINE PHOSPHATASE METHOD

The principles of the alkaline phosphatase anti–alkaline phosphatase (APAAP) technique are the same as those described for the PAP method (Fig. 1–10), except that the PAP complex is replaced with an APAAP complex. The method was first described by Cordell and colleagues,[81] who used a murine monoclonal antibody specific for calf intestinal alkaline phosphatase. The APAAP method has had three major applications: (1) staining of tissues with high levels of endogenous peroxidase, (2) double immunostaining in conjunction with peroxidase, and (3) staining of specific cell types that benefit from the bright red color of alkaline phosphatase substrates.[4]

Alkaline phosphatase labeling may be preferred for tissues rich in endogenous peroxidase, such as bone marrow or lymphoid tissue containing infiltrating myeloid cells, particularly when using frozen sections. Because complete blocking of endogenous peroxidase of myeloid leukocytes in blood and bone marrow smears may be difficult, and because blocking procedures may denature some of the antigenic determinants, the APAAP method has proved useful in staining bone marrow. For example, Erber and McLachlan[82] studied 72 cases of routinely processed and decalcified paraffin-embedded bone marrow trephine tissue using the APAAP method with a panel of 14 monoclonal antibodies; this report provides an excellent resource for those wishing to adopt this method.

For double immunostaining, it is convenient to use the APAAP method in conjunction with an immunoperoxidase stain (Appendix B). The use of alkaline phosphatase as the second label has the advantage of avoiding the cross-reactivity that may occur when two immunoperoxidase procedures are used together. In addition, a simultaneous double immunostaining procedure may be carried out us-ing heterospecific antibodies, such as polyclonal and monoclonal antibodies, as the two primary antibodies under investigation (see Fig. 1–10). Sequential double immunostaining with the APAAP method may also be achieved using fast red and fast blue stains.[83] In the latter case, care must be taken to avoid mixed-color staining (i.e., having the initial red color change to purple); to this end, the weaker staining antigen should be tested first, and the second antibody applied may be developed for a shorter time (10 to 15 minutes, monitored by microscopy).

In some cases, the bright red color produced by alkaline phosphatase substrates (fast red or new fuchsin) may provide more distinct staining than the conventional peroxidase chromogens. The APAAP method may be used successfully, for example, to demonstrate nuclear antigens or to stain cell smears in which only a few cells stain positive. Wong and colleagues,[84] in a study of estrogen receptors (ERs) in 48 human breast carcinomas, demonstrated improved detection of ERs with the APAAP method because of the distinct red color of the alkaline phosphatase chromogen compared with the brown reaction product of diaminobenzidine (DAB). These immunohistochemical results correlated well with the cytosol-based dextran-coated charcoal (DCC) method. In another example, Vardiman and coworkers[85] reported the detection of a small number of hairy cells using monoclonal antibody Leu-M5 (CD11c) to stain peripheral blood and bone marrow preparations from patients with hairy cell leukemia.

It should be remembered that the advantages cited earlier for the APAAP method are conferred by the alkaline phosphatase enzyme label and thus apply equally to the ABC or B-SA methods that use alkaline phosphatase–conjugated avidin or streptavidin. In general, the technical considerations discussed earlier for the PAP method also

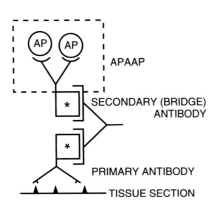
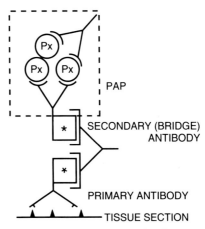

Figure 1–10. Alkaline phosphatase anti–alkaline phosphatase (APAAP) and PAP methods showing the feasibility of double staining by the use of different primary and secondary antibodies, for example, mouse antivimentin, horse antimouse IgG, mouse APAAP *(left);* rabbit antikeratin (polyclonal goat antirabbit IgG, rabbit PAP *(right).* AP, alkaline phosphatase; Px, peroxidase. From Taylor RT, Cote RJ. Immunomicroscopy: A Diagnostic Tool for the Surgical Pathologist, 2nd ed. Philadelphia: WB Saunders, 1994, p 32.

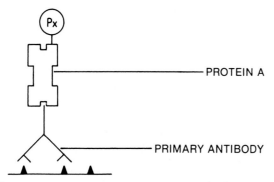

Figure 1–11. Protein A conjugate method. Protein A, labeled with peroxidase, binds to the Fc component of the primary antibody. Px, peroxidase label. From Taylor RT, Cote RJ. Immunomicroscopy A Diagnostic Tool for the Surgical Pathologist, 2nd ed. Philadelphia: WB Saunders, 1994, p 14.

apply to the APAAP method. The specificity of the APAAP reagent must be considered and the optimal concentration determined by titration, as described for the PAP complex. Unlike the PAP complex, in which three molecules of antigen (peroxidase) are bound to two molecules of antibody, the APAAP complex consists of two molecules of antigen (alkaline phosphatase) bound to a single molecule of antibody. This configuration resembles the normal binding interaction of a bivalent antibody, and the APAAP complexes are stable for prolonged periods in storage.

There are two ways to increase the immunostaining intensity of the APAAP labeling method. The first approach is the "double bridge" technique, which can also be used for the PAP method, in which one simply repeats the second and third steps of the immunostaining procedure (i.e., one again adds the secondary [bridge] antibody and the labeling complex.[86, 87] In the context of the APAAP method, the increase in sensitivity is not attributable to the formation of a double bridge per se but probably is due to additional binding to residual unoccupied primary antibody. A second approach to achieving enhanced sensitivity is to combine the APAAP technique with the avidin-biotin–alkaline phosphatase complex (ABAP) method, as described by Davidoff and associates.[88] This amplification procedure is carried out, after primary antibody incubation, by adding sequentially biotinylated antimouse IgG (Vector) and mouse APAAP (DAKO), followed by labeling with the ABAP complex (Vector). In this study, the authors performed immunolocalization of desmin and vimentin in frozen sections of human testis and found that the combination of the APAAP and ABAP methods revealed smaller quantities of these antigens in myofibroblasts of the lamina propria than could be demonstrated by either the APAAP or ABAP method used alone.

PROTEIN A METHODS

Protein A, derived from *Staphylococcus,* has the remarkable ability to bind with the constant (Fc) portion of immunoglobulin molecules from several different species. The only absolute requirement is that the primary antibody binds with protein A; most IgG molecules bind protein A, although affinity varies among different IgG subclasses and in different species (Figs. 1–11 and 1–12). The protein A–peroxidase and related protein A-PAP methods do not match the sensitivity of the PAP, ABC, or streptavidin-based techniques, but they do have advantages that may warrant their use in specific circumstances.

ENZYME-LABELED ANTIGEN METHOD

The enzyme-labeled antigen method (Fig. 1–13) was devised as perhaps the ultimate in specificity among immunoperoxidase techniques. The principles of application of this method are illustrated in Figure 1–13. Only one antibody is used; the method exploits the fact that an antibody molecule possesses two valencies, one of which may be bound to the antigen under study, with the second valency left free to bind with additional molecules of antigen added subsequently. The additional antigen is presented in a form that is directly conjugated with horseradish peroxidase; thus, this is a labeled antigen procedure.

The primary antibody is generally used at a relatively high concentration. This method therefore is

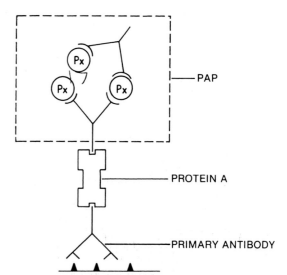

Figure 1–12. Protein A-PAP method. The protein A is used to link the primary antibody (Fc) to the antibody (Fc) within the PAP complex. Px, peroxidase label. From Taylor RT, Cote RJ. Immunomicroscopy: A Diagnostic Tool for the Surgical Pathologist, 2nd ed. Philadelphia: WB Saunders, 1994, p 14.

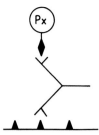

Figure 1–13. Labeled antigen method. The antibody is added in excess so that one valency is bound to the antigen in the section, leaving the second valency free to bind the labeled antigen that is added subsequently. Px, peroxidase label. From Taylor RT, Cote RJ. Immunomicroscopy: A Diagnostic Tool for the Surgical Pathologist, 2nd ed. Philadelphia: WB Saunders, 1994, p 14.

not economical in use of the primary antibody and is best applied for the detection of antigens in which both antigen and antibody are in good supply. One major advantage is that the primary antibody need not be particularly pure because antibodies of irrelevant specificity will not be detected by this technique, even if they bind to the tissue section; lacking specificity for A antigen, they will not bind the A antigen–peroxidase conjugate and thus will not be visualized.

This method has proved particularly suitable for double-staining techniques whereby one seeks to stain two antigens simultaneously within the same section (Fig. 1–14), using- two labeled antigens (e.g., kappa-peroxidase and lambda–alkaline phosphatase) together.

POLYMERIC LABELING TWO-STEP METHOD

The demand for more sensitive, more reliable and simpler methods for IHC continues to escalate. Simplification of conventional multistep detection systems, producing shorter protocols without compromising detection sensitivity, has long been desirable, but it is technically challenging. In practice, reduction of the number of steps has always been accompanied by reduced sensitivity. New approaches, such as catalyzed reporter deposition or tyramine signal amplification (TSA),[7, 8] immuno–polymerase chain reaction (immuno-PCR),[89] and end-product amplification,[90] which give improved detection sensitivity, are accompanied by even more complicated protocols, and often by high or unacceptable nonspecific staining. Other methods that use natural or synthetic polymer carriers to increase the numbers of enzymes or ligands that are coupled to linker antibodies have also been reported as described earlier.

Development of simpler one- or two-step detection methods with amplification is reflective of an encouraging trend toward simplification, which should facilitate standardization of IHC and is consistent with the overall philosophy that, with all other things being equal, simple techniques are better than complicated ones.

A novel polymeric labeling two-step method has been developed to provide great amplification with a relatively simple IHC staining procedure. In 1995, a polymer-enhanced two-step IHC detection system (EnVision, DAKO, Carpinteria, CA) was reported and evaluated.[12, 16, 19] However, the high molecular weight of the dextran carrier used for the conjugation of enzymes to linker antibodies appeared to create spatial hindrance, thus compromising the penetrative ability of the detection reagent. In 1999, we tested a new polymeric labeling reagent named PowerVision (ImmunoVision Technologies, Daly City, CA) in a comparative study with a number of available multistep detection systems.[91] We found that the detection efficiency of the PowerVision reagent was superior, as exemplified by the observation that at a dilution of 1:320, a moderate staining intensity could be achieved by using the PowerVision system, whereas other methods showed faintly positive or negative results. Using the AR technique combining this new two-step detection system, the IHC staining of long-stored archival paraffin sections for monoclonal antibodies to p53 (Pab-1801), $p27^{Kip1}$ and $p21^{WAF1}$ could be restored to a similar level as that obtained by using freshly cut paraffin sections.

The PowerVison system is based on a compact enzyme-linker antibody conjugate, with a high number of enzyme molecules attached to each linker antibody. Molecular size is minimized by use of small linear or minimally branched multifunctional reagents, which are able to polymerize with linker antibodies and enzymes in a tight, compact size (Fig. 1–15).[91] Advantages of this two-step detection system include simplicity and excellent sensitivity.

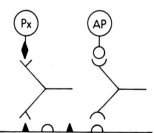

Figure 1–14. Labeled antigen double stain. Two different antibodies recognize their respective antigens in the tissue section and subsequently bind only the corresponding labeled antigen (labeled with peroxidase [Px] or alkaline phosphatase [AP]). From Taylor RT, Cote RJ. Immunomicroscopy: A Diagnostic Tool for the Surgical Pathologist, 2nd ed. Philadelphia: WB Saunders, 1994, p 15.

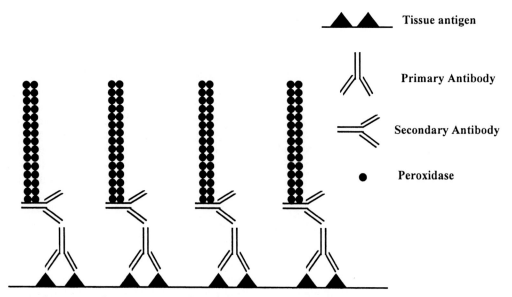

Tissue antigen

Primary Antibody

Secondary Antibody

● Peroxidase

Figure 1–15. Schematic of PowerVision detection system. The enzyme-linker antibody has a more compact molecular shape than other polymer carrier-based conjugates and thus allows the attachment of multiple conjugates in close proximity to each other. The abundant conjugated enzymatic molecules are deposited in each antigenic location, which resembles a big city skyline. (From Shi SR, et al. Appl Immunohistochem Mol Morphol 7:201–208, 1999.)

Successful application of any "ultrasensitive" detection system raises the possibility that it may be necessary to retitrate primary reagents to a higher working dilution in order to avoid nonspecific staining.

TYRAMINE SIGNAL AMPLIFICATION

Based on the principle of enzyme amplification methods for enzyme immunoassays adopted in the 1980s, Bobrow and associates[8, 92] developed a catalyzed reporter deposition technique (CARD) to achieve amplified signal for solid-phase immunoassay system and membrane immunoassays. Subsequently, this CARD technique was introduced to IHC in 1992.[7]

Signal amplification in the CARD method is based on biotinylated tyramine deposition through free radical formation, which is catalyzed by oxidizing horseradish peroxidase. It is postulated that radicalized biotinylated tyramine will be covalently attached to electron-rich moieties (tyrosine, phenylalanine, tryptophan, and so on), resulting in additional biotinylated molecules being deposited at the site of antigen-antibody reaction, that is, amplification of the signal (Fig. 1–16).

Application of this TSA for IHC has achieved positive immunostaining for some "hard-to-detect" antigens in archival paraffin-embedded tissue sections.[93] Several commercial TSA reagents are available (NEN Life Science Products, Boston, MA; CSA system, DAKO, Carpinteria, CA). With use of these TSA kits, additional staining steps are performed after a regular horseradish peroxidase–conjugated detection system, that is, incubation of slides with

a biotinylated tyramine reagent, followed by washing thoroughly, and then incubating slides with horseradish peroxidase–conjugated streptavidin. Finally, chromogen (DAB, amino-ethyl carbazole

Binding of peroxidase conjugated antibody or streptavidin-POX to the labeled hybrid and H_2O_2 radicalization of tyramine-reporter

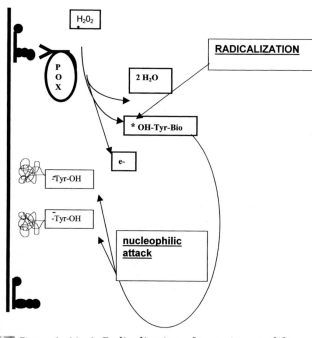

Figure 1–16. *A,* Radiculization of tyramine amplification.

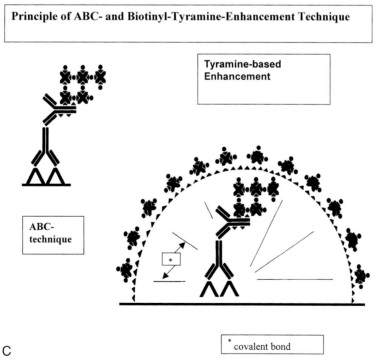

Figure 1–16. Continued. B, Tyramine-reporter deposition. **C,** Comparison with the ABC method. (From Merz H, et al. Chapter 14. In: Shi S-R, Giu J, Taylor CR, eds. Antigen Retrieval Techniques: Immunohistochemistry and Molecular Morphology. Natick, MA, Eaton, 2000:228–229.

Table 1–1. Representative Dilution Titration to Determine Optimal Titer of Antibody for Use in Direct Conjugate Method

	Serial Dilutions of Primary Antibody →					
Intensity of Staining* of:	*1/5*	*1/20*	*1/80*	*1/320*	*1/1280*	*1/2560*
(a) Unwanted background†	+ +	+	±	±	±	±
(b) Specific antigens‡	+ + +	+ + + +	+ + + +	+ + +	+ +	+

* Intensity of staining scored on a semiquantitative scale 0 to + + + +; ± indicates faint positivity of uncertain significance.
† Unwanted background staining may result from several different mechanisms (see text).
‡ Intensity of staining of specific antigen (e.g., with titration of anti-kappa antibody, specific staining would be present in plasma cells).
Adapted from Taylor CR; Cote RJ. Immunomicroscopy: A Diagnostic Tool for the Surgical Pathologist, 2nd ed. Philadelphia: WB Saunders, 1994:23.

[AEC], and so on) is used to visualize the amplified signal in the tissue sections.

Although this TSA method has achieved satisfactory results in terms of significantly increasing intensity of IHC and ISH, it has not been widely applied in diagnostic pathology for several reasons,[94] including the following:

- Additional steps make the method more time-consuming.
- Nonspecific background staining may increase as the signal increases.
- Optimal AR treatment with existing methods may achieve equivalent results.[95]

The so-called ImmunoMax technique recommended a combination of optimized AR with the TSA system for certain hard-to-detect antigens or for expensive primary reagents in using much higher dilution of the primary antibody.[96]

Titration of Primary Antibody and Detection System

The optimal dilution for use of an antibody in immunohistology is defined as that dilution at which the greatest contrast is achieved between the desired (specific) positive staining and any unwanted (nonspecific) background staining. Selection is subjective and is based not simply on the greatest intensity but rather on the greatest useful contrast. Titration is relatively straightforward in the direct method with only a single antibody (Table 1–1). In two- and three-layer methods, exemplified by the indirect conjugate and PAP methods, respectively, each of the separate immune reagents must be applied at optimal dilution. In addition, the dilutions of the primary and secondary (and tertiary) antibodies are interdependent in terms of contrast developed by the procedure as a whole. This fact necessitates comparison of the results obtained using several dilutions of the labeling reagent (secondary antibody) with several different dilutions of the primary antibody; comparison is achieved by checkerboard or chessboard titration (Tables 1–2 and 1–3).

NONCONJUGATE PROCEDURES: SO-CALLED NONLABELED ANTIBODY METHODS

The principles used are similar for all multistep methods and are illustrated here with reference to the three-step PAP method.

Titration of Peroxidase Antiperoxidase Reagent. Given the widespread commercial availability of

Table 1–2. Determination of Optimal Titers for Indirect Immunoperoxidase Method—Checkerboard Titration

		Dilutions of Primary Antibody →					
		1/5	*1/20*	*1/80*	*1/320*	*1/1280*	*Negative Control**
Dilutions of secondary antibody (conjugate) ↓	1/10	slide 1 + + +† (+ +)	slide 2 + + + (+ +)	slide 3 + + + (+ +)	slide 4 + + (+ +)	slide 5 + (+ +)	slide 16 ± (+ +)
	1/40	slide 6 + + + (+)	slide 7 + + + (+)	slide 8 + + + + (+)	slide 9 + + + + (±)	slide 10 + + (±)	slide 17 − (±)
	1/160	slide 11 + + (+)	slide 12 + + (±)	slide 13 + (±)	slide 14 ± (−)	slide 15 ± (−)	slide 18 − (−)

Example of an 18-slide titration
* Negative control (omit primary antibody, replace with preimmune serum, or serum with irrelevant specificity; see negative controls).
† Intensity of specific staining is indicated on a scale of 0 to + + + +; nonspecific background is given in the same scale in parentheses
{ 0 to + + + +; e.g., + + + / (+) } indicates strong specific staining (+ + +) with moderate background (+).
Note: In this example, the optimal result is achieved with slide 9.
Adapted from Taylor CR, Cote RJ. Immunomicroscopy: A Diagnostic Tool for the Surgical Pathologist, 2nd ed. Philadelphia: WB Saunders, 1994:29.

Table 1–3. Checkerboard Titration for Peroxidase-Antiperoxidase Method*

Primary Antibody Dilution (e.g., Rabbit Antiinsulin)	Secondary Antibody Dilution (e.g., Swine Antirabbit IgG)	PAP Dilution (Rabbit PAP)		
		1/20	1/80	1/160
		(Slide Numbers)		
1/80	1/10	1	2	3
	1/40	4	5	6
	1/160	7	8	9
1/320	1/10	10	11	12
	1/40	13	14	15
	1/160	16	17	18
1/1280	1/10	19	20	21
	1/40	22	23	24
	1/160	25	26	27
Control (omit primary antibody)	1/10	28	29	30
	1/40	31	32	33
	1/160	34	35	36

* A 36-slide checkerboard is shown; optimal dilutions of reagents are selected on the basis of that slide giving greatest useful contrast. With experience, it may be possible to reduce the complexity of this titration, omitting some of the dilutions that experience (i.e., previous use of similar reagents from the same source) has shown are unlikely to be optimal.

Adapted from Taylor CR, Cote RJ. Immunomicroscopy: A Diagnostic Tool for the Surgical Pathologist, 2nd ed. Philadelphia: WB Saunders, 1994:29.

PAP reagents, it is necessary to titrate the reagent of choice to determine the dilution that gives optimal staining in a system in which each of the other reagents have also been optimized (see Table 1–3). Ideally, all titrations should be in terms of micrograms of active reagent; in practice, this desired goal is rarely achieved, and we must content ourselves with expression of dilutions, meaning of course that the dilutions used in one laboratory (and reported in one paper) with a particular set of reagents cannot be transferred automatically for use in a second laboratory unless all reagents are identical.

Once optimal dilutions have been determined, the stock of undiluted reagent should be divided into convenient aliquots for the preparation of working dilutions immediately before use. Generally speaking, it is not wise to store reagents in a highly diluted form unless additional protein or stabilizers are added to conserve activity, since reactivity may decline unpredictably. That stability of highly diluted reagents can be achieved is evidenced by the availability of commercial immunostaining kits that do contain prediluted reagents and have a shelf life of 1 year or more.

A principal reason for the use of reagents freshly prepared from aliquots is the need to avoid repeated sampling of a single reagent tube (or bottle), as with a Pasteur pipette, since this practice almost invariably results in bacterial contamination and loss of reactivity that is both unpredictable and aggravating. Here the "pure" scientists might learn a lesson from their often maligned cousins in the commercial sector, who have to a large extent overcome the contamination problem by providing diluted reagents in sealed dropper bottles so that the reagent can be dropped directly from the reagent bottle. We have unashamedly borrowed this technique in our laboratory, and whenever we make up new dilutions of reagents for use over a period of several days we use these small plastic dropper bottles.

Quality Control

Quality control as defined by the College of American Pathologists is "the aggregate of processes and techniques so derived to detect, reduce and correct deficiencies in an analytic process".[97] It is an integral component of a laboratory's quality assurance program, focusing mainly on procedural and technical aspects of the test under question. As it pertains to IHC, quality control standards address and define each step of the "total IHC test," including tissue procurement, fixation, processing, sectioning, staining and, finally, the interpretation and reporting of the staining results. As part of a laboratory's quality control program, all steps of the test are described separately, and parameters of each step are established and monitored in order to ensure consistency of performance and reproducibility of results. Daily records of control results are maintained, and corrective actions are undertaken and documented when results are unacceptable. In this section, we discuss quality control issues as they pertain to the validation of antibodies and the use of controls.

The use of reference standards for the quality control of reagents in the clinical laboratory is well established. For example, serum assay results can be validated by large standardized serum pools, such as those established by the College of American Pathologists' "Check Sample" program. More recently, the development of reference standard controls for IHC has been under consideration.

However, this undertaking is not as simple. Unlike serum samples, pathologic tissues cannot be pooled, and the supply of tissue samples is not infinite. Moreover, morphologically similar tumors are not necessarily antigenically identical. The use of multitissue blocks alleviates some of these problems, but these too contain only a limited amount of tissue, which will eventually become depleted as well. To overcome this, the development of infinite standard reference controls composed of artificial tumors or human tumor cell lines has been proposed.[98]

Validation studies are required for each test and antibody (including each new lot of antibody) that is used by a laboratory. (Such testing is not required for "ready to use" pretested reagents, i.e., those that are part of a kit.) Such studies are imperative because the reagents may be of uncertain origin, composition, or concentration or specificity, or both.[99] Performance parameters to be addressed by these studies include the sensitivity, specificity, precision, accuracy, and reproducibility of the results. It is recommended that these studies be carried out on multitissue control blocks containing both known positive and known negative normal and tumor tissues. The results obtained are reviewed and attest to the specificity and precision of the antibody under study. The specificity of antibody staining is shown by the expected absence of staining in certain cells, tissues, and tumors within the multitissue control blocks. Precision, in contrast, attests to the validity of the entire procedure and is shown by the presence of both positive and negative elements, as expected on the same control slide. A sensitive test is one that detects a small amount of antigen. This is shown by positive results using tissue with known weak positive staining. Accuracy is determined by the evaluation of nonspecific background staining. A negative reagent control can be used in place of the primary antibody to determine this. Finally, if there is no run-to-run variation in the results obtained, the test is reproducible.

The Biologic Stain Commission (BSC), in conjunction with the Food and Drug Administration (FDA), published a set of guidelines for reagent package inserts, which includes recommendations to the manufacturers for the testing and marketing of reagents as well as for the use and purpose of positive and negative controls (Table 1–4).[100] Because of the variability of tissue fixation, processing, and embedding, which are inherent aspects of the IHC test, the Biologic Stain Commission concluded that it was unable to establish a single universal staining protocol. This, therefore, necessitates the concurrent performance and interpretation of controls in conjunction with the tests. These controls ensure proper technique and specificity of the staining method used and are, therefore, essential for correct interpretation of immunohistochemical results.

Both positive and negative controls should be

Table 1–4. Types and Purposes of Daily Quality Control Materials for Immunohistochemistry

Type of Control	Antigen (Analyte)	Antibody (Reagent)	Purpose
Positive	Nonpatient tissue or cells containing antigen to be detected and quantified	Antibody reagent (of the kit) constituted in same way as intended for patient sample	Control of all steps of the analysis
	Known expected result		Training user for appearance of positive reaction; comparison for semiquantitation of reaction
	Fixed-processed in same way as a patient sample		Validates all steps of analysis, including fixation and processing
	Fixed-processed in manner shown to preserve antigen under analysis		Validates all steps of analysis, except fixation or processing used by individual laboratory
Negative (specific)	Tissues or cells expected to be negative by antibody (of kit)	Antibody reagent (of kit) constituted in same way as intended for patient sample	Detection of unintended antibody cross-reactivity to cells or cellular components
	Processed in same way as patient sample		
	May be portion of patient sample		
Negative (nonspecific)	Patient tissue with components that are the same as tissue to be studied	Diluent (as used with antibody) without antibody	Detection of unintended background staining
	Processed in same way as patient sample	Antibody not specific for antigen of interest in same diluents as used with kit antibody	

Adapted from Taylor CR, Cote RJ. Immunomicroscopy: A Diagnostic Tool for the Surgical Pathologist, 2nd ed. Philadelphia: WB Saunders, 1994:27.

used. A positive control is one that is known to contain the antigen under question. These controls should be fixed and processed in a manner that is analogous to the tissue being tested. This is necessary to prevent false-negative reporting on the test specimen. For example, if the test tissue is over-fixed, resulting in diminished or absent antigenicity, yet the control tissue is optimally fixed, a false-negative test result can occur. For this reason, the manufacturers' positive control slides cannot be used as a substitute for positive control slides made "in house" because they are not necessarily processed in the same manner as the tissue being tested. They merely validate reagent performance but cannot verify proper tissue fixation and processing.

From a general standpoint, the best positive controls are those that are processed in house. It is most cost-effective to use surgical tissue controls that have been fixed and processed along with the regular work day's surgical specimens. Tumor tissue is usually preferable for control use, because normal tissue tends to contain more antigen than its neoplastic counterpart. Therefore, the use of normal tissue as a control may result in false-negative results on the tumor tissue in question. Moreover, the ideal positive control should not show uniformly intense positive staining. Rather, the intensity of staining should be variable, with weak staining in many areas. These weakly staining areas can therefore detect subtle changes in primary antibody sensitivity. This, too, helps to decrease the incidence of false-negative results.

Many types of tissue can be used as positive controls. From a general standpoint, surgical material is preferable to autopsy tissue, as the latter may contain areas of autolysis that can affect staining results. For immunocytologic testing of body fluids and fine needle aspiration material, cytospins can be prepared and stored unfixed, or cell blocks can be fixed and embedded to be used as cytologic control material. The most important considerations in the selection of the appropriate control tissue are that it contain the antigen under question and that it is fixed and processed using the same protocol as the test specimen.

Negative controls are used to confirm the specificity of the method used and to assess the presence of nonspecific background staining. This is defined by staining the test tissue in the absence of the primary antibody. This can be accomplished in different ways. Absorption controls are negative controls produced by absorbing the primary antibody with the highly purified protein or peptide antigen that was used to generate the antibody. The original objective of this control technique was to eliminate the binding of the antibody to the protein in the tissue. However, studies have shown that the absorption control cannot determine whether the protein bound in the tissue is the same protein that is used for absorption. The monoclonal antibody may instead recognize a sim-

ilar epitope of unrelated protein, particularly after tissue fixation. Absorption controls, therefore, do not provide the specificity of the antibody for the protein in the tissue.[101–103]

Other negative controls include the substitution of the primary antibody with antibody diluent (buffer plus bovine serum albumin carrier protein) or with nonimmune immunoglobulin, which is derived from the same species and is at the same dilution. The substitution of an irrelevant antibody can also be used as a negative control. To this effect, some authors believe that when a panel of different antibodies are being tested on the same tissue, the results obtained from the different primary antibodies can be used as negative controls for each other (provided that the antibodies are of the same isotype, are derived from the same species, and are of similar concentrations). Finally, with regard to negative controls, if more than one protocol is used on a particular day (i.e., microwave AR pretreatment, protease-trypsin digestion), separate negative control slides should be run for each in accordance with each protocol used.

Another useful control method is the use of multitissue control slides. Each multitissue control slide contains samples of tissues that are arranged in either a checkerboard or sausage pattern. Checkerboard control slides include maps designating the types of tissues present and their specific locations. Sausage control slides are accompanied by a more general map showing the whereabouts of different tissue types, which are often arranged in clusters. As mentioned previously, multitissue control slides are particularly useful for validation studies of new reagents. However, they may also be used for routine quality control purposes. Their disadvantage is their cost and the inability to control how the specimens were fixed and processed.[104, 105]

Internal controls are present when the tissue being tested contains the antigen under question in adjacent normal tissue. The presence of positive internal control staining in the expected cells indicates appropriate immunoreactivity. For ubiquitous antigens, such as vimentin, positive internal control staining may be used as this antibody's positive control. Moreover, because of its ubiquity, staining for vimentin is also helpful as a reporter molecule, that is, to assess fixation and processing of the tissue.[106] As discussed previously, variation in staining results can result from overfixation or underfixation, or both. It has been shown that various epitopes of vimentin are particularly sensitive to overfixation and may, therefore, become altered or destroyed by this process. A monoclonal vimentin antibody, V9, recognizes this sensitive epitope. The intensity of staining with V9 can, therefore, be used to assess the degree of formalin fixation. It can also be used to monitor the recovery from formalin overfixation by AR. To extrapolate further from this concept, the variation of intensity of vimentin internal control staining can be used to identify variations of fixation within a tissue section that can adversely affect test results.

From this discussion, it can be seen that the understanding and application of appropriate positive and negative controls is one of the most important yet often misunderstood aspects of IHC. The proper use of these controls is essential for correct interpretation of immunohistochemical results.

Tissue Fixation, Processing, and Antigen Retrieval Techniques

Tissue preparation consists of fixation, subsequent dehydration, and embedment in paraffin wax to provide a rigid matrix for sectioning. Tissues that are to be embedded in paraffin wax are first "fixed" in order to optimize preservation, a process that profoundly affects the morphologic and immunohistologic results. The ideal fixative for IHC studies should not only be readily available but should also be in widespread use to maximize the range and number of samples available for IHC studies. The fixative should preserve antigenic integrity and should limit extraction, diffusion, or displacement of antigen during subsequent processing. Also, it should give good preservation of morphologic details after embedment in a support medium (e.g., paraffin).

Common fixatives used in histopathology are divided into two groups: coagulant fixatives, such as ethanol, and cross-linking fixatives, such as formaldehyde. Both types of fixative can cause changes in the steric configuration of proteins, which may mask antigenic sites (epitopes) and adversely affect binding with antibody. It is well recognized that cross-linking fixatives alter the IHC results for a significant number of antigens, whereas coagulant fixatives, especially ethanol, have been reported to produce lesser changes.[34, 107–109] In most surgical pathology laboratories, the fixative used is 10% neutral buffer formalin (NBF) (a cross-linking fixative). Subsequent processing usually includes a period in 100% ethanol; thus, tissues are effectively "double fixed" in both formalin and ethanol. For tissues fixed in formalin, the immunostaining intensity is known to be fixation time–dependent for many antigens.[107, 109, 110] A long history of using formalin as a standard tissue fixative has revealed the following advantages:

1. There is good preservation of morphology for a variety of tissues, even after prolonged fixation; in this case "good" is a somewhat subjective term encompassing the various artifactual changes that result in the presentation of the morphologic features that "please" the pathologist, based on previous experience and the manner of fixation-processing to which the pathologist has become accustomed.
2. Formalin is an economical chemical, much cheaper than most alternatives.

3. Formalin fixation can sterilize tissue specimens in a more reliable way than precipitating fixatives, particularly for viruses.
4. Carbohydrate antigens are better preserved.[111]
5. There is preservation of many antigens through cross-linking of protein in situ, thereby avoiding leaching out of proteins that may diffuse in water or alcohol. Many low molecular weight antigens (peptides) are extracted by non–cross-linking fixatives such as alcohol-, or methanol-based solutions, but they are well preserved in tissue by formalin in the form of cross-linked derivatives.[28] Traditionally, non–cross-linking precipitating fixatives are believed to be superior to aldehyde fixation in order to retain immunoreactivity for certain larger proteins, such as intermediate filaments and immunoglobulins.

Formalin may be regarded as a satisfactory fixative for both morphology and IHC provided that a simple and effective AR technique is available to recover those antigens that are diminished or modified.

ANTIGEN RETRIEVAL

A simple heat-induced AR technique (heating tissue section in water) is now widely applied in pathology.[38, 39, 55, 57] Successful application of the AR technique for routine IHC staining of formalin-fixed tissues in diagnostic pathology has rendered the search for alternative fixatives to replace formalin less urgent. In 1997, Prento and Lyon[112] compared the performance of six commercial fixatives offered as "formalin substitutes" and concluded that the best immunostaining was obtained by combining formalin fixation with AR technique, and that none of the six proposed substitutes for formalin was adequate for histopathologic use (i.e., they did not give the "good" morphologic features to which pathologists had become accustomed).

Williams and coworkers[113] performed a careful study to investigate the effect of tissue preparation on IHC staining by using tonsil tissues that were subjected to variations in fixation, processing, and section preparation, as well as storage. They demonstrated that the microwave AR technique ameliorated the problems resulting from variations in fixation, processing, and section preparation. They reported that 10% neutral buffered formalin, 10% zinc formalin, and 10% formal saline gave the most consistent results overall and showed excellent antigen preservation. In contrast, 10% formal acetic acid, B5, and Bouin's fixative all showed poor antigen preservation, even after AR treatment. Reduced effectiveness of AR when used with other fixatives has also been documented by others.[114–116]

Although storage of cut tissue sections was not an issue in the study of Williams and associates,[113] others have reported that decreased intensity of staining may occur for some antigens in slides stored for protracted periods.[117–121,123] It is our experience that "storage-induced" decreases in IHC staining are relatively uncommon, and most of these adverse effects can be recovered by AR treatment. For example, combination of the AR treatment and use of a sensitive polymeric labeling two-step detection system achieves satisfactory results for antibodies to p53 (Pab-1801), p21[WAF1] (Ab-1, Oncogene) and p27[Kip1] (DCS-72.F6, NeoMarkers),[17, 91] even after prolonged storage.

The AR technique has utility not only for enhancement of IHC staining on archival tissue sections but also for standardization of routine IHC.[17, 38, 39, 91] A key element in the appropriate use and standardization of the AR technique for IHC is understanding major factors that influence the effectiveness of AR.

In general, major factors that influence the quality of results of AR-IHC include heating temperature and heating time (heating condition T × t) and the pH value of the AR solution. The chemical components and molarity of the AR solution are cofactors that may influence the effectiveness of AR-IHC in certain instances.

Heating Conditions. As noted previously, the heating AR-IHC method is based on biochemical studies of Fraenkel-Conrat and coworkers, who documented that the chemical reactions that occur between protein and formalin may be reversed, at least in part, by high temperature heating or strong alkaline hydrolysis.[31–33] We demonstrated that the use of conventional heating at 100°C may achieve results similar to those obtained by microwave heating and also that distilled water could be used as the AR solution, albeit with slightly less effect.[34] Subsequently, several publications reported similar results by using conventional heating.[38, 39, 125, 126] Malmstrom and colleagues[122] performed AR-IHC on proliferating cell nuclear antigen (PCNA) (PC10 and 19F4) using distilled water as the AR solution on routinely processed paraffin sections of urinary bladder carcinoma and obtained good results.

The chemical reactions occurring during the formalin fixation process remain obscure. Mason and O'Leary[124] demonstrated that the process of cross-linking does not result in discernible alteration of protein secondary structure, at least as determined by calorimetric and infrared spectroscopic investigation. They also noted that significant denaturation of unfixed purified proteins occurred at temperature ranges from 70°C to 90°C, whereas similar temperatures had virtually no adverse effect on formalin-fixed proteins (i.e., formalin-fixed proteins are more heat-stable). Thus, the AR heating technique, using high temperature heating of tissue sections fixed in formalin, may take advantage of the fact that the cross-linkage of protein produced by formalin fixation may "protect" the primary and secondary structure of formalin-modified protein from denaturation during the heating phase, while allowing some reduction of cross-linkages at the surface of the molecule, thereby restoring antigenicity. Although the mechanism of action of the

AR technique is not clear, it appears unlikely, based on the preceding observation that "protein denaturation alone is the mechanism" as advocated by Cattoretti and colleagues.[43]

In general, the heating conditions appear to be the most important factor in the effectiveness of AR.[37–41, 54–56, 125–130] The evidence may be summarized as follows:

- Significant enhancement of immunohistochemical staining can be achieved by using high-temperature heating of routinely processed paraffin-embedded tissue sections in pure distilled water.[34, 125, 131–133]
- Higher temperatures in general yield superior results.[38, 39, 55–57, 125, 128] An optimal result for AR-IHC is correlated with the product of the heating temperature and the time of AR heating treatment (T [temperature of heating AR procedure] × t [period of heating time]).[110, 129]
- An equivalent intensity of AR-IHC can be obtained using different buffers as AR solutions if the pH value of AR solutions are monitored in a comparable manner, thereby demonstrating that individual specific chemical constituents are not necessary factors in yielding a satisfactory result.[47–49]
- Our early experience that even prolonged exposure of paraffin sections in citrate buffer solution (or indeed any buffer) without heating gave no noticeable AR effect has subsequently been confirmed by numerous studies.[52, 54, 134]

pH and Chemical Composition of the Antigen Retrieval Solution. The pH value of the AR solution is important for some antigens. From a 1995 comparative study,[49, 50] we concluded that antigens fell into three broad categories with respect to the importance of pH on AR:

1. Most antigens showed no significant variation using AR solutions with pH values ranging from 1.0 to 10.0.
2. Certain other antigens, especially nuclear antigens (e.g., MIB1, ER) showed a dramatic decrease in the intensity of the AR-IHC at middle-range pH values, but optimal results at low pH.
3. A small group of antigens (MT1, HMB-45) showed negative or very weak focally positive immunostaining with a low pH (1.0 to 2.0) but excellent results in the high-pH range (Figs. 1–17 and 1–18).

Evers and Uylings[127] also found that the AR-IHC is pH- and temperature-dependent. They tested two antibodies, MAP-2 and SMI-32, and indicated that the optimal pH values were pH 4.5 for MAP-2, and pH 2.5 for SMI-32. They also concluded that it is not important what kind of solution is used as long as the pH is at an appropriate level.

In conclusion, major factors that influence the results of AR IHC stain include heating temperature and heating time (heating condition T × t) and the pH value of the AR solution. The chemical composition and molarity of the AR solution are cofactors that may influence the effectiveness of

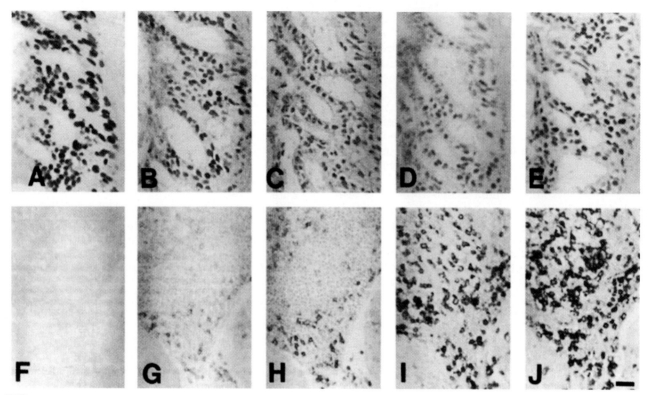

Figure 1–17. Comparisons of the intensity of AR immunostaining in routinely formalin-fixed, paraffin-embedded tissue sections with a monoclonal antibody (MAb) to ER in breast tissue *(A–E)* and Mab MT1 in lymph node *(F–J)*. Sodium diethylbarbiturate-HCl (SDH) buffer was used as the AR solution for both antibodies. The pH values of AR solution were pH 2, 3, 4, 6, and 8, which correspond to staining intensity of ++++, +++, +, ++, +++, respectively, for ER with a type B pattern *(A–E)*. *F–J* show a type C pattern with SDH as the AR solution with a pH of 2, 3, 4, 6, 8, and intensity of staining −, +, ++, +++, ++++, respectively, for MT1. Some nuclei showed very weak false nuclear staining *(F)*. DAB was the chromogen and hematoxylin was the counterstain (original magnification ×100; bar = 20 µm.) (Reproduced, with permission, from Shi S-R, Imam SA, Young, L, et al. Antigen retrieval immunohistochemistry under the influence of pH using monoclonal antibodies. Journal of Histochemistry & Cytochemistry 43:193–201, 1995.)

AR-IHC in certain instances and should be explored when satisfactory results cannot be obtained with the solutions usually used.[39, 40, 55–57, 135]

Test Battery Approach for Antigen Retrieval Technique. A test battery may be defined as a preliminary test of AR technique examining the two major factors, heating condition (T × t) and pH value, which is performed to establish an optimal protocol for the antigen being tested.

Typically, three levels of heating conditions and pH values—low, moderate, and high—may be applied to screen for a potential optimal protocol of AR-IHC for a particular antigen of interest, as indicated in Table 1–5. The test battery method can also be performed in two sequential steps: (1) testing three AR solutions at different pH values, as listed earlier, with one standard temperature (100°C for 10 minutes) in order to find the optimal pH value of AR solution and (2) the testing optimal heating conditions based on the established pH value.

We have demonstrated that different heating methods, including microwave, microwave and pressure cooker, steam, and autoclave heating methods,[38, 39] can be evaluated in a similar fashion and adjusted to yield a similar satisfactory intensity of staining by AR-IHC.

The test battery serves as a rapid screening approach to identify an optimal protocol for each antibody-antigen to be tested. The goal is to establish the "maximal retrieval" level for formalin-masked antigens after undefined fixation times in order to standardize immunostaining results.[47–50] In addition, the use of a test battery may identify false-negative or false-positive AR-IHC staining results.

TECHNIQUES OF IMMNOHISTOCHEMICAL STAINING

The following description is focused on immunostaining techniques for archival paraffin-embedded tissue sections. The basic principles and protocols for fresh frozen tissue sections are the same as those for paraffin section except that the AR and dewaxing procedures are not required for frozen

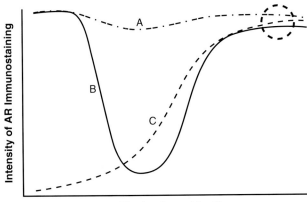

Figure 1–18. Schematic diagram of the three patterns of pH-influenced AR immunostaining. Line A (pattern of type A) shows a stable pattern of staining with only a slight decrease in staining intensity between pH 3 and pH 6. Line B (pattern of type B) shows a dramatic decrease in staining intensity between pH 3 and pH 6. Line C (pattern of type C) exhibits an ascending intensity of AR immunostaining that correlated with increasing pH values of the AR solution. Circle *(right)* indicates the advantage of using an AR solution of higher pH value. (Reproduced, with permission, from Shi S-R, Imam SA, Young L, et al. Antigen retrieval immunohistochemistry under the influence of pH using monoclonal antibodies. Journal of Histochemistry & Cytochemistry 43:193–201, 1995.)

tissue sections. Titration (dilutions) may also differ.

Because the success of the IHC staining method depends on the correct application of both histologic and immunologic techniques, it is recommended that the user be familiar with the literature concerning the antigen under investigation before performing IHC staining. In particular, it is important to know the following:
• The cellular localization of the antigen base
• The specificity of the primary antibody
• The results of previous IHC staining tests (from the literature, and especially from the experience of the performing laboratory), with respect to any

adverse influence on the antigen from tissue fixation processing, and the value of any pretreatment procedure such as heat-induced AR

In addition, detailed information regarding the reagents, particularly the primary antibody and detection system—such as the manufacturer, clone number of monoclonal antibody, and recommended concentration—is helpful in achieving a successful result.

Antigen Retrieval Protocol

MICROWAVE HEATING METHOD
(Shi et al., 1991)[34]
1. Deparaffinized slides are placed in plastic Coplin jars containing AR solution; it is recommended that the same number of slides be used every time, using "blanks if necessary" to ensure consistent heating.
2. Jars are covered with loose-fitting screw caps and heated in the microwave oven for 10 minutes. The 10-minute heating time is divided into two 5-minute cycles with an interval of 1 minute between cycles to check the fluid level in the jars. If necessary, more AR solution is added after the first 5 minutes to avoid drying out the tissue sections. It is recommended that the heating time be standardized by beginning to count the time only after the solution has reached boiling in order to avoid discrepancies among laboratories when using various microwave ovens.
3. After completion of the heating phase, the Coplin jars are removed from the oven and allowed to cool for 15 minutes.
4. Slides are then rinsed twice in distilled water and in phosphate-buffered saline (PBS) for 5 minutes and are ready for IHC staining.

Various heating methods, including conventional heating in water bath, pressure cooker, steamer, and autoclave, may be used and may achieve results similar to those with IHC. Our studies have demonstrated that different heating methods can

Table 1–5. Test Battery Suggested for Screening an Optimal Antigen Retrieval Protocol

TRIS-HCl Buffer	pH 1 to 2	pH 7 to 8	pH 10 to 11
Super high, 120°C*	Slide No. 1	Slide No. 4	Slide No. 7
High, 100°C for 10 minutes	Slide No. 2	Slide No. 5	Slide No. 8
Mid-high, 90°C for 10 minutes†	Slide No. 3	Slide No. 6	Slide No. 9

* The temperature of super high at 120°C may be reached by either autoclaving or microwave heating with longer time.
† The temperature of mid-high at 90°C may be obtained by either a water bath or a microwave oven monitored with a thermometer.
Note: One more slide may be used for control without AR treatment. The citrate buffer pH 6.0 may be used to replace TRIS-HCl buffer pH 7 to 8, as the results are the same.
Adapted from Shi, S-R, Cote RJ, Taylor CR. Antigen retrieval immunohistochemistry: Past, present, and future. J Histochem Cytochem 1997;45:327–343.

yield similar intensities of immunostaining if the heating conditions are adjusted appropriately.[38, 39]

Blocking Nonspecific Binding

Quenching endogenous peroxidase by an H_2O_2-methanol solution is performed immediately after the dewaxing procedure. Blocking of endogenous biotin may be performed before the biotin-conjugated link by using the avidin-biotin blocking reagent, or using skim milk as an alternative blocking reagent (incubate for 10 minutes).[115]

Normal serum taken from the same species as the secondary (link) antibody should be used to block nonspecific binding sites, as discussed previously.

Washing Steps

Thorough washing is critical for each step, except the blocking step of normal serum. PBS, 0.01 M at pH 7.4 (PBS) is widely used, with the washing procedure carried out in a jar containing PBS and immersing slides for two 5-minute periods (total of 10 minutes). Alternatively, PBS may be flooded onto the slides in a humidity chamber for 10 minutes with one change. With automation of IHC staining technique, the washing procedure is also automated, and multiple washes are used.

Incubation of Primary Antibody

The time of incubation depends on the sensitivity and concentration of the primary antibody used, as well as the quality of the tissue section. Concentration of the primary antibody is based on a titration test as described previously, with reference to the manufacturer's instructions. In general, frozen tissue sections require less incubation time than do archival paraffin tissue sections. A commonly used incubation period is 30 minutes at room temperature. With multistage methods, such as the PAP method, successive incubation periods and washings result in a lengthy overall procedure. Some attempt has been made to shorten the procedure by performing incubations at 37°C in a hot plate humidity chamber; the incubation for each step may then be 10 minutes or less. Humidity chambers may be placed in an oven at 37°C, which is a less effective method than the hot plate because of the longer time needed for reagents to reach a temperature of 37°C. Some automated stainers also accelerate the process by operating at 37°C or 42°C. Microwave acceleration of the IHC staining technique has also been described for rapid IHC staining,[136–139] but generally it is not convenient.

Incubation of slides in a humidity chamber is essential at 37°C and is advisable at room temperature. In practice, if a slide treated with antibody is permitted to dry, excessive nonspecific background staining invariably occurs. Even when total drying does not occur, evaporation of the antibody solution on the slide may result in an effective increase in antibody concentration, again producing unwanted background staining. Humidity chambers containing level slide racks may be purchased or can be made rather easily from glass rods and plexiglass or glass plates glued together with water-resistant bonds. Staining racks on which slides rest during incubation should be level to avoid drainage of antibody off the section to other areas of the slide.

Overnight (or extended) incubation may also be used in certain circumstances; here again, a humidity chamber partially filled with water is essential. We have used overnight staining to permit the use of a primary antibody at very high dilutions and have often achieved good results with reduced nonspecific background staining (i.e., take an antibody that gives satisfactory results when incubated for 30 minutes, dilute it 10- or even 100-fold, and then incubate for 12 to 24 hours). This approach conserves precious antibody and reduces background staining due to decreased nonspecific attachment of antibody (the antibody is present at a much lower concentration, favoring binding by high-affinity immunologic reactions). With this method, only the primary antibody is given prolonged incubation; other reagents are used normally. Overnight incubation of primary antibody is a practical consideration for many service laboratories and has the advantages of convenience of working schedule and reduced costs for expensive antibodies based on a higher dilution of primary antibodies.

Incubation of Detection Reagents

As noted previously, titration may be necessary. A good place to begin is by following the manufacturer's instructions for concentration of each reagent and the exact protocol for the detection system. Incubation is carried out carefully, usually at room temperature for 30 minutes for each step (link and label). Dropping reagents on each slide to cover the tissue section completely is a simple but critical procedure. Caution must be taken to confirm that the whole tissue section is immersed in the reagent, including the margins, and that no air bubbles exist, particularly when using automation (e.g., the capillary action–based procedure).

Substrate and Chromogen

Several different chromogens (color-producing substrate systems) are available (Table 1–6). With horseradish peroxidase, DAB may be preferred because the brown reaction product is alcohol-fast and thus is suitable for use with a wide range of counterstains and mountants. AEC, which gives a red color, has become more widely used. Although

Table 1–6. Immunohistochemistry: Commonly Used "Chromogens" or Reaction Products*

Procedure	Color	Solubility in Alcohol
Peroxidase		
Diaminobenzidine (DAB)	Brown	Insoluble
DAB with enhancement	Black	Insoluble
3-Amino-9-ethyl carbazole (AEC)	Red†	Soluble
4-Chloro-1-naphthol (4-CN)	Blue-black	Soluble
Hanker-Yates reagent	Blue	Insoluble
Alpha-naphthol pyronin	Red	Soluble
3,3',5,5'-tetramethylbenzidine (TMB)	Blue	Insoluble
Alkaline Phosphatase		
Fast blue BB	Blue	Soluble
Fast red TR	Red	Soluble
New fuchsin	Red	Insoluble
BCIP-NBT	Blue	Insoluble
Glucose Oxidase		
Tetrazolium	Blue	Insoluble
Tetranitoblue tetrazolium (TNBT)	Black	Insoluble
Immunogold		
With silver enhancement	Black	Insoluble

* Other proprietary "chromogens" are available, but those listed are those that are well documented. Various commercial products can be found in catalogs from several companies.
† AEC has two reaction sites: In the presence of enzyme excess both react, the color passing from red to green-brown.
Adapted from Taylor CR, Cote RJ. Immunomicroscopy: A Diagnostic Tool for the Surgical Pathologist, 2nd ed. Philadelphia: WB Saunders, 1994:67.

it is alcohol-soluble, it is generally considered a lower risk carcinogen than DAB and thus has been favored by commercial suppliers of immunohistologic reagents.

For general purposes, we routinely use DAB or AEC. AEC produces a crisp red color that contrasts well with a hematoxylin counterstain (note that a "progressive" nonalcoholic hematoxylin should be used [e.g., Mayer's, not Harris'] to avoid removal of the colored product, which is alcohol-soluble). At high concentrations of antigen-antibody-enzyme, AEC may produce a brown-yellow color (AEC has two reactive sites: when one is converted it turns red; if both react with peroxidase a green-brown product results). It may be helpful to maintain the acetic acid buffer at pH 4.8 to minimize this effect. Sections must be mounted in an aqueous medium (e.g., 80% glycerol). Aquamount contains small amounts of organic solvent and may cause slow diffusion or loss of stain. Dehydration through alcohol must be avoided. Glycerol-mounted preparations may be made permanent by sealing the edges of the cover slip with nail varnish.

DAB may be used for specific purposes; it is alcohol-resistant and may be subject to staining, dehydration, and mounting in Permount. It is also valuable for the electron microscopist because it is electron-dense. For light microscopy, some investigators advocate osmication of the DAB reaction product, giving a more intense color. We have not found this necessary for light microscopy; indeed, we feel it may be a disadvantage because background staining is also enhanced, and the end result may be diminished contrast despite the more intense staining. A similar effect may be achieved by post-treatment with nickel sulfate or cobalt chloride, which produces excellent contrast.[140, 141]

If DAB is used, solutions should be prepared under a hood by a masked, gloved technician. Unused solution should be disposed of with an excess of water. At the working dilution used, the danger is considered minimal; it is the powdered form that evokes concern. Preweighed aliquots in sealed tubes are available from some manufacturers but are expensive. Ready-to-use liquid DAB is now provided commercially. It has the advantages of convenience, safety, and less environmental pollution.

Alpha-naphthol pyronine (pink), 4-chloro-l-naphthol (blue), and Hanker-Yates reagent are other alternatives, together with a variety of "broad" chromogens (see Table 1–6). A range of substrates is also available for alkaline phosphatase. Some substrates contribute to the sensitivity of the alkaline phosphatase systems by continuing to convert at the enzyme site, resulting in a granular accumulation of the colored product. If carried to excess, this granularity may obscure morphologic definition.

COUNTERSTAINING AND MOUNTING SLIDES

The final step in the process is counterstaining and mounting slides. Hematoxylin is used as the nuclear counterstain for most routine IHC staining. In the case of nuclear antigen immunolocalization, caution must be taken to avoid overdevelopment of the hematoxylin stain (a light hematoxylin stain is critical to allow any nuclear localization of chromogen to be discerned). In our experience, the time of exposure to hematoxylin depends in part on how fresh the dye solution is (a freshly prepared solution of hematoxylin requires a much shorter time than does exposure in an old solution). It may be necessary to monitor the development of the stain by microscopy in order to determine the optimal time of counterstaining. For alcohol-soluble stains (e.g., AEC or fast red), an aqueous mounting medium is used. The mounting medium is warmed on a heating block until it liquefies. One of two methods is used: either one drop is placed on the tissue section and a cover slip is lowered slowly onto the slide or the cover slip is placed on a paper towel, one drop is placed in the center of the cover slip, and the inverted slide is lowered slowly onto the coverslip. In either case, care should be taken to avoid trapping an air bubble between the cover slip and the tissue section. For alcohol-insoluble stains (e.g., DAB or new fuchsin), a permanent mounting medium, such as Permount, may be used. The tissue section is first dehydrated by immersing the slide in graded alcohols: 90% and 100%, twice for each, followed by clearing in xylene (twice for 3 minutes each). Mount the cover slip on the slide as described earlier for aqueous mounting medium. Notice that xylene and Permount should be used in a fume hood.

A step-by-step protocol of routine IHC staining is included in Appendix A of this chapter.

Double Immunoenzymatic Techniques

The identification of two antigens in fixed paraffin-embedded tissues is usually accomplished by immunoperoxidase staining of adjacent serial sections (Fig. 1–19). Although this approach suffices for general use, on occasion it may be difficult to identify with certainty the pattern of staining of a particular cell population in adjacent sections, especially if the cells under study are small or are scattered among other cells (Fig. 1–20).

Double immunoenzymatic techniques permit the demonstration of two antigens concurrently within a single section and have been adapted from both the conjugate antibody method and unlabeled antibody method. As an example of these procedures, the first sequence of staining for one antigen is completed with the development of the peroxidase reaction using DAB as the substrate. Staining for the second antigen is then carried out with a primary antibody of different specificity and a second, different substrate system for the peroxidase

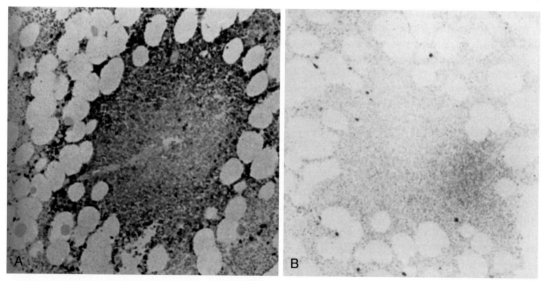

Figure 1–19. *A* and *B*, B5-fixed section of bone marrow aspirate depicting a small solitary nodule consisting of lymphocytes and occasional plasmacytoid lymphocytes, with scattered plasma cells around it. Many of the lymphoid and plasmacytoid cells reacted strongly with anti-lambda antibody *(A)*. Anti-kappa reacted only with scattered plasma cells outside the nodule *(B, small black dots)*. This patient eventually was shown to have a solitary plasmacytoid lymphocytic lymphoma in the small intestine (also lambda type). Paraffin sections, DAB with hematoxylin counterstain (×125) There was no serum paraprotein detectable at this time; presumably the number of tumor cells was insufficient for production of a detectable paraprotein; however, a "monoclonal" IgM appeared later in the course. From Taylor RT, Cote RJ. Immunomicroscopy: A Diagnostic Tool for the Surgical Pathologist, 2nd ed. Philadelphia: WB Saunders, 1994, p 59.

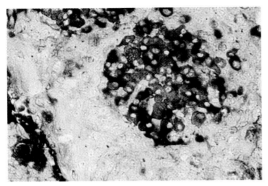

Figure I–20. Double staining for kappa *(brown)* and lambda *(blue)* in paraffin section of a reactive lymph node using sequential horseradish peroxidase and alkaline phosphase methods.

enzyme, for example, 4-chloro-1-naphthol; this produces a contrasting blue reaction product.

The relative merits of elution of the first sequence of antibodies (after reaction with DAB) before titrating the second sequence of antibodies have been much debated. If desired, elution can be accomplished by incubating the sections with acid solutions (usually glycine–hydrochloric acid buffer at pH 2.2 or 1 N hydrochloric acid for 1 hour) or with an oxidizing solution (0.15 mol $KMnO_4$, and 0.01 N H_2SO_4 in 140 V of distilled water at pH 1.8), followed by reduction with 1% $NaSO_4$, for 1 minute. However, Sternberger and Joseph[18] were able to demonstrate two antigens simultaneously without elution of the first set of reagents, despite the fact that the second primary antibody was of the same species as that used for the first antigen and the same PAP labeling reagents were used for both; the success of this system may be due to the fact that the polymerized product of DAB oxidation (used for the first antigen—PAP method) blocks the catalytic site of peroxidase in the first PAP complexes while also obscuring the antigenic reactivity of the first sequence of antibodies, thereby preventing interactions with the second sequence of antibodies and the second substrate system.

Lan and colleagues[142] developed a simple, reliable, and sensitive method for multiple IHC staining by adding a microwave heating procedure (10 minutes) between each sequence of IHC staining (for elution of the previous sequence of IHC staining reagents), an approach that appears to ensure complete blocking of antibody cross-reactivity.

The possibility of cross-reaction of the second sequence of antibodies with the first sequence may be eliminated by the use of a double immunoenzymatic method in which two specific primary antibodies, produced in two different species, are used in combination with separate species-specific secondary antibodies coupled with different enzymes (e.g., peroxidase and glucose oxidase, or peroxidase and alkaline phosphatase). This approach also

has the advantage of expediency in that some of the reagents (e.g., the primary antibodies) can be added simultaneously.[143]

The double-labeled antigen method also allows simultaneous performance of the two staining procedures and is very rapid.[144] Behringer and colleagues[145] developed a hapten-antihapten bridge (HAB) technique to accompany the ABC method for simultaneous double immunostaining. However, a higher concentration of primary antibody is required to obtain a comparable intensity of immunostaining by these last two methods.

When one uses double immunoenzymatic staining, it is sometimes difficult to recognize double staining of individual cells because the colored reaction product of one label may overwhelm the other. In these circumstances, an interrupted technique may prove useful: one antigen is stained when the sections are examined and photographed, and the second antigen is then stained in a contrasting color. Sections are then re-examined, and identical fields are rephotographed for comparison.

Considerable ingenuity has been manifested in adopting and adapting these techniques. For example, it is possible to demonstrate six different antigens on the same section.[146] Combinations of immunogold-silver staining (black) with immunoperoxidase-AEC (red-brown) or immunoalkaline phosphatase–fast red or fast blue produce excellent double or triple stains.[147] A combination of immunoperoxidase-AEC (red) with immunoalkaline phosphatase–fast blue (blue) provides excellent contrasting colors. In general, it is important to check carefully and control the development of the second (and third colors) by microscopy and to use detection systems of comparable sensitivity to obtain the best contrast of multiple colors in the same section. In practice, it is our recommendation that double staining is best for diagnostic use when the pathologist has available suitable computer-assisted image analysis methods for accurate interpretation of the intensity and localization of the double stain. In this respect "spectral image analysis" is a particularly powerful and useful method that of itself renders double stains both practical and useful.[148]

One practical approach to double staining with monoclonal antibodies is given in Appendix B.

Automation

Because of the great variability of specimen fixation and processing among laboratories, it has not been possible to establish a universal standard protocol for IHC. Instead, the goal has become the standardization of protocols within a single laboratory. As discussed earlier, this is accomplished by the rigorous application of proper controls as well as by strict adherence to all aspects of the test, including the preparation of slides, the preparation and application of reagents, the monitoring of incubation times, and so on. Such in-house standardization serves to ensure run-to-run reproducibility of accurate results. This requirement for standardized and reproducible tests, combined with the increasing demand for medically timely and accurate results, calls for automation.

Automated immunostaining devices started to appear in the early 1980s in order to bring this tool that was once limited to the research laboratory into more widespread use. This became necessary in order to meet increased diagnostic demands. Through pilot studies, improvement in software design, and innovations of hardware, this technology, although still evolving, is ready and in use in most of the IHC laboratories in the United States. Other automated devices, such as automated cellular imaging systems and automated AR systems, have been introduced and will also be discussed briefly.

With regard to the staining procedure itself, most of the steps of the manual staining methods are technician-dependent, and specific care by a skilled technician is required during each step to ensure the quality of the results obtained. These steps include the preparation of slides and reagents, the application of reagents and antibodies, the monitoring of incubation times, the washing and wiping of slides, and so on. Moreover, many of these steps are rather slow and repetitive. Because of this method's large number of operator-dependent steps, the likelihood of technical error is increased. For example, a step may be accidentally omitted or performed in the incorrect sequence. The specimens may retain water after rinsing or, conversely, become dry during staining. Incubation times may be too short or too long, the antibody too dilute or too concentrated, or the substrate underdeveloped or overdeveloped. In addition to these technical variables, there are reagent variables to be considered as well. These include the proper selection and use of antibodies with variable avidities as well as the selection of different chromogens, buffers, and enzymes. All these variables must be considered when using a manual staining method. With the advent of automation, most of these issues have already been addressed and standardized as discussed further on.

Automated instruments are designed to imitate the manual staining methods. Those steps of the staining procedure that lend themselves to automation include the application of reagents, the incubation of the tissues, and the rinsing of the slides. From a broad standpoint, this can be accomplished in one of three ways.[149] The slides may be arranged vertically and the reagents applied from above using gravity and top-to-bottom capillary action, which displaces the liquid that is contained between a vertically positioned slide and its cover plate. Conversely, the reagents can climb up from a reagent-containing basin by bottom-to-top capillary action between two adjacent and clamped vertical slides. Using this second technique, the liquids are then eliminated by blotting the bottom of the slides. With the third method, the slides are arranged horizontally on a platform. Reagents and buffers are administered from above by a probe, disposable tip, or reagent test pack, and a horizontally administered air jet eliminates them.

The efficiency of a capillary gap stainer is related to the ability of the capillary gap to fill or empty. This depends, to some extent, on the surface tension of the fluid being used. Aqueous solutions with greater surface tension have more difficulty filling the gap than do alcoholic solutions. This can result in insufficient reagent ascent, which will, of course, affect staining results. Therefore, one needs to monitor for this problem when using capillary gap machines that collect the reagent from below. For this reason, it is advisable that double-mounted slides be used, with the control tissue placed at the top end. This can be used to verify the upper limit of reagent ascent. For obvious reasons, this is less of a problem with capillary gap devices that administer reagents from above with the assistance of gravity. With this type of machine, the control tissue is best placed at the bottom of the slide in order to serve as a monitor for sufficient reagent delivery. A drawback of both these types of the capillary gap technique is their intolerance for the presence of thick, loose, or folded sections that may affect the proper spacing of the gap and result in poor staining or the presence of bubbles. For this reason, some capillary gap machines require the use of specific slides, which, when clamped together, create a precise gap space.

Depending on the need of the individual laboratory, there is a variety of automated immunostainers with different methods, analytic flexibility, and productivity.[150] From a general standpoint, certain performance criteria should be met by all. First, before putting an automated immunostainer to use, parallel studies should be performed to confirm that the results obtained by automated technique are comparable to or better than those obtained previously by the manual method. Furthermore, staining results obtained from the automated instrument, using the same tissue and the same antibody (for example, the positive controls) should show intralaboratory run-to-run reproducibility. Optimally, the machine should also permit the use of multiple antibodies and detection systems and provide random access to accommodate the diversity of antigens and recipes. Its software should allow flexible programming and be user-friendly. Moreover, the ideal instrument should be easy to use and require minimal technician attention during a run. Should a problem occur, the machine must have an error tracking program and be able to report the problem. Regarding the dispensing of reagents, precise and reproducible microliter quantities of each reagent should be dispensed, resulting in complete tissue coverage.

Moreover, the evaporative loss and carry over of reagents should also be kept to a minimum. Many manufacturers supply proprietary reagents, enzymes, chromogens and counterstains that must be used in conjunction with their instrument. Protocols requiring the strict use of proprietary reagents are not as flexible and cannot be customized. Moreover, these reagents tend to be more costly. However, the use of ready-to-use bar codes permits computer-driven tracking and monitoring of reagent volume, lot number, and expiration date. These reagents, therefore, assist with matters pertaining to quality control. Open automated systems, in contrast, are more flexible and allow for the use of other reagents and protocols. These protocols can be customized and stored for use at any time.

The application of automation for immunostaining offers several advantages. The true value of automation is that it offers a uniform and standardized microenvironment, resulting in intralaboratory run-to-run assay consistency. The cost and inconvenience of repeated procedures are, therefore, avoided. Moreover, small microliter amounts of expensive reagents can be dispensed accurately. This saves not only expensive immunologic reagents but also money. Moreover, automation allows for walk-away function and thereby frees not only the time but also the cost of skilled technicians. The use of automated instrumentation may also decrease the amount of technical training that is required through a user-friendly software interface. From a safety standpoint, the use of a consolidated and enclosed automated work station increases biosafety by reducing exposure to, and facilitating the disposal of, hazardous chemicals and carcinogenic reagents. Other benefits of automation include increased throughput and decreased turnaround time by increasing the speed of reactions with heat and mixing. Finally, most systems also offer computer-driven accountability and reportability of each step of the staining procedure.[151, 152]

Automated AR systems have very recently been introduced. Antigen retrieval has been in use since the early 1990s. Nevertheless, because of the multiple variables inherent in this technique, standardization has been a challenge. These variables include the size and power of the microwave, the temperature of the retrieval solution, the duration of the retrieval, and the rate of cooling. Other variables include the number of slides and containers in the microwave as well as the size, color, and material of these containers. With this new automation, all these variables are controlled, and this results in reproducible standardized results.

As mentioned earlier, the automation of quantitative IHC has also become available. The results of these tests are useful for diagnosis, prognosis, and therapy. Automated cellular imaging systems can be used for the detection of molecular markers, hormone receptors, or occult micrometastases.[153, 154] This automation uses standard immunocytochemical staining methods and reagents, along with automated microscopy. The latter is accomplished by the evaluation of the target cells using greater than 100 different morphometric parameters. The results are quantitative and based on standardized scoring and reporting. Moreover, images of the cells, as well as the results, are stored permanently for later review or confirmation, or both, if necessary.

Despite the advent of these exciting new automated technologies, not all problems are corrected by automation. It cannot overcome the improper selection of tissue to be examined, faulty tissue fixation, or problems with processing or sectioning, all of which can compromise antigen detection and interpretation. It cannot replace a pathologist's expertise when selecting the appropriate tests to be performed or when interpreting tissue sections. It is, therefore, by no means a panacea for laboratories with poor quality control standards. Only a laboratory with high standards can operate an automated machine effectively. However, it can and does provide reproducible, standardized, and uniform results and serves as a prelude to quantitative IHC and computerized image analysis. It is time for the morphology and chemistry of tissue diagnosis to unite, not only for diagnosis but also for prognosis and therapy.

Technical Problems

Immunohistochemistry is a multistep diagnostic procedure involving the proper selection, fixation, processing, and staining of tissue. The final interpretation of the results is the responsibility of an experienced pathologist. It is based on the presence, pattern, and intensity of colored chromogen products, which are deposited on the tissue as the result of specific antibody-antigen reactions in the cells. The resultant pattern of staining can be focal or diffuse, nuclear, cytoplasmic, or membranous. When the expected results are not obtained, one must troubleshoot the problem in a systematic way, and each single variable of this multistep diagnostic procedure should be addressed separately, one at a time (Table 1–7).

From a general standpoint, technical problems can be classified into two main categories: those that occur before staining and those that are related to staining. Effects of delayed fixation, overfixation, underfixation, or uneven fixation are well studied and have already been discussed. Conversely, the effects of tissue processing are less studied and less well understood. Currently, processing after fixation is accomplished in most laboratories by automated devices. Other than errors introduced by personnel handling or machine malfunction, the influence of processing on immunostaining results has not been studied thoroughly. One of the few problems in this area that has been described is that due to inadequate tissue dehydra-

Table 1-7. Troubleshooting Variables

Tissue	Pretreatment	Detection System
Patient tissue	Xylene	Link and label
Fixation	Alcohol	Compatibility
Processing	Water	Expiration date
Control tissue	Antigen retrieval	Chromogen
Fixation		Preparation
Processing		Incubation time
		Expiration date
Fixation	**Blocking**	**Results of Test**
Optimal fixation	Peroxidase block	Positive staining
Overfixation	Biotin block	Negative staining
Underfixation	Background block	Focal or weak staining
Delayed fixation		Background staining
		Artifactual staining
Processing	**Antibodies**	**Results of Control**
Dehydration	Prediluted-concentrated	Positive staining
Embedding	Expiration date	Negative staining
Sectioning	Storage	Background staining
Mounting	Contamination	Artifactual staining
Slides	Incubation	

tion before paraffin embedding. This can be prevented by preparing fresh alcohol solutions on a more frequent and regular basis. Other processing problems include the use of incorrect slides, which can result in loss of tissue adherence. Imprecise sectioning can cause crinkling or folding of the tissue, which may result in reagent trapping and uneven staining patterns. Subsequent to processing, other non–staining-related problems pertain to pretreatment protocols (i.e., enzyme digestion or AR, or both). During pretreatment, technical problems are also unavoidable because of the variables involved.

The recognition of inappropriate staining can be divided into five main categories based on the pattern of staining results on the test tissue as well as the pattern of staining results on the positive control.[151] Troubleshooting considerations for each of these patterns are discussed. The five staining patterns to be discussed include:

- Absence of staining of both the test tissue and the positive control
- Absence of staining of the test tissue with appropriate positive staining of the positive control
- Weak staining of the test tissue with appropriate staining of the positive control
- The presence of background staining on the test tissue or the positive control, or both
- The presence of artifactual staining on the test tissue or the positive control, or both

ABSENCE OF STAINING OF BOTH SPECIMEN AND CONTROL

When neither the specimen nor the control stains, one must check to see if the procedure was

followed correctly, that is, that all the steps of the staining process were performed in the correct order, that the incubation times were sufficient, and that no reagents were accidentally omitted. Antibody titrations and dilutions should also be reviewed. This is particularly important for the primary antibody. One should also check the expiration dates and storage of the reagents. Using reagents beyond their expiration date can result in false-negative results. Moreover, antibodies stored in self-defrosting freezers are exposed to repeated freezing and thawing, and this can result in antibody breakdown. The rinse buffer should also be checked, because it may be incompatible with the reaction reagents. The buffer pH must be appropriate, and sodium azide should not be present in buffers that are used with peroxidase enzyme. The drying out of specimens can also result in absence of staining, and one needs to confirm that this did not occur. Was sufficient reagent applied to the sample to prevent dehydration? Was a humidity chamber used? Other possible causes of absence of staining include problems with the chromogen. One must confirm that the chromogen solution was properly prepared and that it is working. This can be accomplished by adding the labeling reagent to the small amount of the prepared chromogen and confirming that a color change occurs. It should be kept in mind that chromogen solutions tend to deteriorate quickly. Finally, lack of staining can also occur because of improper pretreatment before IHC staining, counterstaining, or cover slipping. For example, AEC should not be used with counterstains or mounting media containing alcohol, xylene, or toluene, because these chemicals can dissolve the soluble colored precipitates formed by the reaction of AEC chromogen and substrate.

ABSENCE OF STAINING OF SPECIMEN WITH APPROPRIATE POSITIVE STAINING OF POSITIVE CONTROL

If the positive control slide shows appropriate positive staining of the expected cells, one can assume that the procedure was performed correctly and that the reagents were working properly. In such instances, the problem is prestaining-related, rather than an aspect of the staining procedure itself. It may, therefore, be the result of improper tissue fixation, processing, or pretreatment, or a combination.

Problems with formalin fixation include delay of fixation, overfixation, underfixation, and variable fixation.[155] For some antibodies, depending on the resistance of their target antigens to autolysis, a delay in fixation may cause loss of immunoreactivity and absence of staining. For this reason, fixation should begin as soon as possible, preferably within 30 minutes of removing the specimen. Overfixation can result in absence of staining as well. Causes of this include the cross-linking of antigens as well as the presence of contaminant in the fixative. For these reasons, one should avoid formalin fixation in excess of 48 hours. In instances of underfixation, only the periphery of the tissue has time to absorb the fixative. Toward the center of the specimen, the tissue will remain unfixed and raw. In these center areas, the specimen may undergo coagulative fixation by alcohol during tissue dehydration. This will result in variable staining, with more intense staining at either the center or the periphery of the specimen, depending on which has occurred, what antibody was used, and whether AR was used.

Absence of staining can also result from processing problems, although such problems are less studied and seemingly less important than those due to fixation. Potential processing factors include inadequate dehydration from the use of old alcohol reagents. Moreover, heat-sensitive epitopes can be lost by embedding with paraffin that is too hot. Therefore, the temperature of the paraffin should be monitored so as not to exceed 56°C (Table 1–8).

WEAK STAINING OF SPECIMEN WITH APPROPRIATE STAINING OF POSITIVE CONTROL

Improper fixation or processing of the test tissue, or both, may also cause weak staining of the specimen, whereas the control stains positively. All the causes explained previously for "absence of staining" apply to a lesser degree to the situation of "weak staining." This serves to emphasize further the need for the control slides and the test tissues to be fixed and processed in an identical manner whenever possible. Other factors that may cause weak staining with appropriate positive control staining include a low concentration of antigen in the test tissue. If antibody concentration is found

Table 1–8. Technical Problems and Solutions: Absence of Staining or Weak Staining

Problem	Solution
Inadequate fixation	Avoid delay of fixation (>30 mins) or overfixation (>48 hr)
Incomplete dehydration during processing	Check protocol for processing; perform regular reagent changes (i.e., alcohol)
Paraffin too hot	Monitor temperature of paraffin (<56°C)
Prolonged or excessive heating	Optimize antigen retrieval time
Staining steps not followed	Review procedure manual
Reagents not working	Check expiration dates; check storage parameters; check compatibility with other reagents; check pH
Antibody too dilute	Check antibody titration; increase concentration; lengthen incubation time; increase temperature of reaction; check amount of rising buffer left on slide
Drying out of tissue during processing	Keep specimen moist as indicated by procedure manual; prevent evaporation with humidity chamber
Insufficient incubation time	Lengthen incubation time to achieve desired intensity of staining; add heat; increase concentration of antibody
Chromogen not working	Add chromogen to labeling solution and monitor for change in color

to be too low for the test tissue that had been fixed improperly, one can increase its concentration, lengthen the incubation time, or increase the temperature of the reaction. Any of these measures may intensify the weak staining and provide adequate results. Inappropriately diluted antibody can also be the result of leaving too much buffer rinse on the slide before the antibody is applied (see Table 1–8).

BACKGROUND STAINING

Any positive staining that is not the result of antibody-antigen reaction is termed *nonspecific background staining*. Such staining is demonstrated as inappropriate positive staining on the test tissue or the positive control. However, it is best confirmed by positivity on the negative control. There are a number of conditions that can cause this, the most common of which is the nonspecific ionic binding of antibodies to charged connective tissue elements in the specimen, such as collagen. In these instances, such nonspecific staining can be alleviated by the use of nonimmune serum from the same animal species as the secondary antibody. The addition of salt to the

Table 1–9. Technical Problems and Solutions: Background Staining

Problem	Solution
Nonspecific protein binding	Use nonimmune serum from same animal species as secondary antibody; add salt to buffer
Incomplete removal of paraffin	Use only completely deparaffinized slides
Poorly fixed or necrotic tissue	Make sure tissue is properly fixed; avoid sampling of necrotic areas
Thick preparation	Cut sections at 3 to 5 μm; prepare cytospins that are monolayer in thickness
Inappropriately concentrated antibody	Check titration; decrease concentration; decrease incubation time; decrease temperature of reaction
Endogenous biotin	Block with avidin
Incomplete rinsing of slides	Follow protocol for proper slide rinsing
Chromogen staining too intense	Monitor timing of chromogen-substrate reaction; filter the chromogen; decrease the chromogen concentration

buffer may also help. Another common cause of background staining is the presence of peroxidase in the tissue being studied. If this peroxidase is not removed, positive staining will be found in red blood cells (pseudoperoxidase) and white blood cells (endogenous peroxidase).[156] Endogenous biotin is also found in certain tissues (i.e., liver and kidney) and may cause false-positive signals. This can be avoided in such situations by changing to another detection system that is free of avidin-biotin or by preincubation of the tissue with avidin. Poorly fixed tissues and areas of necrosis will also show background staining in these areas, as will tissue sections that are cut too thick. Some other causes of background positivity pertain to the antibody solution itself. Examples include solutions that contain particulates or inappropriately high concentrations of antibodies. In the former instance, the accumulation of particulates can be due to repeated freezing and thawing of the antibodies. Other less common causes of background staining involve problems related to tissue processing such as the incomplete removal of paraffin. This is recognized by diffuse background positivity that extends beyond the borders of the specimen. Background staining can also result from the incomplete rinsing of slides between steps or by the use of contaminated buffers. Finally, one other consideration that can cause nonspecific positivity is overdevelopment of the chromogen-substrate reaction. This can result from incomplete dissolution or excess concentration of chromogen. Appropriate troubleshooting measures for these problems include filtering of the chromogen solution or decreasing its concentration (Table 1–9).

ARTIFICIAL STAINING

The presence of certain artifacts can result in unexpected and nonspecific results. Artifacts include undissolved precipitates of chromogen or counterstain. The presence of these artifacts can be corrected by filtering. Sometimes, in B5-fixed tissues, black precipitates that are spread across the specimen are encountered. This results from incomplete dezenkerization of the tissue and can be corrected by removing the mercury from the tissue before staining. Not uncommonly, endogenous pigments, such as hemosiderin or melanin, are confused with true histochemical positivity. However, the presence of these pigments will also be seen on the negative control. If a negative control is not available for comparison, the use of a chromogen of contrasting color (such as AEC, which stains red) can be helpful in providing this distinction. Finally, other artifacts worth considering are the presence of microbial contaminants, such as yeast or bacteria (Table 1–10).

Because of the multistep nature of the immunohistochemical procedure, there are numerous technical problems that can arise. Fortunately, many of these can be managed fairly logically and easily with adherence to quality control guidelines and the strict application of positive and negative controls. This is necessary for the correct interpretation of the results and for the avoidance of diagnostic pitfalls. For some examples of the staining problems discussed, see Figures 1–21 to 1–36.

Standardization and Quantitative Immunohistochemistry

Standardization of IHC should be the essence of semiquantitative or quantitative methods and therefore has received increasing attention in both basic and clinical research. Translational research in IHC has relied heavily on retrospective studies, allowing the use of specimens and clinical data from previously published series in which clinical outcome is known and long-term follow up available. In particular, application of the method to archival tissues stored in pathology files world-

Table 1–10. Technical Problems and Solutions: Artifactual Staining

Problem	Solution
Presence of chromogen or counterstain deposits	Filter the chromogen or counterstain
Black deposits in B5-fixed tissue	Remove the mercury before staining
Endogenous pigments confused with specific positive staining	Check the negative control for the presence of these pigments; use a chromogen of contrasting color
Microbiologic contamination	Change reagents often; use fresh reagents; check expiration dates

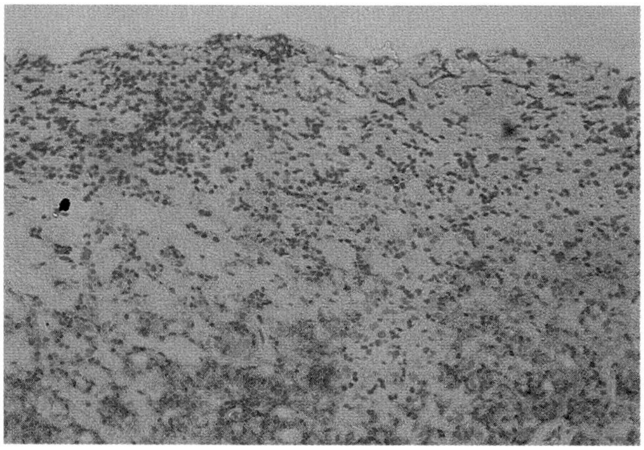

wide has played a critical role in facilitating IHC studies of prognostic markers, with an exponential increase in publications.

"Standardization" is a great challenge, easier said than done because many factors play a part, from fixation and processing of the tissue, through AR, the selection of the IHC staining reagents and protocol, to the final steps of "scoring" and evaluation of the significance of the findings. One approach to the standardization of IHC is to adopt a "total test" strategy as advocated by our group at the University of Southern California.[2] In essence, this approach "requires" that the pathologist pay attention to each and every step of the whole procedure, from the moment that the biopsy specimen is taken, to the type and duration of fixation, the AR method used, the selection of reagents, the performance of the IHC staining,

Figure 1–21. Section stained with autostainer using capillary action principle illustrating insufficient ascent of reagent.

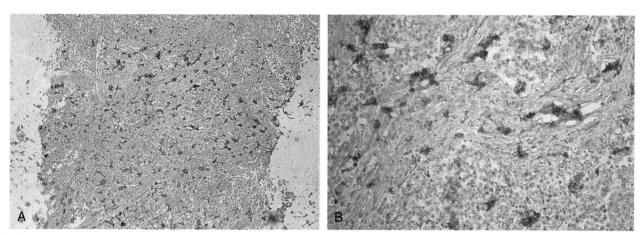

Figure 1–22. *A* and *B,* "Chromogen freckles," which is an artifact that resulted from undissolved precipitates of chromogen.

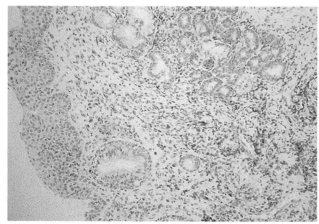

Figure 1–23. Section of parotid gland stained with CD3 showing scattered T-lymphocyte and nonspecific cytoplasmic granular staining in the glandular epithelium.

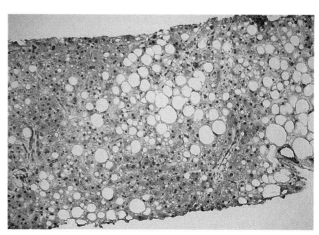

Figure 1–24. Section of liver illustrating endogenous biotin resulting in nonspecific background staining.

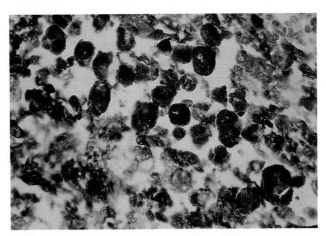

Figure 1–25. Pigmented melanophages, not to be confused with chromogen.

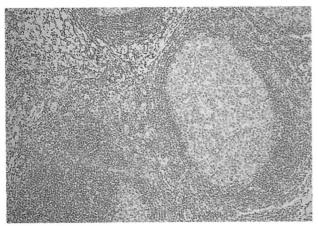

Figure 1–26. Section of lymph node with no primary antibody.

incorporating proper controls, and the interpretation and validation of the staining result (Table 1–11).

From a practical point of view, one of the most difficult issues in the standardization of IHC for use on archival tissues is the adverse influence of formalin, and the degree to which this effect may be reversed by AR. Optimization of the AR process by use of a test battery approach has already been discussed. A standardized AR process contributes greatly to overall standardization of the IHC method, as described.

Another critical issue concerning standardization of IHC is the selection and optimal application of one of the numerous commercially available detection and amplification systems. In general, we have grouped amplification and enhancement systems into three categories (Table 1–12), namely, *predetection phase* (before primary incubation), *detection phase* (from primary incubation to label incubation), and *postdetection phase* (after label incubation) amplification.[91]

PREDETECTION AMPLIFICATION

In effect, the AR technique is an effective and simple technique of predetection-phase amplification.[38, 39, 54–56, 91] It is generally accepted, although not well understood, that AR-induced amplification of signal is the result of increased antigenicity contingent on restoration of certain epitopes in the formalin-modified protein structure.[58, 59] To the extent that the AR technique serves to restore the natural antigen-antibody reaction, it favors specific binding and does not aggravate nonspecific background staining, thereby providing the potential for an enhanced signal-to-noise ratio.

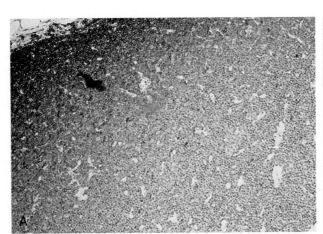
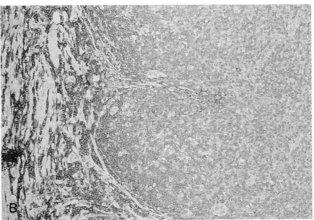

Figure 1–27. Section of lymph node stained with CD45 *(A* and *B)* showing variable fixation artifact. Well-defined cytoplasmic membrane staining is seen in the subcapsular region *(A)* and toward the periphery of the section *(B),* where the tissue is adequately fixed.

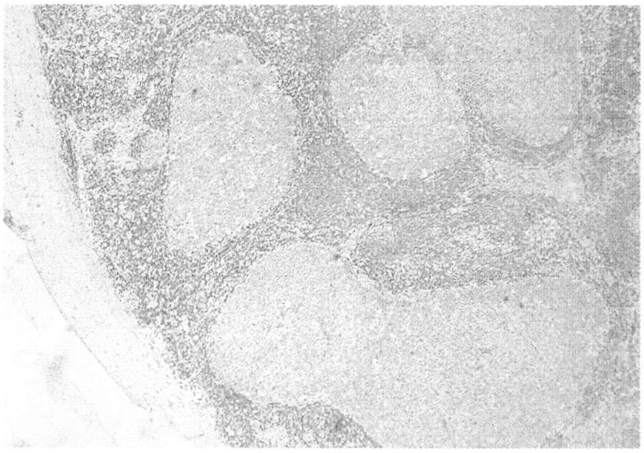

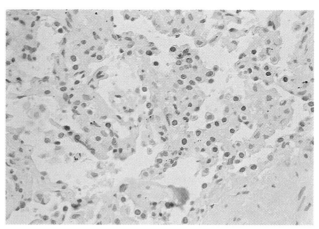

Figure 1–31. Section of normal lung tissue stained with TTF-1 (thyroid transcription factor), exhibiting specific nuclear positivity of the alveolar lining cells (pneumocytes).

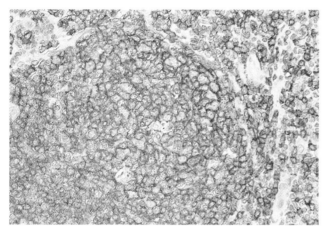

Figure 1–28. Another lymph node section stained with bcl-2 showing similar variable fixation artifact with gradual loss of staining appreciated toward the center of the node.

DETECTION PHASE AMPLIFICATION

As described earlier, development of staining methods has continued apace, reflective of drawbacks intrinsic to the currently available three-step detection systems, including complex time-consuming protocols, difficulties in standardization, inefficient demonstration of certain hard to detect antigens, and endogenous biotin or endogenous enzyme activity. In addition, several computer-assisted automated stainers have been manufactured to address the issues of consistency, high labor intensity, and cost, and have led to remarkable improvements in reproducibility as mentioned earlier. However, to some extent, the proliferation of automated stainers has added to the problem of overall reproducibility of results, because now

Figure 1–29. Sections of lymph node stained with CD20 showing bright cytoplasmic membrane staining of the B cells in the germinal center.

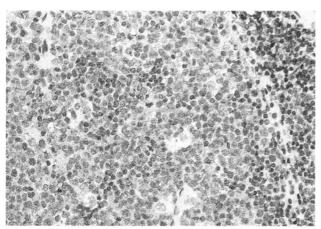

Figure 1–30. Similar lymph node section stained with CD20 showing suboptimal weak staining of the B cells in the germinal center, which is recognized by the presence of scattered tingible body macrophages.

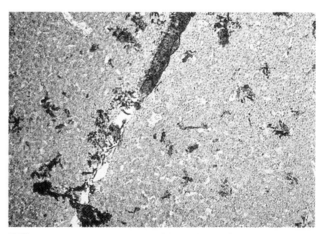

Figure 1–32. Section of lymph node stained with CD43 demonstrating processing problem with cleavage and folding of the tissue, which subsequently resulted in variable staining intensity and precipitation of the chromogen. All these artifacts can adversely affect interpretation.

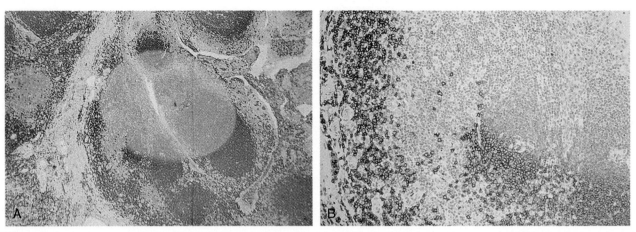

Figure 1–33. *A* and *B,* Section of lymph node stained with CD20 showing low- and high-power views with "bubble artifact." This is the result of microscopic hydrophobic bubbles formed during staining process.

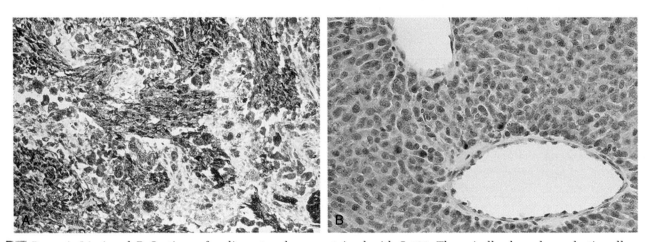

Figure 1–34. *A* and *B,* Sections of malignant melanoma stained with S-100. The spindle-shaped neoplastic cells on the left are overstained to the extent that it is difficult to appreciate true nuclear staining. Similarly, spindle-shaped malignant cells around the blood vessels (on the right) show a gradation with different intensity of staining, resulting in more readily appreciated nuclear positivity.

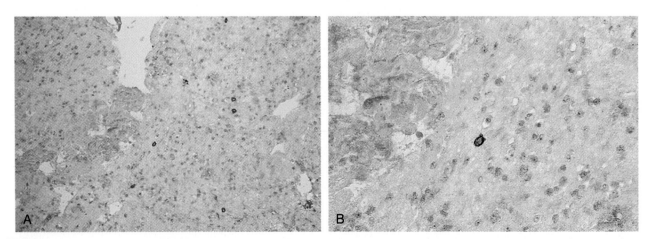

Figure 1–35. *A* and *B,* Cell block section stained with CD20. There is high background staining of the amorphous proteinaceous material. The high power view in *B* highlights positive B lymphoid cells and aberrant nucleolar positivity of scattered T lymphoid cells, which are negative for CD20.

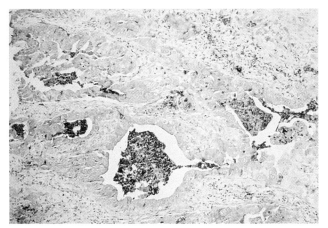

Figure 1–36. Section of adenocarcinoma stained with CEA demonstrating positive polymorphonuclear neutrophils showing strong endogenous peroxidase staining, which are also seen scattered in the stroma.

"any laboratory" can perform immunostaining with little underlying basic knowledge, forcing a total reliance on the automated staining protocols and quality control methods.

POSTDETECTION AMPLIFICATION

Methods of postdetection phase amplification seek to intensify the chromogen reaction. The two principal drawbacks are an increase in the complexity of the immunostaining procedure (with additional steps that are difficult to control) and a general increase in nonspecific background staining. This latter effect often means that although the intensity of the stain is increased, the signal-to-noise ratio is not improved, and interpretation may even be more difficult. In general, we do not recommend this approach for routine use.

DEVELOPMENT OF "REFERENCE STANDARDS" AND STANDARD CURVES FOR CALCULATION OF ANTIGEN CONTENT IN TISSUE SECTION

Currently, in-house controls are used as discussed previously. If properly used, these results enhance quality within any laboratory, but because they are "local" in production and availability, they do not ensure reproducibility among different laboratories. Theoretically, it is possible to develop preparations of purified protein (antigen), which can be diluted to produce a series of known reference standards for both Western blotting and, when suitably prepared, for IHC. The technique of "matrix models"[157] may be applied to create what is in effect an artificial control tissue for the protein (antigen) in question (see further on). In this way, a conversion formula may be developed from a "standard curve" to determine the exact amount of antigen present in formalin-fixed, paraffin-embedded tissue sections under various conditions of immunostaining, including AR pretreatment. Such antigen preparations may also be used as a "pretest" to establish a standardized protocol of IHC and may also serve practical reference standards for quality control of IHC staining. With the certain introduction of computer-assisted image analysis or "spectral imaging," or both, in the not-too-distant future, the need to develop such "reference" standards becomes ever more pressing.

ANTIGEN MATRIX MODEL: AN ARTIFICIAL POSITIVE TISSUE CONTROL

In order to control the quality of immunostaining performed at different times and in different laboratories by different technicians, it is desirable to have a "universal" positive control or "reference standard." A simulated tissue that could serve in this capacity may be prepared using the purified protein-matrix model system to produce a "faux tissue" that may be formalin-fixed, paraffin-

Table 1–11. Components of the "Total Test" in Immunohistochemistry

Elements of Testing Process	Quality Assurance Issues	Responsibility
Clinical question, test selection	Indications for immunohistochemistry; selection of stains	Surgical pathologist; sometimes clinician
Specimen acquisition and management	Specimen collection, fixation, processing, sectioning	Pathologist-technologist
Analytic issues	Qualifications of staff; intra- and interlaboratory proficiency testing of procedures	Pathologist-technologist
Results validation and reporting	Criteria for positivity-negativity in relation to controls; content and organization of report; turnaround time	Pathologist/technologist
Interpretation, significance	Experience-qualifications of pathologist; proficiency testing of interpretational aspects; diagnostic, prognostic significance; appropriateness-correlation	Surgical pathologist or clinician, or both

Adapted from Taylor CR Biotech Histochem 1992;67:110–117.

Table 1–12. Classification of Three Basic Signal Amplification Approaches for Immunohistochemistry

Classification	Basic Principles and Mode of Action	Advantages and Problems
Predetection amplification: Antigen retrieval (AR)	Restoration of formalin-induced modification of protein structure, resulting in dramatic amplification of signal while reducing the background simultaneously	Simplest and cheapest procedure (heating) among all methods of amplification, not effective for some antibodies-antigens
Detection amplification: Multi-step detection systems; PAP, ABC, APAAP, B-SA	Increase the accumulation of labeling signal (enzyme or others) PAP, 2- to 50-fold; ABC, 2- to 100-fold increase	The polylabeling technique and polymer-based amplification systems are simpler, cheaper, and faster than other multistep detection systems; as a biotin-free detection system, avoids the problem of the endogenous biotin reaction
Stepwise amplification	Repeating cycles of detection	
Polymeric and polylabeling amplification	Currently available kits of EnVision, PowerVision and EPOS; average further dilution of primary antibody: 2- to 5-fold, our test: 1:160 further dilution of PCNA	
Postdetection amplification: Enhanced DAB by metal, imidazole, and so on	Enhance the color reaction	Procedures are complicated, involving repeating cycles of reactions; labor and costs may be a drawback to widespread application; background staining increasing with amplification of signal
CARD	HRP catalyzes deposition of biotinylated tyramine at the site of HRP	
Anti–end product (EP)	Anti-EP + biotinylated link + HRP label, 16-fold increase of signal	
Gold-silver enhancement method	Silver enhancement	

PAP, peroxidase-antiperoxidase; ABC, avidin-biotin conjugate; APAAP, alkaline phosphatase anti–alkaline phosphatase; B-SA, biotin-sptreptavidin; PCNA, proliferating cell nuclear antigen; EPOS, enhanced polymer one-step staining (DAKO); Card, catalyzed reporter deposition; HRP, horseradish peroxidase.

Adapted from Shi S-R, Guo J, Cote RJ, et al. Sensitivity and detection efficiency of a novel two-step detection system (PowerVision) for immunohistochemistry. Appl Immunohistochem Mol Morphology 1999; 7:201–208.

embedded, and processed in a manner identical to unknown test specimens for each batch of IHC staining. The intensity of immunohistochemical staining of this positive control tissue section (containing known amounts of antigen) may then be used for calculation of the amount of antigen in test sections.

This matrix model has several advantages over an alternative "Quicgel" method developed by Battifora's group, who created an artificial tissue control block using a breast cancer cell line, which is then added to the tissue cassette containing the clinical biopsy specimen.[158] The advantages of the matrix model include the following:

1. Quicgel requires the availability of suitable cell lines, expressing the antigen in question, which must show consistent behavior under cell culture and storing.
2. The purified protein-matrix model has the potential for achieving consistency in terms of amount of antigen present, based on exact determinations of quantity at various dilutions. The matrix model tissue could be processed and stored in the same way as routine paraffin-embedded specimens, as described for the Quicgel approach. Either of these methods add value; neither is widely used at present.

CONCLUSION

The widespread application of IHC has transformed diagnostic surgical pathology "from something resembling an art into something more closely resembling a science,"[3] However, as described, all is not entirely well. An ongoing major drawback of IHC is the lack of objective quantitative measurement for target antigens under investigation, especially in light of the fact that quantitative IHC is increasingly necessary in both clinical and research pathology, and indeed really is essential for proper use of the prognostic markers that are described elsewhere in this book. It is worth noting that much of what has been written regarding standardization of IHC is equally applicable to the use of ISH methods in surgical pathology. We pathologists have already been practicing molecular morphology (microscopic localization of protein, DNA, and RNA) since the late 1970s. To take the next leap forward, we now need to "do it right," a goal that requires a demonstrable level of standardization, coupled with the use of computer-assisted analysis of the reaction product, to give reliable and true quantitation.

Appendix I-A. Simplified Procedure

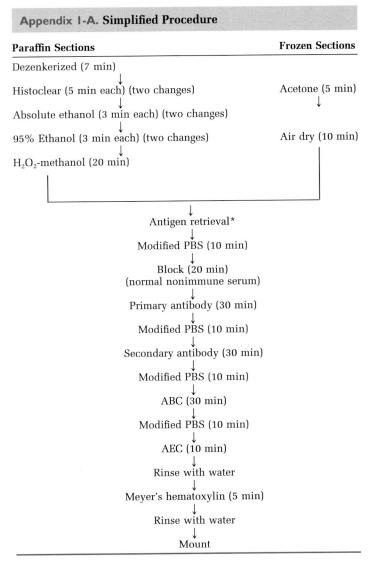

Paraffin Sections   **Frozen Sections**

Dezenkerized (7 min)
↓
Histoclear (5 min each) (two changes)   Acetone (5 min)
↓   ↓
Absolute ethanol (3 min each) (two changes)
↓
95% Ethanol (3 min each) (two changes)   Air dry (10 min)
↓
H$_2$O$_2$-methanol (20 min)

↓
Antigen retrieval*
↓
Modified PBS (10 min)
↓
Block (20 min)
(normal nonimmune serum)
↓
Primary antibody (30 min)
↓
Modified PBS (10 min)
↓
Secondary antibody (30 min)
↓
Modified PBS (10 min)
↓
ABC (30 min)
↓
Modified PBS (10 min)
↓
AEC (10 min)
↓
Rinse with water
↓
Meyer's hematoxylin (5 min)
↓
Rinse with water
↓
Mount

* Optional
PBS, phosphate-buffered saline; ABC, avidin-biotin conjugate; AEC, amino-ethyl carbazole.
Adapted from Taylor CR, Cote RJ. Immunomicroscopy: A Diagnostic Tool for the Surgical Pathologist, 2nd ed. Philadelphia: WB Saunders, 1994, p 422.

Appendix I–B. Double Staining

A satisfactory double-staining method using mouse monoclonal antibodies has been in "routine" use in our laboratory for some time. The method is applicable both to frozen sections and to cytocentrifuge preparations.

Briefly, the procedure involves the sequential application of two different staining systems, both using a mouse monoclonal primary antibody. The first is an indirect ABC peroxidase procedure, using biotinylated horse antimouse IgG linked to ABC peroxidase, with AEC as the substrate. The second is an indirect conjugate method using goat antimouse IgG linked with alkaline phosphatase, and fast-blue as substrate. Controls reveal that there is no detectable binding of the second labeling system (goat antimouse Ig–alkaline phosphatase) to the first monoclonal antibody; this circumstance presumably is due to steric interference. Mounting is in buffered glycerol jelly in deference to the use of AEC, which is alcohol soluble.

ABC, avidin-biotin conjugate; AEC, amino-ethyl carbazole.
Adapted from Taylor CR, Cote RJ. Immunomicroscopy: A Diagnostic Tool for Surgical Pathologists, 2nd ed. Philadelphia: WB Saunders, 1994:424.

References

1. Coons AH, Creech HJ, Jones RN. Immunological properties of an antibody containing a fluorescent group. Proc Soc Exp Biol Med 1941;47:200.
2. Taylor CR. The current role of immunohistochemistry in diagnostic pathology. Adv Pathol Lab Med 1994;7:59.
3. Taylor CR. An exaltation of experts: Concerted efforts in the standardization of immunohistochemistry. Hum Pathol 1994;25:2.
4. Taylor CR, Cote RJ, eds. Immunomicroscopy: A Diagnostic Tool for the Surgical Pathologist, 2nd ed. Philadelphia, WB Saunders, 1994.
5. Avrameas S. Enzyme markers: Their linkage with proteins and use in immunohistochemistry. Histochem J 1972;4: 321.
6. Nakane PK, Pierce GBJ. Enzyme-labeled antibodies for the light and electron microscopic localization of tissue antigens. J Cell Biol 1967;33:307.
7. Adams JC. Biotin amplification of biotine and horseradish peroxidase signals in histochemical stains. J Histochem Cytochem 1992;40:1457.
8. Bobrow MN, Harris TD, Shaughnessy KJ, et al. Catalyzed reporter deposition: A novel method of signal amplification: Application to immunoassays. J Immunol Methods 1989;125:279.
9. Colvin RB, Bhan AK, McCluskey RT, eds. Diagnostic Immunopathology, 2nd ed. New York, Raven Press, 1995.
10. DeLellis RA, Sternberger LA, Mann RB, et al. Immunoperoxidase technics in diagnostic pathology: Report of a workshop sponsored by the National Cancer Institute. Am J Clin Pathol 1979;71:483.
11. Elias JM, ed. Immunohistopathology: A Practical Approach to Diagnosis. Chicago, American Society of Clinical Pathologits Press, 1990.
12. Heras A, Roach CM, Key ME. Enhnced polymer detection system for immunohistochemistry. Mod Pathol 1995;8: 165A.
13. Hsu SM, Raine L, Fanger H. A comparative study of the peroxidase-antiperoxidase method and an avidin-biotin complex method for studying polypeptide hormones with radioimmunoassay antibodies. Am J Clin Pathol 1981;75: 734.
14. Hsu S-M, Raine L, Fanger H. Use of avidin-biotin-peroxidase complex (ABC) in immunoperoxidase techniques: A comparison between ABC and unlabeled antibody (PAP) procedures. J Histochem Cytochem 1981;29:577.
15. Polak JM, van Noorden S, eds. Immunocytochemistry: Modern Methods and Applications, 2nd ed., Bristol, Wright, 1986.
16. Sabattini E, Bisgaard K, Ascani S, et al. The EnVision system: A new immunohistochemical method for diagnostics and research: Critical comparison with the APAAP, ChemMate· CSA, LABC, and SABC techniques. J Clin Pathol 1998;51:506.
17. Shi S-R, Cote RJ, Taylor CR. Standardization and further development of antigen retrieval immunohistochemistry: Strategies and future goals. J Histotechnol 1999;22:177.
18. Sternberger LA, Joseph SA. The unlabeled antibody method: Contrasting color staining of paired pituitary hormones without antibody removal. J Histochem Cytochem 1979;27:1424.
19. Vyberg M, Nielsen S. Dextran polymer conjugate two-step visualization system for immunohistochemistry. Appl Immunohistochem 1998;6:3.
20. Kohler G, Milstein C. Continuous cultures of fused cells secreting antibody of predefined specificity. Nature 1975; 256:495.
21. Leong AS-Y. Commentary: Diagnostic immunohistochemistry—problems and solutions. Pathology 1992;24:1.
22. Taylor CR, Burns J. The demonstration of plasma cells and other immunoglobulin containing cells in formalin-fixed, paraffin-embedded tissues using peroxidase labeled antibody. J Clin Pathol 1974;27:14.
23. Taylor CR. The nature of Reed-Sternberg cells and other malignant "reticulum" cells. Lancet 1974;2:802.
24. Taylor CR. A history of the Reed-Sternberg cell. Biomedicine 1978;28:196.
25. Taylor CR, Kledzik G. Immunohistologic techniques in surgical pathology: A spectrum of new special stains. Hum Pathol 1981;12:590.
26. Pinkus GS. Diagnostic immunocytochemistry of paraffin-embedded tissues. Hum Pathol 1982;13:411.
27. Swanson PE. Editorial: Methodologic standardization in immunohistochemistry: A doorway opens. Appl Immunohistochem 1993;1:229.
28. Larsson L-I, ed. Immunocytochemistry: Theory and Practice. Boca Raton, FL, CRC Press, 1988.
29. Huang S-N. Immunohistochemical demonstration of hepatitis B core and surface antigens in paraffin sections. Lab Invest 1975;33:88.
30. Leong AS-Y, Milios J, Duncis CG. Antigen preservation in microwave-irradiated tisses: A comparison with formaldehyde fixation. J Pathol 1988;156:275.
31. Fraenkel-Conrat H, Brandon BA, Olcott HS. The reaction of formaldehyde with proteins. IV: Participation of indole groups. J Biol Chem 1947;168:99.
32. Fraenkel-Conrat H, Olcott HS. The reaction of formaldehyde with proteins. V: Cross-linking between amino and primary amide or guanidyl groups. J Am Chem Soc 1948; 70:2673.
33. Fraenkel-Conrat H, Olcott HS. Reaction of formaldehyde with proteins. VI: Cross-linking of amino groups with phenol, imidazole, or indole groups. J Biol Chem 1948;174: 827.
34. Shi SR, Key ME, Kalra KL. Antigen retrieval in formalin-fixed, paraffin-embedded tissues: An enhancement method for immunohistochemical staining based on microwave oven heating of tissue sections. J Histochem Cytochem 1991;39:741.
35. Shi SR, Tandon AK, Cote C, et al. S-100 protein in human inner ear: Use of a novel immunohistochemical technique on routinely processed, celloidin-embedded human temporal bone sections. Laryngoscope 1992;102:734.
36. Shi SR, Tandon AK, Haussmann RR, et al. Immunohistochemical study of intermediate filament proteins on routinely processed, celloidin-embedded human temporal bone sections by using a new technique for antigen retrieval. Acta Otolaryngol (Stockh) 1993;113:48.
37. Shi SR, Cote C, Kalra KL, et al. A technique for retrieving antigens in formalin-fixed, routinely acid-decalcified, celloidin-embedded human temporal bone sections for immunohistochemistry. J Histochem Cytochem 1992;40:787.
38. Taylor CR, Shi SR, Chen C, et al. Comparative study of antigen retrieval heating methods: Microwave, microwave and pressure cooker, autoclave, and steamer. Biotech Histochem 1996;71:263.
39. Taylor CR, Shi S-R, Cote RJ. Antigen retrieval for immunohistochemistry: Status and need for greater standardization. Appl Immunohistochem 1996;4:144.
40. Boon ME, Kok LP. Breakthrough in pathology due to antigen retrieval. Mal J Med Lab Sci 1995;12:1.
41. Evers P, Uylings HB, Suurmeijer AJ. Antigen retrieval in formaldehyde-fixed human brain tissue. Methods 1998;15: 133.
42. Gown AM, de Wever N, Battifora H. Microwave-based antigenic unmasking: A revolutionary new technique for routine immunohistochemistry. Appl Immunohistochem 1993;1:256.
43. Cattoretti G, Pileri S, Parravicini C, et al. Antigen unmasking on formalin-fixed, paraffin-embedded tissue sections. J Pathol 1993;171:83.
44. Leong AS-Y, Milios J. An assessment of the efficacy of the microwave antigen-retrieval procedure on a range of tissue antigens. Appl Immunohistochem 1993;1:267.
45. Merz H, Rickers O, Schrimel S, et al. Constant detection of surface and cytoplasmic immunoglobulin heavy and light chain expression in formalin-fixed and paraffin-embedded material. J Pathol 1993;170:257.

46. Shi SR, Chaiwun B, Young L, et al. Antigen retrieval using pH 3.5 glycine-HCl buffer or urea solution for immunohistochemical localization of Ki-67. Biotech Histochem 1994; 69:213.

47. Shi S-R, Cote RJ, Yang C, et al. Development of an optimal protocol for antigen retrieval: A "test battery" approach exemplified with reference to the staining of retinoblastoma protein (pRB) in formalin-fixed paraffin sections. J Pathol 1996;179:347.

48. Shi SR, Cote RJ, Young L, et al. Use of pH 9.5 TRIS-HCl buffer containing 5% urea for antigen retrieval immunohistochemistry. Biotech Histochem 1996;71:190.

49. Shi SR, Imam SA, Young L, et al. Antigen retrieval immunohistochemistry under the influence of pH using monoclonal antibodies. J Histochem Cytochem 1995;43:193.

50. Shi S-R, Gu J, Kalra KL, et al. Antigen retrieval technique: A novel approach to immunohistochemistry on routinely processed tissue sections. Cell Vision 1995;2:6.

51. Suurmeijer AJ, Boon ME. Notes on the application of microwaves for antigen retrieval in paraffin and plastic tissue sections. Eur J Morphol 1993;31:144.

52. Taylor CR, Shi S-R, Chaiwun B, et al. Strategies for improving the immunohistochemical staining of various intranuclear prognostic markers in formalin-paraffin sections: Androgen receptor, estrogen receptor, progesterone receptor, p53 protein, proliferating cell nuclear antigen, and Ki-67 antigen revealed by antigen retrieval techniques. [see comments] Hum Pathol 1994;25:263.

53. von Wasielewski R, Werner M, Nolte M, et al. Effects of antigen retrieval by microwave heating in formalin-fixed tissue sections on a broad panel of antibodies. Histochemistry 1994;102:165.

54. Shi SR, Cote RJ, Taylor CR. Antigen retrieval immunohistochemistry: Past, present, and future. J Histochem Cytochem 1997;45:327.

55. Shi S-R, Cote RJ, Young LL, Taylor CR. Antigen retrieval immunohistochemistry: Practice and development. J Histotechnol 1997;20:145.

56. Shi S-R, Gu J, Kalra KL, et al. Antigen retrieval technique: A novel approach to immunohistochemistry on routinely processed tissue sections. In Gu J, eds. Analytical Morphology: Theory, Applications & Protocols. Natick, MA: Eaton, 1997:1–40.

57. Shi Y, Li G-D, Liu W-P. Recent advances of the antigen retrieval technique. Linchuang yu Shiyan Binglixue Zazhi (J Clin Exp Pathol) 1997;13:265.

58. Shi S-R, Gu J, Taylor CR, eds. Antigen Retrieval Techniques: Immunohistochemistry and Molecular Morphology. Natick, MA: Eaton, 2000.

59. Shi S-R, Gu J, Turrens F, et al. Development of the antigen retrieval technique: Philosophy and theoretical base. In: Shi S-R, Gu J, Taylor CR, eds. Antigen Retrieval Techniques: Immunohistochemistry and Molecular Morphology. Natick, MA: Eaton Publishing, 2000: 17–39.

60. Mann G, ed. Physiologic Histology. Oxford, Oxford University Press, 1902.

61. van Regenmortel MHV. The recognition of proteins and peptides by antibodies. In: van Oss CJ, van Regenmortel MHV, eds. Immunochemistry. New York: Marcel Dekker, 1994:277–300.

62. Barlow DJ, Edwards MS, Thornton JM. Continuous and discontinuous protein antigenic determinants. Nature 1986;322:747.

63. Johnson CW. Issues in immunohistochemistry. Toxicol Pathol 1999;27:246.

64. Streefkerk JG. Inhibition of erythrocyte pseudoperoxidase activity by treatment with hydrogen peroxide following methanol. J Histochem Cytochem 1972;29:829.

65. Burns J. Background staining and sensitivity of the unlabeled antibody-enzyme (PAP) method: Comparison with the peroxidase-labeled antibody sandwich mehtod using formalin-fixed paraffin embedded material. Histochemistry 1975;43:291.

66. Weir EE, Pretlow TG, Pitts A. Destruction of endogenous peroxidase activity in order to locate cellular antigens by peroxidase-labeled antibodies. J Histochem Cytochem 1974;22:51.

67. McMillan EM, Martin D, Wasik R, et al. Demonstration in situ of "T" cells and "T" cell subsets in lichen planus using monoclonal antibodies. J Cutan Pathol 1981;8:228.

68. Straus W. Phenylhydrazine as inhibitor of horseradish peroxidase for use in immunoperoxidase procedures. J Histochem Cytochem 1972;20:949.

69. Straus W. Use of peroxidase inhibitors for immunoperoxidase procedures. In: Feldman R, eds. First International Symposium on Immunoenzymatic Techniques. Amsterdam, Holland), 1976: p 117.

70. Andrew SM, Jasani B. An improved method for the inhibition of endogenous peroxidase non-deleterious to lymphocyte surface markers: Application to immunoperoxidase studies on eosinophil-rich tissue preparations. Histochem J 1987;35:426.

71. Li C-Y, Zeismer SC, Lacano-Villareal O. Use of azide and hydrogen peroxide as an inhibitor for endogenous peroxidase method. J Histochem Cytochem 1987;35:1457.

72. Schmid KW, Hittmair A, Schmidhammer H, et al. Non-deleterious inhibition of endogenous peroxidase activity (EPA) by cyclopropanone hydrate: A definitive approach. J Histochem Cytochem 1989;37:473.

73. Robinson G, Dawson I. Immunochemical studies of the endocrine cells of the gastrointestinal tract. I: The use and value of peroxidase-conjugated antibody techniques for the localization of gastrin-containing cells in human pyloric antrum. Histochem J 1975;7:321.

74. Heyderman E. Immunoperoxidase technique in histopathology: Applications, methods, and controls. J Clin Pathol 1979;32:971.

75. Heyderman E, Neville MA. A shorter immunoperoxidase technique for the demonstration of carcinoembryonic antigen and other cell products. J Clin Pathol 1977;30:138.

76. Lillie RD, Pizzolato P. Histochemical use of borohydride as aldehyde blocking reagent. Stain Technol 1976;13:16.

77. Kelly J, Whelan CA, Weir DG, et al. Removal of endogenous peroxidase visualization of monoclonal antibodies. J Immunol Methods 1987;96:127.

78. Hittmair A, Schmid KW. Inhibition of endogenous peroxidase for the immunocytochemical demonstration of intermediate filament proteins (IFP). J Immunol Methods 1989; 116:199.

79. Mason TE, Phifer RF, Spicer SS, et al. An immunoglobulinenzyme bridge method for localizing tissue antigens. J Histochem Cytochem 1969;17:573.

80. Sternberger LA, ed. Immunocytochemistry. Englewood Cliffs, NJ: Prentice-Hall, 1974.

81. Cordell JL, Falini B, Erber WN, et al. Immunoenzymatic label of monoclonal antibodies using immune complexes of alkaline phosphatase and monoclonal anti-alkaline phosphatase (APAAP complexes). J Histochem Cytochem 1984;32:219.

82. Erber WN, McLachlan J. Use of APAAP technique on paraffin wax embedded bone marrow trephines. J Clin Pathol 1989;42:1201.

83. Wagner L, Worman CP. Color-contrast staining of two different lymphocyte subpopulations: A two-color modification of alkaline phosphatase monoclonal anti-alkaline phosphatase compex technique. Stain Technol 1988;63:129.

84. Wong SY, Carrol EDS, Ah-See SY, et al. Detection of estrogen receptor proteins in breast tumors using an improved APAAP immunohistochemical technique. Cancer 1988;62: 2171.

85. Vardiman JW, Gilewski TA, Ratain MJ, et al. Evaluation of Leu-M5 (CDIIc) in hairy cell leukemia by the alkaline phosphatase anti– phosphatase technique. Am J Clin Pathol 1988;90:250.

86. Ordronneau P, Lindstrom D, Petrusz P. Four unlabeled antibody bridge techniques: A comparison. J Histochem Cytochem 1984;32:172.

87. Vacca LL, Hewett D, Woodson G. A comparison of methods using diaminobenzidine (DAB) to localize peroxidases

in erythrocytes, neutrophils, and peroxidase-anti-peroxidase complex. Stain Technol 1978;53:331.

88. Davidoff MS, Schulze W, Holstein AF. Combination of alkaline phosphatase anti–alkaline phosphatase (APAAP) and avidin-biotin–alkaline phosphatase complex (ABAP)—techniques for amplification of immunocytochemical staining of human testicular tissue. Andrologia 1991;23:353.

89. Sano T, Smith CL, Cantor CR. Immuno-PCR: Very sensitive antigen detection by means of specific antibody-DNA conjugates. Science 1992;258:120.

90. Chen B-X, Szabolcs MJ, Matsushima AY, et al. A strategy for immunohistochemical signal enhancement by end-product amplification. J Histochem Cytochem 1996;44:819.

91. Shi S-R, Guo J, Cote RJ, et al. Sensitivity and detection efficiency of a novel two-step detection system (Power-Vision) for immunohistochemistry. Appl Immunohistochem Mol Morphol 1999;7:201.

92. Bobrow MN, Shaughnessy KJ, Litt GJ. Catalyzed reporter deposition, a novel method of signal amplification. II: Application to membrane immunoassays. J Immunol Methods 1991;137:103.

93. Toda Y, Kono K, Abiru H, et al. Application of tyramide signal amplification system to immunohistochemistry: A potent method to localize antigens that are not detectable by ordinary method. Pathol Int 1999;49:479.

94. Mengel M, Werner M, von Wasielewski R. Concentration dependent and adverse effects in immunohistochemistry using the tyramine amplification technique. Histochem J 1999;31:195.

95. Kawai K, Osamura RY. Antigen retrieval versus amplification techniques in diagnostic immunohistochemistry. In: Shi S-R, Gu J, Taylor CR, eds. Antigen Retrieval Techniques: Immunohistochemistry and Molecular Morphology. Natick, MA: Eaton, 2000:249–253..

96. Merz H, Ottesen K, Meyer W, et al. Combination of antigen retrieval techniques and signal amplification of immunohistochemistry in situ hybridization and FISH techniques. In: Shi S-R, Gu J, Taylor CR, eds. Antigen Retrieval Techniques: Immunohistochemistry and Molecular Morphology. Natick, MA: Eaton, 2000:219–248.

97. College of American Pathologists: Standard for Laboratory Accreditation. Skokie, IL: 1987.

98. Taylor CR. The total test approach to standardization of immunohistochemistry. [editorial] Arch Pathol Lab Med 2000;124:945.

99. Cote RJ, Taylor CR. Immunohistochemistry and related marking techniques. In: Damjanov I, Linder J, eds. Anderson's Pathology, 10th ed. St. Louis: CV Mosby, 1996:136–175.

100. Taylor CR. Report of the Immunohistochemistry Steering Committee of the Biological Stain Commission. "Proposed format: Package insert for immunohistochemistry products." Biotech Histochem 1992;67:323.

101. Burry RW. Specificity controls for immunocytochemical methods. J Histochem Cytochem 2000;48:163.

102. Swaab DF, Pool CW, VanLeenwen FW. Can specificity ever be proven in immunocytochemical staining? J Histochem Cytochem 1977;25:388.

103. Willingham MC. Conditional epitopes: Is your antibody always specific? J Histochem Cytochem 1999;47:1233.

104. Battifora H. The multitumor (sausage tissue block): Novel method for immunohistochemical antibody testing. Lab Invest 1986;55:244.

105. Battifora H, Mehta P. The checkerboard tissue block: An improved multitissue control block. Lab Invest 1990;63:722.

106. Battifora H. Assessment of antigen damage in immunohistochemistry: The vimentin internal control. Am J Clin Pathol 1991;96:669.

107. Battifora H, Kopinski M. The influence of protease digestion and duration of fixation on the immunostaining of keratins: A comparison of formalin and ethanol fixation. J Histochem Cytochem 1986;34:1095.

108. Cuevas EC, Bateman AC, Wilkins BS, et al. Microwave antigen retrieval in immunocytochemistry: A study of 80 antibodies. J Clin Pathol 1994;47:448.

109. Leong AS-Y, Gilham PN. The effects of progressive formaldehyde fixation on the preservation of tissue antigens. Pathology 1989;21:266.

110. Shi S-R, Cote RJ, Chaiwun B, et al. Standardization of immunohistochemistry based on antigen retrieval technique for routine formalin-fixed tissue sections. Appl Immunohistochem 1998;6:89.

111. Yokoo H, Nakazato Y. A monoclonal antibody that recognizes a carbohydrate epitope of human protoplasmic astrocytes. Acta Neuropathol 1996;91:23–30.

112. Prento P, Lyon H. Commercial formalin substitutes for histopathology. Biotech Histochem 1997;72:273.

113. Williams JH, Mepham BL, Wright DH. Tissue preparation for immunocytochemistry. J Clin Pathol 1997;50:801.

114. Allison RT, Best T. p53, PCNA and Ki-67 expression in oral squamous-cell carcinomas—the vagaries of fixation and microwave enhancement of immunocytochemistry. J Oral Pathol Med 1998;27:434.

115. Miller RT, Kubier P, Reynolds B, et al. Blocking of endogenous avidin-binding activiry in immunohistochemistry. Appl Immunohistochem Mol Morphol 1999;7:63.

116. Zhang PJ, Wang H, Wrona EL, et al. Effects of tissue fixatives on antigen preservation for immunohistochemistry: A comparative study of microwave antigen retrieval on Lillie fixative and neutral buffered formalin. J Histotechnol 1998; 21:101.

117. Cote RJ, Shi Y, Groshen S, et al. Association of p27^{kip1} levels with recurrence and survival in patients with stage C prostate carcinoma. J Natl Cancer Inst 1998;90:916.

118. Grabau KA, Nielsen O, Hansen S. Influence of storage temperature and high-temperature antigen retrieval buffers on results of immunohistochemical staining in secitons stored for long periods. Appl Immunohistochem 1998;6:209.

119. Jacobs TW, Prioleau JE, Stillman IE, et al. Loss of tumor marker-immunostaining intensity on stored paraffin slides of breast cancer. J Natl Cancer Inst 1996;88:1054.

120. Kato J, Sakamaki S, Niitsu Y. More on p53 antigen loss in stored paraffin slides. N Engl J Med 1995;333:1507.

121. Prioleau J, Schnitt SI. p53 antigen loss in stored paraffin slides. N Engl J Med 1995;332:1521.

122. Malmstrom PU, Wester K, Vasko J, et al. Expression of proliferative cell nuclear antigen (PCNA) in urinary bladder carcinoma: Evaluation of antigen retrieval methods. APMIS 1992;100:988.

123. Wester K, Wahlund E, Sundstrom C, et al. Paraffin section storage and immunohistochemistry. Appl Immunohistochem Mol Morphol 2000;8:61.

124. Mason JT, O'Leary TJ. Effects of formaldehyde fixation on protein secondary structure: A calorimetric and infrared spectroscopic investigation. J Histochem Cytochem 1991; 39:225.

125. Igarashi H, Sugimura H, Maruyama K. Alteration of immunoreactivity by hydrated autoclaving, microwave treatment, and simple heating of paraffin-embedded tissue sections. APMIS 1994;102:295.

126. Kawai K, Serizawa A, Hamana T, et al. Heat-induced antigen retrieval of proliferating cell nuclear antigen and p53 protein in formalin-fixed, paraffin-embedded sections. Pathol Int 1994;44:759.

127. Evers P, Uylings HB. Microwave-stimulated antigen retrieval is pH and temperature dependent. J Histochem Cytochem 1994;42:1555.

128. Lucassen PJ, Ravid R, Gonatas NK, et al. Activation of the human supraoptic and paraventricular nucleus neurons with aging and in Alzheimer's disease as judged from increasing size of the Golgi apparatus. Brain Res 1993;632: 105.

129. Shi SR, Cote RJ, Taylor CR. Antigen retrieval immunohistochemistry used for routinely processed celloidin-embedded human temporal bone sections: Standardization and development. Auris Nasus Larynx 1998;25:425.

130. Werner M, Von Wasielewski R, Komminoth P. Antigen retrieval, signal amplification and intensification in immunohistochemistry. Histochem Cell Biol 1996;105:253.

131. Katoh A, Breier S. Nonspecific antigen retrieval solutions. J Histotechnol 1994;17:378.

132. O'Reilly PE, Raab SS, Niemann TH, et al. p53, proliferating cell nuclear antigen, and Ki-67 expression in extrauterine leiomyosarcomas. Mod Pathol 1997;10:91.

133. Shin R-W, Iwaki T, Kitamoto T, Tateishi J. Hydrated autoclave pretreatment enhances TAU immunoreactivity in formalin-fixed normal and Alzheimer's disease brain tissues. Lab Invest 1991;64:693.

134. Biddolph SC, Jones M. Low-temperature, heat-mediated antigen retrieval (LTHMAR) on archival lymphoid sections. Appl Immunohistochem Mol Morphol 1999;7:289.

135. Miller RT, Swanson PE, Wick MR. Fixation and epitope retrieval in diagnostic immunohistochemistry: A concise review with practical considerations. Appl Immunohistochem Mol Morphol 2000;8:228.

136. Boon ME, Kok LP, Moorlag HE, et al. Accelerated immunogold-silver and immunoperoxidase staining of paraffin sections with the use of microwave irradiation: Factors influencing results. Am J Clin Pathol 1989;91:137.

137. Chiu KY. Use of microwaves for rapid immunoperoxidase staining of paraffin sections. Med Lab Sci 1987;44:3.

138. Choi T-S, Whittlesey MM, Slap SE, et al. Advances in temperature control of microwave immunohistochemistry. Cell Vision 1995;2:151.

139. Leong AS-Y, Milios J. Rapid immunoperoxidase staining of lymphocyte antigens using microwave irradiation. J Pathol 1986;148:183.

140. Adams JC. Heavy metal intensification of DAB-based HRP reaction product. J Histochem Cytochem 1981;29:775.

141. Hsu SM, Soban E. Color modification of diaminobenzidine (DAB) precipitation by metallic ions and its application for double immunohistochemistry. J Histochem Cytochem 1982;30:1079.

142. Lan HY, Mu W, Nikolic-Paterson DJ, et al. A novel, simple, reliable, and sensitive method for multiple immunoenzyme staining: Use of microwave oven heating to block antibody crossreactivity and retrieve antigens. J Histochem Cytochem 1995;43:97.

143. Mason DY, Sammons R. Alkaline phosphatase and peroxidase for double immunoenzymatic labelling of cellular constituents. J Clin Pathol 1978;31:454.

144. Falini B, De Solas I, Halverson C. Double-labeled antigen method for demonstration of intracellular antigens in paraffin-embedded tissues. J Histochem Cytochem 1982;30:21.

145. Behringer DM, Meyer KH, Veh RW. Antibodies against neuroactive amino acids and neuropeptides. II: Simultaneous immunoenzymatic double staining with labeled primary antibodies of the same species and a combination of the ABC methods and the hapten-anto-hapten bride (HAB) technique. J Histochem Cytochem 1991;39:761.

146. Van Rooijen N. Six methods for separate detection of two different antigens in the same tissue section. J Histochem Cytochem 1980;28:716.

147. Krenacs T, Laszik Z, Dobo E. Application of immunogold-silver staining and immunoenzymatic methods in multiple labeling of human pancreatic Langerhans islet cells. Acta Histochem 1989;85:79.

148. Lehr HA, van der Loos CM, Teeling P, et al. Complete chromogen separation and analysis in double immunohistochemical stains using Photoshop-based image analysis. J Histochem Cytochem 1999;47:119.

149. Herman GE, Elfont EA, Floyd AD. Overview of automated immunostainers. Methods Mol Biol 1994;34:383.

150. Le Neel T, Moreau A, Laboisse C, et al. Comparative evaluation of automated systems in immunohistochemistry. Clin Chim Acta 1998;278:185.

151. Fetsch PA, Abati A. Overview of the clinical immunohistochemistry laboratory: Regulations and troubleshooting guidelines. Methods Mol Biol 1999;115:405.

152. Moreau A, Le Neel T, Joubert M, et al. Approach to automation in immunohistochemistry. Clin Chim Acta 1998;278:177.

153. Bauer KD, Hawes D, de la Torre-Bueno J, et al. Analysis of occult bone marrow metastases using automated cellular imaging. Mod Pathol 2000;13:220A.

154. Makarewicz K, McDuffe L, Shi S-R, et al. Immunohistochemical detection of occult metastases using an automated intelligent microscopy system. Presented at the 88th annual meeting of the American Association of Cancer Research, San Diego, CA, 1997:269.

155. Martin W, Chon A, Fabiono A, et al. Effect of formalin tissue fixation and processing on immunohistochemistry. Am J Surg Pathol 2000;24:1016.

156. Rickers RR, Malinisk RM. Intralaboratory quality assurance of immunohistochemical procedures: Recommended practices for daily application. Arch Pathol Lab Med 1989;113:673.

157. van der Ploeg M, Duijndam WAL. Matrix models: Essential tools for microscopic cytochemical research. Histochemistry 1986;84:283.

158. Riera J, Simpson JF, Tamayo R, et al. Use of cultured cells as a control for quantitative immunocytochemical analysis of estrogen receptor in breast cancer: The Quicgel method. Am J Clin Pathol 1999;111:329.

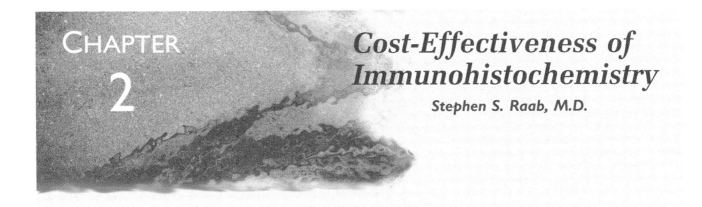

CHAPTER 2

Cost-Effectiveness of Immunohistochemistry

Stephen S. Raab, M.D.

Immunohistochemistry has profoundly shaped the practice of anatomic pathology.[1-9] In the early 21st century, it is difficult to conceive of an anatomic pathology laboratory that does not use immunohistochemistry. Since the 1980s, researchers have focused on determining optimal immunohistochemistry staining panels for diagnostic, prognostic, or predictive purposes.[1, 10-12] The fruits of this research are presented throughout this book. Paralleling the growth of immunohistochemistry research has been the growth of patient-centered outcomes research which has focused on patient endpoints such as survival, morbidity, satisfaction, preference, and cost.[13] Although not implicitly stated, the majority of immunohistochemistry studies are examples of outcomes studies, because they focus on patient life expectancy or survival as the endpoint. Presumably, immunohistochemistry would not be judged useful if it did not positively affect patient care.[1] How immunohistochemistry affects patient outcomes other than survival has rarely been studied. This chapter explores cost-effectiveness, another patient outcome, by first summarizing the principles of cost-effectiveness analysis and then applying these principles to immunohistochemistry.

WHY PERFORM COST-EFFECTIVENESS ANALYSIS?

Cost-effectiveness analysis is a method used in health policy decision making.[1, 14-19] Cost-effectiveness analysis is performed because there is an increased desire on the part of purchasers of health care to know exactly what they are purchasing. This desire is related to (1) the rising costs of health care, (2) variations in medical practice, and (3) financial incentives.[14]

The cost of health care in the United States is approaching $1 trillion per annum and composes more than 15% of the gross national product.[14] This rising cost is attributable to the increasing expansion of medical services (secondary to the growing numbers of insured people), a higher than average medical inflation rate, and the increasing use of new technologies.

The second reason for the increased focus on costs, or variations in medical practice, has been studied by Wennberg and other investigators.[15-24] These authors showed that there are regional variations in practice patterns that may result in higher costs of care in some regions when compared with other regions.[15-24] These variations appear to be unrelated to the clinical characteristics of the respective patient populations. For example, Chassen and coworkers and Wennberg and Gittelsohn showed a fourfold difference in radical prostatectomy rates in adjacent counties that had similar patient demographics and, presumably, disease prevalence.[20-22] It may be assumed that the adjacent counties had differences in medical expenditures for prostate disease. Regional variations in laboratory services such as immunohistochemistry have not been studied.

A third reason for the increased focus on costs is data showing differences in clinical behavior based on financial incentives.[25, 26] Hillman and colleagues examined the radiograph ordering behavior in two groups of physicians, one of which used its own radiographic equipment and the other of which referred patients to radiologists.[26] The group that owned its own equipment was more than four times as likely to order a radiologic test for patients with the same presenting complaint as the group that referred the patients to radiologists.[26] There is little published literature related to pathology ordering behavior and incentive,[27] although incentive-driven test ordering could be seen with some ancillary anatomic pathology tests, such as immunohistochemistry. Because pathologists may bill separately for immunohistochemical tests and decide when immunohistochemistry is warranted, there is an underlying financial incentive for them to order such studies.

WHAT IS COST-EFFECTIVENESS ANALYSIS?

Cost-effectiveness analysis is an analytic method to determine the clinical and economic consequences of various possible actions.[14–16] Cost-effectiveness analysis cannot tell the "correct" action to take, only the consequences of different actions.[14, 19] Users of cost-effectiveness analysis must determine the importance of the different consequences. Cost-effectiveness analysis measures the consequences of two or more alternatives, such as alternative procedures, tests, or treatments. Each alternative has different associated costs and outcomes. It is assumed that cost-effectiveness analysis is performed because there are not infinite financial resources to spend on health care. Cost-effectiveness analysis helps to determine how to spend limited resources wisely.

The term *cost-effective* is often misunderstood in pathology. In a study of the medical literature, Doubilet and associates examined how the term was used and found that cost-effectiveness studies did not conform to the same standards.[28] For example, although many authors used the term *cost-effective,* they may not have compared two or more procedures and simply concluded that a new procedure or test was "effective" and therefore cost-effective. Others have used cost-effective to mean less expensive and have not examined the clinical consequences of different actions. Yet others have shown that one procedure adds benefit, despite its added cost, and assumed that this more beneficial procedure also is more cost-effective. *Cost-effectiveness analysis* refers to a specific type of analysis and tests should not be referred to as *cost-effective* unless this analysis has been performed.[19]

TYPES OF COST-EFFECTIVENESS ANALYSIS

Cost-effectiveness analysis is a form of cost analysis, related to other forms of cost analysis, including cost-minimization, cost-consequence, and cost-benefit analysis.[14, 17, 18] These types of analysis are related because they all measure costs, although they measure the utilities or effectiveness in different metrics. In cost-minimization analysis, the utilities of different tests are assumed to be equal.[14] In this type of analysis, the determination of the superior test depends solely on the comparative costs. For example, suppose a clinical laboratory wanted to determine which flow cytometer should be purchased, and two flow cytometers were equally efficacious. Using cost-minimization analysis, the choice of the "better" flow cytometer would depend solely on cost.

In cost-consequence analysis, the outcomes of different tests are calculated separately and not combined.[14] For example, suppose one wanted to compare, using a cost-consequence analysis, transthoracic fine needle aspiration with sputum cytology as a means to diagnose a patient with a lung lesion. Outcomes that could be measured would include the number of false-negative diagnoses, number of false-positive diagnoses, patient satisfaction, cost of procedure, and complications. Cost is only one of the outcomes measured. In a cost-consequence analysis, these outcomes would all be listed separately. If there were more false-negative results with sputum cytology but also greater patient satisfaction and fewer complications, the choice of the optimal test would still be up to the user of the study and would be based on which outcomes were deemed more important.

In cost-effectiveness analysis, costs and other outcomes are measured in the same metric across all alternatives. Different tests may be compared in terms of cost per life year gained, cost per false-negative diagnosis, or cost per gain in practice productivity. These expressions of cost-effectiveness analysis are known as *cost-effectiveness ratios.*[19] One method of performing cost-effectiveness analysis is with decision analysis, a normative method for using existing probabilistic data to calculate outcomes.[27] Cost-utility analysis is a special type of cost-effectiveness analysis in which the outcomes other than costs are expressed in terms of values or utilities.[29–35] This method requires that patient desires or preferences be measured and is more difficult to perform than cost-effectiveness analysis. In cost-utility analysis, different tests may be compared in terms of quality-adjusted life years.[29–35]

In cost-benefit analysis, all outcomes are expressed in terms of cost.[14, 35] This method is much more common in economics than in health care. A difficulty with this method is that monetary values must be placed on all variables including human life, and this is not always intuitive. An advantage of this type of analysis is that tests or programs may be compared across a variety of social concerns. For example, using cost-benefit analysis, the utility of immunohistochemistry could be compared to the utility of educational or environmental initiatives.

ESSENTIALS OF COST-EFFECTIVENESS STUDIES

In 1993, an expert panel of 13 health researchers and academics was appointed by the United States Public Health Service to review the state of the science of cost-effectiveness analysis and foster consensus regarding the standardization and conduct of studies.[14, 18, 19, 36] The panel advised that cost-effectiveness studies should conform to six specific standards: (1) a statement of perspective, (2) a description of benefits, (3) a description of costs, (4) appropriate use of discounting, (5) use of sensitivity analysis, and (6) a report of summary measures.

The perspective of a cost-effectiveness study is the point of view from which the study is conducted.[14] The choice of perspective affects how the results are to be used. Perspectives include society, health care providers, individual patients, and hospitals. Many published cost-effectiveness studies are performed from the societal perspective, and studies performed from the societal perspective usually are the most broad. Societal perspectives may be used to determine resource allocation on a national level. If cost-effectiveness analyses are performed on an individual patient perspective, many costs, such as those incurred by third party payers, may be ignored. By ignoring or including different costs and outcomes, depending on the perspective, different conclusions may be reached.

How different tests or procedures are compared in terms of benefits and costs often is controversial.[37–39] For example, comparing new Papanicolaou (Pap) smear technologies only in terms of increases in patient life expectancy could arguably not be the best metric.[40] Other benefits include a decrease in patient anxiety in terms of a false-negative result (although this could be accounted for in cost-utility analysis), an increase in cytotechnologist job satisfaction, and a decrease in per slide screening time, resulting in productivity increases. Costs that are included in cost-effectiveness analyses include direct, indirect, and intangible costs (such as the cost of pain and suffering or the loss of function). Direct costs include medical (e.g., reagent and glassware cost), nonmedical (e.g., patient parking or transportation), and time (e.g., patient waiting time or histotechnologist time). Indirect costs may be attributable to organizations (e.g., cost of the physical plant or electricity) or to patients (e.g., loss of work because of illness).[14] One difficulty in cost-effectiveness analysis is actually obtaining true costs; in some instances charges instead of costs are used, despite the fact that they are not equal.[41]

In cost-effectiveness analysis, a cost-effectiveness ratio may be expressed as follows:

cost-effectiveness ratio = [cost (test A) − cost (test B)]/[benefit (test A) − benefit (test B)][15]

Thus, the cost of performing test A instead of test B is divided by the benefit of performing test A instead of test B.

Benefits and costs should be appropriately discounted before comparisons are made. Discounting is a process by which future benefits and costs are compared with present benefits and costs.[14, 19] Discounting is performed because researchers believe a life year saved tomorrow has a lot more value than a life year in the future and discounting takes into account this difference. Many studies perform

discounting at a rate of 3%, although others advocate discounting at rates of 5%, 7%, or higher.[19] The rate chosen may have considerable impact on the study results.

Sensitivity analyses are performed to measure how variations in the analytic assumptions affect outcomes. For example, suppose that a study showed that sputum cytology was more cost-effective than pulmonary fine needle aspiration. A sensitivity analysis could determine the robustness of this result, assuming that costs, sensitivities, or patient satisfaction varies.[14, 19] Thus, sensitivity analysis may reflect different practice conditions, geographic locations, or patient demographics.

It is important to remember that cost-effectiveness analysis does not show that a procedure should be performed instead of another procedure but only that it provides a metric to compare these procedures.[42] For example, cost-effectiveness analysis may show that a cost-effectiveness ratio of $70,000 per life year gained results if procedure 1 is performed instead of procedure 2. This means that procedure 1 is more costly but provides a greater benefit than does procedure 2. In order to get the benefit of gaining a life year per patient by performing procedure 1 instead of procedure 2, $70,000 would have to be spent. Cost-effectiveness analysis does not determine if spending this amount of money is worthwhile. Instead, the literature and society have chosen cost-effectiveness thresholds by which the cost-effectiveness of procedures may be compared. By choosing a cost-effectiveness threshold, it is assumed that a cost may be placed on a life year and this cost may be specifically quantified.[27] A difficulty in cost-effectiveness analysis is that there is no generally agreed upon level of expenditure that is necessarily cost-effective. In some cost-effectiveness studies, the threshold value of a life year has been assumed to be $50,000.[27, 43] If a procedure costs less than $50,000 per patient life year gained, it is cost-effective. If a procedure costs more than $50,000 per patient life year gained, it is not cost-effective. In the preceding example, procedure 1, when compared with procedure 2, would not be considered cost-effective. Other researchers have argued for higher life-year threshold values such as $75,000 or $100,000.[14] At either of these thresholds, procedure 1 would be cost-effective compared with procedure 2.

Cost-effectiveness analysis is fraught with difficulties. Its overall complexity may be daunting. This makes it difficult to perform and understand. Other pitfalls lie in the methods used to perform cost-effectiveness analysis. For example, a problem with life-year valuations is that all life years may not have equal worth.[14] Some researchers think that extending the life expectancy of a pediatric patient by 50 years is worth more than gaining an additional year of life expectancy in 50 chronically ill elderly patients.[14] Cost-effectiveness analysis often treats these gains as equivalent. This is a philosophical issue, and cost-effectiveness analysis cannot provide the answer.

BENEFIT AND COST STUDIES OF IMMUNOHISTOCHEMISTRY

There have been few cost studies of immunohistochemistry and virtually no investigations of the cost-effectiveness of immunohistochemistry. Most published studies of immunohistochemistry have focused on benefits other than costs.[1-12, 44, 45] The reasons for this are multifactorial and only partially related to the complexity of cost-effectiveness modeling. In a review of the impact of immunohistochemistry on patient outcomes, Wick and coworkers stressed that the major determinants of the clinical benefit of immunohistochemistry are the differences in therapy based on the use of immunohistochemistry.[1] It may be argued that the benefits of immunohistochemistry should be gains in particular patient outcomes, such as life expectancy, that may rest on changes in therapy.[27, 45] In this context, the benefits of immunohistochemistry include the identification of specific infectious agents[46, 47] (e.g., *Pneumocystis carinii*[48]), patient identification[1, 49] (e.g., immunostaining for ABH blood group antigens to identify floaters), determination of tumor types and subtypes[1, 3, 10-12] (e.g., hematologic malignancies), separation of benign processes from neoplasms[1, 3, 10-12] (e.g., immunostaining pleural fluids), and its use as predictors and prognostic indicators in neoplasia[1, 50-57] (e.g., predictive immunostaining for progesterone and estrogen receptor proteins and c-*erb*-B2 [HER-2/ *neu*] protein in breast cancer).

Wick and associates stressed that although immunohistochemistry is widely used in many clinical scenarios, the benefits have not been well studied and are even questionable.[1] For example, one common scenario in which immunohistochemistry is used is the determination of a primary site for patients with metastatic carcinoma of unknown origin.[1, 58, 59] Except, perhaps, in patients with metastatic breast cancer, there are no site-specific treatments for metastatic carcinoma of unknown origin.[60-62] Therefore, determining the site of origin by immunohistochemistry probably does not result in increased patient survival. In these patients, survival depends more on overall performance status, age, sites of metastasis, and other variables than it does on determining the likely site of tumor origin.[1, 61, 62] Although immunohistochemistry may be more cost-effective than other diagnostic work-up studies[58, 63] (e.g., bone scans or computed tomography scans), it still may not be clinically useful because of the overall poor response of patients who have metastatic carcinoma of unknown origin to currently available treatment regimens. However, measurement of the cost-effectiveness of performing immunohistochemistry compared with not performing immunohistochemistry in this patient population has not been performed.

Only a handful of immunohistochemistry cost studies have been published. Raab and colleagues examined the cost-effectiveness of fine needle aspiration with immunohistochemistry in the work-up of patients with lung masses and a previous history of malignancy.[63] Depending on the clinical scenario, fine needle aspiration with immunohistochemistry often was more cost-effective than other diagnostic tests (e.g., thoracotomy).[63] Researchers have examined immunohistochemistry use patterns and have argued that immunohistochemistry often is overutilized.[64, 65] These studies have examined costs but have not performed cost-effectiveness analyses.

COST-EFFECTIVENESS MODELING OF IMMUNOHISTOCHEMISTRY

My laboratory developed a decision model[27, 66] to determine the cost-effectiveness of using immunohistochemistry compared with not using immunohistochemistry in different clinical scenarios.[45] The perspective of this study was that of society. These scenarios depicted situations in which the added cost of immunohistochemistry was balanced with various benefits. Specifically, these benefits were (1) increased patient life expectancy provided by a more accurate diagnosis that therefore led to more appropriate therapy, (2) increased diagnostic certainty, and (3) increased ability to predict patient outcome (regardless of treatment). These benefits are not mutually exclusive, and immunohistochemistry provides other benefits not listed here.[1, 10-12] The benefits were separated to simplify the analysis and to create a framework for discussion relating to the interaction among cost and the various benefits. A cost-effectiveness ratio[19, 27] was calculated for each scenario (i.e., cost per increase in life expectancy, cost per increase in diagnostic certainty, and cost per increase in ability to predict prognosis). This analysis is theoretical and serves as a basis to determine if actually measuring immunohistochemistry costs and benefits is warranted in actual practice situations.[67] The cost-effectiveness analysis for the specific scenarios is presented in the following sections.[45]

Scenario 1: Increased Patient Life Expectancy. A 55-year-old man has a 3 cm–diameter pancreatic head mass. A laparotomy is performed, and there is no evidence of disease other than the mass. A needle core biopsy is performed of the mass, and on light microscopic examination of the permanent hematoxylin and eosin (H&E)-stained sections, dense fibrous tissue surrounds rare atypical cells. The differential diagnosis of the atypical cells includes histiocytes and reactive fibroblasts in a case of chronic pancreatitis versus malignant cells in a pancreatic adenocarcinoma. Immunohistochemistry may be used to separate these two entities.[10-12, 68, 69] It is assumed that without a definitively benign diagnosis, a Whipple procedure would be performed and, in this scenario, if the patient has pancreatitis there would be higher mortality associated with undergoing a Whipple procedure. If immunohistochemistry correctly establishes a benign diagnosis, there would be an increase in patient life expectancy.

In this scenario, the use of immunohistochemistry may or may not be effective in increasing patient life expectancy. Immunohistochemistry may not be effective in increasing patient life expectancy for several reasons (e.g., the immunohistochemical stains may not have been technically satisfactory, the stains may have been incorrectly interpreted, or the findings simply may not result in increased patient life expectancy).[10-12] In the analysis, the effectiveness of the immunohistochemical test is expressed as the percentage of the cases with an increase in life expectancy over the total number of cases using immunohistochemistry.[27, 70] For example, if immunohistochemistry is 50% effective, in 50% of cases in which it is used there is an increased life expectancy. If life expectancy is increased, it may be increased to a different extent (e.g., 2 months versus 2 years). The goal of this analysis was to determine the tradeoff between the threshold incidence of effectiveness of immunohistochemistry and the gain in patient life expectancy if immunohistochemistry was performed.[27]

In this analysis, it is implicit that the cost per patient for performing immunohistochemistry is more than the cost per patient for not performing immunohistochemistry. If the cost per patient for immunohistochemistry is less than the cost-effectiveness threshold, performing immunohistochemistry is cost-effective.[19, 71] A cost-effectiveness threshold of $50,000 per life year gained is assumed.[37, 43] If performing immunohistochemistry costs less than $50,000 per patient to gain a year of life expectancy, immunohistochemistry is cost-effective. If performing immunohistochemistry costs more than $50,000 per patient to gain a year of life expectancy, immunohistochemistry is not cost-effective compared with not performing immunohistochemistry.

In the analysis, the cost of an immunohistochemistry test depends on two variables: (1) the cost per immunohistochemical antibody and (2) the number of antibodies ordered per test. The cost per antibody was varied to reflect regional cost or charge variations and included technical, overhead, and interpretive components. In a previous analysis,[63] the technical charge per antibody at the University of Iowa was $90 and the cost was $37 ($27 if overhead was excluded). Allegheny General Hospital had a similar per antibody cost. A sensitivity analysis[18, 72] varying the cost per antibody from $10 to $100 was performed. In the initial analysis, it was assumed that a five-antibody panel was used, which reflects the average number of antibodies ordered per case in 1999 at Allegheny General Hospital. Thus, the cost of the immunohistochemical test could vary from $50 to $500, which reflects potential practice variations in North America. The specific antibodies ordered is not a focus of this study, and it is not necessarily assumed that these antibodies are those recommended by "expert" immunohistochemists.[10-12]

For any given cost of the immunohistochemical test, there is an incidence of test effectiveness above which the test is cost-effective or the use of the test is warranted. This incidence of immunohistochemical test effectiveness is plotted against the years of theoretical life expectancy gained. For example, suppose that the cost per antibody is $50 and there is a 1-year gain in population life expectancy because immunohistochemistry is used. Assuming a cost-effectiveness threshold of $50,000 per life year gained, the threshold incidence of immunohistochemical test effectiveness is 0.005. In other words, the use of immunohistochemistry would have to be effective in gaining a life year in 1 or more of 200 cases in order to be cost-effective (alternatively, 2 of 100 patients could have a life-year gain of 6 months each). If there is a 2-year gain in population life expectancy, the threshold incidence of immunohistochemical test effectiveness is 0.0025. A sensitivity analysis varying the cost-effectiveness threshold from $50,000 to $500,000 per life year gained was performed. Varying this threshold indicates that the societal value of a year of life expectancy changes. For example, a threshold value of $500,000 indicates that society places a very high value on a patient life year.

The threshold incidence of effectiveness of immunohistochemistry is plotted against the gain in per patient life expectancy in Figure 2–1 (again, it is assumed that there are five antibodies per test and a life year is valued at $50,000). The incidences of effectiveness of immunohistochemistry that lie above the curves compose the region in which immunohistochemistry is cost-effective. The three curves represent variations in the antibody cost. Figure 2–1 may be interpreted as follows. Suppose the cost per antibody is $50 and the use of immunohistochemistry resulted in a 0.5-year increase in the population life expectancy. The incidence of effectiveness at which immunohistochemistry is cost-effective is that point on the $50 curve for which there is a 0.5-year gain in life expectancy. This value is 0.01%. Thus, immunohistochemistry would have to be effective in 1 of 100 cases to be cost-effective. If immunohistochemistry is more effective (i.e., results in an increase in life expectancy of 0.5 years in more than 1 per 100 patients), immunohistochemistry also would be cost-effective. As the gain in population life expectancy increases, immunohistochemistry becomes cost-effective at lower incidences of test effectiveness. For example, if the cost per antibody is $50, and there is a 1-year gain in population life expectancy, the incidence of test effectiveness that

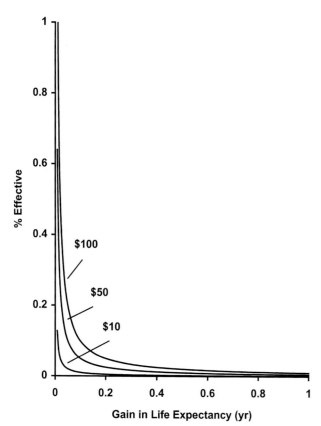

Figure 2–1. Percent effectiveness of immunohisto-chemistry versus gain in patient life expectancy. The percent effectiveness of immunohistochemistry is the incidence with which immunohistochemistry produces the benefit of increasing patient life expectancy. The different curves represent the cost per antibody.

Table 2–1. Incidence of Effectiveness of Immunohistochemistry for Immunohistochemistry to Be Cost-Effective

Cost per Antibody ($)	Life-Year Value		
	$50,000	*$100,000*	*$500,000*
10	1000	2000	10,000
25	400	800	4000
50	200	400	2000
100	100	200	1000

It is assumed that five antibodies are used per test.

mass. A modified radical mastectomy had been performed at another institution; the slides of the breast cancer are not available for review. A hepatic fine needle aspiration is performed and shows clusters of malignant cells. Alpha-fetoprotein levels are not elevated. The differential diagnosis includes a hepatocellular carcinoma versus a metastatic adenocarcinoma of mammary origin. If the diagnosis is hepatocellular carcinoma, a resection will be performed, whereas if the diagnosis is metastatic adenocarcinoma, the patient will receive chemotherapy. Immunohistochemistry may help in differentiating primary from metastatic liver cancer.[10–12, 73–75] Based on the light microscopic examination, the pathologist is approximately 75% certain that the diagnosis is metastatic adenocarcinoma. If immunohistochemistry is performed, the certainty of the diagnosis probably will change.

In scenario 2, the use of immunohistochemistry may be effective in increasing diagnostic certainty. The goal in this scenario is to determine the cost-effectiveness ratio reflecting the cost per gain in diagnostic certainty by using immunohistochemistry. This ratio may then serve as a basis for future discussion regarding the optimal cost-effectiveness threshold.[37, 39, 43]

It is assumed that following the light microscopic examination, the pathologist could express the diagnosis probabilistically.[76] The use of immunohistochemistry may shift the diagnostic probability. In the specific example in this scenario, the pathologist could state that he or she is 75% certain that the diagnosis is metastatic adenocarcinoma. Depending on the immunohistochemical staining profile, this probability could be either increased or decreased. In a theoretical case, the largest potential shift in probability would be 100%, assuming that the pathologist was 100% certain the diagnosis was benign or malignant, and the immunohistochemical results caused a shift to the opposite diagnosis with 100% certainty.

Research in cost-effectiveness has not previously examined the relationship between the cost of a test and the increase in diagnostic certainty. There is no established framework to evaluate the cost-effectiveness ratio of cost per percentage gain in diagnostic certainty.[27] Consequently, there is no established cost-effectiveness threshold. It is uncer-

is cost-effective is 0.005 (i.e., 1 or more per 200 tests would have to produce a 1-year gain in life expectancy for immunohistochemistry to be cost-effective).

In Table 2–1, the cost-effective threshold incidence of immunohistochemistry effectiveness is shown. This incidence varies as the cost per antibody and the cost value per life year varies. For all calculations, it is assumed that five antibodies per case are used and immunohistochemistry results in a 1-year gain in life expectancy. As the cost per antibody or the life-year value increases, the cost-effectiveness threshold incidence of immunohistochemical test effectiveness decreases. If the cost per life year is valued at $100,000 and the cost per antibody is $25, immunohistochemistry would have to be effective in 1 of every 800 tests to be cost-effective. Even if the cost per antibody is high ($100) and a life year is valued relatively low ($50,000), immunohistochemistry would have to be effective in only 1 of every 100 cases to be cost-effective.

Scenario 2: Increased Diagnostic Certainty. The patient is a 58-year-old woman who has a history of breast cancer and cirrhosis and a 2-cm liver

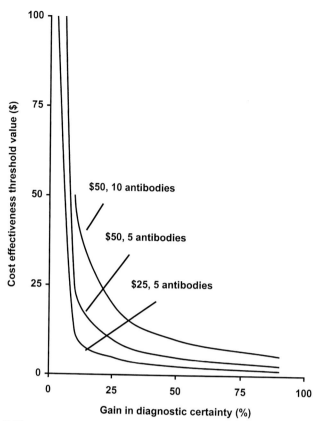

Figure 2–2. Cost-effectiveness threshold value versus gain in diagnostic certainty. The cost-effectiveness threshold value is the cost per percentage gain of diagnostic certainty. The different curves represent different per antibody costs and different numbers of antibodies used.

ical panel. The immunohistochemical test would cost $250, assuming a $50 cost per antibody. If there is a 10% gain in diagnostic certainty, the cost-effectiveness ratio is $25 (cost per percentage gain in diagnostic certainty ratio = test cost/gain in diagnostic certainty = $250/10%). If society (or pathologist, payer, and so on) thinks that spending $25 or more per percentage gain in diagnostic certainty is cost-effective, immunohistochemistry would be cost-effective if, in every case, it demonstrated a 10% gain in diagnostic certainty.

In Figure 2–2, the immunohistochemical cost-effectiveness threshold value is plotted against the gain in diagnostic certainty if immunohistochemistry is used. The curves represent different costs per antibody and different numbers of antibodies used per test. The graph may be interpreted as follows. Suppose the cost per antibody is $50 and five antibodies are used. If the gain in diagnostic certainty is 25%, the cost-effectiveness threshold value would be $10 per percentage gain in diagnostic certainty. This means that the value associated with each percentage gain in diagnostic certainty would have to be $10 or more for immunohistochemistry to be cost-effective. If the payer valued each percentage gain of diagnostic certainty at, for example, $6, immunohistochemistry would not be cost-effective. As the gain in diagnostic certainty increases for any given curve, the cost-effectiveness threshold value decreases. If there is a 25% gain in diagnostic certainty for all curves, the cost-effectiveness threshold value is less than $25 per percentage of diagnostic certainty (i.e., if the per percentage gain in diagnostic certainty is valued at greater than $25, immunohistochemistry would be cost-effective).

In Table 2–2, the incidence of immunohistochemical test effectiveness is calculated as the cost-effectiveness threshold value and the percentage gain in diagnostic certainty vary. It is assumed that five antibodies per test are used and that the cost per antibody is $50. Table 2–2 may be interpreted as follows. Suppose the gain in diagnostic certainty by using immunohistochemistry is 10% (e.g., shifted the certainty of diagnosis from 65% to 75%) and the value placed on a per percentage gain in diagnostic certainty is $1000. If immuno-

tain how much pathologists, providers, or patients are willing to pay (e.g., $1, $100, $100,000) for an increase in diagnostic certainty. Regardless of whether the analysis shows that the cost-effectiveness ratio is $5 or $1000 per percentage gain in diagnostic certainty, the value of the resulting diagnostic certainty is arguable.

The following example illustrates the determination of the cost-effectiveness ratio. Suppose there is a 10% gain in diagnostic certainty as a consequence of using a five-antibody immunohistochem-

Table 2–2. The Incidence of Immunohistochemical Test Effectiveness as the Percentage Gain in Diagnostic Certainty and the Cost-Effectiveness Threshold Value Vary

Cost-Effectiveness Threshold Value ($ per gain in % diagnostic certainty)	Percentage Gain in Diagnostic Certainty		
	10%	*50%*	*100%*
100,000	4000	20,000	36,000
10,000	400	2000	3600
1000	40	200	360
100	4	20	36
10	—	2	3.6
1	—	—	—

histochemistry is effective in 1 of 40 tests, immunohistochemistry is cost-effective. At high cost-effectiveness threshold values (e.g., $100,000 per percentage gain in diagnostic certainty), the incidence of immunohistochemical test effectiveness could be low and immunohistochemistry still would be cost-effective. As the cost-effectiveness threshold value decreases, the incidence of immunohistochemical test effectiveness would have to increase for immunohistochemistry to be cost-effective. If the cost-effectiveness threshold value is $1, regardless of the gain in diagnostic certainty, immunohistochemistry could not be cost-effective, because the incidence of immunohistochemical test effectiveness would be less than 1.0.

Scenario 3: Increased Ability to Predict Patient Outcome (or Prognosis). The patient is a 37-year-old woman who has a 1.5-cm, nonpalpable breast mass. A needle biopsy is performed and shows an invasive ductal carcinoma of high nuclear grade. Immunostains for the estrogen and progesterone receptor proteins[10–12, 77–80] and the *c-erb*-B2 (HER-2/*neu*) protein[10–12, 54, 55] are performed. Based on the staining pattern, the clinician is able to predict patient outcome and therefore prognosis (patient survival).[1] In this scenario, immunohistochemistry is examined solely for its ability to predict outcome and not its ability to affect treatment.

In scenario 3, the use of immunohistochemistry may be effective in increasing the ability to predict patient outcome, regardless of treatment, and therefore establish a more accurate prognosis. The goal in this scenario is to determine the tradeoff between the gain in prognostic accuracy and the effectiveness of immunohistochemistry.

Similar to the analysis in scenario 2, there is no established framework to evaluate the cost-effectiveness ratio of the cost per increase in prognostic accuracy. Consequently, there is no established cost-effectiveness threshold. In this analysis, different cost-effectiveness thresholds are evaluated to reflect possible societal valuations. The calculations are similar to those performed in scenario 1, although the measure of the difference in patient prognosis (or the knowledge of good versus poor patient prognosis) is substituted for the actual gain in patient life expectancy. Immunohistochemistry is assumed to vary in effectiveness from 0 to 100%. The ability of immunohistochemistry to predict patient outcome is expressed as the difference (in years) between the prognosis if immunohistochemistry is not performed and the prognosis if immunohistochemistry is performed. An example calculation follows. Suppose the cost-effectiveness threshold is $10,000 per gain in predicted year of patient survival, the cost per antibody is $50, and a five-antibody panel is performed. If immunohistochemistry predicts an improved prognosis by 1 year (compared with the prognosis if no immunohistochemistry is performed), immunohistochemistry would have to be 40% effective to be cost-effective. In other words, immunohistochemis-

try would have to predict either a prolonged or decreased survival in 4 of every 10 patients in order to be cost-effective.

In Figure 2–3, the incidence of immunohistochemical test effectiveness is plotted against the difference in prognosis if immunohistochemistry is used. The different curves represent different cost-effectiveness thresholds, or values per gain in ability to predict prognosis accurately. For all curves, it is assumed that five antibodies per test are used and the cost per antibody is $50. As the cost value per life year increases and the gain in difference in prognosis remains the same, immunohistochemistry is cost-effective at a lower incidence of effectiveness. For example, at a life-year value of $1000 and a difference in prognosis of 0.5 years, the incidence of immunohistochemical test effectiveness that is cost-effective is 0.5% (one of two tests would have to be effective or produce this difference in prognosis). In contrast, at a life-year value of $50,000, the incidence of immunohistochemical test effectiveness that is cost-effective is 0.01% (1 of 100 tests would have to be effective).

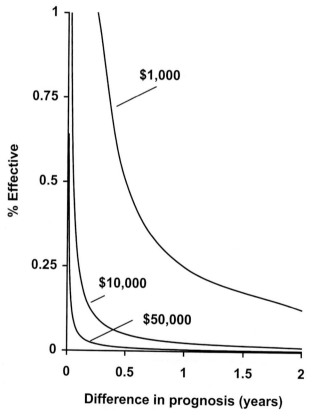

Figure 2–3. Percent effectiveness of immunohistochemistry versus difference in prognosis. The percent effectiveness of immunohistochemistry is the incidence with which immunohistochemistry produces the benefit of predicting a difference in prognosis (compared with immunohistochemistry not being used). The different curves represent different valuations of a prognostic life year.

CONCLUSIONS

The results of this cost-effectiveness modeling indicate that even if immunohistochemistry is rarely efficacious, it still would be cost-effective. This conclusion is true even assuming high immunohistochemistry costs.

A problem in performing cost-effectiveness analyses in anatomic pathology is that the benefits of pathology tests are difficult to identify and quantify in understandable or appropriate metrics.[27, 70] Cost per increase in patient life expectancy, the most commonly used metric in cost-effectiveness analyses,[72] may not be an appropriate measure of anatomic pathology tests, which provide information[27] rather than directly increase life expectancy. Regardless of the validity of this statement, this study evaluated several other cost-effectiveness metrics (e.g., cost per increased ability to predict patient prognosis accurately and cost per increased diagnostic certainty). The motivations driving immunohistochemistry use and whether these metrics correctly capture the utility of immunohistochemistry have not been rigorously investigated. Clearly, immunohistochemistry provides benefits other than those investigated in this cost-effectiveness model.[1]

One reason why immunohistochemistry appears to be so cost-effective is that the benefit to cost ratio of immunohistochemistry is relatively low compared with the same ratio in other medical procedures. Changes in medical care attributable to immunohistochemistry use may take place at a cost of only a few hundred dollars. This raises the possibility that immunohistochemistry is considerably undervalued, like other anatomic pathology tests such as the Pap smear. Studies demonstrating immunohistochemistry efficacy in actual practice situations are necessary.

References

1. Wick MR, Ritter JH, Swanson PE. The impact of diagnostic immunohistochemistry on patient outcomes. Clin Lab Med 1999;19:797–814.
2. Schapira DV, Jarrett AR. The need to consider survival, outcome, and expense when evaluating and treating patients with unknown primary carcinoma. Arch Intern Med 1995;155:2050–2054.
3. Leong ASY, Wick MR, Swanson PE. Immunohistology and Electron Microscopy of Anaplastic and Pleomorphic Tumors. Cambridge, UK: Cambridge University Press, 1997:209–240.
4. Gatter KC, Mason DY. The use of monoclonal antibodies for histopathological diagnosis of human malignancy. Semin Oncol 1982;9:517–525.
5. Dehner LP. On trial: A malignant small cell tumor in a child: Four wrongs do not make a right. Am J Clin Pathol 1998;109:662–668.
6. Gatter KC, Alcock C, Heryet A, Mason DY. Clinical importance of analyzing malignant tumors of uncertain origin with immunohistological techniques. Lancet 1985;1:1302–1305.
7. Wick MR, Loy T, Mills SE, et al. Malignant epithelioid pleural mesothelioma versus peripheral pulmonary adeno-
carcinoma: A histochemical, ultrastructural, and immunohistochemical study of 103 cases. Hum Pathol 1990;21:759–766.
8. Glickman JN, Torres C, Wang HH, et al. The prognostic significance of lymph node micrometastasis in patients with esophageal carcinoma. Cancer 1999;85:769–778.
9. Warnke RA, Gatter KC, Falini B, et al. Diagnosis of human lymphoma with monoclonal antileukocyte antibodies. N Engl J Med 1983;309:1275–1281.
10. Wick MR, Siegal GP. Monoclonal Antibodies in Diagnostic Immunohistochemistry. New York: Marcel Dekker, 1988.
11. Colvin RB, Bhan AK, McCluskey RT. Diagnostic Immunopathology. New York: Raven Press, 1994.
12. Jennette MC. Immunohistology in Diagnostic Pathology. Boca Raton, FL: CRC Press, 1989.
13. Raab SS. Outcomes analysis in anatomic pathology. In: Bissell MG, ed. Laboratory-Related Measures of Patient Outcomes: An Introduction. San Mateo, CA: AACP Press, in press.
14. Raab SS. Cost-effectiveness analysis in pathology. Clin Lab Med 1999;19:757–771.
15. Detsky AS, Naglie IG. A clinician's guide to cost-effectiveness analysis. Ann Intern Med 1990;113:147–154.
16. Roper WL, Winkenwerder W, Hackbarth GM, Krakauer H. Effectiveness in health care: An initiative to evaluate medical practice. N Engl J Med 1988;319:1197–1202.
17. Weinstein MC. Challenges for cost-effectiveness research. Med Decis Making 1986:6:194–198.
18. Weinstein MC, Siegel JE, Gold MR, et al. Recommendations of the Panel on Cost-Effectiveness in Health and Medicine. JAMA 1996;276:1253–1258.
19. Siegel J, Weinstein M, Torrance G. Reporting cost-effectiveness studies and results. In: Gold M, Siegel J, Russell L, Weinstein M, eds. Cost-Effectiveness in Health and Medicine. New York: Oxford University Press, 1996:276–303.
20. Chassin MR, Brook RH, Park RE, et al. Variations in the use of medical and surgical services by the Medicare population. N Engl J Med 1986;314:285–290.
21. Chassin MR, Kosecoff J, Park RE, et al. Does inappropriate use explain geographic variations in the use of health care services? A study of three procedures. JAMA 1987;258:2533–2537.
22. Wennberg J, Gittelsohn A. Small area variations in health care delivery: A population based health information system can guide planning and regulatory decision-making. Science 1973;182:1102–1108.
23. Nattinger AB, Gottlieb MS, Veum J, et al. Geographic variation in the use of breast-conserving treatment for breast cancer. N Engl J Med 1992;326:1102–1107.
24. Farrow DC, Hunt WC, Samet JM. Geographic variation in the treatment of localized breast cancer. N Engl J Med 1992;326:1097–1101.
25. Morreim EH. Conflicts of interest: Profits and problems in physician referrals. JAMA 1989;262:390–394.
26. Hillman BJ, Joseph CA, Mabry MR, et al. Frequency and costs of diagnostic imaging in office practice—a comparison of self-referring and radiologist-referring physicians. N Engl J Med 1990;323:1604–1608.
27. Raab SS. The cost-effectiveness of routine histologic examination. Am J Clin Pathol 1997;108:525–536.
28. Doubilet P, Weinstein MC, McNeil BJ. Use and misuse of the term "cost-effective" in medicine. N Engl J Med 1986;314:253–256.
29. Carr-Hill RA. Background material for the workshop on QALYs. Soc Sci Med 1989;3:469–477.
30. Froberg DG, Kane RL. Methodology for measuring health state preferences. II: Scaling methods. J Clin Epidemiol 1989;42:459–471.
31. Guyatt GH, Veldhuyzen Van Zanten SJ, Feeny DH, et al. Measuring quality of life in clinical trials: A taxonomy and review. Can Med Assoc J 1989;140:1441–1448.
32. Hollen PJ, Gralla RJ, Kris MG, et al. Measurement of quality of life in patients with lung cancer in multicenter trials of new therapies. Cancer 1994;73:2087–2098.

33. Kaplan RM. Quality of life assessment for cost/utility studies in cancer. Cancer Treat Rev 1993;19(Suppl 3):85–96.

34. Loomes G, McKenzie L. The use of QALYs in health care decision making. Soc Sci Med 1989;28:299–308.

35. Torrance GW. Measurement of health state utilities for economic appraisal: A review. J Health Econ 1986;5:1–30.

36. Luce B, Manning W, Siegel J, et al. Estimating costs in cost-effectiveness analysis. In: Gold M, Siegel J, Russell L, Weinstein M, eds. Cost-Effectiveness in Health and Medicine. New York: Oxford University Press, 1996:176–213.

37. Laupacis A, Feeny D, Detsky AS, et al. Tentative guidelines for using clinical and economic guidelines revisited. Can Med Assoc J 1993;148:927–929.

38. Leaf A. Cost-effectiveness as a criterion for Medicare coverage: Sounding board. N Engl J Med 1989;321:989–990.

39. Naylor CD, Williams JI, Basinski A, et al. Technology assessment and cost-effectiveness analysis: Misguided guidelines? Can Med Assoc J 1993;148:921–924.

40. Brown AD, Garber AM. Cost-effectiveness of 3 methods to enhance the sensitivity of Papanicolaou testing. JAMA 1999;281:347–353.

41. Finkler SA. The distinction between costs and charges. Ann Intern Med 1982;96:102–109.

42. Russell LB. Some of the tough decisions required by a national health plan. Science 1989;246:892–896.

43. Owens DK, Sanders GD, Harris RA, et al. Cost-effectiveness of implantable cardioverter defibrillators relative to amiodarone for prevention of sudden cardiac death. Ann Intern Med 1997;126:1–12.

44. Leong ASY, Wright J. The contribution of immunohistochemical staining in tumor diagnosis. Histopathology 1987;11:1295–1305.

45. Raab SS. The cost-effectiveness of immunohistochemistry. Arch Pathol Lab Med 2000;124:1185–1191.

46. Masood S, Hosein I, Pitcher M, et al. Potential value of immunoperoxidase technique in assessment of genital herpes. J Fla Med Assoc 1990;77:516–519.

47. White JM, Poupard JA, Knight RA, Miller LA. Evaluation of two commercially available test methods to determine feasibility of testing for respiratory syncytial virus in a community hospital laboratory. Am J Clin Pathol 1988;90:175–180.

48. Travis WD, Pittaluga S, Lipschik GY, et al. Atypical pathologic manifestations of Pneumocystis carinii pneumonia in the acquired immune deficiency syndrome: Review of 123 lung biopsies from 76 patients with emphasis on cysts, vascular invasion, vasculitis, and granulomas. Am J Surg Pathol 1990;14:615–625.

49. Ritter JH, Sutton TD, Wick MR. Use of immunostains to ABH blood group antigens to resolve problems in identity of tissue specimens. Arch Pathol Lab Med 1994;118:293–297.

50. Wick MR. Oncogene analysis in diagnostic pathology: A current perspective. Am J Clin Pathol 1992;97:S1–S3.

51. Frew A, Ralfkiaer N, Ghosh AK, et al. Immunocytochemistry in the detection of bone marrow metastasis in patients with primary lung cancer. Br J Cancer 1986;53:555–556.

52. Mathieu MC, Friedman S, Bosq J, et al. Immunohistochemical staining of bone marrow biopsies for detection of occult metastasis in breast cancer. Breast Cancer Res Treat 1990;15:21–26.

53. Lacueva FJ, Teruel A, Calpena R, et al. Detection of p-glycoprotein in frozen and paraffin-embedded gastric adenocarcinoma tissues using a panel of monoclonal antibodies. Histopathology 1998;32:328–334.

54. Makris A, Powles TJ, Dowsett M, et al. Prediction of response to neoadjuvant chemoendocrine therapy in primary breast carcinomas. Clin Cancer Res 1997;3:593–600.

55. Ross JS, Fletcher JA. The Her-2/neu oncogene in breast cancer: Prognostic factor, predictive factor, and target for therapy. Stem Cells 1998;16:413–428.

56. Yang X, Uziely B, Groshen S, et al. MDR1 gene expression in primary and advanced breast cancer. Lab Invest 1999;79:271–280.

57. Pegram MD, Lipton A, Hayes DF, et al. Phase II study of receptor-enhanced chemosensitivity using recombinant humanized anti-p185HER2/neu monoclonal antibody plus cisplatin in patients with HER2/neu–overexpressing metastatic breast cancer refractory to chemotherapy treatment. J Clin Oncol 1998;16:2659–2671.

58. Schapira DV, Jarrett AR. The need to consider survival, outcome, and expense when evaluating and treating patients with unknown primary carcinoma. Arch Intern Med 1995;155:2050–2054.

59. Perchalski JE, Hall KL, Dewar MA. Metastasis of unknown origin. Prim Care 1992;19:747–752.

60. Blumenschein GR, DiStefano A, Caderao J, et al. Multimodality therapy for locally advanced and limited stage IV breast cancer: The impact of effective non–cross-resistance late-consolidation chemotherapy. Clin Cancer Res 1997;3:2633–2637.

61. Alberts AS, Falkson G, Falkson HC, et al. Treatment and prognosis of metastatic carcinoma of unknown primary: Analysis of 100 patients. Med Pediatr Oncol 1989;17:188–192.

62. Fizazi K, Culine S. Metastatic carcinoma of unknown origin. Bull Cancer 1998;85:609–617.

63. Raab SS, Slagel DD, Hughes JH, et al. Sensitivity and cost-effectiveness of fine needle aspiration and immunocytochemistry in the evaluation of patients with a pulmonary malignancy and a history of cancer. Arch Pathol Lab Med 1997;121:695–700.

64. Liu Y, Sturgis CD, Silverman JF, Raab SS. The utility of immunocytochemistry (ICC) in cytopathology practice. Acta Cytol 1999;43:967.

65. Grzybicki DM, Liu YL, Silverman JF, Raab SS. Utility of diagnostic immunohistochemistry in surgical pathology. Mod Pathol, in press.

66. Raab SS. The cost-effectiveness of cervical-vaginal rescreening. Am J Clin Pathol 1997;108:525–536.

67. Hornberger J, Brown B, Halpern J. Designing a cost-effective clinical trial. Stat Med 1995;14:2249–2259.

68. Bätge B, Bosslet K, Sedlacek H, et al. Monoclonal antibodies against CEA-related components discriminate between pancreatic duct type carcinomas and nonneoplastic duct lesions as well as nonduct type neoplasias. Virchows Arch [A] 1986;408:361–374.

69. Shimizu M, Saitoh Y, Ohyanagi H, Itoh H. Immunohistochemical staining of pancreatic cancer with CA19-9, KM01, unabsorbed CEA, and absorbed CEA: A comparison with normal pancreas and chronic pancreatitis. Arch Pathol Lab Med 1990;114:195–200.

70. Netser JC, Robinson RA, Smith RJ, et al. Value-based pathology: A cost-benefit analysis of the examination of routine and nonroutine tonsil and adenoid specimens. Am J Clin Pathol 1997;108:158–165.

71. Warner K, Luce B. Cost-Benefit and Cost-Effectiveness Analysis in Health Care: Principles, Practice and Potential. Ann Arbor, MI: Health Administration Press, 1982:1–100.

72. Udvarhelyi IS, Colditz GA, Rai A, et al. Cost-effectiveness and cost-benefit analyses in the medical literature. Ann Intern Med 1992;116:238–244.

73. Brumm C, Schulze C, Charels K, et al. The significance of alpha-fetoprotein and other tumor markers in differential immunocytochemistry of primary liver tumors. Histopathology 1989;14:503–513.

74. Koelma IA, Nap M, Huitema S, et al. Hepatocellular carcinoma, adenoma, and focal nodular hyperplasia. Comparative histopathologic study with immunohistochemical parameters. Arch Pathol Lab Med 1986;110:1035–1040.

75. Ma CK, Zarbo RJ, Frierson HF Jr, et al. Comparative immunohistochemical study of primary and metastatic carcinomas of the liver. Am J Clin Pathol 1993;99:530–532.

76. Raab SS, Thomas PA, Lenel JC, et al. Pathology and probability: Likelihood ratios and receiver operating characteristic curves in the interpretation of bronchial brush specimens. Am J Clin Pathol 1995;103:588–593.

77. Hawkins RA, Roberts MM, Forrest APM. Oestrogen recep-

tors and breast cancer: Current status. Fr J Surg 1980;67:162–165.

78. Fisher ER, Redmond CK, Liu H, et al. Correlation of estrogen receptor and pathologic characteristics of invasive breast cancer. Cancer 1980;45:349–353.

79. Lee SH. Cancer cell estrogen receptor of human mammary carcinoma. Cancer 1979;44:1–12.

80. Brooks JJ, LiVolsi VA, Pietra GG. Mesothelial cell inclusions in mediastinal lymph nodes mimicking metastatic carcinoma. Am J Clin Pathol 1990;93:741–748.

Part II

Organ Systems and Diseases

Immunohistology of Soft Tissue and Osseous Neoplasms

Lisa A. Cerilli, M.D.
Mark R. Wick, M.D.

Soft tissue tumors are an incredibly diverse family of lesions, the categorization of which continues to evolve as more insight is gained into the subtleties of their differentiation patterns. As such, the classification of soft tissue neoplasia is an increasingly complex subject, which is aided by an understanding of the immunohistology of this area. This chapter is a practical summary of that topic, but it does not purport to be an encyclopedic or all-inclusive treatise. Moreover, we emphasize the fact that immunohistologic evaluation of soft tissue tumors is merely an adjunct to thorough morphologic evaluation, not a substitute for it.

IMMUNOHISTOLOGIC MARKERS OF INTEREST IN SOFT TISSUE AND BONE PATHOLOGY

Intermediate Filament Proteins

The intermediate filament proteins (IFPs) are structural components of all human cells, together with microfilaments and microtubules.[1, 2] They are 7 to 10 nm in diameter and are often arranged in skeins or bundles in the cytoplasm. Parallel aggregation of IFPs often is observed in epithelial cells that are rich in high molecular weight keratins, yielding the structures known to electron microscopists as *tonofilaments* or *tonofibrils*.[3] Otherwise, the IFPs as a family are not morphologically distinguishable from one another at an ultrastructural level. They are composed of at least six distinct moieties, on biochemical and functional grounds— keratins, vimentin, desmin, neurofilament proteins (NFPs), glial fibrillary acidic protein (GFAP), and the lamins (nuclear envelope proteins).[4] Only the first five of these entities have been well characterized in diagnostic pathology and are discussed here.

All the IFPs share structural homologies,[5] but their precise natures vary considerably. Molecular weights vary between 40 and 200 kd. The IFPs also have dissimilar isoelectric pH values, and, more importantly, characteristic distribution patterns in non-neoplastic cells and human tumors.[2] Two members of the IFP family, the keratins and NFPs, appear to be composed of heteropolymeric aggregations of two or more proteins, whereas the other representatives of this group are homopolymers containing only one protein isoform.[6] The IFPs are encoded by a multiplicity of genes on various chromosomes (e.g., chromosomes 12q and 17q for the keratins, chromosome 2q for desmin, chromosome 10p for vimentin, and chromosome 17q for GFAP),[7-10] a situation that is somewhat counterintuitive in light of their shared biochemical attributes.

Initially, IFPs were thought to serve a purely structural role in muscle cells, in keeping with their proposed "cytoskeletal" nature. It was hypothesized that the function of these proteins was to keep other cytoplasmic proteins in proper relationship with one another, as well as to anchor the cytoplasmic contractile apparatus to the cell membrane. However, subsequent developments in cell biology cast considerable doubt on this premise.[11] The intermediate filaments are now known to serve a nucleic acid–binding function; moreover, they are susceptible to processing by calcium-activated proteases and are substrates for cyclic adenosine monophosphate–dependent protein kinases. Thus, it has been proposed that all IFPs serve as modulators between extracellular influences governing calcium flux into the cell (and subsequent protease activation) and nuclear function at a transcriptional or translational level.[12] Their morphologic associations with cell membranes and the perinuclear cytoplasm are consistent with this theory and relegate a "cytoskeletal" role to a secondary level. Present opinion favors the view that fibrils of the IFPs are formed not as cellular "buttresses" but rather to restrict the availability of their nucleic acid–binding domains in accord with cell cycle activity. The fact that some of the IFPs insert into intercellular, desmoplakin-containing desmosomes, which are responsible for maintaining tissue integrity, does not necessarily assign a structural biologic role to these filaments, because intercellular junctions may be points of "biochemical communication" with the extracellular milieu.[13]

KERATINS

As the essential IFPs of epithelial cells and epithelial neoplasms, keratins have a high degree of specificity and sensitivity for the diagnosis of carcinoma among malignant tumors. Cytokeratins typically are expressed by any given cell type in pairs, representing an acidic ("type I") and a basic ("type II") keratin.[14] These vary in molecular weight from 40 to 67 kd and have been given numerical catalog designations by Moll and colleagues such that they are numbered, within each respective type grouping, from lowest to highest molecular weight.[15] There are 12 type I keratins with acidic isoelectric points, and 8 type II proteins with basic biochemical attributes. As described by Miettinen, cytokeratins generally tend to pair themselves during cell development so that a type I keratin is associated with a type II keratin that is 7 to 9 kd larger.[14] However, this is not an inviolate rule; for example, cytokeratin 19 (40 kd) has no basic keratin "mate" and exists alone in cells that synthesize it. Moreover, some cell types manifest simple patterns of keratin expression, with only one pair, whereas others may demonstrate up to five pairs.

The particular keratin types that can be detected in given tissues or neoplasms follow predictable, known patterns of gene expression that serve, in part, to identify the cells composing them (Table 3–1). With particular reference to nonepithelial cells, selected cytokeratins (CK8 and CK18 and occasionally CK19) are, in fact, demonstrable in the physiologic state, but the use of special techniques is usually necessary to preserve or detect extremely low densities of those IFPs (e.g., acetone fixation, frozen section immunohistology, or amplified immunodetection methods). Selected mesenchymal neoplasms may likewise exhibit keratin reactivity, which is a bit broader in its scope. For example, CK7, CK13, and CK19 have been observed in synovial sarcomas, in addition to CK8 and CK18.[14] Other soft tissue or bone tumors that are regularly cytokeratin-immunoreactive include epithelioid sarcoma (CK8, CK18, and CK19); chordoma (CK8, CK18, and CK19, with or without CK4 and CK5); parachordoma (CK8); and intraosseous adamantinoma (CK19 [and others?]).[14–18] Thus, together with synovial sarcoma, those neoplasms constitute a group of lesions that some authors have suggested are primary "carcinosarcomas" of soft tissue and bone.

In reference to still other mesenchymal neoplasms, experience since the 1990s has shown that under some circumstances, selected tumors that are typically devoid of keratins may synthesize those IFPs in an "aberrant" fashion (Table 3–2). Indeed, at this point, virtually all sarcoma morphotypes have been reported to show this behavior potentially. Nevertheless, it should be emphasized that "aberrant" keratin reactivity is most common in a narrow spectrum of malignant mesenchymal neoplasms that are studied under usual diagnostic conditions, principally leiomyosarcoma (LMS), malignant peripheral nerve sheath tumor (MPNST), epithelioid angiosarcoma and, to a lesser degree, Ewing's sarcoma/primitive neuroectodermal tumor (ES/PNET).[19] In keeping with the comments made previously, CK8, CK18, and CK19 are expected in this scenario. We would like to stress the fact that aberrancy of IFP synthesis is not a frequent event overall. Many reports on this phenomenon actually represent idiosyncrasies or flaws in immunohisto-

Table 3–1. Cytokeratin Subclasses and Non-neoplastic Cell Types Expressing Them

| Type II (Basic) Cytokeratins* | | | Type I (Acid) Cytokeratins* | |
(Moll Catalog No.)	(Molecular Wt.)	Distribution	(Moll Catalog No.)	(Molecular Wt.)
—	—	Epidermis of palms and soles	CK9	64 kd
CK1	67 kd	Epidermis and keratinizing squamous epithe-	CK10	56.5 kd
CK2	65 kd	lia in all other locations	CK11	56 kd
CK3	63 kd	Cornea	CK12	55 kd
CK4	59 kd	Nonkeratinizing epithelia of internal viscera	CK13	51 kd
CK5	58 kd	Basal cells of squamous and glandular epithe- lia, myoepithelial cells, and mesothelium	CK14	50 kd
CK6	56 kd	Squamous epithelia	CK16	48 kd
CK7	54 kd	Simple epithelia	—	—
—	—	Basal cells of glandular epithelia and myoepi- thelial cells	CK17	46 kd
CK8	52 kd	Simple epithelia	CK18	45 kd
—	—	Simple epithelia; most glandular and some squamous epithelial cells	CK19	40 kd
—	—	Simple epithelial cells of gastrointestinal tract; Merkel cells of skin	CK20	46 kd

*Cytokeratin pairs that typically are coexpressed together in the same cell types are shown on the same line.

Table 3–2. Cytokeratin Subclasses Expressed "Aberrantly" in Mesenchymal Cells and Tumors

Moll Cytokeratin Catalog No.	Recognized by MoAb Clones	Potential Distribution
8	CAM5.2 (Becton-Dickinson) AE3 (PROGEN) KL1 (Serotec) F12-19 (Biogenesis) RCK102 (Biogenesis) DC10 (BioGenex) MAK-6 (Medac) 5D3 (Biogenesis) NCL-5D3 (Medac) 6D7/3F3 (Medac) 2A4 (Biohit) M20 (Accurate) KS8.7 (Paesel) NCL-CK8 (Novocastra) UCD/AB6.01 (ATCC) C22 (Biogenesis) 4.1.18 (BioGenex) H1 (Bioprobe) C51 (Neomarkers) 34BH11 (Enzo) Lu5 (Sera-Lab) C11 (Neomarkers)	Fetal fibroblasts; subserosal fibroblasts; myometrium; vascular smooth muscle; fetal myocardium; vascular endothelial cells; selected reticulum cells of lymphatic organs; neoplastic plasma cells and CD30+ lymphoid cells (very rarely); selected leiomyosarcomas, epithelioid hemangioendotheliomas, epithelioid angiosarcomas, primitive neuroectodermal tumors and Ewing's sarcomas, malignant peripheral nerve sheath tumors, and clear cell sarcomas
18	MFN116 (Axcel) PKK1 (LabSystems) CK18 (Novocastra) KS18.4 (Paesel) KS18.8 (Biotest) DC10 (BioGenex) K918.04 (Cymbus) KS-B17.2 (Sigma) 4B11 (Biohit) DA7 (Bioprobe) KS18.18 (Camon) 34BH11 (DiagBiosys) F12-19 (Biogenesis) C11 (Neomarkers) LP34 (Medac)	Fetal fibroblasts; myometrium; vascular smooth muscle; fetal myocardium; vascular endothelial cells; selected reticulum cells of lymphatic organs; some CD30+ lymphoid cells (rarely); selected leiomyosarcomas, epithelioid hemangioendotheliomas, epithelioid angiosarcomas, primitive neuroectodermal tumors and Ewing's sarcomas, malignant peripheral nerve sheath tumors, and clear cell sarcomas
19	AE1 (BM; ICN) PKK1 (LabSystems) CK19 (Novocastra) RCK108 (BioGenex) BA17 (DAKO) KS19.1 (Serotec) F12-19 (Biogenesis) MAK-6 (Medac)	Myometrium; fetal myocardium; selected neoplastic myeloid cells; some leiomyosarcomas; rare primitive neuroectodermal tumors and Ewing's sarcomas

chemical technique, wherein antikeratin antibodies are used at inappropriately high concentration or with especially sensitive detection procedures. Inasmuch as the IFPs are structurally interrelated,[20] it should not be surprising that cross-labeling of vimentin, desmin, NFPs, or GFAP can be obtained spuriously with many antikeratin reagents. Using information on the interspecies relatedness of intermediate filaments and their similarities to one another, Geisler and Weber[21] outlined the different classes of monoclonal antibodies that may be raised against them:

- Tissue-specific (intermediate filament–discriminating) but broadly reactive across species
- Tissue- and species-specific
- Tissue-nonspecific and species-specific
- Tissue- and species-nonspecific

From a comparative biologic point of view, all these reagents are of interest. However, only the first two categories have potential use as discriminants in surgical pathology.

This brings our discussion to a crucial philosophical point having to do with methodology. At this juncture, a large body of clinical literature exists on the IFP profiles of human neoplasms. If one wishes to benefit from the value of its contents in a diagnostic setting, the techniques used in obtaining those data must be retained. Thus, in a practical sense, substituting "new and improved" immunodetection protocols for old ones, without attention to the effect which that step will have on final interpretations, is inadvisable. Put simply, our goal as diagnostic pathologists is not to identify each and every molecule of a particular IFP—no matter how sparse—in any given tumor, but rather to establish and maintain the "windows" of immunodetection so that overlap between related moieties is minimized and diagnostic utility is maximized. If these maxims are heeded, the incidence of "aberrant" keratin expression in mesenchymal neoplasia should be low when using routinely processed (paraffin-embedded) clinical substrates.

DESMIN

Desmin is a cytoplasmic IFP that is characteristically found in muscle cells and in the neoplasms associated with them.[22-24] In smooth muscle cells, it is seen with cytoplasmic dense bodies and subplasmalemmal dense plaques; in striated muscle, desmin filaments are linked to sarcomeric Z disks.

Small and Sobieszek were the first to recognize desmin as a distinct biochemical moiety in 1977.[25] They found that it represented a residual filamentous protein in muscle cells depleted of actin and myosin in vitro and assigned to it the provisional designation "skeletin." It was observed to have an isoelectric point of approximately 4 and to be heat-stable and insoluble in salt-rich solutions. Amino acid analysis revealed a high concentration of glutamate and aspartate and a significant chemical homology with glial and NFPs. A notable finding in that study was that muscle cells depleted of skeletin (desmin) were still able to contract in response to adenosine triphosphate and calcium. This point led the authors to conclude that the protein in question played no role in contractility but rather served to keep actin and myosin filaments in register and to anchor them to the plasmalemma.

These observations have been confirmed and expanded by others.[26-28] Desmin is now known to have a molecular weight of 53 kd, with a mass per unit of 36 to 37 kd/nm. It is composed of an N-terminal "headpiece" and a C-terminal "tailpiece," both of which are nonhelical in conformation. These bracket an alpha helical middle domain of approximately 300 amino acid residues. The former are greatly variable in biochemical constitution from species to species, but the helical segment is highly "conserved," meaning that interspecies homology in this domain is striking. Chicken and porcine desmin demonstrate less than a 9% biochemical divergence. In fact, this similarity supersedes that which is exhibited between different IFPs in the same species; nevertheless, all five IFPs show an amino acid sequence homology of approximately 30%.[28]

Like other intermediate filaments, desmin displays a 20- to 22-nm axial periodicity. Ip and Heuser showed that it forms heteropolymers that aggregate in a cross-linked, fibrillar, tetrameric fashion.[29] These are arranged side by side in staggered half-unit register, such that the headpiece of one filament is associated with the middle domain of its neighbor. The helical segment composition of desmin allows it to form "coiled coils," with respect to the tertiary structure of the molecule; indeed, such a conformation would be predicted by biochemical models. Hydrophobic amino acid residues are thereby exposed, explaining the ability of desmin to associate with nuclear and plasmalemmal membranes, which are nonhydrophilic.

Desmin appears in developing striated muscle cells at the myotube-forming stage, in which myoblasts fuse with one another.[30] It replaces vimentin, at least in large measure, since the latter is the intermediate filament that is first expressed by virtually all embryonic mesenchymal cells. Desmin filaments are oriented in a longitudinal fashion initially, but as the muscle cell matures, they become concentrated around Z disks.[31] An analysis of desmin immunoreactivity in embryonic and adult muscle cells has been performed by Fischman and Danto[32] using monoclonal antibodies (D3 and D76). D3 recognizes embryonic cellular desmin but does not react with adult cells; D76 displays the reverse of this pattern. These data suggest that either desmin is biochemically altered during cellular development or different epitopes are masked in fetal and adult cells, respectively.

Although desmin is most often expressed by myogenous cells, in vitro studies of chicken embryo and hamster kidney fibroblasts have also revealed its presence.[33] This finding is best explained by implicating a "myofibroblastic" nature for such cells. Other immunofluorescence assessments of intact myofibroblastic tissues have reportedly shown no desmin reactivity, however. Also, not all muscular cells contain desmin. For example, Schmid and colleagues documented three separate cell types in mammalian vascular (aortic) smooth muscle—those that display vimentin only, others that express vimentin and desmin concurrently, and a third group exhibiting only desmin.[34] Immunoelectron microscopic analyses have documented the binding of suitably specific antidesmins to the intermediate filaments of muscle cells and their neoplasms.[35] There should be no cross-reactivity of such reagents with associated contractile proteins, such as actin and myosin; this is particularly important because these three proteins appear to share some epitopes.

The three most well-characterized monoclonal antibodies to desmin are designated D33, DER-11, and DEB-5. By the Western blot technique, they have been shown to recognize desmin epitopes between residues 324 and 415 and to have no cross-reactivity with other IFPs. These reagents show tissue-specificity but species-nonspecificity.

In general, desmin is, as expected, a specific marker for myogenic differentiation among soft tissue tumors. As such, it is seen in the majority of rhabdomyomas, leiomyomas, rhabdomyosarcomas, and LMSs.[22-24, 36-38] Because myofibromatoses also have a partially myogenous nature ultrastructurally, it is understandable that lesions such as desmoid tumors and myofibromas are likewise potentially desmin-reactive.[39] Nonetheless, myoepithelial cells typically lack desmin. Desmin may also be coexpressed by neoplasms with "divergent" phenotypes, examples of which include primitive neuroectodermal tumors (PNETs), "desmoplastic small cell tumors" (variants of PNETs), epithelioid sarcomas, MPNSTs, and malignant "rhabdoid" tumors.[40–44]

VIMENTIN

Vimentin is a 57-kd protein that was initially isolated from a mouse fibroblast culture.[2, 45] Its name derives from the Latin *vimentum,* describing an array of flexible rods. This IFP is considered to be the "primordial" member of the intermediate filament family, because it is present in most, if not all, fetal cells early in development. Moreover, when two or more IFPs are coexpressed by a cell line or neoplasm, vimentin is virtually always one of them.[46] Accordingly, vimentin is not considered to be cell type–specific. From the perspective of mesenchymal tumor pathology, it is of interest that vimentin shows a greater amino acid homology to desmin, NFPs, and GFAP than it does to the keratins.[21, 45]

The ubiquity of vimentin in soft tissues limits its diagnostic use in the setting of tumor pathology. However, it does serve a useful "control marker" function—to ensure that the tissue has been properly preserved and processed.[47] If vimentin cannot be easily detected in non-neoplastic endothelial cells, fibroblasts, and other mesenchymal elements that are routinely present in any tissue section, the reactivity or nonreactivity of accompanying neoplastic cells cannot be properly determined. Occasionally, the pattern of vimentin expression is also distinctive. For example, in malignant "rhabdoid" tumors of the soft tissues, that IFP usually assumes a densely globular cytoplasmic configuration, indenting the nuclei of the neoplastic cells.[44] A listing of characterized commercially available antibodies to vimentin, the most widely used of which are clones V9 and 3B4,[46, 48–53] is provided in Tables 3–3 to 3–7.

NEUROFILAMENT PROTEINS

The NFPs are composed of three basic subunits with molecular weights of 68 kd, 150 kd, and 200 kd.[54, 55] Hence, they are clearly larger than all other IFPs. Each of the three NFPs appears to be a separate gene product, rather than derivatives of the other two.[56] Expression of this family of IFPs is correlated with the differentiation of neurogenic "blast" cells into committed neurons in the developing embryo or in neoplasia.[57, 58] Another peculiarity of the NFPs that is not shared by other intermediate filament classes, except for GFAP, is

that each of the three neurofilament isoforms may be either phosphorylated or nonphosphorylated in vivo.[59] Correspondingly, antibodies to the NFPs may be specific for only one of those two configurations.[60, 61]

Practically speaking, NFPs are generally not well detected in formalin-fixed, paraffin-embedded tissues, even with modern immunohistochemical methods and commercial antibodies. Among these, our experience has been that the "SMI" series of monoclonal antibodies[62] is most consistently active against routinely processed surgical pathology specimens. It is known that among soft tissue neoplasms, neuroblastoma variants, ganglioneuromas, paragangliomas, and metastatic neuroendocrine carcinomas are the only lesions that are potentially labeled for NFPs.[63–66]

GLIAL FIBRILLARY ACIDIC PROTEIN

GFAP is not an IFP that figures into the diagnosis of soft tissue tumors in a very meaningful manner. This 51-kd protein is the major component of astrocytes, ependymal cells, and retinal Müller cells and is not typically expressed by mature oligodendroglia.[66–68] Nonglial tissues with putative GFAP-reactivity include Schwann cells, Kupffer cells, and some chondrocytes.[68] It is therefore not unexpected that selected neoplasms including such elements (peripheral nerve sheath tumors and chondroid tumors)[69–74] may occasionally demonstrate immunolabeling for GFAP. Nevertheless, this is a rather rare occurrence and does not, in our estimation, justify the routine application of anti-GFAP reagents to diagnostic problems in soft tissue pathology.

Epithelial Membrane Antigen

Epithelial membrane antigen (EMA) is one of several human milk fat globule proteins (HMFGPs) that are derived from the mammary epithelium. The HMFGPs are greatly variable in molecular weight (51 kd to >1000 kd), and they are predominantly glycoproteinaceous.[75] They compose part of the plasmalemma of epithelial cells in areas of the cell membrane overlying tight junctions.[76] In addition, because HMFGPs are packaged in the Golgi apparatus, globular labeling of that structure may be seen immunohistologically.[76] The function of the HFMGPs, including EMA, is still not absolutely certain. It is thought that they serve a role in secretion or, alternatively, have a protective function for the cell.[75]

The distribution of HMFGPs is such that most, but not all, non-neoplastic human epithelial cells express at least one member of this protein family. Exceptions include the gastrointestinal surface epithelium, endocervical epithelium, prostatic acinar epithelium, epididymis, germ cells, hepatocytes,

Text continued on page 69

Table 3–3. Antibody Reagents Used by the Authors in the Study of Soft Tissue Tumors

Reagent	Source	Dilution	Protocol	Principal Diagnostic Use
Antikeratins (M)				Recognition of epithelioid sarcoma, synovial sarcoma, and "divergent" epithelial differentiation in selected other soft tissue sarcomas
AE1/AE3	Boehringer-Mannheim	1:150	MWER	
CAM5.2	Becton-Dickinson	1:200	MWER	
MAK-6	Medac	1:75	MWER	
DC10	BioGenex	1:50	MWER	
CK18	Novocastra	1:50	MWER	
CK19	Novocastra	1:50	MWER	
CK7	BioGenex	1:75	MWER	
Antidesmin (M)	BioGenex	1:2000	MWER	Recognition of smooth muscle and striated muscle tumors
Antivimentin (M)	BioGenex	1:2000	MWER	Ubiquitous intermediate filament in soft tissue neoplasms; serves as a positive specimen control
Anti–epithelial membrane antigen (M)	DAKO	1:400	NT	Recognition of epithelioid sarcoma, synovial sarcoma, and selected peripheral nerve sheath tumors
Anti–muscle-specific actin (clone HHF-35) (M)	Enzo	1:8000	MWER	Recognition of smooth muscle and striated muscle tumors as well as myofibroblastic differentiation
Anti–alpha isoform actin (clone 1A4) (M)	DAKO	1:200	MWER	Recognition of smooth muscle tumors and myofibroblastic differentiation
Antimyoglobin (P)	DAKO	1:800	MWER	Recognition of striated muscle tumors
Anti-MyoD1 (M)	DAKO	1:10	MWER	Recognition of striated muscle tumors
Antimyogenin (M)	Novocastra	1:30	MWER	Recognition of striated muscle tumors
Anti–h-caldesmon (M)	DAKO	1:200	MWER	Recognition of smooth muscle tumors
Anti–S-100 protein (P)	DAKO	1:1000	NT	Recognition of melanocytic, Schwannian, and cartilage neoplasms
Anti-CD57 (M)	Becton-Dickinson	1:20	MWER	Recognition of Schwannian tumors
Anti–collagen type IV (M)	BioGenex	1:40	MWER	Recognition of synovial, myogenous, peripheral nerve sheath, and endothelial neoplasms
Antilaminin (M)	Sigma	1:20	MWER	Recognition of synovial, myogenous, peripheral nerve sheath, and endothelial neoplasms
Anti–factor VIII–related antigen (M)	DAKO	1:20	MWER	Recognition of endothelial neoplasms
Anti-CD34 (M)	DAKO	1:800	MWER	Recognition of endothelial tumors, dermatofibrosarcoma protuberans, solitary fibrous tumors, and selected peripheral nerve sheath tumors and epithelioid sarcomas
Anti-CD31 (M)	DAKO	1:40	MWER	Recognition of endothelial tumors
Antithrombomodulin (M)	DAKO	1:200	MWER	Recognition of endothelial tumors and mesotheliomas
Anti-*Ulex europaeus I* lectin (P)	DAKO	1:4000	NT	Recognition of endothelial tumors via binding of *Ulex europaeus I* lectin
Ulex europaeus I (lectin)	DAKO	1:1000	NT	Recognition of endothelial tumors
Anti-CD68	DAKO	1:800	MWER	Putative marker of fibrohistiocytic tumors (see text)
Antiosteonectin (M)	BioDesign	1:100	MWER	Sensitive marker of possible osteoblastic differentiation
Antiosteocalcin (M)	Biogenesis	1:100	MWER	Specific marker of osteoblastic differentiation
Antisynaptophysin (M)	BioGenex	1:40	MWER	Detection of neuroectodermal differentiation
Anti-CD99 (M)	DAKO	1:20	MWER	Recognition of virtually all primitive neuroectodermal tumors and Ewing's sarcomas; labels roughly 50% of synovial sarcomas and malignant peripheral nerve sheath tumors; also present in lymphoblastic lymphomas-leukemias presenting in soft tissue

M, monoclonal; P, polyclonal (heteroantiserum); MWER, microwave-enhanced epitope retrieval; NT, no pretreatment of tissue sections.

Table 3-4. Percentages of Positivity for Pertinent Immunoreactants in Malignant Small Round Cell Tumors of Soft Tissue and Bone*

Antigen/Tumor	KER	EMA	VIM	DES	MSA	MYOGN	SYN	CD57	S-100P	CD45	CD99	OCN
RMS	<10†	<1†	93	94	96	92	0	17	7	0	19	0
ES/PNET	7	0	75	<1†	<1†	<1†	65	30	<10†	0	91	0
PSRCT	50†	30†	75†	50†	50†	50†	75†	30†	<10†	0	90§	0
MCS	<5†	0	98	0	0	0	0	58	97‖	0	13	0
SCOS	<1†	0	100	<1	<5†	0	0	50†	33	0	35	73
ML/LEUK	0	0	75†	0	0	0	0	<5†	0	98	50†	0
SCSS	75**	75	100	0	0	0	0	90	30†	0	0	0

*All figures in this table represent percentages of immunoreactive cases in each tumor category; unless specified otherwise, the source of these data is the Internet site entitled "Immunoquery" (Author: Frisman D; URL = *http://www.immunoquery.com*).

†Data derived from authors' experience.

‡Peripheral neuroectodermal tumors expressing DES, MSA, or MYOGN are classified as polyphenotypic small round cell tumor by many observers.

§Desmoplastic small round cell tumor variants of polyphenotypic small round cell tumors are generally negative for CD99.

‖S-100 protein is seen only in the chondroid islands of mesenchymal chondrosarcoma.

**Keratins 7, 13, and 19 are seen in 45 to 50% of cases of small cell synovial sarcoma, but less than 10% of differential diagnostic alternatives.

KER, keratin, as detected with a mixture of antibodies CAM5.2, MAK-6, and AE1/AE3; EMA, epithelial membrane antigen; VIM, vimentin; DES, desmin; MSA, muscle-specific actin; MYOGN, myogenin; SYN, synaptophysin; S-100P, S-100 protein; OCN, osteocalcin; RMS, embryonal and alveolar rhabdomyosarcomas; ES/PNET, Ewing's sarcoma/primitive neuroectodermal tumor; PSRCT, polyphenotypic small round cell tumor; MCS, mesenchymal chondrosarcoma; SCOS, small cell osteosarcoma; ML/LEUK, malignant lymphoma/leukemia; SCSS, small cell poorly differentiated synovial sarcoma.

65

Table 3-5. Percentages of Positivity for Pertinent Immunoreactants in Malignant Spindle Cell Tumors of Soft Tissue and Bone*

Antigen/Tumor	KER	EMA	VIM	DES	MSA	SMA	CALD	S-100P	CD57	Collagen Type IV	LM	CD34	CD31	UL	CD99	OCN
SCRMS	<10†	<1†	95	95	96	25	<1	7	17	98†	100	0	0	0	20	0
FS	0	0	100	0	0	<5†	0	0	0	0	0	0	0	0	0	0
LMS	<10†	0	91	75†	90	88	75	8	50	75	63	16	<1†	0	20	0
MPNST	<10†	20	100	11	18	<1	<1	63	43	83	80	9	0	0	50†	0
MSS	76	75	100	0	0	12	<1†	30†	90	100	95	0	0	0	50†	0
SCAS	<5†	0	100	0	<10†	<10†	<5†	<1†	0	10	55	80	80	70	0	0
KS	0	0	100	0	0	100	<5†	0	0	50†	50†	86	53	10	0	0
FOS	<1†	0†	100	<1†	<1†	<1†	<1†	10†	50†	0	0	0	0	0	0	80†

*All figures in this table represent percentages of immunoreactive cases in each tumor category; unless specified otherwise, the source of these data is the Internet site entitled "Immunoquery" (Author: Frisman D; URL = *http://www.immunoquery.com*).

†Data derived from authors' experience.

KER, keratin, detected by a mixture of CAM5.2, MAK-6, and AE1/AE3; EMA, epithelial membrane antigen; VIM, vimentin; DES, desmin; MSA, muscle-specific actin; SMA, "smooth muscle" (alpha isoform) actin; CALD, h-caldesmon; S-100P, S-100 protein; OCN, osteocalcin; LM, laminin; UL, *Ulex europaeus I* lectin binding; FS, fibrosarcoma; SCRMS, spindle cell rhabdomyosarcoma; LMS, leiomyosarcoma; MPNST, malignant peripheral nerve sheath tumor; MSS, monophasic spindle cell synovial sarcoma; SCAS, spindle cell angiosarcoma; KS, Kaposi's sarcoma; FOS, fibroblastic osteosarcoma.

Table 3–6. Percentages of Positivity for Pertinent Immunoreactants in Malignant Epithelioid Tumors of Soft Tissue and Bone*

Antigen/ Tumor	KER	EMA	VIM	DES	MSA	SMA	CALD	S-100P	CD57	HMB-45	TY	M1	CD31	CD34	Collagen Type IV	OCN
EPS	100	96	100	10	39	33	25*	<5*	0	0	0	0	<1†	52	50†	0
EPSS	95†	99†	100	0	0	0	0	10†	50†	0	0	0	0	0	100	0
EAS	10†	0	100	0	0	0	0	<1†	0	0	0	0	80	80	65†	0
EMPNST	<10†	20	100	11	18	<1	<1	63	43	<1†	<1†	<1†	0	9	83	0
CCS	<1†	0	100	0	30	0	0	90†	17	85	90†	70†	0	4	0	0
SEFS	<1†	0†	100†	0†	0†	0†	0†	0†	0†	0†	0†	0†	0†	0†	0†	0†
ELMS	<10†	0	90	75	90	85	75	8	50†	0	0	0	0	16	75	0
ASPS	0	0	50†	20	<10†	0†	0	30	0	0	0	0	0	0	0	0
HMFH	<1†	0	100	<10†	17	18	<5†	<1†	0†	0	0	0	0	0	0	0
EOS	<1†	0†	100	<1†	<1†	<1†	0	<5†	50†	0	0	0	0	0	0	82

*All figures in this table represent percentages of immunoreactive cases in each tumor category; unless specified otherwise, the source of these data is the Internet site entitled "Immunoquery" (Author: Frisman D; URL = *http://www.immunoquery.com*).

†Data derived from authors' experience.

KER, keratin, as detected by a mixture of CAM5.2, MAK-6, and AE1/AE3; EMA, epithelial membrane antigen; VIM, vimentin; DES, desmin; MSA, muscle-specific actin; SMA, "smooth muscle" (alpha isoform) actin; CALD, h-caldesmon; S-100P, S-100 protein; TY, tyrosinase; M1, MART-1 (melan-A); OCN, osteocalcin; EPS, epithelioid sarcoma; EPSS, epithelioid synovial sarcoma; EAS, epithelioid angiosarcoma; EMPNST, epithelioid malignant peripheral nerve sheath tumor; CCS, clear cell sarcoma; SEFS, sclerosing epithelioid fibrosarcoma; ELMS, epithelioid leiomyosarcoma; ASPS, alveolar soft part sarcoma; HMFH, histiocytic malignant fibrous histiocytoma; EOS, epithelioid osteosarcoma.

Table 3–7. Percentages of Positivity for Pertinent Immunoreactants in Malignant Pleomorphic Tumors of Soft Tissue and Bone*

Antigen/Tumor	KER	EMA	VIM	DES	MSA	SMA	CALD	S-100P	CD57	Collagen Type IV	LM	CD34	CD31	UL	CD99	OCN
PRMS/	<10†	<1†	100	95	96	25	<1	7	17	98†	100	0	0	0	20	0†
PLPS/DLPS	0	0	100	0	<1†	<1†	<1†	70†‡	0	20†	10†	0	0	0	0	0†
PLMS/DLMS	<10†	0	91	75†	90	88	75	8	50	75	63	16	<1†	0	20	0†
MPNST	<10†	20	100	11	18	<1	<1	63	43	83	80	9	0	0	10†	0†
DMSS	76‡	75‡	100	0	0	12	<1†	30†	90‡	100‡	95‡	0	0	0	50‡	0†
MFH	<1†	0	100	<10†	17	18	<5†	<1†	0†	0	0	0	0	0	0	0†
DCHOR	100‡	94‡	100	3	0	0	0	88‡	32‡	13	10	0	0	10†‡	0	0†
DCHS	<1†	0†	100	0	0	0	0	97‡	58‡	10†‡	5†‡	0	0	0	0	0†
POGS	<1†	<1†	100	11	0	50	0	32‡	50†	0	0	0	0	0	35	82

*All figures in this table represent percentages of immunoreactive cases in each tumor category; unless specified otherwise, the source of these data is the Internet site entitled "Immunoquery" (Author: Frisman D; URL = *http://www.immunoquery.com*).

†Data derived from authors' experience.

‡Reactivity for specified determinants is focal only.

KER, keratin, detected by a mixture of CAM5.2, MAK-6, and AE1/AE3; EMA, epithelial membrane antigen; VIM, vimentin; DES, desmin; MSA, muscle-specific actin; SMA, "smooth muscle" (alpha isoform) actin; CALD, h-caldesmon; S-100P, S-100 protein; LM, laminin; UL, *Ulex europaeus I* lectin binding; OCN, osteocalcin; PRMS, pleomorphic rhabdomyosarcoma; PLPS/DLPS, pleomorphic and "dedifferentiated" liposarcoma; PLMS/DLMS, pleomorphic and "dedifferentiated" leiomyosarcoma; MPNST, pleomorphic malignant peripheral nerve sheath tumor; DMSS, "dedifferentiated" monophasic spindle cell synovial sarcoma; MFH, malignant fibrous histiocytoma; DCHOR, "dedifferentiated" chordoma; DCHS, "dedifferentiated" chondrosarcoma; POGS, pleomorphic osteosarcoma.

adrenal cortical cells, rete testis, squamous cells of the epidermis, and thyroid follicular epithelium.[77]

The most well-characterized monoclonal antibody to EMA (which is the most widely used HMFGP) is E29. It labels a glycoprotein of approximately 450 kd. In specific reference to the soft tissues, the notochord, perineurial fibroblasts, and plasma cells are the only non-neoplastic elements capable of EMA-positivity.[78–80] Nevertheless, neoplastic processes that may be EMA-immunoreactive are somewhat more numerous. Synovial sarcoma, epithelioid sarcoma, selected peripheral nerve sheath tumors ("perineuriomas" and some "neurothekeomas"), chordomas, parachordomas, and selected plasmacytomas are commonly labeled.[81] It should be stressed that "true" EMA-reactivity (i.e., that which generally equates with epithelial differentiation) must be cell membrane–based. Purely cytoplasmic labeling without a membrane component is a spurious pattern that should be ignored for diagnostic purposes.[82]

Nonintermediate Filament Myogenic Markers

ACTINS

Aside from desmin, as discussed earlier, the next most useful group of cytoplasmic determinants for the definition of myogenous differentiation is the protein family of the actins.[24, 83] There are six major isoforms of these microfilamentous contractile polypeptides, which have been designated skeletal muscle alpha, smooth muscle alpha and gamma, cardiac muscle alpha, and nonmyogenous beta and gamma actins.[83, 84] Alpha and gamma muscle isoforms are seen in tissues with "pure" myogenic differentiation, but they are also demonstrable in cells with myofibroblastic or myoepithelial features.[85–88] All these biochemical moieties cluster around 45 kd, and they may be labeled with antibodies that recognize conserved amino acid sequences in each of them or, alternatively, by isoform-selective reagents.[83–85] Obviously, from a diagnostic perspective, only the latter are desirable. However, because of inevitable problems that arise in the immunohistologic detection of heteropolymeric proteins, even some of those antiactins are not truly specific for "pure" myogenous differentiation. This is true of one commonly used commercial reagent, clone 1A4, which is widely known as *anti–smooth muscle actin*.[86] In reality, it decorates other cell types besides those of the smooth muscle, myofibroblastic tissues, or myoepithelium. Another antibody designated *HHF-35*, or *anti–muscle-specific actin*, shows more muscle-restricted immunoreactivity in routinely processed human specimens.[24, 85]

OTHER SARCOMERIC CONTRACTILE PROTEINS

The contractile mechanism in skeletal muscle is effected by a complex of proteins that include my-

osin II (molecular weight 460 kd), actin, tropomyosin (molecular weight 70 kd), and troponin. The troponin molecule has three subunits, called troponin I, troponin T, and troponin C, with molecular weights between 18 kd and 35 kd.[89] Myosin is an actin-binding protein; it has two globular heads and an elongated tail. In particular, myosin II is composed of two heavy chains and four light (two phosphorylatable and two basic) chains. These combine with N-terminal portions of the myosin heavy chains to form globular heads, each of which has an actin-binding site and an enzymatic locus that hydrolyzes adenosine triphosphate. The heads of the myosin molecules form cross-bridges to actin.[90] Myosin molecules are configured in a symmetric fashion on either side of the center of the sarcomere. Sarcomeric thin filaments are polymers composed of two actin chains arranged in a double helix. Tropomyosin molecules, in turn, are situated in the groove between the two chains of actin. Troponins are interspersed along the tropomyosin.[91] Troponin T melds other troponin components with tropomyosin; troponin I inhibits the interaction of myosin and actin, and troponin C contains binding sites for calcium in the initiation of muscle contraction. Actinin, a 190-kd moiety, binds actin to the Z lines of the sarcomere. Another protein, titin, connects Z lines to M lines and provides the base on which thick filaments may form.[92] Because of their relatively poor sensitivity, all the markers in this section are used uncommonly for diagnostic purposes at present.[93–98]

MYOGLOBIN

Myoglobin is a 17.8-kd protein that is found exclusively in skeletal muscle and that forms complexes with iron molecules.[99] The concentration of this molecule is highest in muscles that undergo sustained contraction. Because myoglobin appears relatively late in the maturational sequence of striated muscle, it is typically undetectable immunohistologically in embryonic neoplasms that show differentiation toward that tissue. Accordingly, pleomorphic "adult"-type rhabdomyosarcoma and rhabdomyoma are the soft tissue tumors in which myoglobin is identified most often.[93, 94, 96, 100–106]

MYO-D1 AND MYOGENIN

A "superfamily" of transcription factors that regulates cell lineage–specific proliferation is represented in striated muscle by several moieties, known as the *Myo-D family*.[107–109] They are encoded by genes that reside on chromosomes 1, 11, and 12 and are part of a polypeptide complex called the *basic helix–loop helix (BHLH) motif*, all of which are rather small proteins composed of 220 to 320 amino acids. Two members of this intranuclear protein group, Myo-D1 and myogenin, have been used as specific markers of striated muscle differentiation in human neoplasms since the 1990s.[107–110] They activate their own transcription and that of other BHLH proteins and, in concert with the retinoblastoma gene, govern the exit from the cell cycle and the initiation of striated muscle differentiation.

Because antibodies to Myo-D1 and myogenin must gain access to the nucleoplasm, they have been difficult to use in routine surgical specimens. However, modifications of "antigen retrieval" solutions and the use of heat-mediated epitope enhancement have allowed these reagents to enter diagnostic use.[109] It must be stressed that, like hormonal receptor proteins, both Myo-D1 and myogenin are strictly localized to cellular nuclei; hence, background cytoplasmic labeling—which has been a consistent problem with antibodies to Myo-D1 especially—must be ignored as a spurious pattern of staining.

CALDESMON

Caldesmon is a cytoplasmic protein with two isoform classes, one of which is found predominantly in smooth muscle cells and other cell types with partial myogenic differentiation. High molecular weight isoforms with molecular weights between 89 and 93 kd are capable of binding to actin, tropomyosin, calmodulin, myosin, and phospholipids, and they function to counteract actin-tropomyosin–activated myosin-adenosine triphosphatase (ATPase). As such, they are mediators for the inhibition of calcium-dependent smooth muscle contraction.[111]

Commercial antibodies to caldesmon are now being applied to diagnostic problems in surgical pathology. They appear to be specific for smooth muscle, myofibroblastic, and myoepithelial differentiation and, as such, are useful adjuncts to desmin and actin immunostains.[111, 112]

Potential Markers of Schwannian Differentiation

S-100 PROTEIN

S-100 protein derives its name from the fact that it is soluble in saturated (100%) ammonium sulfate solution. It was first isolated from the central nervous system but is now known to have a wide distribution in human tissues, including glia, neurons, chondrocytes, Schwann cells, melanocytes, fixed phagocytic or antigen-presenting mononuclear cells, Langerhans' histiocytes, myoepithelial cells, notochord, and various epithelia (especially those in the breast, salivary glands, sweat glands, and female genital system).[113] S-100 protein is dimeric in nature, with alpha and beta subunits. Hence, it has three isoforms—S-100ao (alpha dimer); S-100a (alpha-beta isoform); and S-100b (beta dimer). The two subunits of this protein have molecular weights approximating 10.5 kd each, and the function of S-100 protein is essentially that of a calcium flux regulator.[114]

Both monoclonal antibodies and heteroantisera to S-100 protein are available for diagnostic use. Some of the former reagents are monospecific for the alpha or beta subunits; therefore, they exhibit relatively narrower spectra of reactivity than seen with polyclonal antisera. For example, beta subunit–specific antibodies preferentially label glial cells and Schwann cells.[115] Those antibodies have not enjoyed widespread use among clinically oriented pathologists and, at present, heteroantisera to S-100 protein are the most commonly used in hospital practice. In the proper context, as part of panels of antibodies designed to evaluate several possible lineages of differentiation in a morphologically indeterminate neoplasm, reagents against S-100 protein are still valuable indicators of Schwannian, melanocytic, or chondrocytic identity in tumors of the soft tissues and bone.[116–120]

CD57 (LEU7; HNK-1)

CD57 is a membrane antigen seen in approximately 20% of peripheral blood mononuclear leukocytes, a proportion of which have "natural killer" activity. It has a molecular weight of 95 kd. Antibodies in this cluster designation, the prototype of which is HNK-1 (subsequently renamed Leu7),[121] also react with several neural molecules having a variety of molecular weights that vary from 19 to 72 kd.[122–125] Some of these moieties are associated with 5′-nucleotidase activity,[124] whereas others are myelin-associated glycoproteins (MAGs).[122, 125] The largest of the MAGs (MAG-72) is related structurally to the immunoglobulin superfamily gene products, as well as neural adhesion molecules and the autophosphorylation site of epidermal growth factor receptor. MAGs are integral cell membrane proteins that are found normally in oligodendroglia. Their function is believed to involve mediation of interaxonal or axonal-glial interaction during myelination and, as such, their additional association with Schwann cells and neural neoplasms should not be surprising. Nevertheless, HNK-1 reactivity has also been documented in perineurial (non-Schwannian) peripheral nerve sheath lesions.[126] In general, CD57 is used as a potential marker not only of peripheral nerve sheath tumors but also of ESs and PNETs, in which matrical proteins of neurosecretory granules and synaptic vesicles are thought to contain a target protein for HNK-1.[70, 72, 127–135]

It must be stressed that CD57 is not restricted to nerve sheath cells or neuroectodermal elements among all soft tissue tumors, but rather is most often observed in those cell types. Synovial sarcomas, LMSs, and some metastatic carcinomas also may be labeled by HNK-1.[127] Thus, inclusion of CD57 antibodies in panels that are designed to detect myogenous, epithelial, and neural differentiation is the proper approach to their use. The most common settings in which CD57 is valuable concern the differential diagnostic separation of fibrosarcoma versus MPNST, malignant fibrous histiocytoma (MFH) versus MPNST, and myxoid nerve sheath tumors (both benign and malignant) versus non-neural myxoid neoplasms.

COLLAGEN TYPE IV AND LAMININ

Volumetrically, the predominant component of basement membranes—regardless of which cell types they invest—is collagen type IV. It is a triple helical molecule weighing 550 kd, with globular end regions and two noncollagenous domains. One of the latter is located 330 nm from the carboxy end of the molecule, at which point there is a "bending point" that gives the moiety a "hockey stick" configuration overall.[136] Type IV collagen differs from other collagen types because it does not form fibrils, shows interruptions of its helical structure, and has a different amino acid constituency. Genes coding for the helical chains of this molecule are located on chromosome 13q.[137]

Laminin is another important component of basement membranes. It is a 1000-kd molecule, the three short forms and one long arm of which have globular end regions. Laminin binds to glycosaminoglycans, acting as a bridge for attachment of collagen type IV in basement membranes to the surrounding matrix.[138] The exact location of laminin in basement membranes has been contentious, with some investigators claiming that it is part of the lamina densa, others suggesting that is resides in the lamina lucida, and still others believing that it is codistributed between these two compartments.[139] Beyond simple "boundary" and anchoring functions, laminin probably also influences intercellular interactions and contributes to alterations in cellular morphology.[140]

In the soft tissues, complete basement membranes are formed around endothelial cells, smooth muscle cells, and Schwann cells.[141, 142] Thus, reagents directed against collagen type IV and laminin are useful inclusions in antibody panels aimed at detecting those lineages. In particular, however, fibrosarcoma and MFH are often difficult to distinguish from MPNSTs, because not all MPNSTs are reactive for either S-100 protein or CD57. Immunoreactivity for either collagen type IV or laminin would greatly favor the interpretation of a peripheral nerve sheath tumor in those differential diagnoses, and we use both markers most often in that specific setting. Hence, they have been included in this section as adjuvant "neural" determinants.

Endothelial Markers

Several determinants that are associated with endothelial cells have been applied to the recognition of vascular neoplasms of soft tissue. These have varying degrees of sensitivity and specificity, as discussed subsequently.

FACTOR VIII–RELATED ANTIGEN (VON WILLEBRAND FACTOR)

Factor VIII–related antigen, or von Willebrand factor (vWF), is a very large polymeric protein that is synthesized exclusively by endothelial cells and megakaryocytes. It consists of three multimeric subunits that are greater than 10,000 kd in molecular weight; physiologically, they undergo proteolysis to yield substantially smaller fragments that can be found in plasma.[143] The function of vWF is twofold. First, it forms circulating complexes with antihemophilic factor, also known as *factor VIII coagulant protein.* The latter moiety is a 265-kd protein that affects the activation of factor X in the intrinsic coagulation pathway; it is manufactured by hepatocytes. Second, vWF plays a crucial role in platelet aggregation so that patients who have low levels or dysfunctional variants of this protein have the clinical bleeding diathesis known as *von Willebrand's syndrome.*[144]

In the context of soft tissue pathology, vWF is used principally to distinguish vascular neoplasms from their morphologic simulants.[145–147] Because vWF is packaged within Weibel-Palade bodies (WPBs) in endothelial cells, it is logical to expect that immunoreactivity for that analyte would parallel the ultrastructural presence of such organelles. That is indeed the case, and because WPBs are rare in poorly differentiated neoplasms of the blood vessels, it explains why the sensitivity of vWF is as low as it is (approximately 10 to 15%) for the recognition of lesions such as high-grade angiosarcoma.[146, 147] Accordingly, this marker has much more utility in the spectrum of benign and borderline endothelial tumors, such as hemangioma variants and the family of "hemangioendotheliomas."[148]

CD34

CD34, or the human hematopoietic progenitor cell antigen, is recognized by several monoclonal antibodies including My10, QBEND-10, and BI-3C5.[149–152] It is a 110-kd protein that, as its name suggests, is expressed by embryonic cells of the hematopoietic system,[150, 153] including lymphoid and myelogenous elements and also endothelial cells. Correspondingly, again in the setting of soft tissue tumors, CD34 is a potential indicator of vascular differentiation. It is highly sensitive for endothelial differentiation, regardless of tumor grade, and recognizes greater than 85% of angiosarcomas and Kaposi's sarcomas (KSs).[148–150, 152] Nevertheless, the specificity of CD34 is a problem, inasmuch as it has been reported in some LMSs, peripheral nerve sheath tumors, and epithelioid sarcomas,[150, 153, 154] which could potentially simulate variants of angiosarcoma or hemangioendothelioma. In addition, CD34 is so commonly present in dermatofibrosarcoma protuberans (and its variants), spindle cell lipoma, and solitary fibrous tumor that it is regularly used as an adjunct for the diagnosis of those tumors.[155–157] Thus, as endothelial markers, antibodies to CD34 are best used in a panel of reagents that is designed to account for these other diagnostic possibilities.

CD31

The platelet-endothelial cell adhesion molecule-1 (PECAM-1) is also known as CD31.[158] It is a 130-kd transmembrane glycoprotein that is shared by vascular lining cells, megakaryocytes, platelets, and selected other hematopoietic elements, as recognized by monoclonal antibody JC/70A.[159] This marker is highly restricted to endothelial neoplasms among all tumors of the soft tissue, and its sensitivity is also excellent.[160] In our hands, virtually 100% of angiosarcomas are CD31+, regardless of grade or histotype, and the same statement applies to hemangioma and hemangioendothelioma variants.[161, 162] It must be acknowledged, however, that KS is labeled more consistently for CD34 than for CD31,[162] the reasons being unknown.

THROMBOMODULIN

Thrombomodulin (TMN) is a 75-kd cytoplasmic glycoprotein that is distributed among endothelial cells, mesothelial cells, osteoblasts, mononuclear phagocytic cells, and selected epithelia.[163–168] Its physiologic role is to convert thrombin from a coagulant protein to an anticoagulant.[165] Because of the potential presence of TMN in some metastatic carcinomas and most mesotheliomas,[167, 168] both of which may be confused with epithelioid angiosarcomas, it cannot be used as a single marker for vascular neoplasms. Nevertheless, TMN has proved to be a sensitive indicator of endothelial differentiation, particularly in poorly differentiated vascular malignancies.[166, 169] KS is likewise consistently immunoreactive for this determinant.[170] Thus, its inclusion in antibody panels is certainly worthwhile.

ULEX EUROPAEUS I AGGLUTININ

Ulex europaeus I (UEAI) agglutinin is not an antibody reagent, but instead represents a lectin that is produced by the gorse plant. It recognizes the Fuc-alpha-1–2-Gal linkage in fucosylated oligosaccharides, which compose portions of various glycoproteins.[171] In particular, the H blood group antigen and CEA regularly bind to UEAI, as does a separate fucosylated protein that is expressed by endothelial cells.[147, 166, 171] Biotinylated *Ulex* may be used a histochemical reagent in surgical pathology or, alternatively, unlabeled lectin can be used, with its binding to tissue subsequently detected by application of biotinylated anti-*Ulex* and avidin-biotin-peroxidase complex. Because of the nonspecificity of UEAI for endothelial differentiation, as mentioned earlier, it is absolutely necessary to use this lectin as part of a histochemical-immunohistochemical panel. For example, epithelioid sarcoma and various metastatic carcinomas may also bind *Ulex,* in addition to vascular neoplasms.[172, 173] However, the extremely high sensitivity of UEAI justifies its continued use as a potential endothelial determinant.

"Fibrohistiocytic" Markers

A variety of monoclonal antibodies and heteroantisera have been advanced since 1985 as "histiocytic" or "fibrohistiocytic" markers in paraffin sections, to be used in the identification of lesions such as benign or malignant fibrous histiocytomas, atypical fibroxanthomas, and "histiocytomas" of skin and soft tissue. The targets of these reagents include moieties such as alpha-1-antitrypsin, muramidase (lysozyme), alpha-1-antichymotrypsin, cathepsin B, CD68, factor XIIIa, and the HAM 56 antigen.[174–183]

Although it is true that a majority of fibrohistiocytic neoplasms do label for the specified determinants, the specificity of those markers is poor. Carcinomas, melanomas, and other sarcoma morphotypes also potentially express them with relatively high frequency.[184, 185] The current approach to the diagnosis of fibrohistiocytic tumors is one of ultimate exclusion, in recognition of the fact that neoplasms of other lineages may demonstrate morphologic appearances that are strikingly similar to them. Thus, a putatively fibrohistiocytic lesion is interpretable as such only when epithelial, myogenous, neural, and endothelial differentiation has been excluded in a vimentin-reactive tumor by application of suitable immunostains or performance of electron microscopy. In that context, the application of additional antibodies to "histiocytic" markers is superfluous and may even be misleading. Therefore, we do not advocate their use.

Markers of Osteoblastic Differentiation

One of the greatest challenges in the realm of bone and soft tissue tumor pathology is the reliable recognition of osseous matrix production in malignant lesions. Because the contextual presence of true osteoid equates with a diagnosis of osteosarcoma, this is an important issue. Since the late 1990s, a number of putatively osteoblast-specific markers have been advanced in the pertinent literature, including bone morphogenetic protein, type I collagen, COL-I-C peptide, decorin, osteocalcin

(OCN), osteonectin (ONN), osteopontin, proteoglycans I and II, bone sialoprotein, and bone glycoprotein 75.[186] Among these, only two—ONN and OCN—have been associated with sufficiently good performance in paraffin sections to merit their inclusion in diagnostic immunohistologic studies.

OSTEOCALCIN

OCN is one of the most prevalent noncollagenous intraosseous proteins, and it is predominantly localized to osteoblasts. This 9-kd cytoplasmic protein contains abundant gamma carboxyglutamic acid residues. Its expression is down-regulated by helix-loop-helix–type transcription factors and up-regulated by vitamin D analogs, such as 1,25 dihydroxyvitamin D_2 and 24-epi-1,25 dihydroxyvitamin D_2, in the final steps of osteoblastic differentiation and osteoid formation.[186–192] Various heteroantisera and monoclonal antibodies to OCN have been used in immunohistochemical analyses;[187, 190, 193–196] these have shown that fibroblasts in several anatomic locations appear to express epitopes that cross-react with polyclonal anti-OCN reagents, leading to the conclusion that monoclonal antibodies with selective peptide recognition are preferred for diagnostic work.[193] OCN generally has a reasonable level of sensitivity for osteoblastic differentiation (approximately 70%) and is, for practical purposes, virtually completely specific for bone-forming cells and tumors.[195, 196] Thus, it can be used with reasonable success as a single marker to detect such neoplasms.

OSTEONECTIN

ONN is a protein that is concerned with regulating the adhesion of osteoblasts and platelets to their extracellular matrix, as well as early stromal mineralization. ONN is modified differently at a post-translational level in bone cells and megakaryocytes to yield molecules with different oligosaccharide substructures; sequences of ONN-related genomic DNA, intranuclear RNA, and mRNA are identical in those two-cell types.[186, 195–201] It would also appear that several other cells may synthesize ONN-associated epitopes; in one assessment, fibroblasts, vascular pericytes, endothelia, chondrocytes, selected epithelial cells, and nerves were also immunoreactive for this determinant.[196] Overall, a sensitivity of 90% and a specificity of 54% has been reported for ONN relative to the diagnosis of osteoblastic neoplasms.[195, 196] Again, because of potential problems concerning cross-reactivity of available antisera to this marker,[196, 202–204] monoclonal antibodies should be used diagnostically. Even then, since ONN does not demonstrate the selectivity of expression that is associated with OCN, it must be used only as part of a panel of reagents that are directed at several lineage-related proteins.

Other Markers of Interest in Soft Tissue Tumors

There are several other determinants that often figure into differential diagnosis in the sphere of soft tissue tumor pathology. They include melanocyte-related markers such as melan-A (MART-1), tyrosinase, and HMB-45;[205–210] neuroendocrine and neuroectodermal products such as synaptophysin, neuron-specific (gamma dimer) enolase, protein gene product 9.5, and NB84;[211–217] and hematopoietic determinants such as CD1a, CD45, HLA-DR, and light-chain immunoglobulins.[218–224] Because these reactants are covered in detail elsewhere in this book, in sections dealing with the skin, the endocrine organs, and the hematopoietic system, they will simply be mentioned here. A bit more commentary is justified in reference to yet another lymphoreticular marker, CD99, which is also known as p30/32 glycoprotein or MIC2 protein.[225–227] It is a cell surface protein that is encoded by genes on the X and Y chromosomes.[228, 229] CD99 is expressed in a membranous pattern by a high proportion of ESs and PNETs, but may be expressed in a less distinct pattern in lymphoblastic lymphomas and synovial sarcomas, as well as other mesenchymal neoplasms and selected epithelial lesions.[223, 225, 226, 230–237] Available commercial monoclonal antibodies to this determinant include 12E7, O13, and HBA-71 (see Table 3–3).

SOFT TISSUE TUMORS

Benign Tumors of Soft Tissue

PROLIFERATIVE FIBROBLASTIC LESIONS

Fibromatoses are characterized by parallel fascicles of slender fibroblasts separated by variable amounts of collagen. Several forms of fibromatosis are recognized, including congenital myofibromatoses and several adult varieties, which differ substantively only in location—abdominal, penile, plantar, and palmar. Other rare forms include hyaline, gingival, and digital fibromatoses. These lesions may appear similar to hemangiopericytoma, leiomyoma, fibroma, and peripheral nerve sheath tumors. Separation of these entities continues to rely largely on the histopathologic and clinical impression, given that these "fibroblastic" entities do not harbor any unique immunophenotype. As expected, all show uniform strong vimentin positivity, but a subset may also stain for desmin (Fig. 3–1) and muscle-selective isoforms of actin. Reproducible reactivity for S-100 protein among peripheral nerve sheath tumors (neurofibroma, schwannoma) is useful to distinguish them from fibroblastic lesions.

Fibroma of tendon sheath and collagenous fibroma (desmoplastic fibroblastoma) are usually suf-

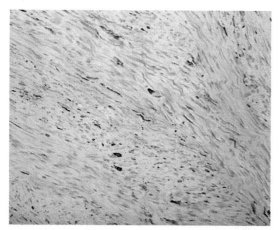

Figure 3–1. Desmoid tumor showing multifocal reactivity for desmin.

ficiently distinct clinically to separate them from fibromatosis. They often react either diffusely or focally for muscle-specific actin[238] and smooth muscle actin[239] and may even show faint S-100 positivity.[240] Desmin, however, is not found.[238, 240] In addition to sharing an immunophenotypic profile, fibroma of tendon sheath and collagenous fibroma have been observed to harbor the same abnormality of chromosome 11q12.[241]

PERIPHERAL NERVE SHEATH TUMORS

The most common peripheral nerve sheath tumors in both children and adults are neurofibromas and schwannomas. The differential diagnostic considerations differ somewhat between neurofibroma and schwannoma: Neurofibromas are commonly confused with myxomas, nonpigmented spindle cell or "neurotizing" melanocytic nevi, or cellular and organizing scar tissue, whereas schwannomas are more likely to be confused with leiomyomas.

S-100 protein is extremely useful in this context, as it is strongly expressed by schwannomas and variably expressed by neurofibromas. The majority of peripheral nerve sheath tumors are also positive for the Leu7 antigen. The diagnostic mimics, melanocytic nevi and leiomyomas, may also show reactivity for both S-100 protein and Leu7 antigen. In these instances, the lack of HMB-45, tyrosinase, and myogenic determinants, including desmin and muscle-associated actins, is useful to separate melanocytic nevi and leiomyomas, respectively. A consistent exception to the utility of HMB-45 is psammomatous melanotic schwannoma, a tumor that arises in the gut, soft tissue, and bone composed of melanosome-laden cells that are otherwise typical of peripheral nerve sheath elements. Nearly all 31 examples in a series by Carney were HMB-45 reactive.[242] In difficult cases, the distinction between neurofibroma and melanocytic nevi is

facilitated by the presence of factor XIIIa, which is found only in neurofibroma.

The perineurial cells within neurofibroma contain EMA, which may be detectable by immunohistochemical analysis in a small population of cells in these tumors. EMA may also be of some value in the diagnosis of neurothekeoma because of the persistence of perineurial elements around most tumor clusters. Nerve sheath neoplasms are occasionally labeled by antibodies to GFAP, whereas other benign soft tissue tumors are not. Myelin basic protein may also be of some value in the diagnosis of neurilemmal tumors, although there has been some disagreement in the literature on this point. Currently, we do not advocate a practical role for either of these markers in the immunophenotypic analysis of benign soft tissue tumors.

SPINDLE CELL LIPOMA

Although the diagnosis of spindle cell lipoma is usually straightforward, selected cases resemble other spindle cell proliferations. Spindle cell lipoma is strongly CD34+,[243, 244] a feature shared by some of its histologic mimics, including solitary fibrous tumor, neurofibroma, dermatofibrosarcoma protuberans, and angiolipoma. Lack of S-100 protein staining in the spindle cells is useful to distinguish it from neurofibroma. Additionally, strong BCL-2 reactivity is found in spindle cell lipoma, also a feature of some cases of solitary fibrous tumor. Identification is usually possible using a panel of immunostains and close attention to the histologic features.

LEIOMYOMAS

Certain markers with specificity for muscle differentiation may be useful in recognizing leiomyomas, beyond desmin and muscle-associated actins, but their application in diagnostic immunohistopathology is not generally considered routine. Smooth muscle myosin and Z-band protein have been advocated by some, particularly when either the histologic pattern is unusual (such as myxoid or hyalinized lesions) or the interpretation of a myogenous lesion is not corroborated by desmin or muscle-specific actin stains.

GRANULAR CELL TUMOR

Granular cell tumor, a benign neoplasm with an only rarely recognized clinicopathological malignant counterpart, has been intensely studied by immunohistochemical means. In addition to resembling histiocytic lesions, granular change is a recognized variant of leiomyoma[245] and certain carcinomas such as renal cell carcinoma. Granular cell tumors of the adult type show consistent diffuse positivity for S-100 protein (nuclear and cytoplasmic), NSE, vimentin, and CD68.[246-249] A major subset is also reactive for the Leu7 antigen or myelin basic protein, or both.[246]

A histologically identical lesion occurs almost exclusively in female newborns or infants along the alveolar ridge, designated *congenital granular cell tumor;* this tumor differs from the adult variety by its complete lack of S-100 protein and NSE reactivity. Both the adult and congenital types share positivity for alpha-1-antitrypsin, CD68, and vimentin. Although traditionally regarded as a "histiocytic" marker, CD68 positivity is related to the abundance of phagolysosomes, a distinctive feature of granular cell tumors. Therefore, it is not possible to distinguish true granular cell tumors from granular cell alterations–granular histiocytic proliferations using only CD68.

HEMANGIOMA

Benign vascular lesions showing a dense cellularity and relatively little overt canalization may prove diagnostically troublesome. Both capillary juvenile hemangioma and epithelioid hemangioma can be confused with low-grade angiosarcoma, epithelioid sarcoma, or hemangiopericytoma. When the diagnosis of epithelioid sarcoma is under consideration, several endothelial markers should be applied, because that tumor is often reactive with the UEAI lectin. The absence of factor VIII–related antigen and CD31 is helpful in this regard. Epithelial markers, which are characteristically positive in epithelioid sarcoma, are uniformly absent in vascular proliferations. Hemangiopericytoma may be easily separated by its lack of selective endothelial markers.

The potential of GLUT1 as a marker for juvenile hemangioma is interesting and requires further study to determine its reliability. Increased expression of GLUT1 has been reported in a variety of solid human tumors.[250-253] One study of vascular lesions found intense endothelial GLUT1 immunoreactivity in 97% (139 of 143) of juvenile hemangiomas, and complete absence in 66 vascular malformations.[252] To date, there are no substantiated immunohistochemical means of differentiating hemangiomas from histologically similar examples of angiosarcoma.

RHABDOMYOMAS

Rhabdomyomas are benign tumors with striated muscle differentiation that may assume "adult," "juvenile," or "fetal" variants microscopically; the adult type shows abundant eosinophilic cytoplasm within tumor cells, whereas the fetal type consists of small, rather undifferentiated cells admixed with others having the appearance of fetal muscle. The juvenile form is a histologic hybrid of these patterns and may represent a lesion in transition. The differential diagnosis sometimes includes granular cell tumor, hibernoma, paraganglioma, and rhabdomyosarcoma.

In our experience, all forms of rhabdomyoma stain for vimentin, desmin, muscle-specific actin, Myo-D1, myogenin and, to varying degrees, myoglobin. Smooth muscle actin, vimentin, GFAP, Leu7 antigen, CD68, cytokeratin, and EMA are generally absent, although one investigator noted rare SMA+ cells.[254-256] Focal CD56 positivity has been observed in one case.[257] Although S-100 protein has been observed in some cases of rhabdomyoma, its presence is focal and rare[254] and therefore not likely to be confused with the pattern of S-100 reactivity in paraganglioma and granular cell tumor. The presence of myogenic determinants and a lack of CD68 are also useful in the recognition of rhabdomyomas. As with vascular tumors, immunohistochemical distinction between benign skeletal muscle tumors and their malignant counterparts is impossible. In most cases, standard clinicopathologic evaluation is sufficient for their unequivocal separation.

ANGIOMYOFIBROBLASTOMA

Angiomyofibroblastoma is a relatively recently described entity of the superficial soft tissues with a marked predilection for the vulvar region. These tumors show reactivity for vimentin, desmin (Fig. 3–2), actin (Fig. 3–3), and estrogen receptor protein.[258, 259] Additional studies support these findings[260-262] and also elucidate a subset of cases with CD34 and progesterone receptor positivity.[260, 261] There is no staining for factor XIIIa, keratin, S-100 protein, Leu7, GFAP, and CD68.[260] These findings are shared with smooth muscle tumors, but not most other myxoid tumors including myxoid liposarcoma, myxoid MFH, myxoid neurofibroma, and myxoid MPNST.

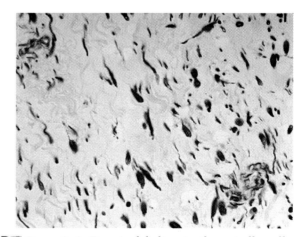

Figure 3–2. Desmin labeling in the spindle cells of angiomyofibroblastoma.

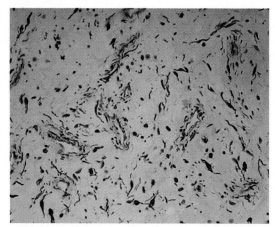

Figure 3–3. Alpha isoform ("smooth muscle") actin is seen in the spindle cells and blood vessels of angiomyofibroblastoma.

Although the clinical features of angiomyofibroblastoma may overlap considerably with aggressive angiomyxoma, usually morphologic differences are sufficient for their separation. Angiomyofibroblastomas are usually smaller, well-circumscribed lesions, which contrasts with the obvious infiltrative, sometimes deeper seated aggressive angiomyxoma. The perivascular accentuation of stromal cells typical of angiomyofibroblastoma is not found in aggressive angiomyxoma. In contrast to angiomyofibroblastomas that show desmin reactivity, aggressive angiomyxomas generally lack this determinant. Therefore, immunohistochemistry may be helpful in a limited manner, although the distinction rests generally on recognizing conventional morphologic differences. This separation is important because aggressive angiomyxoma has a significant recurrence potential that is not a feature of angiomyofibroblastoma.

Borderline Tumors of Soft Tissue

HEMANGIOPERICYTOMA

Hemangiopericytoma is an uncommon neoplasm characterized by a spindle cell proliferation embedded within a staghorn vascular pattern. However, occasional examples are composed largely of plump, ovoid cells that may cause confusion with other soft tissue tumors (Fig. 3–4). The immunophenotype of these neoplasms is neither unique nor characteristic. In general, the diagnosis of hemangiopericytoma remains one of histologic pattern recognition, with immunohistochemistry aiding in excluding other diagnoses.

The spindle cells in hemangiopericytoma consistently react with vimentin, although there is notable variation in intensity from tumor to tumor.[263] Normal pericytes express factor XIIIa and HLA-DR, determinants that are also found in approximately 50% of hemangiopericytomas.[264–266] Factor XIIIa is seen in some fibrohistiocytic proliferations, but is

consistently lacking in meningioma and glomus tumor, which are not infrequently under differential consideration. A few cases have demonstrated focal reactivity for muscle-associated actins[267] and Leu7 antigen. Desmin, CD31, cytokeratin, and S-100 are uniformly negative.[264, 266] The diagnosis of hemangiopericytoma continues to rest on histopathology alone, with the finding of factor XIIIa positivity in some cases corroborating the impression.

Overexpression of the insulin-like growth factor-II (IGF-II) is found in hemangiopericytoma and is believed to play a role in tumor-related hypoglycemia. The IGF-II peptide can be detected by immunohistochemical means using antigen retrieval. Whether detection of this peptide is useful clinically is the subject of current investigations.

SOLITARY FIBROUS TUMOR

Originally described in 1931 as a mesenchymal pleural tumor,[268] solitary fibrous tumor was recognized increasingly in extrapulmonary sites during the 1990s. Some cases of "hemangiopericytoma" may in fact represent solitary fibrous tumor that was previously unrecognized outside the pleural cavity. Other histologic differential diagnoses include synovial sarcoma, cellular angiofibroma, neurofibroma, and spindle cell lipoma. The spindle cells of solitary fibrous tumors are strongly CD34+ (Fig. 3–5) and vimentin-positive, frequently BCL-2 positive, and uniformly cytokeratin-negative, CD31−, and actin-negative.[157, 269–271] This tumor is also added as part of the growing list of tumors showing strong, diffuse CD99 (O13) reactivity.[272]

A broad panel of immunostains, including BCL-2 and CD34, is necessary to exclude other spindle cell proliferations that mimic solitary fibrous tumor. Neurofibromas may be BCL-2+ and CD34+,

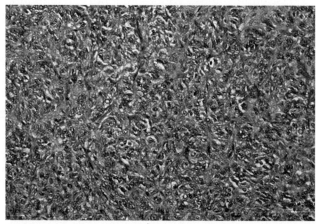

Figure 3–4. Hemangiopericytoma composed of ovoid tumor cells. This histologic image is potentially shared by a number of neoplasms of disparate lineages.

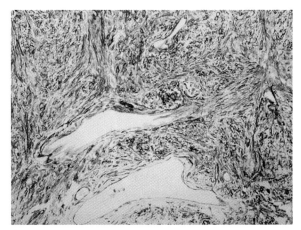

Figure 3–5. Solitary fibrous tumor, demonstrating uniform immunoreactivity for CD34.

but the absence of S-100 protein staining in solitary fibrous tumor helps in this distinction. BCL-2 reactivity is also common in synovial sarcoma,[270] but synovial sarcoma lacks CD34 staining and often focally reacts for epithelial antigens.[157] Spindle cell lipoma, another CD34+ tumor, requires close histologic examination for accurate diagnosis. The cellular variant of spindle cell lipoma sometimes manifests a proliferative vascular pattern that simulates that of solitary fibrous tumor. A strong predilection for the upper extremities, a highly bundled quality to the collagen, and admixed lipocytes are features of spindle cell lipoma that may prove useful in certain cases.

The myxoid variant of solitary fibrous tumor is easily mistaken for other myxoid lesions such as low-grade fibromyxoid sarcoma, myxoid liposarcoma, and myxoid MPNST. Close attention to mitotic activity, overall cellularity, and atypia is usually sufficient to separate these entities. S-100 protein immunostaining may assist in the recognition of myxoid MPNST; negative staining should be interpreted in the overall context of the histologic impression and does not necessarily exclude the latter diagnosis.

OSSIFYING FIBROMYXOID TUMOR OF SOFT PARTS

Ossifying fibromyxoid tumor of soft parts is a recently described mesenchymal lesion originally defined as a borderline or low-grade malignant tumor. It is slow-growing, and has a propensity to arise in the extremities within the deep subcutis or skeletal muscle. Microscopically, ossifying fibromyxoid tumors of soft parts are composed of lobulated nests of small, cytologically bland round cells within a stroma that may vary from myxoid to densely hyalinized. An incomplete shell of lamellar bone is a usual feature, but may be lacking in some cases.

The spindle cells stain strongly and diffusely for

S-100 protein and vimentin.[273–279] Most stain for Leu7 and NSE[273, 277] and occasionally for synaptophysin[273] and GFAP.[274, 276] In addition, myogenous differentiation is found in many cases, as evidenced by desmin and alpha smooth muscle actin immunostaining.[273, 274, 279] Cytokeratin, EMA,[275, 276, 279] and HMB-45[276] are not found.

EPITHELIOID HEMANGIOENDOTHELIOMA

Epithelioid hemangioendothelioma (EHE) is believed to behave intermediately in the epithelioid vascular tumor spectrum, between epithelioid hemangioma and the highly aggressive epithelioid angiosarcoma. These are angiocentric tumors showing primitive vascular differentiation with a predilection for the skin and soft tissues, as well as the liver and lungs (Fig. 3–6). An essential criterion for the diagnosis of EHE is immunohistochemical evidence of endothelial differentiation. It is necessary to use multiple vascular markers such as factor VIII–related antigen, CD31, UEAI lectin, and CD34, because these tumors may show heterogeneity of expression of vascular antigens. EHEs are usually labeled by the UEAI lectin[280, 281] and, unlike angiosarcomas, are usually reactive for factor VIII–related antigen.[281] In our experience to date, EHEs are generally positive for CD31.

Carcinoma may be confused with this tumor because the primitive intracellular vacuoles that typify EHE may mimic mucin vacuoles of adenocarcinoma. Sarcomas with an epithelioid appearance are frequently considered, but perhaps the best microscopic mimic of this tumor is epithelioid sarcoma. Both epithelioid sarcoma and EHE share the features of a nodular growth pattern and plump eosinophilic cells surrounding cores of necrotic debris. The presence of the keratin in EHE has been a point of debate. There are convincing reports of coexpression of endothelial and epithelial markers in EHE, mainly those arising within bone.[282, 283] In

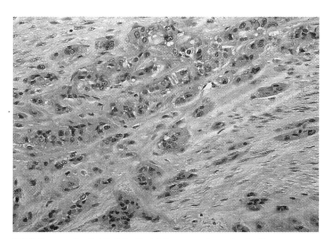

Figure 3–6. Epithelioid hemangioendothelioma composed of plump polygonal cells with bland cytologic features and intracellular lumen formation.

a study by Gray and associates, staining for CAM5.2, MAK-6, and AE1/AE3 was observed in the majority of tumors in frozen section material.[282] Inadequate tissue was available for keratin studies of paraffin-embedded counterparts, however. A study of 30 cases from the skin and soft tissue found focal staining with at least one of three different antikeratins (MNF-116, CAM5.2) in 26% of cases.[284] The finding of keratin-positive cases underscores the need to include additional epithelial markers in the evaluation of such tumors. The lack of EMA or CEA in EHE is useful.

KAPOSIFORM HEMANGIOENDOTHELIOMA

Kaposiform hemangioendothelioma was first thought to arise exclusively in children and infants[285] but is now recognized as an usual tumor that may also affect adults.[284] Many of the original nine cases were associated with lymphangiomatosis and Kasabach-Merritt syndrome (a consumption coagulopathy syndrome). These tumors show a nodular vascular proliferation reminiscent of KS and hemangioma, admixed with scattered nests of larger epithelioid cells containing abundant eosinophilic cytoplasm, hemosiderin, hyaline droplets, and vacuoles. The differential diagnosis includes capillary hemangioma (of infancy), angiosarcoma, KS, and spindle cell hemangioendothelioma.

The spindle cells of kaposiform hemangioendothelioma manifest expression of some, but not all, the typical endothelial markers. CD34 is generally found, but factor VIII−related antigen and UEA1 are absent.[285] Larger "feeder" vessels along the periphery display obvious endothelial differentiation, however. KS−associated herpesvirus (KSHV, or HHV 8) has not been found using polymerase chain reaction (PCR) techniques.[285, 286] Although immunohistochemistry is an interesting adjunct, the diagnosis largely rests on the clinical situation and the characteristic histologic features of kaposiform hemangioendothelioma.

AGGRESSIVE ANGIOMYXOMA

Aggressive angiomyxoma is a peculiar neoplasm of the pelvic and perineal soft tissues that most commonly affects women. It is composed of loosely arranged, bland stellate cells embedded in a myxoid matrix punctuated by numerous venule- and capillary-sized blood vessels reminiscent of myxoid liposarcoma (Fig. 3−7). The vascular pattern lacks the fine "chicken wire" appearance that characterizes its malignant mimics. Morphologic and immunophenotypic features of aggressive angiomyxoma also may overlap those of intramuscular myxoma.[287−288] However, the clinicopathologic features of the latter are sufficiently distinct from aggressive angiomyxoma to allow for their confident separation.

Initial immunohistochemical analyses revealed

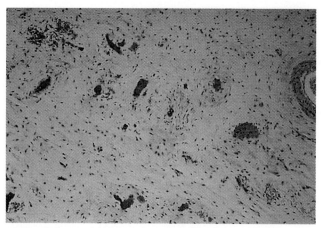

Figure 3–7. Aggressive angiomyxoma of pelvic soft tissues—a lesion for which differential diagnostic considerations include angiomyofibroblastoma, myxoid smooth muscle tumors, peripheral nerve sheath tumors, and myxoid liposarcoma. Immunohistology assists in eliminating only purely myogenous and neurogenic lesions.

reactivity for actin, but not for S-100 protein or factor VIII−related antigen in the stellate cell population of angiomyxoma, suggesting a myogenic or myofibroblastic pattern of differentiation.[289] Subsequent studies, including those in our laboratory, demonstrate variable reactivity for muscle-specific actin, vimentin, and generally absence of desmin. Ultrastructural studies[287] support a fibroblastic-myofibroblastic phenotype. Although recent investigations fail to reproduce either muscle-specific actin or desmin staining,[288, 289] the general assumption of myofibroblastic differentiation remains generally accepted.

Malignant Tumors of Soft Tissue

Sarcomas may be divided into four groups based on their primary histologic growth pattern. These groups include small round cell tumors, epithelioid polygonal cell tumors, spindle cell neoplasms, and pleomorphic lesions. For each category, immunohistologic attributes are correlated with "idealized" immunophenotypes and an algorithm-based approach to their interpretation.

SMALL ROUND CELL NEOPLASMS
(Fig. 3–8; Table 3–4)

The small round cell tumors of soft tissue compose a heterogeneous group of neoplasms that predominate in childhood and adolescence and share similar morphologic features. Rhabdomyosarcoma, PNETS, ES, and lymphoma-leukemia are the prototypic members of this group. Other entities include intra-abdominal desmoplastic small round cell tumor and rhabdoid tumor.

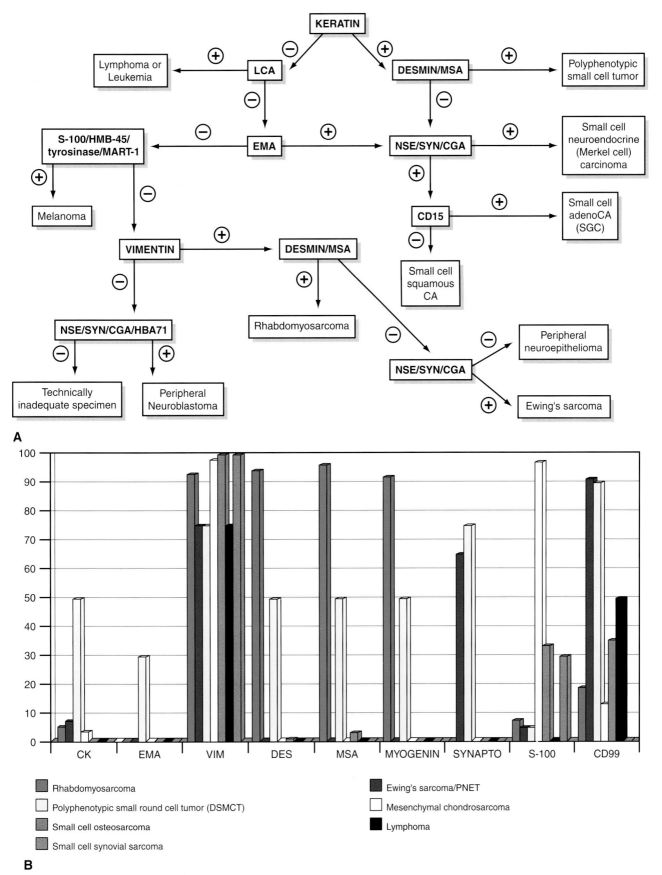

A

B

Figure 3–8. A, Algorithmic immunohistologic diagnosis of malignant small round cell tumors. *B,* Graphic representation of the frequency of reactivity for small round cell tumors against commonly used immunoreactants. CK, cytokeratin; EMA, epithelial membrane antigen; VIM, vimentin; DES, desmin; MSA, muscle-specific actin; SYNAPTO, synaptophysin.

RHABDOMYOSARCOMA

Embryonal rhabdomyosarcoma (E-RMS) accounts for more than half of all rhabdomyosarcomas and is the most problematic to diagnose. The morphology of E-RMS varies widely, depending on the degree of cellular differentiation, cellularity, and pattern of growth. Strap cells, large eosinophilic myoblasts, and myxoid stroma may be seen focally in E-RMS but not in its microscopic mimics. However, a significant number of E-RMS cases consist only of densely packed undifferentiated small blue cells (Fig. 3–9) that evoke a broad differential diagnosis list. Diagnostic considerations include neuroblastoma, esthesioneuroblastoma, ES, synovial sarcoma, rhabdoid tumor, melanoma, melanotic neuroectodermal tumor of infancy, granulocytic sarcoma, and malignant lymphoma. Furthermore, it may be confused with the solid variant of alveolar rhabdomyosarcoma (Fig. 3–10), which has prognostic implications. When the patient is older, small cell carcinoma and poorly differentiated small cell angiosarcoma also become considerations.

It is with the poorly differentiated variants of E-rhabdomyosarcoma that immunohistochemical analysis proves to be most helpful. E-RMS expresses markers in a cumulative and consistent sequence (vimentin, desmin, fast myosin, and myoglobin), which evolves with morphologic differentiation and follows a pattern similar to normal myogenesis. Therefore, vimentin is uniformly present, although its diagnostic utility is minimal. Among myogenic-selective markers, desmin is the most consistently detectable in paraffin-embedded specimens, showing appreciable staining in virtually all cases of E-rhabdomyosarcoma as well as in the alveolar and pleomorphic histologic subtypes (Fig. 3–11).[23] Other small round cell tumors, with the notable exception of intraabdominal desmoplastic small round cell tumors, lack desmin staining. Because a large number of tumor cells in rhabdomyosarcoma are normally

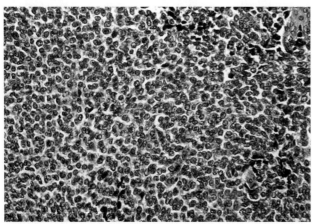

Figure 3–9. The "solid" form of primitive embryonal or alveolar rhabdomyosarcoma represents a prototypical small round cell malignancy for which several adjunctive studies are necessary.

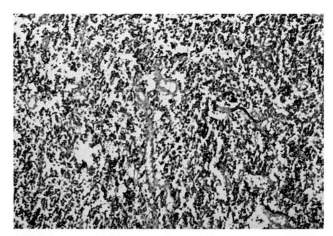

Figure 3–10. The typical image of alveolar rhabdomyosarcoma.

stained, desmin is particularly helpful in small biopsy material in which the diagnosis is often the most challenging.

MyoD1 is touted as highly specific and sensitive for E-rhabdomyosarcoma, showing nuclear expression in 82 to 100% of cases.[110, 290–292] This myogenic regulatory protein is a DNA-binding nuclear regulatory protein that initiates myogenesis in mesenchymal stem cells. The staining pattern shows marked heterogeneity among E-RMS cells, as well as differential nuclear staining.[291] Positive labeling is more intense in small, primitive tumor cells, whereas larger cells exhibiting obvious evidence of skeletal muscle differentiation generally do not show clearly positive nuclear staining.[110] On occasion, MyoD1 has been shown to cross-react with unknown cytoplasmic antigens, showing variable fibrillary, cytoplasmic immunoreactivity in neuroblastoma and ES/PNET.[109] Additionally, primitive childhood tumors that harbor the EWS/FLI1 fusion gene may coexpress myogenic and neuroectodermal determinants.[292]

Among other muscle-related determinants, myogenin is probably the most frequently detected in E-RMS. Positive nuclear staining for myogenin is stronger than that for MyoD1 when there are abundant differentiated tumor cells, but is less prominent when small, primitive tumor cells predominate.[110] The sensitivity of this marker, in our experience, still falls well short of that seen for desmin and muscle-associated actins. LMS, ES/peripheral PNETs did not show expression in preliminary studies[110] and may be reasonably excluded in instances with strong anti-MyoD1 positivity. Using the highly sensitive technique of PCR, however, myogenin mRNA has been noted in the majority of other normal tissues and childhood tumors.[293]

The microfilament-associated protein vinculin is a major component of muscle tissue, in which it is believed to function in the alignment of sarcomeric myofibrils. Among the different histologic subtypes of rhabdomyosarcoma, antivinculin expression is most prominent in differentiated tumors; a focal

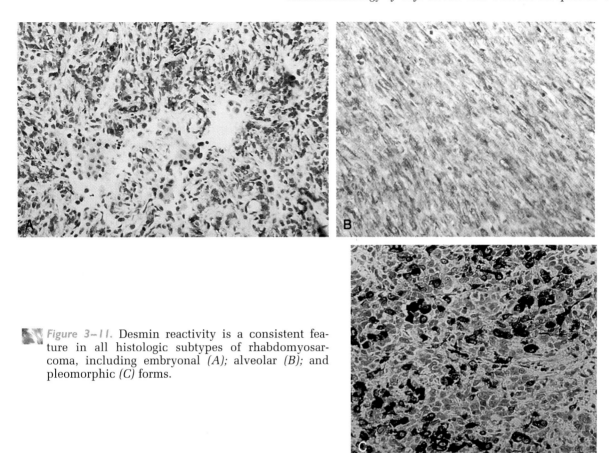

Figure 3–11. Desmin reactivity is a consistent feature in all histologic subtypes of rhabdomyosarcoma, including embryonal *(A)*; alveolar *(B)*; and pleomorphic *(C)* forms.

staining pattern has been observed showing a high degree of correlation with the presence of differentiating rhabdomyoblasts, whereas a diffuse staining pattern has been observed in small, poorly differentiated cells.[294] Vinculin immunoreactivity has also been observed in leiomyosarcoma. Along with other myogenic markers, vinculin may be useful in the differential diagnosis of anaplastic, poorly differentiated sarcomas.[294]

Dystrophin, the protein product of the Duchenne muscular dystrophy locus, is a major cytoskeleton protein in skeletal muscle cells. The investigation of the utility of this marker in the diagnosis of rhabdomyosarcoma is limited to one study focusing on frozen section material.[295] Dystrophin was found in 8 of 9 cases of rhabdomyosarcoma, and was lacking in other small cell tumors, including lymphoma, PNET, and Wilms' tumor.[295] A case of "clear cell rhabdomyosarcoma" confirmed as myogenic by striated muscle features on electron microscopy has also been reported as showing desmin, muscle actin, and dystrophin positivity.[296]

Myriad preliminary markers are available that have been touted as useful in the differential diagnosis of "undifferentiated" phenotypes of rhabdomyosarcoma. Undifferentiated rhabdomyosarcoma, as defined by a small cell tumor lacking desmin reactivity but showing MyoD1 reactivity, has been diagnosed using various other markers.

Nestin is an IFP expressed in immature skeletal muscle cells as well as in tumors of the central and peripheral nervous system, endothelial cells, and in some muscle cells adjacent to tumors.[297] Preliminary studies suggest that nestin recognizes very undifferentiated cases of rhabdomyosarcoma that are desmin-negative.[297] We believe the latter contention requires further evidence before advocating the use of this marker to define undifferentiated rhabdomyosarcoma. Insulin-like growth factor II (IGF-II) also has potential for use in the differential diagnosis of undifferentiated rhabdomyosarcoma. IGF-II expression has been found to be inversely correlated with the degree of rhabdomyosarcoma differentiation by in situ hybridization, identifying occasional desmin-negative tumors.[298] The fetal form of the acetylcholine receptor may also be useful for discriminating rhabdomyosarcoma, with a low degree of differentiation from other small cell tumors. By reverse PCR methods, this moiety has been detected in all embryonal and alveolar rhabdomyosarcoma (n = 16) but not in other nonrhabdomyosarcomatous tumors (n = 45). In these same tumors evaluated by immunohistochemistry, the fetal form of the acetylcholine receptor (AChR) was identified in the majority of embryonal tumors and approximately half of alveolar rhabdomyosarcomas.[299] Although many of the myogenic markers such as myogenin react with normal skeletal muscle, fetal-type AChR does not. PCR evaluation for fetal AChR may become potentially useful to detect small amounts of residual disease. Of note, when evaluating undifferentiated rhabdomyosarcoma, the expression of neural cell adhesion molecules (NCAMs) and neurofilament isoforms has been noted on frozen tissue, which, by itself, does not signify a neural tumor or mitigate against the diagnosis of rhabdomyosarcoma.[300]

Therapy has been shown to cause tumor cytodifferentiation and decreased mitotic activity in all histologic categories of rhabdomyosarcoma. Unchanged or increased post-therapeutic proliferative activity as assessed by MIB-1 immunostaining has been regarded as evidence for a more aggressive biologic potential for E-RMS. However, myoid marker expression has not been found to change after therapy.[301] Immunohistochemical analysis for proliferation markers might be useful for highlighting foci of less-differentiated rhabdomyosarcoma.

The only interpretative pitfall engendered by a reliance on myogenic markers involves the inclusion of "polyphenotypic" small round cell tumors showing myogenic differentiation. These lesions are characterized by the apparent coexpression of divergent or multilineage differentiation, and are discussed in more detail later in this section. The solution to this diagnostic challenge, as a model for all immunophenotypic analyses in soft tissue neoplasms, is the inclusion of several different lineage-selective markers in a broad panel of diagnostic immunostains. Of course, this approach has its limitations as well, because E-RMS may occasionally be labeled by antibodies to "neuroectodermal" determinants such as NSE and the CD57 antigen (Leu7) (Fig. 3–12) (see further on).

EXTRASKELETAL EWING'S SARCOMA AND PERIPHERAL PRIMITIVE NEUROECTODERMAL TUMORS

The Ewing's family of tumors is composed of bone and soft tissue small round cell neoplasms

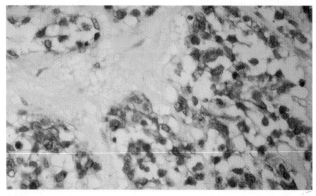

Figure 3–12. CD57 reactivity is infrequently observed in small cell rhabdomyosarcomas.

that are, in part, defined by the chromosomal aberration t(11;22)(q24;q12) and its closely related variants. Since the early 1990s, considerable attention has been paid to growing evidence that ES and peripheral PNET are closely related neoplastic proliferations. A fundamental relationship between ES and PNET is clearly evident on the basis of the shared reciprocal translocation t(11;22), the potential for "classic" ES to exhibit neuroectodermal features in tissue culture, and similarities in proto-oncogene expression. When classically defined, ES can be distinguished from PNET by the absence of pseudorosettes and the lack of ultrastructurally or immunohistochemically detectable neuroectodermal features. However, neuroectodermal antigens (NSE, Leu7, 200-kd neurofilament) have been found not only in the majority of PNETs but also in over half of cases of ES.[215, 302, 303] In one study of ES, an atypical light microscopic appearance correlated with the presence of neuroectodermal features in most instances.[302] These data support the concept that ES and PNET are both peripheral primitive neuroectodermal neoplasms, differing only in the extent of neuroectodermal phenotype and morphologic differentiation.

Some immunohistochemical differences are apparent between ES and PNET. ES stains more readily for vimentin, whereas PNET is more often characterized by the presence of neurofilaments. Most examples of classic ES are heavily laden with glycogen and fail to exhibit ultrastructural features of neuroectodermal differentiation.

The identification of the EWS and FLI-1 genes flanking the translocation break point by reverse transcriptase (RT)-PCR has allowed for detection of the chimeric transcription factor mRNA produced by the fusion gene.[304, 305] Transcripts have not been detected in non-ES/PNET small cell tumors, whereas approximately three fourths of ES with intact mRNA successfully yield chimeric transcripts.[304, 305] Exceptional tumors demonstrate biphenotypic expression of EWS-FLI1 and PAX3-FKHR transcripts, specific for Ewing's family tumors and alveolar rhabdomyosarcoma, respectively.[306] Preliminary evidence suggests that ES showing EWS/FLI1 gene expression may lose this phenotype after chemotherapy and radiation, which is attributed to apparent therapy-induced differentiation in the residual tumor.[307]

The Ewing's family of tumors is characterized by high MIC2/CD99 expression, a glycoprotein detected by various monoclonal antibodies, including HBA71, 12E7, RFB-1[308] and O13 (see Table 3–3). It is diffusely present in almost all cases of ES with a distinctly membranous pattern[308, 309] and is also identified in the overwhelming majority of PNETs. MIC2 is also a sensitive marker for PNET/ES in specimens from formalin-fixed cell blocks, air-dried, and alcohol-fixed cytologic material.[310] Although initially touted as specific for ES, CD99 has been identified in a variety of other tumors, although staining is generally weaker and lacks the membranous pattern found in ES/PNET. In the proper histologic context, MIC2 still represents a useful marker for discriminating among small cell tumors.

ES is negative for chromogranin, cytokeratin, glial fibrillary protein, desmin, muscle-specific actin, myoglobin, factor VIII-RA, and leukocyte common antigen.[311, 312] In a study of 50 cases confirmed by molecular evidence of the specific translocation, cytokeratin expression, which was frequently intense, was present in 10 cases (20%) of ES (in 5 diffusely and in 5 focally).[313]

Integrins are a large heterogeneous family of membrane glycoproteins that show a complex expression pattern of some subunits among different types of small cell tumors of childhood. Notably, ES/PNET show a beta 1+, alpha 1−, alpha 3−, alpha 5+, and alpha 6− pattern.[314] This overlaps considerably with rhabdomyosarcoma, although it is distinct from neuroblastoma, which shows beta 1+, alpha 1+, alpha 3+, alpha 5−, and alpha 6−. ILK (beta 1-integrin linked kinase) is a protein kinase that interacts with the cytoplasmic domain of the beta 1-integrin repeats. Using a polyclonal antibody against ILK, one study found ILK expression in all ES and PNET cases and one third of neuroblastomas that were studied.[315] In contrast, other small cell tumors of childhood did not stain, suggesting that ILK may be a novel marker for tumors with primitive neural differentiation. Trk receptors are a family (A, B, C) of receptors showing differential expression in ES compared with neuroblastoma. ES tumors contain Trk A transcripts (A+/B−/C+) by immunohistochemistry, whereas neuroblastoma shows a (A−/B−/C+) phenotype. Therefore, the expression patterns of integrins and Trk receptors may assist in the discrimination of ES from neuroblastoma.

MESENCHYMAL CHONDROSARCOMA

Mesenchymal chondrosarcoma (MCS) is a particularly aggressive cartilaginous neoplasm that is seen most often in young adults and commonly occurs in extraskeletal locations. It is typified by a small cell population that is virtually indistinguishable from that of classic ES, except that MCS is punctuated by islands of primitive cartilage that appear to arise from the small cells in a manner that simulates embryonic chondrogenesis. Other histologic features of MCS include the presence of hemangiopericytoma-like vasculature; nonetheless, the cytologic similarities between small cells of MCS and ES have led to speculation that the former represents chondroblastic differentiation in a neuroectodermal or Ewing's-type neoplasm.

MCS is a rare tumor and, as such, is not as extensively characterized by immunohistochemistry. One noteworthy distinction is that unlike other forms of chondrosarcoma, staining for S-100 protein is not found in the small cells of MCS but is limited to chondroblastic islands.[316, 317] All components stain for Leu7 antigen, and most cases are also reactive for NSE.[316] Our experience confirms this finding, showing reactivity for NSE and Leu7 in the small cell population, the latter marker also being apparent in chondroid areas. Factor XIIIa has been shown to label MCS strongly.[317] MCS arising in the central nervous system is alleged by some to show cytokeratin and GFAP reactivity in 25% of cases.[318]

MCS does not react with antibodies to desmin, actin, cytokeratin, and EMA.[316] Unlike PNET, MCS is not reactive for synaptophysin.[316] Given that the majority of MCS cases show strong CD99 reactivity in more than 50% of the cells, MSC cannot be reliably distinguished from ES/PNET on the basis of CD99 reactivity.[319] Thus, immunohistochemical studies are not especially helpful in the differential diagnosis of MCS in small biopsies.

POLYPHENOTYPIC SMALL ROUND CELL TUMORS

There is considerable evidence that divergent differentiation characterizes a proportion of small round cell tumors in both adults and children. We have encountered 15 examples of tumors that are phenotypically indistinct from ES or PNET that are nonetheless immunoreactive for epithelial and myogenic determinants in addition to neuroectodermal markers. They are generally even more aggressive neoplasms than PNET and ES, an observation that mandates a broad immunophenotypic analysis of all small round cell tumors in our practice. Other investigators have described variations on this theme, either by documenting histologic evidence of divergent differentiation (including gland-like structures in PNET) or by describing morphologic attributes that are peculiar to a particular site.[320–322] We advocate the term *polyphenotypic small round cell tumor* to describe the variable and divergent immunohistochemical attributes of these lesions.

The "desmoplastic abdominal small round cell tumor" (DSRT) is the most widely recognized polyphenotypic tumor and is characterized by the EWS/WT1 chimeric transcript resulting from t(11;22)(p31;q12). It is a primitive-appearing tumor characterized by massive reactive fibrosis surrounding nests of tumor cells (Fig. 3–13), which reveal a broadly reactive immunoprofile, with frequent staining for keratin (86%), EMA (93%), NSE (81%), vimentin (97%), and desmin (90%).[323] Interestingly, strong membranous CD99 reactivity is seen in only a subset of cases.[40, 323, 324] Actin, myogenin, and chromogranin are generally not present, although there are some exceptions.

In our own experience with DSRT, 47% of cases arose in the peritoneal or retroperitoneal tissues. They generally were not reactive for muscle-specific actin and did not stain for MIC2. Although such attributes are reproducible in this anatomic location, we are as yet unconvinced that they es-

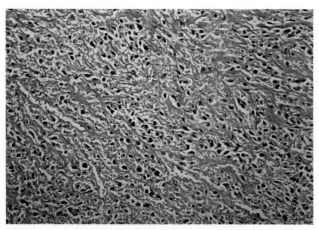

Figure 3–13. Desmoplastic small round cell tumor is a distinctive small round cell malignancy that manifests a densely fibrogenic stroma.

tablish the desmoplastic small cell tumor of the abdomen as an entity distinct from polyphenotypic neoplasms in other sites. In fact, we have observed progression from a phenotypically characteristic PNET to a desmoplastic polyphenotypic neoplasm in one of our cases. Therefore, tumors showing the typical phenotype described, but demonstrating either the EWS/ERS fusion chimeric transcript characteristic of ES/PNET, or biphenotypic expression of EWS-FLI1 and PAX3-FKHR transcripts, bring to light the highly variable patterns of differentiation that have become a recognized feature of this category of tumors.

POORLY DIFFERENTIATED SYNOVIAL SARCOMA, SMALL CELL VARIANT

The small cell variant of poorly differentiated synovial sarcoma (PD-SS) can easily be mistaken on morphologic grounds for other small round cell tumors such as ES, as well as high-grade MPNST. To further complicate this situation, there are reports of tumors harboring the distinctive t(X;18), resulting in the SSX/SYT fusion transcript, that also show distinct neural differentiation and may contain Homer-Wright rosettes and cytoplasmic fibrillary processes.[325, 326] CD99 reactivity may further complicate the diagnostic interpretation if one is not aware of its frequent presence in the small cell variant of synovial sarcoma. Although CD99 labeling may be intense in some cases, it does not demonstrate the characteristic membranous pattern that typifies ES/PNET. Subsets of cytokeratins may be contributory when strongly positive; CK7 has been reported in up to 50% of PD-SS cases, but is absent in PNET.[327]

HEMATOLYMPHOID MALIGNANCIES

Hematopoietic neoplasms only rarely present as soft tissue masses, and this phenomenon is partic-

ularly atypical in pediatric patients in whom other forms of small round cell tumors are most common. Because of the virtually uniform presence of LCA (CD45) in hematopoietic cells, and its absence on other human cells, including neoplastic populations, this marker has considerable utility in most instances. Although not all antibodies raised against CD45 identify determinants that survive routine tissue-processing protocols, the monoclonal "cocktail" PD7/26;2B11 (see Table 3–3), among other commercially available products, is sensitive in paraffin-embedded materials.

Reactivity for CD45, for all practical purposes, is diagnostic of a hematopoietic lineage; conversely, apart from expected staining for vimentin in some lymphoid cell populations, these neoplasms do not generally react with antibodies to other lineage-selective markers. However, it should be noted that lymphoblastic small cell lymphomas commonly label for CD99, thereby presenting a potential pitfall in interpretation. The most crucial part of evaluating an enigmatic lesion is to remember to include LCA in the panel, as lymphomas may present in a variety of unexpected morphologies, such as with signet ring cells,[328] a myxoid background,[329] or a fibrillary matrix.[330]

SARCOMAS WITH A SPINDLED APPEARANCE (Fig. 3–14)

The spindle cell sarcomas of the deep soft tissues include fibrosarcoma, LMS, MPNST, monophasic spindle cell synovial sarcoma, MFH, and angiosarcoma. Despite the advancements of immunohistochemistry and the ever-increasing armamentarium of markers, distinction among these types remains challenging.

Fibrosarcoma

In the late 1990s, fibrosarcoma was perhaps the most commonly diagnosed soft tissue malignancy. The diagnostic criteria for fibrosarcoma have evolved considerably, making it among the rarest of soft tissue sarcomas. The recognition of entities such as MFH, fibromatosis, and nodular fasciitis, as well as the introduction of immunohistochemistry, largely account for this change. Fibrosarcoma most often presents as a slowly growing mass arising anywhere in the body in patients in middle adulthood. As such, the tumor clinically and microscopically overlaps with the fibromatoses. Fibrosarcomas may also arise in infants, but are considered a separate entity because of their markedly better clinical behavior.

The histologic diagnosis of fibrosarcoma rests on the characteristic herringbone pattern of intersecting fascicles of fibroblasts in conjunction with the lack of other specific morphologic differentiation. By definition, such lesions display vimentin reactivity but do not stain for other lineage-selective

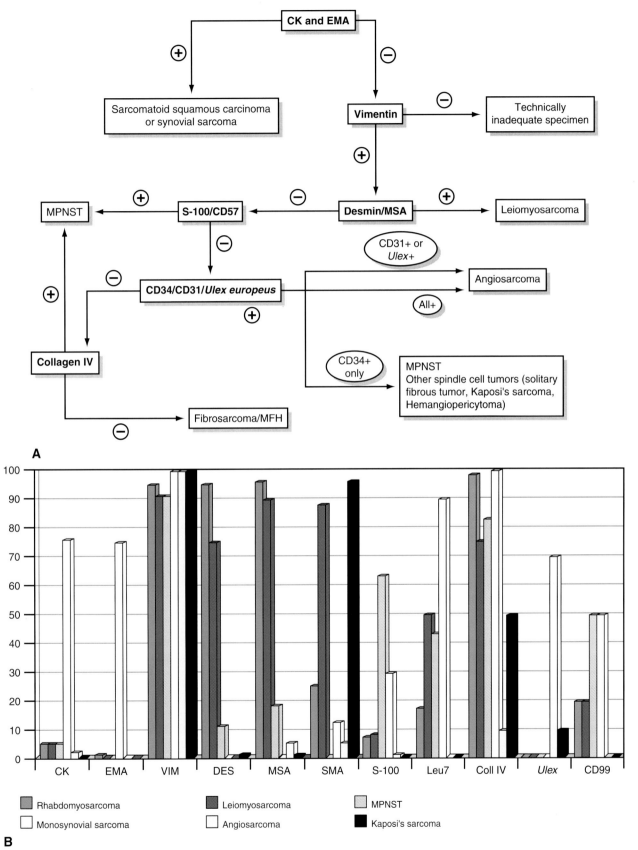

Figure 3–14. *A* and *B,* Sarcomas with a spindled appearance.

markers. In contrast, inflammatory fibrosarcoma of the mesentery and retroperitoneum shows evidence of myofibroblastic differentiation, with frequent actin positivity.[331]

Leiomyosarcoma

LMSs are most commonly found in the retroperitoneum, in adults of middle age or older. They rarely occur in the deep soft tissues of the extremities but may be seen in more superficial sites, particularly in the dermis and subcutis. The differential diagnosis of LMS traditionally includes other sarcomas composed of intersecting fascicles, including fibrosarcoma, MPNST, and occasionally synovial sarcoma and rhabdomyosarcoma. Conditions such as inflammatory pseudotumor, neurofibroma, and hemangiopericytoma (see Fig. 3–4) are often considerations for LMS showing minimal atypia.

Currently, the immunohistochemical confirmation of smooth muscle differentiation in LMS is based on the demonstration of desmin (see Fig. 3–14) and alpha smooth muscle actin. Desmin also reacts with skeletal muscle and is not present in all smooth muscle tumors; similarly, alpha smooth muscle actin is also detectable in myoepithelial cells. Some studies have indicated that actin may be more sensitive than desmin in detecting myogenic differentiation in smooth muscle neoplasms, emphasizing the need to assess both that marker and desmin. Although initial studies reported poor recognition by anti–smooth muscle antibodies of LMS, the general consensus today is that currently available commercial reagents that detect this marker are sufficiently sensitive for smooth muscle differentiation. In our experience, more general muscle-specific reagents are better as screening tools, but when non–smooth muscle myogenic differentiation may be a consideration, the inclusion of more selective markers (e.g., desmin and SMA) is indicated. For example, rare cases of rhabdomyosarcoma may assume a spindle cell appearance (usually in paragenital locations); hence, in somatic lesions of children, particularly in the extremities or the head and neck region, selective staining for smooth muscle actins (or, conversely, for striated muscle markers) has diagnostic value.

Immunophenotypic overlap with other soft tissue is not uncommon in LMS, in that S-100 protein and Leu7 may be encountered. However, coexpression of S-100 protein and Leu7 is infrequent. Likewise, LMS may sometimes react with antibodies to "histiocyte-selective" markers such as alpha-1-antichymotrypsin and CD68 and may be stained with antibodies to CD34, a marker traditionally regarded as "endothelial-selective." CD30 has been reported in approximately half of leiomyomas and LMSs,[332] but the diagnostic utility of CD30 among other spindle cell lesions is limited because it has also been found in fibromatosis, rhabdomyosarcomas, fibrosarcoma, synovial sarcoma, and MFH.[332]

Two cytoskeleton-associated actin-binding proteins, calponin and h-caldesmon, are novel putative smooth muscle markers that have not been extensively studied in soft tissue tumors. h-Caldesmon is a muscle-specific protein that combines with actin and tropomyosin to regulate cellular contraction.[111] Calponin is a smooth muscle–specific protein that is developmentally expressed in up to four isoforms and binds strongly to actin in a calcium-independent manner.[333] Both markers are expressed in parenchymal and vascular smooth muscle cells, and calponin is also present in myofibroblasts of desmoplastic stroma.[334] Leiomyoma, angioleiomyoma, LMS, and glomus tumor show intense and extensive immunoreactivity for h-caldesmon, whereas rhabdomyosarcoma and desmoid tumors are negative.[111] Controversy continues about whether that marker is useful to differentiate MFH from LMS.[111, 334] Although synovial sarcoma shows focal calponin positivity,[334] a panel that includes several muscle-specific markers should differentiate this tumor from LMS.

LMS has been conclusively shown to express low molecular weight cytokeratins.[335, 336] LMS on occasion may react strongly with antibodies to MIC2 with a dot-like cytoplasmic staining pattern.[336] In addition to well-known reactivity for estrogen and progesterone receptors in uterine LMS, LMS of vascular and retroperitoneal origin may also show positivity.[336, 337] Hence, caution must be exercised when using hormone receptor status to interpret whether a metastatic LMS is of uterine or extrauterine origin.

Increased expression of GLUT-1 glucose transporter protein has been reported in many human cancers, including non–small cell lung cancer,[338] colorectal cancer,[339] angiosarcoma,[340] and carcinoma of the thyroid.[341] A high proportion of tumor cells showing GLUT-1 overexpression has been associated with a high incidence of lymph node metastases[339] and overall poorer survival.[338] Some uterine LMS and up to one half of extrauterine LMS exhibit GLUT-1 positivity, whereas leiomyomas are uniformly negative.[337] Although data are limited, evidence suggests that GLUT-1 positivity correlates with distant metastases in LMS, confirming earlier studies.[337] We find these observations interesting, but currently the utility of GLUT-1 in soft tissue tumor diagnosis requires more scrutiny.

Studies indicate that both benign and malignant smooth muscle tumors may be more common in human immunodeficiency virus (HIV)-infected individuals. Smooth muscle tumors in immunocompromised individuals occur in unusual locations and exhibit evidence of latent infection by clonal Epstein-Barr virus (EBV).[342] Several EBV antigens are expressed in LMS, including latent antigen EBNA-1, immediate-early antigen BZFL1, and early antigen EA-D, as well as late antigens, including viral capsid antigen p160, gp 125, and membrane antigen gp 350.[343] These findings confirm that EBV is capable of lytic infection of smooth muscle cells and supports a role for EBV in oncogenesis. Adjacent non-neoplastic tissues and KS lesions demonstrate an absence of detectable EBV infection.[342]

Malignant Peripheral Nerve Sheath Tumor

MPNST (also known as neurofibrosarcoma, malignant schwannoma, and neurogenic sarcoma) is a sarcoma that may range in appearance from tumors that are indistinguishable from fibrosarcoma to others showing obvious Schwannian differentiation, making them one of the most challenging diagnoses among the soft tissue tumors. Many MPNSTs are recognizable on histologic grounds alone, although some show overlapping histologic features with other high-grade sarcomas. Tumors showing a nerve trunk association represent a minority of cases.

Determinants associated with normal nerve sheath or benign peripheral nerve sheath tumors are frequently detected in MPNSTs. MPNST shows reactivity for S-100 protein, a marker that typifies normal Schwann cells. Even so, most studies indicate that only 50 to 70% of these lesions are S-100–reactive, with positive cases often showing reactivity in a small proportion of cells.[43] CD57 (Leu7) is a determinant that in part composes MAGs and is found in neural-associated cell adhesion molecules. More than half of MPNSTs are CD57-reactive (Fig. 3–15).[72] Myelin basic protein is less commonly encountered in MPNST. Of course, none of these three nerve sheath–associated determinants by themselves is definitive in the identification of MPNST. However, among S-100, myelin basic protein, and Leu7, two thirds of MPNSTs will show reactivity against at least one marker.[43] Conjoint reactivity for S-100/Leu7, S-100/myelin basic protein, and myelin basic protein/Leu7 has been seen in 34%, 34%, and 24% of cases, respectively.[43] This coexpression of antigens is important, because none of them in isolation is immunospecific for nerve sheath tumors. Importantly, MPNST rarely reacts for epithelial determinants.

MPNST can usually be separated from LMS on histologic grounds, but occasionally this will be a source of confusion. LMS also has the potential for S-100 protein and Leu7 reactivity.[344, 345] Rare examples of LMS may be positive for myelin basic protein or NSE, markers that may also occasionally be seen in MPNST.[344, 345]

Another spindle cell sarcoma that shares overlapping histologic immunophenotypic features with MPNST is monophasic synovial sarcoma. The frequent (40%) finding of focal S-100 staining among spindle cell synovial sarcomas further complicates their separation.[346] Differential diagnosis is also confounded by the occasional presence of focal desmin and actin reactivity among nonrhabdomyoblastic elements in MPNST. Cytokeratin subsets may prove useful in difficult cases, as the vast majority of monophasic synovial sarcomas are reactive for CK7 or CK19, or both.[346] Most MPNSTs, including those that are EMA– or keratin+, do not express these cytokeratin subsets.

Reports of MPNSTs with vascular differentiation have been described.[347] Such tumors may occur in patients with or without neurofibromatosis. Immunohistochemical analysis confirms the presence of endothelial differentiation in those cases.

One particularly difficult area is distinguishing some forms of spindle cell malignant melanoma from MPNST, especially in metastatic sites.[348] That this occurs is not surprising because there are numerous well-known histologic associations between peripheral nerve sheath cells and melanocytes, as represented by pigmented neurofibromas and schwannoma, neurotropic melanoma, epithelioid MPNST resembling melanoma, and the combined occurrence of epithelioid blue nevi and psammomatous melanotic schwannoma in Carney's syndrome. Features that argue against MPNST include proximity to a lymph node, lack of continuity with a nerve, and a history of melanoma. Tumors with an appearance similar to MPNST but showing strong diffuse S-100 protein reactivity should be considered malignant melanoma until proved otherwise.

Despite the production of collagen type IV by nerve sheath cells, the immunohistochemical detection of this marker is of limited value in the diagnosis of nerve sheath neoplasms; cells displaying smooth muscle, endothelial, and fibroblastic differentiation may also be reactive for this and other matrical proteins. The potential confusion that results from these overlapping patterns of reactivity is largely avoidable in the context of specific clinicopathologic evaluation and a rational panel-oriented approach to immunohistochemical analysis.

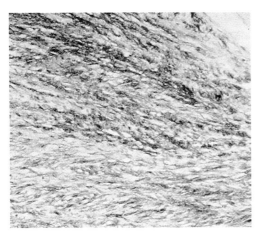

Figure 3–15. CD57 in malignant peripheral nerve sheath tumor (MPNST). Reactivity for S-100 protein, CD57, myelin basic protein, or collagen type IV is observed in greater than 85% of MPNSTs.

Monophasic Spindle Cell Synovial Sarcoma

Monophasic spindle cell ("fibrous") synovial sarcomas represent one extreme of the morphologic spectrum of these neoplasms. Classic biphasic synovial sarcoma is usually not a problem in identification, whereas the monophasic spindle cell form continues to be more challenging in the differential diagnosis of spindle cell neoplasms. This pattern may easily be confused with fibrosarcoma, MPNST, hemangiopericytoma (see Fig. 3–4), and LMS.

The presence of cytokeratin and EMAs is typical of the monophasic spindle cell form of synovial sarcoma (Fig. 3–16). Unlike biphasic variants, spindle cell–predominant lesions are only focally and inconsistently reactive for cytokeratin; in particular, the spindle cells of monophasic spindle cell synovial sarcoma show immunoreactivity for CK5/CK6, CK7, CK8, CK18, and CK19.[349] EMA staining is found in a larger subset of cases that may or may not react for keratin. Although CEA may occasionally be found in the epithelial components of biphasic synovial sarcoma, it is typically absent from the spindle cell component in both the biphasic and monophasic variants.[350] Even in cases that histologically appear entirely spindled, we recommend the use of epithelial markers and collagen type IV in an effort to delineate more overtly the epithelial components that may be obscured.

CD99 may be present in synovial sarcoma,[251, 351] but this marker is potentially shared by a number of other spindle cell neoplasms. The membranous pattern of CD99 staining characteristic of ES/PNET has not been found in synovial sarcoma.[352] A minority of monophasic synovial sarcomas also react for CD57 and S-100 protein.[350]

Strong positivity for BCL-2 has been noted in the spindle cell component of synovial sarcoma.[353, 354] In a study of spindle cell sarcomas in which fluorescence in situ hybridization (FISH) analysis confirmed t(X;18), 79% of synovial sarcoma cases were positive for BCL-2, but all other spindle cell sarcomas were negative, including 20 LMSs, 4 MPNSTs, and 4 fibrosarcomas.[354] Strong positivity for BCL-2 has also been observed in a variety of other soft tissue tumors, notably spindle cell li-

poma, KS, solitary fibrous tumor, and gastrointestinal stromal tumors.[353] These lesions, unlike synovial sarcomas, have as a common denominator the frequent presence of CD34, which may therefore be a useful discriminator if necessary.

Spindle Cell Angiosarcoma

Although the diagnosis of angiosarcoma is often relatively straightforward, its rarity and histologic variability may lead to uncertainty in diagnosis. Evaluation of commonly used endothelial markers has illustrated that spindle cell angiosarcomas label with UEAI in the vast majority of cases, whereas fewer than 30% demonstrate factor VIII-RA reactivity. All angiosarcomas are vimentin-reactive. Although UEAI binding characterizes spindle cell angiosarcomas, it may also be demonstrated in occasional examples of monophasic synovial sarcoma. EMA, myogenic- and nerve sheath–associated markers are lacking in spindle cell angiosarcoma.

The lack of sensitivity displayed by antibodies to factor VIII-RA has generated development of a variety of contemporary "endothelial-specific" antibodies, including PAL-E, FICA, EN4, E92, and TMN. Nonetheless, most of these antibodies have proved less than optimal, either because of poor performance in routinely processed materials or because of a wide range of reactivity among nonendothelial neoplasms. The utility of other newer markers is addressed subsequently in discussions on poorly differentiated and epithelioid angiosarcoma.

Kaposi's Sarcoma

KS occurs in four clinical forms—the chronic (Mediterranean), lymphadenopathic, transplantation-associated, and acquired immunodeficiency syndrome (AIDS)-related, among which microscopic differences are negligible. In its developed state, KS shows a cellular and mitotically active proliferation of spindle cells, which may be con-

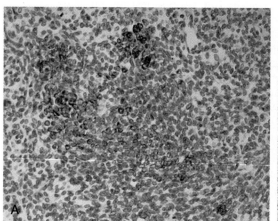
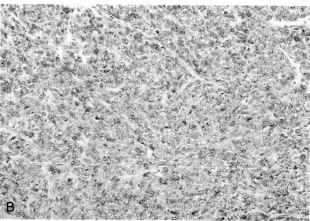

Figure 3–16. Synovial sarcoma showing immunoreactivity for keratin *(A)* and epithelial membrane antigen *(B)*.

fused with spindle cell angiosarcoma as well as spindle cell hemangioendothelioma. KS is positive for CD34 and variably reacts with other endothelial markers. Therefore, distinction from other vascular tumors remains largely clinical, with careful examination for subtle microscopic clues. The presence of cavernous vessels and epithelioid endothelial cells allows for recognition of spindle cell hemangioendothelioma. Overt cytologic atypia and clinical findings usually aid in the differential diagnosis with angiosarcoma.

SARCOMAS WITH AN EPITHELIOID APPEARANCE (Fig. 3–17; Table 3–6)

A number of soft tissue sarcomas are composed of large epithelioid or polygonal-shaped cells, yielding an appearance not unlike that of carcinomas. These lesions include epithelioid sarcoma, epithelioid monophasic synovial sarcoma, clear cell sarcoma, alveolar soft part sarcoma, epithelioid LMS, epithelioid angiosarcoma, epithelioid MPNST, malignant granular cell tumors, and "histiocytic" MFH. Many of the latter lesions only differ histologically from "histogenetically similar" spindle cell lesions; however, the algorithmic approach to their immunophenotypic characterization is a bit different.

Epithelioid Sarcoma

Epithelioid sarcoma demonstrates a characteristic histologic growth pattern, characterized by multinodular and coalescing nodules with central necrosis. This pattern may simulate necrobiotic granuloma, nodular fasciitis, melanoma, or metastatic carcinoma. The occasional presence of cytoplasmic vacuoles simulating vascular lumina also raises the possibility of EHE. Hemorrhage and cystic change in such lesions may mimic features of angiosarcoma.[355] Rare tumors present with atypical histologic patterns such as chondroid differentiation[356] or a rhabdoid appearance.[357]

The most striking immunophenotypic attribute of epithelioid sarcoma is a prominent and often intense perinuclear zone of vimentin staining (Fig. 3–18), attributable to perinuclear collections of intermediate filaments identified on ultrastructural analysis. Virtually all reports of epithelioid sarcoma have been vimentin-rich, and the coexpression of vimentin and keratin is considered a characteristic feature in these tumors. The degree of cytokeratin reactivity may be heterogeneous within a given tumor, often staining more intensely in overtly epithelioid areas (Fig. 3–19). Although initially reported otherwise, CD34 positivity in epithelioid sarcoma is found in a sizable subgroup.[154, 358] Furthermore, cases showing CD31 reactivity have been recorded as well.[358] The presence of the latter marker in some cases suggests that, at least in part, ES shows divergent differentiation toward endothelium. Single reports of ES ex-

pressing neurofilaments have also been made.[359, 360] Occasional immunophenotypic heterogeneity in these cases reiterates the possibility of divergent differentiation in high-grade neoplasms.

Epithelioid sarcoma shares many immunohistologic traits with synovial sarcoma, in that both are reactive for cytokeratin and EMA, showing an "epithelial" membrane-based pattern for the latter marker. In addition, both may occasionally display reactivity for CEA. Epithelioid sarcoma may occasionally react for S-100 protein, whereas synovial sarcoma is usually negative. Epithelioid sarcoma may be extensively degenerative, and as such, interpretation of S-100 protein results in necrotic tissue has been found to be unreliable.[361] In contrast, cytokeratin appears to be far less affected by extensive tissue necrosis.

Immunohistochemical studies do not allow for the separation of epithelioid sarcoma from metastatic carcinomas within soft tissue. However, such a distinction can usually be made on clinical grounds alone. Most cases of ES strongly express cadherins, a feature that may contribute to their epithelioid appearance.[362] The immunoexpression of VE-cadherin by the majority of cases, in the absence of E-cadherin, is also consistent with an element of mesenchymal differentiation. Immunohistochemistry may be useful for distinguishing epithelioid sarcoma from isolated necrobiotic granuloma. A granuloma would manifest reactivity for CD45, whereas epithelioid sarcoma does not; unlike ES, necrobiotic granulomas also are neither EMA+ nor cytokeratin+. In contrast, the separation of epithelioid sarcoma from epithelioid hemangioendothelioma may be somewhat problematic, since ES is characteristically reactive with the UEAI lectin and occasionally with CD34 or CD31, or both, as well. Epithelioid vascular tumors have likewise shown keratin reactivity, as mentioned earlier.

Epithelioid Monophasic Synovial Sarcoma

In its classic biphasic form, synovial sarcoma rarely poses a diagnostic problem, but when the epithelioid component dominates, its microscopic features widely overlap with other, more frequently encountered sarcomas. Given the apparent similarities between epithelioid sarcoma and synovial sarcoma in general, it would follow that "pure" epithelioid variants of the latter would be difficult to recognize by immunophenotypic analysis. However, as our limited experience with these lesions indicates, epithelioid synovial sarcomas faithfully reproduce the phenotype of polygonal elements in biphasic variants.

Epithelioid Angiosarcoma

Apart from more typical images in angiosarcoma, an epithelioid pattern is not uncommonly encountered as the sole pattern and, as such, may be

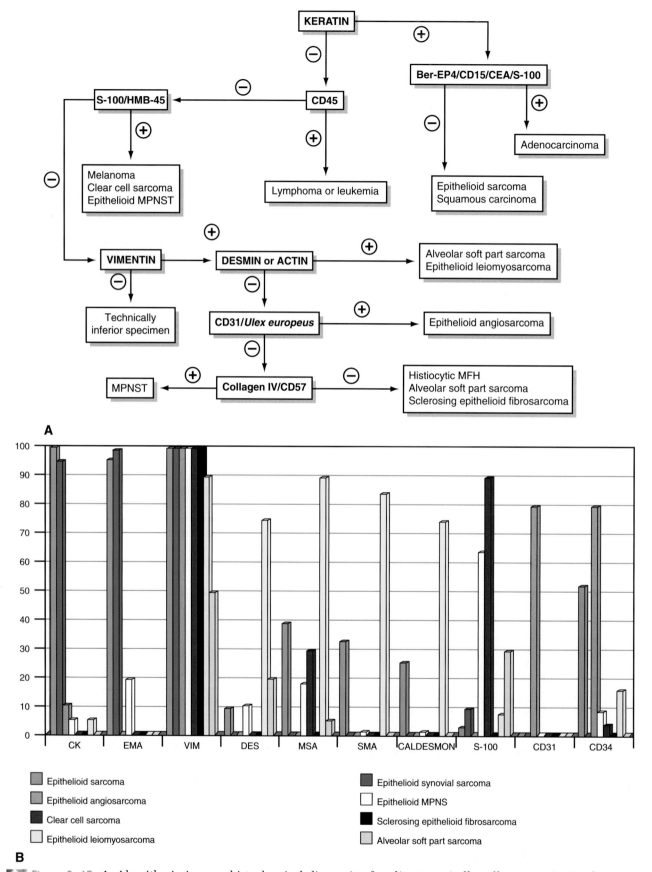

Figure 3–17. *A*, Algorithmic immunohistochemical diagnosis of malignant spindle cell tumors. *B*, Graphic representation of the frequency of reactivity for malignant spindle cell tumors against commonly used immunoreactants. MPNST, malignant peripheral nerve sheath tumor; MFH, malignant fibrous histiocytoma; CK, cytokeratin; EMA, epithelial membrane antigen; VIM, vimentin; DES, desmin; MSA, muscle-specific actin; SMA, smooth muscle actin.

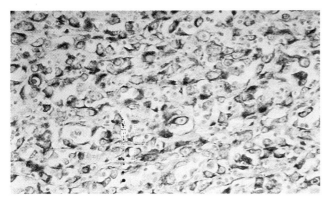

Figure 3–18. Epithelioid sarcoma showing intense immunoreactivity for vimentin, with perinuclear accentuation.

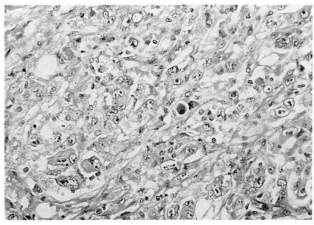

Figure 3–20. Epithelioid angiosarcoma is potentially confused diagnostically with metastatic malignant melanoma or poorly differentiated carcinoma in the soft tissues.

difficult to interpret. Epithelioid variants of angiosarcoma are recognized clinicopathologically as distinct from epithelioid hemangioendothelioma, and they typically involve deep soft tissues. Differential diagnostic considerations often include amelanotic melanoma, poorly differentiated carcinoma, and other epithelioid sarcomas (Fig. 3–20).

Different immunoreactivity patterns have been noted in epithelioid angiosarcoma compared with well-differentiated angiosarcoma. Anti-CD31 and UEAI have been found to be sensitive markers, staining typical vasoformative tumors as well as purely epithelioid variants.[160, 363, 364] Anti–factor VIII-RA and anti-CD34 stain undifferentiated tumors less often. A positive reaction has been found for CD31, CD34, UEAI (Fig. 3–21), or factor VIII-RA, in up to 86% of tumors.[160]

Analyses of the tissue distribution of hematopoietic progenitor cell antigen (CD34) initially suggested that in soft tissue, reactivity for this substance was selective and sensitive for endothelial neoplasms. However, the presence of CD34 in virtually every other form of polygonal cell neoplasm in soft tissue, including epithelioid LMS and

MPNST, clear cell sarcoma, epithelioid sarcoma, and "histiocytic" MFH, has diminished its potential utility as a single marker.[363] We have observed that epithelioid angiosarcoma may often be reactive for the tumor-associated glycoprotein TAG-72 (recognized by the monoclonal antibody B72.3). To date, we have not encountered B72.3 reactivity in any nonendothelial epithelioid soft tissue lesions. Furthermore, none of 10 EHEs has labeled with that marker. The biologic significance of this observation remains unclear. We suggest that conjoint positivity for endothelial markers CD31 and UEAI with B72.3 is diagnostic of epithelioid angiosarcoma.

Clear Cell Sarcoma

Our current understanding of clear cell sarcoma is that it represents the primary soft tissue counterpart of cutaneous malignant melanoma. Local recurrences are common and may precede distant metastases. This neoplasm is typified by a uniform

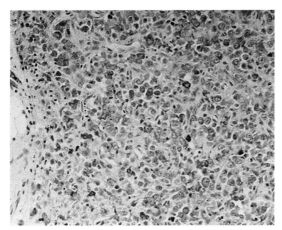

Figure 3–19. Keratin positivity is seen in this epithelioid sarcoma.

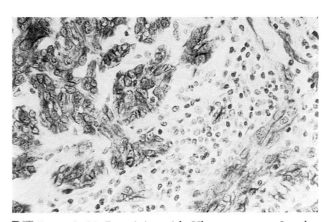

Figure 3–21. Reactivity with *Ulex europaeus I* agglutinin in epithelioid angiosarcoma.

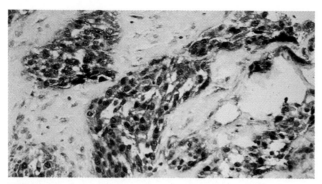

Figure 3–22. Clear cell sarcoma labels for S-100 protein in accord with the contention that it is a malignant melanoma of soft tissues.

pattern of polygonal cells tightly packed by a delicate fibrous network. The cells show clear or lightly eosinophilic cytoplasm that contains glycogen; melanin pigment may or may not be observed.

The immunohistochemical attributes of clear cell sarcoma strengthen its relationship to malignant melanoma. These include reactivity for vimentin, S-100 protein (Fig. 3–22), tyrosinase, and HMB-45 (Fig. 3–23) and the absence of staining for cytokeratin and EMA. Muscle, nerve sheath, or endothelial-selective markers are not found in clear cell sarcoma. Generally, epithelial markers are also negative, although one study reported 7 of 24 clear cell sarcomas with keratin expression using the antibodies CAM5.2, LP 34, and MNF-116.[366]

Although melanoma and clear cell sarcoma share immunophenotypical features, preliminary evidence suggests cytogenetic differences between the two tumors. The t(12;22)(q13;q12) translocation, yielding the formation of a hybrid EWS/ATF-1 gene characteristic of clear cell sarcoma, has been found lacking in cutaneous malignant melanoma.[367, 368] Therefore, our understanding of this tumor continues to evolve, as alternations at the molecular level may eventually serve as useful adjunctive tools for diagnosis.

Epithelioid Malignant Peripheral Nerve Sheath Tumors

Epithelioid MPNST is an extremely rare variant that bears histologic resemblance to melanoma, carcinoma, and rhabdoid tumor (Fig. 3–24). The lack of palisaded or fascicular growth leaves histologic features for separation from other epithelioid tumors of soft tissue, including clear cell sarcoma and rhabdoid tumor. As a result of these factors, epithelioid MPNST is an underrecognized diagnostic entity. Immunohistochemistry is helpful, however, in excluding several other soft tissue tumors.

There are a number of antigens that may be useful in defining the nerve sheath differentiation, including S-100 protein, CD57, and myelin basic protein. S-100 protein reactivity is slightly more frequent than in conventional MPNST and is found in at least 70% of cases.[369] The majority of cases also express NSE.[369] CD57 (Fig. 3–25) and myelin basic protein staining is less frequent. Despite an epithelioid appearance, cytokeratin and CEA are lacking; however, rare examples are focally positive for EMA. The uniform lack of reactivity for UEAI, factor VIII-RA, and CD31 aids in distinguishing this lesion from epithelioid angiosarcoma; desmin and muscle-specific actin, and HMB-45 negativity are also notable.

Rare pigmented variants of peripheral nerve sheath tumors, some with epithelioid features, have shown HMB-45 reactivity; in such cases, separation from metastatic malignant melanoma or clear cell sarcoma may be facilitated by demonstrating collagen type IV reactivity. Immunostains for type IV collagen define linear staining around single cells and small groups of cells in epithelial MPNST and are often negative in epithelioid me-

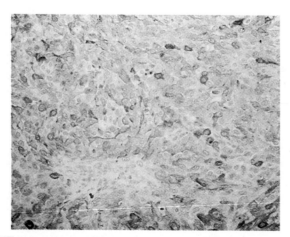

Figure 3–23. HMB-45 immunoreactivity in clear cell sarcoma.

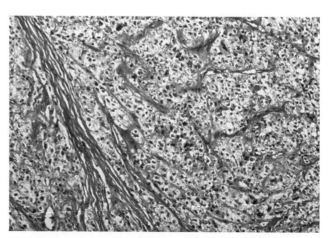

Figure 3–24. Epithelioid MPNST lacks distinguishing histologic features and requires intensive adjunctive study for proper diagnosis.

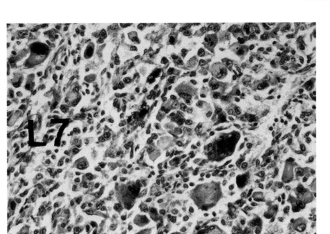

Figure 3-25. Reactivity for CD57 in epithelioid MPNST.

lanocytic proliferations. In the absence of collagen IV staining, however, such cases may be problematic, even with ultrastructural analysis. At a practical level, if an HMB-45–positive epithelioid tumor is deeply seated, with no cutaneous component, and does not have the clinicopathologic features of clear cell sarcoma, a diagnosis of epithelioid MPNST is most probable.

Sclerosing Epithelioid Fibrosarcoma

Sclerosing epithelioid fibrosarcoma is a variant of fibrosarcoma that presents in deeply seated locations and is intimately associated with deep fascia, periosteum, or skeletal muscle.[370] The lesions demonstrate infiltrative small cords or nests of uniform small polygonal cells with clear cytoplasm. Prominent matrical collagen with an osteoid-like configuration is invariably present. These tumors also display zones characteristic of conventional fibrosarcoma, and some also show a storiform pattern or myxoid zones. The differential diagnosis is rather broad, including a variety of benign fibrous proliferations (nodular fasciitis, myositis ossificans, desmoid, hyalinizing leiomyoma) as well as less common entities such as sclerosing lymphoma, metastatic lobular carcinoma, ossifying fibromyxoid tumor, monophasic synovial sarcoma, clear cell sarcoma, small cell osteosarcoma, and extraskeletal myxoid chondrosarcoma.

Immunohistochemical data is sparse on this entity, limited to a study of 25 cases, which yielded a relatively consistent profile. Most tumors were strongly reactive for vimentin, which tended to localize within the cytoplasm.[370, 371] Scattered tumor cells stained weakly and focally for EMA in approximately one half of the cases examined. S-100 protein, found in 29% of cases, demonstrated a similar weak and focal immunoreactive pattern. Cytokeratin, as evaluated by CAM5.2 and AE1/AE3, and NSE were found rarely. None of the studied cases stained for LCA, HMB-45, CD68, or

desmin.[370] In most instances, immunostains were principally used for excluding other entities, rather than specifically defining this tumor.

Epithelioid Leiomyosarcoma

Epithelioid changes may occasionally occur in smooth muscle tumors as a focal feature, or less frequently as the predominant pattern. Such tumors have previously been designated *leiomyoblastoma,* but current information indicates that even relatively bland tumors harbor metastatic potential. The term *epithelioid LMS* has been adopted to refer to smooth muscle tumors composed of sheets and clusters of epithelioid cells with vacuolated or granular cytoplasm.

We have studied eight examples of epithelioid LMS, six of which were retroperitoneal, with the remainder located in deep musculature of the trunk. All tumors were vimentin-reactive. In each case, either muscle-specific actin or desmin was also detected; however, in contrast to spindle cell variants of LMS, only two epithelioid lesions were coreactive for both muscle-specific actin and desmin, an observation noted by other investigators in single case reports of such lesions.[372] This finding parallels ultrastructural evidence of diminished or poorly organized myofilament structures in many of these lesions. Despite the inhomogeneous expression of desmin and muscle-specific actin, epithelioid LMSs are uniformly negative for markers of a nonmyogenic phenotype. None has displayed reactivity for S-100 protein, cytokeratin, EMA, UEAI lectin, factor VIII-RA, CD31, or CEA.[372, 373]

Alveolar Soft Part Sarcoma

There has been considerable controversy regarding the cellular nature of differentiation in alveolar soft part sarcoma ever since its first description in 1952. Advances in immunohistochemistry and electron microscopy have helped elucidate the differentiation of these peculiar neoplasms. Electron microscopy shows a paucity of filaments, and distinctive cytoplasmic crystals. Despite attempts to prove a neuroectodermal or endocrine lineage of differentiation, the most recent studies endorse a myogenic phenotype.

The presence of positive immunostaining for several muscle-associated proteins, such as desmin, actins, myosin, Z-band protein, B-enolase, and the MM isozyme of creatine kinase, provide some evidence that these tumors show skeletal muscle differentiation and may in fact represent a form of rhabdomyosarcoma.[374, 375] Desmin positivity with absent actin staining or isolated actin immunoreactivity has been observed in a number of studies.[109] Immunoelectron microscopy studies have demonstrated desmin and vimentin localized on whorled bundles of intermediate filaments in the perinuclear cytoplasm. The presence of desmin in alveolar soft part sarcoma has also been confirmed by demonstrating such filaments using Western blotting techniques. Because desmin is an intermediate filament of both striated and smooth muscle cells, its presence does not alone indicate whether the phenotypic expression of alveolar soft part sarcoma is rhabdomyogenic or leiomyogenic. Desmin positivity also has been identified in a number of nonmyogenic tumors, including mesothelioma and rhabdoid tumors.[24, 100, 376] Both alpha sarcomeric actin and alpha smooth muscle actin immunoreactivity have been described in alveolar soft part sarcoma.[377–379]

Recent studies have evaluated the presence of the myogenic regulatory proteins MyoD1 and myogenin.[378, 380, 381] Rhabdomyosarcomas show characteristic nuclear staining with these antibodies. One large study of alveolar soft part sarcoma found the complete absence of nuclear staining for MyoD1, although this finding remains controversial.[382, 383] Granular cytoplasmic reactivity with the anti-MyoD1 antibody 5.8A, which is sometimes pronounced, is found in the majority of cases of alveolar soft part sarcoma, but is regarded as nonspecific.

None of the seven cases we studied has been positive for NSE, CD57, cytokeratin, chromogranin, or S-100 protein. Similarly, EMA, factor VIII-RA, CD31, UEAI, and CEA are uniformly absent in alveolar soft part sarcoma. The antibody HMB-45 has only occasionally been included in immunohistochemical studies, but has been reported as negative in seven cases.[375]

"Histiocytic" Malignant Fibrous Histiocytoma

Occasional examples of MFH are entirely composed of uniform polygonal cells with a sheet-like growth pattern (Fig. 3–26). Such lesions are representative of a "histiocytic" variant of this neoplasm. Because of the considerable controversy over the nature of MFH in general, a more detailed discussion of the immunohistochemical attributes of these lesions is offered in the following section on pleomorphic tumors of soft tissue. With special reference to the differential diagnostic context being considered here, none of the examples of histiocytic MFH that we have studied has displayed lineage-selective markers other than vimentin. This reactivity has been accompanied by staining for the relatively nonselective proteolytic enzymes alpha-1-antitrypsin, alpha-1-antichymotrypsin, and cathepsin B, and the "histiocyte-selective" but diagnostically nonspecific markers MAC387, CD68, and HAM 56.

PLEOMORPHIC TUMORS OF SOFT TISSUE
(Fig. 3–27; Table 3–7)

Soft tissue sarcomas that may display a pleomorphic microscopic appearance include MFH, pleo-

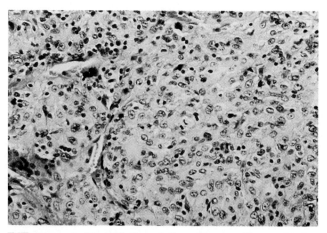

Figure 3–26. "Histiocytic" malignant fibrous histiocytoma (MFH) composed of sheets of relatively monomorphic epithelioid cells. The differential diagnosis of this entity is broad.

morphic rhabdomyosarcoma, pleomorphic and dedifferentiated liposarcoma, dedifferentiated LMS, and MPNST. Most of the lineage-selective determinants described in this chapter are often only unreliably displayed in "dedifferentiated" or pleomorphic areas of these soft tissue neoplasms, with the conspicuous exception of pleomorphic rhabdomyosarcoma and MPNST.

Malignant Fibrous Histiocytoma

As a histologic pattern, MFH remains the most common form of soft tissue sarcoma in adults. Reactivity for alpha-1-antitrypsin, alpha-1-antichymotrypsin (Fig. 3–28), and ferritin, and binding of the peanut agglutinin are associated with "fibrohistiocytic" differentiation and partly support its original designation. Other proteolytic enzymes, such as lysozyme, cathepsin B, and "nonspecific" esterase have been touted as similarly selective for MFH. More advanced immunohistochemical determinants have since disproved the purely "histiocytic" differentiation of these tumors that was originally described before 1970. Subsequent analyses with improved histiocytic markers such as CD68 have failed to demonstrate a relationship. Roholl and colleagues suggested a phenotype for MFH that was more closely allied with that of myofibroblasts.[384] This observation has been supported by analyses, including our own, that identify populations of muscle specific–, actin-, and desmin-reactive cells in MFH. The ultrastructural characterization of myofibroblast-like elements and the detection of intermediate filaments by the more sensitive method of immunoblotting corroborates this view.

From a practical view, most examples of MFH are still best defined by the presence of vimentin in the absence of other evidence of lineage-specific differentiation. Pleomorphic neoplasms with overt

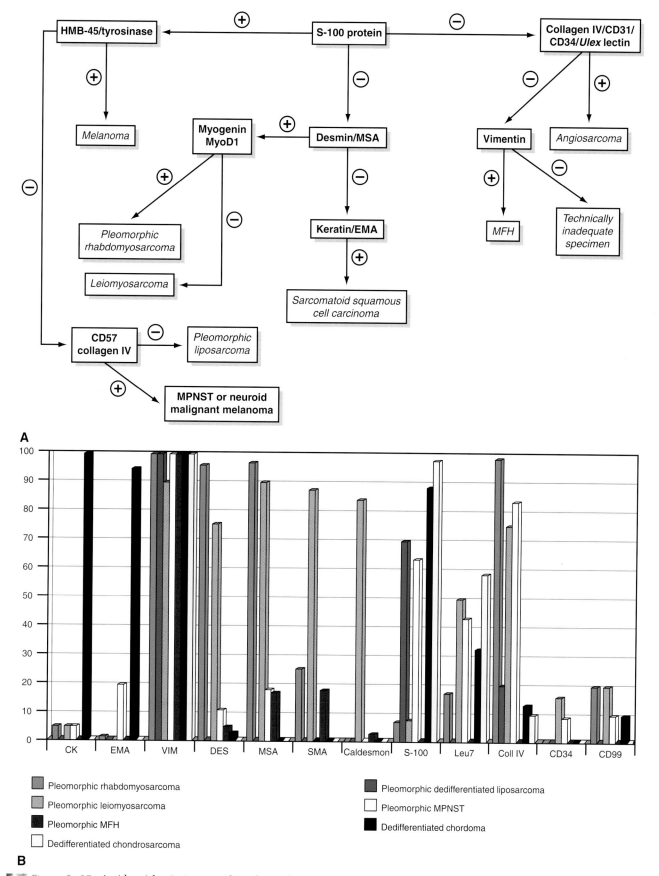

Figure 3–27. *A,* Algorithmic immunohistologic diagnosis of malignant pleomorphic tumors. *B,* Graphic representation of the frequency of reactivity for pleomorphic tumors against commonly used immunoreactants. MSA, muscle-specific actin; EMA, epithelial membrane antigen; MFH, malignant fibrous histiocytoma; MPNST, malignant peripheral nerve sheath tumor; CK, cytokeratin; VIM, vimentin; DES, desmin; MSA, muscle-specific actin; SMA, smooth muscle actin.

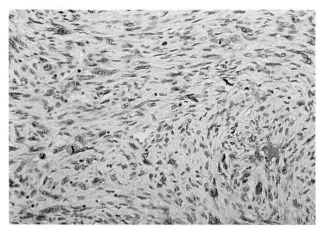

Figure 3-28. MFH labels for several determinants that are associated with mononuclear phagocytic cells, such as alpha-1-antichymotrypsin, as shown here. However, those markers are completely nonspecific, and it is much more important to undertake systematic *elimination* of several lineage-related markers as the first step in the diagnosis of MFH.

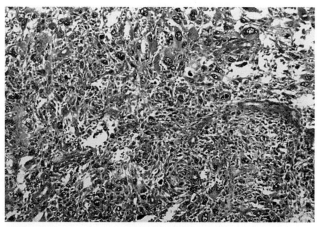

Figure 3-29. Pleomorphic rhabdomyosarcoma, shown here, is often indistinguishable from MFH on conventional morphologic studies.

lineage-selective staining patterns (e.g., muscle- or neural-associated markers) are thus readily distinguished in most cases from MFH.

The question of whether MFHs compose a unified group of neoplasms has lingered since the advent of more lineage-specific detection methods. It has become apparent that MFH-like areas may evolve in tumors that are otherwise typical examples of neurogenic, myogenic, or lipoblastic neoplasms. This observation, together with the relatively nonspecific immunoprofile that characterizes MFH, has given credence to the suggestion that MFH reflects a common final pathway of differentiation ("dedifferentiation") among soft tissue sarcomas in general. This hypothesis has gained morphologic support from studies in cultured cell lines and as tumor cells explanted in nude mice. Phenotypically uniform examples of MFH in the latter studies developed other immunophenotypes once explanted; some exhibited a myogenic profile, whereas others became reactive for S-100 protein. A similar phenomenon may account for the presence of epithelial markers in rare examples of this neoplasm.

Pleomorphic Rhabdomyosarcoma

Among the various forms of rhabdomyosarcoma, the pleomorphic type is the most uncommon and is confined to adults (Fig. 3–29). Nevertheless, it is relatively easy to diagnose immunohistochemically because of the presence of the myogenic determinants desmin, muscle-specific or sarcomeric actin, myosin, or myoglobin (Fig. 3–30) in most examples.[385] These proteins are readily detected in tumor foci bearing the characteristic "strap" cells but may also be identified in spindle cell or pleomorphic foci. The latter observations have in fact suggested that the relative frequency of this neoplasm among pleomorphic sarcomas in adults (many of which have been histologically classified as MFH) is perhaps greater than previously acknowledged. Because MFH may occasionally display reactivity for desmin and muscle-specific actin, this conclusion has its critics, but we would emphasize that in MFH, in contrast to rhabdomyosarcoma, reactivity for these determinants is generally extremely focal. Pleomorphic rhabdomyosarcomas do not generally exhibit the nerve sheath markers such as S-100 protein, Leu7 antigen, or myelin basic protein, but they may be reactive for proteolytic enzymes, again emphasizing the lack of specificity of the latter reactants.

Pleomorphic and "Dedifferentiated" Liposarcomas

Pleomorphic liposarcoma is defined as a neoplasm that resembles MFH except for the regular interspersion of lipoblasts. "Dedifferentiated" liposarcoma presents a similar histologic appearance

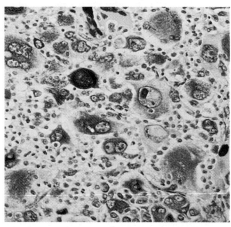

Figure 3-30. Reactivity for myoglobin in pleomorphic rhabdomyosarcoma.

but differs from the pleomorphic variant in that the pleomorphic foci show an abrupt transition from well-differentiated liposarcoma; the pleomorphic area in this latter variant may be represented by any of a variety of other sarcoma morphotypes, but is most commonly MFH-like. The "dedifferentiated" variant often signifies a recurrence-related change in a well-differentiated liposarcoma and does not represent actual dedifferentiation of differentiated cells, but rather anaplastic overgrowth of primitive mesenchymal cells. Hence, it is not unexpected that pleomorphic and dedifferentiated liposarcomas manifest a potential for reactivity with most of the determinants seen in MFH, including sporadic staining for CD68[386] and generalized reactivity for proteolytic enzymes. Unlike MFH, these adipose tissue tumors also exhibit S-100 protein staining in their lipoblastic or well-differentiated components. In contrast to peripheral nerve sheath tumors, these sarcomas are uniformly nonreactive with antibodies to myelin-associated substances (CD57 and myelin basic protein). In our experience, myoglobin, desmin, and muscle-specific actin are also absent in poorly differentiated liposarcomas.

Pleomorphic Malignant Peripheral Nerve Sheath Tumor

In addition to its spindle cell and epithelioid forms, MPNST may assume a pleomorphic appearance. In most cases, the pleomorphic variant shows patterns of reactivity for S-100 protein, CD57, and myelin basic protein that are essentially similar to those exhibited by better differentiated forms of this neoplasm.[387] Unlike spindle cell variants of MPNST, pleomorphic subtypes have not been shown to be desmin-reactive.

Other Primary Neoplasms of Soft Tissue

Some primary tumors of the soft tissues do not fit neatly into one of the foregoing categories. Malignant rhabdoid tumor, chordoma, extraosseous myxoid chondrosarcoma ("chordoid" sarcoma), extraskeletal osteosarcoma, aggressive angiomyxoma, and some liposarcoma and angiosarcoma variants are included in this group.

GRANULAR CELL ANGIOSARCOMA

The granular cell variant of angiosarcoma is extremely rare. It is characterized by cells with abundant granular pink cytoplasm, simulating those of granular cell tumor (Fig. 3–31).[388] Immunohistochemistry demonstrates UEAI and factor VIII-RA positivity, confirming its endothelial nature. Unlike other angiosarcomas, CD31 and CD34 may be absent. CD68 has been demonstrated to stain the cytoplasmic granules.

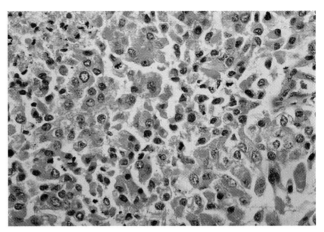

Figure 3–31. Granular cell angiosarcoma is an uncommon lesion with a differential diagnosis that includes granular cell tumor, metastatic melanoma, and epithelioid leiomyosarcoma.

RHABDOID TUMOR

Tumors that are histologically identical to the "malignant rhabdoid tumor" (a well-accepted tumor of the kidney in childhood) may occur in a wide variety of extrarenal sites in both children and adults.[389] The hallmarks of this neoplasm are hyaline cytoplasmic eosinophilic inclusions, an eccentric, rounded nucleus with vesicular chromatin and a prominent nucleolus (Fig. 3–32), which characteristically manifest a complex immunophenotype.

As observed in some other high-grade soft tissue tumors, such as synovial sarcoma, epithelial sarcoma, and MPNST, rhabdoid tumors show divergent epithelial differentiation, and thus may cause diagnostic confusion. In a study of 18 strictly defined cases, the overwhelming majority showed reactivity for EMA (Fig. 3–33) and keratin (Fig. 3–34).[390, 391] Almost all rhabdoid tumors react for vimentin,[390] with a tendency for perinuclear accentuation within the cytoplasm. Three fourths of cases colabel for vimentin and epithelial markers. Reactivity to muscle-specific actin, CEA, SMA, CD99, synaptophysin, CD57, NSE, and S-100 protein may be detected in a few cases. HMB-45, chromogranin, myoglobin, and CD34 are not found. Although the immunophenotype of rhabdoid tumor overlaps with those of other sarcomas and poorly differentiated carcinomas, the morphologic appearance of this tumor is generally sufficiently distinct for accurate diagnosis.

LIPOSARCOMA VARIANTS

Liposarcoma is easily recognized by most pathologists in its well-differentiated form. Nevertheless, myxoid and round cell variants of this neoplasm show few, if any, discernible lipoblasts and may therefore be difficult to discriminate from a variety of other tumors.

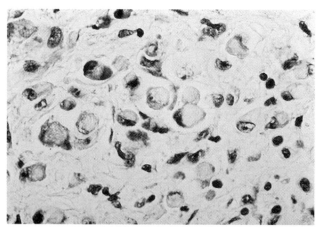

Figure 3–32. The histologic image of extrarenal malignant rhabdoid tumor features large cells with eosinophilic cytoplasm, eccentric vesicular nuclei, and prominent nucleoli.

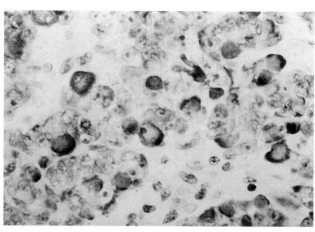

Figure 3–34. Keratin in rhabdoid tumor, raising diagnostic concern for another type of soft tissue sarcoma or metastatic carcinoma.

Myxoid liposarcoma expresses vimentin and S-100 protein, with the latter confined to lipoblastic elements. In addition, a subset of tumors with the characteristic t(12;16) have been found to express muscle markers, including desmin, muscle-specific actin, and alpha-SMA, which is focal in distribution.[392] Myelin basic protein, CD34 and CD57 are not detectable, allowing for a distinction from myxoid nerve sheath tumors, in conjunction with the morphologic features.

Round cell liposarcoma is itself a heterogeneous neoplasm that may resemble either chondrosarcoma or cellular peripheral nerve sheath tumors. S-100 protein and vimentin reactivity are common to all three tumors, but CD57 is seen only in chondrosarcoma. MPNSTs that are similar microscopically to round cell liposarcoma differ in their reactivity for myelin basic protein.

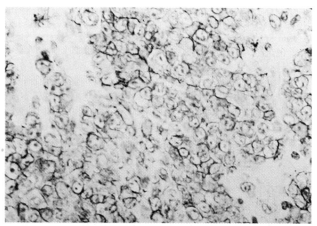

Figure 3–33. Epithelial membrane antigen may be seen in extrarenal rhabdoid tumor, potentially causing confusion with variants of epithelioid sarcoma or metastatic carcinoma.

CHONDROID TUMORS (Fig. 3–35)

Chordoma

Chordoma is a malignant tumor that occurs in close relation to the axial skeleton. It is well known to show such epithelioid features and a syncytial, sometimes lobulated arrangement of plump, vacuolated cells. The differential diagnosis of chordoma includes a variety of tumors, including adenocarcinoma, chondrosarcoma, myxopapillary ependymoma, and EHE. Rarely, chordoma may arise in the peripheral soft tissues.[393]

The expression of keratin confirms its epithelial nature but does not allow for reliable separation from metastatic adenocarcinoma. The expression patterns of cytokeratins of chordoma are broad and include labeling with CAM5.2 (reacting with CK8/CK18, CK19) and AE1/AE3 (reacting with CK1 to CK8, CK10, CK14 to CK16, CK19) (Fig. 3–36).[394] Further complicating the distinction from carcinoma is the capacity of chordoma to express EMA (Fig. 3–37).[395, 396] However, reactivity for these determinants is indeed useful to separate chordoma from chondrosarcoma, which is uniformly negative for epithelial markers; both tumor types share S-100 expression. Most studies show that chordoma does not react for GFAP. Although both chordoma and EHE have the ability to show cytokeratin reactivity, EHE shows factor VIII-RA positivity and is negative for S-100. Chordomas do not react with antibodies to desmin, neurofilaments, NSE, or chromogranin.[18]

Chordoma Variants

In 1973, Heffelfinger and associates described a variant of chordoma with cartilaginous areas that were indistinguishable from chondrosarcoma.[397, 398] They designated these lesions as *chondroid chordomas* and believed they showed a better prognosis than did conventional chordoma. The immu-

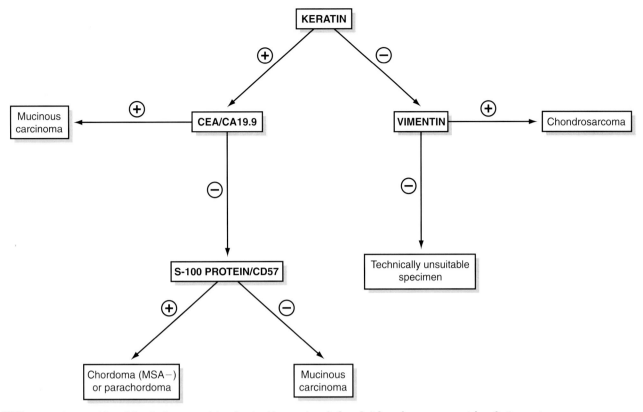

Figure 3–35. Algorithmic immunohistologic diagnosis of chordoid and mucomyxoid soft tissue tumors.

nohistochemical staining pattern with positivity for cytokeratin, EMA, and CEA can be helpful in distinguishing it from chondrosarcoma.[396, 398–400] Chondrosarcoma and chondroid chordoma both show S-100 protein and vimentin reactivity.

In the "dedifferentiated" form of chordoma (Fig. 3–38), the poorly differentiated component assumes an immunophenotype that is characteristic of MFH. Nonetheless, an occasional S-100–positive cell persists, whereas cytokeratins are less commonly retained in spindle cell or pleomorphic areas of dedifferentiated chordoma (Fig. 3–39).

Parachordoma

Parachordoma is an exceptionally rare, slowly growing tumor that arises in the deep soft tissues of the extremities. The differential diagnosis primarily includes extraskeletal myxoid chondrosarcoma and chordoma, although chondroid lipoma, ossifying fibromyxoid tumor, myoepitheliomas, and subcutaneous sacrococcygeal myxopapillary ependymoma may occasionally be considered. Parachordoma shows a distinct immunohistochemical profile from extraskeletal myxoid chondrosarcoma

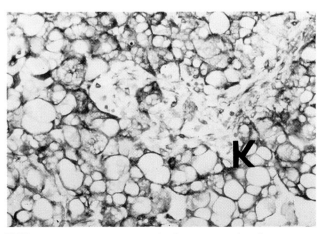

Figure 3–36. Reactivity for keratin in chordoma.

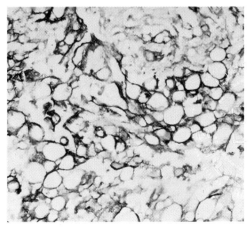

Figure 3–37. Immunoreactivity for epithelial membrane antigen in chordoma.

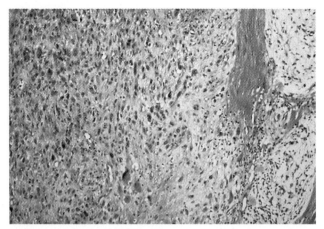

Figure 3-38. Rare examples of chordoma undergo anaplastic transformation ("dedifferentiation"), in which the undifferentiated foci acquire an immunophenotype that is closely similar to that of MFH.

and chordoma. Parachordomas are almost always positive for CK8/CK18 (CAM5.2), EMA, S-100 protein, type IV collagen, and vimentin.[16, 401-404] In contrast, extraskeletal myxoid chondrosarcoma is generally negative for CK8/CK18.[16] Extraskeletal myxoid chondrosarcoma is infrequently collagen IV–positive as well, in contrast to parachordoma, in which this determinant frequently delineates nests of tumor cells.

Although parachordoma and chordoma may show immunophenotypic overlap in regard to CK8/CK18, EMA, vimentin, and S-100 protein reactivity, parachordomas lack CK1/CK10 (34βE12), CK19, and type IV collagen, in contrast to chordoma.[16]

Chondroblastoma

Chondroblastoma is a relatively infrequently encountered entity that may be confused with aneurysmal bone cyst, giant cell reparative granuloma, giant cell tumor, and clear cell chondrosarcoma (CCC). Chondroblastoma is usually strongly reactive for vimentin, NSE, and S-100 protein.[405-407] In

particular, the proliferating stromal cells show strong S-100 protein positivity, facilitating differentiation from giant cell tumor of bone, or aneurysmal bone cyst, which is negative.[407] Rare stromal cells in CCC may show S-100 protein reactivity, which should be remembered when this differential diagnosis is under consideration or in small biopsy material.[408] Collagen type IV has been noted focally around individual tumor cells in chondroblastoma and is always seen in the chondroid matrix.[406]

Aberrant cytokeratin expression is a potential feature of chondroblastoma, as evidenced by labeling for CK8, CK18, CK19, and, to a lesser extent, CK7.[407, 409] The mononuclear chondroblastic tumor cells do not stain with macrophage-associated antibodies, including CD68.[406, 410] A subset of chondroblastomas showed distinct cytoplasmic muscle-specific actin positivity in the tumor chondroblasts in one study.[411]

Conventional Chondrosarcoma

The differential diagnosis of conventional myxoid chondrosarcoma includes reactive and benign cartilaginous tumors (e.g., enchondroma), chondroblastic osteosarcoma, EHE, and chordoma. Chondrosarcoma shows reactivity for vimentin and S-100 protein. We have studied 28 cases that additionally showed NSE and CD57 positivity, but none stained for keratin, EMA, CEA, or desmin (unpublished data). Chondrosarcoma of the conventional type does not stain for ONN except for foci undergoing ossification.[206] Immunohistochemistry cannot distinguish conventional chondrosarcoma from other cartilaginous lesions, but it can help differentiate it from EHE and chordoma. EHE is negative for S-100 protein and expresses endothelial determinants. Chordomas, unlike chondrosarcoma, stain for epithelial markers.

Extraskeletal Myxoid Chondrosarcoma

Although similar light microscopic features are noted in skeletal and extraskeletal myxoid chon-

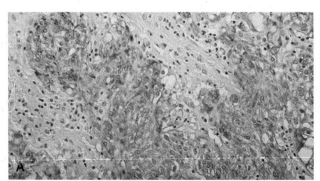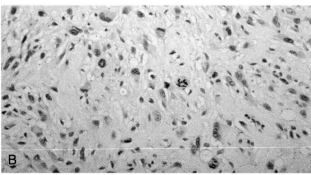

Figure 3-39. Reactivity for keratin in well-differentiated areas *(A)* of "dedifferentiated" chordoma, and negativity for the same marker *(B)* in anaplastic foci.

drosarcoma, there are fundamental differences at the ultrastructural and molecular levels, suggesting that these tumors represent distinct entities. Extraskeletal myxoid chondrosarcoma is a low-grade sarcoma showing cartilaginous differentiation and has been found, in most cases, to contain reciprocal t(9;22), resulting in fusion of the EWS and CHN genes.[412–414] Immunohistochemically, examples may be negative or only focally reactive for S-100 protein, with negativity for cytokeratin (AE1/AE3), factor VIII-RA, and CD31.

Clear Cell Chondrosarcoma

CCC is a rare tumor characterized by special histologic features, slow growth, and relatively good prognosis, which serve to separate it from conventional chondrosarcoma. The histologic pattern is that of clear cells arranged in lobules; the frequent presence of areas mimicking other primary bone tumors often obscures the diagnosis. Similar to conventional chondrosarcoma and chondroblastoma, the tumor cells of CCC show reactivity for S-100 protein, vimentin, alpha-1-antichymotrypsin, and lysozyme.[413] Some examples show strong ONN expression in clear cell, chondroid, and osseous areas, the latter generally associated with osteosarcoma. This presence of ONN in CCC contrasts with its absence in conventional chondrosarcoma and mesenchymal chondrosarcoma,[415, 416] suggesting that CCC has cartilaginous as well as osteogenic differentiation.

OSSEOUS TUMORS

Osteosarcoma

Soft tissue osteosarcoma is a highly unusual tumor outside the skeletal system in which the mesenchymal tumor cells elaborate "malignant" osteoid. Like their skeletal counterparts, extraskeletal osteosarcomas show a variety of histologic patterns, including fibroblastic, chondroblastic, small cell, and telangiectatic patterns. Clinically, extraskeletal osteosarcoma can mimic other neoplasms such as ES/PNET, chondroblastoma, and angiosarcoma. Compared with its osseous counterpart, extraskeletal osteosarcoma occurs mainly in individuals older than age 30, a feature that may be useful in differential diagnosis.

Immunohistochemistry shows few characteristic features and is used primarily to exclude other lesions under consideration. Extraskeletal osteosarcomas consistently are strongly reactive for vimentin, with reactivity of the osteoid matrix for CD57. The majority of cases of extraskeletal osteosarcoma express alpha smooth muscle actin focally, with a subset of these also coexpressing desmin.[417] S-100 protein positivity is typically seen in areas showing cartilaginous differentiation, but may be present focally in osteoblasts as well.[417] Epithelial

markers rarely may be observed.[417–419] When present, they are weak and focal. GFAP and neurofilament are absent.

The presence of strong alkaline phosphatase labeling is useful to differentiate extraskeletal osteosarcoma from other pleomorphic sarcomas.[415] The exceptions in which alkaline phosphatase reactivity may be lacking are cases of extraskeletal osteosarcoma dominated by a MFH-like pattern. The major drawback of this marker is that it must be assessed using cryostat sections or imprint smears.

The bone matrix proteins ONN and osteocalcin have generated much interest lately, but their efficacy in identifying osteosarcoma needs to be further substantiated. A strongly positive stain for ONN is found in the neoplastic components of osteosarcoma, as well as in osteoblastoma. Weaker labeling of the mononuclear cells in giant cell tumor and chondroblastoma has been observed.[420] Pleomorphic and fibrosarcomatous osteosarcomas react focally as well.[421] This latter finding may be related to the fact that ONN production is an early event in the differentiation of cells of the osteoblastic lineage. The specificity of ONN and OCN is 39 to 40% and 91 to 100% for bone-forming tumors.[197, 198] These markers may be useful in a broad panel of immunostains for corroborating the diagnosis of extraskeletal osteosarcoma.

Giant Cell Tumor of Bone and Giant Cell Tumor of Soft Tissue

Giant cell tumor of bone is a locally aggressive tumor that typically involves the epiphysis and metaphysis of long tubular bones. The tumors consist of a mixture of mononuclear cells showing vesicular, oval nuclei and uniformly distributed osteoclast-like, multinucleated giant cells. A morphologically similar tumor may also arise in the soft tissue, generally associated with a tenosynovial region. The terms *giant cell tumor of soft parts, malignant giant cell tumor of soft parts,* and *MFH, giant cell type* have been used to refer to extraosseous giant cell tumors. These lesions are presumably different from tenosynovial giant cell tumors because they lack dense stromal collagen, siderophages, and xanthoma cells. Their immunohistochemical profiles, however, are the same.

Immunohistochemistry of these tumors has focused largely on identifying the nature of the mononuclear stromal and multinucleate giant cells in giant cell tumors. The giant cells stain strongly for CD68.[422–425] The mononuclear (stromal) cells are also CD68+, albeit with weaker intensity. They also label for smooth muscle actin (HHF-35) and lack CD45, S-100 protein, desmin, and lysozyme.[422, 424] The frequent occurrence of vascular invasion without distant metastasis in giant cell tumor has prompted interest in their synthesis of matrix metalloproteinases (MMPs) and tissue inhibitors (TIMPs), which are believed to play a role in wound healing, neoplastic invasion, and metastases. MMP-9 (gelatinase B) is highly expressed in the giant cells and focally in the mononuclear cells.[422, 427, 428] Furthermore, a relative increase in TIMPs compared with MMPs in recurrent and metastatic tumors has been found in two investigations.[422, 429]

References

1. Denk H, Krepler R, Artlieb U, et al. Proteins of intermediate filaments: An immunohistochemical and biochemical approach to the classification of soft tissue tumors. Am J Pathol 1983;110:193–208.
2. Lazarides E. Intermediate filaments: A chemically heterogeneous, developmentally regulated class of proteins. Annu Rev Biochem 1982;51:219–250.
3. Erlandson RA. Diagnostic Transmission Electron Microscopy of Tumors. New York: Raven, 1994:165.
4. Osborn M, Weber K. Biology of disease: Tumor diagnosis by intermediate filament typing: A novel tool for surgical pathology. Lab Invest 1983;48:372–394.
5. Anderton BH. Intermediate filaments: A family of homologous structures. J Muscle Res Cell Motil 1981;2:141–166.
6. Hermann H, Aebi U. Intermediate filaments and their associates: Multitalented structural elements specifying cytoarchitecture and cytodynamics. Curr Opin Cell Biol 2000;12:79–90.
7. Mischke D. The complexity of gene families involved in epithelial differentiation: Keratin genes and the epidermal differentiation complex. Subcell Biochem 1998;31:71–104.
8. Saavedra-Matiz CA, Chapman NH, Wijsman EM, et al. Linkage of hereditary distal myopathy with desmin accumulation to 2q. Hum Hered 2000;50:166–170.
9. Ferrari S, Cannizzaro LA, Battini R, et al. The gene encoding human vimentin is located on the short arm of chromosome 10. Am J Hum Genet 1987;41:616–626.
10. Yoshime T, Maruno M, Kumura E, et al. Stochastsic determination of the chromosomal region responsible for expression of human glial fibrillary acidic protein in astrocytic tumors. Neurosci Lett 1998;247:29–32.
11. Goldman R, Goldman AE, Green K, et al. Intermediate filaments: Possible functions as cytoskeletal connecting links between the nucleus and the cell surface. Ann NY Acad Sci 1985;455:1–17.
12. Osborn M: Summary: Intermediate filaments 1984. Ann NY Acad Sci 1985;455:669–681.
13. Vandenburgh HH. Cell shape and growth regulation in skeletal muscle: Exogenous versus endogenous factors. J Cell Physiol 1983;116:363–371.
14. Miettinen M. Keratin immunohistochemistry: Update of applications and pitfalls. Pathol Annu 1993;28(Pt. 2):113–143.
15. Moll R, Franke WW, Schiller DL, et al. The catalogue of human cytokeratins: Patterns of expression in normal epithelia, tumors, and cultured cells. Cell 1982;31:11–24.
16. Folpe AL, Agoff SN, Willis J, Weiss SW. Parachordoma is immunohistochemically and cytogenetically distinct from axial chordoma and extraskeletal myxoid chondrosarcoma. Am J Surg Pathol 1999;23:1059–1067.
17. Fisher C, Miettinen M. Parachordoma: A clinicopathologic and immunohistochemical study of four cases of an unusual soft tissue neoplasm. Ann Diagn Pathol 1997;1:3–10.
18. O'Hara BJ, Paetau A, Miettinen M. Keratin subsets and monoclonal antibodies HBME-1 in chordoma: Immunohistochemical differential diagnosis between tumors simulating chordoma. Hum Pathol 1998;29:119–126.
19. Swanson PE, Dehner LP, Sirgi KE, Wick MR. Cytokeratin immunoreactivity in malignant tumors of bone and soft tissue. Appl Immunohistochem 1994;2:103–112.
20. Pruss RM, Mirsky R, Raff MC, et al. All classes of intermediate filaments share a common antigenic determinant defined by a monoclonal antibody. Cell 1981;27:419–428.
21. Geisler N, Weber K. Comparison of the proteins of two immunologically distinct intermediate-sized filaments by amino acid sequence analysis: desmin and vimentin. Proc Natl Acad Sci U S A 1981;78:4120–4123.
22. Wick MR. Antibodies to desmin in diagnostic pathology. In: Wick MR, Siegal GP, eds. Monoclonal Antibodies in Diagnostic Immunohistochemistry. New York: Marcel Dekker, 1988:93–114.
23. Truong LD, Rangdaeng S, Cagle P, et al. The diagnostic utility of desmin: A study of 584 cases and review of the literature. Am J Clin Pathol 1990;93:305–314.
24. Rangdaeng S, Truong LD. Comparative immunohistochemical staining for desmin and muscle specific actin: A study of 576 cases. Am J Clin Pathol 1991;96:32–45.
25. Small JV, Sobieszek A. Studies on the function and composition of the 10-nm (100 A) filaments of vertebrate smooth muscle. J Cell Sci 1977;23:243–268.
26. Geisler N, Weber K. Purification of smooth muscle desmin and a protein-chemical comparison of desmins from chicken gizzard and hog stomach. Eur J Biochem 1980;111:425–433.
27. Lazarides E, Balzer DR Jr. Specificity of desmin to avian and mammalian muscle cells. Cell 1978;14:429–438.
28. Geisler N, Weber K. The amino acid sequence of chicken muscle desmin provides a common structural model for intermediate filament proteins. EMBO J 1982;1:1649–1656.
29. Ip W, Heuser JE. Subunit structure of desmin and vimentin protofilaments and how they assemble into intermediate filaments. Ann NY Acad Sci 1985;455:185–199.
30. Ngai J, Capetanaki YG, Lazarides E. Expression of the genes encoding for the intermediate filament proteins vimentin and desmin. Ann NY Acad Sci 1985;455:144–155.
31. Tokuyasu KT, Maher PA, Dutton AH, Singer SJ. Intermediate filaments in skeletal and cardiac muscle tissue in embryonic and adult chicken. Ann NY Acad Sci 1985;455:200–212.
32. Fischman DA, Danto SI. Monoclonal antibodies to desmin: Evidence for stage-dependent intermediate filament immunoreactivity during cardiac and skeletal muscle development. Ann NY Acad Sci 1985;455:167–184.
33. Tuszynski GP, Frank ED, Damsky CD, et al. The detection of smooth muscle desmin-like protein in BHK21/C13 fibroblasts. J Biol Chem 1979;254:6138–6143.
34. Schmid E, Osborn M, Rungger-Brandle E, et al. Distribution of vimentin and desmin filaments in smooth muscle tissue of mammalian and avian aorta. Exp Cell Res 1982;137:329–340.
35. Richardson FL, Stromer MH, Huiatt TW, Robson RM. Immunoelectron and immunofluorescence localization of desmin in mature avian muscles. Eur J Cell Biol 1981;26:91–101.
36. Daste G, Gioanni J, Lauque D, et al. GC12, marker of cells of mesodermal origin: Value and application to cytodiagnosis of serous effusions. Arch Anat Cytol Pathol 1997;45:185–191.
37. Pollock L, Rampling D, Greenwald SE, Malone M. Desmin expression in forms: Influence of the desmin clone and immunohistochemical method. J Clin Pathol 1995;48:535–538.
38. Chang TK, Li CY, Smithson WA. Immunocytochemical study of small round cell tumors in routinely processed specimens. Arch Pathol Lab Med 1989;113:1343–1348.
39. Granter SR, Badizadegan K, Fletcher CDM. Myofibromatosis in adults, glomangiopericytoma, and myopericytoma: A spectrum of tumors showing perivascular myoid differentiation. Am J Surg Pathol 1998;22:513–525.
40. Ordi J, de Alava E, Torne A, et al. Intraabdominal desmoplastic small round-cell tumor with EWS/ERG fusion transcripts. Am J Surg Pathol 1998;22:1026–1032.
41. Parham DM, Dias P, Kelly DR, et al. Desmin positivity in primitive neuroectodermal tumors of childhood. Am J Surg Pathol 1992;16:483–492.
42. Manivel JC, Wick MR, Dehner LP, Sibley RK. Epithelioid

sarcoma: An immunohistochemical study. Am J Clin Pathol 1987;87:319–326.

43. Wick MR, Swanson PE, Scheithauer BW, Manivel JC. Malignant peripheral nerve sheath tumor: An immunohistochemical study of 62 cases. Am J Clin Pathol 1987;87:425–433.

44. Fanberg-Smith JC, Hengge M, Hengge UR, et al. Extrarenal rhabdoid tumors of soft tissue: A clinicopathologic and immunohistochemical study of 18 cases. Ann Diagn Pathol 1998;2:351–362.

45. Geisler N, Plessmann U, Weber K. Amino acid sequence characterization of mammalian vimentin, the mesenchymal intermediate filament protein. FEBS Lett 1983;163: 22–24.

46. Gereben B, Leuheiber K, Rausch WD, et al. Inverse hierarchy of vimentin epitope expression in primary cultures of chicken and rat astrocytes: A double immunofluorescence study. Neurobiology 1998;6:141–150.

47. Battifora H. Assessment of antigen damage in immunohistochemistry: The vimentin internal control. Am J Clin Pathol 1991;96:669–671.

48. Gereben B, Gerics B, Galfi P, et al. Species specificity of glial vimentin, as revealed by immunocytochemical studies with the VIM3B4 and V9 monoclonal antibodies. Neurobiology 1995;3:151–164.

49. Olah I, Glick B. Anti-vimentin monoclonal antibodies differentiate two resident cell populations in chicken spleen. Dev Comp Immunol 1994;18:67–73.

50. Heatley M, Whiteside C, Maxwell P, Toner P. Vimentin expression in benign and malignant breast epithelium. J Clin Pathol 1993;46:441–445.

51. Bohn W, Wiegers W, Beuttenmuller M, Traub P. Species-specific recognition patterns of monoclonal antibodies directed against vimentin. Exp Cell Res 1992;201:1–7.

52. Carbone A, Gloghini A, Volpe R, Boiocchi M. Anti-vimentin antibody reactivity with Reed-Sternberg cells of Hodgkin's disease. Virchows Arch A 1990;417:43–48.

53. Meyer SA, Ingraham CA, McCarthy KD. Expression of vimentin by cultured astroglia and oligodendroglia. J Neurosci Res 1989;24:251–259.

54. Dahl D. Immunohistochemical differences between neurofilaments in perikarya, dendrites, and axons: Immunofluorescence study with antisera raised to neurofilament polypeptides (200 kd, 150 kd, and 70 kd) isolated by anion exchange chromatography. Exp Cell Res 1983;149:397–408.

55. Hickey WF, Lee V, Trojanowski JQ, et al. Immunohistochemical application of monoclonal antibodies against myelin basic protein and neurofilament triplet protein subunits: Advantage over antisera and technical limitations. J Histochem Cytochem 1983;31:1126–1135.

56. Shaw G. Neurofilaments: Abundant but mysterious neuronal structures. Bioessays 1986;4:161–166.

57. Tapscott SJ, Bennett GS, Toyama Y, et al. Intermediate filament proteins in the developing chick spinal cord. Dev Biol 1981;86:40–54.

58. Tremblay GF, Lee VMY, Trojanowski JQ. Expression of vimentin, glial filament, and neurofilament proteins in primitive childhood brain tumors: A comparative immunoblot and immunoperoxidase study. Acta Neuropathol 1985;68:239–244.

59. Lee VMY, Carden MJ, Trojanowski JQ. Novel monoclonal antibodies provide evidence for the in-situ existence of a non-phosphorylated form of the large neurofilament subunit. J Neurosci 1986;6:850–858.

60. Brown A. Contiguous phosphorylated and non-phosphorylated domains along axonal neurofilaments. J Cell Sci 1998;111:455–467.

61. Sternberger LA, Sternberger NH. Monoclonal antibodies distinguish phosphorylated and non-phosphorylated forms of neurofilaments in situ. Proc Natl Acad Sci USA 1983; 80:6126–6130.

62. Ulfig N, Nickel J, Bohl J. Monoclonal antibodies SMI311 and SMI312 as tools to investigate the maturation of nerve cells and axonal patterns in human fetal brain. Cell Tissue Res 1998;291:433–443.

63. Trojanowski JQ, Lee VMY. Anti-neurofilament monoclonal antibodies: Reagents for the evaluation of human neoplasms. Acta Neuropathol 1983;59:155–158.

64. Trojanowski JQ, Lee VMY, Schlaepfer WW. An immunohistochemical study of central and peripheral nervous system tumors with monoclonal antibodies against neurofilaments and glial filaments. Hum Pathol 1984;15:248–257.

65. Trojanowski JQ, Lee VMY. Expression of neurofilament antigens by normal and neoplastic human adrenal chromaffin cells. N Engl J Med 1985;313:101–104.

66. Osborn M, Altmannsberger M, Shaw G, et al. Various sympathetic derived human tumors differ in neurofilament expression: Use in diagnosis of neuroblastoma, ganglioneuroblastoma, and pheochromocytoma. Virchows Arch B Cell Pathol 1982;40:141–156.

67. Shaw G, Weber K. The intermediate filament complement of the brain: A comparison between different mammalian species. Eur J Cell Biol 1984;33:95–104.

68. Trojanowski JQ. Neurofilament and glial filament proteins. In: Wick MR, Siegal GP, eds. Monoclonal Antibodies in Diagnostic Immunohistochemistry. New York: Marcel Dekker, 1988:115–146.

69. Dolman CL. Glial fibrillary acidic protein and cartilage. Acta Neuropathol 1989;79:101–103.

70. Yasuda T, Sobue G, Ito T, et al. Human peripheral nerve sheath neoplasms: Expression of Schwann cell–related markers and their relation to malignant transformation. Muscle Nerve 1991;14:812–819.

71. Lodding P, Kindblom LG, Angervall L, et al. A clinicopathologic study of 29 cases. Virchows Arch A 1990;416: 237–248.

72. Giangaspero F, Fratamico FC, Ceccarelli C, Brisigotti M. Malignant peripheral nerve sheath tumors and spindle cell sarcomas: An immunohistochemical analysis of multiple markers. Appl Pathol 1989;7:134–144.

73. Kawahara E, Oda Y, Ooi A, et al. Expression of glial fibrillary acidic protein (GFAP) in peripheral nerve sheath tumors: A comparative study of immunoreactivity of GFAP, vimentin, S100 protein, and neurofilament in 38 schwannomas and 18 neurofibromas. Am J Surg Pathol 1988;12: 115–120.

74. Memoli VA, Brown EF, Gould VE. Glial fibrillary acidic protein (GFAP) immunoreactivity in peripheral nerve sheath tumors. Ultrastruct Pathol 1984;7:269–275.

75. Swanson PE. Monoclonal antibodies to human milk fat globule proteins. In: Wick MR, Siegal GP, eds. Monoclonal Antibodies in Diagnostic Immunohistochemistry. New York: Marcel Dekker, 1988:227–283.

76. Petersen OW, VanDeuers B. Characterization of epithelial membrane antigen expression in human mammary epithelium by ultrastructural immunoperoxidase cytochemistry. J Histochem Cytochem 1986;34:801–809.

77. Sloane JP, Ormerod MG. Distribution of epithelial membrane antigen in normal and neoplastic tissues and its value in diagnostic tumor pathology. Cancer 1981;47: 1786–1795.

78. Ormerod MG, Steele K, Westwood JH, Mazzini MN. Epithelial membrane antigen: Partial purification, assay, and properties. Br J Cancer 1983;48:533–541.

79. Heyderman E, Strudley I, Powell G, et al. A new monoclonal antibody to epithelial membrane antigen (EMA)—E29: A comparison of its immunocytochemical reactivity with polyclonal anti-EMA antibodies and another monoclonal antibody, HMFG-2. Br J Cancer 1985;52:355–361.

80. Cordell J, Richardson TC, Pulford KAF, et al. Production of monoclonal antibodies against human epithelial membrane antigen for use in diagnostic immunocytochemistry. Br J Cancer 1985;52:347–354.

81. Wick MR, Swanson PE, Manivel JC. Immunohistochemical analysis of soft tissue sarcomas: Comparisons with electron microscopy. Appl Pathol 1988;6:169–196.

82. Swanson PE, Manivel JC, Scheithauer BW, Wick MR. Epi-

thelial membrane antigen in human sarcomas: An immunohistochemical study. Surg Pathol 1989;2:313–322.

83. Miettinen M. Antibody specificity to muscle actins in the diagnosis and classification of soft tissue tumors. Am J Pathol 1988;130:205–215.

84. Schurch W, Skalli O, Seemayer TA, Gabbiani G. Intermediate filament proteins and actin isoforms as markers for soft tissue tumor differentiation and origin. I: Smooth muscle tumors. Am J Pathol 1987;128:91–103.

85. Tsukada T, McNutt MA, Ross R, Gown AM. HHF35, a muscle actin-specific monoclonal antibody. II: Reactivity in normal, reactive, and neoplastic human tissue. Am J Pathol 1987;127:389–402.

86. Jones H, Steart PV, DuBoulay CE, Roche WR. Alpha-smooth muscle actin as a marker for soft tissue tumors: A comparison with desmin. J Pathol 1990;162:29–33.

87. Cintorino M, Vindigni C, DelVecchio MT, et al. Expression of actin isoforms and intermediate filament proteins in childhood orbital rhabdomyosarcomas. J Submicrosc Cytol Pathol 1989;21:409–419.

88. Bussolati G, Papotti M, Foschini MP, Eusebi V. The interest of actin immunocytochemistry in diagnostic histopathology. Basic Appl Histochem 1987;31:165–176.

89. Ogut O, Granzier H, Jin JP. Acidic and basic troponin-T isoforms in mature fast-twitch skeletal muscle and effect on contractility. Am J Physiol 1999;276:C1162–C1170.

90. Lutz GJ, Lieber RL. Skeletal muscle myosin-II structure and function. Exerc Sport Sci Rev 1999;27:63–77.

91. Lefevre G. Troponins: Biological and clinical aspects. Ann Biol Clin 2000;58:39–48.

92. Atkinson RA, Joseph C, Dal Piaz F, et al. Binding of alpha-actinin to titin: Implications for Z-disk assembly. Biochemistry 2000;39:5255–5264.

93. Dodd S, Malone M, McCulloch W. Rhabdomyosarcoma in children: A histological and immunohistochemical study of 59 cases. J Pathol 1989;158:13–18.

94. Lai R, Tian Y, An J, et al. A comparative study on morphology and immunohistochemistry of rhabdomyosarcoma and embryonal skeletal muscles. Chin Med J 1997;110:392–396.

95. Gruchala A, Niezabitowski A, Wasilewska A, et al. Rhabdomyosarcoma: Morphologic, immunohistochemical, and DNA study. Gen Diagn Pathol 1997;142:175–184.

96. Carter RL, Jameson CF, Philp ER, Pinkerton CR. Comparative phenotypes in rhabdomyosarcoma and developing skeletal muscle. Histopathology 1990;17:301–309.

97. Saku T, Tsuda N, Anami M, Okabe H. Smooth and skeletal muscle myosins in spindle cell tumors of soft tissue: An immunohistochemical study. Acta Pathol Jpn 1985;35:125–136.

98. Osborn M, Hill C, Altmannsberger M, Weber K. Monoclonal antibodies to titin in conjunction with antibodies to desmin separate rhabdomyosarcomas from other tumor types. Lab Invest 1986;55:101–108.

99. Moczygemba C, Guidry J, Wittung-Stafshede P. Heme orientation affects holo-myoglobin folding and unfolding kinetics. FEBS Lett 2000;470:203–206.

100. Parham DM, Webber B, Holt H, et al. Immunohistochemical study of childhood rhabdomyosarcomas and related neoplasms: Results of an Intergroup Rhabdomyosarcoma Study project. Cancer 1991;67:3072–3080.

101. Carter RL, McCarthy KP, Machin LG, et al. Expression of desmin and myoglobin in rhabdomyosarcomas and in developing skeletal muscle. Histopathology 1989;15:585–595.

102. Coindre JM, deMascarel A, Trojani M, et al. Immunohistochemical study of rhabdomyosarcoma: Unexpected staining with S100 protein and cytokeratin. J Pathol 1988;155:127–132.

103. Seidal T, Kindblom LG, Angervall L. Myoglobin, desmin, and vimentin in ultrastructurally proven rhabdomyomas and rhabdomyosarcomas: An immunohistochemical study utilizing a series of monoclonal and polyclonal antibodies. Appl Pathol 1987;5:201–219.

104. Brooks JJ. Immunohistochemistry of soft tissue tumors: Myoglobin as a tumor marker for rhabdomyosarcoma. Cancer 1982;50:1757–1763.

105. Tsokos M, Howard R, Costa J: Immunohistochemical study of alveolar and embryonal rhabdomyosarcoma. Lab Invest 1983;48:148–155.

106. Kraevsky NA: Use of immunohistochemical methods in the diagnosis of myogenous tumors. Acta Histochem Suppl 1984;30:79–80.

107. Hosoi H, Sugimoto T, Hayashi Y, et al. Differential expression of myogenic regulatory genes, MyoD1 and myogenin, in human rhabdomyosarcoma sublines. Int J Cancer 1992;50:977–983.

108. Newsholme SJ, Zimmerman DM. Immunohistochemical evaluation of chemically induced rhabdomyosarcomas in rats: Diagnostic utility of MyoD1. Toxicol Pathol 1997;25:470–474.

109. Wang NP, Marx J, McNutt MA, et al. Expression of myogenic regulatory proteins (myogenin and MyoD1) in small blue round cell tumors of childhood. Am J Pathol 1995;147:1799–1810.

110. Cui S, Hano H, Harada T, et al. Evaluation of new monoclonal anti-MyoD1 and anti-myogenin antibodies for the diagnosis of rhabdomyosarcoma. Pathol Int 1999;49:62–68.

111. Dias P, Chen B, Dilday B, et al. Strong immunostaining for myogenin in rhabdomyosarcoma is significantly associated with tumors of the alveolar subclass. Am J Pathol 2000;156:399–408.

112. Watanabe K, Kusakabe T, Hoshi N, et al. h-Caldesmon in leiomyosarcoma and tumors with smooth muscle-like differentiation: Its specific expression in the smooth muscle cell tumors. Hum Pathol 1999;30:392–396.

113. Huber PA. Caldesmon. Int J Biochem Cell Biol 1997;29:1047–1051.

114. Shiro B, Siegal GP. The use of monoclonal antibodies to S100 protein in diagnostic immunohistochemistry. In: Wick MR, Siegal GP, eds. New York: Marcel Dekker, 1988:455–503.

115. Fujii T, Machino K, Andoh H, et al. Calcium-dependent control of caldesmon-actin interaction by S100 protein. J Biochem 1990;107:133–137.

116. Loeffel SC, Gillespie GY, Mirmiran SA, et al. Cellular immunolocalization of S100 protein within fixed tissue sections by monoclonal antibodies. Arch Pathol Lab Med 1985;109:117–122.

117. Masui F, Ushigome S, Fujii K. Clear cell chondrosarcoma: A pathological and immunohistochemical study. Histopathology 1999;34:447–452.

118. Abramovici LC, Steiner GC, Bonar F. Myxoid chondrosarcoma of soft tissue and bone: A retrospective study of 11 cases. Hum Pathol 1995;26:1215–1220.

119. Swanson PE, Wick MR. Clear cell sarcoma: An immunohistochemical analysis of six cases and comparison with other epithelioid neoplasms of soft tissue. Arch Pathol Lab Med 1989;113:55–60.

120. Kahn HJ, Marks A, Thom H, Baumal R. Role of antibody to S100 protein in diagnostic pathology. Am J Clin Pathol 1983;79:341–347.

121. Van den Berg LH, Sadiq SA, Thomas FP, Latov N. Characterization of HNK-1 bearing glycoproteins in human peripheral nerve myelin. J Neurosci Res 1990;25:295–299.

122. Weiss SW, Langloss JM, Enzinger FM. Value of S100 protein in the diagnosis of soft tissue tumors, with particular reference to benign and malignant Schwann cell tumors. Lab Invest 1983;49:299–308.

123. Hammer JA, O'Shannessy DJ, DeLeon M, et al. Immunoreactivity of PMP-22, P0, and other 19 to 28 kd glycoproteins in peripheral nerve myelin of mammals and fish with HNK-1 and related antibodies. J Neurosci Res 1993;35:546–558.

124. Merkouri E, Matsas R. Monoclonal antibody BM89 recognizes a novel cell surface glycoprotein of the L2/HNK-1 family in the developing mammalian nervous system. Neuroscience 1992;50:53–68.

125. Vogel M, Kowalewski HJ, Zimmermann H, et al. Association of the HNK-1 epitope with 5-nucleotidase from To marmorata (electric ray) electric organ. Biochem J 1991;278:199–202.

126. Abo T, Balch CM. A differentiation antigen of human NK and killer cells, identified by a monoclonal antibody (HNK-1). J Immunol 1981;127:1024–1029.

127. Hirose T, Scheithauer BW, Sano T. Perineurial malignant peripheral nerve sheath tumor (MPNST): A clinicopathologic, immunohistochemical, and ultrastructural study of seven cases. Am J Surg Pathol 1998;22:1368–1378.

128. Swanson PE, Manivel JC, Wick MR. Immunoreactivity for Leu7 in neurofibrosarcoma and other spindle cell sarcomas of soft tissue. Am J Pathol 1987;126:546–560.

129. Michels S, Swanson PE, Robb JA, Wick MR. Leu7 in small cell neoplasms: An immunohistochemical study. Cancer 1987;60:2958–2964.

130. Amann G, Zoubek A, Salzer-Kuntschik M, et al. Relation of neurological marker expression and EWS gene fusion types in MIC2/CD99-positive tumors of the Ewing family. Hum Pathol 30:1058–1064.

131. Abe S, Imamura T, Park P, et al. Small round cell type of malignant peripheral nerve sheath tumor. Mod Pathol 1998;11:747–753.

132. Gardner LJ, Polski JM, Fallon R, Dunphy CH. Identification of CD56 and CD57 by flow cytometry in Ewing's sarcoma or primitive neuroectodermal tumor. Virchows Arch A 1998;433:35–40.

133. Sangueza OP, Requena L. Neoplasms with neural differentiation: A review. Part II: Malignant neoplasms. Am J Dermatopathol 1998;20:89–102.

134. Devaney K, Vinh TN, Sweet DE. Small cell osteosarcoma of bone: An immunohistochemical study with differential diagnostic considerations. Hum Pathol 1993;24:1211–1225.

135. Pettinato G, Manivel JC, d'Amore ESG, et al. Melanotic neuroectodermal tumor of infancy: A reexamination of a histogenetic problem based on immunohistochemical, flow cytometric, and ultrastructural study of 10 cases. Am J Surg Pathol 1991;15:233–245.

136. Salzer JL, Holmes WP, Colman DR. The amino acid sequences of the myelin-associated glycoproteins: Homology to the immunoglobulin gene superfamily. J Cell Biol 1987; 104:959–965.

137. Dixit SN, Mainardi CL, Beachey EH, Kang AH. 7S domain constitutes the amino-terminal end of type IV collagen: An immunohistochemical study. Coll Rel Res 1983;3:263–273.

138. Griffin CA, Emanuel BS, Hansen JR, et al. Human collagen genes encoding basement membrane alpha-1 (IV) and alpha-2 (IV) chains map to the distal long arm of chromosome 13. Proc Natl Acad Sci U S A 1987;84:512–516.

139. Terranova VP, Rohrbach DH, Martin GR. Role of laminin in the attachment of PAM212 (epithelial) cells to basement membrane collagen. Cell 1980;22:719–726.

140. Foidart JM, Bere EW, Yaar M Jr, et al. Distribution and immunoelectron microscopic localization of laminin, a noncollagenous basement membrane glycoprotein. Lab Invest 1980;42:336–342.

141. McGarvey ML, Baron-Van Evercooren BV, Kleinman KH, et al. Synthesis and effects of basement membrane components in cultured rat Schwann cells. Dev Biol 1984;105: 18–28.

142. Nigar E, Dervan PA. Quantitative assessment of basement membranes in soft tissue tumors: Computerized image analysis of laminin and type IV collagen. J Pathol 1998; 185:184–187.

143. Ogawa K, Oguchi M, Yamabe H, et al. Distribution of collagen type IV in soft tissue tumors: An immunohistochemical study. Cancer 1986;58:269–277.

144. d'Ardenne AJ, Kirkpatrick P, Sykes BC. Distribution of laminin, fibronectin, and interstitial collagen type III in soft tissue tumors. J Clin Pathol 1984;37:895–904.

145. Fischer BE, Thomas KB, Schlokat U, Doruer F. Triplet structure of human von Willebrand factor. Biochem J 1998;331:483–488.

146. Kaufman RJ, Pipe SW. Regulation of factor VIII expression and activity by von Willebrand factor. Thromb Haemost 1999;82:201–208.

147. Mukai K, Rosai J. Factor VIII-related antigen: An endothelial marker. In: DeLellis RA, ed. Diagnostic Immunohistochemistry. New York: Masson, 1984:243–261.

148. Sehested M, Hou-Jensen K. Factor VIII-related antigen as an endothelial cell marker in benign and malignant diseases. Virchows Arch A 1981;391:217–225.

149. Ordonez NG, Batsakis JG. Comparison of *Ulex europaeus I*

lectin and factor VIII-related antigen in vascular lesions. Arch Pathol Lab Med 1984;108:129–132.

150. Swanson PE, Wick MR. Immunohistochemical evaluation of vascular neoplasms. Clin Dermatol 1991;9:243–253.

151. Ramani P, Bradley NJ, Fletcher CDM. QBEND10, a new monoclonal antibody to endothelium: Assessment of its diagnostic utility in paraffin sections. Histopathology 1990; 17:237–242.

152. Traweek ST, Kandalaft PL, Mehta P, Battifora H. The human hematopoietic progenitor cell antigen (CD34) in vascular neoplasms. Am J Clin Pathol 1991;96:25–31.

153. Sirgi KE, Wick MR, Swanson PE. B72.3 and CD34 immunoreactivity in malignant epithelioid soft tissue tumors: Adjuncts in the recognition of endothelial neoplasms. Am J Surg Pathol 1993;17:179–185.

154. Miettinen M, Lindenmayer AE, Chanbal A. Endothelial cell markers CD31, CD34, and BNH9 antibody to H- and Y-antigens: Evaluation of their specificity and sensitivity in the diagnosis of vascular tumors and comparison with von Willebrand factor. Mod Pathol 1994;7:82–90.

155. Natkunam Y, Rouse RV, Zhu S, et al. Immunoblot analysis of CD34 expression in histologically diverse neoplasms. Am J Pathol 2000;156:21–27.

156. Arber DA, Kandalaft PL, Mehta P, Battifora H. Vimentin-negative epithelioid sarcoma: The value of an immunohistochemical panel that includes CD34. Am J Surg Pathol 1993;17:302–317.

157. Harvell JD, Kilpatrick SE, White WL. Histologic relations between giant cell fibroblastoma and dermatofibrosarcoma protuberans: CD34 staining showing the spectrum and a simulator. Am J Dermatopathol 1998;20:339–345.

158. Templeton SF, Solomon AR Jr. Spindle cell lipoma is strongly CD34-positive: An immunohistochemical study. J Cutan Pathol 1996;23:546–550.

159. Hasegawa T, Matsuno Y, Shimoda T, et al. Extrathoracic solitary fibrous tumors: Their histological variability and potentially aggressive behavior. Hum Pathol 1999;30:1464–1473.

160. Metzelaar MJ, Korteweg J, Sizma JJ, Nieuwenhuis HK. Biochemical characterization of PECAM-1 (CD31 antigen) on human platelets. Thromb Haemost 1991;66:700–707.

161. Parums DV, Cordell JL, Michlein K, et al. JC70: A new monoclonal antibody that detects vascular endothelium associated antigen on routinely processed tissue sections. J Clin Pathol 1990;43:752–757.

162. Ohsawa M, Naka N, Tomita Y, et al. Use of immunohistochemical procedures in diagnosing angiosarcomas: Evaluation of 98 cases. Cancer 1995;75:2867–2874.

163. DeYoung BR, Wick MR, Fitzgibbon JF, et al. CD31: An immunospecific marker for endothelial differentiation in human neoplasms. Appl Immunohistochem 1993;1:97–100.

164. DeYoung BR, Swanson PE, Argenyi ZB, et al. CD31 immunoreactivity in mesenchymal neoplasms of the skin and subcutis. J Cutan Pathol 1995;22:215–222.

165. Takahashi Y, Hosaka Y, Niina H, et al. Soluble thrombomodulin purified from human urine exhibits a potent anticoagulant effect in vitro and in vivo. Thromb Haemost 1995;73:805–811.

166. Kurosawa S, Galvin JB, Esmon NC, Esmon CT. Proteolytic formation and properties of functional domains of thrombomodulin. J Biol Chem 1987;262:2206–2212.

167. Karmochkine M, Boffa MC. Thrombomodulin: Physiology and clinical applications. Rev Med Interne 1997;18:119–125.

168. Yonezawa S, Maruyama I, Sakae K, et al. Thrombomodulin as a marker for vascular tumors: Comparative study with factor VIII and *Ulex europaeus I* lectin. Am J Clin Pathol 1987;88:405–411.

169. Kim SJ, Shiba E, Ishii H, et al. Thrombomodulin is a new biological and prognostic marker for breast cancer: An immunohistochemical study. Anticancer Res 1997;17:2319–2323.

170. Ordonez NG. Value of thrombomodulin immunostaining in the diagnosis of mesothelioma. Histopathology 1997;31: 25–30.

171. Appleton MA, Attanoos RL, Jasani B. Thrombomodulin as

a marker of vascular and lymphatic tumors. Histopathology 1996;29:153–157.

172. Zhang YM, Bachmann S, Hemmer C, et al. Vascular origin of Kaposi's sarcoma: Expression of leukocytic adhesion molecule-1, thrombomodulin, and tissue factor. Am J Pathol 1994;144:51–59.

173. Holthofer H, Virtanen I, Kariniemi AL, et al. *Ulex europaeus I* lectin as a marker for vascular endothelium in human tissues. Lab Invest 1982;47:60–66.

174. Leader M, Collins M, Patel J, Henry K. Staining or factor VIII–related antigen and *Ulex europaeus I* (UEA-I) in 230 tumors: An assessment of their specificity for angiosarcoma and Kaposi's sarcoma. Histopathology 1986;10:1153–1162.

175. Wick MR, Manivel JC. Epithelioid sarcoma and epithelioid hemangioendothelioma: An immunohistochemical and lectin-histochemical comparison. Virchows Arch A 1987;410:309–316.

176. DuBoulay CEH. Demonstration of alpha-1-antitrypsin and alpha-1-antichymotrypsin in fibrous histiocytomas using the immunoperoxidase technique. Am J Surg Pathol 1982;6:559–564.

177. Kindblom LG, Jacobsen GK, Jacobsen M. Immunohistochemical investigations of tumors of supposed fibroblastic-histiocytic origin. Hum Pathol 1982;13:834–840.

178. Meister P, Nathrath W. Immunohistochemical characterization of histiocytic tumors. Diagn Histopathol 1981;4:79–87.

179. Pulford KAF, Rigney EM, Micklem KJ, et al. KP1: A new monoclonal antibody that detects a monocyte/macrophage–associated antigen in routinely processed tissue sections. J Clin Pathol 1989;42:414–421.

180. Gloghini A, Volpe R, Carbone A. Ki-M6 immunostaining in routinely processed sections of reactive and neoplastic human lymphoid tissue. Am J Clin Pathol 1990;94:734–741.

181. Gown AM, Tsukada T, Ross R. Human atherosclerosis. II: Immunocytochemical analysis of the cellular composition of human atherosclerotic lesions. Am J Pathol 1986;125:191–207.

182. Takeya M, Yamashiro S, Yoshimura T, Takahashi K. Immunophenotypic and immunoelectron microscopic characterization of major constituent cells in malignant fibrous histiocytoma using human cell lines and their transplanted tumors in immunodeficient mice. Lab Invest 1995;72:679–688.

183. Nemes Z, Thomazy V. Factor XIIIa and the classic histiocytic markers in malignant fibrous histiocytoma: A comparative immunohistochemical study. Hum Pathol 1988;19:822–829.

184. Reid MB, Gray C, Fear JD, Bird CC. Immunohistologic demonstration of factors XIIIa and XIIIs in reactive and neoplastic fibroblastic and fibrohistiocytic lesions. Histopathology 1986;10:1171–1178.

185. Thewes M, Engst R, Boeck K, Ring J. Expression of cathepsins in dermal fibrous tumors: An immunohistochemical study. Eur J Dermatol 1998;8:86–89.

186. Gloghini A, Rizzo A, Zanette I, et al. KP1/CD68 expression in malignant neoplasms including lymphomas, sarcomas, and carcinomas. Am J Clin Pathol 1995;103:425–431.

187. Doussis IA, Gatter KC, Mason DY. CD68 reactivity of non-macrophage-derived tumors in cytological specimens. J Clin Pathol 1993;46:334–336.

188. Schulz A, Loreth B, Battmann A, et al. Bone matrix production in osteosarcoma. Verh Dtsch Ges Pathol 1998;82:144–153.

189. Park YK, Yang MH, Kim YW, Park HR. Osteocalcin expression in primary bone tumors: In situ hybridization and immunohistochemical study. J Korean Med Sci 1995;10:263–268.

190. Lian JB, Stein GS. Development of the osteoblast phenotype: Molecular mechanisms mediating osteoblast growth and development. Iowa Orthop J 1995;15:118–140.

191. Tamura T, Noda M. Identification of a DNA sequence involved in osteoblast-specific gene expression via interaction with helix-loop-helix (HLH)-type transcription factors. J Cell Biol 1994;126:773–782.

192. Garnero P, Grimaux M, Seguin P, Delmas PD. Characterization of immunoreactive forms of human osteocalcin generated in vivo and in vitro. J Bone Miner Res 1994;9:255–264.

193. Mahonen A, Jaaskelainen T, Maenpaa PH. A novel vitamin D analog with two double bonds in its side chain: A potent inducer of osteoblastic cell differentiation. Biochem Pharmacol 1996;51:887–892.

194. Arbour NC, Darwish HM, DeLuca HF. Transcriptional control of the osteocalcin gene by 1/25 dihydroxyvitamin D-2 and its 24-epimer in rat osteosarcoma cells. Biochim Biophys Acta 1995;1263:147–153.

195. Bradbeer JN, Virdi AS, Serre CM, et al. A number of osteocalcin antisera recognize epitopes on proteins other than osteocalcin in cultured skin fibroblasts: Implications for the identification of cells of the osteoblastic lineage in vitro. J Bone Miner Res 1994;9:1221–1228.

196. Takada J, Ishii S, Ohta T, et al. Usefulness of a novel monoclonal antibody against human osteocalcin in immunohistochemical diagnosis. Virchows Arch A 1992;420:507–511.

197. Fanburg JC, Rosenberg AE, Weaver DL, et al. Osteocalcin and osteonectin immunoreactivity in the diagnosis of osteosarcoma. Am J Clin Pathol 1997;108:464–473.

198. Fanburg-Smith JC, Bratthauer GL, Miettinen M. Osteocalcin and osteonectin immunoreactivity in extraskeletal osteosarcoma: A study of 28 cases. Hum Pathol 1999;30:32–38.

199. Naylor SL, Helin-Davies D, Charoenworawat P, et al. The human osteonectin gene (OSN) has Taq I and Msp I polymorphisms. Nucleic Acids Res 1989;17:6753.

200. Rodan GA, Noda M. Gene expression in osteoblastic cells. Crit Rev Eukaryot Gene Expr 1991;1:85–98.

201. Villarreal XC, Grant BW, Long GL. Demonstration of osteonectin mRNA in megakaryocytes: The use of the polymerase chain reaction. Blood 1991;78:1216–1222.

202. Kelm RJ Jr, Hair GA, Mann KG, Grant BW. Characterization of human osteoblast and megakaryocyte-derived osteonectin (SPARC). Blood 1992;80:3112–3119.

203. Kamihagi K, Katayama M, Ouchi R, Kato I. Osteonectin/SPARC regulates cellular secretion rates of fibronectin and laminin extracellular matrix proteins. Biochem Biophys Res Commun 1994;200:423–428.

204. Serra M, Morini MC, Scotlandi K, et al. Evaluation of osteonectin as a diagnostic marker of osteogenic bone tumors. Hum Pathol 1992;23:1326–1331.

205. Wuisman P, Roessner A, Bosse A, et al. Osteonectin in osteosarcomas: A marker for differential diagnosis and/or prognosis? Ann Oncol 1992;3(Suppl 2):S33–S35.

206. Bosse A, Vollmer E, Bocker W, et al. The impact of osteonectin for differential diagnosis of bone tumors: An immunohistochemical approach. Pathol Res Pract 1990;186:651–657.

207. Fetsch PA, Marincola FM, Filie A, et al. Melanoma-associated antigen recognized by T-cells (MART-1): The advent of a preferred immunocytochemical antibody for the diagnosis of metastatic malignant melanoma with fine needle aspiration. Cancer 1999;87:37–42.

208. Kaufmann O, Koch S, Burghardt J, et al. Tyrosinase, melan-A, and KBA62 as markers for the immunohistochemical identification of metastatic amelanotic melanomas in paraffin sections. Mod Pathol 1998;11:740–746.

209. Zelger BG, Steiner H, Wambacher B, Zelger B. Malignant melanomas simulating various types of soft tissue tumors. Dermatol Surg 1997;23:1047–1054.

210. Fetsch JF, Michal M, Miettinen M. Pigmented (melanotic) neurofibroma: A clinicopathologic and immunohistochemical analysis of 19 lesions from 17 patients. Am J Surg Pathol 2000;24:331–343.

211. Cangul IT, van Garderen E, Van der Poel HJ, et al. Tyrosinase gene expression in clear cell sarcoma indicates a melanocytic origin: Insight from the first reported canine case. APMIS 1999;107:982–988.

212. Papas-Corden P, Zarbo RJ, Gown AM, Crissman JD. Immunohistochemical characterization of synovial, epithelioid, and clear cell sarcomas. Surg Pathol 1989;2:43–58.

213. Gould VE, Wiedenmann B, Lee I, et al. Synaptophysin expression in neuroendocrine neoplasms as determined by immunocytochemistry. Am J Pathol 1987;126:243–257.

214. Ladanyi M, Heinemann FS, Huvos AG, et al. Neural differentiation in small round cell tumors of bone and soft tissue with the translocation t(11;22)(q24;q12): An immunohistochemical study of 11 cases. Hum Pathol 1990;21:1245–1251.

215. Parham DM, Hijazi Y, Steinberg SM, et al. Neuroectodermal differentiation in Ewing's sarcoma family of tumors does not predict tumor behavior. Hum Pathol 1999;30:911–918.

216. Roessner A, Jurgens H. Round cell tumors of bone. Pathol Res Pract 1993;189:111–136.

217. Dierick AM, Roels H, Langlois M. The immunophenotype of Ewing's sarcoma: An immunohistochemical analysis. Pathol Res Pract 1993;189:26–32.

218. Wang AR, May D, Bourne P, Scott G. PGP9.5: A marker for cellular neurothekeoma. Am J Surg Pathol 1999;23:1401–1407.

219. Miettinen M, Chatten J, Paetau A, Stevenson A. Monoclonal antibody NB84 in the differential diagnosis of neuroblastoma and other small round cell tumors. Am J Surg Pathol 1998;22:327–332.

220. Gerbig AW, Zala L, Hunziker T. Tumor-like eosinophilic granuloma of the skin. Am J Dermatopathol 2000;22:75–78.

221. Stefanato CM, Andersen WK, Calonje E, et al. Langerhans cell histiocytosis in the elderly: A report of three cases. J Am Acad Dermatol 1998;39:375–378.

222. Knowles DM II. Lymphoid cell markers: Their distribution and usefulness in the immunopathologic analysis of lymphoid neoplasms. Am J Surg Pathol 1985;9(Suppl):85–108.

223. Weiss LM, Bindl JM, Picozzi VJ, et al. Lymphoblastic lymphoma: An immunophenotypic study of 26 cases with comparison to T-cell acute lymphoblastic leukemia. Blood 1986;67:474–478.

224. Picker LJ, Weiss LM, Medeiros LJ, et al. Immunophenotypic criteria for the diagnosis of non-Hodgkin's lymphoma. Am J Pathol 1987;128:181–201.

225. Ozdemirli M, Fanburg-Smith JC, Hartmann DP, et al. Precursor B-lymphoblastic lymphoma presenting as a solitary bone tumor and mimicking Ewing's sarcoma: A report of four cases and review of the literature. Am J Surg Pathol 1998;22:795–804.

226. Petruch UR, Horny HP, Kaiserling E. Frequent expression of hematopoietic and non-hematopoietic antigens by neoplastic plasma cells: An immunohistochemical study using formalin-fixed, paraffin-embedded tissue. Histopathology 1992;20:35–40.

227. Robertson PB, Neiman RS, Worapongpaiboon S, et al. O13 (CD99) positivity in hematologic proliferations correlates with TdT positivity. Mod Pathol 1997;10:277–282.

228. Soslow RA, Bhargava V, Warnke RA. MIC2, TdT, bcl-2, and CD34 expression in paraffin-embedded high-grade lymphoma/acute lymphoblastic leukemia distinguishes between distinct clinicopathologic entities. Hum Pathol 1997;28:1158–1165.

229. Hibshoosh H, Lattes R. Immunohistochemical and molecular genetic approaches to soft tissue tumor diagnosis: A primer. Semin Oncol 1997;24:515–525.

230. Smith MJ, Goodfellow PN. MIC2R: A transcribed MIC2-related sequence associated with a CpG island in the human pseudoautosomal region. Hum Mol Genet 1994;3:1575–1582.

231. Smith MJ, Goodfellow PJ, Goodfellow PN. The genomic organization of the human pseudoautosomal gene MIC2 and the detection of a related locus. Hum Mol Genet 1993;2:417–422.

232. Fellinger EJ, Garin-Chesa P, Su SL, et al. Biochemical and genetic characterization of the HBA-71 Ewing's sarcoma cell surface antigen. Cancer Res 1991;51:336–340.

233. Amann G, Zoubek A, Salzer-Kuntschik M, et al. Relation of neurological marker expression and EWS gene fusion types in MIC2/CD99-positive tumors of the Ewing family. Hum Pathol 1999;30:1058–1064.

234. Renshaw AA: O13 (CD99) in spindle cell tumors: Reactivity with hemangiopericytoma, solitary fibrous tumor, synovial sarcoma, and meningioma, but rarely with sarcomatoid mesothelioma. Appl Immunohistochem 1995;3:250–256.

235. Soslow RA, Wallace M, Goris J, et al. MIC2 gene expression in cutaneous neuroendocrine carcinoma (Merkel cell carcinoma). Appl Immunohistochem 1996;4:235–240.

236. Lumadue JA, Askin FB, Perlman EJ. MIC2 analysis of small cell carcinoma. Am J Clin Pathol 1994;102:692–694.

237. Nicholson SA, McDermott MB, Swanson PE, Wick MR. CD99 and cytokeratin-20 in small-cell and basaloid tumors of the skin. Appl Immunohistochem Mol Morphol 2000;8:37–41.

238. Eckert F, Schaich B. Tenson sheath fibroma: A case report with immunohistochemical studies. Hautarzt 1992;43:92–96.

239. Ide F, Shimoyama T, Horie N, Tanaka H. Collagenous fibroma (desmoplastic fibroblastoma) presenting as a parotid mass. J Oral Pathol Med 1999;28:465–468.

240. Neilsen GP, O'Connell JX, Dickersin GR, Rosenberg AE. Collagenous fibroma (desmoplastic fibroblastoma): A report of seven cases. Mod Pathol 1996;9:781–785.

241. Sciot R, Samson I, van der Berghe H, et al. Collagenous fibroma (desmoplastic fibroblastoma): Genetic link with fibroma of tendon sheath? Mod Pathol 1999;12:565–568.

242. Carney JA: Psammomatous melanotic schwannoma: A distinctive, heritable tumor with special associations, including cardiac myxoma and the Cushing syndrome. Am J Surg Pathol 1990;14:206–222.

243. Templeton SF, Solomon AR Jr. Spindle cell lipoma is strongly CD34 positive: An immunohistochemical study. J Cutan Pathol 1996;23:546–550.

244. Suster S, Fisher C. Immunoreactivity for the human hematopoietic progenitor cell antigen (CD34) in lipomatous tumors. Am J Surg Pathol 1997;21:195–200.

245. Shimokama T, Watanabe T. Leiomyoma exhibiting a marked granular change: Granular cell leiomyoma versus granular cell schwannoma. Hum Pathol 1992;23:327–331.

246. Mazur MT, Shultz JJ, Myers JL. Granular cell tumor: Immunohistochemical analysis of 21 benign tumors and one malignant tumor. Arch Pathol Lab Med 1990;114:692–696.

247. Cavaliere A, Sidoni A, Ferri I, Falini B. Granular cell tumor: An immunohistochemical study. Tumori 1994;80:224–228.

248. Kurtin PJ, Bonin DM. Immunohistochemical demonstration of the lysosome-associated glycoprotein CD68 (KP-1) in granular cell tumors and schwannomas. Hum Pathol 1994;25:1172–1178.

249. Filie AC, Lage JM, Azumi N. Immunoreactivity of S100 protein, alpha-1-antitrypsin, and CD68 in adult and congenita granular cell tumors. Mod Pathol 1996;9:888–892.

250. Younes M, Lechago LV, Lechago J. Overexpression of the human erythrocyte glucose transporter occurs as a late event in human colorectal carcinogenesis and is associated with an increased incidence of lymph node metastases. Clin Cancer Res 1996;2:1151–1154.

251. Haber RS, Weiser KR, Pritsker A, et al. GLUT1 glucose transporter expression in benign and malignant thyroid nodules. Thyroid 1997;7:363–367.

252. North PE, Waner M, Mizeracki A, Mihm MC Jr. GLUT1: A newly discovered immunohistochemical marker for juvenile hemangiomas. Hum Pathol 2000;31:11–22.

253. Younes M, Brown RW, Stephenson M, et al. Overexpression of Glut1 and Glut3 in stage I nonsmall cell lung cancer is associated with poor survival. Cancer 1997;80:1046–1051.

254. Kapadia SB, Meis JM, Frisman DM, et al. Fetal rhabdomyoma of the head and neck: A clinicopathological and immunophenotypic study of 24 cases. Hum Pathol 1993;24:754–765.

255. Tanda F, Rocca PC, Bosincu L, et al. Rhabdomyomas of the tunica vaginalis of the testis: A histologic, immunohistochemical, and ultrastructural study. Mod Pathol 1997;10:608–611.
256. Bastian BC, Brocker EB. Adult rhabdomyoma of the lip. Am J Dermatopathol 1998;20:61–64.
257. Gibas Z, Miettinen M. Recurrent parapharyngeal rhabdomyoma: Evidence of neoplastic nature of the tumor from cytogenetic study. Am J Surg Pathol 1192;16:721–728.
258. Ockner DM, Sayadi H, Swanson SE, et al. Genital angiomyofibroblastoma: Comparison with aggressive angiomyxoma and other myxoid neoplasms of skin and soft tissue. Am J Clin Pathol 1997;107:36–44.
259. Fletcher CDM, Tsang WTW, Fisher C, et al. Angiomyofibroblastoma of the vulva: A benign neoplasm distinct from aggressive angiomyxoma. Am J Surg Pathol 1992;16:373–382.
260. Neilsen GP, Rosenberg AE, Young RH, et al. Angiomyofibroblastoma of the vulva and vagina. Mod Pathol 1996;9:284–291.
261. Granter SR, Nucci MR, Fletcher CD. Aggressive angiomyxoma: Reappraisal of its relationship to angiomyofibroblastoma in a series of 16 cases. Histopathology 1997;30:3–10.
262. Laskin WB, Fetsch JF, Tavassoli FA. Angiomyofibroblastoma of the female genital tract: Analysis of 17 cases including a lipomatous variant. Hum Pathol 1997;28:1046–1055.
263. Enzinger FM, Weiss SW. Fibrous tumors of infancy and childhood. In: Enzinger FM, Weiss SW, eds. Soft Tissue Tumors. St Louis, Mosby–Yearbook, 1995:722.
264. Nemes Z. Differentiation markers in hemangiopericytoma. Cancer 1992;69:133–140.
265. Molnar P, Nemes Z. Hemangiopericytoma of the cerebellopontine angle: Diagnostic pitfalls and the diagnostic value of the subunit A of factor XIII as a tumor marker. Clin Neuropathol 1995;14:19–24.
266. Catalano PJ, Brandwein M, Shah DK, et al. Sinonasal hemangiopericytomas: A clinicopathologic and immunohistochemical study of seven cases. Head Neck 1996;18:42–53.
267. Middleton LP, Duray PH, Merino MJ. The histological spectrum of hemangiopericytoma: Application of immunohistochemical analysis including proliferative markers to facilitate diagnosis and predict prognosis. Hum Pathol 1998;29:636–640.
268. Klempreer P, Rabin CB. Primary neoplasms of the pleura: A report of five cases. Arch Pathol 1931;11:385–412.
269. Hanau CA, Miettinen M. Solitary fibrous tumor: Histological and immunohistochemical spectrum of benign and malignant variants presenting at different sites. Hum Pathol 1995;26:440–449.
270. Hasegawa T, Matsuno Y, Shimoda T, et al. Frequent expression of bcl-2 protein in solitary fibrous tumors. Jpn J Clin Oncol 1998;28:86–91.
271. Brunnemann RB, Ro JY, Ordonez NG, et al. Extrapleural solitary fibrous tumor: A clinicopathologic study of 24 cases. Mod Pathol 1999;12:1034–1042.
272. de Saint Aubain Somerhausen N, Rubin BP, Fletcher CD. Myxoid solitary fibrous tumor: A study of seven cases with emphasis on differential diagnosis. Mod Pathol 1999;12:463–471.
273. Matsumoto K, Yamamoto T, Min W, et al. Ossifying fibromyxoid tumor of soft parts: Clinicopathologic, immunohistochemical and ultrastructural study of four cases. Pathol Int 1999;49:742–746.
274. Ekfors TO, Kulju T, Aaltonen M, Kallajoki M. Ossifying fibromyxoid tumour of soft parts: Report of four cases including one mediastinal and one infanile. APMIS 1998;106:1124–1130.
275. Yang P, Hirose T, Hasegawa T, et al. Ossifying fibromyxoid tumor of soft parts: A morphological and immunohistochemical study. Pathol Int 1994;44:448–453.
276. Miettinen M. Ossifying fibromyxoid tumor of soft parts: Additional observations of a distinctive soft tissue tumor. Am J Clin Pathol 1991;95:142–149.
277. Fukunaga M, Ushigome S, Ishikawa E. Ossifying subcutaneous tumor with myofibroblastic differentiation: A variant of ossifying fibromyxoid tumor of soft parts? Pathol Int 1994;44:727–734.
278. Schofield JB, Krausz T, Stamp GW, et al. Ossifying fibromyxoid tumour of soft parts: Immunohistochemical and ultrastructural analysis. Histopathology 1999;22:101–112.
279. Williams SB, Ellis GL, Meis JM, Heffner DK. Ossifying fibromyxoid tumour (of soft parts) of the head and neck: A clinicopathological and immunohistochemical study of nine cases. J Laryngol Otol 1993;107:75–80.
280. Hamakawa H, Omori T, Sumida T, Tanioka H. Intraosseous epithelioid hemangioendothelioma of the mandible: A case report with an immunohistochemical study. J Oral Pathol Med 1999;28:233–237.
281. Siddiqui MT, Evans HL, Ro JY, Ayala AG. Epithelioid haemangioendothelioma of the thyroid gland: A case report and review of literature. Histopathology 1998;32:473–476.
282. Gray MH, Rosenberg AE, Dickerson GR, Bhan AK. Cytokeratin expression in epithelioid vascular neoplasms. Hum Pathol 1990;21:212–217.
283. Van Haelst UJ, Pruszczynski M, ten Cate LN, Mravunac M. Ultrastructural and immunohistochemical study of epithelioid hemangioendothelioma of bone: Coexpression of epithelial and endothelial markers. Ultrastruct Pathol 1990;14:141–149.
284. Mentzel T, Beham A, Calonje E, et al. Epithelioid hemangioendothelioma of skin and soft tissues: Clinicopathologic and immunohistochemical study of 30 cases. Am J Surg Pathol 1997;21:363–374.
285. Zukerberg LR, Nickoloff BJ, Weisee SW. Kaposiform hemangioendothelioma of infancy and childhood: An aggressive neoplasm associated with Kasaback-Merritt syndrome and lymphangiomatosis. Am J Surg Pathol 1993;17:321–328.
286. Hisaoka M, Hashimoto H, Iwamasa T. Diagnostic implication of Kaposi's sarcoma–associated herpesvirus with special reference to the distinction between spindle cell hemangioendothelioma and Kaposi's sarcoma. Arch Pathol Lab Med 1998;122:72–76.
287. Begin LR, Clement PB, Kirk ME, et al. Aggressive angiomyxoma of pelvic soft parts: A clinicopathologic study of nine cases. Hum Pathol 1985;16:621–628.
288. Sementa AR, Gambini C, Borgiani L, Comes P. Aggressive angiomyxoma of the pelvis and perineum: Report of a case with immunohistochemical and electron microscopic study. Pathologica 1989;81:463–469.
289. Sementa AR, Gambini C, Borgiani L, Comes P. Aggressive angiomyxoma of the pelvis and perineum: Report of a case with immunohistochemical and electron microscopic study. Pathologica 1989;81:463–469.
290. Tsang WY, Chan JK, Lee KC, et al. Aggressive angiomyxoma: A report of four cases occurring in men. Am J Surg Pathol 1992;16:1059–1065.
291. Tallini G, Parham DM, Dias P, et al. Myogenic regulatory protein expression in adult soft tissue sarcomas: A sensitive and specific marker of skeletal muscle differentiation. Am J Pathol 1994;144:693–701.
292. Dias P, Parham DM, Shapiro DN, et al. Myogenic regulatory protein (MyoD1) expression in childhood solid tumors: Diagnostic utility in rhabdomyosarcoma. Am J Pathol 1990;13:1283–1291.
293. Sorensen PH, Shimada H, Liu XF, et al. Biphenotypic sarcomas with myogenic and neural differentiation express the Ewing's sarcoma EWS/FLI1 fusion gene. Cancer Res 1995;15:1385–1392.
294. Gattenlohner S, Muller-Hernelink HK, Marx A. Polymerase chain reaction-based diagnosis of rhabdomyosarcomas: Comparison of fetal type acetylcholine receptor subunits and myogenin. Diagn Mol Pathol 1998;7:129–134.
295. Meyer T, Brinck U. Immunohistochemical detection of vinculin in human rhabdomyosarcomas. Gen Diagn Pathol 1997;142:191–198.
296. Pinto A, Paslawski D, Sarnat HB, Parham DM. Immunohistochemical evaluation of dystrophin expression in small round cell tumors of childhood. Mod Pathol 1993;6:679–683.

297. Bowman F, Champigneulle J, Schmitt C, et al. Clear cell rhabdomyosarcoma. Pediatr Pathol Lab Med 1996;16:951–959.

298. Kobayshi M, Sjoberg G, Soderhall S, et al. Pediatric rhabdomyosarcomas express the intermediate filament nestin. Pediatr Res 1998;43:86–92.

299. Yun K. A new marker for rhabdomyosarcoma: Insulin like growth factor II. Lab Invest 1992;67:653–664.

300. Gattenlohner S, Vincent A, Leuschner I, et al. The fetal form of the acetylcholine receptor distinguished rhabdomyosarcomas from other childhood tumors. Am J Pathol 1998;152:437–444.

301. Molenaar WM, Muntinghe FL. Expression of neural adhesion molecules and neurofilament protein isoforms in skeletal muscle tumors. Hum Pathol 1998;29:1290–1293.

302. Coffin CM, Rulon J, Smith L, et al. Pathologic features of rhabdomyosarcoma before and after treatment: A clinicopathologic and immunohistochemical analysis. Mod Pathol 1997;10:1175–1187.

303. Navarro S, Cavazzana AO, Llombart-Bosch A, Triche TJ. Comparison of Ewing's sarcoma of bone and peripheral neuroepithelioma: An immunocytochemical and ultrastructural analysis of two primitive neuroectodermal neoplasms. Arch Pathol Lab Med 1994;118:608–615.

304. Lizard-Nacol S, Justrabo E, Mugneret F, et al. Immunocytologic study of light cell lines established in vitro from Ewing's sarcoma: Identification of neural markers. C R Seances Soc Biol Fil 1988;182:118–125.

305. Lee CS, Southey MC, Waters K, et al. EWS/FLI-1 fusion transcript detection and MIC2 immunohistochemical staining in the detection of Ewing's sarcoma. Pediatr Pathol Lab Med 1996;16:379–392.

306. Scotlandi K, Serra M, Manara MC, et al. Immunostaining of the p30/32MIC2 antigen and molecular detection of EWS rearrangements for the diagnosis of Ewing's sarcoma and peripheral neuroectodermal tumor. Hum Pathol 1996;27:408–416.

307. de Alava E, Lozano MD, Sola I, et al. Molecular features in a biphenotypic small cell sarcoma with neuroectodermal and muscle differentiation. Hum Pathol 1998;29:181–184.

308. Knezevich SR, Hendson G, Methers JA, et al. Absence of detectable EWS/FLI1 expression after therapy-induced neural differentiation in Ewing sarcoma. Hum Pathol 1997;29:289–294.

309. Ambros IM, Ambros PF, Strehl S, et al. MIC2 is a specific marker for Ewing's sarcoma and peripheral primitive neuroectodermal tumors: Evidence for a common histogenesis of Ewing's sarcoma and peripheral primitive neuroectodermal tumors from MIC2 expression and specific chromosome aberration. Cancer 1991;67:1886–1893.

310. Fellinger EJ, Garin-Chesa P, Triche TJ, et al. Immunohistochemical analysis of Ewing's sarcoma cell surface antigen p30/32MIC2. Am J Pathol 1991;139:317–325.

311. Halliday BE, Slagel DD, Elsheikh TE, Silverman JF. Diagnostic utility of MIC-2 immunocytochemical staining in the differential diagnosis of small blue cell tumors. Diagn Cytopathol 1998;19:410–416.

312. Miettinen M, Lehto VP, Virtanen J. Histogenesis of Ewing's sarcoma: An evaluation of intermediate filaments and endothelial cell markers. Virchows Arch Cell Pathol 1988;41:277.

313. Navas-Palacios JJ, Aparicio-Duque R, Valdes MD. On the histogenesis of Ewing's sarcoma: An ultrastructural, immunohistochemical, and cytochemical study. Cancer 1984;53:1882.

314. Gu M, Antonescu CR, Guiter G, et al. Cytokeratin immunoreactivity in Ewing's sarcoma: Prevalence in 50 cases confirmed by molecular diagnostic studies. Am J Surg Pathol 1999;24:410–416.

315. Barth T, Moller P, Mechtersheimer G. Differential expression of beta 1, beta 3, beta 4 integrins in sarcomas of the small round blue cell category. Virchows Arch 1995;426:19–25.

316. Chung DH, Lee JI, Kook MC, et al. ILK (beta 1 integrin-linked protein kinase): A novel immunohistochemical marker for Ewing's sarcoma and primitive neuroectodermal tumour. Virchows Arch 1998;433:113–117.

317. Swanson PE, Lillemoe TJ, Manivel JC, Wick MR. Mesenchymal chondrosarcoma: An immunohistochemical study. Arch Pathol Lab Med 1990;114:943–948.

318. Kurotaki H, Tateoka H, Takeuchi M, et al. Primary mesenchymal chondrosarcoma of the lung: A case report with immunohistochemical and ultrastructural features. Acta Pathol Jpn 1992;42:364–371.

319. Rushing EJ, Armonda RA, Ansari Q, Mena H. Mesenchymal chondrosarcoma: A clinicopathologic and flow cytometric study of 13 cases presenting in the central nervous system. Cancer 1996;77:1884–1891.

320. Granter SR, Renshaw AA, Fletcher CD, et al. CD99 reactivity in mesenchymal chondrosarcoma. Hum Pathol 1996;27:1273–1276.

321. Lyon DB, Dortzbach RK, Gilbert-Barness E. Polyphenotypic small-cell orbitocranial tumor. Arch Ophthalmol 1991;111:1402–1408.

322. Pearson JM, Harris M, Eyden BP, Banerjee SS. Divergent differentiation in small round-cell tumours of the soft tissues with neural features—an analysis of 10 cases. Histopathology 1993;23:1–9.

323. Frydman CP, Klein MJ, Abdelwahab IF, Zwass A. Primitive multipotential primary sarcoma of bone: A case report and immunohistochemical study. Mod Pathol 1991;4:768–772.

324. Gerald WL, Ladanyi M, de Alava E, et al. Clinical, pathologic, and molecular spectrum of tumors associated with t(11;22)(p13;q12): Desmoplastic small round-cell tumor and its variants. J Clin Oncol 1998;16:3028–3036.

325. Katz RL, Quezado M, Senderowicz AM, et al. An intra-abdominal small round cell neoplasm with features of primitive neuroectodermal and desmoplastic round cell tumor and a EWS/FLI-1 fustion transcript. Hum Pathol 1997;28:502–509.

326. Noguera R, Navarro S, Cremades A, et al. Translocation (X;18) in a biphasic synovial sarcoma with morphologic features of neural differentiation. Diagn Mol Pathol 1998;7:16–23.

327. Masui F, Matsuno Y, Yokoyama R, et al. Synovial sarcoma, histologically mimicking primitive neuroectodermal tumor/Ewing's sarcoma at distant sites. Jpn J Clin Oncol 1999;29:438–441.

328. Machen SK, Fisher C, Gautam RS, et al. Utility of cytokeratin subsets for distinguishing poorly differentiated synovial sarcoma from peripheral primitive neuroectodermal tumour. Histopathology 1998;33:501–507.

329. Ramnani D, Lindberg G, Gokaslan ST, Albores-Saavedra J. Signet-ring cell variant of small lymphocytic lymphoma with a prominent sinusoidal pattern. Ann Diagn Pathol 1999;3:220–226.

330. Tse CC, Chan JK, Yuen RW, Ng CS. Malignant lymphoma with myxoid stroma: A new pattern in need of recognition. Histopathology 1991;18:31–35.

331. Tsang WY, Chan JK, Tang SK, et al. Large cell lymphoma with a fibrillary matrix. Histopathology 1992;29:80–82.

332. Meis JM, Enzinger FM. Inflammatory fibrosarcoma of the mesentery and retroperitoneum: A tumor closely simulating inflammatory pseudotumor. Am J Surg Pathol 1991;15:1146–1156.

333. Mechtersheimer G, Moller P. Expression of Ki-1 antigen (CD30) in mesenchymal tumors. Cancer 1990;66:1732–1737.

334. Winder SJ, Walsh MP. Calponin: Thin filament-linked regulation of smooth muscle contraction. Cell Signal 1993;5:677–686.

335. Miettinen MM, Sarloma-Rikala M, Kovatich AJ, Lasota J. Calponin and h-caldesmon in soft tissue tumors: Consistent h-caldesmon immunoreactivity in gastrointestinal stromal tumors indicates traits of smooth muscle differentiation. Mod Pathol 1999;12:756–762.

336. Kaddu S, Baham A, Cerroni L, et al. Cutaneous leiomyosarcoma. Am J Surg Pathol 1997;21:970–987.

337. Oliai BR, Tazelaar HD, Lloyd RV, et al. Leiomyosarcoma

of the pulmonary veins. Am J Surg Pathol 1999;23:1082–1088.

338. Rao UN, Finkelstein SD, Jones MW. Comparative immunohistochemical and molecular analysis of uterine and extrauterine leiomyosarcomas. Mod Pathol 1999;12:1001–1009.

339. Younes M, Brown RW, Stephenson M, et al. Overexpression of Glut1 and Glut2 in stage I nonsmall cell lung carcinoma is associated with poor survival. Cancer 1997; 80:1046–1051.

340. Younes M, Lechago LV, Lechago J. Overexpression of the human erythrocyte glucose transporter occurs as a late event in human colorectal carcinogenesis and is associated with an increased incidence of lymph node metastases. Clin Cancer Res 1996;2:1151–1154.

341. North PE, Waner M, Mizeracki A, Mihm MC. GLUT1: A newly discovered immunohistochemical marker for juvenile hemangiomas. Hum Pathol 2000;31:11–22.

342. Haber RS, Weiser KR, Pritsker A, et al. GLUT1 glucose transported expression in benign and malignant thyroid nodules. Thyroid 1997;7:363–367.

343. Bowman F, Gultekin H, Dickman PS. Latent Epstein-Barr virus infection demonstrated in low-grade leiomyosarcomas of adults with acquired immunodeficiency syndrome, but not in adjacent Kaposi's lesion or smooth muscle tumors in immunocompetent patients. Arch Pathol Lab Med 1997;121:834–838.

344. Jenson HB, Montalvo EA, McClain KL, et al. Characterization of natural Epstein-Barr virus infection and replication in smooth muscle cells from a leiomyosarcoma. J Med Virol 1999;57:36–46.

345. Swanson PE, Wick MR, Dehner LP. Leiomyosarcoma of somatic soft tissues in childhood: An immunohistochemical analysis of six cases with ultrastructural correlation. Hum Pathol 1991;22:569–577.

346. Swanson PE, Stanley MW, Scheihauer BW, Wick MR. Primary cutaneous leiomyosarcoma: A histological and immunohistochemical study of 9 cases, with ultrastructural correlation. J Cutan Pathol 1988;15:129–141.

347. Smith TA, Machen SK, Fisher C, Goldblum JR. Usefulness of cytokeratin subsets for distinguishing monophasic synovial sarcoma from malignant peripheral nerve sheath tumor. Am J Clin Pathol 1999;112:641–648.

348. Morphopoulos GD, Banerjee SS, Ali HH, et al. Malignant peripheral nerve sheath tumour with vascular differentiation: A report of four cases. Histopathology 1996;28:401–410.

349. King R, Busam K, Rosai J. Metastatic malignant melanoma resembling malignant peripheral nerve sheath tumor: Report of 16 cases. Am J Surg Pathol 1999;23:1499–1505.

350. Lopes JM, Bjerkehagen B, Holm R, et al. Immunohistochemical profile of synovial sarcoma with emphasis on the epithelial-type differentiation: A study of 49 primary tumours, recurrences, and metastases. Pathol Res Pract 1994; 190:168–177.

351. Machen SK, Fisher C, Gautam RS, et al. Utility of cytokeratin subsets for distinguishing poorly differentiated synovial sarcoma from peripheral primitive neuroectodermal tumour. Histopathology 1998;33:501–507.

352. Ordonez NG, Mahfouz SM, MacKay B. Synovial sarcoma: An immunohistochemical and ultrastructural study. Hum Pathol 1990;21:733–749.

353. Nicholson AG, Goldstraw P, Fisher C. Synovial sarcoma of the pleura and its differentiation from other primary pleural tumours: A clinicopathological and immunohistochemical review of three cases. Histopathology 1998;33:508–513.

354. Suster S, Fisher C, Moran CA. Expression of bcl-2 oncoprotein in benign and malignant spindle cell tumors of soft tissue, skin, serosal surfaces, and gastrointestinal tract. Am J Surg Pathol 1998;22:863–872.

355. Hirakawa N, Naka T, Yamamoto I, et al. Overexpression of bcl-2 protein in synovial sarcoma: A comparative study of other soft tissue spindle cell sarcomas and an additional analysis by fluorescence in situ hybridization. Hum Pathol 1996;27:1060–1065.

356. Von Hochstetter AR, Meyer VE, Grant JW, et al. Epitheli-

oid sarcoma mimicking angiosarcoma: The value of immunohistochemistry in the differential diagnosis. Virchows Arch A Pathol Anat Histopathol 1991;418:271–278.

357. Chetty R, Slavin JL. Epithelioid sarcoma with extensive chondroid differentiation. Histopathology 1994;24:400–401.

358. Guillou L, Wadden C, Coindre JM, et al. "Proximal type" epithelioid sarcoma: A distinctive aggressive neoplasm showing rhabdoid feature: Clinicopathologic, immunohistochemical, and ultrastructural study of a series. Am J Surg Pathol 1997;21:130–146.

359. Gerharz CD, Moll R, Meister P, et al. Cytoskeletal heterogeneity of an epithelioid sarcoma with expression of vimentin, cytokeratins, and neurofilaments. Am J Surg Pathol 1990;14:274–283.

360. Domagala W, Weber K, Osborn M. Diagnostic significance of coexpression of intermediate filaments in fine needle aspiration. Acta Cytol 1988;32:49–59.

361. Judkins AR, Montone KT, LiVolsi VA, van de Rijn M. Sensitivity and specificity of antibodies on necrotic tumor tissue. Am J Clin Pathol 1997;110:641–646.

362. Smith ME, Brown JI, Fisher C. Epithelioid sarcoma: Presence of vascular-endothelial cadherin and lack of epithelial cadherin. Histopathology 1998;33:425–431.

363. Cerilli LA, Huffman HT, Anand A. Primary renal angiosarcoma: A case report with immunohistochemical, ultrastructural, and cytogenetic features and review of the literature. Arch Pathol Lab Med 1998;122:929–935.

364. Poblet E, Gonzalez-Palacios F, Jimenez FJ. Different immunoreactivity of endothelial markers in well and poorly differentiated areas of angiosarcomas. Virchows Arch 1996; 428:217–221.

365. Natkunam Y, Rouse RV, Zhu S, et al. Immunoblot analysis of CD34 expression in histologically diverse neoplasms. Am J Pathol 2000;156:21–27.

366. Mooi Wj, Deenik W, Peterse JL, Hogendoorn PC. Keratin immunoreactivity in melanoma of soft parts (clear cell sarcoma). Histopathology 1995;27:61–65.

367. Hiraga H, Nojima T, Abe S, et al. Establishment of a new continuous clear cell sarcoma cell line: Morphological and cytogenetic characterization and detection of chimaeric EWS/ATF-1 transcripts. Virchows Arch 1997;431:45–51.

368. Stenman G, Kindblom LG, Angervall L. Reciprocal translocation t(12;22)(q13;q13) in clear-cell sarcoma of tendons and aponeuroses. Genes Chromosomes Cancer 1992;4:122–127.

369. Laskin WB, Weiss SW, Bratthauer GL. Epithelioid variant of malignant peripheral nerve sheath tumor (malignant epithelioid schwannoma). Am J Surg Pathol 1991;15:1136–1145.

370. Meis-Kindblom JM, Kindblom LG, Enzinger FM. Sclerosing epithelioid fibrosarcoma: A variant of fibrosarcoma simulating carcinoma. Am J Surg Pathol 1995;19:979–993.

371. Eyden BP, Manson C, Banerjee SS, et al. Sclerosing epithelioid fibrosarcoma: A study of five cases emphasizing diagnostic criteria. Histopathology 1998;33:354–360.

372. Suster S. Epithelioid leiomyosarcoma of the skin and subcutaneous tissue: Clinicopathologic, immunohistochemical, and ultrastructural study of five cases. Am J Surg Pathol 1994;18:232–240.

373. Lopez-Barea F, Rodriguez-Peralto JL, Sanchez-Herrera S, et al. Primary epithelioid leiomyosarcoma of bone: Case report and literature review. Virchows Arch 1999;434:367–371.

374. Mukai M, Torikata C, Iri H, et al. Histogenesis of alveolar soft-part sarcoma: An immunohistochemical and biochemical study. Am J Surg Pathol 1986;10:212–218.

375. Miettinen M, Ekfors T. Alveolar soft part sarcoma: Immunohistochemical evidence for muscle cell differentiation. Am J Clin Pathol 1990;93:32–38.

376. Hurlimann J. Desmin and neural marker expression in mesothelial cells and mesotheliomas. Hum Pathol 1994;25: 753–757.

377. Foschini MP, Ceccarelli C, Eusebi V, et al. Alveolar soft-part sarcoma: Immunological evidence of rhabdomyoblastic differentiation. Histopathology 1988;13:101–108.

378. Foschini MP, Eusein V. Alveolar soft part sarcoma: A new

type of rhabdomyosarcoma? Semin Diagn Pathol 1994;4:58–68.

379. Hirose T, Kudo E, Hasaegawa T, et al. Cytoskeletal properties of alveolar soft part sarcoma. Hum Pathol 1990;21:204–211.

380. Menesce LP, Eyden BP, Edmondson D, Harris M. Immunophenotype and ultrastructure of alveolar soft part sarcoma. J Submicrosc Cytol Pathol 1993;2593:377–387.

381. Rosai J, Dias P, Parham DM, et al. MyoD1 protein expression in alveolar soft part sarcoma as confirmatory evidence of its skeletal muscle nature. Am J Surg Pathol 1991;15:974–981.

382. Nakano H, Tateishi A, Imamura T, et al. RT-PCR suggests human skeletal muscle × 4 origin of alveolar soft part sarcoma. Oncology 2000;58:319–323.

383. Ordonez NG, Mackay B. Alveolar soft-part sarcoma: A review of the pathology and histogenesis. Ultrastruct Pathol 1998;22:275–292.

384. Roholl PJ, Prinsen I, Rademakers LP, et al. Two cell lines with epithelial cell–like characteristics established from malignant fibrous histiocytomas. Cancer 1991;68:1963–1972.

385. Gaffney EF, Dervan PA, Fletcher CD. Pleomorphic rhabdomyosarcoma in adulthood: Analysis of 11 cases with definition of diagnostic criteria. Am J Surg Pathol 1993;17:601–609.

386. Gloghini A, Rizzo A, Zanette I, et al. KP1/CD68 expression in malignant neoplasms including lymphomas, sarcomas, and carcinomas. Am J Clin Pathol 1995;103:425–431.

387. Fisher C, Carter RL, Ramachandra S, Thomas DM. Peripheral nerve sheath differentiation in malignant soft tissue tumours: An ultrastructural and immunohistochemical study. Histopathology 1992;20:115–125.

388. Hitchcock MG, Hurt MA, Santa Cruz DJ. Cutaneous granular cell angiosarcoma. J Cutan Pathol 1994;21:256–262.

389. Kodet R, Newton WA Jr, Sachs N, et al. Rhabdoid tumors of soft tissues: A clinicopathologic study of 26 cases enrolled on the Intergroup Rhabdomyosarcoma Study. Hum Pathol 1991;22:674–684.

390. Fanburg-Smith JC, Hengge M, Hengge UR, et al. Extrarenal rhabdoid tumors of soft tissue: A clinicopathologic and immunohistochemical study of 18 cases. Ann Diagn Pathol 1998;2:351–362.

391. Perrone T, Swanson PE, Twiggs L, et al. Malignant rhabdoid tumor of the vulva: Is distinction from epithelioid sarcoma possible? A pathologic and immunohistochemical study. Am J Surg Pathol 1989;13:848–858.

392. Gibas Z, Miettinen M, Limon J, et al. Cytogenetic and immunohistochemical profile of myxoid liposarcoma. Am J Clin Pathol 1995;103:20–26.

393. Miettinen M, Gannon FH, Lackman R. Chordomalike soft tissue sarcoma in the leg: A light and electron microscopic and immunohistochemical study. Ultrastruct Pathol 1992;16:577–586.

394. Naka T, Iwamoto Y, Shinohara N, et al. Cytokeratin subtyping in chordomas and the fetal notochord: An immunohistochemical analysis of aberrant expression. Mod Pathol 1997;10:545–551.

395. Hu Y, Gao Y, Zhang X. A clinicopathological and immunohistochemical study of 34 cases of chordoma. Chung Hua Ping li Hsueh Tsa Chih 1996;25:142–144.

396. Mi C. An immunohistochemical and ultrastructural study of 20 chordomas. Chung Hua Ping li Hsueh Tsa Chih 1992;21:106–108.

397. Heffelfinger MJ, Dahlin DC, MacCarty CS, Beabout JW. Chordomas and cartilaginous tumors at the skull base. Cancer 1973;32:410–420.

398. Rosenberg AE, Brown GA, Bhan AK, Lee JM. Chondroid chordoma—a variant of chordoma: A morphologic and immunohistochemical study. Am J Clin Pathol 1994;101:36–41.

399. Wojno KJ, Hruban RH, Garin-Chesa P, Huvos AG. Chondroid chordomas and low-grade chondrosarcomas of the craniospinal axis: An immunohistochemical analysis of 17 cases. Am J Surg Pathol 1992;16:1144–1152.

400. Ishida T, Dorfman HD. Chondroid chordoma versus low-grade chondrosarcoma of the base of the skull: Can immu-

nohistochemistry resolve the controversy? J Neurooncol 1994;18:199–206.

401. Niezabitowski A, Limon J, Wasilewska A, et al. Parachordoma—a clinicopathologic, immunohistochemical, electron microscopic, flow cytometric, and cytogenetic study. Gen Diagn Pathol 1995;141:49–55.

402. Wiebe BM, Jensen K, Laursen H. Parachordoma of the sacrococcygeal region—a neuroepithelial tumor. Clin Neuropathol 1995;14:343–346.

403. Karabela-Bouropoulou V, Skourtas C, Liapi-Avgeri G, Mahaira H. Parachordoma: A case report of a very rare soft tissue tumor. Pathol Res Pract 1996;192:972–978.

404. Ishida T, Oda H, Oka T, et al. Parachordoma: An ultrastructural and immunohistochemical study. Virchows Arch A Pathol Anat Histopathol 1993;422:239–245.

405. Nakamura Y, Becker LE, Marks A. S-100 protein in tumors of cartilage and bone: An immunohistochemical study. Cancer 1983;52:1820–1824.

406. Posl M, Amling M, Ritzel H, et al. Morphologic characteristics of chondroblastoma: A retrospective study of 56 cases of the Hamburg bone tumor register. Pathologe 1996;17:26–34.

407. Semmelink HJ, Pruszczynski M, Wiersma-van Tilburg A, et al. Cytokeratin expression in chondroblastomas. Histopathology 1990;16:257–263.

408. Monda L, Wick MR. S-100 protein immunostaining in the differential diagnosis of chondroblastoma. Hum Pathol 1985;16:287–293.

409. Edel G, Ueda Y, Nakanishi J, et al. Chondroblastoma of bone: A clinical, radiological, light and immunohistochemical study. Virchows Arch A Pathol Anat Histopathol 1992;421:355–366.

410. Brecher ME, Simon MA. Chondroblastoma: An immunohistochemical study. Hum Pathol 1988;19:1043–1047.

411. Povysil C, Tomanova R, Matejovsky Z. Muscle-specific actin expression in chondroblastoma. Hum Pathol 1997;28:316–320.

412. Kilpatrick SE, Inwards CY, Fletcher CD, et al. Myxoid chondrosarcoma (chordoid sarcoma) of bone: A report of two cases and review of the literature. Cancer 1997;79:1903–1910.

413. Antonescu CR, Argani P, Erlandson RA, et al. Skeletal and extraskeletal myxoid chondrosarcoma: A comparative clinicopathologic, ultrastructural, and molecular study. Cancer 1998;83:1504–1521.

414. Orndal C, Carlen B, Akerman M, et al. Chromosomal abnormality t(9;22)(q22;q12) in an extraskeletal myxoid chondrosarcoma characterized by fine needle aspiration cytology, electron microscopy, immunohistochemistry and DNA flow cytometry. Cytopathology 1991;2:261–270.

415. Wang LT, Liu TC. Clear cell chondrosarcoma of bone: A report of three cases with immunohistochemical and affinity histochemical observations. Pathol Res Pract 1993;189:411–415.

416. Bosse A, Ueda Y, Wuisman P, et al. Histogenesis of clear cell chondrosarcoma: An immunohistochemical study with osteonectin, a non-collagenous structure protein. J Cancer Res Clin Oncol 1991;117:43–49.

417. Lidang Jensen LM, Schumacher B, Jensen MO, et al. Extraskeletal osteosarcomas: A clinicopathologic study of 25 cases. Am J Surg Pathol 1998;22:588–594.

418. Dardick I, Schatz JE, Colgan TJ. Osteogenic sarcoma with epithelial differentiation. Ultrastruct Pathol 1992;16:463–474.

419. Hasegawa T, Hirose T, Hizawa K, et al. Immunophenotypic heterogeneity in osteosarcomas. Hum Pathol 1991;22:583–590.

420. Serra M, Morini MC, Scotlandi K, et al. Evaluation of osteonectin as a diagnostic marker of osteogenic bone tumors. Hum Pathol 1992;23:1326–1331.

421. Schulz Z, Jundt G, Berghauser KH, et al. Immunohistochemical study of osteonectin in various types of osteosarcoma. Am J Pathol 1988;132:233–238.

422. Masui F, Ushigome S, Fujii K. Giant cell tumor of bone: An immunohistochemical comparative study. Pathol Int 1998;48:355–361.

423. Fornasier VL, Protzner K, Zhang I, Mason L. The prognos-

tic significance of histomorphometry and immunohisto-chemistry in giant cell tumors of bone. Hum Pathol 1996; 27:754–760.

424. Watanabe K, Tajino T, Kusakabe T, et al. Giant cell tumor of bone: Frequent actin immunoreactivity in stromal tumor cells. Pathol Int 1997;47:680–684.

425. Paulino AF, Spiro RH, O'Malley B, Huvos AG. Giant cell tumour of the retropharynx. Histopathology 1998;33:344–348.

426. Folpe AL, Weiss SW, Fletcher CD, Gown AM. Tenosynovial giant cell tumors: Evidence for a desmin-positive dendritic cell subpopulation. Mod Pathol 1998;11:939–944.

427. Ueda Y, Imai K, Tsuchiya H, et al. Matrix metalloproteinase 9 (gelatinase B) is expressed in multinucleated giant cells of human giant cell tumor of bone and is associated with vascular invasion. Am J Pathol 1996;148:611–622.

428. Rao VH, Singh RK, Delimont DC, et al. Transcriptional regulation of MMP-9 expression in stromal cells of human giant cell tumor of bone by tumor necrosis factor-alpha. Int J Oncol 1999;14:291–300.

429. Schoedel DE, Greco MA, Stetler-Stevenson WG, et al. Expression of metalloproteinases and tissue inhibitors of metalloproteinases in giant cell tumor of bone: An immunohistochemical study with clinical correlation. Hum Pathol 1996;27:1144–1148.

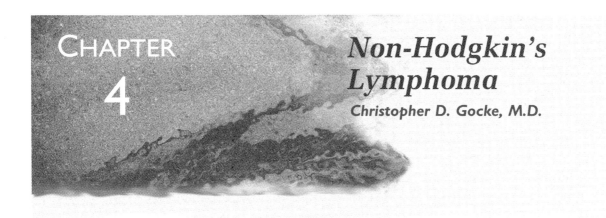

CHAPTER 4

Non-Hodgkin's Lymphoma

Christopher D. Gocke, M.D.

The development of immunohistochemistry as a diagnostic discipline has been intimately linked to the non-Hodgkin's lymphomas. In part, this is attributable both to the lymphocyte's role as a producer of reagents for immunologic studies and to the ready availability of lymphocytes from humans and animals as targets of study. This interaction has been mutually reinforcing: The understanding of lymphocyte development and lymphoma nosology has created a need for more diagnostic reagents, and the rapidly expanding pool of reagents has assisted with finer distinctions among non-Hodgkin's lymphomas.

Since the early 1990s, a number of changes have been made to the diagnostic schemas for non-Hodgkin's lymphoma. The Kiel and Lukes-Collins classifications and a de facto classification, the Working Formulation, were replaced by the Revised European American Lymphoma (REAL) classification in 1994.[1] In this effort, an international group of expert hematopathologists compiled a list of recognizable disease entities in the area of lymphoid neoplasms. These diseases were defined on the basis of their morphologic, immunophenotypic, and genetic features, with occasional reference to clinical presentation. The contribution that each of these features makes to the diagnosis of a particular entity varies so that many lymphoid diseases can be recognized by morphology alone, whereas others require additional molecular or immunologic information. Although not without its dissenters,[2–4] the REAL classification has gained adherents and has demonstrated its clinical utility.[5, 6]

Also since the early 1990s, planning for a revision of the REAL classification has taken place. Under the auspices of the European Association for Hematopathology and the North American–based Society for Hematopathology, a larger group of hematopathologists has been preparing a similar disease-based listing of all hematologic malignancies while making minor modifications to the lymphoma classification.[7, 8] The efforts of this group will be published soon as the World Health Organization Classification of Tumours of Haemopoietic and Lymphoid Tissues.[9] Because of the general acceptance that the parent REAL classification has gained, and because the system is based explicitly (if only partially) on immunophenotyping, this chapter approaches non-Hodgkin's lymphoma immunophenotyping using the World Health Organization (WHO) classification as a guide. Recognized variants are addressed when they differ significantly from the main disease.

The use of antibody panels in immunohistochemistry is well accepted. This is particularly true in hematolymphoid diagnostics, in which the combination of cytologic-histologic characteristics and a single antibody result may not be sufficient to distinguish benign from malignant or one form of lymphoma from another.[10, 11] No single panel suffices for all situations, but a number of proposed panels using a modest number of antibodies can often provide the needed information. As in other areas of pathology, lymphoma immunohistochemistry usually serves an adjunctive role to morphology. Hematopathologists also have at their disposal, and need to judiciously use, a number of other aids to diagnosis, such as molecular testing, flow cytometry, and cytogenetics. It must be emphasized that correlation of the patient's history with the laboratory data can be invaluable.

The terminology for lymphoma immunophenotyping differs slightly from that of many other tumor types. The cell surface antigens of leukocytes have been assigned cluster of differentiation (CD) designations, each of which may bind with any number of diagnostic antibodies.[12] To the average pathologist's chagrin, the CD nomenclature has not been organized by cell or tissue type; consequently, widely separated numbers may refer to similar cell types, for example, B cell–restricted epitopes CD20 and CDw75. In addition to being designated by reference to their CD target, antibodies are also often given an arbitrary clone designation (e.g., 4C7) or one related to the place of origin (e.g., Ki-1 from Kiel, Germany).

Much of the early work in diagnostic hematopathology required frozen tissue or acetone-fixed frozen tissue because the available antibodies failed to recognize epitopes preserved by cross-linking fixatives. Because of the level of expertise involved in preparing and interpreting frozen section immunohistochemistry, few routine pathology laboratories offered such diagnostic services. More recently, there has been success in developing monoclonal antibodies that recognize fixed tissue antigens. An increasing number of such reagents, useful for tissue preserved with either formalin or mercuric fixatives, are now commercially available. This chapter deals primarily with immunohistochemistry performed using antibodies effective on fixed, paraffin-embedded material. This technology is easily handled in most pathology laboratories and results in excellent cytologic evaluation that is not always obtainable with frozen sections. Partial digestion of proteins with enzymes provides better immunolabeling results for some antibodies.[13] A variety of antigen unmasking or retrieval procedures has also assisted in the move to fixed tissue analysis.[14, 15] Of course, snap frozen tissue may always be preserved and transferred to a reference laboratory for further study if necessary.

An understanding of the development, maturation, and migration of lymphocytes provides a rationale for lymphoma immunophenotyping, since stages in lymphocyte maturation are defined, in part, by the macromolecules they produce. Reviews of the topic are provided in standard pathology texts,[16, 17] and more detailed treatments are available.[18–21] Malignancies of lymphocytes certainly express antigen complements that bear a resemblance to different developmental stages. In fact, both the Lukes and Collins and Kiel classifications of lymphoma explicitly rely on the stages of normal lymphocyte differentiation as organizing principles.[22–24] Lymphomas are commonly thought of as being composed of cells arrested in development at certain stages.[25] This is a useful concept, although the many exceptions suggest that it is not a perfect representation of reality.

ANTIBODIES WITH UTILITY IN NON-HODGKIN'S LYMPHOMA DIAGNOSIS

B Cell

CD19. CD19 is the earliest immunochemical marker of B-lineage differentiation. No paraffin-reactive antibody is available.

CD20. The CD20 epitope is acquired late in the pre–B cell stage of maturation and remains on cells throughout most of their differentiation, although it is lost at the plasma cell stage. As recognized by the antibody L26, CD20 is strongly positive on approximately half of lymphoblastic lymphoma-leukemias, almost all mature B-cell lymphomas (plasma cell lesions excepted), Reed-

Sternberg cells in roughly one quarter of the cases of classic Hodgkin's disease, and almost no T-cell lymphomas (Fig. 4–1).

CD21. The CD21 antibody cluster recognizes the receptor for complement component C3d, which mediates the phagocytosis of complement-coated particles. It is found on follicular dendritic cells and some B lymphocytes. It may be useful in outlining the follicular dendritic cell network in follicular lymphomas and helps identify the hyperplastic islands of dendritic cells in angioimmunoblastic T-cell lymphoma.

CD22. CD22 is a transmembrane molecule that may perform an intracellular signaling function. Its expression roughly parallels that of CD19. It is strongly expressed in hairy cell leukemia.

CD23. CD23 is a membrane protein that exhibits weak binding of IgE and regulates cytokine release from monocytes. It is most useful in distinguishing B-cell chronic lymphocytic leukemia/small lymphocytic lymphoma (CLL/SLL) from other entities and remains present in CLL/SLL that has undergone large cell transformation.

CD79a. A relatively recent entry to the diagnostic armamentarium, antibodies to CD79a work well in detecting B cells on paraffin sections (Fig. 4–2A).[26] The antigen is associated with the immunoglobulin molecule and is expressed early in ontogeny. Nearly all the assayed precursor B-cell lymphoblastic lymphoma-leukemias are positive, with no T-cell staining. Mature B-cell lymphomas also stain with CD79a.

DBA.44. DBA.44 is a B subset antibody that strongly stains the cytoplasm of most hairy cell leukemias. However, it is not specific for hairy cell leukemia, since it is also found in some marginal zone lymphomas (MZLs) and large cell lymphomas.

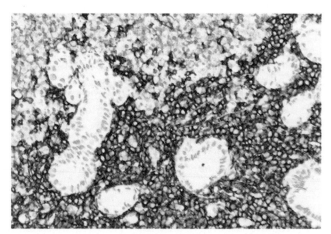

Figure 4–1. CD20 immunolabeling of marginal zone B-cell lymphoma of mucosa-associated lymphoid tissue type. Cytoplasmic staining of B cells infiltrating among gastric glands. Note the weaker or absent staining in the plasmacytic component toward the luminal surface *(top)*.

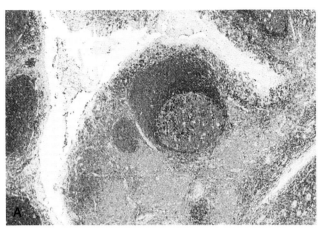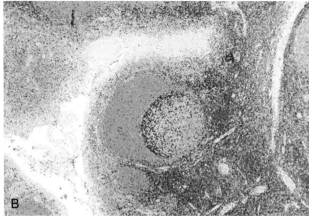

Figure 4–2. *A*, CD79a in a normal lymph node. The mantle lymphocytes, most germinal center cells, and scattered interfollicular B lymphocytes mark for this early B-cell antigen. *B*, CD2 in a normal lymph node. Most interfollicular lymphocytes as well as scattered T cells in the light zone of the germinal centers mark for this early T-cell antigen.

T Cell

CD2. CD2, the E-rosette receptor, is an extremely broad T-cell marker. Antibodies to it immunolabel the vast majority of T- and natural killer (NK)–cell malignancies, but signal amplification by the Immunomax method may be required for paraffin section use.[27] Some thymic B cells are also CD2+ (Fig. 4–2*B*).

CD3. The T-cell antigen receptor binds to the CD3 protein complex at the cell membrane. A commercially available anti-CD3 antibody is polyclonal and reacts with most T-cell lymphomas in fixed tissue, the exceptions being some anaplastic large cell lymphomas and NK leukemia-lymphomas. CD3 is very specific for T-cell derivation.

CD4. The CD4 molecule interacts with HLA class II during antigen recognition and defines a helper-inducer subset of T cells. It is also found on a variety of monocyte-derived cells, including Langerhans' and other dendritic cells. The CD4 epitope is absent from immature thymocytes and is expressed during T-cell development. Precursor T–lymphoblastic lymphomas are therefore variable in their expression of CD4, but most mature T-cell lymphomas are positive, with the exception of aggressive NK-cell leukemia, extranodal NK-cell lymphoma, gamma delta T-cell lymphoma, subcutaneous panniculitis-like T-cell lymphoma, and enteropathy-type T-cell lymphoma. The antibody available for use on paraffin sections is not as sensitive as those for flow cytometry or frozen tissue.[28] Antibodies for paraffin section detection of Th1 and Th2 subsets are not currently available.

CD5. CD5 is a signal transduction molecule present on the surface of most thymocytes and immature peripheral T cells. It is also detectable on a small subset of circulating B cells, and its primary use in diagnostic immunohistochemistry is in the detection of malignancies derived from those cells:

B-cell CLL/SLL and mantle cell lymphoma. Antigen retrieval is necessary.

CD7. CD7 has the distinction of being the most frequently lost T-subset marker, particularly on MF.[29] It is also present on non–T-cell malignancies, including NK tumors and acute myeloid leukemia. It is detectable on paraffin sections only with difficulty.

CD8. The CD8 antigen defines the suppressor-cytotoxic T-cell subset. It is expressed in concert with CD4 in thymocytes, but this state persists in only a small population of circulating cells. CD4/CD8 ratios are not analogous to immunoglobulin light chain ratios in B-cell malignancies; infectious and inflammatory conditions can markedly skew the normal 2:1 ratio. The beta chain of CD8 detected in fixed tissue has nearly the sensitivity of flow cytometry.

Other Antibodies with Utility in Non-Hodgkin's Lymphoma Diagnosis

ALK. ALK is the protein product of the anaplastic lymphoma kinase gene, first identified as a partner in the t(2;5) characteristic of anaplastic large cell lymphoma (ALCL). The protein is not normally detectable outside the central nervous system. In ALCL, its expression is up-regulated by fusion to the NPM gene, resulting in one of the few tumor-specific markers in hematopathology. Expression in lymphomas is limited to ALCL and rare diffuse large B-cell lymphomas.[30] Antibodies useful in fixed tissue localize both to the cytoplasm and to the nucleus of tumor cells.[31] Nearly all ALK+ tumors are also CD30+ and EMA+ and CD115− (Fig. 4–3).

Cyclin D1. The cyclin D1 protein, also known as bcl-1 and PRAD 1, is a cell cycle regulatory pro-

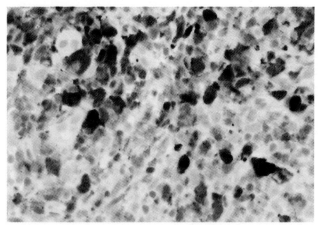

Figure 4–3. ALK antibody highlighting both cytoplasm and nuclei of malignant cells in lymphohistiocytic variant of anaplastic large cell lymphoma, T-cell, primary systemic type. Intervening small lymphs and histiocytes are negative.

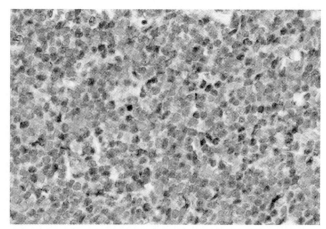

Figure 4–4. Cyclin D1 in a mantle cell lymphoma. Note nuclear positivity.

tein identified through the t(11;14) translocation of its gene in mantle cell lymphomas. It is a nuclear protein detectable in paraffin sections and is found in the majority of mantle cell lymphomas (Fig. 4–4). Hairy cell leukemia and plasmacytoma may also express cyclin D1, albeit with a weaker signal. Nonspecific cytoplasmic staining is seen in many B-cell lymphomas and does not correlate with mRNA expression.

BCL-2. bcl-2 was the first of the translocation-associated proteins to be identified in lymphoma. Approximately three quarters of follicular lymphomas bear a t(14;18) translocation that juxtaposes the bcl-2 gene to the immunoglobulin heavy chain gene, resulting in bcl-2 overexpression (Fig. 4–5). The protein is part of a heterodimeric complex that is regulated by binding with one of several partners and carries out a poorly understood "anti-apoptotic" function. bcl-2 is normally present in the cytoplasm of follicular mantle B lymphocytes, occasional germinal center cells, and many T lymphocytes. It is abundant in most lymphomas of small lymphocytes, including approximately 80% of follicular lymphoma. Its presence in other lymphomas is attributable to up-regulation unrelated to t(14;18).

BCL-6. bcl-6 protein is expressed normally in germinal center lymphocytes[32] and serves as a transcriptional regulatory protein. In the normal node, it is distributed in a pattern reciprocal to that of bcl-2. Localized to the nucleus of tumor cells, it is expressed in a variety of B-cell neoplasms and is lost with follicular lymphoma progression. It is also detected in the lymphocytic and histiocytic variants of nodular lymphocyte-predominant Hodgkin's disease.

CD1a. CD1a is a transmembrane antigen normally found on cortical thymocytes and Langerhans' cells. It is associated with β_2-macroglobulin and may have a role in thymocyte development. It

is found on a subset of precursor T-lymphoblastic lymphoma-leukemia.

CD10. Also known as the common ALL antigen (CALLA), CD10 is a zinc metallopeptidase expressed in early lymphoid progenitors and normal germinal center cells. It is almost always present on the surface of precursor B-lymphoblastic and Burkitt's lymphomas and much less frequently on precursor T-lymphoblastic leukemia-lymphoma. Many follicular lymphoma and some diffuse large B-cell lymphomas, along with multiple myeloma, are positive.

CD15. CD15, the X hapten or Lewis X antigen, can be identified with the LeuM1 antibody. Originally noted as a monocyte-myeloid cell marker, it was recognized as a marker for the Reed-Sternberg cells of classic Hodgkin's disease. It is negative in most non-Hodgkin's lymphomas, with the exception of some primary cutaneous ALCLs and other peripheral T-cell lymphomas. The pattern of stain-

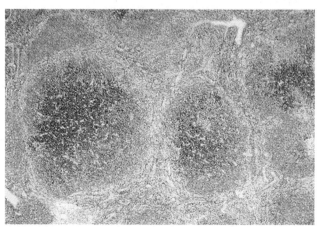

Figure 4–5. bcl-2 in a follicular lymphoma. The malignant follicles stain with an antibody to bcl-2, whereas most surrounding lymphocytes are negative. The pattern is reversed in lymph nodes exhibiting follicular hyperplasia.

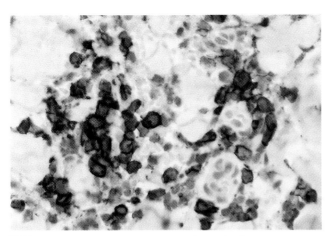

Figure 4–6. CD30 labeled with antibody BerH2 in an anaplastic large cell lymphoma, T-cell, primary cutaneous type. Some cells exhibit paranuclear Golgi staining *(center)* in addition to strong membrane positivity.

ing is typically membranous, with a paranuclear dot-like, Golgi localization. The surgical pathologist will note that this antibody is also used to stain adenocarcinomas.

CD25. The interleukin-2 receptor is designated CD25. Originally isolated from T lymphocytes, it is now known to be expressed on hairy cell leukemia and adult T-cell leukemia-lymphoma. There are no antibodies useful on paraffin sections.

CD30. The CD30 antigen is part of the tumor necrosis factor–receptor superfamily and has pleiotropic effects on cells carrying it. An increase in soluble CD30 in a variety of diseases has been noted. In the surgical pathology laboratory, CD30 may be recognized in frozen tissue with the Ki-1 antibody or in paraffin sections with BerH2. The accepted staining pattern is membranous or paranuclear dot-like; cytoplasmic staining should be viewed skeptically (Fig. 4–6). Scattered large and small "activated" lymphs are positive in normal nodes and tonsils, particularly at the edge of ger-

minal centers. Almost by definition, CD30 is present in ALCL and lymphomatoid papulosis and is seen in 95% of classic Hodgkin's disease cases in some (like CD15, not necessarily all) Reed-Sternberg cells. CD30 also marks sporadic nonanaplastic lymphoma cells. It has been noted in germ cell tumors and some melanomas, and so is neither tumor-specific nor lymphoma-specific.

CD43. CD43 appears to function as an antiadhesion molecule, mediating repulsion among leukocytes. Also called *leukosialin,* the modified protein is expressed on the surface of all leukocytes except for some resting B cells. CD43 expression in lymphomas is highly correlated with CD5; thus, most T-cell malignancies and a group of small lymphocyte B-cell malignancies (CLL/SLL, mantle cell lymphoma, prolymphocytic leukemia [PLL]) are often positive, whereas follicular lymphoma is rarely positive (Fig. 4–7). The broad expression pattern on most leukocytes makes CD43 unuseful as a lineage marker, but a very sensitive indicator of aberrant B-cell populations.

CD45. CD45 is a membrane protein tyrosine phosphatase found on all leukocytes in a number of isoforms. Antibodies such as 2B11 recognize epitopes common to all isoforms and are known as antileukocyte common antigen (LCA). These mark almost all circulating and fixed white cells. Alternate mRNA splicing leads to isoforms RA, RB, and RC, as well as a form without any of the spliced exons (RO). A number of antibodies have been identified as being specific for restricted (isoform-limited) epitopes of CD45. The RB form is widespread on cells, so antibodies to it (such as PD7/26) are also commonly referred to as panleukocyte antibodies, although their spectrum is not as broad as anti-CD45 antibodies. CD45RA is present predominantly in B lymphocytes, whereas CD45RO is localized to myeloid and T cells. LCA is useful in identifying most lymphomas, except roughly 30% of ALCL and most Hodgkin's disease. An anti-CD45RA antibody, 4KB5, is not as sensitive for B-cell lymphomas as CD20 and marks approxi-

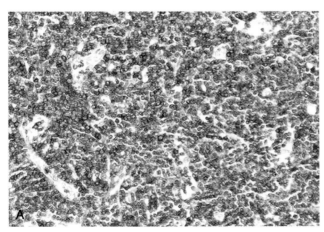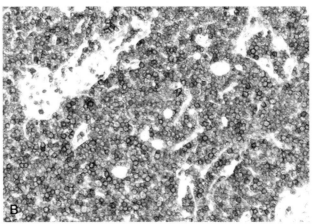

Figure 4–7. Coexpression of antibodies to CD43 *(A)* and CD20 *(B)* in a small lymphocytic lymphoma.

mately 5% of T-cell lymphoma cases. CD45RO antibodies, such as OPD4 and UCHL1, mark many T-cell lymphomas but also identify histiocytes and some B cells.

CD56. Neural cell adhesion molecule is designated CD56. CD56 is the prototypic NK-cell marker but is also found on subsets of CD4+ and CD8+ T cells. Many of the extranodal peripheral T-cell and NK-cell leukemia-lymphomas express CD56 regardless of their state of activation. Some benign and malignant plasma cells are also positive.

CD57. CD57 cluster antibodies also identify normal NK cells as well as a T-cell subset. Thus, malignancies that are CD57+ include a minority of T-lymphoblastic leukemia-lymphomas, roughly three quarters of the indolent T-cell large granular lymphocytic leukemias, and a surprisingly small portion of NK-cell lymphomas.[33] Thus, a typical phenotype for an NK cell is CD3−, CD5−, CD56+, CD57−.[34]

CD99. The MIC2 gene product is labeled CD99 and serves to regulate the interactions between intercellular adhesion molecules. It is found in many lymphoblastic leukemia-lymphomas, in acute myeloid leukemias, in some low-grade B-cell lymphomas, and in a variety of solid tumors.

Epstein-Barr Virus Latent Membrane Protein. Latent membrane protein (LMP-1) is a viral protein that protects infected cells from apoptosis through up-regulation of bcl-2. As such, it serves as a marker of Epstein-Barr virus (EBV) infection. The correlation of LMP-1 by immunohistochemistry to EBV RNA by in situ hybridization is reportedly good for many diseases but is poor for NK/T-cell lymphomas. This may be attributable to the latency state of the virus.

T Cell–Restricted Intracellular Antigen (TIA-1). TIA-1 is a cytotoxic granule-associated protein expressed in NK cells and cytotoxic T lymphocytes. It is expressed regardless of the state of activation of the cell. B-cell malignancies are uniformly negative, whereas NK cell and some T-cell lymphomas have a granular, cytoplasmic positivity.

Perforin-Granzyme B. This pair of granule-associated proteins is also localized to cytotoxic T- and NK-cells. They are essential for both apoptosis and immune-mediated cell death of target cells via induction of cell membrane perforation. However, their expression is assumed to be evidence of an activated state. They mark subcutaneous panniculitis-like T-cell lymphoma, aggressive NK-cell leukemia, and extranodal NK/T-cell lymphoma, nasal type.

Ki-67. Ki-67 antibodies recognize a nuclear protein involved in the proliferative portion of the cell cycle. They can be used as a measure of the growth fraction by dividing the number of positive cells by all cells present. This index roughly correlates with tumor grade and is important in the differential diagnosis of some tumors (e.g., Burkitt's lymphoma). Correlations between Ki-67 in-

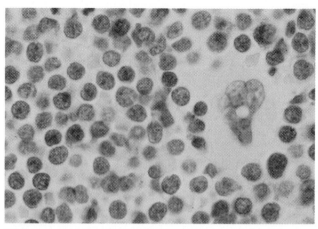

Figure 4–8. Antibody to terminal deoxynucleotidyl transfer (TDT) marking precursor B-lymphoblastic leukemia in a nuclear pattern.

dex and outcome have been made for mucosa-associated lymphoid tissue (MALT) lymphomas and diffuse large cell lymphomas.

Terminal Deoxynucleotidyl Transferase. Terminal deoxynucleotidyl transferase (TdT) is a DNA polymerase that is active during the process of immunoglobulin and T-cell receptor gene rearrangement early in a precursor B or T cell's life. Only normal early B and T lymphoblasts mark for TdT. The staining pattern is nuclear. TdT is a sensitive and specific antibody for lymphoblastic lymphoma-leukemia, since only a small proportion of myeloid leukemia cases are positive (Fig. 4–8).

GENERAL ISSUES

Non-Hodgkin's Lymphoma Versus Reactive Conditions

It is probably safe to say that no other area in hematopathology causes as much anxiety and sleeplessness for pathologists as the distinction between an atypical reactive lymphoid process and lymphoma.[35] One of the most common dilemmas is an obviously nodular process in a node, with a differential diagnosis of follicular lymphoma and marked follicular hyperplasia. When the usual morphologic clues have failed to resolve the issue, a small panel of antibodies may provide great assistance. bcl-2 is characteristically expressed in the cytoplasm of follicular lymphoma cells (74 to 97% of cases, depending on grade, according to one large study[36]) and is absent from the centrocytes and centroblasts of a hyperplastic follicle.[37] It should be cautioned that both normal mantle lymphocytes and many T cells express bcl-2 (although generally less intensely than follicular lymphoma cells) so that occasional positive cells within reactive follicles are expected and should not be over-interpreted. Conversely, in some follicular lymphomas, the large transformed cells may not mark with bcl-2, and this should not invalidate the diagnosis. CD10 is positive in most follicular lymphomas and not in hyperplasias,[38, 39] although weak reactivity in the latter has been noted by flow cytometry,[40] so care should be exercised. Immunoglobulin light-chain restriction is helpful as an indicator of malignancy[41]; unfortunately, this is relatively infrequent in follicular lymphomas studied by paraffin section immunohistochemistry. Antibodies to CD45RA have been reported to separate follicular lymphoma from follicular hyperplasia with a distribution pattern similar to that of bcl-2.[42]

KEY DIAGNOSTIC POINTS

- bcl-2 positivity *in* enlarged follicles is seen in lymphoma; bcl-2 positivity *around* follicles is typical of hyperplasia.
- Immunoglobulin light-chain staining usually is not helpful in distinguishing follicular processes.
- Beware bcl-2+ benign, small, primary follicles and intrafollicular T cells.

Interfollicular reactive processes are more frequent in the differential diagnosis of Hodgkin disease, but some bear resemblance to non-Hodgkin's lymphomas. Monocytoid cell aggregates or Langerhans' cell histiocytosis may occasionally raise concern for partial nodal involvement by MZL. Again, bcl-2 positivity is an important guide, as 79% of MZLs are positive and hyperplasias are not.[36] Malignant Langerhans' cells are typically S-100+ and CD1a+.[43] A florid paracortical immunoblastic proliferation as seen, for example, with infectious mononucleosis may raise concern for a non-Hodgkin's lymphoma as well as for Hodgkin's disease. Examination with pan-B− and pan-T−cell markers may be helpful, particularly if small sheets of B cells are identified.[11] Reactive processes typically show a mixture of B and T immunoblasts or a predominance of T immunoblasts. T-cell−rich B-cell lymphoma, a variant of diffuse large B-cell lymphoma, may be mistaken for a benign condition, but can typically be properly diagnosed with a series of pan−B-cell markers and immunoglobulin light-chain antibodies.[44]

Non-Hodgkin's Lymphoma Versus Other Malignancies

Non-Hodgkin's lymphoma is sometimes part of the differential diagnosis in poorly differentiated large cell malignancies. Most forms of lymphoma can be ruled in or out by the use of antibodies to CD45RB (LCA), S-100, and cytokeratin (such as the AE1/AE3 mixture or CAM5.2). Pitfalls to avoid pertain particularly to ALCL, which may mimic an epithelial malignancy in its sinusoidal distribution, apparent cohesive growth pattern, and cytologic characteristics (especially when monomorphic). LCA is frequently absent,[45, 46] many cases are null cell (express neither T- nor B-cell epitopes),[46] and EMA is present—albeit focally—in as many as 80% of cases.[47] If the pathologist maintains an index of suspicion for ALCL, CD30 will typically resolve the issue. Vimentin is positive in a large variety of tissue types and, although useful as a control for antigen preservation,[48] has little role in lymphoma diagnosis.

CLASSIFICATION OF THE NON-HODGKIN'S LYMPHOMAS

The initial distinction in the WHO classification separates lymphomas into B cell, T cell, and Hodgkin's types (see Chapter 5). Although this separation is an immunologic one, it may not require immunohistochemistry or flow cytometry to be made. For example, follicular lymphomas are uniformly B-cell malignancies and generally do not require immunophenotyping for diagnosis. This is significant for both turnaround time and financial reasons, since the plurality of lymphomas in the United States are follicular lymphomas.[49] Other entities may be strongly suspected on the basis of routine morphologic study and require only confirmatory immunologic work-up. It is a rare case that progresses sequentially through the immunohistochemistry laboratory from proof of lymphoid nature, through lineage assignment, to a final subclassification.

B-Cell Neoplasms

B- and T-cell neoplasms are divided into precursor disorders (lymphoblastic leukemias and lymphomas) with normal counterparts in the earliest bone marrow and thymus compartments and mature, or "peripheral," malignancies akin to normal extrathymic, nodal, splenic, or circulating lymphocytes. This discussion is focused on those malignancies commonly diagnosed using immunohistochemistry, that is, "solid" tumors.

PRECURSOR B-CELL NEOPLASMS

Precursor B-Cell Lymphoblastic Leukemia-Lymphoma

Typical Phenotype: CD19+, CD79a+, CD20−/+, CD22+/−, CD10+, TDT+, immunoglobulin-negative

Lymphoblastic lymphoma and acute lymphoblastic leukemia are morphologically and immunophenotypically the same disease and are distinguished on clinical grounds.[50] Although the majority of lymphoblastic leukemias are of B lineage, only approximately 20% of lymphoblastic lymphomas express B-cell markers.[51, 52] Practically all cases of lymphoblastic leukemia-lymphoma produce an enzyme, TDT, that is involved in gene rearrangement.[53–57] TDT marks the nucleus of lymphoblasts. CD19 is expressed in almost all precursor B-cell lymphoblastic lymphomas but is not detectable in paraffin sections. CD20 is not found reliably,[54–56, 58] nor is LCA (CD45RB).[59] Both CD74 (LN2)[60] and CD79a[55] antibodies are useful markers of B-cell or pre–B-cell lymphoblastic lymphomas. Antibodies to CD43 are often thought of as T-cell markers, but their specificity is quite broad. Most examples of precursor B-cell lymphoblastic lymphoma-leukemia express CD43 but are CD3–.[55] The MIC2 gene product, CD99, parallels the expression distribution of TDT in lymphoblastic lymphomas,[61, 62] although the antigen pattern is membranous rather than nuclear. Of course, other small round cell tumors, particularly in children, are also positive with anti-CD99. The majority of precursor B-cell neoplasms are CD10 positive, but some precursor T-cell tumors also express CD10.[63] Other antigens that are sometimes found in precursor B-cell lymphoma include CD34,[57] cytokeratin,[54] the NK-cell antigen CD56,[64] and the Fas ligand.[65] bcl-2 is frequently found in the cytoplasm and has been noted to assist in the differential diagnosis with Burkitt's lymphoma–leukemia[66]; however, other "blastic" lymphoid neoplasms such as the blastoid variant of mantle cell lymphoma may also be bcl-2+.

KEY DIAGNOSTIC POINTS

- CD20 and LCA may be negative in precursor B-cell lymphoblastic lymphoma-leukemia.
- TDT is almost always present in the nucleus of lymphoblastic lymphoma cells (although it may also be found in biphenotypic and some myeloid leukemias).
- CD10 and CD99 are usually present.

MATURE B-CELL NEOPLASMS

B-Cell Chronic Lymphocytic Leukemia/Small Lymphocytic Lymphoma

Typical Phenotype: CD20+, CD23+, CD79a+, CD5+, CD43+

As with lymphoblastic leukemia-lymphoma, the immunophenotypes of B-cell CLL and SLL are practically indistinguishable. These malignancies of mature small B lymphocytes commonly have an indolent course. They are pan–B-cell marker–positive, although CD20 may have weaker cytoplasmic intensity than do other B-cell lymphomas. An early study found expression of Leu22 (CD43) in only 39% of cases,[41] but other authors have more recently identified CD43 in 79 to 100% of cases.[38, 67, 68] With the advent of CD5 antibodies useful in fixed tissue (in particular, clone 4C7 used with antigen retrieval methods), most SLL could be shown to be positive, although some cases exhibited weak or incomplete staining of cells.[69, 70] Although CD5 negativity by flow cytometry is often a cause for re-examining a diagnosis of B-cell CLL/SLL,[71] this is not yet true of paraffin immunohistochemistry. When present, CD23 (BU38) is useful in distinguishing this entity from mantle cell lymphoma,[38, 68, 72–75] but it should be recalled that both follicular dendritic cells and follicular lymphomas may also express CD23. CD23 expression appears to be maintained even after large cell transformation of SLL.[76] bcl-2 is positive.[74] Pertinent negative findings in B-cell CLL/SLL include CD10,[38, 77] cyclin D1,[74, 78–81] and bcl-6.[82] Elevated levels of the oncoprotein p53, although infrequently encountered, have been associated with a poor clinical outcome.[83] The chemokine receptor CXCR3 was shown to be expressed in 37 of 39 cases of CLL/SLL and absent in mantle cell, follicular, and small noncleaved–cell lymphomas.[84]

KEY DIAGNOSTIC POINTS

- CD20 and bcl-2 mark mantle cell and follicular lymphomas, and some MZLs, along with B-cell CLL/SLL.
- B-cell CLL/SLL can be distinguished from mantle cell lymphoma by CD23 (present) and cyclin D1 (absent).
- B-cell CLL/SLL can be distinguished from follicular lymphoma by CD10 (absent) and CD5/CD43 (present).

B-Cell Prolymphocytic Leukemia

Typical Phenotype: Same as B-cell CLL/SLL, but may be CD5–, CD22+

B-cell PLL rarely presents as a diagnostic dilemma in a lymph node, and although splenic involvement may raise the possibility of a splenic lymphoma, the elevated white blood cell count and typical smear make this unlikely. B-cell PLL may be CD5– and CD23–[75] and is more likely to be CD22+ than B-cell CLL/SLL.[85] Unsurprisingly, measures of mitotic index—such as Ki-67[86]—are higher in B-cell PLL.

Lymphoplasmacytic Lymphoma

Typical Phenotype: Immunoglobulin (usually IgM)-positive (focal), CD20+, CD22+, CD79a+, CD5–, CD10–, CD43+/–

This tumor of small lymphocytes and plasmacytoid lymphs is the pathologic correlate of the clinical syndrome Waldenström's macroglobulinemia. As would be expected, immunoglobulin heavy chain in the cytoplasm of the more plasmacytic cells is typically of the IgM isotype.[87] Immunoglobulin light-chain restriction is almost always demonstrable, again particularly in the more differentiated cells.[88, 89] CD20 is positive, but CD23 and CD43 (present in only 20 to 40% of cases[67, 68, 77, 90]) are far more frequently absent than in B-cell CLL/SLL. CD5 and CD10 are normally negative, but exceptions have been noted.[88] CD138 (syndecan, a marker of normal and malignant plasma cells) was absent from all 17 cases of B-cell PLL tested.[91] The Fas ligand is weakly expressed,[65] but Fas itself (CD95, a transmembrane receptor in the tumor necrosis factor–receptor superfamily) is often present.[92] BCL-2 is reported to be positive in 80% of cases.[11]

Splenic Marginal Zone B-Cell Lymphoma (With or Without Villous Lymphocytes)

Typical Phenotype: Immunoglobulin-negative or immunoglobulin-positive, B-cell antigen–positive, CD5−, CD10−, CD23−, CD43−/+, CD11c+/−

Splenic marginal zone B-cell lymphoma (SMZL) is one of the primary splenic lymphomas and may have a peripheral blood component of "villous" lymphocytes.[93] The cytoplasm projections of these villous cells may lead to confusion with hairy cell leukemia, but the immunophenotypes are different. Mature B-cell antigens are typically present (CD20, CD79a), but DBA.44 (CD72)—a B-cell marker found on a variety of low-grade B-cell lymphoma cells and most closely associated with hairy cell leukemia—is found in the cytoplasm of only 30% of SMZL cases.[94] CD43 is rarely present.[67] CD11c is present in approximately half the patients with SMZL,[95–98] compared with nearly all cases of hairy cell leukemia, but antibodies are effective for only flow cytometry or frozen sections. Ki-67 is typically low.[99, 100] BCL-2 is reportedly positive in most cases,[94, 101, 102] whereas cyclin D1 is uniformly negative.[80, 100, 103] An antibody that detects tartrate-resistant acid phosphatase (TRAP) in fixed tissues has been developed and is reportedly sensitive for hairy cell leukemia,[104, 105] but only a few cases of SMZL, showing weak expression, have been published.[106]

Hairy Cell Leukemia

Typical Phenotype: B-cell antigen–positive, CD5−, CD10−, CD23−, CD11c+ (strong), CD25+, FMC7+, CD103+

The lack of white pulp involvement in the spleen of leukemic patients makes confusion with primary splenic lymphomas uncommon, but bone marrow involvement is constant and may be exten-

sive. An aspirate is often unobtainable; the pathologist may be called on to discriminate between hairy cell leukemia and other low-grade B-cell malignancies in the marrow trephine biopsy. LCA, as well as most pan–B-cell antigens, is present[107]; T-cell markers and CD43 are negative.[108, 109] A marker such as CD20 may be useful in detecting minimal residual disease in the bone marrow.[110] As mentioned earlier, DBA.44 is frequently (50 to 100%) positive in hairy cell leukemia.[106, 111, 112] TRAP positivity by immunohistochemistry is also more frequent and more intense than in SMZL and MALT lymphomas (although one report notes that not all hairy cells in a given case stain,[106]) and the combination of TRAP and DBA.44 positivity is reported to be specific for hairy cell leukemia.[106, 113] Cyclin D1 is overexpressed in many cases of hairy cell leukemia, although at lower levels than in mantle cell lymphoma.[114, 115] Some authors report weak immunoreactivity in most or all cases of hairy cell leukemia,[115] whereas others fail to detect cyclin D1.[80, 81]

Plasma Cell Myeloma-Plasmacytoma

Typical Phenotype: Cytoplasmic immunoglobulin-positive (strong), CD19−, CD20−, CD22−, CD79a+/−, CD45RB−/+, EMA−/+, CD43+/−, CD56+/−, CD30+

Most myelomas and plasmacytomas do not present a diagnostic dilemma. They contain abundant intracellular immunoglobulin. Light-chain antibodies establish monotypia and separate them from reactive or infectious conditions, whereas the strong light-chain positivity and absence of CD20 and (usually) LCA distinguish plasmacytoma-myeloma from large B-cell lymphoma (Fig. 4–9). CD138 can provide support, as it is quite sensitive and specific for plasmacytic differentiation.[91, 116] BCL-2 is frequently present.[117]

KEY DIAGNOSTIC POINTS

- Antigens such as CD45RB and CD20, commonly associated with mature B lymphocytes, are absent from many plasma cells.
- In immature or anaplastic myeloma, do not be misled by EMA positivity.
- Similarly, CD30 positivity (typically cytoplasmic rather than membranous or paranuclear) should not occasion a diagnosis of ALCL.

Marginal Zone B-Cell Lymphoma of Mucosa-Associated Lymphoid Tissue Type

Typical Phenotype: Immunoglobulin-positive (40%, may be either the lymphoid or plasma cell

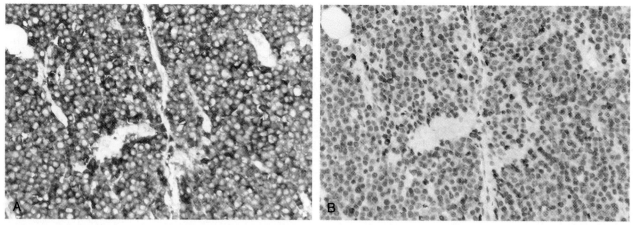

Figure 4–9. Lambda *(A)* and kappa *(B)* immunoglobulin light-chain antibodies demonstrate the clear monotypia of the plasma cells in this multiple myeloma.

component, or both), CD20+, CD79a+, CD5−, CD10−, CD23−, CD43−/+, CD11c+/−

The extranodal marginal zone B-cell lymphoma or MALT-type lymphoma presents in adults with localized disease, most commonly in the gastrointestinal tract, less frequently in other mucosa-bearing sites—such as the lacrimal gland, lung, and breast—and occasionally in nonmucosal sites like the skin and thyroid gland. It presents a heterogeneous cytologic picture, with abundant small marginal zone ("centrocyte-like") cells, monocytoid B cells with more abundant cytoplasm and reniform nuclei, and plasma cells. The small cells frequently infiltrate glandular epithelium to form lymphoepithelial lesions, which may be highlighted by a cytokeratin antibody. Immunostaining for light chains may provide assistance in distinguishing a reactive gastritis or similar condition, a common problem on small endoscopic biopsies. Light-chain monotypia is reported in 40% or more of cases[1, 118]; cutaneous extranodal MZL has been reported to be monotypic 70% of the time.[119] Both the small cell component and the plasma cell component should be examined for monotypia; lymphocyte staining may be weak so that careful comparison of the two antibodies and attention to the cytoplasm, not the surrounding interstitial staining, is necessary. The plasma cells are commonly found in a subepithelial location. In up to 40% of cases, they are monotypic and are usually easier to diagnose than the small cell component.[1] Dutcher bodies may be present. In the balance of cases, plasma cells are reactive and do not demonstrate light-chain monotypia.

The extranodal MZLs, with rare exception, do not express either CD5 or CD43[120, 121]; those that do may exhibit more aggressive disease.[122] They can be discriminated from follicular lymphoma because they are CD10−.[121] Like other lymphomas comprising small lymphocytes, extranodal MZLs are bcl-2+[123–127]; however, "high-grade" or MZLs with areas of transformed large cells are positive much less often.[124] Conversely, p53 is more fre-

quently overexpressed, and proliferation-related antigens like Ki-67 are more abundant in high-grade MALT lymphomas than in low-grade ones.[124, 128, 129] bcl-6, an oncoprotein regulator of lymphocyte differentiation found to be overexpressed in a subset of large cell lymphomas, can be identified in the large transformed lymphocytes of some high-grade MALT lymphomas.[128] Germinal centers are a common element in MALT lymphomas and may be made more apparent by immunostaining for CD21, particularly in cases of follicular colonization. The chemokine receptor CXCR3 is present in the monocytoid and plasmacytic cells of extranodal MZLs.[84]

Immunoproliferative small intestine disease is a disorder related to extranodal MALT lymphoma that is prevalent in populations living around the Mediterranean Sea. Although mucosal plasma cells expressing IgA without light chains predominate, at different stages immunoproliferative small intestine disease has marginal zone lymphocytes or large transformed lymphs similar to non-Mediterranean cases of MALT lymphoma.[130]

Nodal Marginal Zone B-Cell Lymphoma With or Without Monocytoid B Cells

Typical Phenotype: Immunoglobulin-positive, CD20+, CD79a+, CD5−, CD10−, CD23−, CD43−/+, CD11c+/−

The cytologic and immunophenotypic composition of nodal MZL is fundamentally the same as its extranodal counterpart, although some cases may be particularly rich in medium-sized monocytoid cells and relatively devoid of the smaller nodal marginal zone cells. As in the gastrointestinal tract, immunoglobulin light-chain analysis is frequently productive, with approximately 30% of cases showing monotypia.[41, 131, 132] Monotypia can be particularly helpful in favoring a diagnosis of nodal MZL over a reactive follicular hyperplasia with monocytoid B cells. CD5, CD10, and CD23 are rarely positive,[39, 70, 77, 133–135] excluding diagnoses of B-cell CLL/SLL and follicular lymphoma. Also, CD43 is expressed in 20 to 40% of the tumors.[67] The absence of cyclin D1[39, 135] essentially excludes mantle cell lymphoma. As with MALT lymphoma, most nodal examples overexpress bcl-2 (79% in one large study[36]), albeit more weakly than follicular lymphoma with which this entity may coexist.[136] Also as in the extranodal counterpart, p53 is immunohistochemically detectable in a small fraction of tumors (although point mutations in the gene are absent, indicating another mechanism of up-regulation).[137] This is in contradistinction to splenic MZLs, which frequently harbor p53 mutations.[97, 138] MZL has a phenotype similar to that of hairy cell leukemia, with the exception that DBA.44 is not expressed in most cases.[111]

Follicular Lymphoma

Typical Phenotype: B-cell antigen–positive, CD10+/−, CD5−, CD23−/+, CD43−, CD11c−

Follicular lymphoma is the most common form of non-Hodgkin's lymphoma in North America.[49] Fortunately, in most instances its characteristic morphology makes distinction from reactive conditions and other lymphomas straightforward. When small sample size or other limitations make diagnosis more difficult, the characteristic immunophenotype can resolve the issue. Pan-B−cell antigens such as CD20 and CD79a are always present, and CD10 is expressed in 90 to 95% of cases using formalin-fixed tissue.[38, 139] The latter is pertinent to the differential diagnosis of mantle cell and SLL; also helpful is the infrequency (<5% of cases) of CD43 and CD5 positivity in follicular lymphoma.[38, 39, 41, 67, 70, 71, 140] Light-chain monotypia has been noted in 28% of cases and is generally not helpful in distinguishing follicular lymphoma from other lymphomas.[41]

The bcl-2 protein was first isolated from follicular lymphomas and has played a large role in our understanding of non-Hodgkin's lymphoma in general. Now, bcl-2 has been pressed into service as a diagnostic tool for the disease. bcl-2 forms heterodimers with a number of related proteins, including bcl-x; the *bcl-2* gene is on chromosome 18 and is involved in the translocation of chromosomes 14 and 18 characteristic of follicular lymphoma. The majority of tumors overexpress the bcl-2 protein as a result of the translocation, ranging from 97% of grade I neoplasms through 83% of grade II neoplasms to 74% of grade III neoplasms.[36, 141–144] Even follicular lymphomas without an identifiable translocation overexpress bcl-2, although at a lower frequency,[145] suggesting another mechanism of up-regulation. Staining is typically more intense in the small cleaved cells, and not all small cells may stain.[146] Even variant forms of follicular lymphoma mark with anti-bcl-2 antibodies.[147] Although bcl-2 status changes with grade, it has been shown not to predict clinical outcome.[148] Like normal follicle center cells,[82] most follicular lymphomas also express bcl-6,[145, 149] a regulator of gene transcription. Transformation of follicular lymphoma to diffuse large B-cell lymphoma is accompanied by a decrease in bcl-6 expression.[150]

Cyclin D1, the hallmark of mantle cell lymphoma, is not found in follicular lymphoma.[79, 80] Tumor suppressor gene products like p53[141, 142] and RB (the retinoblastoma protein)[141] and the p53 binding protein MDM2[151] are present in more high-grade follicular lymphomas than in low-grade follicular lymphomas. Other points potentially useful in diagnosis include the rarity of CD57+ T cells in follicular lymphoma (compared with nodular lymphocyte−predominant Hodgkin's disease),[152] the generally intact meshwork of follicular dendritic cells in follicular lymphoma as demonstrated by anti-CD21 antibodies,[153] the absence of CXCR3,[84] and the frequent presence of CD30+ cells, particularly at the periphery of the follicles.[154, 155] Finally, bcl-2 has been used as an indicator of minimal residual disease in the bone marrow of follicular lymphoma patients when staining is strong and uniform.[156]

KEY DIAGNOSTIC POINTS

- bcl-2 expression is sensitive for follicular lymphoma, but not specific.
- The addition of CD43 or CD5, cyclin D1, and CD10 effectively separates the lymphomas of small lymphocytes.

Mantle Cell Lymphoma

Typical Phenotype: Surface IgM/D+, B-cell antigen−positive, CD5+, CD10−/+, CD23−, CD43+, CD11c−

With the normal counterpart believed to arise from the lymphocytes found in the inner follicle mantle, it is no surprise that the usual mature B-cell markers (CD20, CD79a) are strongly positive (although DBA.44 may be present in only a minority of cases[106]). Immunoglobulin light chains can be detected in about 40% of the cases in paraffin.[41] CD23, found in a subset of activated B lymphocytes and follicular dendritic cells, is characteristically negative in mantle cell lymphoma, although approximately 5 to 10% of tumors are positive.[38, 39, 68, 73–75, 157–159] CD10 is infrequently present.[39, 157, 160] The most useful findings in paraffin section immunohistochemistry are the presence in the nucleus of cyclin D1 protein (76 to 100% of cases) and in the cytoplasm of CD5 (73 to 100%, but some cases are weak).* As with other small lymphocyte lymphomas, CD43 is frequently co-expressed with CD5.[38, 41, 67, 68, 74] Uncommon forms of

---

*References 38, 39, 70, 74, 78, 80, 81, 157, 158, 161.

mantle cell lymphoma, including the blastoid variant (characterized by larger cells with more dispersed chromatin) and tumors localized to the mucosa[159, 160, 162] express the same antigenic pattern as the standard type, permitting distinction from precursor B-cell lymphoblastic lymphoma[57, 163] and transformed SLL.[76] In addition, TDT and CD99 are not found in the blastoid variant of mantle cell lymphoma but are in lymphoblastic lymphoma/leukemia.[57] Approximately 90% of tumors are bcl-2 producing, requiring the pathologist to be alert to the possibility of follicular lymphoma or SLL.[74, 159] Mutation in the p53 gene may result in overexpression,[164] which may in turn correlate with a more aggressive course.[165–167] The Ki-67 index can be quite variable, ranging from 5–40%.[168]

KEY DIAGNOSTIC POINTS

- Cyclin D1 is only rarely expressed by lymphomas other than mantle cell.
- Mantle cell lymphomas are often not as intensely positive for cyclin D1 as parathyroid or breast control tissues.

Diffuse Large B-Cell Lymphoma

Typical Phenotype: B-cell antigen–positive, CD45RB+ (except some anaplastic and mediastinal lymphomas), CD5−/+, CD10−/+

There are a variety of morphologic patterns to diffuse large B-cell lymphoma, and the immunophenotype is varied as well.[169, 170] The following observations have been made on a wide range of different large cell lymphomas: CD5 is generally negative,[70] although there are exceptions that do not seem to derive from mantle cell lymphoma or SLL[171]; bcl-2 (24 to 74%) and BAX expression correlate with poor outcome,[37, 172–176] as may CD44[177] and caspase expression[178]; CD43 is present in 15 to 30%[41, 67] of typical B-cell antigen–positive cases, and DBA.44[106] and CD99 are identified in some.[62] The Ki-67 index is high relative to lymphomas of small lymphocytes.[179] bcl-6, the protein associated with development of follicle center cells and with transformation of follicular lymphoma,[82, 149] is detectable in 70 to 80% of diffuse large B-cell lymphomas.[176, 180] CD10 is present about half the time.[180] Cytokeratin has rarely been identified in large cell lymphoma.[181] CD30+ large B-cell lymphomas, anaplastic or otherwise, are not currently distinguished from other diffuse large B-cell lymphomas in the WHO classification because there is no proven prognostic significance.[182]

T-cell–rich B-cell lymphomas are not immunophenotypically distinct from other diffuse large B-cell lymphomas,[183] except that they may be EMA+. Comments about the immunophenotype of recognized subtypes of diffuse large B-cell lymphoma follow.

Mediastinal Large B-Cell Lymphoma.[184] This unique entity presents in the mediastinum and is currently believed to have, as a normal counterpart, thymic medullary B cells. These lymphomas are CD20+ and CD22+, but CD21−.[185–187] CD43 is not coexpressed.[185] Typically, CD20 immunolabeling is strong. CD30 is expressed in more than half of cases[188]; staining may be diffuse cytoplasmic rather than punctate.

Primary Effusion Lymphoma.[189] A neoplasm induced by human herpes virus 8 (Kaposi's sarcoma–associated herpesvirus), this large cell lymphoma is limited to the pleural, peritoneal, and pericardial spaces of immunosuppressed patients who are virally infected. Most cases fail to express either B- or T-cell markers and are frequently CD30+.[190, 191]

Intravascular Large B-Cell Lymphoma.[192, 193] The majority of cases express B-cell markers,[194] although T cells have been reported. A variety of lymphocyte homing receptors have been discovered on the cell surface, allowing one to hypothesize about the mechanism of restriction of the lymphoma cells to the intravascular space.[193, 195]

KEY DIAGNOSTIC POINTS

- CD45RB and either CD20 or CD79a, along with S-100, cytokeratin, CD3, and CD30, form a useful panel for large cell neoplasms.
- CD30 positivity in large B-cell lymphomas is usually present in a minority of B cells, may be related to plasmacytic differentiation,[196] and has no prognostic significance.
- Sheets of large B cells are unusual in reactive conditions and should raise strong concern for lymphoma.[29]

Burkitt's Lymphoma–Burkitt's Cell Leukemia

Typical Phenotype: B-cell antigen–positive, CD10+/−, CD5−

Burkitt's and Burkitt-like lymphoma are difficult to categorize reproducibly on morphology alone (although their natural histories may be distinctive), and have been collapsed into one category in the WHO classification.[8] CD19, CD20, and CD79a are all present, and CD5 and CD23 usually are not. In an important difference from lymphoblastic lymphoma-leukemia, TDT is not found in the nuclei of Burkitt's cells.[197] Ki-67 is highly expressed (not unexpectedly given the growth fraction), and Burkitt's lymphoma has been defined as having a Ki-67 index of nearly 100%.[8] bcl-2 and CD10 have a roughly reciprocal relationship in the two variants of Burkitt's lymphoma-leukemia: The incidence of CD10 positivity is high in Burkitt's and low in Burkitt-like lymphoma, whereas bcl-2 positivity is high in Burkitt-like and low in Burkitt's lymphoma.[36] CD43 also serves to distinguish the two immunophenotypically: It is almost always present in Burkitt's and present less than half the time in Burkitt-like lymphoma.[67]

T-Cell and NK-Cell Neoplasms

PRECURSOR T-CELL NEOPLASMS

Precursor T-Lymphoblastic Leukemia-Lymphoma

Typical Phenotype: CD1a+/−, CD2+/−, CD3+ (always cytoplasmic CD3+), CD4+/CD8+ or CD8−/CD8−, CD5+/−, CD7+, CD10−/+, TDT+, CD16−/+, CD57−/+, B antigen−negative

Lymphoblasts of this disease are morphologically indistinguishable from precursor B-lymphoblastic lymphoma-leukemia and require immunologic analysis. TDT is uniformly expressed. In addition to the usual B- and T-lineage–specific antibodies, both the TAL-1 (SCL) protein and the c-kit receptor can be used to distinguish the nature of the malignancy. Antibodies to each of these proteins detect approximately 40 to 50% of T-lymphoblastic tumors and none of the B-lineage cases.[198, 199] The differential diagnosis with other blastic malignancies is usually straightforward: The blastoid variant of mantle cell lymphoma is TDT− and marks as a mature B-cell tumor, whereas granulocytic sarcomas are TDT− and frequently myeloperoxidase or lysozyme positive. Note that CD43, in addition to identifying T-cell malignancies, also marks many myelogenous processes.[198] CD99 expression is almost universal in precursor T-cell acute lymphoblastic leukemia[62]; this fact must be borne in mind when considering the differential diagnosis of pediatric small cell tumors.

MATURE T-CELL NEOPLASMS

Immunohistochemical analysis can be extremely helpful in the diagnosis and classification of peripheral (or mature) T-cell neoplasms. Although there are no immunologic markers of T-cell clonality analogous to immunoglobulin light chains, there are aberrant patterns of antigen expression that are rarely, if ever, found in normal mature T cells.[29, 200] Cells that are "double positive" for CD4 and CD8 (express both) or are "double negative" (express neither) are normally very minor populations outside the thymus. Similarly, loss of one or more pan–T-cell antigens such as CD2, CD3, CD5, TCRαβ or, most frequently, CD7, is supportive of a diagnosis of T-cell lymphoma. There are, of course, benign cases that serve as exceptions to the rule. Most of these analyses can be carried out only on fresh or frozen tissue and so are of limited use in the average pathology laboratory. Flow cytometry or consultation with a reference laboratory may be necessary.

Several of the mature T-cell leukemias are so rarely seen in surgical pathology specimens that only their usual phenotypes are supplied.

T-Prolymphocytic Leukemia

Typical Phenotype: CD2+, CD3+, CD4+ (65%), CD5+, CD7+, CD4+/CD8+ (21%), CD25−

T-Cell Large Granular Lymphocytic Leukemia

Typical Phenotype: CD2+, CD3+, CD4−, CD5−, CD7−, CD8+, TCRαβ+, CD16+, CD56−, CD57+/−, CD25−

Aggressive NK-Cell Leukemia

Typical Phenotype: CD2+, CD3−, CD4−, CD8+/−, TCRαβ−, CD16+, CD56+/−, CD57+/−

These leukemias may express the cytotoxic granule-associated protein TIA-1, which is normally found in NK cells and cytotoxic T lymphocytes, regardless of their state of activation.[201] The tumor cells are commonly infected with EBV.[202]

Adult T-Cell Lymphoma-Leukemia

Typical Phenotype: CD2+, CD3+, CD4+ (most cases), CD5+, CD7−, CD25+

Another virally induced leukemia-lymphoma (this one attributable to human T-lymphotropic virus 1 [HTLV-1]), adult T-cell lymphoma-leukemia commonly presents with an elevated white blood cell count but also has a pure lymphomatous form. In either case, the diagnosis is most convincingly made by demonstration of clonal viral DNA in tumor cells by molecular biologic methods. The histologically heterogeneous pattern makes this tumor practically indistinguishable from unspecified peripheral T-cell lymphomas absent the characteristic clinical presentation.[203] CD25 expression is typically strong. A CD30+ version of the malignancy accounting for approximately 20% of cases frequently presents extranodally and lacks leukemic manifestations, but has similar survival as CD30− cases.[204]

Extranodal NK/T-Cell Lymphoma, Nasal Type

Typical Phenotype: CD2+, CD3−, CD4−/+, CD8−/+, CD5−/+, CD7−/+, CD56+, CD43+, TCRαβ−, EBV-LMP-1+/−

As with most of the T-cell lymphomas, the distinct clinical presentation (aggressive extranodal disease, often midfacial, with necrosis [found more often in Asia]) is crucial to the diagnosis of this entity,[202] formerly known as *angiocentric lymphoma* or *lymphomatoid granulomatosis*. Angiocentricity and angioinvasiveness (leading to infarctive necrosis) are frequent, but not specific, features. This disease is intimately related to EBV infection (proven molecularly), and some cases may carry the EBV latent membrane protein (LMP-1) in tumor cells, demonstrable by paraffin section immunohistochemistry.[205–207] The expression of cytotoxic granule antigens (also detectable immunohistochemically) such as TIA-1, granzyme B, and perforin implies that this lymphoma is derived from an activated NK cell or, less commonly, a cytotoxic T-cell precursor.[201, 208–210] Pulmonary cases appear more convincingly to be B-cell large cell lymphomas.[211]

Enteropathy-Type Intestinal T-Cell Lymphoma

Typical Phenotype: CD3+, CD4−, CD7+, CD8+/−, CD56−/+, CD103+

Intestinal T-cell lymphoma most often occurs in patients with gluten-sensitive enteropathy and presents with refractory, perforating ulcers in the jejunum. A mass may or may not be evident. The histologic appearance is heterogeneous, although a subset of cases comprises monomorphic medium-sized cells—tropism for the epithelium is usually marked. Most of the intestinal lymphocytes exhibit a cytotoxic T-cell phenotype (TIA-1+ and granzyme B+), with CD56 expression relatively infrequent.[201, 212, 213] EBV infection as assessed either immunohistochemically or by in situ hybridization is infrequent.[214] ALCL involving the gastrointestinal tract has been described[215] but it is not clear that these tumors belong to the enteropathy-type category. p53 is almost universally overexpressed.[216] CD103, an integrin alpha chain that is present on more than 90% of normal intestinal intraepithelial lymphocytes and likely plays a role in homing to epithelia, is present on all enteropathy-type T-cell lymphomas. The B-ly-7 antibody recognizing this epitope is not useful in fixed tissue.

Hepatosplenic γδ T-Cell Lymphoma

Typical Phenotype: CD2+, CD3+, CD4−, CD5−, CD7+, CD8+/−, CD56+/−, TCRγδ+ (some TCRαβ+), EBV-LMP-1−

This rare primary hepatic lymphoma is composed of CD56+ T cells, most in a nonactivated state as assessed by the presence of TIA-1 and absence of perforin and granzyme B.[208, 209, 217] An unusual feature of these lymphomas is the expression of T-cell receptors of the gamma delta type, rather than the more common alpha beta heterodimer.[218] This can be determined on fixed, paraffin-embedded material now that satisfactory antibodies are available (βF1 and TCRγδ).

Subcutaneous Panniculitis-Like T-Cell Lymphoma

Typical Phenotype: CD3+, CD4−, CD8+/−, CD30−/+, CD43+, CD45RO+, CD56−/+, TIA-1+, perforin-positive, granzyme B−positive, TCRαβ+

Subcutaneous panniculitis-like lymphoma, as the name indicates, has a distinct site of involvement and morphologic pattern. The epidermis is usually spared, the tumor cells surround the dermal fat cells but do not efface them, and there is often angioinvasion by lymphocytes but no substantial infarction. Most cases are of the CD8 type and generally do not express CD56.[219, 220] All have an activated cytotoxic T-cell profile, but CD30 is only infrequently identified.[220] Immunologic distinction from other T-cell lymphomas that may involve the panniculus, such as nasal-type NK/T-cell lymphoma, may be based in part on the absence of CD56 (although some cutaneous angiocentric lymphomas are CD56− and not EBV-related)[221] and in part on the absence of an epidermal component or angiodestruction. Primary cutaneous ALCL may extend to the subcutis and mimic subcutaneous panniculitis-like T-cell lymphoma, but judicious interpretation of CD30 can assist in separating them.

Mycosis Fungoides–Sézary Syndrome

Typical Phenotype: CD2+, CD3+, CD4+, CD5+, CD7−/+, CD8−, CD25−, TCRαβ+

Mycosis fungoides and its leukemic counterpart, Sézary syndrome, are nearly indistinguishable from one another immunophenotypically, and together they form the bulk of T-cell lymphomas seen in the United States. The primary difficulty in diagnosing MF lies in the distinction from reactive or pseudolymphomas of any cause. In addition to the standard morphologic clues and molecular testing for T-cell gene rearrangements, immunohistochemistry can provide some guidance. MF frequently exhibits one or more aberrations in phenotype compared with normal T cells: CD7 is often lost,[222] approximately two thirds of cases lose another antigen (CD2, CD3, or CD5, or a combination),[223] and βF1 and CD3 (normally coexpressed) may be discordant.[224] Admixtures of B cells and CD8+ lymphocytes are also much more common in reactive conditions than in MF.[223] Characteristically, S-100+ and CD1a+ Langerhans' and interdigitating reticulum cells accompany the MF cells,[225] both in the dermis and in Pautrier's microabscesses. Large cell transformation of MF may be correlated with p53 expression detected immunohistochemically.[226]

KEY DIAGNOSTIC POINTS

- Pan−T-cell antigen loss may be demonstrable on many cases of MF, particularly if frozen section immunology is available.
- Abundant B cells or CD8+ T cells argue against MF.

Anaplastic Large Cell Lymphoma, T/Null Cell, Primary Cutaneous Type

Typical Phenotype: CD3+, CD4+, CD8−, CD15+, CD30+, EMA+, ALK−

The presence of the CD30 molecule is crucial to the recognition of this entity and the related CD30+ lymphoproliferative disorder, lymphomatoid papulosis.[227, 228] The distinction is important for patient management, as these proliferations do remarkably well with conservative therapy. The anaplastic cells may be monomorphous or polymorphous and range in number from few (in lymphomatoid papulosis type A) to numerous or sheet-like (in lymphomatoid papulosis type C and primary cutaneous ALCL). Although CD4+ and CD8−, the lymphocytes have the phenotype of activated cytotoxic cells in their expression of TIA-1 and granzyme B.[229, 230] EMA and ALK (anaplastic lymphoma kinase; the gene is involved in the t(2;5) translocation in roughly 40 to 80% of ALCL) may be found in cutaneous CD30+ ALCL. However, ALK+ ALCLs in the skin are typically not primary to the skin. CD30− large cell lymphoma also may not belong in the primary cutaneous ALCL disease category, since it exhibits a poorer outcome.[233, 234] EBV infection, as assessed by LMP-1, does not play a role in this disease.[235] The antibody HECA-452 detects an antigen on most normal skin-resident lymphocytes; the antigen is found on nearly half of primary cutaneous ALCL but no nodal ALCL.[47]

Peripheral T-Cell Lymphoma, Not Otherwise Characterized

Typical Phenotype: T-cell antigens variable, CD4+ ≥ CD8+ (may be double negative), rare B antigen−positive

A "wastebasket" category of post-thymic T-cell lymphomas,[203] this group is best defined by what it is not, that is, one of the specific peripheral T-cell lymphomas. Cytologically, there is a spectrum of T-cell sizes and sometimes an admixture of histiocytes or eosinophils. Distinction from a reactive process may be difficult immunohistochemically unless frozen tissue can be examined for antigenic loss or inappropriate expression characteristic of T-cell lymphoma.[29, 224, 236, 237] TIA-1 is present in a minority of cases, particularly those in extranodal sites,[201] and LMP-1 expression is infrequent.[238]

Angioimmunoblastic T-Cell Lymphoma

Typical Phenotype: CD2+, CD3+, CD4+, CD8−/+, CD21+ and CD23+ (in proliferated follicular dendritic cells)

It is primarily the characteristic clinical features (prominent systemic symptoms, modest systemic lymphadenopathy, polyclonal gammopathy and complications from autoantibodies and infections) that separate this entity from other peripheral T-cell lymphomas. Morphologically, there is a prominent, arborizing network of high endothelial vessels, a generalized paucity of lymphocytes, hyperplastic dendritic cell islands, and clusters of medium-sized lymphs with pale cytoplasm. The latter mark as CD4+ T cells, with no evidence of cytotoxic differentiation.[201, 209] The islands of proliferated follicular dendritic cells are characteristic of the entity and can be highlighted by antibodies to CD21 and CD23.[239] Large B cells may be found scattered throughout the node; these should not be mistaken for T-cell−rich B-cell lymphoma. Approximately two thirds of cases show LMP-1 positivity, with both B and T cells infected.[240] There are data to suggest that EBV infection is not causative but is related to the immunosuppression of the disorder; B-cell clones driven by EBV infection may explain the occasional B-cell immunoblastic lymphoma that develops in these cases.[241]

Anaplastic Large Cell Lymphoma, T/Null Cell, Primary Systemic Type

Typical Phenotype: CD45RB+/−, CD3−/+, T-cell antigens variable, CD15−/+, CD21−, CD25+/−, CD30+, CD43−/+, CD45RO−/+, EMA+/−, CD68−, lysozyme-negative, ALK+/−

The systemic form of ALCL is one of the more common types of non-Hodgkin's lymphoma, but because of its early sinusoidal localization in nodes and its pleomorphic cellular composition, it may not be recognized as a lymphoma at all. The anaplastic lymphoma cells are large, with prominent nucleoli, convoluted, Reed-Sternberg−like nuclei, and a somewhat cohesive appearance. The phenotype is readily recognizable but may present some difficulty to the unwary.[45, 242] LCA is present in most cases; one review indicated a frequency of 70 to 80%, but paraffin-embedded tissue may yield a lower fraction.[243] The lineage is more frequently T cell than null cell (lacking both B- and T-cell markers). ALCL has a T-cell lineage in 70% of cases, a B-cell lineage in 15% (these are considered diffuse large B-cell lymphomas), a B- and T-cell lineage in 5%, and a null cell lineage in 10%.[242] CD30 is, by definition, expressed in these tumors, with CD15 generally not seen.[46, 244] CD30 decorates the cell membrane and marks the Golgi area in a paranuclear dot-like fashion; diffuse cytoplasmic positivity may represent nonspecific background staining or staining of benign, large, transformed cells. EMA is focal in many cases, and antibodies to cytokeratin are reported to stain the perinuclear area of rare cases.[244] As mentioned earlier, the cutaneous lymphocyte antibody HECA-452 marks fewer than 20% of primary systemic cases.[47] Detection of the latent membrane protein of EBV has been variable.[46, 245] The small cell variant and lymphohistiocytic variant each have fewer large cells than prototypical cases, but the malignant cells maintain the expected phenotype.[246–248] The ALK protein is overexpressed in 43 to 75% of tumors; its presence correlates with EMA expression and increased patient survival.[249–252] Like many other mature T-cell lymphomas, primary systemic ALCL often exhibits a cytotoxic T-cell phenotype because of its production of TIA-1 and granzyme B.[201, 253–255] p53 is evident in the cytoplasm (>60% of cases), but mutations in the gene have not been isolated.[256, 257] CD30 and EMA expression has been used as an immunohistochemical marker of minimal disease in the bone marrow.[258]

Hodgkin's lymphoma is the most frequent differential in the diagnosis of systemic ALCL. Immunophenotyping can be invaluable if the typical LCA+/CD15-/T-cell marker−positive/EMA+/ALK+ picture is present. There are, however, borderline cases that may be difficult to resolve even after molecular analysis. Carcinomas may be distinguished from ALCL by the presence of cytokeratins (rare in lymphoma) and the absence of common and lineage-specific lymphocyte antigens. CD30 has been reported in germ cell tumors and melanoma. Melanoma, of course, may be excluded by its expression of S-100 and HMB-45.

KEY DIAGNOSTIC POINTS

- Most cases of systemic ALCL are LCA+, CD3+, CD43+, and CD30+.
- Look for CD30 in a Golgi and cell membrane pattern.
- EMA and ALK positivity, along with T-lineage markers, help distinguish ALCL from Hodgkin's lymphoma; fascin is usually negative in ALCL.

References

1. Harris NL, Jaffe ES, Stein H, et al. A revised European-American classification of lymphoid neoplasms: A proposal from the International Lymphoma Study Group. Blood 1994;84:1361–1392.
2. Poppema S. Lymphoma classification proposal. Blood 1996;87:412–413.
3. Meijer CJ, van der Valk P, de Bruin PC, Willemze R. The revised European-American lymphoma (REAL) classification of non-Hodgkin's lymphoma: A missed opportunity? Blood 1995;85(7):1971–1972.
4. Rosenberg SA. Classification of lymphoid neoplasms. Blood 1994;84:1359–1360.
5. Pittaluga S, Bijnens L, Teodorovic I, et al. Clinical analysis of 670 cases in two trials of the European Organization for the Research and Treatment of Cancer Lymphoma Cooperative Group subtyped according to the Revised European-American Classification of Lymphoid Neoplasms: A comparison with the Working Formulation. Blood 1996;87:4358–4367.
6. A clinical evaluation of the International Lymphoma Study Group classification of non-Hodgkin's lymphoma. The Non-Hodgkin's Lymphoma Classification Project. Blood 1997;89:3909–3918.
7. Jaffe ES, Harris NL, Diebold J, Muller-Hermelink HK. World Health Organization Classification of lymphomas: A work in progress. Ann Oncol 1998;9(Suppl 5):S25–30.
8. Harris NL, Jaffe ES, Diebold J, et al. The World Health Organization classification of hematological malignancies. Report of the Clinical Advisory Committee Meeting, Airlie House, Virginia, November, 1997. Mod Pathol 2000;13:193–207.
9. Jaffe ES, Harris NL, Stein H, Vardiman JW, eds. World Health Organization Classification of Tumours: Pathology and Genetics of Tumours of Haemopoietic and Lymphoid Tissues. Lyon: IARC Press, in press.
10. Abbondanzo SL. Paraffin immunohistochemistry as an adjunct to hematopathology. Ann Diagn Pathol 1999;3:318–327.
11. Chu PG, Chang KL, Arber DA, Weiss LM. Practical applications of immunohistochemistry in hematolymphoid neoplasms. Ann Diagn Pathol 1999;3:104–133.
12. Kishimoto T, Goyert S, Kikutani H, et al, eds. Leucocyte Typing VI: White Cell Differentiation Antigens. New York: Garland, 1997.
13. Pileri SA, Roncador G, Ceccarelli C, et al. Antigen retrieval techniques in immunohistochemistry: Comparison of different methods. J Pathol 1997;183:116–123.
14. Shi SR, Key ME, Kalra KL. Antigen retrieval in formalin-fixed, paraffin-embedded tissues: An enhancement method for immunohistochemical staining based on microwave oven heating of tissue sections. J Histochem Cytochem 1991;39:741–748.
15. Shi SR, Cote RJ, Taylor CR. Antigen retrieval immunohistochemistry: Past, present, and future. J Histochem Cytochem 1997;45:327–343.
16. Johnson K, Chensue S, Ward P. Immunopathology. In: Rubin E, Farber J, eds. Pathology. 3rd ed. Philadelphia: Lippincott-Raven, 1999:104–153.
17. Inghirami G, Knowles D. The immune system: Structure and function. In: Knowles D, ed. Neoplastic Hematopathology. Baltimore: Williams & Wilkins, 1992:27–72.
18. Benoist C, Mathis D. T lymphocyte differentiation and biology. In: Paul W, ed. Fundamental Immunology. 4th ed. Philadelphia: Lippincott-Raven, 1999:367–410.
19. DeFranco A. B lymphocyte activation. In: Paul W, ed. Fundamental Immunology. 4th ed. Philadelphia: Lippincott-Raven, 1999:225–261.
20. Melchers F, Rolink A. B-lymphocyte development and biology. In: Paul W, ed. Fundamental Immunology. 4th ed. Philadelphia: Lippincott-Raven, 1999:183–224.
21. Rudin CM, Thompson CB. B-cell development and maturation. Semin Oncol 1998;25:435–446.
22. Lennert K, Feller A. Histopathology of Non-Hodgkin's Lymphomas. 2nd ed. Berlin: Springer-Verlag, 1992.
23. Lukes R, Collins R. A functional approach to the classification of malignant lymphoma. Recent Results Cancer Res 1974;46:18–30.
24. Lukes RJ, Collins RD. Immunologic characterization of human malignant lymphomas. Cancer 1974;34(4 Suppl):1488–1503.
25. Stetler-Stevenson M, Medieros L, Jaffe E. Immunophenotypic methods and findings in the diagnosis of lymphoproliferative diseases. In: Jaffe E, ed. Surgical Pathology of the Lymph Nodes and Related Organs. 2nd ed. Philadelphia: WB Saunders, 1995:22–57.
26. Mason DY, Cordell JL, Brown MH, et al. CD79a: A novel

marker for B-cell neoplasms in routinely processed tissue samples. Blood 1995;86:1453–1459.

27. Malisius R, Merz H, Heinz B, et al. Constant detection of CD2, CD3, CD4, and CD5 in fixed and paraffin-embedded tissue using the peroxidase-mediated deposition of biotin-tyramide. J Histochem Cytochem 1997;45:1665–1672.

28. Macon WR, Salhany KE. T-cell subset analysis of peripheral T-cell lymphomas by paraffin section immunohistology and correlation of CD4/CD8 results with flow cytometry. Am J Clin Pathol 1998;109:610–617.

29. Picker LJ, Weiss LM, Medeiros LJ, et al. Immunophenotypic criteria for the diagnosis of non-Hodgkin's lymphoma. Am J Pathol 1987;128:181–201.

30. Delsol G, Lamant L, Mariame B, et al. A new subtype of large B-cell lymphoma expressing the ALK kinase and lacking the 2;5 translocation. Blood 1997;89:1483–1490.

31. Falini B, Bigerna B, Fizzotti M, et al. ALK expression defines a distinct group of T/null lymphomas ("ALK lymphomas") with a wide morphological spectrum. Am J Pathol 1998;153:875–886.

32. Falini B, Fizzotti M, Pileri S, et al. Bcl-6 protein expression in normal and neoplastic lymphoid tissues. Ann Oncol 1997;8 Suppl 2:101–104.

33. Arber D, Weiss L. CD57: A review. Appl Immunohistochem 1995;3:137–152.

34. Frizzera G, Wu CD, Inghirami G. The usefulness of immunophenotypic and genotypic studies in the diagnosis and classification of hematopoietic and lymphoid neoplasms: An update. Am J Clin Pathol 1999;111(1 Suppl 1):S13–39.

35. Troxel DB, Sabella JD. Problem areas in pathology practice: Uncovered by a review of malpractice claims. Am J Surg Pathol 1994;18:821–831.

36. Lai R, Arber DA, Chang KL, et al. Frequency of bcl-2 expression in non-Hodgkin's lymphoma: A study of 778 cases with comparison of marginal zone lymphoma and monocytoid B-cell hyperplasia. Mod Pathol 1998;11:864–869.

37. Wang T, Lasota J, Hanau CA, Miettinen M. Bcl-2 oncoprotein is widespread in lymphoid tissue and lymphomas but its differential expression in benign versus malignant follicles and monocytoid B-cell proliferations is of diagnostic value. APMIS 1995;103:655–662.

38. de Leon ED, Alkan S, Huang JC, Hsi ED. Usefulness of an immunohistochemical panel in paraffin-embedded tissues for the differentiation of B-cell non-Hodgkin's lymphomas of small lymphocytes. Mod Pathol 1998;11:1046–1051.

39. Kurtin PJ, Hobday KS, Ziesmer S, Caron BL. Demonstration of distinct antigenic profiles of small B-cell lymphomas by paraffin section immunohistochemistry. Am J Clin Pathol 1999;112:319–329.

40. Almasri NM, Iturraspe JA, Braylan RC. CD10 expression in follicular lymphoma and large cell lymphoma is different from that of reactive lymph node follicles. Arch Pathol Lab Med 1998;122:539–544.

41. Gelb AB, Rouse RV, Dorfman RF, Warnke RA. Detection of immunophenotypic abnormalities in paraffin-embedded B-lineage non-Hodgkin's lymphomas. Am J Clin Pathol 1994;102:825–834.

42. Browne G, Tobin B, Carney DN, Dervan PA. Aberrant MT2 positivity distinguishes follicular lymphoma from reactive follicular hyperplasia in B5- and formalin-fixed paraffin sections. Am J Clin Pathol 1991;96:90–94.

43. Emile JF, Wechsler J, Brousse N, et al. Langerhans' cell histiocytosis: Definitive diagnosis with the use of monoclonal antibody O10 on routinely paraffin-embedded samples. Am J Surg Pathol 1995;19:636–641.

44. Ng CS, Chan JK, Hui PK, Lau WH. Large B-cell lymphomas with a high content of reactive T cells. Hum Pathol 1989;20:1145–1154.

45. Falini B, Pileri S, Stein H, et al. Variable expression of leucocyte-common (CD45) antigen in CD30 (Ki1)-positive anaplastic large-cell lymphoma: Implications for the differential diagnosis between lymphoid and nonlymphoid malignancies. Hum Pathol 1990;21:624–629.

46. Clavio M, Rossi E, Truini M, et al. Anaplastic large cell lymphoma: A clinicopathologic study of 53 patients. Leuk Lymphoma 1996;22:319–327.

47. de Bruin PC, Beljaards RC, van Heerde P, et al. Differences in clinical behaviour and immunophenotype between primary cutaneous and primary nodal anaplastic large cell lymphoma of T-cell or null cell phenotype. Histopathology 1993;23:127–135.

48. Battifora H. Assessment of antigen damage in immunohistochemistry: The vimentin internal control. Am J Clin Pathol 1991;96:669–671.

49. Anderson JR, Armitage JO, Weisenburger DD. Epidemiology of the non-Hodgkin's lymphomas: Distributions of the major subtypes differ by geographic locations: Non-Hodgkin's Lymphoma Classification Project. Ann Oncol 1998;9:717–720.

50. Medeiros L. Intermediate and high-grade diffuse non-Hodgkin's lymphomas in the Working Formulation. In: Jaffe E, ed. Surgical Pathology of the Lymph Nodes and Related Organs. 2nd ed. Philadelphia: WB Saunders, 1995:283–343.

51. Weiss LM, Bindl JM, Picozzi VJ, et al. Lymphoblastic lymphoma: An immunophenotype study of 26 cases with comparison to T cell acute lymphoblastic leukemia. Blood 1986;67:474–478.

52. Cossman J, Chused TM, Fisher RI, et al. Diversity of immunological phenotypes of lymphoblastic lymphoma. Cancer Res 1983;43:4486–4490.

53. Braziel RM, Keneklis T, Donlon JA, et al. Terminal deoxynucleotidyl transferase in non-Hodgkin's lymphoma. Am J Clin Pathol 1983;80:655–659.

54. Ozdemirli M, Fanburg-Smith JC, Hartmann DP, et al. Precursor B-lymphoblastic lymphoma presenting as a solitary bone tumor and mimicking Ewing's sarcoma: A report of four cases and review of the literature. Am J Surg Pathol 1998;22:795–804.

55. Iravani S, Singleton TP, Ross CW, Schnitzer B. Precursor B lymphoblastic lymphoma presenting as lytic bone lesions. Am J Clin Pathol 1999;112:836–843.

56. Chimenti S, Fink-Puches R, Peris K, et al. Cutaneous involvement in lymphoblastic lymphoma. J Cutan Pathol 1999;26:379–385.

57. Soslow RA, Zukerberg LR, Harris NL, Warnke RA. BCL-1 (PRAD-1/cyclin D-1) overexpression distinguishes the blastoid variant of mantle cell lymphoma from B-lineage lymphoblastic lymphoma. Mod Pathol 1997;10:810–817.

58. Soslow RA, Baergen RN, Warnke RA. B-lineage lymphoblastic lymphoma is a clinicopathologic entity distinct from other histologically similar aggressive lymphomas with blastic morphology. Cancer 1999;85:2648–2654.

59. Van Eyken P, De Wolf-Peeters C, Van den Oord J, et al. Expression of leukocyte common antigen in lymphoblastic lymphoma and small noncleaved undifferentiated non-Burkitt's lymphoma: An immunohistochemical study. J Pathol 1987;151:257–261.

60. Taubenberger JK, Cole DE, Raffeld M, et al. Immunophenotypic analysis of acute lymphoblastic leukemia using routinely processed bone marrow specimens. Arch Pathol Lab Med 1991;115:338–342.

61. Robertson PB, Neiman RS, Worapongpaiboon S, et al. O13 (CD99) positivity in hematologic proliferations correlates with TdT positivity. Mod Pathol 1997;10:277–282.

62. Riopel M, Dickman PS, Link MP, Perlman EJ. MIC2 analysis in pediatric lymphomas and leukemias. Hum Pathol 1994;25:396–399.

63. Sheibani K, Nathwani BN, Winberg CD, et al. Antigenically defined subgroups of lymphoblastic lymphoma: Relationship to clinical presentation and biologic behavior. Cancer 1987;60:183–190.

64. Tsang WY, Chan JK, Ng CS, Pau MY. Utility of a paraffin section–reactive CD56 antibody (123C3) for characterization and diagnosis of lymphomas. Am J Surg Pathol 1996;20:202–210.

65. Mullauer L, Mosberger I, Chott A. Fas ligand expression in nodal non-Hodgkin's lymphoma. Mod Pathol 1998;11:369–375.

66. Soslow RA, Bhargava V, Warnke RA. MIC2, TdT, bcl-2, and CD34 expression in paraffin-embedded high-grade lymphoma/acute lymphoblastic leukemia distinguishes between distinct clinicopathologic entities. Hum Pathol 1997;28:1158–1165.

67. Lai R, Weiss LM, Chang KL, Arber DA. Frequency of CD43 expression in non-Hodgkin lymphoma: A survey of 742 cases and further characterization of rare CD43+ follicular lymphomas. Am J Clin Pathol 1999;111:488–494.

68. Kumar S, Green GA, Teruya-Feldstein J, et al. Use of CD23 (BU38) on paraffin sections in the diagnosis of small lymphocytic lymphoma and mantle cell lymphoma. Mod Pathol 1996;9:925–929.

69. Kaufmann O, Flath B, Spath-Schwalbe E, et al. Immuno-histochemical detection of CD5 with monoclonal antibody 4C7 on paraffin sections. Am J Clin Pathol 1997;108:669–673.

70. Dorfman DM, Shahsafaei A. Usefulness of a new CD5 antibody for the diagnosis of T-cell and B-cell lymphoproliferative disorders in paraffin sections. Mod Pathol 1997;10:859–863.

71. Huang JC, Finn WG, Goolsby CL, et al. CD5− small B-cell leukemias are rarely classifiable as chronic lymphocytic leukemia. Am J Clin Pathol 1999;111:123–130.

72. Orazi A, Cattoretti G, Polli N, et al. Distinct morphophenotypic features of chronic B-cell leukaemias identified with CD1c and CD23 antibodies. Eur J Haematol 1991;47:28–35.

73. Singh N, Wright DH. The value of immunohistochemistry on paraffin wax embedded tissue sections in the differentiation of small lymphocytic and mantle cell lymphomas. J Clin Pathol 1997;50:16–21.

74. Aguilera NS, Chu WS, Andriko JA, Abbondanzo SL. Expression of CD44 (HCAM) in small lymphocytic and mantle cell lymphoma. Hum Pathol 1998;29:1134–1139.

75. Dorfman DM, Pinkus GS. Distinction between small lymphocytic and mantle cell lymphoma by immunoreactivity for CD23. Mod Pathol 1994;7:326–331.

76. Dunphy CH, Wheaton SE, Perkins SL. CD23 expression in transformed small lymphocytic lymphomas/chronic lymphocytic leukemias and blastic transformations of mantle cell lymphoma. Mod Pathol 1997;10:818–822.

77. Watson P, Wood KM, Lodge A, et al. Monoclonal antibodies recognizing CD5, CD10 and CD23 in formalin-fixed, paraffin-embedded tissue: Production and assessment of their value in the diagnosis of small B-cell lymphoma. Histopathology 2000;36:145–150.

78. Swerdlow SH, Yang WI, Zukerberg LR, et al. Expression of cyclin D1 protein in centrocytic/mantle cell lymphomas with and without rearrangement of the BCL1/cyclin D1 gene. Hum Pathol 1995;26:999–1004.

79. Yang WI, Zukerberg LR, Motokura T, et al. Cyclin D1 (Bcl-1, PRAD1) protein expression in low-grade B-cell lymphomas and reactive hyperplasia. Am J Pathol 1994;145:86–96.

80. Vasef MA, Medeiros LJ, Koo C, et al. Cyclin D1 immunohistochemical staining is useful in distinguishing mantle cell lymphoma from other low-grade B-cell neoplasms in bone marrow. Am J Clin Pathol 1997;108:302–307.

81. Zukerberg LR, Yang WI, Arnold A, Harris NL. Cyclin D1 expression in non-Hodgkin's lymphomas: Detection by immunohistochemistry. Am J Clin Pathol 1995;103:756–760.

82. Raible MD, Hsi ED, Alkan S. Bcl-6 protein expression by follicle center lymphomas: A marker for differentiating follicle center lymphomas from other low-grade lymphoproliferative disorders. Am J Clin Pathol 1999;112:101–107.

83. Aguilar-Santelises M, Magnusson KP, Wiman KG, et al. Progressive B-cell chronic lymphocytic leukaemia frequently exhibits aberrant p53 expression. Int J Cancer 1994;58:474–479.

84. Jones D, Benjamin RJ, Shahsafaei A, Dorfman DM. The chemokine receptor CXCR3 is expressed in a subset of B-cell lymphomas and is a marker of B-cell chronic lymphocytic leukemia. Blood 2000;95:627–632.

85. Bennett JM, Catovsky D, Daniel MT, et al. Proposals for the classification of chronic (mature) B and T lymphoid leukaemias: French-American-British (FAB) Cooperative Group. J Clin Pathol 1989;42:567–584.

86. de Melo N, Matutes E, Cordone I, et al. Expression of Ki-67 nuclear antigen in B and T cell lymphoproliferative disorders. J Clin Pathol 1992;45:660–663.

87. Harris NL, Bhan AK. B-cell neoplasms of the lymphocytic, lymphoplasmacytoid, and plasma cell types: Immunohistologic analysis and clinical correlation. Hum Pathol 1985;16:829–837.

88. Hall PA, D'Ardenne AJ, Richards MA, Stansfeld AG. Lymphoplasmacytoid lymphoma: An immunohistological study. J Pathol 1987;153:213–223.

89. Zukerberg LR, Medeiros LJ, Ferry JA, Harris NL. Diffuse low-grade B-cell lymphomas: Four clinically distinct subtypes defined by a combination of morphologic and immunophenotypic features. Am J Clin Pathol 1993;100:373–385.

90. Tworek JA, Singleton TP, Schnitzer B, et al. Flow cytometric and immunohistochemical analysis of small lymphocytic lymphoma, mantle cell lymphoma, and plasmacytoid small lymphocytic lymphoma. Am J Clin Pathol 1998;110:582–589.

91. Chilosi M, Adami F, Lestani M, et al. CD138/syndecan-1: A useful immunohistochemical marker of normal and neoplastic plasma cells on routine trephine bone marrow biopsies. Mod Pathol 1999;12:1101–1106.

92. Nguyen PL, Harris NL, Ritz J, Robertson MJ. Expression of CD95 antigen and Bcl-2 protein in non-Hodgkin's lymphomas and Hodgkin's disease. Am J Pathol 1996;148:847–853.

93. Catovsky D, Matutes E. Splenic lymphoma with circulating villous lymphocytes/splenic marginal-zone lymphoma. Semin Hematol 1999;36:148–154.

94. Hammer RD, Glick AD, Greer JP, et al. Splenic marginal zone lymphoma: A distinct B-cell neoplasm. Am J Surg Pathol 1996;20:613–626.

95. Matutes E, Morilla R, Owusu-Ankomah K, et al. The immunophenotype of hairy cell leukemia (HCL): Proposal for a scoring system to distinguish HCL from B-cell disorders with hairy or villous lymphocytes. Leuk Lymphoma 1994;14(Suppl 1):57–61.

96. Matutes E, Morilla R, Owusu-Ankomah K, et al. The immunophenotype of splenic lymphoma with villous lymphocytes and its relevance to the differential diagnosis with other B-cell disorders. Blood 1994;83:1558–1562.

97. Baldini L, Fracchiolla NS, Cro LM, et al. Frequent p53 gene involvement in splenic B-cell leukemia/lymphomas of possible marginal zone origin. Blood 1994;84:270–278.

98. Rosso R, Neiman RS, Paulli M, et al. Splenic marginal zone cell lymphoma: Report of an indolent variant without massive splenomegaly presumably representing an early phase of the disease. Hum Pathol 1995;26:39–46.

99. Piris MA, Mollejo M, Campo E, et al. A marginal zone pattern may be found in different varieties of non-Hodgkin's lymphoma: The morphology and immunohistology of splenic involvement by B-cell lymphomas simulating splenic marginal zone lymphoma. Histopathology 1998;33:230–239.

100. Mollejo M, Lloret E, Menarguez J, et al. Lymph node involvement by splenic marginal zone lymphoma: Morphological and immunohistochemical features. Am J Surg Pathol 1997;21:772–780.

101. Wu CD, Jackson CL, Medeiros LJ. Splenic marginal zone cell lymphoma: An immunophenotypic and molecular study of five cases. Am J Clin Pathol 1996;105:277–285.

102. Pawade J, Wilkins BS, Wright DH. Low-grade B-cell lymphomas of the splenic marginal zone: A clinicopathological and immunohistochemical study of 14 cases. Histopathology 1995;27:129–137.

103. Savilo E, Campo E, Mollejo M, et al. Absence of cyclin D1 protein expression in splenic marginal zone lymphoma. Mod Pathol 1998;11:601–606.

104. Janckila AJ, Cardwell EM, Yam LT, Li CY. Hairy cell identification by immunohistochemistry of tartrate-resistant acid phosphatase. Blood 1995;85:2839–2844.

105. Janckila AJ, Lear SC, Martin AW, Yam LT. Epitope enhancement for immunohistochemical demonstration of tartrate-resistant acid phosphatase. J Histochem Cytochem 1996;44:235–244.

106. Hoyer JD, Li CY, Yam LT, et al. Immunohistochemical demonstration of acid phosphatase isoenzyme 5 (tartrate-resistant) in paraffin sections of hairy cell leukemia and other hematologic disorders. Am J Clin Pathol 1997;108: 308–315.

107. Stroup R, Sheibani K. Antigenic phenotypes of hairy cell leukemia and monocytoid B-cell lymphoma: An immunohistochemical evaluation of 66 cases. Hum Pathol 1992;23: 172–177.

108. Kreft A, Busche G, Bernhards J, Georgii A. Immunophenotype of hairy-cell leukaemia after cold polymerization of methyl-methacrylate embeddings from 50 diagnostic bone marrow biopsies. Histopathology 1997;30:145–151.

109. Segal GH, Stoler MH, Fishleder AJ, Tubbs RR. Reliable and cost-effective paraffin section immunohistology of lymphoproliferative disorders. Am J Surg Pathol 1991;15: 1034–1041.

110. Hakimian D, Tallman MS, Kiley C, Peterson L. Detection of minimal residual disease by immunostaining of bone marrow biopsies after 2-chlorodeoxyadenosine for hairy cell leukemia. Blood 1993;82:1798–1802.

111. Ohsawa M, Kanno H, Machii T, Aozasa K. Immunoreactivity of neoplastic and non-neoplastic monocytoid B lymphocytes for DBA.44 and other antibodies. J Clin Pathol 1994;47:928–932.

112. Hounieu H, Chittal SM, al Saati T, et al. Hairy cell leukemia: Diagnosis of bone marrow involvement in paraffin-embedded sections with monoclonal antibody DBA.44. Am J Clin Pathol 1992;98:26–33.

113. Yaziji H, Janckila AJ, Lear SC, et al. Immunohistochemical detection of tartrate-resistant acid phosphatase in non-hematopoietic human tissues. Am J Clin Pathol 1995;104: 397–402.

114. Bosch F, Campo E, Jares P, et al. Increased expression of the PRAD-1/CCND1 gene in hairy cell leukaemia. Br J Haematol 1995;91:1025–1030.

115. de Boer CJ, Kluin-Nelemans JC, Dreef E, et al. Involvement of the CCND1 gene in hairy cell leukemia. Ann Oncol 1996;7:251–256.

116. Costes V, Magen V, Legouffe E, et al. The Mi15 monoclonal antibody (anti-syndecan-1) is a reliable marker for quantifying plasma cells in paraffin-embedded bone marrow biopsy specimens. Hum Pathol 1999;30:1405–1411.

117. Hamilton MS, Barker HF, Ball J, et al. Normal and neoplastic human plasma cells express bcl-2 antigen. Leukemia 1991;5:768–771.

118. Diss TC, Wotherspoon AC, Speight P, et al. B-cell monoclonality, Epstein Barr virus, and t(14;18) in myoepithelial sialadenitis and low-grade B-cell MALT lymphoma of the parotid gland. Am J Surg Pathol 1995;19:531–536.

119. Baldassano MF, Bailey EM, Ferry JA, et al. Cutaneous lymphoid hyperplasia and cutaneous marginal zone lymphoma: Comparison of morphologic and immunophenotypic features. Am J Surg Pathol 1999;23:88–96.

120. Berger F, Felman P, Thieblemont C, et al. Non-MALT marginal zone B-cell lymphomas: A description of clinical presentation and outcome in 124 patients. Blood 2000;95: 1950–1956.

121. Arends JE, Bot FJ, Gisbertz IA, Schouten HC. Expression of CD10, CD75 and CD43 in MALT lymphoma and their usefulness in discriminating MALT lymphoma from follicular lymphoma and chronic gastritis. Histopathology 1999;35: 209–215.

122. Ferry JA, Yang WI, Zukerberg LR, et al. CD5+ extranodal marginal zone B-cell (MALT) lymphoma: A low grade neoplasm with a propensity for bone marrow involvement and relapse. Am J Clin Pathol 1996;105:31–37.

123. Cerroni L, Signoretti S, Hofler G, et al. Primary cutaneous marginal zone B-cell lymphoma: A recently described entity of low-grade malignant cutaneous B-cell lymphoma. Am J Surg Pathol 1997;21:1307–1315.

124. Nakamura S, Akazawa K, Kinukawa N, et al. Inverse correlation between the expression of bcl-2 and p53 proteins in primary gastric lymphoma. Hum Pathol 1996;27:225–233.

125. Chetty R, O'Leary JJ, Biddolph SC, Gatter KC. Immunohistochemical detection of p53 and Bcl-2 proteins in Hashimoto's thyroiditis and primary thyroid lymphomas. J Clin Pathol 1995;48:239–241.

126. Ashton-Key M, Biddolph SC, Stein H, et al. Heterogeneity of bcl-2 expression in MALT lymphoma. Histopathology 1995;26:75–78.

127. Navratil E, Gaulard P, Kanavaros P, et al. Expression of the bcl-2 protein in B cell lymphomas arising from mucosa associated lymphoid tissue. J Clin Pathol 1995;48: 18–21.

128. Omonishi K, Yoshino T, Sakuma I, et al. Bcl-6 protein is identified in high-grade but not low-grade mucosa-associated lymphoid tissue lymphomas of the stomach. Mod Pathol 1998;11:181–185.

129. Nakamura S, Akazawa K, Yao T, Tsuneyoshi M. A clinicopathologic study of 233 cases with special reference to evaluation with the MIB-1 index. Cancer 1995;76:1313–1324.

130. Isaacson PG. Gastrointestinal lymphomas of T- and B-cell types. Mod Pathol 1999;12:151–158.

131. Davis GG, York JC, Glick AD, et al. Plasmacytic differentiation in parafollicular (monocytoid) B-cell lymphoma: A study of 12 cases. Am J Surg Pathol 1992;16:1066–1074.

132. Nizze H, Cogliatti SB, von Schilling C, et al. Monocytoid B-cell lymphoma: Morphological variants and relationship to low-grade B-cell lymphoma of the mucosa-associated lymphoid tissue. Histopathology 1991;18:403–414.

133. Ballesteros E, Osborne BM, Matsushima AY. CD5+ low-grade marginal zone B-cell lymphomas with localized presentation. Am J Surg Pathol 1998;22:201–207.

134. Dierlamm J, Pittaluga S, Wlodarska I, et al. Marginal zone B-cell lymphomas of different sites share similar cytogenetic and morphologic features. Blood 1996;87:299–307.

135. Campo E, Miquel R, Krenacs L, et al. Primary nodal marginal zone lymphomas of splenic and MALT type. Am J Surg Pathol 1999;23:59–68.

136. Hernandez AM, Nathwani BN, Nguyen D, et al. Nodal benign and malignant monocytoid B cells with and without follicular lymphomas: A comparative study of follicular colonization, light chain restriction, bcl-2, and t(14;18) in 39 cases. Hum Pathol 1995;26:625–632.

137. Levy V, Miller C, Koeffler HP, Said JW. p53 in lymphomas of mucosal-associated lymphoid tissues. Mod Pathol 1996; 9(3):245–248.

138. Baldini L, Guffanti A, Cro L, et al. Poor prognosis in non-villous splenic marginal zone cell lymphoma is associated with p53 mutations. Br J Haematol 1997;99:375–378.

139. McIntosh GG, Lodge AJ, Watson P, et al. NCL-CD10-270: A new monoclonal antibody recognizing CD10 in paraffin-embedded tissue. Am J Pathol 1999;154:77–82.

140. Contos MJ, Kornstein MJ, Innes DJ, Ben-Ezra J. The utility of CD20 and CD43 in subclassification of low-grade B-cell lymphoma on paraffin sections. Mod Pathol 1992;5:631–633.

141. Nguyen PL, Zukerberg LR, Benedict WF, Harris NL. Immunohistochemical detection of p53, bcl-2, and retinoblastoma proteins in follicular lymphoma. Am J Clin Pathol 1996;105:538–543.

142. Cooper K, Haffajee Z. bcl-2 and p53 protein expression in follicular lymphoma. J Pathol 1997;182:307–310.

143. Ashton-Key M, Diss TC, Isaacson PG, Smith ME. A comparative study of the value of immunohistochemistry and the polymerase chain reaction in the diagnosis of follicular lymphoma. Histopathology 1995;27:501–508.

144. Gaulard P, d'Agay MF, Peuchmaur M, et al. Expression of the bcl-2 gene product in follicular lymphoma. Am J Pathol 1992;140:1089–1095.

145. Skinnider BF, Horsman DE, Dupuis B, Gascoyne RD. Bcl-6 and Bcl-2 protein expression in diffuse large B-cell lymphoma and follicular lymphoma: Correlation with 3q27

and 18q21 chromosomal abnormalities. Hum Pathol 1999; 30:803–808.

146. Logsdon MD, Meyn RE Jr, Besa PC, et al. Apoptosis and the Bcl-2 gene family—patterns of expression and prognostic value in stage I and II follicular center lymphoma. Int J Radiat Oncol Biol Phys 1999;44:19–29.

147. Goates JJ, Kamel OW, LeBrun DP, et al. Floral variant of follicular lymphoma: Immunological and molecular studies support a neoplastic process. Am J Surg Pathol 1994; 18:37–47.

148. Pezzella F, Jones M, Ralfkiaer E, et al. Evaluation of bcl-2 protein expression and 14;18 translocation as prognostic markers in follicular lymphoma. Br J Cancer 1992;65: 87–89.

149. Cattoretti G, Chang CC, Cechova K, et al. BCL-6 protein is expressed in germinal-center B cells. Blood 1995;86: 45–53.

150. Szereday Z, Csernus B, Nagy M, et al. Somatic mutation of the 5' noncoding region of the BCL-6 gene is associated with intraclonal diversity and clonal selection in histological transformation of follicular lymphoma. Am J Pathol 2000;156:1017–1024.

151. Moller MB, Nielsen O, Pedersen NT. Oncoprotein MDM2 overexpression is associated with poor prognosis in distinct non-Hodgkin's lymphoma entities. Mod Pathol 1999; 12:1010–1016.

152. Kamel OW, Gelb AB, Shibuya RB, Warnke RA. Leu 7 (CD57) reactivity distinguishes nodular lymphocyte predominance Hodgkin's disease from nodular sclerosing Hodgkin's disease, T-cell-rich B-cell lymphoma and follicular lymphoma. Am J Pathol 1993;142:541–546.

153. Scoazec JY, Berger F, Magaud JP, et al. The dendritic reticulum cell pattern in B cell lymphomas of the small cleaved, mixed, and large cell types: An immunohistochemical study of 48 cases. Hum Pathol 1989;20:124–131.

154. Miettinen M. CD30 distribution: Immunohistochemical study on formaldehyde-fixed, paraffin-embedded Hodgkin's and non-Hodgkin's lymphomas. Arch Pathol Lab Med 1992;116:1197–1201.

155. Piris M, Gatter KC, Mason DY. CD30 expression in follicular lymphoma. Histopathology 1991;18:25–29.

156. Chetty R, Echezarreta G, Comley M, Gatter K. Immunohistochemistry in apparently normal bone marrow trephine specimens from patients with nodal follicular lymphoma. J Clin Pathol 1995;48:1035–1038.

157. Kurtin PJ. Mantle cell lymphoma. Adv Anat Pathol 1998;5: 376–398.

158. Pittaluga S, Wlodarska I, Stul MS, et al. Mantle cell lymphoma: A clinicopathological study of 55 cases. Histopathology 1995;26:17–24.

159. Lavergne A, Brouland JP, Launay E, et al. Multiple lymphomatous polyposis of the gastrointestinal tract: An extensive histopathologic and immunohistochemical study of 12 cases. Cancer 1994;74:3042–3050.

160. Fraga M, Lloret E, Sanchez-Verde L, et al. Mucosal mantle cell (centrocytic) lymphomas. Histopathology 1995;26: 413–422.

161. Yatabe Y, Suzuki R, Tobinai K, et al. Significance of cyclin D1 overexpression for the diagnosis of mantle cell lymphoma: A clinicopathologic comparison of cyclin D1-positive MCL and cyclin D1-negative MCL-like B-cell lymphoma. Blood 2000;95:2253–2261.

162. Kumar S, Krenacs L, Otsuki T, et al. Bc1-1 rearrangement and cyclin D1 protein expression in multiple lymphomatous polyposis. Am J Clin Pathol 1996;105:737–743.

163. Singleton TP, Anderson MM, Ross CW, Schnitzer B. Leukemic phase of mantle cell lymphoma, blastoid variant. Am J Clin Pathol 1999;111:495–500.

164. Gronbaek K, Nedergaard T, Andersen MK, et al. Concurrent disruption of cell cycle associated genes in mantle cell lymphoma: A genotypic and phenotypic study of cyclin D1, p16, p15, p53 and pRb. Leukemia 1998;12:1266–1271.

165. Chang CC, Liu YC, Cleveland RP, Perkins SL. Expression of c-Myc and p53 correlates with clinical outcome in diffuse large B-cell lymphomas. Am J Clin Pathol 2000;113: 512–518.

166. Louie DC, Offit K, Jaslow R, et al. p53 overexpression as a marker of poor prognosis in mantle cell lymphomas with t(11;14)(q13;q32). Blood 1995;86:2892–2899.

167. Hernandez L, Fest T, Cazorla M, et al. p53 gene mutations and protein overexpression are associated with aggressive variants of mantle cell lymphomas. Blood 1996;87:3351–3359.

168. Fiel-Gan MD, Almeida LM, Rose DC, et al. Proliferative fraction, bcl-1 gene translocation, and p53 mutation status as markers in mantle cell lymphoma. Int J Mol Med 1999; 3:373–379.

169. Stein H, Lennert K, Feller AC, Mason DY. Immunohistological analysis of human lymphoma: Correlation of histological and immunological categories. Adv Cancer Res 1984;42:67–147.

170. Doggett RS, Wood GS, Horning S, et al. The immunologic characterization of 95 nodal and extranodal diffuse large cell lymphomas in 89 patients. Am J Pathol 1984;115:245–252.

171. Taniguchi M, Oka K, Hiasa A, et al. De novo CD5+ diffuse large B-cell lymphomas express VH genes with somatic mutation. Blood 1998;91:1145–1151.

172. Fang JM, Finn WG, Hussong JW, et al. CD10 antigen expression correlates with the t(14;18)(q32;q21) major breakpoint region in diffuse large B-cell lymphoma. Mod Pathol 1999;12:295–300.

173. Martinka M, Comeau T, Foyle A, et al. Prognostic significance of t(14;18) and bcl-2 gene expression in follicular small cleaved cell lymphoma and diffuse large cell lymphoma: Clinical and investigative medicine. Med Clin Exp 1997;20:364–370.

174. Gascoyne RD, Krajewska M, Krajewski S, et al. Prognostic significance of Bax protein expression in diffuse aggressive non-Hodgkin's lymphoma. Blood 1997;90:3173–3178.

175. Gascoyne RD, Adomat SA, Krajewski S, et al. Prognostic significance of Bcl-2 protein expression and Bcl-2 gene rearrangement in diffuse aggressive non-Hodgkin's lymphoma. Blood 1997;90:244–251.

176. Skinnider BF, Horsman DE, Dupuis B, Gascoyne RD. Bcl-6 and Bcl-2 protein expression in diffuse large B-cell lymphoma and follicular lymphoma: Correlation with 3q27 and 18q21 chromosomal abnormalities. Hum Pathol 1999; 30:803–808.

177. Drillenburg P, Wielenga VJ, Kramer MH, et al. CD44 expression predicts disease outcome in localized large B cell lymphoma. Leukemia 1999;13:1448–1455.

178. Donoghue S, Baden HS, Lauder I, et al. Immunohistochemical localization of caspase-3 correlates with clinical outcome in B-cell diffuse large-cell lymphoma. Cancer Res 1999;59:5386–5391.

179. Weiss LM, Strickler JG, Medeiros LJ, et al. Proliferative rates of non-Hodgkin's lymphomas as assessed by Ki-67 antibody. Hum Pathol 1987;18:1155–1159.

180. Dogan A, Bagdi E, Munson P, Isaacson PG. CD10 and BCL-6 expression in paraffin sections of normal lymphoid tissue and B-cell lymphomas. Am J Surg Pathol 2000;24: 846–852.

181. Frierson HFJ, Bellafiore FJ, Gaffey MJ, et al. Cytokeratin in anaplastic large cell lymphoma. Mod Pathol 1994;7:317–321.

182. de Bruin PC, Gruss HJ, van der Valk P, et al. CD30 expression in normal and neoplastic lymphoid tissue: Biological aspects and clinical implications. Leukemia 1995;9:1620–1627.

183. Krishnan J, Wallberg K, Frizzera G. T-cell-rich large B-cell lymphoma: A study of 30 cases, supporting its histologic heterogeneity and lack of clinical distinctiveness. Am J Surg Pathol 1994;18:455–465.

184. Suster S. Primary large-cell lymphomas of the mediastinum. Semin Diagn Pathol 1999;16:51–64.

185. Davis RE, Dorfman RF, Warnke RA. Primary large-cell lymphoma of the thymus: A diffuse B-cell neoplasm presenting as primary mediastinal lymphoma. Hum Pathol 1990;21:1262–1268.

186. Rodriguez J, Pugh WC, Romaguera JE, et al. Primary mediastinal large cell lymphoma is characterized by an inverted pattern of large tumoral mass and low beta 2 mi-

croglobulin levels in serum and frequently elevated levels of serum lactate dehydrogenase. Ann Oncol 1994;5:847–849.

187. Rodriguez J, Pugh WC, Romaguera JE, Cabanillas F. Primary mediastinal large cell lymphoma. Hematol Oncol 1994;12:175–184.

188. Higgins JP, Warnke RA. CD30 expression is common in mediastinal large B-cell lymphoma. Am J Clin Pathol 1999;112:241–247.

189. Knowles DM. Immunodeficiency-associated lymphoproliferative disorders. Mod Pathol 1999;12:200–217.

190. Green I, Espiritu E, Ladanyi M, et al. Primary lymphomatous effusions in AIDS: A morphological, immunophenotypic, and molecular study. Mod Pathol 1995;8:39–45.

191. Nador RG, Cesarman E, Chadburn A, et al. Primary effusion lymphoma: A distinct clinicopathologic entity associated with the Kaposi's sarcoma–associated herpes virus. Blood 1996;88:645–656.

192. DiGiuseppe JA, Nelson WG, Seifter EJ, et al. Intravascular lymphomatosis: A clinicopathologic study of 10 cases and assessment of response to chemotherapy. J Clin Oncol 1994;12:2573–2579.

193. Ferry JA, Harris NL, Picker LJ, et al. Intravascular lymphomatosis (malignant angioendotheliomatosis): A B-cell neoplasm expressing surface homing receptors. Mod Pathol 1988;1:444–452.

194. Domizio P, Hall PA, Cotter F, et al. Angiotropic large cell lymphoma (ALCL): Morphological, immunohistochemical and genotypic studies with analysis of previous reports. Hematol Oncol 1989;7:195–206.

195. Kanda M, Suzumiya J, Ohshima K, et al. Intravascular large cell lymphoma: Clinicopathological, immuno-histochemical and molecular genetic studies. Leuk Lymphoma 1999;34:569–580.

196. Rudinger T, Ott G, Ott M, et al. Reply to: B-cell anaplastic large cell lymphoma—the forgotten entity. Am J Surg Pathol 2000;24:159–160.

197. Suzumiya J, Ohshima K, Kikuchi M, et al. Terminal deoxynucleotidyl transferase staining of malignant lymphomas in paraffin sections: A useful method for the diagnosis of lymphoblastic lymphoma. J Pathol 1997;182:86–91.

198. Chetty R, Pulford K, Jones M, et al. An immunohistochemical study of TAL-1 protein expression in leukaemias and lymphomas with a novel monoclonal antibody, 2TL 242. J Pathol 1996;178:311–315.

199. Sykora KW, Tomeczkowski J, Reiter A. C-kit receptors in childhood malignant lymphoblastic cells. Leuk Lymphoma 1997;25:201–216.

200. Chan J, Tsang W. Reactive lymphadenopathies. In: Weiss L, ed. Pathology of Lymph Nodes. New York: Churchill Livingstone, 1996:81–167.

201. Chan AC, Ho JW, Chiang AK, Srivastava G. Phenotypic and cytotoxic characteristics of peripheral T-cell and NK-cell lymphomas in relation to Epstein-Barr virus association. Histopathology 1999;34:16–24.

202. Chan JK, Sin VC, Wong KF, et al. Nonnasal lymphoma expressing the natural killer cell marker CD56: A clinicopathologic study of 49 cases of an uncommon aggressive neoplasm. Blood 1997;89:4501–4513.

203. Chan JK. Peripheral T-cell and NK-cell neoplasms: An integrated approach to diagnosis. Mod Pathol 1999;12:177–199.

204. Takeshita M, Akamatsu M, Ohshima K, et al. CD30 (Ki-1) expression in adult T-cell leukaemia/lymphoma is associated with distinctive immunohistological and clinical characteristics. Histopathology 1995;26:539–546.

205. Tao Q, Ho FC, Loke SL, Srivastava G. Epstein-Barr virus is localized in the tumour cells of nasal lymphomas of NK, T or B cell type. Int J Cancer 1995;60:315–320.

206. de Bruin PC, Jiwa M, Oudejans JJ, et al. Presence of Epstein-Barr virus in extranodal T-cell lymphomas: Differences in relation to site. Blood 1994;83:1612–1618.

207. Sabourin JC, Kanavaros P, Briere J, et al. Epstein-Barr virus (EBV) genomes and EBV-encoded latent membrane protein (LMP) in pulmonary lymphomas occurring in nonimmunocompromised patients. Am J Surg Pathol 1993;17:995–1002.

208. Kanavaros P, Vlychou M, Stefanaki K, et al. Cytotoxic protein expression in non-Hodgkin's lymphomas and Hodgkin's disease. Anticancer Res 1999;19(2A):1209–1216.

209. Boulland ML, Kanavaros P, Wechsler J, et al. Cytotoxic protein expression in natural killer cell lymphomas and in alpha beta and gamma delta peripheral T-cell lymphomas. J Pathol 1997;183:432–439.

210. Macon WR, Williams ME, Greer JP, et al. Natural killer-like T-cell lymphomas: Aggressive lymphomas of T-large granular lymphocytes. Blood 1996;87:1474–1483.

211. Guinee D Jr, Jaffe E, Kingma D, et al. Pulmonary lymphomatoid granulomatosis: Evidence for a proliferation of Epstein-Barr virus infected B-lymphocytes with a prominent T-cell component and vasculitis. Am J Surg Pathol 1994;18:753–764.

212. Chott A, Vesely M, Simonitsch I, et al. Classification of intestinal T-cell neoplasms and their differential diagnosis. Am J Clin Pathol 1999;111(1 Suppl 1):S68–74.

213. de Bruin PC, Connolly CE, Oudejans JJ, et al. Enteropathy-associated T-cell lymphomas have a cytotoxic T-cell phenotype. Histopathology 1997;31:313–317.

214. Ilyas M, Niedobitek G, Agathanggelou A, et al. Non-Hodgkin's lymphoma, coeliac disease, and Epstein-Barr virus: A study of 13 cases of enteropathy-associated T- and B-cell lymphoma. J Pathol 1995;177:115–122.

215. Carey MJ, Medeiros LJ, Roepke JE, et al. Primary anaplastic large cell lymphoma of the small intestine. Am J Clin Pathol 1999;112:696–701.

216. Murray A, Cuevas EC, Jones DB, Wright DH. Study of the immunohistochemistry and T cell clonality of enteropathy-associated T cell lymphoma. Am J Pathol 1995;146:509–519.

217. Wu H, Wasik MA, Przybylski G, et al. Hepatosplenic gamma-delta T-cell lymphoma as a late-onset posttransplant lymphoproliferative disorder in renal transplant recipients. Am J Clin Pathol 2000;113:487–496.

218. Cooke CB, Krenacs L, Stetler-Stevenson M, et al. Hepatosplenic T-cell lymphoma: A distinct clinicopathologic entity of cytotoxic gamma delta T-cell origin. Blood 1996;88:4265–4274.

219. Salhany KE, Macon WR, Choi JK, et al. Subcutaneous panniculitis-like T-cell lymphoma: Clinicopathologic, immunophenotypic, and genotypic analysis of alpha/beta and gamma/delta subtypes. Am J Surg Pathol 1998;22:881–893.

220. Kumar S, Krenacs L, Medeiros J, et al. Subcutaneous panniculitic T-cell lymphoma is a tumor of cytotoxic T lymphocytes. Hum Pathol 1998;29:397–403.

221. Kinney MC. The role of morphologic features, phenotype, genotype, and anatomic site in defining extranodal T-cell or NK-cell neoplasms. Am J Clin Pathol 1999;111(1 Suppl 1):S104–118.

222. Chang K, Weiss L. CD7: A review. Appl Immunohistochem 1994;2:146–156.

223. Bakels V, van Oostveen JW, van der Putte SC, et al. Immunophenotyping and gene rearrangement analysis provide additional criteria to differentiate between cutaneous T-cell lymphomas and pseudo-T-cell lymphomas. Am J Pathol 1997;150:1941–1949.

224. Picker LJ, Brenner MB, Weiss LM, et al. Discordant expression of CD3 and T-cell receptor beta-chain antigens in T-lineage lymphomas. Am J Pathol 1987;129:434–440.

225. Bani D, Giannotti B. Differentiation of interdigitating reticulum cells and Langerhans cells in the human skin with T-lymphoid infiltrate: An immunocytochemical and ultrastructural study. Arch Histol Cytol 1989;52:361–372.

226. Li G, Chooback L, Wolfe JT, et al. Overexpression of p53 protein in cutaneous T cell lymphoma: Relationship to large cell transformation and disease progression. J Invest Dermatol 1998;110:767–770.

227. Kempf W, Dummer R, Burg G. Approach to lymphoproliferative infiltrates of the skin: The difficult lesions. Am J Clin Pathol 1999;111(1 Suppl 1):S84–93.

228. Krishnan J, Tomaszewski MM, Kao GF. Primary cutaneous CD30-positive anaplastic large cell lymphoma: Report of 27 cases. J Cutan Pathol 1993;20:193–202.

229. Kummer JA, Vermeer MH, Dukers D, et al. Most primary cutaneous CD30-positive lymphoproliferative disorders

have a CD4-positive cytotoxic T-cell phenotype. J Invest Dermatol 1997;109:636–640.

230. Boulland ML, Wechsler J, Bagot M, et al. Primary CD30-positive cutaneous T-cell lymphomas and lymphomatoid papulosis frequently express cytotoxic proteins. Histopathology 2000;36:136–144.

231. Vergier B, Beylot-Barry M, Pulford K, et al. Statistical evaluation of diagnostic and prognostic features of CD30+ cutaneous lymphoproliferative disorders: A clinicopathologic study of 65 cases. Am J Surg Pathol 1998;22:1192–1202.

232. Herbst H, Sander C, Tronnier M, et al. Absence of anaplastic lymphoma kinase (ALK) and Epstein-Barr virus gene products in primary cutaneous anaplastic large cell lymphoma and lymphomatoid papulosis. Br J Dermatol 1997;137:680–686.

233. Beljaards RC, Kaudewitz P, Berti E, et al. Primary cutaneous CD30-positive large cell lymphoma: Definition of a new type of cutaneous lymphoma with a favorable prognosis: A European Multicenter Study of 47 patients. Cancer 1993;71:2097–2104.

234. Brice P, Cazals D, Mounier N, et al. Primary cutaneous large-cell lymphoma: Analysis of 49 patients included in the LNH87 prospective trial of polychemotherapy for high-grade lymphomas: Groupe d'Étude des Lymphomes de l'Adulte. Leukemia 1998;12:213–219.

235. Anagnostopoulos I, Hummel M, Kaudewitz P, et al. Low incidence of Epstein-Barr virus presence in primary cutaneous T-cell lymphoproliferations. Br J Dermatol 1996;134:276–281.

236. Borowitz MJ, Newby S, Brynes RK, et al. Multiinstitution study of non-Hodgkin's lymphomas using frozen section immunoperoxidase: The Southeastern Cancer Study Group experience. Blood 1984;63:1147–1152.

237. Strickler JG, Weiss LM, Copenhaver CM, et al. Monoclonal antibodies reactive in routinely processed tissue sections of malignant lymphoma, with emphasis on T-cell lymphomas. Hum Pathol 1987;18:808–814.

238. Hamilton-Dutoit SJ, Pallesen G. A survey of Epstein-Barr virus gene expression in sporadic non-Hodgkin's lymphomas: Detection of Epstein-Barr virus in a subset of peripheral T-cell lymphomas. Am J Pathol 1992;140:1315–1325.

239. Leung CY, Ho FC, Srivastava G, et al. Usefulness of follicular dendritic cell pattern in classification of peripheral T-cell lymphomas. Histopathology 1993;23:433–437.

240. Anagnostopoulos I, Hummel M, Finn T, et al. Heterogeneous Epstein-Barr virus infection patterns in peripheral T-cell lymphoma of angioimmunoblastic lymphadenopathy type. Blood 1992;80:1804–1812.

241. Nathwani B, Jaffe E. Angioimmunoblastic lymphadenopathy (AILD) and AILD-like T-cell lymphomas. In: Jaffe E, ed. Surgical Pathology of the Lymph Nodes and Related Organs. 2nd ed. Philadelphia: WB Saunders, 1995:390–412.

242. Kadin ME. Primary Ki-1-positive anaplastic large-cell lymphoma: A distinct clinicopathologic entity. Ann Oncol 1994;5 Suppl 1:25–30.

243. Perkins PL, Ross CW, Schnitzer B. CD30-positive, anaplastic large-cell lymphomas that express CD15 but lack CD45: A possible diagnostic pitfall. Arch Pathol Lab Med 1992;116:1192–1196.

244. Biernat W. Ki-1-positive anaplastic large cell lymphoma: A morphologic and immunologic study of 14 cases. Patologia Polska 1994;45:39–44.

245. Brousset P, Rochaix P, Chittal S, et al. High incidence of Epstein-Barr virus detection in Hodgkin's disease and absence of detection in anaplastic large-cell lymphoma in children. Histopathology 1993;23:189–191.

246. Bayle C, Charpentier A, Duchayne E, et al. Leukaemic presentation of small cell variant anaplastic large cell lymphoma: Report of four cases. Br J Haematol 1999;104:680–688.

247. Kinney MC, Collins RD, Greer JP, et al. A small-cell-predominant variant of primary Ki-1 (CD30)+ T-cell lymphoma. Am J Surg Pathol 1993;17:859–868.

248. Piris M, Brown DC, Gatter KC, Mason DY. CD30 expression in non-Hodgkin's lymphoma. Histopathology 1990;17:211–218.

249. Gascoyne RD, Aoun P, Wu D, et al. Prognostic significance of anaplastic lymphoma kinase (ALK) protein expression in adults with anaplastic large cell lymphoma. Blood 1999;93:3913–3921.

250. Hodges KB, Collins RD, Greer JP, et al. Transformation of the small cell variant Ki-1+ lymphoma to anaplastic large cell lymphoma: Pathologic and clinical features. Am J Surg Pathol 1999;23:49–58.

251. Nakagawa A, Nakamura S, Ito M, et al. CD30-positive anaplastic large cell lymphoma in childhood: Expression of p80npm/alk and absence of Epstein-Barr virus. Mod Pathol 1997;10:210–215.

252. Nakamura S, Shiota M, Nakagawa A, et al. Anaplastic large cell lymphoma: A distinct molecular pathologic entity: A reappraisal with special reference to p80(NPM/ALK) expression. Am J Surg Pathol 1997;21:1420–1432.

253. Foss HD, Anagnostopoulos I, Araujo I, et al. Anaplastic large-cell lymphomas of T-cell and null-cell phenotype express cytotoxic molecules. Blood 1996;88:4005–4011.

254. Foss HD, Demel G, Anagnostopoulos I, et al. Uniform expression of cytotoxic molecules in anaplastic large cell lymphoma of null/T cell phenotype and in cell lines derived from anaplastic large cell lymphoma. Pathobiology 1997;65:83–90.

255. Krenacs L, Wellmann A, Sorbara L, et al. Cytotoxic cell antigen expression in anaplastic large cell lymphomas of T- and null-cell type and Hodgkin's disease: Evidence for distinct cellular origin. Blood 1997;89:980–989.

256. Cesarman E, Inghirami G, Chadburn A, Knowles DM. High levels of p53 protein expression do not correlate with p53 gene mutations in anaplastic large cell lymphoma. Am J Pathol 1993;143:845–856.

257. Inghirami G, Macri L, Cesarman E, et al. Molecular characterization of CD30+ anaplastic large-cell lymphoma: High frequency of c-myc proto-oncogene activation. Blood 1994;83:3581–3590.

258. Fraga M, Brousset P, Schlaifer D, et al. Bone marrow involvement in anaplastic large cell lymphoma: Immunohistochemical detection of minimal disease and its prognostic significance. Am J Clin Pathol 1995;103:82–89.

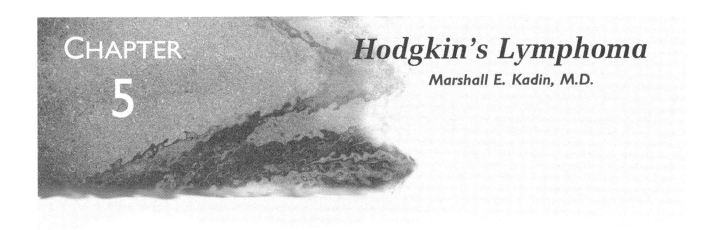

CHAPTER 5

Hodgkin's Lymphoma

Marshall E. Kadin, M.D.

Hodgkin's lymphoma (HL) is widely accepted to be a malignant clonal proliferation of B lymphocytes or, less often, T lymphocytes surrounded by variable numbers of inflammatory cells and fibrosis, resulting in four major histologic types: (1) lymphocyte predominance, (2) nodular sclerosis, (3) mixed cellularity, and (4) lymphocyte depletion (Fig. 5–1).[1] Lymphocyte predominance has been divided into two distinct categories that have different biologic and clinical significance: nodular lymphocyte predominance HL (NLPHL) and lymphocyte-rich classic HL (LRCHL) (Fig. 5–2).[2, 3]

NLPHL is a B-cell neoplasm derived from germinal center B cells that are continually undergoing somatic mutations of the immunoglobulin genes.[3–5] LRCHL belongs to the group of postgerminal center B-cell lymphomas, including nodular sclerosis, mixed cellularity, and lymphocyte depletion types, in which the Hodgkin/Reed-Sternberg cells (H/RSCs) have undergone extensive somatic mutations of immunoglobulin genes.[6] The H/RSCs in NLPHL (also known as *popcorn cells* because of their distinctive morphology) express BCL-6, a transcription factor of germinal center B cells, but not CD138/syndecan-1, a proteoglycan associated with postgerminal center B cells.[7] Conversely, H/RSCs in classic HL are heterogeneous with respect to expression of BCL-6 and CD138, reflecting their mixed germinal center or postgerminal center origin.

In all cases of NLPHL and in a minority of classic HL cases, there is expression of B-cell antigens (CD20, CD79a) by the H/RSCs (Fig. 5–3).[8–11] In addition, the H/RSCs in NLPHL often are surrounded by a population of activated helper-inducer memory T cells (CD4+, CD57+, CD45R+, CD45–), which are normally confined to the light zone of germinal centers of secondary follicles (Fig. 5–4).[4]

In a minority (10 to 20%) of classic HL cases, H/RSCs appear to have a T-cell phenotype with variable expression of T-cell antigens (CD2, CD3, CD4, CD8) and antigens associated with cytotoxic molecules (granzyme B, perforin and TIA-1) (Fig. 5–5).[12–18] A T-cell derivation was proved for H/RSCs by polymerase chain reaction amplification of T-cell receptor genes from single picked H/RSCs in approximately 1 to 2% of classic HL cases.[19–21] However, aberrant T-cell antigen expression was also detected in some classic HLs with immunoglobulin gene rearrangements, presumably of B-cell derivation.[21]

In all cases of classic HL, the tumor cells express CD30, a member of the tumor necrosis factor superfamily (Fig. 5–6).[22–24] Activation of CD30 signaling by native CD30L or Epstein-Barr virus latent membrane protein 1 (EBV-LMP1) results in activation of NFκB transcription factor, which has an antiapoptotic effect, promotes cell proliferation, and causes up-regulation of cytokine production by H/RSCs.[25, 26] H/RSCs also express CD40,[27] a B-cell antigen characteristic of germinal center B cells, activation of which inhibits apoptosis (Fig. 5–7).[28] H/RSCs manifest variable expression of CD25 (Tac, p55), the alpha unit of the receptor for interleukin-2 (IL-2).[29, 30] Finally, H/RSCs in classic HL express CD15 detected by antibody LeuM1 in 60 to 85% of cases, average 68% (Fig. 5–8).[31–34] The antigenic determinant for LeuM1 is a trisaccharide, 3-fucosyl-*N*-acetyllactosamine, which is formed by the 1-3 fucosylation of a type 2 blood group backbone chain (Gal 1-4Glc N Ac); the carbohydrate backbone is identical to that of Lewis X, also known as *X-hapten*.[35] A comparative study by Ree and coworkers, confirmed in our laboratory, showed that anti–Lewis-X (BG-7) from Signet Laboratories (Dedham, MA) is superior to LeuM1 for staining H/RSCs, yielding 87%, versus 68.5% for LeuM1 (Fig. 5–9).[36]

A new sensitive marker, fascin, has been described for H/RSCs in classic HL.[37] Fascin is a 55-kd actin-bundling protein that is localized predominantly in dendritic cells in non-neoplastic tissues. The staining profile for fascin raises the possibility of a dendritic cell derivation, particularly an interdigitating reticulum cell, for the neoplastic cells of HL, notably in nodular sclerosis (Fig. 5–10). However, since fascin expression can

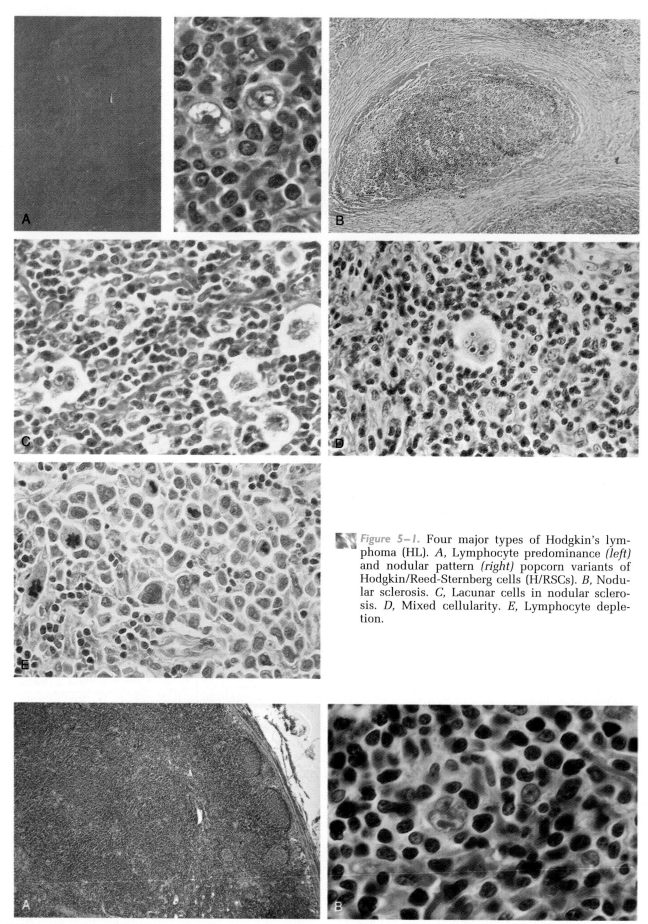

Figure 5–1. Four major types of Hodgkin's lymphoma (HL). *A,* Lymphocyte predominance *(left)* and nodular pattern *(right)* popcorn variants of Hodgkin/Reed-Sternberg cells (H/RSCs). *B,* Nodular sclerosis. *C,* Lacunar cells in nodular sclerosis. *D,* Mixed cellularity. *E,* Lymphocyte depletion.

Figure 5–2. Lymphocyte predominance classic Hodgkin's lymphoma. *A,* Low magnification of histologic appearance. *B,* Hodgkin/Reed-Sternberg cells.

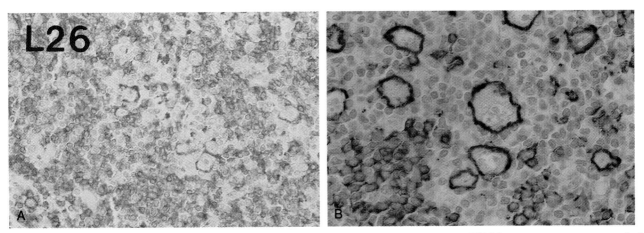

Figure 5–3. B-cell antigen expression in lymphocyte predominance HL. *A*, Large H/RSCs at center are surrounded by nodule of smaller L26+ (CD20+) B lymphocytes. *B*, CD20+ H/RSCs in lymphocyte predominance HL.

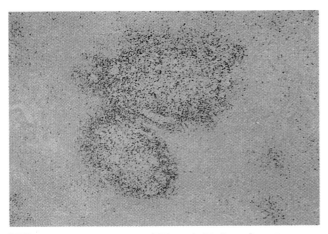

Figure 5–4. Leu7+ (CD57+) T lymphocytes surrounding H/RSCS in nodular lymphocyte predominance HL.

be induced by EBV infection of B cells, the possibility that viral induction of fascin in lymphoid or other cell types must also be considered.[37]

EBV is associated with the etiology of HL and EBV-LMP1, or small RNAs of EBV known as *EBERs* can be detected in about 50% of cases of classic HL (Fig. 5–11).[38] H/RSCs commonly express the EBV gene product latent membrane protein 1 (LMP-1), a transforming protein that can confer a growth advantage on H/RSCs.[39, 40] The frequency of EBV detection in HL is much higher in mixed cellularity and lymphocyte depletion types than in the nodular sclerosis type.[40–42] EBV is frequently detected in classic HL that occurs in immunocompromised patients, such as those infected with human immunodeficiency virus (HIV) and those with post-transplant immunoproliferative disorders.[43] EBV is also detected at higher fre-

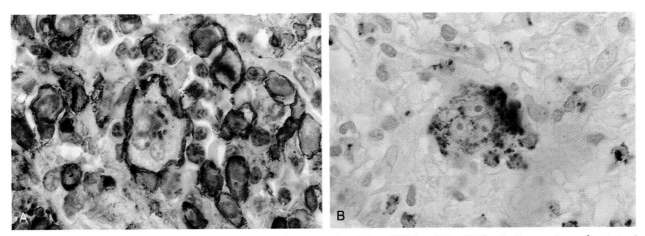

Figure 5–5. HL with T-cell phenotype. *A*, H/RSCs stained for UCHL1 (CD45RO). *B*, Expression of cytotoxic molecule TIA-1 by H/RSCs and smaller surrounding tumor-infiltrating lymphocytes.

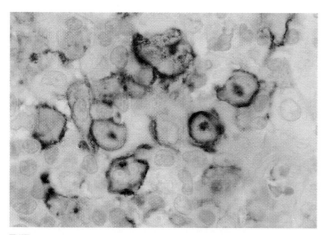

Figure 5–6. H/RSCs stained for CD30 with antibody Ber-H2.

quency in HL patients from developing countries.[41, 42]

In contrast to classic HL, the popcorn cell variants of LPNHL usually do not express CD15, CD25, or CD30. Instead they are often positive for leukocyte common antigen (LCA) or CD45, and for epithelial membrane antigen (EMA) (Fig. 5–12); LCA and EMA are usually absent on H/RSCs in classic HL (Fig. 5–13).[44, 45] The German Hodgkin Study Group showed the importance of using an immunohistochemical analysis for the correct diagnosis of lymphocyte predominance Hodgkin's disease (LPHD). Immunohistochemistry disproved the morphologic diagnosis of LPHD by an expert panel in 25 of 104 cases, whereas 13 cases originally not confirmed as LPHD showed an LPHD-like immunophenotypic pattern with a significantly better survival than classic HL.[46]

ANTIBODIES

The antibodies in most common use for diagnosis of HL are Ber-H2, LeuM1, LCA, fascin, L26, LN1, LN2, UCHL1, CD3, ALK-1, and EBV-LMP1. EMA and CD57 are useful in the recognition of LPNHL. Monoclonal antibody LN1 reacts with H/RSCs in about one third of HL cases, most frequently in cases of nodular lymphocyte predominance Hodgkin's disease (NLPHD) (greater than 75% of cases).[10] Monoclonal antibody LN2, which recognizes the MHC class II–associated invariant chain, reacts with H/RSCs in approximately two thirds of HL cases.[10] All the antibodies mentioned previously can be used in formalin-fixed, paraffin-embedded tissues. Additional antibodies that are useful in the diagnosis of difficult cases are BNH.9[47] and CBF.78[48] (Fig. 5–14 and Table 5–1).

ANTIGEN RETRIEVAL METHOD USED

For antigen retrieval, we have replaced the use of a microwave oven with a steamer that heats the sections to 95°C to 98°C. The slides are immersed in Coplin jars containing citrate buffer (pH 6, 0.01 mol/L) and heated in the steamer for 20 minutes. Afterward, slides are cooled at room temperature for 30 minutes, rinsed in double-distilled water, and then transferred to phosphate-buffered saline, pH 7.4.

IMMUNOSTAINING PITFALLS

Inconsistency of Immunophenotype. An inconsistency of immunophenotype of H/RSCs has been reported in simultaneous and consecutive specimens from the same patients in paraffin sections. Chu and coworkers found that the immuno-

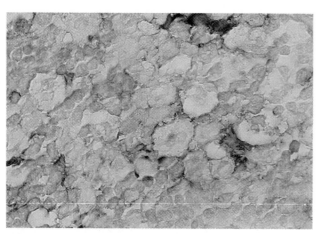

Figure 5–7. H/RSCs expressing CD40.

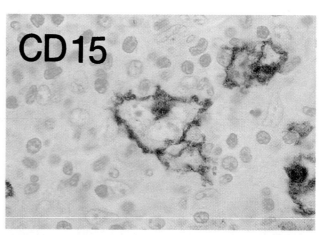

Figure 5–8. H/RSCs expressing CD15 detected by antibody LeuM1.

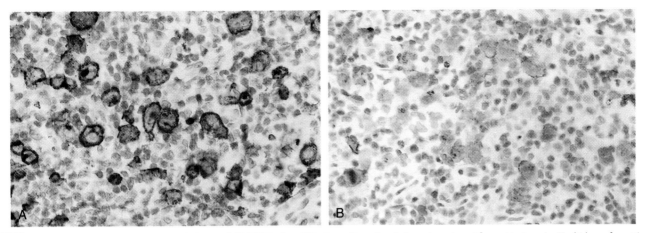

Figure 5–9. Comparative staining of H/RSC for CD15 antigenic determinant with anti–Lewis-X *(A)* and anti–LeuM1 *(B)* antibodies in a case of lymphocyte depletion HL shows increased sensitivity with anti–Lewis-X antibody.

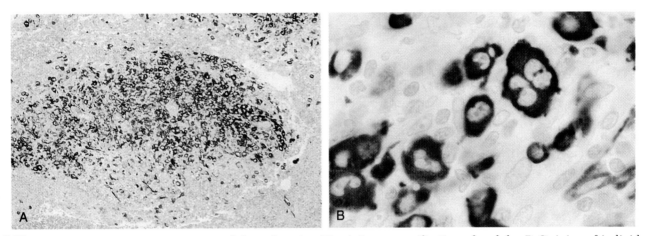

Figure 5–10. Fascin expression in nodular sclerosing HL. *A,* Low magnification of nodule. *B,* Staining of individual H/RSCs at high magnification.

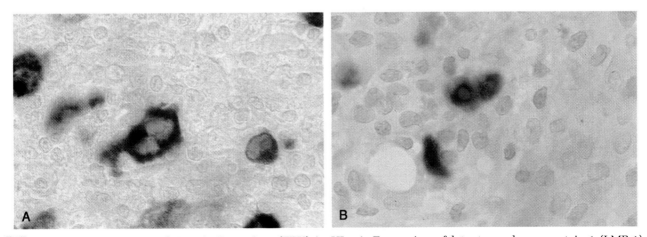

Figure 5–11. Detection of Epstein-Barr virus (EBV) in HL. *A,* Expression of latent membrane protein-1 (LMP-1). *B,* EBV small RNAs (EBERs).

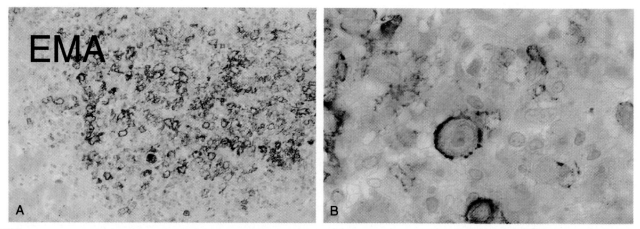

Figure 5–12. Expression of epithelial membrane antigen (EMA) in nodular lymphocyte predominance HL. *A,* Low magnification of nodule. *B,* High magnification of individual H/RSCs.

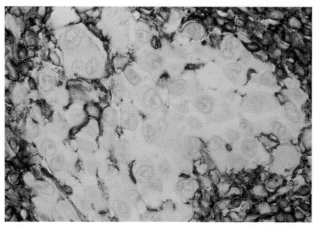

Figure 5–13. Absence of LCA (leukocyte common antigen) on H/RSCs in classic HL.

phenotype of H/RSCs was identical in simultaneous biopsies in only 11 of 39 (28%) patients and remained constant in consecutive biopsies in only 4 of 21 (19%).[49] Major differences were related to cell lineage–specific antigens, whereas minor differences involved mainly CD15 and CD74 antigens.

CD15 Antigen. There can be difficulties when the demonstration of CD15 is relied on to make a diagnosis of HL, because upward of 30% of cases of classic HL will not express CD15 detected by LeuM1 antibody. We and others have found that detection of Lewis-X antigen is more sensitive.[36] It is also important to identify the cells that express CD15 because granulocytes express high levels of CD15[31] and are often present in various tumors other than HL.

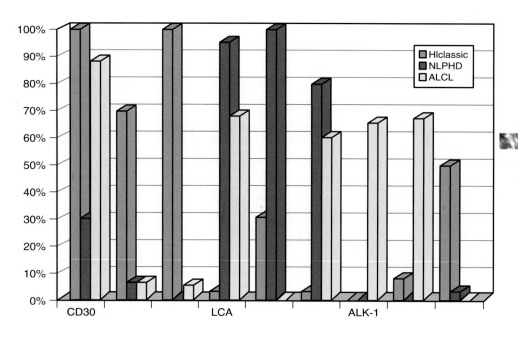

Figure 5–14. Frequency of antigens in classic HL, nodular lymphocyte predominance Hodgkin's disease, and anaplastic large cell lymphoma.

Table 5–1. Antibodies for Detection of Hodgkin's Disease–Associated Antigens

Antibody	Clone	Manufacturer	Dilution	Type of Antigen Retrieval Method
CD30	Ber-H2	DAKO	1:20	Steamer/citrate buffer pH 6, 20 min at 95°C–98°C
CD15	LeuM1	Becton-Dickinson	1:25	Same as CD30
CD45 (LCA)	2B11	DAKO	1:200	Same as CD30
CD20	L26	DAKO	1:100	Same as CD30
CD45RO	UCHL1	DAKO		Pepsin digest 10 min at 37°C
CD3	UCHT1	DAKO		Steamer/citrate buffer pH 6, 20 min at 95°C–98°C
CD40	MAB89	Immunotech	1:40	Same as CD3
ALK-1	ALK-1	DAKO	1:25	Same as CD3
Fascin	55K-2	DAKO	1:75	Same as CD3
Lewis-X type 2 chain (BG-7)	P12	Signet	1:40	Steamer/citrate buffer pH 8, 20 min at 95°C–98°C
EBV-LMP1	CS1-4	DAKO	1:50	Steamer/citrate buffer pH 6, 20 min at 95°C–98°C
BCL-6	PG-B6p	DAKO	1:10	Same as EBV-LMP1
CD57	Leu7	DAKO	1:10	Same as EBV-LMP1
EMA	E29	DAKO	1:50	Pepsin digest, 12 min at 37°C
CDw75	LN1	ICN Biomedicals	Undiluted	Steamer/citrate buffer pH 6, 20 min at 95°C–98°C
CD74	LN2	ICN Biomedicals	Undiluted	Steamer/citrate buffer pH 6, 20 min at 95°C–98°C

Interleukin-2 Receptor. The interleukin-2 receptor (CD25) has been used as a target for immunotherapy protocols to treat HL.[50] A pitfall of these protocols is the difficulty sometimes encountered in demonstrating CD25 expression by H/RSCs against which the therapy is directed. Indeed, CD25 is often expressed on activated tumor-infiltrating lymphocytes (TILs) in HL, and it is important to distinguish them from H/RSCs. We found that this is possible in most cases when a biotinylated tyramine enhancement step[51] is applied to formalin-fixed paraffin-embedded tissues.[30]

CD30 Antigen. The use of monoclonal antibody Ber-H2 together with antigen retrieval methods has enabled sensitive detection of CD30 in formalin-fixed paraffin-embedded tissues. However, some hematopathologists prefer to use B5-fixed tissues, which afford excellent cytomorphology of lymphoid tissues. B5 is a mercuric chloride–containing fixative that requires removal of mercury before immunostaining. This is usually accomplished with Lugol's solution followed by sodium thiosulfate. A study by Facchetti and coworkers showed that omission of the Lugol's treatment is optimal for detection of CD30, even without wet heating with microwave or proteolytic predigestion of sections.[52]

IMMUNOSTAINING IN THE DIFFERENTIAL DIAGNOSIS OF TUMOR LOOK-ALIKES

Nonlymphoid Tumors. CD30, the most consistent marker of H/RSCs, is readily detected in formalin-fixed, paraffin-embedded tissues.[22, 53] However, CD30 can also be expressed by tumor cells in some nonlymphoid maligancies, including embryonal carcinoma, melanoma, and pancreatic cancer.[53, 54] Because sinus infiltration of lymph nodes is characteristic of CD30+ anaplastic large cell lymphomas (ALCLs), there is potential for confusion of ALCLs with the few metastatic carcinomas that express CD30 antigen.[22] Moreover, because malignant melanoma can express CD30, there is the possibility of mistaking a poorly differentiated melanoma for a primary CD30+ ALCL.[54]

CD15 expressed on H/RSCs is also associated with carcinomas.[55] Fortunately, it would be uncommon to encounter a carcinoma that would be mistaken for HL. Conversely, the cohesive tumor cells in the syncytial variant of nodular sclerosing HL might rarely be mistaken for metastatic carcinoma expressing CD15.

Non-Hodgkin's Lymphomas
Anaplastic Large Cell Lymphoma. CD30 is displayed on the tumor cells of ALCL, which is a non-HL with a different natural history than HL.[22, 56–59] Although the histologic features of ALCL, particularly cohesive growth pattern and lymph node sinus infiltration by tumor cells, were thought to be distinguishing characteristics of ALCL, more experience has shown that rare cases of cell-rich HL—particularly those classified as nodular sclerosis type II in the British National Investigation,[60] or the syncytial variant,[61]—and some cases of lymphocyte depletion HL can be confused with ALCL (Fig. 5–15).[62] In these cases, a panel of antibodies can be used to make the distinction (Table 5–2). Perhaps most useful is the

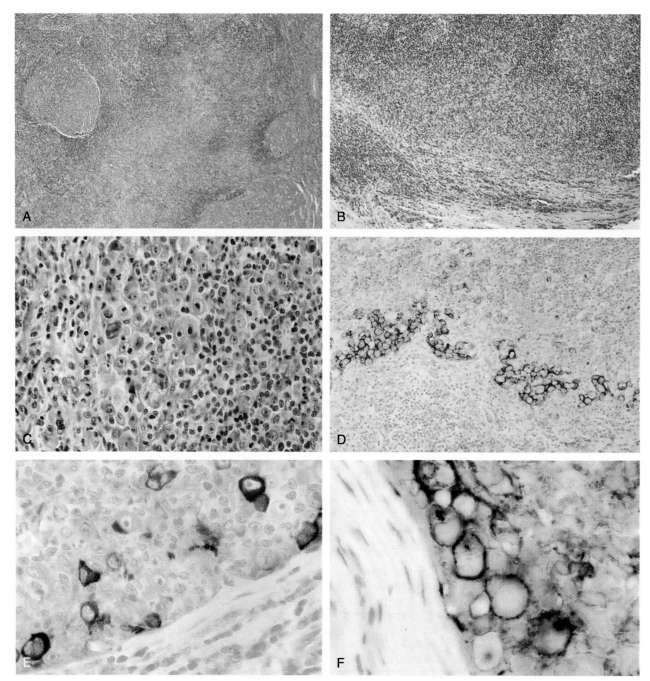

Figure 5–15. Cell-rich classic HL with interfollicular and intrasinus distribution of tumor cells. *A,* Low magnification of interfollicular pattern. *B,* Low magnification of sinus infiltration. *C,* High magnification of H/RSCs within sinus of lymph node. *D,* Expression of CD30 by H/RSCs within sinus. *E,* Expression of fascin by H/RSCs. *F,* Expression of CD40 by H/RSCs within sinus.

polyclonal antibody p80NPM/ALK or monoclonal antibody ALK-1 directed against the NPM/ALK fusion protein resulting from the t(2;5)(p23;q35) and other less frequent chromosomal rearrangements in ALCL (Fig. 5–16).[63, 64] This fusion product is rarely, if ever, expressed in the malignant cells of HL.[62]

Primary Mediastinal B-Cell Large Cell Lymphoma. Primary mediastinal B-cell lymphoma (PMBCL) can be confused with HL because it pre-

sents as a mass in the anterior mediastinum of young adults, often contains H/RS-like cells in a background of collagen sclerosis (Fig. 5–17),[65] and the H/RS-like cells were found to express CD30 in 35 of 51 (69%) cases in one study.[66] However, PMBCL can be distinguished from HL by the strong, uniform expression of CD20, lack of CD15, absence of EBV (EBERs and LMP-1) and lack of an inflammatory background, particularly eosinophils, which is characteristic of HL.

Table 5–2. Antibody Panel for Differential Diagnosis of Hodgkin's Lymphoma

Lymphoma Type	Hodgkin's Lymphoma	Anaplastic Large Cell Lymphoma	Primary Mediastinal B-Cell Large Cell Lymphoma	T-Cell–Rich B-Cell Lymphoma
CD30	+	+	−/+	N
CD15	+	R	N	N
CD20	+/−	N	+	+
CD3	N	+	N	N
CD40	+	N	+	+
CD45 (LCA)	N	+/−	+	+
EBV–LMP-1	+/−	N	N	N
ALK	N	+	N	N
Fascin	+	N	N	N

+, Nearly all cases positive; +/−, most cases positive; −/+ minority of cases positive; R, rare (<5%); N, no cases positive.

T-Cell–Rich B-Cell Lymphoma. T-cell–rich B-cell lymphoma (TCRBCL) was recognized as a non-HL usually occurring in patients older than 50 years with advanced (stage III or IV) disease. Response to recognized chemotherapy regimens for HL is poor. Therefore, it is important to distinguish TCRBCL from HL, particularly NLPHD or LRCHL (Fig. 5–18).[66, 67] The tumor cells in TCRBCL appear to be negative for CD30 and CD15, as well as for vimentin, all of which are expressed in H/RSCs in classic HL. Furthermore, the reactive inflammatory infiltrate rich in TIA-1+ lymphocytes in both TCRBCL and classic HL is rarely encountered in NLPHD, whereas CD57+ lymphocytes characteristic of NLPHD are not numerous in TCRBCL.[68]

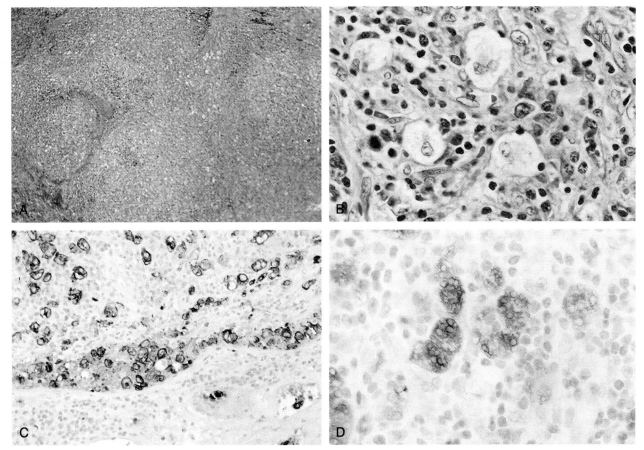

🖎 *Figure 5–16.* Hodgkin's-like anaplastic large cell lymphoma with *(A)* nodular pattern and *(B)* lacunar cells. *C,* CD30 staining of tumor cells within sinus. *D,* Expression of p80NPM/ALK by tumor cells in lacunar spaces.

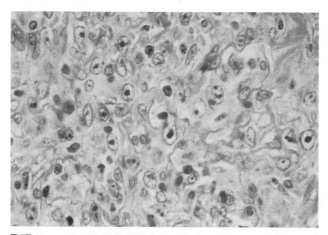

Figure 5–17. H/RSC-like cells in primary mediastinal B-cell large cell lymphoma.

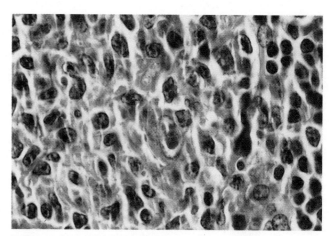

Figure 5–19. H/RSC-like cells in lymph node infected by cytomegalovirus.

IMMUNOSTAINING OF PSEUDONEOPLASTIC LOOK-ALIKES

Infectious Mononucleosis. H/RS-like cells in infectious mononucleosis are similar in most respects to their morphologic counterparts in HL with respect to expression of EBERs, EBV-LMP1, and CD30, and low expression of LCA.[69] However, the H/RSC-like cells in infectious mononucleosis are CD15– and lack the rosette of T lymphocytes characteristic of H/RSCs in HL.[70]

Cytomegalovirus Lymphadenitis. Lymph nodes infected with cytomegalovirus contain H/RSC-like cells that are caused by viral inclusions and are readily distinguished from HL by negative immunohistochemical staining for CD15 and CD30 (Fig. 5–19).

Interfollicular Lymphadenitis. Lymphadenitis mimicking Hodgkin's disease has been described as a benign lymphadenopathy that can mimic interfollicular HL.[71, 72] Cervical lymph nodes are affected most often. There is no progression to

lymphoma. The lymph nodes show follicular hyperplasia with a mottled interfollicular zone with epithelioid histiocytes, lymphocytes, eosinophils, and immunoblasts. Some immunoblasts with prominent nucleoli resemble H/RSCs. However, their nucleoli are typically smaller and basophilic, in contrast to the eosinophilic nucleoli of H/RSCs. Immunohistochemistry distinguishes this disorder from interfollicular HL because the H/RSC-like cells display B- or T-cell antigens and lack CD15.[72, 73]

References

1. Lukes RJ, Butler JJ. The pathology and nomenclature of Hodgkin's disease. Cancer Res 1966;26:1311.
2. Harris NL, Jaffe ES, Stein H, et al. A revised European-American classification of lymphoid neoplasms: A proposal from the International Lymphoma Study Group. Blood 1994;84:1361.
3. Mason DY, Banks PM, Chan J, et al. Nodular lymphocyte predominance Hodgkin's disease: A distinct clinicopathologic entity. Am J Surg Pathol 1994;18:526.
4. Poppema S. The nature of the lymphocytes surrounding Reed-Sternberg cells in nodular lymphocyte predominance and other types of Hodgkin's disease. Am J Pathol 1989; 135:351.
5. Marafioti T, Hummel M, Anagnostopoulos I, et al. Origin of nodular lymphocyte predominance Hodgkin's disease from a clonal expansion of highly mutated germinal center B cells. N Engl J Med 1997;337:453.
6. Kanzler H, Kuppers R, Hansmann ML, et al. Hodgkin and Reed-Sternberg cells in Hodgkin's disease represent the outgrowth of a dominant tumor clone derived from (crippled) germinal center B cells. J Exp Med 1996;184:1495.
7. Carbone A, Gloghini A, Gaidano G, et al. Expression status of Bcl-6 and syndecan-1 identifies distinct histogenetic subtypes of Hodgkin's disease. Blood;1998:2220.
8. Pinkus GS, Said JW. Hodgkin's disease, lymphocyte predominance type, nodular—further evidence for a B cell derivation: L&H variants of Reed-Sternberg cells express L26, a pan B cell marker. Am J Pathol 1988;133:211.
9. Epstein AL, Marder RJ, Winster JN, et al. Two new monoclonal antibodies (LN-1, LN-2) reactive in B5 formalin-fixed, paraffin-embedded tissues with follicular center and mantle zone human B lymphocytes and derived tumors. J Immunol 1984;133:1028.
10. Marder RJ, Variokojis D, Silver J, et al. Immunohistochemical analysis of human lymphomas with monoclonal anti-

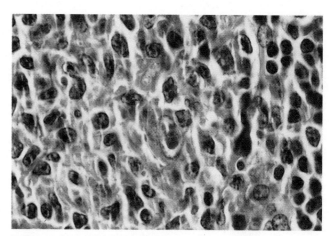

Figure 5–18. H/RSC-like cells in T-cell–rich B-cell lymphoma.

bodies to B cell and Ia antigens reactive in paraffin sections. Lab Invest 1985;52:497.

11. Korkopoulou P, Cordell J, Jones M, et al. The expression of B-cell marker mb-2 (CD79a) in Hodgkin's disease. Histopathology 1994;24:511.

12. Kadin ME, Muramoto L, Said J. Expression of T cell antigens on Reed-Sternberg cells in a subset of patients with nodular sclerosing and mixed cellularity Hodgkin's disease. Am J Pathol 1988;130:345.

13. Casey TT, Olson SJ, Cousar JB, et al. Immunophenotypes of Reed-Sternberg cells: A study of 19 cases of Hodgkin's disease in plastic embedded sections. Blood 1989;74:2624.

14. Dallenbach FE, Stein H. Expression of T-cell receptor beta chain in Reed-Sternberg cells. Lancet 1989;2:828.

15. Oka K, Mori N, Kojima M. Anti-Leu-3a antibody reactivity with Reed-Sternberg cells of Hodgkin's disease. Arch Pathol Lab Med 1988;112:139.

16. Oudejans JJ, Kummer JA, Jiwa M, et al. Granzyme B expression in Reed-Sternberg cells of Hodgkin's disease. Am J Pathol 1996;148:233.

17. Krenacs L, Wellmann A, Sorbara L, et al. Cytotoxic cell antigen expression in anaplastic large cell lymphomas of T-cell and null-cell type and Hodgkin's disease: Evidence for a distinct cellular origin. Blood 1997;89:980.

18. Felgar RE, Macon WR, Kinney MC, et al. TIA-1 expression in lymphoid neoplasms. Am J Pathol 1997;150:1893.

19. Muschen M, Rajewsky K, Brauninger A, et al. Rare occurrence of classical Hodgkin's disease as a T cell lymphoma. J Exp Med 2000;191:387−394.

20. Hummel M, Ziegler S, Marifioti T, et al. Detection of clonal T-cell receptor gamma-chain gene-rearrangements in Reed-Sternberg cells of Hodgkin's disease. Blood, 2000;95:302.

21. Willenbrock K, Ichinohasama R, Kadin ME, et al. Clonal rearrangement of TCR-β chain gene in a cutaneous T cell lymphoma and classical Hodgkin's disease of the same patient: Further evidence from single cell PCR, manuscript in preparation.

22. Stein H, Mason DY, Gerdes J, et al. The expression of the Hodgkin's disease associated antigen Ki-1 in reactive and neoplastic lymphoid tissue: Evidence that Reed-Sternberg cells and histiocytic malignancies are derived from activated lymphoid cells. Blood 1985;66:848.

23. Durkop H, Latza U, Hummel M, et al. Molecular cloning and expression of a new member of the nerve growth factor receptor family that is characteristic of Hodgkin's disease. Cell 1992;68:421.

24. Smith CA, Gruss HJ, Davis T, et al. CD30 antigen, a marker for Hodgkin's lymphoma, is a receptor whose ligand defines an emerging family of cytokines with homology to TNF. Cell 1993;73:1349.

25. Bargou RC, Emmerich F, Krappmann D, et al. Constitutive nuclear factor-kβ-Rel A activation is required for proliferation and survival of Hodgkin's disease tumor cells. J Clin Invest 1997;100:2961.

26. Bargou RC, Leng C, Krappmann D. High level nuclear NF-kβ and Oct-2 is a common feature of cultured Hodgkin/ Reed-Sternberg cells. Blood 1996;87:4340.

27. Carbone A, Gloghini A, Gattei V, et al. Expression of functional CD40 antigen on Reed-Sternberg cells and Hodgkin's disease cell lines. Blood 1995;85:780.

28. Banchereau J, Bazan F, Blanchard D, et al. The CD40 antigen and its ligand. Annu Rev Immunol 1994;12:881.

29. Hsu SM, Chien-te KT, Hsu PL. Expression of p55 (Tac) interleukin-2 receptor (IL-2R) but not p75IL-2R, in cultured H-RS cells and H-RS cells in tissues. Am J Pathol 1990;136:735.

30. Levi E, Butmarc J, Kourea HP, et al. Detection of interleukin-2 receptors on tumor cells in formalin-fixed, paraffin-embedded tissues. Appl Immunohistochem 1997;5:234.

31. Stein H, Uchanska-Ziegler B, Gerdes J, et al. Hodgkin's and Sternberg-Reed cells contain antigens specific to late cells of granulopoiesis. Int J Cancer 1982;29:283.

32. Hsu SM, Jaffe ES. Leu M1 and peanut agglutinin stain the neoplastic cells of Hodgkin's disease. Am J Clin Pathol 1984;82:29.

33. Pinkus GS, Thomas P, Said JW. Leu-M1—A marker for Reed-Sternberg cells in Hodgkin's disease: An immunoperoxidase study of paraffin-embedded tissues. Am J Pathol 1985;119:244.

34. Von Wasielewski R, Mengel M, Fischer R, et al. Classical Hodgkin's disease: Clinical impact of the immunophenotype. Am J Pathol 1997;151:1123.

35. Gooi HC, Feizi T, Kapadia A, et al. Stage-specific embryonic antigen involves (1-3) fucosylated type 2 blood group chains. Nature 1981;292:156.

36. Ree HJ, Teplitz C, Khan A. The Lewis antigen: A new paraffin section marker for Reed-Sternberg cells. Cancer 1991; 67:1346.

37. Pinkus GS, Pinkus JL, Langhoff E, et al. Fascin, a sensitive new marker for Reed-Sternberg cells of Hodgkin's disease: Evidence for a dendritic or B cell derivation? Am J Pathol 1997;150:543.

38. Weiss LM, Mohaven LA, Wanke RA, et al. Detection of Epstein-Barr viral genomes in Reed-Sternberg cells of Hodgkin's disease. N Engl J Med 1989;320:502.

39. Wang D, Liebowitz D, Kieff E. An EBV membrane protein expressed in immortalized lymphocytes transforms established rodent cells. Cell 1985;43:831.

40. Pallesen G, Hamilton-Dutoit MR, Young LS. Expression of Epstein-Barr viruses latent gene products in tumor cells of Hodgkin's disease. Lancet 1991;337:320.

41. Ambinder RF, Browning PJ, Lorenzana I, et al. Epstein-Barr virus in childhood Hodgkin's disease in Honduras and the United States. Blood 1993;81:462.

42. Gulley ML, Eagan PA, Quintanilla-Martinez L, et al. Epstein-Barr virus DNA is abundant and monoclonal in the Reed-Sternberg cells of Hodgkin's disease: Association with mixed cellularity subtype and Hispanic American ethnicity. Blood 1994;83:1595.

43. Herndier BG, Sanchez HC, Chang KL, et al. High prevalence of Epstein-Barr virus in the Reed-Sternberg cells of HIV-associated Hodgkin's disease. Am J Pathol 1993;142:1073.

44. Dorfman RF, Gatter KC, Pulford KAF, et al. An evaluation of the utility of anti-granulocyte and anti-leukocyte monoclonal antibodies in the diagnosis of Hodgkin's disease. Am J Pathol 1986;123:508.

45. Chittal SM, Caveriviere P, Schwarting R, et al. Monoclonal antibodies in the diagnosis of Hodgkin's disease: The search for a rational panel. Am J Surg Pathol 1988;12:9.

46. von Wasilewski R, Werner M, Fischer R, et al. Lymphocyte predominant Hodgkin's disease: An immunohistochemical analysis of 208 reviewed Hodgkin's cases from the German Hodgkin Study Group. Am J Pathol 1997;150:793.

47. Delsol G, Blancer A, Al Saati T. Antibody BNH.9 detects red blood cell−related antigens on anaplastic large cell (CD30+) lymphomas. Br J Cancer 1991;64:321.

48. Al Saati T, Tkaczuk J, Krissansen G, et al. A novel antigen detected by CBF.78 antibody further distinguishes anaplastic large cell lymphoma from Hodgkin's disease. Blood 1996;88:2741.

49. Chu WS, Abbondanzo SL, Frizzera G. Inconsistency of the immunophenotype of Reed-Sternberg cells in simultaneous and consecutive specimens from the same patients: A paraffin section evaluation in 56 patients. Am J Pathol 1992; 141:11.

50. Tepler I, Schwartz G, Parker K, et al. Phase I trial of an IL-2 fusion toxin (DAB486IL-2) in hematologic malignancies: Complete response in a patient with Hodgkin's disease refractory to chemotherapy. Cancer 1994;73:1276.

51. Merz H, Malisius R, Mannveiler S, et al. Immunomax: A maximized immunohistochemical method for the retrieval and enhancement of hidden antigens. Lab Invest 1995;73:149.

52. Facchetti F, Alebardi O, Vermi W. Omit iodine and CD30 will shine: A simple technical procedure to demonstrate CD30 antigen on B5-fixed material. [letter] Am J Surg Pathol 2000;24:319.

53. Schwarting R, Gerdes J, Durkop H, et al. Ber-H2: A new anti−Ki-1 (CD30) monoclonal antibody directed at a formol-resistant epitope. Blood 1989;74:1678.

54. Polski JM, Janney CG. Ber-H2 (CD30) immunohistochemical staining in malignant melanoma. Mod Pathol 1999;12:903.

55. Sheibani K, Battifora H, Burke JS, et al. Leu-M1 antigen in human neoplasms: An immunohistochemical study. Am J Surg Pathol 1986;12:227.

56. Kadin ME, Sako D, Berlin N, et al. Childhood Ki-1 lymphoma presenting with skin lesions and peripheral lymphadenopathy. Blood 1986;68:1042.

57. Nakamura S, Takagi N, Kojima M, et al. Clinicopathologic study of large cell anaplastic lymphoma (Ki-1-positive large cell lymphoma) among Japanese. Cancer 1991;68:118.

58. Gascoyne RD, Aoun P, Wu D, et al. Prognostic significance of anaplastic lymphoma kinase (ALK) protein expression in adults with anaplastic large cell lymphoma. Blood 1999;93:3913.

59. Falini B, Pileri S, Zinzani PL, et al. ALK+ lymphoma: Clinico-pathological findings and outcome. Blood 1999;93:2697.

60. Haybittle JL, Hayhoe FGJ, Easterling MJ, et al. Review of British National Lymphoma Investigation studies of Hodgkin's disease and development of a prognostic index. Lancet 1985;1:967.

61. Strickler JG, Michie SA, Warnke RA, et al. The "syncytial variant" of nodular sclerosing Hodgkin's disease. Am J Surg Pathol 1986;10:470.

62. Rudiger T, Jaffe ES, Delsol G, et al. Workshop report on Hodgkin's lymphoma and related diseases (grey zone lymphoma). Ann Oncol 1998;Suppl 5:531.

63. Shiota M, Fujimotoa J, Takenaga M, et al. Diagnosis of t(2;5)(p23;q35)−associated Ki-1 lymphoma with immunohistochemistry. Blood 1994;84:3648.

64. Pulford K, Lamant L, Morris SW, et al. Detection of anaplastic lymphoma kinase (ALK) and nucleolar protein nucleophosmin (NPM)−ALK proteins I normal and neoplastic cells with monoclonal antibody ALK1. Blood 1997;89:1394.

65. Paulli M, Strater J, Gianelli U, et al. Mediastinal B-cell lymphoma: A study of its histomorphologic spectrum based on 109 cases. Hum Pathol 1999;30:178.

66. Higgins JP, Warnke RA. CD30 expression is common in mediastinal large B-cell lymphoma. Am J Clin Pathol 1999;112:241.

67. Chittal SM, Brousset P, Voigt JJ, et al. Large B-cell lymphoma rich in T cells and simulating Hodgkin's disease. Histopathology 1991;19:221.

68. Rudiger T, Ott G, Ott MM, et al. Differential diagnosis between classic Hodgkin's lymphoma, T-cell-rich B-cell lymphoma, and paragranuloma by paraffin immunohistochemistry. Am J Surg Pathol 1998;22:1184.

69. Strickler JG, Fedeli F, Horwitz CA, et al. Infectious mononucleosis in lymphoid tissue: Histopathology, in situ hybridization, and differential diagnosis. Arch Pathol Lab Med 1993;117:269.

70. Reynolds DJ, Banks PM, Gulley ML. New characterization of infectious mononucleosis and a phenotypic comparison with Hodgkin's disease. Am J Pathol 1995;146:379.

71. Fellbaum CH, Hansmann ML, Lennert K. Lymphadenitis mimicking Hodgkin's disease. Histopathology 1988;12:153.

72. Doggett RS, Colby TV, Dorfman RF. Interfollicular Hodgkin's disease. Am J Surg Pathol 1983;7:145.

73. Chan JKC, Tsang WYW. Reactive lymphadenopathies. In: Weiss LM, ed. Pathology of Lymph Nodes. Contemporary Issues in Surgical Pathology, Vol. 21. Philadelphia: Churchill Livingstone, 1996.

CHAPTER 6

Immunohistologic Features of Melanocytic Neoplasms

Mark R. Wick, M.D.

Malignant melanoma (MM) continues to be one of the greatest diagnostic challenges in surgical pathology. Both as a primary lesion in the skin and in metastatic sites, this neoplasm is capable of assuming many different macroscopic and histologic guises. Recognized microscopic phenotypes of MM include superficial spreading, nodular, lentiginous, balloon (clear) cell, pleomorphic-sarcomatoid, spindle cell/desmoplastic/neuroid, small cell (neuroendocrine-like), hemangiopericytoid, signet ring cell, myxoid, adenoid-pseudopapillary, metaplastic, rhabdoid, and "nevoid" forms (Figs. 6–1 to 6–3).[1–3] Because all those images may be amelanotic in nature, the differential diagnostic considerations in such cases are truly protean. Accordingly, electron microscopy, immunohistology, and cytogenetic analysis have become exceedingly important in the accurate recognition of melanoma. This discussion focuses on immunohistology and is directed principally at diagnostic questions concerning melanocytic tumors in general. However, brief consideration is also given to "prognostic" markers for MM.

FILAMENTOUS PROTEINS IN MELANOCYTIC NEOPLASMS

Intermediate filament protein (IFP) analysis has been an important cornerstone of immunohistochemical evaluation since the early 1980s. In general terms, it can still be stated with accuracy that immunostains for keratins, vimentin, desmin, neurofilament proteins, and glial fibrillary acidic protein (GFAP) are broadly capable of distinguishing among histologically similar classes of neoplasms with dissimilar lineages.[4, 5] A more detailed discussion of this topic is included in an earlier chapter on soft tissue tumors (Chapter 3).

In specific regard to melanocytic neoplasms, nevi and MMs typically are labeled only for vimentin and lack the other four groups of IFPs (Figs. 6–4 and 6–5).[5–7] Moreover, the density of vimentin in melanogenic tumors is high, yielding intense immunoreactivity for that marker in most instances. Using frozen tissue or specially (nonformalin) fixed specimens, various authors have shown that MMs may, in fact, contain detectable amounts of keratin and other intermediate filaments.[2, 8, 9] However, in a cooperative interinstitutional study, in which I participated, using paraffin sections and modern immunohistochemical methods, less than 3% of melanomas were keratin-positive (Fig. 6–6), and those lesions that expressed that IFP generally did so in a focal fashion. Similarly, GFAP and desmin have been reported in a very small minority (<1%) of MMs.[2] These have usually been tumors that demonstrated "metaplastic" sarcomatoid microscopic features or, conversely, desmoplastic and neuroid characteristics. For practical purposes, and in specific reference to studies of paraffin sections for IFPs, it is still true that greater than 95% of melanocytic neoplasms are labeled solely for vimentin, even after application of current techniques such as heat-mediated epitope retrieval.

Because muscle-specific actin (recognized by monoclonal antibody HHF-35), alpha isoform (smooth muscle) actin (recognized by antibody 1A4), and caldesmon are also preferentially seen in nonepithelial, nonmelanocytic, nonglial tissues, those determinants would be unexpected in melanocytic neoplasms. They are, in fact, rarely detected in such lesions and when observed, they are again restricted to spindle cell melanomas that show evidence of divergent myofibroblastic differentiation.[2]

CELL MEMBRANE PROTEINS

A diversity of proteins associated with cell membranes come into play in relation to the differential diagnosis of MM. Nonetheless, these proteins fall into two broad categories: those associated with epithelial cells and others relating to hematopoietic elements.

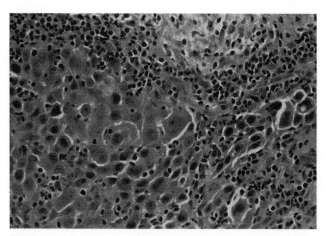

Figure 6–1. Large cell epithelioid amelanotic malignant melanoma, which is the most commonly encountered histologic variant of that tumor.

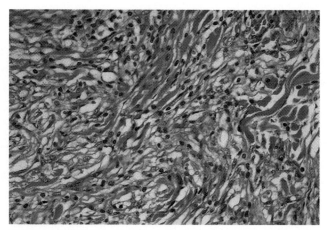

Figure 6–3. Sarcomatoid-desmoplastic amelanotic melanoma, simulating a sarcoma.

Epithelial Determinants

Epithelial Membrane Antigen (EMA). EMA, which is actually a family of glycoproteins that are related to the milk fat globule proteins, is expressed by a variety of somatic epithelia and their neoplasms.[10] The principal exceptions in the latter group include germ cell tumors, adrenocortical proliferations, and hepatocellular neoplasms.[11, 12] An EMA-like moiety also may be observed in selected lymphoid and plasmacellular tumors.[10, 11] Conversely, melanocytic proliferations are consistently nonreactive for this marker.[10–12] It may be observed with a tantalizingly spurious cell membranous distribution in foci of melanomas that border zones of geographic necrosis; however, this pattern of labeling is artifactual and should be disregarded. Purely cytoplasmic reactivity for EMA is similarly discounted interpretatively.

Carcinoembryonic Antigen (CEA). CEA is also a family of glycoproteinaceous cell membrane constituents that are present mainly in tissues and neoplasms with endodermal derivation or differentia-

tion. In the past, it was contended that CEA may be observed in melanomas as well,[13] but that premise is felt to be a reflection of faulty technique and the use of unabsorbed heteroantisera in immunohistologic studies.[14] Such reagents recognize several proteins other than CEA (e.g., nonspecific cross-reacting antigen, biliary glycoprotein), many of which are not restricted to epithelial cells. If monoclonal antibodies are used with suitable specificity to restricted CEA epitopes, melanocytic neoplasms should demonstrate no labeling whatsoever.[15]

Tumor-Associated Glycoprotein-72 (TAG72)/Ber-EP4 Antigen/MOC31 Antigen. TAG72 (recognized by monoclonal antibody B72.3), Ber-EP4, and MOC31 are all cell membrane glycoproteins that are most consistently synthesized by epithelial cells.[16] There are rare exceptions to that statement—for example, the presence of TAG72 in some epithelioid vascular tumors—but they do not include melanocytic neoplasms.[15] Therefore, immunostains against this group of adjunctive epithe-

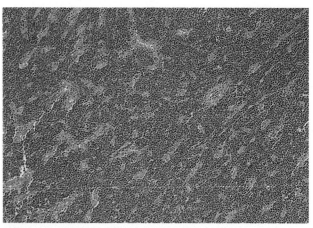

Figure 6–2. Small cell amelanotic melanoma, resembling neuroendocrine carcinoma.

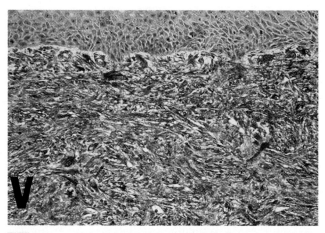

Figure 6–4. Intense vimentin-labeling is typically present in the cells of all malignant melanomas, as shown here.

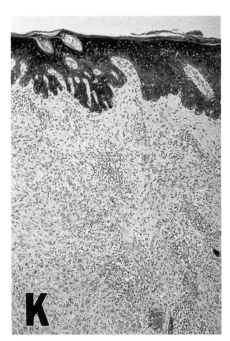

Figure 6–5. Keratin is lacking in greater than or equal to 97% of melanomas in paraffin sections. K, keratin stain.

lial markers are useful supplements to others for keratin, EMA, and CEA in helping to exclude epithelial neoplasms in the differential diagnosis of MMs. One can safely state that virtually all somatic carcinomas should be reactive for at least one of the membrane determinants cited earlier in this discussion, as well as keratin. In contrast, those rare melanomas that can be labeled for keratin lack similar corroborating evidence of epithelial differentiation.

Placenta-like Alkaline Phosphatase (PLAP). PLAP is an isozyme that is commonly synthesized by neoplastic germ cells, as well as selected somatic epithelial malignancies.[17] As such, it is a useful screening marker for gonadal tumors such as seminoma, embryonal carcinoma, and yolk sac carcinoma, all of which may enter the differential diagnosis of MM. In contrast, melanocytic proliferations are consistently nonreactive for PLAP. However, it must be remembered that this determinant is centered in cell membranes; therefore, neoplasms that demonstrate only a cytoplasmic "blush" for PLAP in immunohistologic preparations (including melanomas) should not be regarded as truly positive for that marker.

"Hematopoietic" Markers

Selected cell surface antigens that are typically associated with hematopoietic cells and neoplasms also are potentially seen in melanocytic cells and neoplasms. They include CD10, CD44, CD56, CD57, CD59, CD68, CD74, CD99, CD117 (c-kit protein), CD146, class II major histocompatibility antigens (MHC2A [HLA-DR, HLA-DP, HLA-DQ]), β_2-microglobulin, and bcl-2 protein.[18–26] The author has observed all those markers in selected examples of Spitz (epithelioid and spindle cell) nevus, architecturally disordered ("dysplastic") nevus, and melanoma. Conversely, melanocytes uniformly lack other hematopoietic determinants that may enter into differential diagnostic evaluations of MM, such as terminal deoxynucleotidyl transferase, factor XIIIa, myeloperoxidase, CD15, CD20, CD21, CD23, CD30, CD35, CD43, and CD45.

The expression of MHC2A and β_2-microglobulin by melanocytic proliferations appears to be a property confined to inflamed banal nevi or architecturally disordered nevi, as well as MMs.[27] Clinicians interested in using immunotherapy for melanoma will often request that such a neoplasm be studied immunohistologically for its synthesis of those markers. MMs that "escape" immune surveillance have been noted to down-regulate their expression of β_2-microglobulin and histocompatibility antigens over time[26] through mutations in the corresponding gene complexes and other mechanisms. Because of the immunophenotypic heterogeneity seen in melanocytic lesions (as well as other tumors) for MHC2A and β_2-microglobulin, such determinants should not be used in a differential diagnostic capacity.

The ability of melanomas to be labeled for bcl-2 protein and CD10, CD68, CD56, CD57, CD99, and CD117 creates the possibility that they may be confused with lymphomas, histiocytic lesions, primitive neuroectodermal and neuroendocrine neoplasms, and gastrointestinal stromal tumors, respectively. As usual, the application of carefully

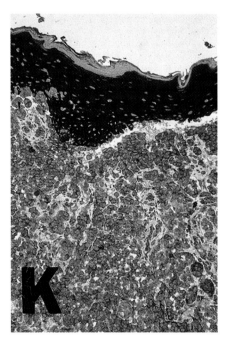

Figure 6–6. Only rare melanomas demonstrate keratin reactivity (shown here) in routinely processed specimens. K, keratin stain.

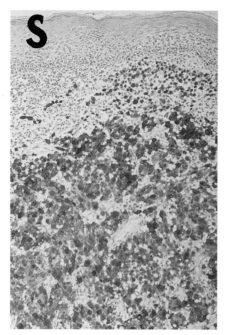

Figure 6–7. Intense nucleocytoplasmic immunoreactivity for S-100 protein (S) in primary cutaneous epithelioid melanoma.

constructed panels of antibody reagents, tailored to specific diagnostic scenarios, should preclude those mistakes.

NB84

NB84 is a monoclonal antibody that was raised against a cell membrane determinant found in neuroblastomas. It is active in paraffin sections and labels not only neuroblastic neoplasms but also a subset of primitive neuroectodermal tumors.[28] Melanocytic proliferations are nonreactive with this reagent. The latter fact is helpful when the differential diagnosis centers around small cell melanoma versus a neuroblastic or neuroectodermal tumor arising in a large congenital nevus or neurocristic hamartoma.[29]

CALCIUM-BINDING PROTEINS

Several proteins that affect intracellular calcium metabolism, including annexin VI, cap-g, annexin V, calmodulin, calretinin, and S-100 protein, can be seen in melanocytic proliferations.[30] Only two of these have definite diagnostic importance and will be discussed further here.

S-100 Protein

One of the first, as well as one of the most enduring, markers for MM is S-100 protein (S-100P). This 21-kd moiety was first detected in glial cells of the central nervous system, and it was given its name because of solubility in 100% saturated ammonium sulfate solution.[31] In 1981, Gaynor and colleagues[32] recognized the fact that S-100P was present in human melanoma cells as well, leading to its subsequent widespread application as a diagnostic indicator for that tumor (Figs. 6–7 and 6–8).

The function of S-100P has never been determined with precision; however, it is thought to function in intracellular calcium trafficking or microtubular assembly, or both.[33, 34] It has a loose physiologic relationship to calmodulin, another calcium flux protein.[30] There are two subunits to S-100P: alpha and beta, yielding three possible dimeric forms: *alpha-alpha, alpha-beta,* and *beta-beta.*[35] Melanocytes synthesize only the first of those combinations. Immunoreactivity for S-100P should be both nuclear and cytoplasmic in order to be regarded as valid. Immunoelectron microscopic studies have verified the presence of this protein in both intracellular compartments in normal and neoplastic melanocytes.[36]

At this point, many antibodies to S-100P have been developed, some of which are dimer-specific monoclonal products.[37] In general practice, however, most clinical laboratories still use heteroantisera against this marker that recognize all three isotypes of the protein. This allows such reagents to be used successfully as high-sensitivity screening tools. In that context, my experience has been that greater than 98% of MM cases can be labeled for S-100P, regardless of histologic subtype. A redaction of the pertinent literature by Smoller[38] yielded a slightly smaller figure (97.4%). Other S-100P+ tumor types that enter into differential diagnostic consideration with melanocytic lesions include various poorly differentiated carcinomas, selected histiocytic proliferations, malignant gliomas, peripheral nerve sheath tumors, and Langerhans' cell lesions.[36, 38, 42] It should be obvious, then, that S-100P is most valuable in this setting as an initial screening reagent for melanocytic tu-

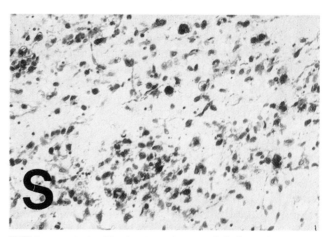

Figure 6–8. Nucleocytoplasmic labeling for S-100 protein (S) in myxoid-sarcomatoid melanoma.

mors, rather than being a specific marker for such neoplasms.

Calretinin

Calretinin is a cytoplasmic 31-kd protein, which again was first isolated from central nervous system tissues.[43, 44] It also is seen in peripheral nerves in the skin and elsewhere.[45] Otherwise, this polypeptide is rather restricted in distribution, having been detected thus far only in mesothelium,[44] germinal surface epithelium of the ovary,[44] and selected adenocarcinomas (most notably a subset in the colon and rectum).[46] Melanocytic tumors are not included in the list of neoplasms that show potential calretinin immunoreactivity.

MELANOCYTE-"SPECIFIC" MONOCLONAL ANTIBODIES

Beginning in the early 1980s, the availability of monoclonal antibody technology was applied to a quest for a "melanoma-specific" reagent, which ideally would be suited not only for diagnostic but also for therapeutic utility.[47] This search continues today and has not yet come to ultimate fruition.

A variety of antimelanocyte hybridoma products have been described, only some of which are applicable to paraffin sections and routinely processed tissue specimens. They have been summarized previously by Smoller.[38] Those whose activity is restricted to frozen tissue substrates include PAL-M1, PAL-M2, 691-13-17, 691-15-Nu4B, and "MEL" series antibodies number 1 through number 4. In contrast, HMSA-2, 2-139-1, 6-26-3, KBA62, 1C11, 7H11, Mel-CAM, Mel-5, and SM5-1 do have immunoreactivity with formalin-fixed, paraffin-embedded specimens.[38, 48, 49] Generally speaking, the markers just listed have not entered or are no longer used in the sphere of diagnostic pathology because of special tissue processing requirements that are associated with them, an unavailability of commercial distribution, or a lack of sensitivity or specificity for malignant melanocytic lesions. Those that have been used in a clinical context are considered in the following sections.

gp100/PMel 17–Related Monoclonal Antibodies

Several monoclonal antibodies have now been raised against a glycoproteinaceous antigenic group that is restricted to cells of melanocytic lineage. This group is designated *gp100,* and corresponding cDNA to it has been cloned.[50, 51] Two proteins are encoded by that nucleic acid sequence—gp100 itself (with a molecular weight of 100 kd) and gp10 (with a molecular weight of 10 kd).[51] The transla-

tional product related to gp100-C1 cDNA is closely homologous, but not identical, to yet another melanocytic protein termed *PMel 17.*[52] Both are localized to the inner membranes of type 1, 2, and 3 premelanosomes; they similarly serve as potential targets for cytotoxic T lymphocytes, probably in concert with MHC2A.[53] Indeed, one marker in this group, MART-1, was named specifically for that property (melanoma antigen recognized by T cells-1); it is recognized by two monoclonal antibodies, A-103 and M2-7C10, and is also known as melan-A (Fig. 6–9).[54–65] Nucleotide sequence analysis performed by Adema and colleagues showed that the cDNAs for gp100 and PMel 17 emanate from a single gene, by alternative splicing.[51] This conclusion gained further support by their observation that gp100 and PMel 17 are consistently expressed concomitantly by both non-neoplastic and neoplastic melanocytic populations.[66] Conversely, Chiamenti and colleagues[67] suggested that the protein target of HMB-45 was a unique premelanosome-related polypeptide, but that proposition has not been confirmed by other investigators.

gp100 *transcripts* are not specific for melanocytes and have been observed in a wide variety of tissue types.[50] Nonetheless, *translation* of the mRNA in question does occur only in melanocytic elements. This finding strongly suggests that immunohistology is the most practical technologic method for assessment of gp100 as a melanocyte marker and that nucleic acid–based procedures (e.g., in situ hybridization, polymerase chain reaction) are likely to be associated with unacceptably low specificity of gp100 for pigment-producing cells.

Antibodies in the gp100/PMel 17 group include NKI-beteb, NKI/C3, HMB-45, HMB-50, and MART-1/melan-A (Figs. 6–10 and 6–11).[51, 52, 54–66, 68–84] These demonstrate variable levels of specificity and sensitivity for melanocytes, nevi, and melanomas, vis-à-vis other cell lineages and tumor types. In practice, HMB-45 and MART-1 have thus far

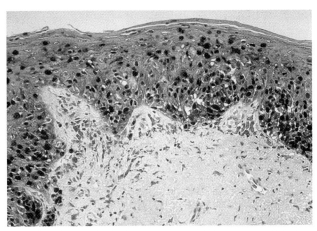

Figure 6–9. Global cytoplasmic immunoreactivity is seen for MART-1 melan-A protein in this primary superficial, spreading melanoma.

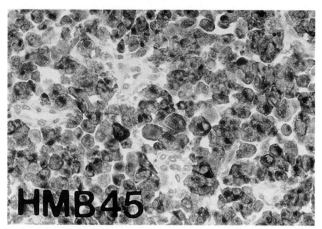

Figure 6–10. Intense cytoplasmic positivity is seen with HMB-45 in epithelioid melanoma metastatic to a lymph node.

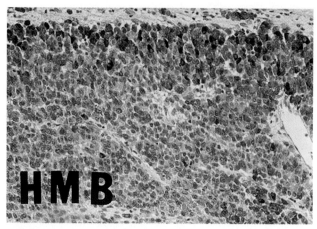

Figure 6–11. Heterogeneous cytoplasmic labeling with HMB-50 (HMB) is seen in metastatic lymph node epithelioid melanoma.

enjoyed the greatest use as agents to confirm the identity of S-100P+ neoplasms as melanocytic in nature.

Unfortunate peculiarities exist that relate to the commercial distribution of HMB-45. I had the opportunity to evaluate the original supernatant product from the HMB-45 clone, which I received as a generous gift from Dr. Allen Gown (one of the developers of the antibody) in the mid-1980s. In a published study that reflected this evaluation, our group found HMB-45 to be greater than 95% sensitive for melanoma and essentially 100% specific for that diagnosis among non–spindle cell malignancies.[76] Afterward, HMB-45 was sold to a commercial firm that marketed an impure form of the hybridoma product. It showed a much lower degree of specificity and was seen to label a variety of tumors other than melanomas.[36, 85–88] When other firms subsequently assumed distributorship of HMB-45, its specificity "recovered." Nevertheless, in a probable effort to maximize profits, many of those companies have now prediluted the "neat" antibody that is provided to users, and its overall sensitivity is now no better than 60% as a result of that manipulation.

Another observation relating to HMB-45, HMB-50, MART-1, and other gp100-related reagents has widely but erroneously been said to reflect "cross-reactivity" with nonmelanocytic cells. This refers to the ability of the cited antibodies to label angiomyolipomas, lymphangioleiomyomatosis, "sugar" tumors (clear cell myomelanocytic tumors) of the lung and other organs, and other examples of proliferations showing epithelioid perivascular cell features (Fig. 6–12).[89–94] These lesions do manifest ultrastructural evidence of premelanosome synthesis and therefore have at least partial melanocytic differentiation.[90, 91] Hence, gp100-related antibodies are not manifesting cross-reactivity in labeling such pathologic entities; that affinity is merely a biologic extension of their specificity for premelanosome-associated proteins.

One true exception to the last statement is represented by the ability of MART-1/melan-A (but not HMB-45, NKI-beteb, or HMB-50) to label the tumor cells of a subset of adrenocortical carcinomas and sex cord tumors of the gonads (Fig. 6–13).[60, 96] No evidence of true melanocytic differentiation has been seen in such neoplasms, and MART-1 antibodies are presumably recognizing an antigenic epitope in those steroidogenic proliferations that is shared with the gp100/PMel 17 molecules.

As alluded to earlier, none of the antibodies considered in this section is effective at labeling more than a small fraction (<10%) of spindle cell/desmoplastic/neuroid melanomas.[61, 76, 77] This "shortcoming" is likely a reflection of the fact that such neoplasms typically manifest clonal evolution from a melanocytic phenotype to a more fibroblastic or schwannian motif, losing in the process their ability to synthesize premelanosomes and proteins related to those organelles.

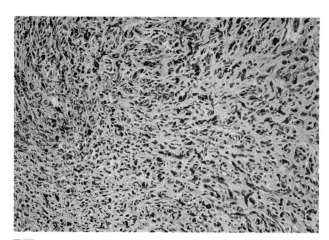

Figure 6–12. Multifocal immunoreactivity is apparent with HMB-45 in this spindle cell–rich angiomyolipoma of the kidney.

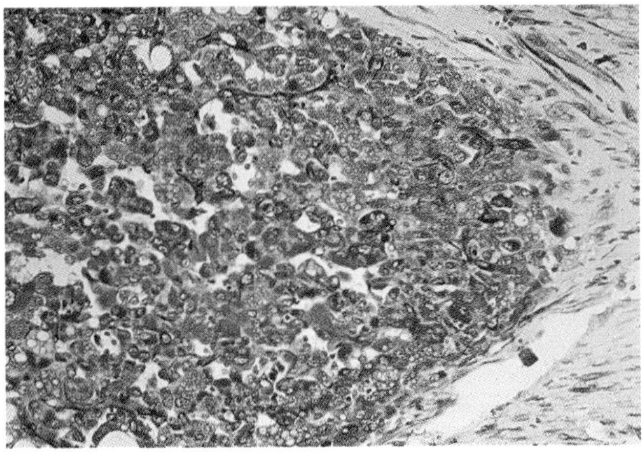

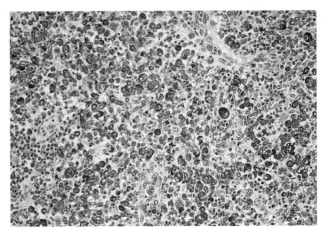

Figure 6–13. Diffuse labeling for MART-1/melan-A (with antibody clone A-103) in adrenocortical carcinoma.

Tyrosinase-Related Antibodies

In normal melaninogenesis, the amino acid tyrosine is hydroxylated to form 3,4-dihydroxyphenylalanine (dopa), which is then oxidized to dopaquinone. The latter moiety is polymerized to form melanin, thereafter combining with melanoprotein to form a stable complex within premelanosomes and melanosomes.[97] Tyrosinase plays a central role in this process by catalyzing the first step in the stated sequence.[98] As such, it is a specific marker for melanocytic differentiation. This premise has been affirmed by studies showing that tyrosinase gene transcripts are strictly confined to melanin-producing cells.[99]

T311 and MAT-1 are the two antityrosinase monoclonal antibodies that have been analyzed best in surgical pathology.[100–109] The second of them is an IgG reagent that was raised using a synthetic peptide corresponding to the carboxy terminus of human tyrosinase as an immunogen.[107] Both antibodies show a high level (>80%) of sensitivity and virtually absolute specificity for melanoma of the non–spindle cell type, among all malignant tumors (Fig. 6–14). Nevi are conversely nonreactive with MAT-1 in many instances, as are non-neoplastic melanocytes.[106] Hence, the epitope it recognizes is presumably related to melanocytic maturation as well as differentiation. In light of that finding, and because of the excellent specificity of antityrosinase antibodies, it would seem logical and permissible to use them diagnostically as mixtures (so-called cocktails).

Microphthalmia Transcription Factor Protein

The microphthalmia gene encodes a transcription factor that is necessary to the survival and development of melanocytes during embryogenesis.[110] Microphthalmia transcription factor protein (MTFP) is a nuclear basic helix-loop-helix leucine zipper moiety that, together with the PAX3 and MSG1 gene products, plays a role in controlling the activity of melanogenic enzymes by up-regulating the cyclic adenosine monophosphate pathway.[111–113] (Incidentally, another related gene, TFE, has similar properties, and its transcription factor may emerge in the future as an additional melanocyte marker.[113]

Although data on the immunoreactivity of MTFP antibodies are preliminary, these reagents appear to be sensitive and specific for the identification of melanocytic proliferations.[114–117] As is true of most other markers in this general category, except for S-100P, MTFP has typically labeled most non-sarcomatoid melanocytic lesions but a substantially lesser proportion of spindle cell/desmoplastic melanomas.[114, 115, 117] In keeping with its known intracellular localization, MTFP should be regarded as truly present immunohistologically only if nuclear reactivity is observed.[116] As additional support for their partially melanocytic nature, angiomyolipoma, lymphangioleiomyomatosis, and sugar tumors share MTFP reactivity with MM.[118, 119]

NEUROENDOCRINE MARKERS IN MELANOCYTIC LESIONS

Because of a conceptual association of both melanocytic and neuroendocrine proliferations with the neuroectoderm, it could be expected that these categories of neoplasia might demonstrate significant immunohistologic homologies. With the passage of time, however, it has become clear that there are both consistent similarities and differences between them.

Proteins that are restricted anatomically to neurosecretory granules and neurosynaptic vesicles, such as chromogranins and synaptophysin, are

Figure 6–14. Multifocal intense positivity for tyrosinase in metastatic epithelioid melanoma in the liver.

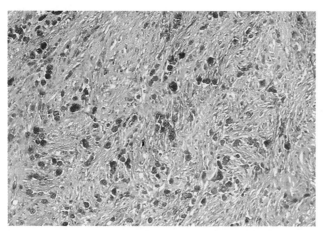

Figure 6–15. "Melanotic" schwannoma, in which a high proportion of the tumor cells demonstrate divergent melanocytic differentiation.

consistently absent in "pure" melanocytic tumors.[120–124] However, it is apparent that selected lesions that are basically neuroendocrine or nonmelanocytic neuroectodermal neoplasms (e.g., neuroendocrine carcinomas, paragangliomas, primitive neuroectodermal tumors, peripheral nerve sheath tumors) may exhibit a variable degree of divergent melanocytic differentiation. This phenomenon yields diagnostic entities such as pigmented carcinoid tumor,[125, 126] pigmented paraganglioma,[127] melanotic neuroectodermal tumor,[128, 129] and melanotic schwannoma[130] (both benign and malignant) (Fig. 6–15). In these lesions, "minor" melanocytic elements have the same immunophenotype as the cells of cutaneous nevi or MMs (i.e., S-100P+, HMB45+, MART-1+, tyrosinase-positive), but the remaining constituents are monodifferentiated epithelial, neural, or schwannian tissues. The latter cells lack melanocytic markers altogether, producing a dimorphic and mutually exclusive immunophenotype.

Other "neuroendocrine" determinants that may be seen in melanoma are, in fact, synthesized by a broad repertoire of cell types. They include, but are not limited to, melanocytes, neuroendocrine epithelial cells, neuroblasts, primitive mesenchymal neuroectodermal cells, and Schwann cells. The markers in question are principally represented by neuron-specific (*gamma* dimer) enolase, CD57, neural cell adhesion molecule (CD56), and CD99 (MIC2 protein).[131–136] With the exception of CD99, they tend to be observed preferentially in melanocytic proliferations with neuroid features, such as neurotized intradermal nevi and "neurotropic" melanomas.[134] Thus, it is obvious that such markers cannot be used to distinguish between truly neuroendocrine and melanocytic neoplasms.

PUTATIVELY PROGNOSTIC MARKERS FOR MELANOMA

Since the early 1990s, several publications have considered adjunctive morphologic pathologic pro-

cedures that have putative prognostic utility in MM. These include immunostaining for mutated p53 protein (a promoter of programmed cell death); Ki-67, proliferating cell nuclear antigen, and Ki-S5 (cell cycle–related indicators of proliferation); heat shock proteins (markers of replicating or "activated" cells); bcl-2 protein (an inhibitor of apoptosis); VLA-4 and alpha-v/beta-3 integrins (intercellular adhesion molecules that correlate with entrance into the vertical growth phase of melanoma); CD26/dipeptidyl-aminopeptidase IV (a membrane-bound protease that facilitates tumor cell invasion); and cyclin-D1, cyclin-D3, and p16INK4-alpha (CDKN2A) gene product (cell cycle regulators).[137–142] Another proposed method uses immunostains for endothelial markers (e.g., von Willebrand factor, CD31, and CD34) to assess stromal vascularity in vertical growth–phase melanomas, with the premise that increased angiogenesis is correlated with an adverse prognosis.[143, 144] In general, the aforementioned markers have not been embraced as clinically relevant tools as yet because of disagreements on interpretative thresholds and methodologic issues attending them.

It is important to note that prognostically adverse results of the analytical techniques just cited appear to be intimately associated with acquisition of the vertical growth phase in melanomas. This reality probably reflects several biologic events that accompany the "malignant eclipse" from radial to vertical growth. They potentially include an increase in autocrine, mitogenic growth factors in vertical growth melanomas (VGMs), decreased rates of apoptosis in VGM tumor cells, an acquired resistance to growth-inhibitory factors in the vertical growth phase, augmented angiogenesis by VGM cells, and loss of the c-kit (CD117) gene product (having tyrosine kinase activity).[145, 146] On a cytogenetic level, it has been shown that the transition between radial and vertical growth phases is paralleled by gains in gene copy numbers on chromosomes 7, 8, 6p, 1q, 20, 17, and 2, in decreasing order of frequency.[147]

At present, nonmorphologic techniques to evaluate the prognosis of MMs must be regarded as investigational and cannot yet be recommended for routine clinical application. All necessary pathologic data, such as tumor location, size, depth, ulceration, mitotic activity, and growth phase, can still be obtained by examination of standard microscopic preparations of melanoma as stained with hematoxylin and eosin.

SPECIFIC DIFFERENTIAL DIAGNOSTIC PROBLEMS CONCERNING MALIGNANT MELANOCYTIC PROLIFERATIONS

Several sections in the foregoing discussion have made reference to selected differential diagnostic issues that revolve around the morphologic and

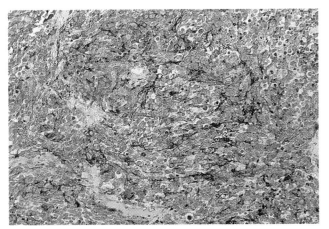

Figure 6–16. Immunolabeling for tyrosinase in sarcomatoid melanoma; less than 10% of examples of this tumor variant stain for melanocytic markers other than S-100 protein.

immunophenotypic variation in MM. These are considered further in the following sections.

Melanoma Versus Melanocytic Nevus Variants

Several articles have appeared on the use of immunohistology for the separation of benign and malignant melanocytic neoplasms of various types. In particular, the differential diagnosis of Spitz nevus versus melanoma has been discussed several times in reference to their relative expression of mutant p16 and p53 proteins, Ki-67, Ki-S5, and other markers relating to cellular transformation or proliferation.[148-152] Although some general trends have emerged from such analyses, there is too much overlap in the immunophenotypes of melanocytic nevi and melanomas for those data to be used meaningfully in individual cases. As I have stated previously, I do not endorse or use that practice.

Melanocytic Neoplasms Versus Histiocytic Proliferations

In the skin and elsewhere, it may be histologically difficult to separate amelanotic melanocytic lesions from histiocytic proliferations such as epithelioid histiocytoma, foam cell–poor xanthogranuloma, atypical fibroxanthoma, and reticulohistiocytoma (reticulohistiocytosis).[153-155] Even though occasional histiocytic tumors may label for S-100P, they are consistently nonreactive with HMB-45, HMB-50, MART-1, antityrosinase, and anti-MTFP. In contrast, histiocytomas and melanocytic neoplasms may both be reactive for factor XIIIa and CD68, which have been loosely (and mistakenly) advanced as histiocytic markers.[23, 158]

Recognition of Rhabdoid and Sarcomatoid Malignant Melanomas

Rhabdoid and sarcomatoid melanomas (including desmoplastic, myxoid, and neurotropic subtypes) may be chosen for special discussion because they demonstrate antigenic deletion or aberrancy in a relatively substantial proportion of cases. Indeed, the first example of rhabdoid melanoma that I encountered was a metastatic keratin-positive, S-100P– tumor in a patient who was known to have had melanoma in the past. That particular variant of melanocytic malignancy loses reactivity for S-100P, HMB-45, MART-1, or tyrosinase in approximately 20% of cases in my experience and acquires positivity for keratin or desmin in roughly 1 to 3% of cases.[2, 159-161] Obviously, an extended panel of reagents, including essentially all the available melanocytic markers, must therefore be used to recognize rhabdoid melanomas with accuracy.

Sarcomatoid melanomas are consistently S-100P+, but only 3 to 10% can be labeled for other, more specific melanocytic determinants (Fig. 6–16).[76, 114, 115, 117, 162] Because a proportion of such lesions becomes transmogrified into spindle cell proliferations with divergent phenotypes, immunoreactivity for CD56, CD57, nerve growth factor receptor, desmin, and actin isoforms is potentially observed in them (Fig. 6–17).[2, 131-136] Especially in the absence of a given history of melanoma, those immunophenotypic quirks represent distinct diagnostic pitfalls for the unwary.

Amelanotic Melanoma Versus Other Epithelioid Malignancies

A classic differential diagnostic question posed by surgical pathologists is that of melanoma versus poorly differentiated carcinoma versus large cell non-Hodgkin's lymphoma or "syncytial" Hodgkin's disease.[163, 164] This is particularly true of tumors

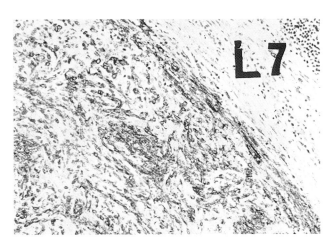

Figure 6–17. CD57/Leu7 (L7) in sarcomatoid-desmoplastic malignant melanoma, likely reflecting neuroid differentiation in that tumor.

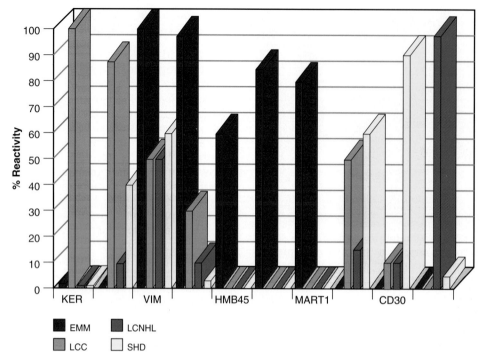

Figure 6–18. Immunoreactivity patterns in large cell undifferentiated malignancies. EMM, epithelioid malignant melanoma; LCC, undifferentiated large cell carcinoma; LCNHL, large cell non-Hodgkin's lymphoma; SHD, syncytial Hodgkin's disease; KER, keratin; VIM, vimentin.

presenting in lymph nodes, when there is no known history of a prior malignancy.

Under such circumstances, applicable antibody panels should include reagents to keratins, EMA, vimentin, S-100P, HMB-45, tyrosinase, MART-1, CD15, CD30, and CD45. Expected results in the specified classes of tumor being considered are depicted in Figure 6–18.

The same basic approach may be used when the differential diagnosis is that of metastatic serosal melanoma versus malignant mesothelioma, except that antibodies to calretinin, thrombomodulin, and HBME-1 should be included. The great majority of mesotheliomas, if not all of them, will express at least one of the latter three determinants, whereas MM is nonreactive for all of them.[165–167]

Neuroendocrine carcinomas may be separated from MM by attention to keratin reactivity patterns and positivity for chromogranins and synaptophysin.[124] As stated earlier, melanocytic lesions lack the latter two markers consistently, whereas at least 50% of neuroendocrine epithelial tumors express at least one of them. Keratin often assumes a dot-like, perinuclear, globular intracytoplasmic pattern of labeling in neuroendocrine carcinomas,[168] but that configuration is not seen in the small minority of keratin-positive MMs.

Metastatic Melanoma Versus Malignant Glioma

In the central nervous system, metastatic amelanotic melanoma may imitate the microscopic ap-

pearance of a high-grade malignant glioma virtually perfectly. This resemblance is further complicated by the common reactivity seen in both lesions for S-100P[131, 169–171] and the potential for a small minority of melanomas to express GFAP as well.[2] Hence, other melanocytic markers such as HMB-45, antityrosinase, and MART-1 are crucial to making this diagnostic distinction. All those determinants are absent in pure glial neoplasms.[170, 171]

Melanoma Versus Soft Tissue Sarcomas

The ability of melanoma to simulate the appearance of varied soft tissue sarcomas is also well documented.[172] These include malignant peripheral nerve sheath tumors, gastrointestinal stromal tumors, epithelioid angiosarcoma, rhabdoid tumors, osteosarcomas, and primitive neuroectodermal tumors, to name a few.[173] The detailed immunophenotypic properties of those lesions are provided elsewhere in this volume. However, none of these sarcomas manifests reactivity for gp100-related melanocytic markers or tyrosinase, making those markers essential to the differential diagnostic process.

A notable exception to the preceding statement is represented by clear cell sarcoma of soft tissue (melanoma of soft parts), which clearly does exhibit true melanocytic differentiation.[174–176] Because the immunohistologic profiles of that tumor and MM are superimposable,[176] other specialized studies are usually necessary to separate them when clinical findings make the diagnosis uncertain. In particular, clear cell sarcoma regularly shows the presence of a t(12;22) chromosomal translocation, which is not present in melanomas.[177, 178]

Uncommonly, primitive neuroectodermal tumors also may demonstrate divergent melanocytic differentiation and thereby imitate the appearance of small cell MM.[2, 120, 128, 129] Furthermore, both lesions have the potential to express CD56, CD57, and CD99. Diffuse reactivity for S-100P, gp100-related markers, or MTFP would argue strongly for an interpretation of melanoma in this setting. Conversely, immunopositivity for FLI-1 protein is restricted to primitive neuroectodermal tumors (PNETs).[179] Again, cytogenetic evaluation is advisable whenever possible in this particular situation, inasmuch as primitive neuroectodermal tumors demonstrate a reproducible t(11;22) chromosomal translocation.[181]

The most difficult diagnostic distinction to make in this context is that of sarcomatoid MM versus superficial malignant peripheral nerve sheath tumor (SMPNST). Indeed, in many ways, the two are nearly identical.[181] Obviously, a history of previous melanoma would be important information to have in such a case, but if that is unavailable, I generally restrict an interpretation of superficial malignant peripheral nerve sheath tumor to lesions that are clearly associated with a large nerve or a pre-existing neurofibroma or to lesions that have occurred in patients with systemic neurofibromatosis.[182]

References

1. Nakhleh RE, Wick MR, Rocamora A, et al. Morphologic diversity in malignant melanomas. Am J Clin Pathol 1990; 93:731–740.
2. Banerjee SS, Harris M. Morphologic and immunophenotypic variation in malignant melanoma. Histopathology 2000;36:387–402.
3. Reed RJ, Martin P. Variants of melanoma. Semin Cutan Med Surg 1997;16:137–158.
4. Battifora H. Clinical application of the immunohistochemistry of filamentous proteins. Am J Surg Pathol 1988; 12(Suppl):24–42.
5. Osborn M. Intermediate filaments as histologic markers: An overview. J Invest Dermatol 1983;81(Suppl 1):104s–109s.
6. Ramaekers FCS, Puts JJ, Moesker O, et al. Intermediate filaments in malignant melanomas: Identification and use as a marker in surgical pathology. J Clin Invest 1983;71: 635–643.
7. Caselitz J, Janner M, Breitbart E, et al. Malignant melanomas contain only the vimentin type of intermediate filaments. Virchows Arch A 1983;400:43–51.
8. Zarbo RJ, Gown AM, Nagle RB, et al. Anomalous cytokeratin expression in malignant melanoma: One- and two-dimensional Western blot analysis and immunohistochemical survey of 100 melanomas. Mod Pathol 1990;3:494–502.
9. Miettinen M, Franssila K. Immunohistochemical spectrum of malignant melanoma: The common presence of keratins. Lab Invest 1989;61:623–628.
10. Swanson PE. Monoclonal antibodies to human milk fat globule proteins. In: Wick MR, Siegal GP, eds. Monoclonal Antibodies in Diagnostic Immunohistochemistry. New York, Marcel Dekker, 1988:227–284.
11. Pinkus GS, Kurtin PJ. Epithelial membrane antigen—a diagnostic discriminant in surgical pathology. Hum Pathol 1985;16:929–940.
12. Sloane JP, Ormerod MG. Distribution of epithelial membrane antigen in normal and neoplastic tissues and its value in diagnostic tumor pathology. Cancer 1981;47: 1786–1795.
13. Selby WL, Nance KV, Park KH. Carcinoembryonic antigen immunoreactivity in metastatic malignant melanoma. Mod Pathol 1992;5:415–419.
14. Ravindranath MH, Shen P, Habal N, et al. Does human melanoma express carcinoembronic antigen? Anticancer Res 2000;20:3083–3092.
15. Ben-Izhak B, Levy R, Weill S, et al. Anorectal malignant melanoma: A clinicopathology study, including immunohistochemistry and DNA flow cytometry. Cancer 1997;79: 18–25.
16. Muraro R, Kuroki M, Wunderlich D, et al. Generation and characterization of B72.3 second generation monoclonal antibodies reactive with the tumor associated glycoprotein-72 antigen. Cancer Res 1988;48:4588–4596.
17. Wick MR, Swanson PE, Manivel JC. Placental alkaline phosphatase-like reactivity in human tumors: An immunohistochemical study of 520 cases. Hum Pathol 1987;18: 946–954.
18. Chorvath B, Hunakova L, Turzova M, et al. Monoclonal antibodies to two adhesive cell surface antigens (CD43 and CD59) with different distribution on hematopoietic and non-hematopoietic tumor cell lines. Neoplasma 1992;39: 325–329.
19. Radka SF, Charron DJ, Brodsky FM. Class II molecules of the major histocompatibility complex considered as differentiation markers. Hum Immunol 1986;16:390–400.
20. Carrel S, Schmidt-Kessen A, Mach JP, Heumann D, Girardet C. Expression of common acute lymphoblastic leukemia antigen (CALLA) on human malignant melanoma cell lines. J Immunol 1983;130:2456–2460.
21. Herbold KW, Zhou J, Haggerty JG, Milstone LM. CD44 expression on epidermal melanocytes. J Invest Dermatol 1996;106:1230–1235.
22. Sarlomo-Rikala M, Kovatich AJ, Barusevicius A, Miettinen M. CD117: a sensitive marker for gastrointestinal stromal tumors that is more specific than CD34. Mod Pathol 1998; 11:728–734.
23. Pernick NL, DaSilva M, Gangi MD, et al. "Histiocytic" markers in melanoma. Mod Pathol 1999;12:1072-1077.
24. Tang NE, Luyten GP, Mooy CM, et al. HNK-1 antigens on uveal and cutaneous melanoma cell lines. Melanoma Res 1996;6:411–418.
25. Weidner N, Tjoe J. Immunohistochemical profile of monoclonal antibody O13. Am J Surg Pathol 1994;18:486–494.
26. Tron VA, Krajewski S, Klein-Parker H, et al. Immunohistochemical analysis of bcl-2 protein regulation in cutaneous melanoma. Am J Pathol 1995;146:643–650.
27. Ruiter DJ, Bhan AK, Harrist TJ, et al. Major histocompatibility antigens and mononuclear inflammatory infiltrate in benign nevomelanocytic proliferations and malignant melanoma. J Immunol 1982;129:2808–2815.
28. Miettinen M, Chatten J, Paetan A, Stevenson A. Monoclonal antibody NB84 in the differential diagnosis of neuroblastoma and other small round cell tumors. Am J Surg Pathol 1998;22:327–332.
29. Mezebish D, Smith K, Williams J, et al. Neurocristic cutaneous hamartoma: A distinctive dermal melanocytosis with an unknown malignant potential. Mod Pathol 1998; 11:573–578.
30. Van Ginkel PR, Gee RL, Walker TM, et al. The identification and differential expression of calcium-binding proteins associated with ocular melanoma. Biochim Biophys Acta 1998;1448:290–297.
31. Ludwin SK, Kosek JC, Eng LF. The topographical distribution of S100 protein and GFA protein in the adult rat brain: An immunohistochemical study using horseradish peroxidase–labeled antibodies. J Comp Neurol 1976;165: 197–208.
32. Gaynor R, Irie R, Morton D, et al. S100 protein: A marker for human malignant melanomas? Lancet 1981;1:869–871.

33. Baudier J, Briving C, Deinum J, et al. Effect of S100 protein and calmodulin on calcium-induced disassembly of brain microtubule proteins in vitro. FEBS Lett 1982;147: 165–168.

34. Stefansson K, Wollmann R, Jerkovic M. S100 protein in soft tissue tumors derived from Schwann cells and melanocytes. Am J Pathol 1982;106:261–268.

35. Takahashi K, Isobe T, Ohtsuki Y, et al. Immunohistochemical study on the distribution of alpha and beta subunits of S100 protein in human normal and neoplastic tissues. Virchows Arch B 1984;45:385–396.

36. Herrera GA, Pena JR, Turbat-Herrera EA, et al. The diagnosis of melanoma: Current approaches addressing tumor differentiation. Pathol Annu 1994;29(Part 1):233–260.

37. Loeffel SC, Gillespie GY, Mirmiram SA, et al. Cellular immunolocalization of S100 protein within fixed tissue sections by monoclonal antibodies. Arch Pathol Lab Med 1985;109:117–122.

38. Smoller BR. Immunohistochemistry in the diagnosis of melanocytic neoplasms. Pathol State Art Rev 1994;2:371–383.

39. Kindblom LG, Lodding P, Rosengren L, et al. S100 protein in melanocytic tumors. Acta Pathol Microbiol Scand 1984;92:219–230.

40. Nakajima T, Watanabe S, Sato Y, et al. An immunoperoxidase study of S100 protein distribution in normal and neoplastic tissues. Am J Surg Pathol 1982;7:715–727.

41. Cochran AJ, Lu HF, Li PX, et al. S100 protein remains a practical marker for melanocytic and other tumors. Melanoma Res 1993;3:325–330.

42. Swanson PE, Wick MR. Immunohistochemistry of cutaneous tumors. In: Leong AS-Y, ed. Applied Immunohistochemistry for the Surgical Pathologist. Cambridge, UK, Edward Arnold, 1993:269–308.

43. Rogers J, Khan M, Ellis J. Calretinin and other calcium binding proteins in the nervous system. Adv Exp Med Biol 1990;269:195–203.

44. Tos AP, Doglioni C. Calretinin: A novel tool for diagnostic immunohistochemistry. Adv Anat Pathol 1998;5:61–66.

45. Schulze E, Witt M, Fink T, et al. Immunohistochemical detection of human skin nerve fibers. Acta Histochem 1997;99:301–309.

46. Gotzos V, Wintergerst ES, Musy JP, et al. Selective distribution of calretinin in adenocarcinomas of the human colon and adjacent tissues. Am J Surg Pathol 1999;23:701–711.

47. Nance KV, Siegal GP. The use of monoclonal antibodies in the search for tumor-specific antigens. In: Wick MR, Siegal GP, eds. Monoclonal Antibodies in Diagnostic Immunohistochemistry. New York, Marcel Dekker, 1988:593–622.

48. Shih IM, Nesbit M, Herlyn M, Kurman RJ. A new MELCAM (CD146)–specific monoclonal antibody, MN-4, on paraffin-embedded tissue. Mod Pathol 1998;11:1098–1106.

49. Trefzer U, Rietz N, Chen Y, et al. SM5-1: A new monoclonal antibody which is highly sensitive and specific for melanocytic lesions. Arch Dermatol Res 2000;292:583–589.

50. Brouwenstijn N, Slager EH, Bakker AB, et al. Transcription of the gene encoding melanoma-associated antigen gp10 tissues and cell lines other than those of the melanocytic lineage. Br J Cancer 1997;76:1562–1566.

51. Adema GJ, deBoer AJ, Vogel AM, et al. Molecular characterization of the melanocyte lineage-specific antigen gp100. J Biol Chem 1994;269:20126–20133.

52. Adema GJ, Bakker AB, deBoer J, et al. PMel17 is recognized by monoclonal antibodies NKI-beteb, HMB-45, HMB-50, and by anti-melanoma cytotoxic T-cells. Br J Cancer 1996;73:1044–1048.

53. Kawakami Y, Nishimura MI, Restifo NP, et al. T-cell recognition of human melanoma antigens. J Immunother 1993;14:88–93.

54. Chen YT, Stockert E, Jungbluth A, et al. Serological analysis of melan-A (MART-1), a melanocyte-specific protein homogeneously expressed in human melanomas. Proc Natl Acad Sci U S A 1996;93:5916–5919.

55. Kawakami Y, Battles JK, Kobayashi T, et al. Production of recombinant MART-1 proteins and specific anti-MART-1 polyclonal and monoclonal antibodies: Use in the characterization of the human melanoma antigen MART-1. J Immunol Methods 1997;202:13–25.

56. Kageshita T, Kawakami Y, Hirai S, Ono T. Differential expression of MART-1 in primary and metastatic melanoma lesions. J Immunother 1997;20:460–465.

57. Nicotra MR, Nistico P, Mangoni A, et al. Melan-A/MART-1 antigen expression in cutaneous and ocular melanomas. J Immunother 1997;20:466–469.

58. Pierard-Franchimont C, Letawe C, Nikkels AF, Pierard GE. Patterns of the immunohistochemical expression of melanoma-associated antigens and density of CD45R0+ activated T-lymphocytes and L1-protein–positive macrophages in primary cutaneous melanomas. Int J Mol Med 1998;2:721–724.

59. Fetsch PA, Marincola FM, Filie A, et al. Melanoma-associated antigen recognized by T-cells (MART-1): The advent of a preferred immunocytochemical antibody for the diagnosis of metastatic malignant melanoma with fine needle aspiration. Cancer 1999;87:37–42.

60. Busam KJ, Jungbluth AA. Melan-A, a new melanocytic differentiation marker. Adv Anat Pathol 1999;6:12–18.

61. Orosz Z. Melan-A/MART-1 expression in various melanocytic lesions and in non-melanocytic soft tissue tumors. Histopathology 1999;34:517–525.

62. Yu LL, Flotte TJ, Tanabe KK, et al. Detection of microscopic melanoma metastases in sentinel lymph nodes. Cancer 1999;86:617–627.

63. Anichini A, Molla A, Mortarini R, et al. An expanded peripheral T-cell population to a cytotoxic T-lymphocyte (CTL)-defined, melanocyte-specific antigen in metastatic melanoma patients impacts on generation of peptide-specific CTLs but does not overcome tumor escape from immune surveillance in metastatic lesions. J Exp Med 1999;190:651–667.

64. Bergman R, Azzam H, Sprecher E, et al. A comparative immunohistochemical study of MART-1 expression in Spitz nevi, ordinary melanocytic nevi, and malignant melanomas. J Am Acad Dermatol 2000;42:496–500.

65. Heegaard S, Jensen OA, Prause JU. Immunohistochemical diagnosis of malignant melanoma of the conjunctiva and uvea: Comparison of the novel antibody against melan-A with S100 protein and HMB-45. Melanoma Res 2000;10:350–354.

66. Adema GJ, deBoer AJ, VantHullenaar R, et al. Melanocyte lineage-specific antigens recognized by monoclonal antibodies NKI-beteb, HMB-50, and HMB-45 are encoded by a single cDNA. Am J Pathol 1993;143:1579–1585.

67. Chiamenti AM, Vella F, Bonetti F, et al. Anti-melanoma monoclonal antibody HMB-45 on enhanced chemiluminescence-Western blotting recognizes a 30–35 kDa melanosome-associated sialated glycoprotein. Melanoma Res 1996;6:291–298.

68. Esclamado RM, Gown AM, Vogen AM. Unique proteins defined by monoclonal antibodies specific for human melanoma. Am J Surg 1986;152:376–385.

69. Gown AM, Vogel AM, Hoak DH, et al. Monoclonal antibodies specific for melanocytic tumors distinguish subpopulations of melanocytes. Am J Pathol 1986;123:195–203.

70. Schaumburg-Lever G, Metzler G, Kaiserling E. Ultrastructural localization of HMB-45 binding sites. J Cutan Pathol 1991;18:432–435.

71. Palazzo JP, Duray PH. Congenital agminated Spitz nevi: Immunoreactivity with a melanoma-associated monoclonal antibody. J Cutan Pathol 1988;15:166–170.

72. Smoller BR, McNutt NS, Hsu A. HMB-45 staining of dysplastic nevi: Support for a spectrum of progression toward melanoma. Am J Surg Pathol 1989;13:680–684.

73. Skelton HG III, Smith KJ, Barrett TL, et al. HMB-45 staining in benign and malignant melanocytic lesions: A reflection of cellular activation. Am J Dermatopathol 1991;131:543–550.

74. Wick MR. HMB-45: A clue to the biology of malignant melanoma? J Cutan Pathol 1991;18:307–308.

75. Smoller BR, Hsu A, Krueger J. HMB-45 monoclonal antibody recognizes an inducible and reversible melanocyte cytoplasmic protein. J Cutan Pathol 1991;18:315–322.

76. Wick MR, Swanson PE, Rocamora A. Recognition of malignant melanoma by monoclonal antibody HMB-45: An immunohistochemical study of 200 paraffin-embedded cutaneous tumors. J Cutan Pathol 1988;15:201–207.

77. Blessing K, Sanders DS, Grant JJ. Comparison of immunohistochemical staining of the novel antibody melan-A with S100 protein and HMB-45 in malignant melanoma and melanoma variants. Histopathology 1998;32:139–146.

78. Vogel AM, Esclamado RM. Identification of a secreted Mr 95,000 glycoprotein in human melanocytes and melanomas by a melanocyte specific monoclonal antibody. Cancer Res 1988;48:1286–1294.

79. Kim RY, Wistow GJ. The cDNA RPE1 and monoclonal antibody HMB-50 define gene products preferentially expressed in retinal pigment epithelium. Exp Eye Res 1992; 55:657–662.

80. Bar H, Schlote W. Malignant melanoma in the CNS: Subtyping and immunocytochemistry. Clin Neuropathol 1997; 16:337–345.

81. Barrett AW, Bennett JH, Speight PM: A clinicopathological and immunohistochemical analysis of primary oral mucosal melanoma. Eur J Cancer B Oral Oncol 1995;31B:100–105.

82. Fernando SS, Johnson S, Bate J. Immunohistochemical analysis of cutaneous malignant melanoma: Comparison of S100 protein, HMB-45 monoclonal antibody, and NKI/C3 monoclonal antibody. Pathology 1994;26:16–19.

83. Bishop PW, Menasce LP, Yates AJ, et al. An immunophenotypic survey of malignant melanomas. Histopathology 1993;23:159–166.

84. Mackie RM, Campbell I, Turbitt M. Use of NKI/C3 monoclonal antibody in the assessment of benign and malignant melanocytic lesions. J Clin Pathol 1984;37:367–372.

85. Friedman HD, Tatum AH. HMB-45 positive malignant lymphoma: A case report with literature review of aberrant HMB-45 reactivity. Arch Pathol Lab Med 1991;115:826–830.

86. Hancock C, Allen BC, Herrera GA. HMB-45 detection in adenocarcinomas. Arch Pathol Lab Med 1991;115:886–890.

87. Unger PD, Hoffman K, Thung SN, et al. HMB-45 reactivity in adrenal pheochromocytomas. Arch Pathol Lab Med 1992;116:151–153.

88. Zimmer CM, Gottschalk J, Goebel S, Cerros-Navarro J. Melanoma-associated antigens in tumors of the nervous system: An immunohistochemical study with the monoclonal antibody HMB-45. Virchows Arch A 1992;420:121–126.

89. Eble JN, Amin MB, Young RH. Epithelioid angiomyolipoma of the kidney: A report of five cases with prominent and diagnostically confusing epithelioid smooth muscle component. Am J Surg Pathol 1997;21:1123–1130.

90. Fetsch PA, Fetsch JF, Marincola FM, et al. Comparison of melanoma antigen recognized by T-cells (MART-1) to HMB-45: Additional evidence to support a common lineage for angiomyolipoma, lymphangiomyomatosis, and clear cell sugar tumor. Mod Pathol 1998;11:699–703.

91. Ribalta T, Lloreta J, Munne A, et al. Malignant pigmented clear cell epithelioid tumor of the kidney: Clear cell ("sugar") tumor versus malignant melanoma. Hum Pathol 2000;31:516–519.

92. Zamboni G, Pea M, Martignoni G, et al. Clear cell "sugar" tumor of the pancreas: A novel member of the family of lesions characterized by the presence of perivascular epithelioid cells. Am J Surg Pathol 1996;20:722–730.

93. Bonetti F, Pea M, Martignoni G, et al. Clear cell ("sugar") tumor of the lung is a lesion strictly related to angiomyolipoma—the concept of a family of lesions characterized by the presence of the perivascular epithelioid cells (PEC). Pathology 1994;26:230–236.

94. Tanaka Y, Ijiri R, Kato K, et al. HMB-45/melan-A and

95. smooth muscle actin-positive clear-cell epithelioid tumor arising in the ligamentum teres hepatis: Additional example of clear-cell "sugar" tumors. Am J Surg Pathol 2000;24:1295–1299.

95. Gaffey MJ, Mills SE, Zarbo RJ, et al. Clear cell tumor of the lung: Immunohistochemical and ultrastructural evidence of melanogenesis. Am J Surg Pathol 1991;15:644–653.

96. Busam KJ, Iversen K, Coplan KA, et al. Immunoreactivity for A103, an antibody to melan-A (MART-1) in adrenocortical and other steroid tumors. Am J Surg Pathol 1998;22:57–63.

97. Lerner AB, Fitzpatrick TB. Biochemistry of melanin formation. Physiol Rev 1950;30:91–126.

98. Fitzpatrick TB, Miyomato M, Iskikawa K. The evolution of concepts of melanin biology. Arch Dermatol 1967;96:305–323.

99. Pellegrino D, Bellina CR, Manca G, et al. Detection of melanoma cells in peripheral blood and sentinel lymph nodes by RT-PCR analysis: A comparative study with immunohistochemistry. Tumori 2000;86:336–338.

100. Orchard GE. Comparison of immunohistochemical labeling of melanocyte differentiation antibodies melan-A, tyrosinase, and HMB-45 with NKI/C3 and S100 protein in the evaluation of benign nevi and malignant melanoma. Histochem J 2000;32:475–481.

101. Jungbluth AA, Iversen K, Coplan K, et al. T311—an anti-tyrosinase monoclonal antibody for the detection of melanocytic lesions in paraffin embedded tissues. Pathol Res Pract 2000;196:235–242.

102. DeVries TJ, Trancikova D, Ruiter DJ, van Muijen GN. High expression of immunotherapy candidate proteins gp100, MART-1, tyrosinase, and TRP-1 in uveal melanoma. Br J Cancer 1998;78:1156–1161.

103. Kaufmann O, Koch S, Burghardt J, et al. Tyrosinase, melan-A, and KBA62 as markers for the immunohistochemical identification of metastatic amelanotic melanomas on paraffin sections. Mod Pathol 1998;11:740–746.

104. Blaheta HJ, Schittek B, Breuninger H, et al. Lymph node micrometastases of cutaneous melanoma: Increased sensitivity of molecular diagnosis in comparison to immunohistochemistry. Int J Cancer 1998;79:318–323.

105. Cormier JN, Abati A, Fetsch P, et al. Comparative analysis of the in vivo expression of tyrosinase, MART-1/Melan-A, and gp100 in metastatic melanoma lesions: Implications for immunotherapy. J Immunother 1998;21:27–31.

106. Sato N, Suzuki S, Takimoto H, et al. Monoclonal antibody MAT-1 against human tyrosinase can detect melanogenic cells on formalin-fixed paraffin-embedded sections. Pigment Cell Res 1996;9:72–76.

107. Takimoto H, Suzuki S, Masui S, et al. MAT-1, a monoclonal antibody that specifically recognizes human tyrosinase. J Invest Dermatol 1995;105:764–768.

108. Chen YT, Stockert E, Tsang S, et al. Immunophenotyping of melanomas for tyrosinase: Implications for vaccine development. Proc Natl Acad Sci U S A 1995;92:8125–8129.

109. Clarkson KS, Sturdgess IC, Molyneux AJ. The usefulness of tyrosinase in the immunohistochemical assessment of melanocytic lesions: Comparison of the novel T311 antibody (anti-tyrosinase) with S100, HMB-45, and A103 (MART-1; melan-A). J Clin Pathol 2001;54:196–200.

110. Takeda K, Yasumoto K, Takada R, et al. Induction of melanocyte-specific microphthalmia-associated transcription factor by Wnt-3a. J Biol Chem 2000;275:14013–14016.

111. Vachtenheim J, Novotna H. Expression of genes for microphthalmia isoforms, Pax3 and MSG1, in human melanomas. Cell Mol Biol 1999;45:1075–1082.

112. Galibert MD, Yavuzer U, Dexter TJ, Goding CR. Pax3 and regulation of the melanocyte-specific tyrosinase-related protein-1 promoter. J Biol Chem 1999;274:26894–26900.

113. Verastegui C, Bertolotto C, Bille K, et al. TFE3, a transcription factor homologous to microphthalmia, is a potential transcriptional activator of tyrosinase and TyrpI genes. Mol Endocrinol 2000;14:449–456.

114. Koch MB, Shih IM, Weiss SW, Folpe AL. Microphthalmia

transcription factor and melanoma cell adhesion molecule expression distinguish desmoplastic/spindle-cell melanoma from morphologic mimics. Am J Surg Pathol 2001; 25:58–64.

115. King R, Googe PB, Weilbaecher KN, et al. Microphthalmia transcription factor expression in cutaneous benign and malignant melanocytic, and nonmelanocytic tumors. Am J Surg Pathol 2001;25:51–57.

116. King R, Weilbaecher KN, McGill G, et al. Microphthalmia transcription factor: A sensitive and specific melanocyte marker for melanoma diagnosis. Am J Pathol 1999;155: 731–738.

117. Miettinen M, Fernandez M, Franssila K, et al. Microphthalmia transcription factor in the immunohistochemical diagnosis of metastatic melanoma: Comparison with four other melanoma markers. Am J Surg Pathol 2001;25:205–211.

118. Zavala-Pompa A, Folpe AL, Jimenez RE, et al. Immunohistochemical study of microphthalmia transcription factor and tyrosinase in angiomyolipoma of the kidney, renal cell carcinoma, and retroperitoneal sarcomas: Comparative evaluation with traditional diagnostic markers. Am J Surg Pathol 2001;25:65–70.

119. Folpe AL, Goodman ZD, Ishak KG, et al. Clear cell myomelanocytic tumor of the faciform ligament/ligamentum teres: A novel member of the perivascular epithelioid cell cell family of tumors with a predilection for children and young adults. Am J Surg Pathol 2000;24:1239–1246.

120. Wick MR, Stanley SJ, Swanson PE. Immunohistochemical diagnosis of sinonasal melanoma, carcinoma, and neuroblastoma with monoclonal antibodies HMB-45 and anti-synaptophysin. Arch Pathol Lab Med 1988;112:616–620.

121. Franquemont DW, Mills SE. Sinonasal malignant melanoma: A clinicopathologic and immunohistochemical study of 14 cases. Am J Clin Pathol 1991;96:689–697.

122. Wiedenmann B, Franke WW, Kuhn C, et al. Synaptophysin: A marker protein for neuroendocrine cells and neoplasms. Proc Natl Acad Sci U S A 1986;83:3500–3504.

123. Lloyd RV, Wilson BS. Specific endocrine tissue marker defined by a monoclonal antibody. Science 1983;222:628–630.

124. Kontochristopoulos GJ, Stavropoulos PG, Krasagakis K, et al. Differentiation between Merkel cell carcinoma and malignant melanoma: An immunohistochemical study. Dermatology 2000;201:123–126.

125. Klemm KM, Moran CA, Suster S. Pigmented thymic carcinoids: A clinicopathological and immunohistochemical study of two cases. Mod Pathol 1999;12:946–948.

126. Gal AA, Koss MN, Hochholzer L, et al. Pigmented pulmonary carcinoid tumor: An immunohistochemical and ultrastructural study. Arch Pathol Lab Med 1993;117:832–836.

127. Moran CA, Albores-Saavedra J, Wenig BM, Mena H. Pigmented extraadrenal paragangliomas: A clinicopathologic and immunohistochemical study of five cases. Cancer 1997;79:398–402.

128. Pettinato G, Manivel JC, d'Amore ESG, et al. Melanotic neuroectodermal tumor of infancy: A reexamination of a histogenetic problem based on immunohistochemical, flow cytometric, and ultrastructural study of 10 cases. Am J Surg Pathol 1991;15:233–245.

129. Kapadia SB, Frisman DM, Hitchcock CL, et al. Melanotic neuroectodermal tumor of infancy: Clinicopathological, immunohistochemical, and flow cytometric study. Am J Surg Pathol 1993;17:566–573.

130. Mennemeyer RP, Hallman KO, Hammar SP, et al. Melanotic schwannoma: Clinical and ultrastructural studies of three cases with evidence of intracellular melanin synthesis. Am J Surg Pathol 1979;3:3–10.

131. Orchard GE, Wilson-Jones E. Immunocytochemistry in the diagnosis of malignant melanoma. Br J Biomed Sci 1994; 51:44–56.

132. Springall DR, Gu J, Cocchia D, et al. The value of S100 immunostaining as a diagnostic tool in human malignant melanomas: A comparison using S100 and neuron-specific enolase antibodies. Virchows Arch A 1983;400:331–343.

133. Dhillon AP, Rode J, Leathem A. Neuron-specific enolase: An aid to the diagnosis of melanoma and neuroblastoma. Histopathology 1982;6:81–92.

134. Reed JA, Finnerty B, Albino AP. Divergent cellular differentiation pathways during the invasive stage of cutaneous malignant melanoma progression. Am J Pathol 1999;155: 549–555.

135. Sangueza OP, Requena L. Neoplasms with neural differentiation: A review. Part II: Malignant neoplasms. Am J Dermatopathol 1998;20:89–102.

136. Mooy CM, Luyten GP, DeJong PT, et al. Neural cell adhesion molecule distribution in primary and metastatic uveal melanomas. Hum Pathol 1995;26:1185–1190.

137. Wick MR. Prognostic factors for cutaneous melanoma. Am J Clin Pathol 1998;110:713–718.

138. Moretti S, Spallanzani A, Chiarugi A, et al. Correlation of Ki-67 expression in cutaneous primary melanoma with prognosis in a prospective study: Different correlation according to thickness. J Am Acad Dermatol 2001;44:188–192.

139. Florenes VA, Faye RS, Maelandsmo GM, et al. Levels of cyclin D1 and D3 in malignant melanoma: Deregulated cyclin expression is associated with poor clinical outcome in superficial melanomas. Clin Cancer Res 2000;6:3614–3620.

140. Straume O, Sviland L, Akslen LA. Loss of nuclear p16 protein expression correlates with increased tumor proliferation (Ki-67) and poor prognosis in patients with vertical growth phase melanoma. Clin Cancer Res 2000;6:1845–1853.

141. Kaleem Z, Lind AC, Humphrey PA, et al. Concurrent Ki-67 and p53 immunolabeling in cutaneous melanocytic neoplasms: An adjunct for recognition of the vertical growth phase in malignant melanomas? Mod Pathol 2000;13:217–222.

142. Henrique R, Azevedo R, Bento MJ, et al. Prognostic value of Ki-67 expression in localized cutaneous malignant melanoma. J Am Acad Dermatol 2000;43:991–1000.

143. Graham CH, Rivers J, Kerbel RS, et al. Extent of vascularization as a prognostic indicator in thin (<0.76 mm) malignant melanomas. Am J Pathol 1994;145:510–514.

144. Vlaykova T, Talve L, Hahka-Kemppinen M, et al. MIB-1 immunoreactivity correlates with blood vessel density and survival in disseminated malignant melanoma. Oncology 1999;57:242–252.

145. Kerbel RS, Kobayashi H, Graham CH, Lu C. Analysis and significance of the malignant "eclipse" during the progression of primary cutaneous human melanomas. J Invest Dermatol Symp Proc 1996;1:183–187.

146. Gutman M, Singh RK, Radinsky R, Bar-Eli M. Intertumoral heterogeneity of receptor-tyrosinase kinase expression in human melanoma cell lines with metastatic capabilities. Anticancer Res 1994;14:1759–1765.

147. Elder D. Tumor progression, early diagnosis, and prognosis of melanoma. Acta Oncol 1999;38:535–547.

148. Nagasaka T, Lai R, Medeiros LJ, et al. Cyclin D1 overexpression in Spitz nevi: an immunohistochemical study. Am J Dermatopathol 1999;21:115–120.

149. Kanter-Lewensohn L, Hedblad MA, Wedje J, Larsson O. Immunohistochemical markers for distinguishing Spitz nevi from malignant melanomas. Mod Pathol 1997;10:917–920.

150. Bergman R, Shemer A, Levy R, et al. Immunohistochemical study of p53 protein expression in Spitz nevi as compared with other melanocytic tumors. Am J Dermatopathol 1995;17:547–550.

151. Penneys NS, Seigfried E, Nahass G, Vogler C. Expression of proliferating cell nuclear antigen in Spitz nevus. J Am Acad Dermatol 1995;32:964–967.

152. Takahashi H, Maeda K, Maeda K, et al. Immunohistochemical characterization of Spitz's nevus: Differentiation from common melanocytic nevi, dysplastic melanocytic nevus, and malignant melanoma. J Dermatol 1987;14:533–541.

153. Glusac EJ, McNiff JM. Epithelioid cell histiocytoma: A si-

mulant of vascular and melanocytic neoplasms. Am J Dermatopathol 1999;21:1–7.

154. Busam KJ, Granter SR, Iversen K, Jungbluth AA. Immunohistochemical distinction of epithelioid histiocytic proliferations from epithelioid melanocytic nevi. Am J Dermatopathol 2000;22:237–241.

155. Busam KJ, Rosai J, Iversen K, Jungbluth AA. Xanthogranulomas with inconspicuous foam cells and giant cells mimicking malignant melanoma: A clinical, histologic, and immunohistochemical study of three cases. Am J Surg Pathol 2000;24:864–869.

156. Ma CK, Zarbo RJ, Gown AM. Immunohistochemical characterization of atypical fibroxanthoma and dermatofibrosarcoma protuberans. Am J Clin Pathol 1992;97:478–483.

157. Diaz-Cascajo C, Borghi S, Bonczkowitz M. Pigmented atypical fibroxanthoma. Histopathology 1998;33:537–541.

158. Gloghini A, Rizzo A, Zanette I, et al. KP1/CD68 expression in malignant neoplasms including lymphomas, sarcomas, and carcinomas. Am J Clin Pathol 1995;103:425–431.

159. Suster S. Tumors of the skin composed of large cells with abundant eosinophilic cytoplasm. Semin Diagn Pathol 1999;16:162–177.

160. Borek BT, McKee PH, Freeman JA, et al. Primary malignant melanoma with rhabdoid features: A histologic and immunocytochemical study of two cases. Am J Dermatopathol 1998;20:123–127.

161. Laskin WB, Knittel DR, Frame JN. S100 protein and HMB-45-negative "rhabdoid" malignant melanoma: A totally dedifferentiated malignant melanoma? Am J Clin Pathol 1995;103:772–773.

162. Anstey A, Cerio R, Ramnarain N, et al. Desmoplastic malignant melanoma: An immunocytochemical study of 25 cases. Am J Dermatopathol 1994;16:14–22.

163. Gatter KC, Alcock K, Heryet A, et al. The differential diagnosis of routinely processed anaplastic tumors using monoclonal antibodies. Am J Clin Pathol 1984;82:33–43.

164. Strickler JG, Michie SA, Warnke RA, Dorfman RF. The "syncytial" variant of nodular sclerosing Hodgkin's disease. Am J Surg Pathol 1986;10:470–477.

165. Ritter JH, Mills SE, Gaffey MJ, et al. Clear cell tumors of the alimentary tract and abdominal cavity. Semin Diagn Pathol 1997;14:213–219.

166. Ordonez NG. Role of immunohistochemistry in differentiating epithelial mesothelioma from adenocarcinoma. Am J Clin Pathol 1999;112:75–89.

167. Mizutani H, Ohyanagi S, Hayashi T, et al. Functional thrombomodulin expression on epithelial skin tumors as a differentiation marker for suprabasal keratinocytes. Br J Dermatol 1996;135:187–193.

168. Battifora H, Silva EG. The use of antikeratin antibodies in the immunohistochemical distinction between neuroendocrine (Merkel cell) carcinoma of the skin, lymphoma, and oat cell carcinoma. Cancer 1986;58:1040–1046.

169. Clark HB. Immunohistochemistry of nervous system antigens: Diagnostic applications in surgical neuropathology. Semin Diagn Pathol 1984;1:309–316.

170. Zimmer C, Gottschalk J, Goebel S, Cervos-Navarro J. Melanoma-associated antigens in tumors of the nervous system: An immunohistochemical study with monoclonal antibody HMB-45. Virchows Arch A 1992;420:121–126.

171. Gottschalk J, Jautzke G, Schreiner C. Epithelial and melanoma antigens in gliosarcoma: An immunohistochemical study. Pathol Res Pract 1992;188:182–190.

172. Lodding P, Kindblom LG, Angervall L. Metastases of malignant melanoma simulating soft tissue sarcoma: A clinicopathological, light- and electron microscopic and immunohistochemical study of 21 cases. Virchows Arch A 1990; 417:377–388.

173. Banerjee SS, Coyne JD, Menasce LP, et al. Diagnostic lessons of mucosal melanoma with osteocartilaginous differentiation. Histopathology 1998;33:255–260.

174. Swanson PE, Wick MR. Clear cell sarcoma: An immunohistochemical analysis of six cases and comparison with other epithelioid neoplasms of soft tissue. Arch Pathol Lab Med 1989;113:55–60.

175. Mechtersheimer G, Tilgen W, Klar E, Moller P. Clear cell sarcoma of tendons and aponeuroses: Case presentation with special reference to immunohistochemical findings. Hum Pathol 1989;20:914–917.

176. Almeida MM, Nunes AM, Frable WJ. Malignant melanoma of soft tissue: A report of three cases with diagnosis by fine needle aspiration cytology. Acta Cytol 1994;38:241–246.

177. Stenman G, Kindblom LG, Angervall L. Reciprocal translocation t(12;22)(q13;q13) in clear-cell sarcoma of tendons and aponeuroses. Genes Chromosomes Cancer 1992;4:122–127.

178. Langezaal SM, Graadt van Roggen JF, Gleton-Jansen AM, et al. Malignant melanoma is genetically distinct from clear cell sarcoma of tendons and aponeuroses (malignant melanoma of soft parts). Br J Cancer 2001;84:535–538.

179. Folpe AL, Hill CE, Parham DM, et al. Immunohistochemical detection of FLI-1 protein expression: A study of 132 round cell tumors with emphasis on mimics of Ewing's sarcoma/primitive neuroectodermal tumor. Am J Surg Pathol 2000;24:1657–1662.

180. Winters JL, Geil JD, O'Connor WN. Immunohistology, cytogenetics, and molecular studies of small round cell tumors of childhood: A review. Ann Clin Lab Sci 1995;25: 66–78.

181. Swanson PE, Scheithauer BW, Wick MR. Peripheral nerve sheath neoplasms: Clinicopathologic and immunochemical observations. Pathol Annu 1995;30(Pt 2):1–82.

182. Wick MR. Malignant peripheral nerve sheath tumors of the skin. Mayo Clin Proc 1990;65:279–282.

CHAPTER 7

Carcinomatous Differentiation and Metastatic Carcinoma of Unknown Primary

David J. Dabbs, M.D.

Despite the number of years that immunohisto-chemistry (IHC) has been practiced in the discipline of surgical pathology, it remains an imperfect science. Surely, the technology, detection systems, and quality assurance procedures have advanced tremendously, but a paucity of specific antibodies remain that allow for "100% unequivocal, definitive diagnosis" in every case. Indeed, it has been said that "it may be dangerous to base any distinction in tumor pathology primarily on the basis of the pattern of immunoreactivity of a given marker, no matter how specific it is purported to be."[1] This statement echoes the philosophy of the standard of practice in surgical pathology in that morphology is the basis of diagnosis in surgical pathology and IHC is a powerful ancillary technique used to obtain more information from the paraffin section.

Even the most specific antibodies (e.g., thyroglobulin and prostate-specific antigen [PSA]) are not entirely site-specific, and we therefore resort to panels of antibodies that give statistical power to our morphologic diagnoses. Relevant diagnostic immunopanels change rapidly based on information from immunohistochemical studies, and we can expect this constant infusion of new data on antibody sensitivity and specificity to impart an uncomfortable state of chronic flux on the discipline of IHC.

METASTATIC CARCINOMA OF UNKNOWN PRIMARY

The task of the pathologist is to diagnose neoplasms correctly so that appropriate therapies can be planned for the patient. This task is complicated by the fact that neoplasms demonstrate a wide variety of tissue patterns, along with different details of cellular morphology.

In surgical pathology and cytopathology, the starting point for diagnostic interpretation is to categorize a neoplasm as a carcinoma, germ cell tumor, sarcoma, lymphoma, or melanoma. For the IHC approach, the starting point becomes an exer-cise in choosing the appropriate antibodies to identify the neoplasm correctly based on cell lines of differentiation. Once the tumor is identified as one of these major categories, further information about the cellular differentiation may be obtained from specific cellular defining maturation markers or tissue-based specific markers, such as differential cytokeratin (CK) staining, hematopoietic specific markers, and so on. In addition, specific cell products may be identified (e.g., neuroendocrine granules), one may identify a battery of expression of maturation markers (e.g., L26 and CD43 coexpression in small cell lymphomas), or the expression of oncofetal antigens may be demonstrated. For a combined IHC-ultrastructural approach to diagnosis, the reader is referred to a review on the subject by Hammar.[2]

This approach to immunohistochemical diagnosis is used for the patient who presents with a metastasis of unknown primary (MUP). By definition, there is no obvious primary neoplastic site giving rise to the clinical metastasis, despite a careful clinical history, physical examination, radiologic imaging, and biochemical or histologic investigations. Patients with MUP account for 5 to 15% of all patients with malignancy.[1, 3–6]

The economic considerations of clinical work-up in these patients has not been extensively studied.

There are little data available on the cost-effectiveness of IHC in surgical pathology. Putti and colleagues, in a retrospective study of 186 cases, observed that IHC was essential for the definitive diagnosis of an undifferentiated neoplasm in 18% of cases, was used to support a diagnosis in 40% of cases, and was used for prognostic information in the remainder of cases.[7] Schapira and Jerrett[6] analyzed the clinical work-ups in a group of 199 patients and concluded that the search for a primary neoplasm incurred an average cost of $17,973, with only 19.6% of patients surviving for more than 1 year. Raab (see Chapter 2) believes that IHC may be used for prognostic purposes or to derive a more accurate diagnosis by which to guide therapy. Using several different models,

Raab concludes that IHC is probably undervalued and is a cost-effective maneuver in the study of tumors.

Radiologic studies themselves have limited value in the management of these patients, and prognosis is not affected.[8, 9] Even autopsies on some of these patients may not detect the primary site of tumor because of small size, extensive dissemination, or regression due to therapy.[10]

In 1988, Le-Chevalier and coworkers studied 302 autopsy specimens from patients who presented with MUP.[11] The primary tumor site was located premortem in 27% of patients, at autopsy in 50% of patients, and remained unidentified in 16% of patients.[11] The most common primary tumor sites in this study included pancreas, lung, kidney, and colon-rectum, a list that includes the two malignancies with the highest incidence in both men and women. Only the number of metastases present in the patients was a prognostic factor, and survival was not related to the premortem discovery of the primary tumor site.[11]

Kirsten and colleagues studied 286 patients with MUP and concluded that the factors that predicted survival were lymph node presentation, good performance status, and body weight loss of less than 10%.[12] Using a panel of antibodies to determine differentiation of tumors in 41 patients with MUP, van der Gaast and associates,[13] concluded that the immunohistochemical panel approach to uncover tumor origin is useful for selecting appropriate treatment of patients, especially those who may benefit from combination chemotherapy.[14]

Others have found that the histologic features of a poorly differentiated carcinoma have no influence on survival.[15] The immunohistochemical studies of MUP have elucidated the origin of tumors in as little as 5% to as many as 70% of patients.[16] Most investigators arrived at the same conclusion: For individual patient therapy, the discovery of the tumor origin is welcome and may be therapeutically useful.

The appropriate work-up for identifying a primary tumor depends on the patient's clinical symptoms, age, history, sex, and the likelihood of finding the primary tumor. The clinician must also take into account the economics of an extensive clinical work-up, as well as the inconvenience or discomfort to which the patient is subjected.[17] Patients with MUP do poorly as a group, and the importance of establishing the diagnosis of the tumor rests with the interventions of hormonal manipulation, chemotherapy, and radiation.[18]

The current clinical approach is an attempt to identify favorable prognostic groups in patients with unknown primary tumors so that they can be managed appropriately.[3, 19–22] This group of tumors includes leukemia-lymphoma, germ cell tumors, small cell carcinoma of the lung, and carcinomas of the breast, ovary, endometrium, and adrenal, thyroid, and prostate glands.[12, 23, 24] When possible,

it is useful to separate regional from distant metastases, because localized disease is more amenable to treatment.[4, 25] Other favorable clinical features that have been described include location of tumor in the retroperitoneum or peripheral lymph nodes, tumor limited to one or two metastatic sites, a negative smoking history, and young age.[4]

The majority of MUPs in adults are adenocarcinomas and undifferentiated carcinomas, but the relative numbers of each differ depending on age and sex.[26, 27]

Huebner and colleagues, in a series of 343 patients, found that 40% had adenocarcinoma, 28% had undifferentiated carcinoma, 14% had squamous cell carcinoma, 3% had small cell carcinoma, and the remainder had poorly defined tumors.[28] Patients with visceral metastasis of carcinoma below the diaphragm did poorly and responded poorly to chemotherapy.[29]

In some studies, adenocarcinomas have accounted for 48 to 60% of carcinomas of unknown primary site.[2, 5, 30, 31] For patients who present with primary lymph node metastases, there may be clues to the primary site of the tumor based on the anatomic site of lymph node involvement.

For the patient who presents with metastatic adenocarcinoma in the neck, the metastatic work-up will probably begin in the lung (males) or breast (females), although gastrointestinal and prostate adenocarcinomas both show a predilection for the left side of the neck.[32, 33]

Undifferentiated carcinomas of the head and neck are the most common primary source for metastatic tumors in head and neck lymph nodes,[5] and the majority of these are of squamous mucosal derivation. The prognosis for this group of patients rests largely on the nodal status, with patients having stage N3 lesions carrying a poor prognosis.[34]

In women presenting with adenocarcinomas in the axillae, the primary tumors are most often found in the ipsilateral breast.[35] In women who present with malignant abdominal effusions, common abdominal sites include ovaries, endometrium, and cervix, whereas men with malignant abdominal effusions typically have primary tumor sites in the gastrointestinal tract, predominantly in the colon, rectum, or stomach.[36] For pleural effusions, the breast is the most common primary site for women, with the lung being the most common site for a primary tumor in men. Malignant lymphomas are seen in both sexes.[37] Metastatic carcinomas in inguinal lymph nodes likely represent metastases from the lower extremities if located in the femoral triangle lymph nodes or metastases from the anorectal-gynecologic organs if the metastatic lesions are in the medial femoral lymph nodes.[5]

Patients presenting with skeletal metastases often have primary carcinomas in the lung, breast, kidney, or urogenital region, and imaging studies have been particularly useful in elucidating the primary tumor.[38]

The liver is one of the single largest repositories for metastatic malignancies of all types, especially for carcinomas. The most common malignancies metastatic to the liver are from the gastrointestinal tract, with colorectal carcinomas leading this group. Lung and breast carcinomas also commonly metastasize to the liver, as do pancreaticobiliary carcinomas. This entire group of adenocarcinomas may appear similar to primary cholangiocarcinoma of the liver and may simulate some hepatocellular carcinomas, particularly the less-differentiated hepatocellular carcinomas. Prostate carcinoma, although unusual, does metastasize to the liver and can be confused with cholangiocarcinoma. Thus, for hepatic metastases of unknown primary in women, colorectal, breast, and lung carcinomas are of primary consideration, whereas in men, colorectal, lung, and prostate carcinomas top the list. Malignant melanoma metastatic to the liver is not uncommon, with the highest frequency of liver metastases seen with primary eye melanomas.[4]

Pisharodi and associates,[39] in a fine needle biopsy study of 200 malignant aspirates of the liver, found that 32% were hepatocellular carcinomas, 49.5% were readily diagnosed as metastatic carcinomas, and 18.5% were problematic. Of this latter group, immunocytochemistry contributed to definitive diagnosis in half the cases.

In the brain, differentiating metastatic adenocarcinoma or poorly differentiated carcinoma from a glial tumor is straightforward, although determining the source of the metastasis may be problematic, especially when the occult primary is unknown.[40–43] Lung carcinomas are the most likely primary to be discovered subsequent to central nervous system (CNS) presentation, and other common primaries include breast, kidney, thyroid, and gastrointestinal tract.[40–44] Patients with other adenocarcinomas, such as ovarian, prostatic, and pancreaticobiliary, rarely present with brain metastases, because there is almost always evidence of widespread dissemination of these tumors before the occurrence of cerebral metastasis. The survival of most patients with carcinomatous brain metastases is in the range of 3 to 11 months.[29, 45, 46] Along with the liver, the lung is a major repository for metastatic carcinomas, especially adenocarcinomas. Identification of the origin of an adenocarcinoma in the lung is a frequent, difficult, and challenging process for the surgical pathologist, because adenocarcinomas not only are the most frequent primary lung tumor but also are the most common metastatic tumor found in the lung. Distinction among these tumor types can be especially challenging on scant biopsy materials, such as transbronchial biopsy or fine needle aspiration biopsy (FNAB). It is important to identify those carcinomas that can be treated by chemotherapy or hormonal manipulation, or both, especially metastatic breast or prostate carcinomas.

THE PATHOLOGIST'S APPROACH TO THE STUDY OF THE UNKNOWN PRIMARY TUMOR

The goal of the surgical pathologist should be to identify metastatic carcinomas that are within the "treatable" group of tumors, namely, carcinomas of breast, prostate, ovary, and endometrium, thyroid and adrenal glands, and germ cell tumors and neuroendocrine carcinomas.[3] The response to cisplatin-based chemotherapy regimens for other carcinomas is less certain,[27] but the identity of the carcinoma, if available, is useful to determine more useful therapeutic regimens for these patients in a prospective manner.[3, 11, 18, 26]

Tissue procurement is the first step in the workup for tumors of unknown primary origin. It is common practice to obtain tissue by FNAB or core tissue biopsy. The sensitivity of FNAB for metastatic carcinoma in a series of 266 superficial lymph nodes was 96.5%, with no false-positive results and nine false-negative results.[47] Tissue from both FNAB and core biopsies can be triaged for ancillary studies in the same manner. There is also great value in the immunocytochemical study of malignant effusions, and often these are the first samples available by virtue of therapeutic evacuation.[48–54] Whatever the method of obtaining tissue, it is ideal to be able to monitor the process so that adequate tissue may be obtained to triage for the patient's problem appropriately, namely, division of the specimen for potential immunocytochemistry, electron microscopy, flow cytometry, and so on. Monitoring the tissue procurement process can be performed with frozen sections, immediate interpretation of FNAB, or tissue imprints. In addition to tissue procurement, the pathologist must define the problem by taking the patient's age, sex, known risk factors, duration of symptoms, and clinical and radiologic findings. Based on this information and the carcinomatous morphologic appearance of the tumor, the quest for the study of tumor origin begins.

In this chapter, the role of diagnostic IHC in diagnosing metastatic carcinoma of unknown primary is emphasized, especially as it occurs in the liver, lung, brain, and lymph nodes. The role of electron microscopic ultrastructure in combination with IHC for patients with MUP has been discussed.[2]

BIOLOGY OF THE CELLULAR ANTIGENS

Of the four main categories of malignant neoplasms, carcinomas compose the largest single group of metastatic tumors from unknown primary sites. Indeed, it is unusual for sarcomas to present as metastases of unknown primary origin, typically because sarcomas are usually bulky neoplasms that cause local symptoms before clinical metastases appear.

The simple and broad spectrum CKs are the initial antibodies of choice for detecting carcinomatous differentiation. More specific subcategorization of the tumor origin is then possible using a variety of site-specific CKs as well as antibodies directed against various cellular products. It is a combination of these cellular antigens that may yield a cost-effective approach to tumor categorization.

The approach to definitive diagnosis of the patient with MUP effectively follows five sequential steps:

1. Determine the cell line of differentiation—carcinoma, lymphoma, melanoma, sarcoma, or germ cell.
2. Determine the CK type or types of distribution in the tumor cells, since some subsets of CKs are unique to certain tumor types.
3. Determine if there is coexpression of vimentin.
4. Determine if there is expression of supplemental antigens of epithelial or germ cell derivation, that is, carcinoembryonic antigen (CEA), epithelial membrane antigen (EMA), or placental alkaline phosphatase (PLAP).
5. Determine if there is expression of cell-specific products, cell-specific structures, or receptors that are unique identifiers of cell types, for example, neuroendocrine granules, peptide hormones, thyroglobulin, PSA, prostate-specific membrane antigen, inhibin, gross cystic disease fluid protein (GCDFP), villin, uroplakins, or thyroid transcription factor-1 (TTF-1).

Cytokeratins: An Overview

The soft epithelial keratin intermediate filaments comprise approximately 20 different keratin polypeptides of the approximately 30 keratin polypeptides.[55-57] These polypeptides, numbered 1 through 20, comprise the type II (basic) keratins and the type I (acidic) keratins (Table 7–1). This family of intermediate filaments is crucial in diagnostic IHC for the identification of carcinomatous differentiation and for identification of specific carcinoma subtypes.

Keratin filaments are formed by tetrameric heteropolymers of two different keratins, two from type I and two from type II, to maintain cellular electrical neutrality. The vast majority of keratins are paired together as acidic and basic types, with rare exception. The classification and numbering system of the keratins is based on the catalog of Moll and associates.[58] The different keratins are identified by their biochemical properties, exemplified by two-dimensional polyacrylamide gel electrophoresis, which separates the filaments on

the basis of isoelectric point, and sodium dodecyl sulfate–polyacrylamide gel electrophoresis (SDS-PAGE), which separates the polypeptides on the basis of molecular weight. There are 12 keratins with more acidic isoelectric points that form type I (acidic) keratins and 8 keratins with more basic isoelectric points, the type II (basic-neutral) keratins.[59] The keratins are products of two gene families: Most genes for type II keratins are localized on chromosome 12 and the genes for type I keratins are localized on chromosome 17.[60-62] Within each group, the CKs are numbered consecutively, from highest to lowest molecular weight in each group. Most low molecular weight (LMW) keratins are typically found in all epithelia except squamous epithelium, whereas high molecular weight (HMW) keratins are typical of squamous epithelium.[58]

The original methods for identification of the different keratin types in tissues relied on tedious biochemical methods, chiefly performed by Franke and Moll and their associates.[58, 63] More recently, the problem of keratin subtyping has been expedited by the development of numerous monoclonal keratin-specific antibodies.[55, 57, 58, 64] This development was crucial for the ease of keratin subtyping that now seems so essential to the diagnostic surgical pathologist.

Distribution of Keratin Antigens in Tissues

SIMPLE EPITHELIAL KERATINS

Simple epithelial keratins are the first keratins to appear in embryonic development, as they are expressed in virtually all simple (nonstratified), ductal, and pseudostratified epithelial tissues.[57, 58] Since these keratins are widespread, they may be useful for the identification of epithelial differentiation. Almost all mesotheliomas and carcinomas,[57, 58] except squamous cell carcinomas, contain the simple keratins 8 and 18. A few visceral organs such as liver contain only keratins 8 and 18.

Although identified by many keratin antibodies that recognize a cocktail of keratin peptides (e.g., pankeratin antibodies AE1 and AE3 antibodies), CAM5.2 and 35βH11 recognize keratins 8 and 18 almost exclusively (Fig. 7–1). This group of antibodies is perhaps the most commonly used to demonstrate the simple keratins in surgical pathology. Since simple keratins are widely distributed in most carcinomas, these antibodies are particularly useful in the initial approach to investigation for carcinomatous differentiation (Table 7–2; see also Table 7–1).

Cytokeratin 19

The lowest molecular weight of the keratin group, CK19 is a simple keratin that has a distribu-

Table 7–1. The Most Common Soft Keratins and Their Distribution

Type II (Basic) Keratin			Type I (Acidic) Keratin	
	Molecular Weight (kd)	**Typical Distribution in Normal Tissues**		*Molecular Weight (kd)*
		Epidermis of palms and soles	CK9	64
CK1	67	Keratinizing squamous epidermis	CK10	56.5
CK2	65	Epithelia, all locations	CK11	56
CK3	63	Cornea	CK12	55
CK4	59	Nonkeratinizing squamous epithelia of internal organs	CK13	51
CK5	58	Basal cells of squamous and glandular epithelia, myoepithelia, mesothelium	CK14	50
		Squamous epithelia	CK15	50
CK6	56	Squamous epithelia, especially hyperproliferative	CK16	48
CK7	54	Simple epithelia	CK17	46
CK8	52	Basal cells of glandular epithelia, myoepithelia	CK18	45
		Simple epithelia		
		Simple epithelia, most glandular and some squamous epithelia (basal)	CK19	40
		Simple epithelia of intestines and stomach, Merkel cells	CK20	46

From Quinlan RA, Schiller DL, Hatzfeld M, et al. Patterns of expression and organization of cytokeratin intermediate filaments. Ann NY Acad Sci 1985;455:282–306.

tion similar to keratins 8 and 18 and is also present in the basal layer of the squamous epithelium of mucosal surfaces and may be seen in epidermal basal cells.[65] CK19 is a good screening marker for epithelial neoplasms because of its

wide distribution in simple epithelia and in many squamous tissues. The monoclonal antibody AE1 (Boehringer-Mannheim, Indianapolis, IN) reacts with CK19 as does the AE1/AE3 cocktail (Boehringer-Mannheim). Also reacting in formalin-fixed tis-

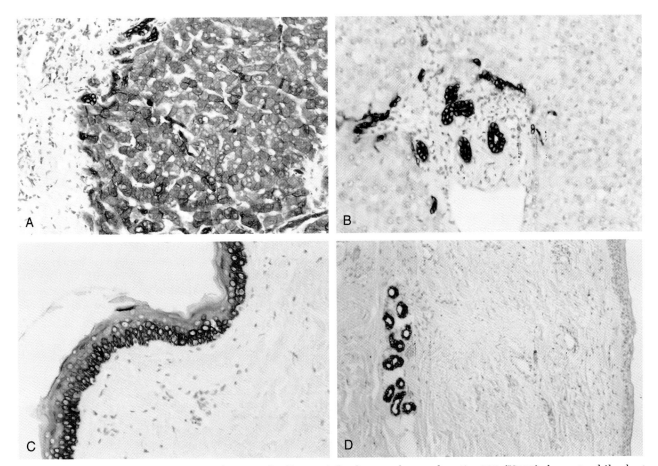

Figure 7–1. *A,* CAM5.2 decorates liver and adjacent bile ducts, whereas keratin 903 (K903) decorates bile ducts *(B)* and stratum corneum of skin *(C). D,* 35βH11 stains only eccrine coils and not epidermis.

Table 7–2. Keratin Antigens and Antibodies

CK Antigen	Antibody Clone	Notes
CK8	35βH11	Carcinomas of simple epithelium
CK8	CAM5.2	Carcinoma of simple epithelium
Pankeratin	AE1/AE3	Carcinomas of simple and complex epithelium
CK1/CK10	34β4	Squamous cell carcinoma
CK7	OV-TL 12/30	Nongastrointestinally derived carcinomas Rare cells in some gastrointestinal carcinomas
CK20	K20	Most gastrointestinal carcinomas; mucinous ovarian tumors; biliary, transitional, and Merkel cell carcinomas
CK19	RCK 108	Most carcinomas; many carcinomas with squamous component; myoepithelial cells
CK1/CK10/CK5/CK14	34βE12	Basal cells of prostate; most duct-derived carcinomas
CK18/CK19	PKK1	Most carcinomas
CK10/CK11/CK13/CK14/CK15/CK16/CK19	AE1	Most squamous lesions and many carcinomas
CK8/CK14/CK15/CK16/CK18/CK19	MAK-6	Most carcinomas

sues is a monoclonal antibody to CK19—RCK108 (DAKO, Carpinteria, CA).[66] CK19 is mostly negative, or rarely is seen focally in hepatoma.[66]

Cytokeratin 7

CK7 is a 54-kd type II simple keratin that has a restricted distribution compared with keratins 8 and 18.

Its presence in many simple, pseudostratified, and ductal epithelia and mesothelia is similar to the distribution of keratins 8 and 18. Much of the data in the literature on CK7 is based on the reactivity patterns of antibody OV-TL 12/30 (DAKO, Carpinteria, CA) in formalin-fixed paraffin-embedded tissues. The OV-TL 12/30 antibody parallels the CK7 immunoreactivity with RCK 105, an antibody for frozen sections[67, 68] (Table 7–3).

Predigestion with protease or heat-induced epitope retrieval (HIER) is required for OV-TL 12/30. The lack or extreme paucity of CK7 distribution in tissues such as colonic epithelium, hepatocytes, and prostatic acinar tissue is useful diagnostically.[67–70] This antibody identifies transitional cell epithelium but does not decorate squamous epithelium.[64] The restricted topography of CK7 makes it especially useful in evaluating the origin of adenocarcinomas, as this keratin is present in most breast,[64] lung,[64] ovarian,[71–77] pancreaticobiliary,[64] and transitional cell carcinomas,[64] but it is either absent or only decorates rare cells in colorectal and prostatic carcinomas[64, 67, 69, 70, 78, 79] (Tables 7–4 and 7–5, and Fig. 7–2). A diagnostic pitfall in the interpretation of CK7 immunostaining is that CK7 decorates subsets of endothelial cells of normal soft tissues, as well as endothelial cells in venules and lymphatics in intestinal mucosa, uterine exocervix, and lymphoid tissue.[80]

Diagnostic Utility of Cytokeratin 7. The specific diagnostic utility of CK7 lies in the fact that there are three dominant patterns of immunostaining:

1. Tumors that are characteristically strongly and diffusely positive include those of the lung, breast, ovary, endometrium, bladder, and thymus, as well as mesotheliomas, neuroendocrine tumors, pancreaticobiliary and parotid adenocarcinomas, and the fibrolamellar variant of hepatoma.[81]

2. Carcinomas that may immunostain a minority of cells include biliary, gastric, and colorectal tumors.

3. Carcinomas that are almost invariably negative but may occasionally show rare CK7-positive cells include hepatomas, duodenal ampulla carcinomas, colorectal carcinomas, and adrenal cortical tumors.

For diagnostic purposes, carcinomas that are metastatic in the lymph nodes, liver, or brain and immunostain strongly with CK7 may have origin in the lung, breast, ovary, endometrium, bladder, or neuroendocrine system. Strong diffuse CK7 immunostaining is a valuable marker in the diagnostic work-up of a carcinoma and may be used as a

Table 7–3. Cytokeratin Immunohistochemistry

Antigen	Clone	Method	Source
CK7	OV-TL 12/30	A, B	Boehringer Mannheim, Indianapolis, IN
CK8	CAM5.2	C	Becton, Dickinson and Co., Franklin Lakes, NJ
CK17	E3	B	Novocastne, Newcastle on Tyne, U.K.
CK19	RCK 108	B	DAKO, Carpinteria, CA
AE1/AE3		A	Boehringer Mannheim, Indianapolis, IN

A, Sigma Protease Type VIII, Sigma Diagnostics Inc., St. Louis, MO. B, Two-Cycle Microwave in Buffer, Ventana Medical Systems, Tucson, AZ. C, Pepsin–Crude Pepsin.

Table 7–4. Dominant CK7/CK20 Immunoprofile in Select Neoplasms

Immunoprofile	Neoplasms
CK7+/CK20+	Transitional cell carcinoma
	Pancreatic carcinoma
	Ovarian mucinous carcinoma
	Merkel cell carcinoma
CK7+/CK20−	Non–small cell carcinoma and adenocarcinoma of lung
	Breast carcinoma, ductal and lobular
	Nonmucinous ovarian carcinoma
	Endometrial adenocarcinoma
	Mesothelioma
CK7−/CK20+	Colorectal adenocarcinoma
CK7−/CK20−	Small cell carcinoma, lung
	Squamous cell carcinoma, lung
	Prostate adenocarcinoma
	Renal cell carcinoma
	Hepatoma

From Wang MP, Zee S, Zarbo RJ, et al. Coordinate expression of cytokeratin 7 and 20 defines unique subsets of carcinomas. Appl Immunohistochem 1995;3:99–107.

starting point for further immunohistochemical study.

Metastatic carcinomas in lung that are CK7 positive must be differentiated from a primary lung carcinoma with a panel of antibodies, and the IHC work-up will be dependent on the patient's age, sex, and presenting findings.

KEY DIAGNOSTIC POINTS FOR CYTOKERATIN 7 (see Tables 7–3 to 7–5)

- Strongly, diffusely positive in most lung, breast, ovarian, endometrial, bladder, thymic, parotid, pancreatic and neuroendocrine carcinomas and mesotheliomas, as well as in fibrolamellar hepatoma
- Mostly negative—perhaps rare positive cells in colorectal and other gastrointestinal carcinomas, hepatoma, prostate and renal cell carcinomas, squamous and small cell carcinomas
- Decorates subsets of endothelial cells in normal tissues

Table 7–5. Immunohistogram Frequency of CK7 Immunostaining of Select Tumors

	25	50	75	100
Lung non–small cell carcinoma			83	
Lung adenocarcinoma				100
Transitional cell carcinoma				100
Mesothelioma		70		
Thymic carcinoma				100
Breast carcinoma				100
Hepatoma	24			
Prostate	16			
Renal cell	24			
Colorectal	10			
Gastric		55		
Pancreatic			74	
Ovary serous/endometrioid				100
Endometrial				100

From Wang MP, Zee S, Zarbo RJ, et al. Coordinate expression of cytokeratin 7 and 20 defines unique subsets of carcinomas. Appl Immunohistochem 1995;3:99–107.

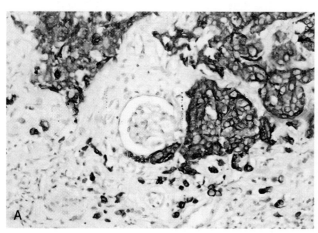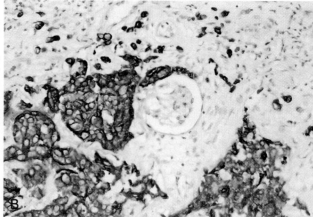

Figure 7–2. Transitional cell carcinoma of the kidney is immunostained by CK7 *(A)* and CK20 *(B).*

Cytokeratin 7 for Differential Diagnosis

- Transitional cell carcinoma—positive versus squamous cell carcinoma—negative
- Colorectal carcinomas (rare to negative [R-N]) versus lung, breast, thymus, and ovarian carcinomas, which all stain positive
- Endometrial and pancreatic carcinomas stain positive, neuroendocrine tumors may stain positive or negative

Cytokeratin 20

CK20 is a 46-kd LMW that was discovered by Moll and associates.[82] The tissue distribution of CK20 is limited predominantly to gastrointestinal epithelium and its tumors, mucinous tumors of the ovary, and Merkel cell neoplasms.[72–74, 83–85] The limited distribution of CK20 in colorectal, pancreatic, and gallbladder carcinomas, Merkel cell carcinomas, and transitional cell carcinomas is useful in the identification of this group of tumors in primary or even metastatic sites.[63, 85, 86] When combined with the specific tissue distribution of other keratins such as CK7, it is possible to identify colon cancer metastases in the lung, distinguish pulmonary small cell carcinoma from Merkel cell carcinoma, and distinguish transitional cell carcinoma from other squamous cell carcinomas and poorly differentiated carcinomas. It is of importance to recognize that CK20 in this subgroup of tumors is most often distributed strongly and diffusely. Rare CK20+ cells may be seen in some other neoplasms. Up to 10% of primary pulmonary adenocarcinomas not otherwise specified (NOS) or bronchoalveolar types may show up to 10 to 20% CK20+ cells (D. Dabbs, unpublished observation). One third of breast carcinomas, especially the papillary and mucinous variants, show CK20 positivity.[87]

Hepatoma and cholangiocarcinoma can be distinguished by the presence of CK7, CK8, CK18, and CK19 in cholangiocarcinomas, with no appreciable immunostaining of hepatoma by CK7 or AE1/AE3 antibodies.[88–90]

Epithelioid hemangioendothelioma (EH) can mimic a carcinoma in the liver, especially since it may be focally positive with AE1/AE3.[91] The use of vascular markers CD31, CD34, or factor VIII would be crucial for this differential diagnosis.

Although the prominent expression of CKs is the essential element of epithelial differentiation, on occasion expression of other lineage-specific markers may cloud the issue. Such is the case of finding keratins in nonepithelial tissues (see further on), and the rare observation of leukocyte common antigen (CD45) in some undifferentiated or neuroendocrine carcinomas[92] and CD30 in embryonal carcinomas.[93] The use of a panel of antibodies and the pattern and intensity of immunostaining is critically important in these confounding situations.

KEY DIAGNOSTIC POINTS FOR SIMPLE CYTOKERATINS

- CAM5.2, 35βH11, AE1/AE3: Broad coverage of carcinomatous differentiation
- CK7 (+): Mesothelioma; transitional, neuroendocrine, and thymic carcinomas; adenocarcinomas of breast, lung, ovary, endometrium, and pancreas; and fibrolamellar hepatoma
- CK7 (R-N): Renal, prostate, squamous, and small cell carcinomas, and hepatoma
- CK20 (+): Colorectal, pancreas, mucinous ovarian, Merkel cell, and transitional cell carcinomas; focally positive in breast (especially papillary and mucinous) and lung adenocarcinomas
- CK20 (N): Hepatoma and renal, prostate, squamous, and small cell carcinomas; rare focal immunostaining in less than 10% of non–small cell lung carcinomas

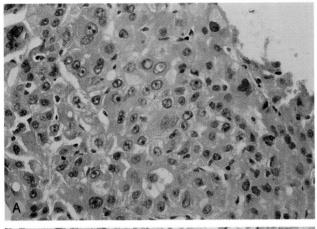

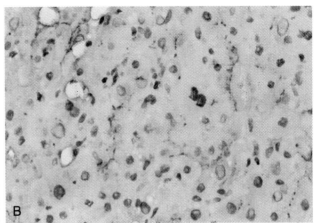

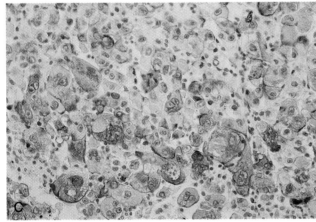

Figure 7–3. Hepatoma *(A)* may show a canalicular polyclonal carcinoembryonic antigen (pCEA) pattern *(B)* and CAM5.2 immunostaining *(C)*.

- Diagnostic pitfall—rare CD45 membrane staining in undifferentiated and neuroendocrine carcinomas

SIMPLE CYTOKERATINS: DIFFERENTIAL DIAGNOSTIC PANELS

Hepatoma Versus Metastatic Carcinoma
(Fig. 7–3)
- Hepatoma: AE1/AE3 (R-N), CK7 (N), CK20 (N), CAM5.2+, 35βH11+
- Fibrolamellar hepatoma variant: CK 7+
- Metastatic carcinoma: AE1/AE3+, CAM5.2+, 35βH11+, variable CK7, CK20

Hepatoma Versus Cholangiocarcinoma
(Fig. 7–4)
- Hepatoma: AE1/AE3 (R-N), CK7 (N), CK20 (N), CAM5.2+, 35βH11+
- Cholangiocarcinoma: AE1/AE3+, CK7+, CK20+, CAM5.2+, 35βH11+
- Hepatoma versus EH
  Hepatoma: AE1/AE3 (R-N); EH AE1/AE3 (negative or positive [−/+])
  EH: CD34/CD31/factor VIII+/− on tumor cells
- Hepatoma: CD34+ in sinusoids, not tumor cells

Lung Adenocarcinoma Versus Metastatic Colorectal-Pancreatic Adenocarcinomas
- Lung: CK7+ in lung, and less than 10% of adenocarcinomas with focal CK20+ cells
- Colorectal: CK20+, CK7−, or very rare positive cells.
- Pancreas: CK20+, CK7+

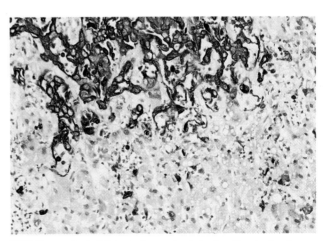

Figure 7–4. Metastatic gastrointestinally derived carcinomas are often CK20+, but hepatic parenchyma is CK20−.

Lung Squamous Cell Carcinoma Versus Metastatic Transitional Cell Carcinoma

- Squamous cell carcinoma: 34βE12+, CK7−, CK20−
- Transitional cell carcinoma: 34βE12+/−, CK7+, CK20+

Keratins of Stratified Epithelia: Complex Keratins

Keratins of HMW are observed in stratified epithelia and generally are not present in the simple visceral-type epithelia. Basal cells of prostate and myoepithelial cell populations of ducts and glandular tissue also contain an abundance of HMW type II keratins and LMW type I keratins. The antibody 34βE12 or keratin 903 (K903)[94–96] identifies a cocktail of keratins including Moll types I, II, V, X, XI, and XIV/XV. The practical diagnostic use of this pattern of expression is to identify basal and myoepithelial cells in their respective organs. For prostate tissue, the decoration of basal cells with K903 can exclude a process of invasive carcinoma.[94–96] Although the absence of basal cell staining in prostate with this antibody supports a diagnosis of carcinoma given other appropriate morphologic data, it cannot be used exclusively to diagnose carcinoma in the absence of staining. In similar fashion, the decoration of myoepithelial cells in glandular organs such as breast is important to distinguish benign from malignant lesions. For example, the decoration of myoepithelial cells in ductal carcinoma in situ or sclerosing adenosis can confirm a benign lesion.[96] This keratin of stratified type is also typically present in squamous epithelium and, using antibody K903, is the single best stain for detecting squamous differentiation in an otherwise poorly differentiated squamous cell carcinoma.

These HMW structural keratins are also commonly seen in duct-derived epithelium (breast, pancreas, biliary tract, lung) and in transitional, ovarian, and mesothelial tissues.[94–96] The degree of immunostaining of these tissues with HMW keratin antibodies is typically strong and diffuse, a feature that is helpful diagnostically, since HMW keratin immunostaining is seen only focally in visceral epithelial tissues such as colon, stomach, kidney, and liver.[94–96]

Keratin 14, as defined by antibody clone LL002 (YLEM, Avezzano, Italy), is a sensitive and specific indicator of oncocytes.[97] The antibody identified oncocytes in normal and neoplastic thyroid tissues as effectively as antibodies to mitochondria. Further studies may be useful to see if the same results can be duplicated with oncocytes and oncocytic tumors in other organs.

KEY DIAGNOSTIC POINTS OF ANTIBODIES TO COMPLEX KERATINS

- Confirms the presence of basal cells of prostate (Fig. 7–5)

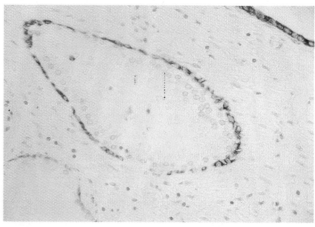

Figure 7–5. Basal cells in this prostate section are seen with K903. Myoepithelial cells can also be seen with K903.

- Confirms the presence of myoepithelial cells of ductal and glandular tissue
- Present in basal cell layer of stratified and squamous epithelium
- Strong and diffuse in squamous epithelial differentiation
- Present in a wide variety of duct-derived carcinomas and mesotheliomas, and most neoplasms that demonstrate tonofilaments ultrastructurally
- CK14 identifies oncocytes

Cytokeratin 5/Cytokeratin 6

CK5/CK6 is useful in the differential diagnosis of metastatic carcinoma in the pleura versus epithelial mesothelioma. Epithelial mesotheliomas are strongly positive in all cases, and pulmonary adenocarcinomas are largely negative or show focal immunostaining[98] (Fig. 7–6).

Almost all squamous cell carcinomas, half of transitional cell carcinomas metastatic in lung, and many undifferentiated large cell carcinomas immunostain with CK5/CK6 in a focal, weak pattern.[99, 100] Nonpulmonary lung carcinomas may express CK5/CK6, but these are mostly of ovarian origin.[100]

Hyperplastic mesothelial cells can be seen on occasion in the sinuses of lymph nodes from the chest or cervical chain.[101] The differential diagnosis in this instance is metastatic carcinoma. The presence of strong, diffuse CK5/CK6 in the cells of these nests should aid in identifying them as mesothelial in origin.

Keratins in Nonepithelial Cells

Keratins have been documented by IHC,[102–108] dot immunoblot,[109] and polymerase chain reaction[110] in several types of tumors in which there is

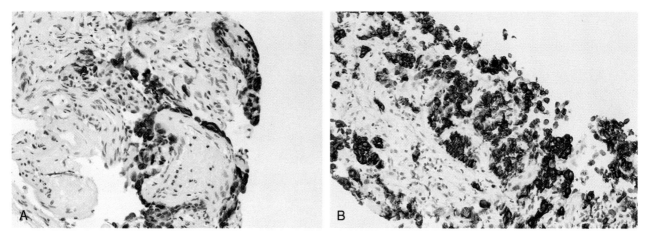

Figure 7–6. Antibodies to CK5/CK6 strongly immunostain reactive mesothelial cells in a pleural biopsy *(A)* and epithelial mesothelioma cells *(B)*.

no morphologic evidence of epithelial differentiation (Table 7–6). This type of keratin immunostaining has been referred to as *anomalous, aberrant, spurious,* and *unexpected.*[109, 111, 112]

The keratins most often found in these nonepithelial mesenchymal tissues or melanocytic lesions are keratins 8 and 18 and, less commonly, keratin 19 (see Table 7–6). Antibodies that detect these LMW keratins have demonstrated positive immunostaining in a variety of formalin-fixed, paraffin-embedded mesenchymal tumors, including leiomyosarcomas (21 to 25%),[104, 113, 114] fibrosarcoma (4%), liposarcoma (21%), rhabdomyosarcoma,[115] malignant peripheral nerve sheath tumors (5%), some malignant fibrous histiocytomas (5%),[116] gastrointestinal stromal tumors (50%), rare solitary fibrous tumors of pleura,[117] angiosarcoma (33%),[118–120] and primitive neuroectodermal tumors (50%).[119–127] Keratin usually decorates scattered cells in this group of tumors in traditional formalin-fixed, paraffin-embedded tissue, whereas carcinomas and sarcomatoid carcinomas are heavily and diffusely stained[128] (Fig. 7–7). In addition, keratin-positive soft tissue and bone tumors with partial epithelial

differentiation are variably decorated with keratin in the epithelial areas as expected. This group includes synovial sarcomas, epithelioid sarcoma, chordoma, malignant peripheral nerve sheath tumor, and adamantinoma of long bones.[129–135] Although some of the soft tissue tumors may mimic metastatic carcinoma morphologically, the finding of sporadic cell immunostaining is unlike the strong, diffuse immunostaining seen in carcinomas, especially when using the broad coverage antibodies. Frozen tissues fixed in acetone or alcohol, including alcohol-fixed cytologic specimens, yield far more keratin-positive cells, and this can be confusing diagnostically, especially cytologic specimens for which alcohol is a standard fixative for needle aspiration specimens.[133]

Malignant melanoma also demonstrates immunostaining for keratins 8 and 18, but in formalin-fixed, paraffin-embedded tissues, the prevalence is around 1% of cases, with focal tumor cell decoration.[136–139] Frozen sections and alcohol-fixed melanomas show substantially more positive tumor cells than do formalin-fixed specimens, and it is important to recognize this to avoid misdiagnosing

Table 7–6. Keratin Immunostaining in Nonepithelial Neoplasms by Immunohistochemistry

Tumor	Keratins	References
Plasmacytoma	8	161
K-1 anaplastic lymphoma	8, 18	149, 158, 162, 163
Reticulum cells in lymph nodes	8, 18	148, 150–155
Malignant fibrous histiocytoma	8	106, 107, 109, 113, 136
Malignant schwannoma	8, 18	130
Angiosarcoma	8, 18	119–121, 123, 124, 126
Smooth muscle–uterine, vascular	8, 18	114, 127, 128
Leiomyosarcoma	8, 18	109, 113, 115
Rhabdomyosarcoma	8, 18	116
Subserosal mesothelial connective tissue progenitor cells	8	99
Malignant melanoma	8, 18	110, 131, 137–140
Astrocytoma	Aberrant	141, 142
Meningioma	8, 18	143–146

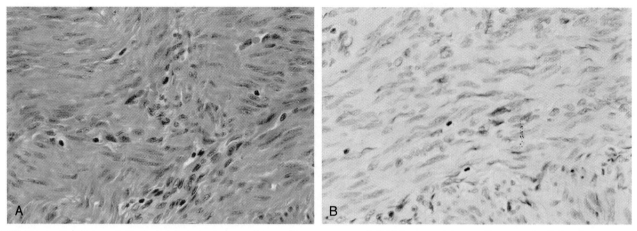

Figure 7–7. *A* and *B*, Smooth muscle neoplasm shows scattered CAM5.2 positive cells, a typical focal pattern of immunostaining for keratin seen in a variety of mesenchymal tumors.

melanoma as a carcinoma, especially in alcohol-fixed cytologic preparations.[109, 133, 140]

The consensus regarding keratin immunostaining of nonepithelioid sarcomas and melanomas is that although the presence of keratin is real as measured by molecular techniques and more sensitive immunohistologic methods (frozen sections, alcohol fixation), the observed nonexpression of keratin staining in these tumors in formalin-fixed tissue is desirable because of its diagnostic usefulness.

Truly "spurious" keratin immunoreactivity has been described in human glial tissue and in some human astrocytomas, especially with antibodies AE1 and 34βE12.[140, 141] In addition, the cocktail AE1/AE3 may cross-react with both normal and neoplastic astrocytes.[141, 142] The spurious keratin immunoreactivity is probably due to cross-reaction with glial cells containing glial fibrillary acidic proteins.[142] The presence of keratin determined by immunologic or molecular methods has not been documented in astrocytes. This is an obvious pitfall for the misdiagnosis of metastatic carcinoma in the brain. The antibody CAM5.2 does not react with astroglial cells, and thus is best used to detect carcinomatous differentiation in the CNS.

Meningiomas, especially the "secretory variant," may express keratin in up to one third of cases.[143–146]

Epithelial differentiation is simulated in lymph nodes with the LMW keratin–positive fibroblastic reticulum cells of the paracortex[147–155] (Fig. 7–8). These dendritic cells immunostain with CAM5.2 and AE1/AE3, revealing an extensive network of extrafollicular dendritic processes in lymph nodes, tonsils, and spleen.[153] These keratin-positive cells are a pitfall for the diagnosis of metastatic carcinoma, because the conventional wisdom had been that keratin-positive cells in a lymph node equated with metastatic carcinoma. The pitfall is twofold[1]:

• When searching for keratin-positive micrometastases in patients with breast carcinoma, one must distinguish the dendritic processes from carcinoma cells that cluster in the subcapsular sinus.[2]

• Needle aspirates and touch prints of lymph nodes may contain keratin-positive cells without containing metastatic carcinoma; one must be aware of the morphologic features of the keratin-positive cells.[150–152, 154]

Keratin-positive cells have been described in plasmacytoma and in K-1 anaplastic large cell lymphoma.[156–162] For anaplastic large cell lymphoma, keratins may be detected in as many as 30% of cases and, along with some EMA-positive anaplastic lymphoma cells, the definitive diagnosis can be confusing. However, adherence to a broad spectrum antibody for keratin immunoreactivity will show only focal rare staining at most in these lymphomas.

Plasmacytomas likewise should be studied with broad coverage antibodies in a panel that includes antibodies to kappa and lambda light chains.

Keratin Immunohistochemistry

The majority of keratin immunostaining is performed on formalin-fixed paraffin-embedded tis-

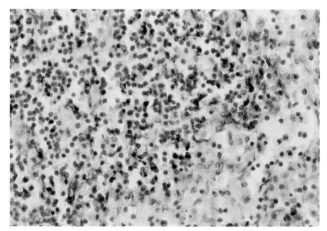

Figure 7–8. In this normal lymph node, interfollicular dendritic cells are CAM5.2+.

sues. The duration of formalin fixation is a key factor when trying to optimize the technical performance of keratin immunoperoxidase stains. The fixation time is closely related to the time required for enzymatic predigestion.[156, 163] Generally, tissue fixed in 10% formalin for more than 2 days requires greater time with enzymatic predigestion, with lesser time required for tissues fixed briefly (hours) in 10% formalin. Most, if not all, keratin antibodies require predigestion with protease for 4 to 16 minutes (depending on antibody and fixation duration) for optimal keratin antibody performance (see Table 7–3).

COMBINED ANTIBODY (PANEL) APPROACH TO SOLVING DIAGNOSTIC PROBLEMS

When antibodies to CK7, CK20, or other keratins are combined in panels with various antibodies to other intermediate filaments (e.g., vimentin), antibodies to supplemental epithelial antigens (e.g., CEA, EMA), or antibodies to specific cell products (e.g., neuroendocrine granules), a more specifc identification of cell type may be rendered.

Carcinoma Subsets with Frequent Vimentin Coexpression

Mesenchymal and endothelial cells regularly immunostain with vimentin, and this immunostaining generally provides a measure of internal quality control for the quality of immunoreactivity.[164] If there is no immunostaining of vessels or stromal cells by vimentin, it denotes significant damage to tissue antigens.

Carcinomas in effusion specimens are universally positive for vimentin (presumably an in vivo fluid effect) and thus have no diagnostic utility.[165]

Initially thought to be an intermediate filament restricted to mesenchymal cells, vimentin has been found in a diverse number of neoplasms, including a variety of carcinomas (Table 7–7). Vimentin decorates any spindle cell neoplasm—mesenchymal spindle neoplasms and sarcomatoid carcinomas included. Vimentin decorates a subset of carcinomas

regularly and to a significant degree, and this can be useful in the context of a panel of antibodies to narrow a differential diagnosis. Carcinomas with frequent (more than 50 to 60%) and strong (more than 25% of cells) vimentin coexpression include spindle cell carcinomas, renal cell carcinomas (except the chromophobe variant), endometrial adenocarcinomas and malignant mixed müllerian tumors, serous ovarian carcinomas, pleomorphic salivary gland tumors, and follicular thyroid carcinomas.[165, 166] Epithelial and sarcomatoid mesotheliomas also regularly demonstrate vimentin.[167]

Certain carcinomas may immunostain with vimentin but with lesser frequency (10 to 20%) and with far less intensity (<10% of cells). This group includes adenocarcinomas of colorectum, lung, breast, and prostate, and nonserous ovarian carcinomas.

Therefore, the finding of substantial coexpression of vimentin in a metastatic carcinoma may aid in narrowing the differential diagnosis and adds value to the rest of the antibody panel (Fig. 7–9).

Vimentin coexpression is especially useful in identifying endometrial and endometrioid carcinoma in curettage specimens of the uterine cervix and corpus, as endometrial and endometrioid carcinomas immunostain strongly for vimentin but endocervical carcinomas stain mostly negative (weak focal staining in up to 13% of endocervical carcinomas).[168, 169]

KEY DIAGNOSTIC POINTS OF VIMENTIN COEXPRESSION IN CARCINOMAS

- Common in renal, endometrial, ovarian serous, salivary gland, follicular thyroid, and sarcomatoid (spindle cell) carcinomas, as well as in malignant mixed müllerian tumors
- May be seen in focal cells in 10 to 20% of colorectal, lung, breast, prostate, and nonserous ovarian adenocarcinomas
- Not diagnostically useful in body cavity effusion specimens
- Epithelial and sarcomatoid mesotheliomas are usually vimentin-positive
- Important internal quality measure for antigen assessment

Combinations of Antibodies to Keratins and Carcinoembryonic Antigen

CEA is a 180-kd glycoprotein that is 50% carbohydrate.[170] There are many CEA antibodies available to a variety of CEA epitopes. The polyclonal antibodies commonly cross-react with tissue-nonspecific cross-reacting antigen and biliary glycoprotein I.[171–174] This older CD66e series of CEA antibodies typically react strongly and diffusely with

Table 7–7. Major Patterns of Coexpression of Cytokeratin-Vimentin in Carcinomas

Coexpression Common (>50%)	Coexpression Uncommon (<10%)
Renal cell carcinoma	Colorectal adenocarcinoma
Endometrial adenocarcinoma	Breast ductal-lobular carcinoma
Spindle cell carcinoma	Lung non–small cell carcinoma
Thyroid follicular carcinoma	Prostate adenocarcinoma
Salivary gland carcinoma	Endocervical adenocarcinoma

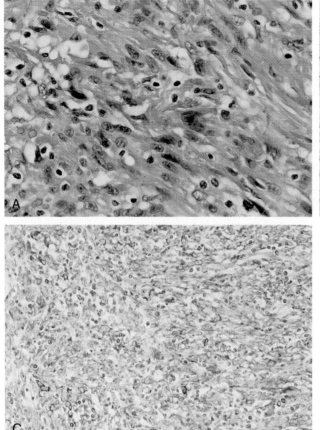

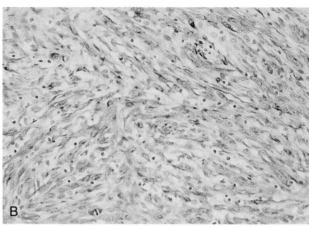

Figure 7–9. This sarcomatoid carcinoma of lung *(A)* richly coexpresses CAM5.2 *(B)* and vimentin *(C)*. Most carcinomas of this type in lung and upper aerodigestive tract are sarcomatoid squamous cell carcinomas.

ductal carcinomas of the breast in addition to lung and colorectal carcinomas. However, the CEAD-14 clone (Enteric Products, Inc., Stony Brook, NY)[175, 176] reacts with only a small subset of carcinomas of the breast (mostly high grade), which is a useful diagnostic point of distinction for breast carcinomas[177] that are metastatic to lung, liver, lymph node, or brain.

Adenocarcinomas of colorectal origin can be distinguished from lung adenocarcinomas, ovarian carcinomas, and ductal carcinomas of the breast, regardless of metastatic site. Primary adenocarcinomas of the lung are typically CK7+, CK20−, and CEAD-14+, whereas colorectal carcinomas are CK7−, CK20+, and CEAD-14+; ductal and lobular breast carcinomas are CK7+, CK20−, and CEAD-14−; and ovarian carcinomas are CK7+, CK20+/−, and CEA−.[68, 71, 74–76, 178–182] Neoplasms that typically are strongly positive for most CEA antibodies include adenocarcinomas of the lung, colon, stomach, biliary tree, pancreas, urinary bladder, endocervix, paranasal sinuses, sweat glands, and breast[177, 183, 184] (Table 7–8).

Neoplasms that are essentially negative with any CEA antibody include adenocarcinomas of prostate, kidney, adrenal gland, and endometrium; serous ovarian tumors; and mesotheliomas.[183]

Liver cell–derived tumors are nonreactive with the monoclonal CEA antibodies but do react with

the polyclonal antibodies in a distinct pattern of pericanalicular decoration, since the polyclonal antibodies cross-react with the hepatic bile canalicular biliary glycoprotein.[185–187] Adenocarcinomas of pulmonary, gastrointestinal, thymic, endocervical, and cholangiobiliary origin typically show strong, although variable, cytoplasmic immunostaining for CEA antibodies.

The EH of liver can mimic carcinoma to perfection. Demonstration of positive CD31/CD34 factor VIII with variable keratin and no CEA staining will separate this entity from carcinoma and hepatoma.[89]

Table 7–8. Carcinoembryonic Antigen Immunostaining of Adenocarcinoma: Polyclonal Carcinoembryonic Antigen or Monoclonal Antibodies

Carcinoembryonic Antigen Common	Carcinoembryonic Antigen Negative
Paranasal sinuses	Prostate
Lung	Kidney
Colon	Adrenal
Stomach	Endometrium
Biliary	Ovary, Serous
Pancreas	
Sweat glands	
Breast	

Unlike normal liver, neoplastic liver sinusoids demonstrate the presence of immunoreactive CD34, and this can be useful in the differential diagnosis of primary liver neoplasm versus metastatic carcinoma and non-neoplastic liver, especially on small biopsy samples[188] (Fig. 7–10).

The antibody HepPar 1 detects a protein of unknown function in liver cells, yet it is 79% specific for hepatic differentiation, and sensitivity is high.[189]

True hepatocellular carcinoma differentiation (polyclonal CEA+, HepPar 1+, sinusoidal cell CD34+) has been described on rare occasions as a component of some adenocarcinomas from urinary bladder and stomach.[190, 191]

Primary Hepatic Tumors Versus Metastatic Adenocarcinoma: Differential Diagnostic Panels

- Hepatoma: Canalicular pattern polyclonal CEA (antibiliary glycoprotein); CAM5.2+, AE1/AE3 (R-N), CK7/CK20 (R-N), CD34+ sinusoids, HepPar 1+/−
- Gastrointestinal, lung, breast, thymus, endocervical, primary cholangiocarcinoma: CEA+, AE1/AE3+, variable CK7/CK20 immunostaining

- Nonseminomatous germ cell tumors AE1/AE3+/−, PLAP+
- Breast carcinomas: CEAD-14 (R-N), CK7+, GCDFP-15+/−
- Prostate, renal, endometrial, adrenal, and serous ovarian tumors and mesothelioma: CEA (N)
- EH: CD31/CD34+, factor VIII+, CAM5.2−/+, CEA (N)

Epithelial Membrane Antigen

Encoded by the MUC1 gene on chromosome 1 and a derivative human antigen, EMA is a transmembrane glycoprotein of the breast mucin complex, and its expression is increased in carcinomas.[192–194] Unlike normal breast in which EMA is present on the apical cell membrane, in neoplasms, EMA is present on the entire circumferential cell membrane.[193] Increased amounts of the large glycoprotein interfere with cell-to-cell and cell-to-matrix adhesion in neoplastic cells.[195]

The utility of EMA antibody is in the detection of epithelial differentiation, as a supplement to the CKs. Spindle cell, small cell, and large cell neoplasms may on rare occasion be decorated with EMA but may be negative for CKs.[196–198]

There are several EMA antibodies available, each of which reacts to different epitopes of the large

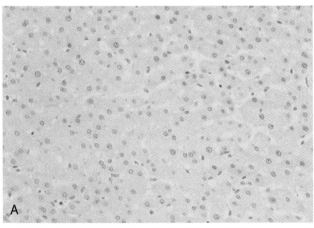

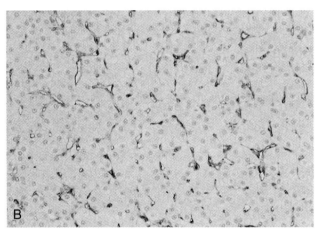

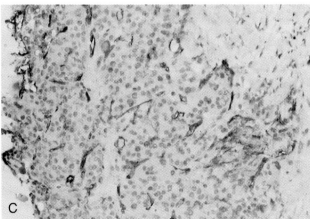

Figure 7–10. Normal liver *(A)* sinusoids do not express CD34, whereas hepatic adenomas *(B)* and hepatic carcinomas *(C)* often show sinusoidal CD34; this is especially helpful on needle aspirates or biopsies to identify primary liver neoplasia.

glycoprotein antigen; they include MAM-6,[199] episialin,[200] polymorphic epithelial mucin,[201] CA15-3,[202] DF3 antigen,[203] and breast epithelial mucin.[204, 205] For neoplastic epithelial differentiation, most antibodies have 85% sensitivity and 89% specificity.[206]

The EMA antibodies decorate skin and adnexa, breast, lung, bile ducts, pancreas, salivary gland, urothelium, endometrium and endocervix, prostate ducts, thyroid, mesothelium, and neoplasms of these tissues (Table 7–9). Many sarcomatoid carcinomas and epithelial and sarcomatoid mesotheliomas are positive.[50, 52, 206] Reactive mesothelium may stain weakly compared with thick membranous staining of mesothelioma.[207, 208] Many types of adenocarcinomas immunostain with EMA and must be distinguished from mesothelial cells in effusions by using a panel of immunostains that includes CK5/CK6, CEA, LeuM1, BerEP4, and B72.3.[50, 98, 209]

Subsets of normal and neoplastic hematopoietic cells express EMA, including plasma cells and erythroblasts,[162, 210] and neoplastic cells including the L&H cells (60% of cases) of lymphocyte-predominant Hodgkin's lymphoma,[211–213] 5% of B-cell lymphomas,[26, 214, 215] 18% of T-cell lymphomas,[216–219] and about 60% of anaplastic large cell lymphomas.[220–224] The EMA antibodies do not have absolute sensitivity and specificity for carcinomas and therefore should always be used with a panel of CKs and other corroborating antibodies such as leukocyte common antigen.[206]

In addition to epithelial neoplasms, a number of sarcomas, CNS tumors, small round cell tumors, and a few germ cell tumors may be positive with EMA.[206] These tumors include malignant nerve sheath tumors, synovial sarcoma, leiomyosarcoma, malignant fibrous histiocytoma, epithelioid sarcoma, and chordoma.[206] With the exception of the last two tumors mentioned, EMA immunostaining is focal.

Choroid plexus neoplasms and meningiomas show strong membranous EMA immunostaining.[206] Germ cell tumors are largely negative except for variable EMA immunostaining in choriocarcinoma and teratoma, whereas the epithelial small round cell tumors of nephroblastoma and hepatoblastoma immunostain with EMA in the majority of cases.[206, 225]

KEY DIAGNOSTIC POINTS OF EPITHELIAL MEMBRANE ANTIGEN

- Used as a supplement to detect epithelial neoplasms because CKs may occasionally be negative in undifferentiated carcinomas
- EMA immunostaining may be membranous or cytoplasmic, or both
- Negative in malignant melanoma
- Negative in germ cell neoplasms except choriocarcinoma and teratoma
- EMA decorates plasma cells, 60% of anaplastic large cell lymphomas, L&H cells of Hodgkin's lymphoma and a few T- and B-cell lymphomas
- Strongly positive in malignant mesothelioma, negative to weak for normal "reactive" mesothelial cells

Germ Cell Neoplasia

It is important to be able to diagnose these germ cell neoplasms correctly because they are highly amenable to treatment, even in advanced stages.[6, 24] They may present as carcinoma of unknown primary, including seminoma and its variants, embryonal carcinoma, endodermal sinus tumor, and choriocarcinoma. A combination of antibodies to simple CKs, EMA, PLAP, alpha-fetoprotein, and human chorionic gonadotropin (hCG) can be used to arrive at the correct diagnosis in most cases.

The PLAP antibodies database from the literature includes M2A, 43-9F, and TRA-1-60.[226–228]

Germ cell tumors are diffusely positive for CAM5.2, except seminoma, which is largely negative in most cases but may demonstrate rare focal

Table 7–9. Epithelial Membrane Antigen Immunostaining in Carcinomas and Nonepithelial Tissues

Typically Positive	Mostly Negative	Focal Presence in Nonepithelial Tissue
Skin and adnexa	Germ cell tumors except choriocarcinoma-teratoma	Plasma cells
Breast		Erythroblasts
Lung		L&H cells of Hodgkin's lymphoma
Bile ducts		Few cells in non-Hodgkin's lymphoma
Pancreas		Anaplastic large cell lymphoma
Salivary gland		Malignant nerve sheath tumors
Urothelium		Synovial sarcoma
Endometrium		Leiomyosarcoma
Endocervix		Malignant fibrous histiocytoma
Prostate ducts		
Thyroid		
Mesothelioma		
Sarcomatoid carcinomas		
Meningiomas		

staining.[229] More than focal keratin staining should raise the suspicion of an embryonal carcinoma component.

The PLAP is strongly positive with crisp membranous decoration and cytoplasmic staining in classic seminoma, negative in the spermatocytic variant,[230, 231] and variably positive in embryonal, yolk sac, and choriocarcinomas.[231–237] The PLAP is not 100% specific for germ cell tumors, as 10 to 15% of non–germ cell carcinomas will immunostain, and this group includes müllerian carcinomas and gastrointestinal, lung, and rare breast and renal carcinomas.[238, 239] However, these carcinomas are EMA-positive, whereas germ cell tumors are negative.

The EMA is negative in all these tumors except choriocarcinoma, in which it decorates about 50% of cases.[229, 231, 240]

Alpha-fetoprotein is present in most yolk sac tumors in patchy distribution, but only focally in some cases of embryonal carcinoma.[229, 231, 240–242]

Hepatoid differentiation in germ cell tumors, especially with yolk sac tumors, typically immunodecorates with alpha-fetoprotein and does not show the immunoprofile of true hepatocytic differentiation, that is, the biliary pattern of immunostaining with polyclonal CEA.[243]

KEY DIAGNOSTIC POINTS OF GERM CELL TUMORS (Table 7–10)

* Seminoma: CAM5.2 (R-N), PLAP+, EMA (N)
* Embryonal carcinoma: CAM5.2+, PLAP+, EMA (N), alpha-fetoprotein (R-N), CD30+
* Yolk sac carcinoma: CAM 5.2+, PLAP+, EMA (N), alpha-fetoprotein+/−
* Choriocarcinoma: CAM5.2+, PLAP+/−, EMA−/+, hCG+
* PLAP immunostains 10 to 15% of non–germ cell carcinomas, but they are also EMA-positive

Focusing on Tumor Differentiation: Cell-Specific Products

Even though the tissue of origin of most metastases can be ascertained with the panel approach of

Table 7–10. Cytokeratin/Carcinoembryonic Antigen in Carcinoma Differential Diagnosis

Tumor/Location	34βE12	CAM5.2	AE1/AE3	CK7	CK20	CEAD-14	CK17	TTF-1
Merkel cell	N	+	+	R-N	+	N	N	N
Small cell carcinoma	N	+	+	−/+	N	−/+	N	+
Lung adenocarcinoma	−/+	+	+	+	R-N	+	−/+	+/−
Breast	−/+	+	+	+	N	R-N	−/+	N
Seminoma	N	R-N	R-N	N	N	N	N	N
Endometrium	−/+	+	+	+	N	N	+/−	N
Bladder	−/+	+	+	+	+	R-N	+	N
Parotid gland	−/+	+	+	+	N	N	N	N
Neuroendocrine tumors	N	+	+	+	N	−/+	+/−	N
Pancreas	−/+	+	+	+/−	−/+	+	+/−	N
Biliary	−/+	+	+	+/−	+/−	+	+/−	N
Gastric	N	+	+	+/−	+/−	+	+/−	N
Colorectal carcinomas	N	+	+	R-N	+	+	N	N
Prostate	N	+	+	−/+	N	N	R-N	N
Renal carcinoma	N	+	+	N	N	N	N	N
Germ cell carcinoma	N	+	+	+	N	−/+	N	N
Hepatocellular carcinoma*	N	+	N	R-N	N	N	N	N
Ovarian mucinous carcinoma	N	+	+	+	+	N	N	N
Ovarian nonmucinous carcinoma	N	+	+	+	N	N	+/−	N
Thyroid gland	−/+	+	+	−/+	+/−	N	−/+	+
Adrenal gland	N	N	N	N	N	N	N	N
Thymus	−/+	+	+	N	N	−/+	N	N
Endocervix	R-N	+	+	+	N	+	N	N

* Canalicular with polyclonal CEA
+, positive; +/−, mostly positive; −/+, mostly negative; R, rare cells show staining; N, negative.

CKs, CEA, EMA, and vimentin, there remains a subset of neoplasms that do not readily lend themselves to definitive identification. The use of additional antibodies to cell-specific products in most instances has a high specificity for certain tissues, enabling the pathologist to "fine focus" the search for the origin of a metastasis.

Some of these antibodies are discussed here, including chromogranin A, synaptophysin, neuron-specific enolase (NSE), thyroglobulin, PSA, inhibin, CD5, melan-A, TTF-1, and GCDFP-15 and villin.

NEUROENDOCRINE ANTIBODIES

Antibodies to neuroendocrine cell components are usually used in the context of trying to distinguish tumor cell types in specific organs such as lung, thyroid, colon, and adrenal gland. The antibodies are not typically used in the initial screening panel of the work-up of an undifferentiated tumor, and there is little literature that deals with this topic.[244] It is critically important to use the following antibody immunostains together as a panel, because no single antibody has perfect specificity and sensitivity.

It is well known that a few "neuroendocrine cells" can be seen with IHC in a wide variety of carcinomas. This is not to be equated with a diagnosis of "neuroendocrine carcinoma." Only after a complete account of the clinical findings, imaging studies, histologic studies, and immunohistochemical findings should a diagnosis be rendered.

Chromogranins

The chromogranins (types A, B, and C) are a group of monomeric proteins that compose the major portion of the soluble protein extract of the neurosecretory granules of neuroendocrine cells; chromogranin A, with a molecular weight of 75 kd, is the most abundantly distributed. There is a strong correlation between the chromogranin cellular immunostaining quantity and the number of neuroendocrine-type secretory granules seen at the level of electron microscopy.[245]

The LK2H10 clone is a monoclonal antibody with abundant representation in the literature.[245-248] Immunostaining intensity decreases with poor differentiation. The specificity of LK2H10 is close to 100%, but sensitivity is closer to 75%.[249]

The lowest sensitivity of LK2H10 is for typical carcinoids (about 50%), but histologic recognition of carcinoid is straightforward.

Synaptophysin

Synaptophysin is a glycoprotein that is an integral part of the neuroendocrine secretory granule membrane[244, 250] and is recognized by monoclonal antibody (SY38) in a variety of neuroendocrine tumors. Synaptophysin is a broad spectrum neuroendocrine marker,[251] with higher sensitivity but lower specificity than antibody to chromogranin. Immunostaining for SY38 has also been documented to be most effective in identifying metastases of neuroendocrine type.[244]

Large cell undifferentiated neuroendocrine carcinoma (LCNEC) can present as an MUP, and it is easy to miss the diagnosis without applying the appropriate neuroendocrine markers. The correct diagnosis of LCNEC is an important distinction, because it carries the same dismal prognosis as does small cell carcinoma, whether in the lung or gastrointestinal tract.[252, 253] Synaptophysin may be the most frequent positive marker in LCNEC.[253]

In one study, small cell lung carcinomas were decorated by synaptophysin in up to 79% of cases, whereas chromogranin was positive in 47 to 60% of cases, bombesin was positive in 45% of cases, and NSE was seen in 33 to 60% of cases.[254] Synaptophysin may be seen in 8% of non–small cell carcinomas.[255]

Leu 7

The CD57 antigen of a human T-cell line generated a monoclonal antibody (HNK-1). The differentiation antigen of the T-cell line is indicative of a natural killer cell activity.[256, 257] The CD57 antibody also recognizes antigen of myelin-associated glycoprotein in the myelin of the central and peripheral nervous systems. CD57 reactivity has also been found in enterochromaffin cells, pancreatic islet cells, islet cell tumors, carcinoid tumors, pheochromocytomas, and small cell carcinoma of the lung.[258-261]

CD57 lacks the high sensitivity and specificity of chromogranin and synaptophysin and therefore should be used as part of a panel that includes these antibodies.

Neuron-Specific Enolase

The enolase enzymes comprise five different forms, each of which is composed of three homodimers and two hybrids. NSE is found in a variety of normal and neoplastic neuroendocrine cells and predominates in the brain.[262-265] Originally believed to be a specific marker for neuroendocrine differentiation, it has subsequently been observed that NSE can be found in virtually any type of neoplasm and because of this, it is a poor antibody to use to screen for neuroendocrine differentiation. Overall a poor marker for detection of neuroendocrine differentiation because of its lack of specificity, NSE may be useful in combination with other more specific antibodies, such as chromogranin and synaptophysin, for the appropriate neuroendocrine morphologic identification and documentation of immunostaining.

Peptide Hormones

Peptide hormones are present in unique, sequestered tissues in the normal state and generally recapitulate the same hormone production in neoplasms. Endocrine neoplasms, with few exceptions, show a characteristic histologic pattern, and therefore the study of hormone production is often of academic interest only.

Poorly differentiated endocrine neoplasms, depending on the site of origin, may produce characteristic peptide hormones. The group of poorly differentiated neuroendocrine tumors and their hormone production include islet cell tumors (insulin, glucagon, somatostatin, gastrin), pulmonary small cell carcinoma (bombesin in 45% of cases),[254] and medullary thyroid carcinoma (calcitonin).

The CK profile of neuroendocrine tumors is somewhat distinctive in that virtually all are positive for keratins 8 and 18 (e.g., CAM5.2) but negative for keratins 7 and 20 and HMW keratin (e.g., K903). Merkel cell carcinomas are characteristically positive for keratin 20 and negative for keratin 7, which is the reverse for immunostaining of small cell carcinomas of lung (CK 7+, CK 20−).

KEY DIAGNOSTIC POINTS OF NEUROENDOCRINE DIFFERENTIATION

- Typical neuroendocrine keratin profile: keratin 8+, keratin 18+, and keratin 7+/−
- Chromogranin and synaptophysin complement each other as part of a diagnostic panel
- Specific peptide (bombesin, glucagon, and so on) may supplement the preceding studies

---

Thyroglobulin

Thyroglobulin, a 670-kd heavily glycosylated protein, provides iodination sites for the production of thyroid hormones and is unique to the thyroid follicular epithelium. The great majority of thyroid carcinomas show immunostaining with thyroglobulin, although most of the positive cases are readily interpreted as follicular or papillary carcinomas. The undifferentiated anaplastic carcinomas may show only rare positive cells. Thyroid carcinomas are almost always negative with monoclonal CEA antibody, which is a helpful feature in differential diagnosis. Thyroglobulin may be seen as scattered positive cells in medullary carcinoma and, conversely, calcitonin-positive cells may be seen in poorly differentiated follicular carcinomas.[266-268] Thyroglobulin may be seen in 10 to 25% of cases of leukemic blast cells in bone marrow.[269]

KEY DIAGNOSTIC POINTS OF THYROGLOBULIN

- Positive in almost all thyroid carcinomas, with reduced or sporadic immunostaining of poorly differentiated or anaplastic types
- Highly specific for thyroid carcinomas, with rare positivity in some leukemic blast cells

---

Thyroid Transcription Factor-1

TTF-1, a nuclear tissue-specific protein transcription factor, is found only in thyroid and thyroid tumors regardless of histologic type, as well as in lung carcinomas, including adenocarcinomas (75%), non–small cell carcinomas (63%), neuroendocrine and small cell carcinomas (>90%), and squamous cell carcinomas (10%).[270-276] Selectively expressed during embryogenesis in the thyroid, the diencephalon of the brain, and in respiratory epithelium, TTF-1 binds to and activates factors for surfactant protein derived from Clara cells.[277, 278]

TTF-1 is rarely seen in carcinomas outside the lung or thyroid[278-280] (Fig. 7–11). Neuroendocrine tumors of the lung, including typical and atypical carcinoids and large cell neuroendocrine carcinomas, are almost always positive with TTF-1, demonstrating a kinship with small cell carcinomas.[279]

The utility of TTF-1 becomes readily apparent in the differential diagnosis of primary versus metastatic carcinomas, especially in the lung. CK7 and CK20, along with TTF-1 and CEA, are the antibodies that best discriminate primary lung carcinoma from metastatic carcinoma to the lung.

KEY DIAGNOSTIC POINTS OF THYROID TRANSCRIPTION FACTOR-1

- Nuclear immunostaining in all carcinomas of thyroid origin of any histologic type
- Nuclear immunostaining of the vast majority of carcinomas of the lung—adenocarcinomas, small cell and non–small cell, and large cell, with a minority of squamous cell carcinomas

---

DIFFERENTIAL DIAGNOSTIC PANELS FOR THYROID TRANSCRIPTION FACTOR-1

- Primary lung versus metastatic breast carcinoma
  Lung: TTF-1+, CK7+, CEAD-14+
  Breast: TTF-1 (N), CK7+, CEAD-14 (R-N)
- Primary lung adenocarcinoma versus malignant epithelial mesothelioma
  Lung: TTF-1+, CK7+, LeuM1+, B72.3+, BerEP4+/−, CEA+, CK5/CK6 (R-N)
  Mesothelioma: TTF-1 (N), CK5/CK6+, CK 7+/−,

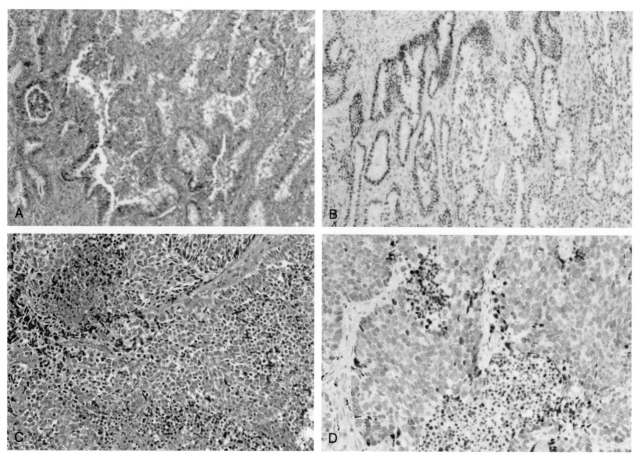

Figure 7–11. Thyroid transcription factor 1 (TTF-1) antibody is helpful because it identifies two thirds of pulmonary adenocarcinomas *(A and B)* and 95% of pulmonary small cell carcinomas *(C and D).*

CK20+/−, LeuM1 (N), B72.3 (N), BerEP4 (N), CEA (N)
- Primary lung versus metastatic thyroid carcinoma of all types
  Lung: TTF-1+, CEA+
  Thyroid: TTF-1+, CEA (N)
- Primary lung versus nonpulmonary metastatic carcinoma
  Lung: TTF-1+
  Other carcinoma: TTF-1 (N)

Villin

Villin is a calcium-dependent actin-binding cytoskeletal protein that is found in the brush border of the intestine and in the proximal renal tubular epithelium. A brush border is characteristic of colorectal carcinomas and is recognized at the ultrastructural level by the presence of microvilli with a dense core of microfilaments, core rootlets, and surface glycocalyx. Up to 33% of pulmonary adenocarcinomas may demonstrate microvillus rootlets by ultrastructure, and their presence correlates closely with villin immunostaining.[281–284] Antibodies to villin are useful for identifying its molecular presence, which is in almost all colorectal carcinomas and in more than 90% of lung carcinomas that have microvillus rootlets.[281–284] CKs are a necessary part of a diagnostic panel to distinguish lung and colon carcinomas, and 90% of lung adenocarcinomas are CK20−, whereas colorectal carcinomas are CK20+.

Prostate Carcinoma Antigens

PROSTATE-SPECIFIC ANTIGEN

Together, antibodies to PSA and prostatic acid phosphatase (PAP) will decorate greater than 95% of prostate carcinomas, but there are some caveats. The immunostaining of tumor cells falls off with increasing Gleason grade with both antibodies, and PAP is found in a wide variety of other tumors, including hindgut carcinoid tumors.[285] PSA has been found as patchy staining in some salivary gland tumors, in up to one third of breast carcinomas and sweat gland tumors, in periurethral glands in men and women, in cystitis glandularis of the bladder, in urachal remnants, and in some anal glands.[286–294] Nevertheless, PSA is highly specific for prostate tissue, as it functions as a serine protease of the seminal fluid,[295, 296] and it decorates the histologic subtypes of tumors, including mucinous, signet ring, and endometrioid carcinomas.[297–299] Metastatic prostate carcinoma may be immunostained to a variable degree in metastatic sites, including lymph nodes.[300–302] Immunoreactivity is not diminished by brief decalcification procedures.

PSA has been found to decorate scattered tumor cells from cutaneous malignant melanoma and its metastases.[303] This should not create a diagnostic dilemma because prostate cancers are strongly, diffusely positive with LMW keratin antibodies such as CAM5.2, which is another illustration of the necessity of examining tumors with a panel of antibodies.

PROSTATE-SPECIFIC MEMBRANE ANTIGEN

Prostate-specific membrane antigen (PSMA), which has a partial homologous structure with the transferrin receptor, is highly specific for prostate cells.[304–307] Unlike PAP, PSMA is up-regulated in prostate carcinoma so that stronger staining is seen in higher grade carcinomas.[305, 306, 308]

There is extraprostatic expression of PSMA as well, occurring in colonic neuroendocrine cells, breast, and salivary gland.[305, 306, 309] The antibodies that have been cited in the literature are 7E11-C5.3[309, 310] and 3F5.4G6.[311]

Prostate as Metastasis of Unknown Primary

- A combination of PSA, PAP, and PSMA would detect virtually all prostate carcinoma in nonprostate (metastatic) sites
- Nonprostate tissues may immunostain with these antibodies, necessitating additional corroborating antibodies in a panel that is relevant to the clinical situation
- The more common nonprostatic lesions for immunostaining with PSA and PSMA include breast carcinomas (rare in males), salivary gland tumors, pancreas, and anal glands
- PSA immunostaining may be seen in metastatic melanoma; one should use appropriate antibody panels to avoid problems

Uroplakins

The asymmetric unit membrane that is unique to the umbrella cells of urinary tract transitional epithelium contains a transmembrane protein that is unique to transitional epithelium. In studies performed thus far, the uroplakins are highly specific for transitional epithelium, with moderate sensitivity,[312, 313] and are not seen in squamous epithelial tissue.

Gross Cystic Disease Fluid Protein

Originally described by Pearlman and colleagues[314] and Haagensen and associates,[315] the prolactin-inducing protein identified by Murphy and coworkers[316] has the same amino acid sequence as GCDFP-15 and is found in abundance in breast cystic fluid and any cell type that has apocrine features.[317–319] The latter, in addition to breast, includes acinar structures in salivary glands, apocrine glands, sweat glands, Paget's disease of skin, vulva, and prostate.[320–324]

Aside from these immunoreactivities, most other carcinomas show no appreciable immunostaining.[324]

The positive predictive value for GCDFP-15 and specificity are both 99%.[324] The sensitivity for the monoclonal antibody clone D6 (Cambridge Research Laboratories, Cambridge, MA) has been reported to be as high as 74%,[324] but the experience of others has been closer to 40 to 50%.[320] Similar results are obtained with the use of antibody BRST-2 (Signet Laboratories, Inc., Dedham, MA).

Since the specificity of GCDFP antibodies for breast carcinoma is so high, this antibody is often used in a screening panel in the appropriate clinical situation, which often turns out to be the presentation of a woman with MUP or a new lung mass in a patient with a history of breast cancer. Others have demonstrated the utility and specificity of GCDFP-15 antibodies in the distinction of breast carcinoma metastatic in the lung.[325, 326]

KEY DIFFERENTIAL DIAGNOSTIC POINTS OF METASTATIC BREAST CARCINOMA

- GCDFP-15 has 99% specificity; 50% sensitivity for breast carcinoma
- Metastatic breast carcinoma in lung
  Breast: GCDFP-15+/−, TTF-1 (N), CEAD-14 (R-N)
  Lung carcinoma: GCDFP-15 (N), TTF-1+, CEAD-14+

Melan-A and Inhibin in Adrenocortical Tumors

Melan-A, a product of the MART-1 gene, is an antigen recognized by antibody A-103, and although its primary utility is in the identification of melanoma cells, it also identifies more than half of adrenocortical neoplasms, especially carcinomas.[327–331] Like inhibin, it also reacts with some sex cord–stromal tumors.[306] The A-103 antibody is more specific for adrenocortical tumors because it does not react with other carcinomas, whereas inhibin is more sensitive.[330] More studies need to be performed on adrenal carcinomas with antibodies to inhibin. However, if melanoma is excluded as a diagnostic possibility, a positive A-103 immunostain is strong evidence in favor of an adrenocortical carcinoma.[329]

CD5

CD5 is a 67-kd glycoprotein receptor that may be present on a variety of T lymphocytes and mantle zone lymphocytes.[332] Hishima and colleagues[333] found CD5 expression in thymic carcinoma, and subsequent reports verified and expanded those findings. In the studies published, the clones of antibodies used include NCL-CD5 (CD5/54/B4),[334, 335] with sensitivities of 29 to 67% for immunostaining of thymic carcinomas[334, 336]; for clone NCL-CD5-4C7, sensitivities of 62 to 100%[336, 337] are reported. For mediastinal carcinomas, the usual differential diagnosis includes metastatic squamous carcinoma and other poorly differentiated metastatic lung carcinomas and germ cell tumors, none of which immunostains with clone NCL-CD5-4C7[337] (Fig. 7–12). Although some normal epithelia and carcinomas of gastrointestinal, breast, and urologic sites react with this clone, this fact is largely irrelevant to the focused study on the mediastinum.[337] A positive CD5 mediastinal tumor is strong evidence for thymic carcinoma, although some atypical thymomas and thymic carcinomas arising in a thymoma are also positive.[337, 338] Spindle cell carcinomas have been nonreactive with CD5 antibody.[339]

KEY DIAGNOSTIC POINTS OF CD5

- Positive in the majority of thymic carcinomas of most histologic types, except spindle cell variants
- Negative in spindle cell thymic carcinoma
- Lung carcinomas are largely negative for CD5

Metastatic Carcinoma in the Pleura Versus Epithelial Mesothelioma

As discussed in the opening of this chapter, the anatomic site of metastasis of a neoplasm is a good starting point in determining the origin of the neoplasm. Neoplasms metastatic to the pleura are most often due to primary lung carcinomas, but may be due to carcinomas originating in other anatomic sites. Therefore, the differential diagnosis of a malignant epithelial neoplasm in the pleura includes metastatic lung carcinoma, metastatic nonpulmonary carcinoma, and malignant mesothelioma.

The single best antibody to use to make the discrimination between lung carcinoma and mesothelioma is TTF-1, which has a high sensitivity and very high specificity for lung carcinomas, especially adenocarcinoma, non–small cell carcinoma, and small cell carcinoma.[272, 274, 276] In addition, CK5/CK6, which is largely restricted to mesothelial cells, may stain lung carcinomas and nonpulmonary carcinomas to a focal degree. A discussion of additional antibodies and complete antibody panels that may be useful in this discrimination follows.

CARCINOEMBRYONIC ANTIGEN

The antibody clones CEJO65, A5B7, and D14 are positive in up to 95% of lung carcinomas and nonpulmonary carcinomas, except those of prostate, kidney, breast, and liver.[340]

B72.3

The B72.3 antibody reacts with tumor-associated glycoprotein, which is commonly expressed in a wide variety of adenocarcinomas and, with current techniques, reacts only focally with 2 to 5% of mesotheliomas.[341–346]

LeuM1

LeuM1 is a cluster designate that reacts with the Lewis (x) antigen and was reported by Sheibani

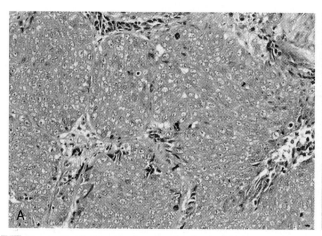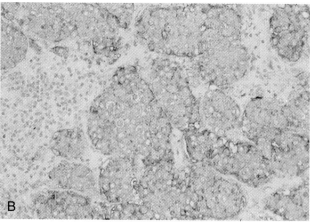

Figure 7–12. Carcinoma in the lung *(A)* in a patient with a history of thymic carcinoma proved to be CD5+ *(B)*, consistent with metastasis to the lung.

and colleagues in 1986 to react mostly with adeno-carcinomas.[347] More recent studies demonstrate immunoreactivity in the range of 70 to 75% for adeno-carcinomas from all sites, whereas positive staining is seen in 2 to 10% of mesotheliomas.[344, 345, 348–351]

BG8

BG8 is an anti-Lewis (y) antibody, described by Jordon and colleagues[352] in 1989, that was shown to react predominantly with adenocarcinomas of the lung and focally or weakly with epithelial meso-theliomas. A further study by Riera and cowork-ers[345] confirmed immunostaining in 93% of lung adenocarcinomas, with only focal or weak staining in 9% of epithelial mesotheliomas.

BerEP4

The monoclonal antibody BerEP4 has stirred some controversy regarding its utility in separating lung adenocarcinomas from mesothelioma because of the wide variation of interpretation of a positive result.[353–355] More recent work[355] demonstrates diffuse positive staining in 92% of pulmonary adeno-carcinomas and focal or weak immunostaining in 26% of mesotheliomas. In the same study, BerEP4 staining of nonpulmonary adenocarcinomas was erratic, and as a result it was considered to be a poor discriminator between mesothelioma and non-pulmonary adenocarcinomas.

MOC31

Reacting with a 38-kd membrane glycoprotein, MOC31 reacts with 89 to 98% of adenocarcinomas of various origins, typically with strong staining patterns.[351, 356–360] Only 5% of mesotheliomas show focal or weak staining.[360]

CALRETININ

Calretinin is a 29-kd intracellular calcium-binding protein that has been described in a variety of cells, including neurons, steroid-producing cells, renal convoluted tubules, eccrine glands, thymic keratinized cells, and mesothelial cells.[361, 362] There has been a difference in immunostaining results depending on the antibody used, with the greater specificity seen with the Zymed clone.[363] Calretinin staining in adenocarcinomas in various sites is almost always focal or weak.

To summarize, the recommended panels of immunostains based on ability to discriminate between adenocarcinomas (including lung) metastatic to the pleura and epithelial mesothelioma include TTF-1, calretinin, CK5/CK6, CEA, MOC31, B72.3, and BG8.[100, 364] Additional antibodies that may be useful, but have lower sensitivities or specificities include LeuM1, Ber-EP4, and thrombomodu-lin.[365]

KEY DIAGNOSTIC POINTS OF METASTATIC CARCINOMA IN PLEURA VERSUS EPITHELIAL MESOTHELIOMA

- TTF-1+ in lung carcinomas, TTF-1− in other carcinomas and mesothelioma
- CK5/CK6+ in epithelial mesothelioma, (R-N) in lung carcinomas, −/+ in other carcinomas—chiefly squamous, transitional, and ovarian carcinomas
- Calretinin+ in epithelial mesothelioma
- CEA, MOC31, B72.3, BG8 all − in mesothelioma, +/− in adenocarcinomas
- Possible useful adjuncts: LeuM1, BerEP4, thrombomodulin

HORMONE RECEPTORS (ESTROGEN/PROGESTERONE)

Intuitively, it would seem as though the estrogen receptor/progesterone receptor (ER/PR) would be confined to hormone-responsive tissues such as breast, but even the recent literature on this topic is controversial. Although some authors conclude that ER/PR is found only in subsets of breast carcinomas and carcinomas of the ovary and endometrium,[325, 366, 367] others have observed mostly ER, and rarely PR, in carcinomas of the lung,[368–372] stomach, and thyroid.

Vargas and colleagues[372] demonstrated the estrogen-related protein p29 in 98% of non–small cell lung cancers by IHC, suggesting that the estrogen axis may be important in this group of malignancies. In the study by Vargas and associates, these same tumors were all negative with the commercially available antibody ER1D5 (DAKO, Carpinteria, CA). Survival of this group of patients differed for men versus women, suggesting some gender-specific p29-associated factor influence.

In a personal study (D. Dabbs, unpublished observations), ER was observed using antibody 6F11 (Ventana, Tucson, AZ) with HIER in 67% of lung adenocarcinomas, but no immunostaining of the same carcinomas was seen with ER1D5. As a result of these findings, I am reluctant to use the presence of ER in an adenocarcinoma of lung as definitive evidence of a metastatic breast carcinoma with antibody ER6F11. Other investigators have arrived at the same conclusion regarding the low specificity of ER in carcinomas of unknown primary.[366]

PAGET'S DISEASE

Paget's disease occurs as a mammary form and extramammary (EM) form. Paget's disease of the breast is almost always indicative of an underlying breast carcinoma,[373–375] whereas EM Paget's disease may be an indicator of metastatic carcinoma.

Paget's disease of the breast manifests as CK7+

malignant cells infiltrating the epidermis of the nipple. Tumor cells are conspicuous by their infiltrative "shotgun" pattern, large size, abundant cytoplasm, signet ring forms, and, sometimes, mucin positivity. Epidermal keratinocytes are negative with CK7. Most Paget's cases are CK7+, GCDFP-15+, and CEA+, characteristic of breast, but occasional cases may be CK7− (Fig. 7–13). Toker cells are CK7+ and may be present in the skin of the normal nipple, but generally they are inconspicuous compared with Paget cells[376] and should not cause diagnostic problems.

The Paget cells may be assessed for ER[377] or the neu-oncoprotein.[378]

The EM forms of Paget's disease occur predominantly in females as vulvar or perianal disease but may also occur in males and at other sites.

Primary vulvar Paget's disease is a localized carcinoma of sweat duct origin that may be in situ or invasive; histologically, it is composed of large cytoplasmic cells that are mucin-positive and universally CK7+ and GCDFP-15+.[316]

The extravulvar form of the disease presents in the perianal areas as metastatic disease from sites that may include the rectum or urinary bladder.[316] Therefore, the diagnostic problem inherent with a histologic diagnosis of extravulvar Paget's disease is the differential diagnosis of adnexal skin neoplasm versus metastatic carcinoma from rectum or urinary bladder.

Colorectal carcinomas presenting as Paget's disease are often mucin-positive with signet ring forms and intraluminal "dirty" necrosis[320]; they are GCDFP-15−, CEA+, strongly positive for CK20, and may be focally or weakly positive for CK7.[316–323]

Transitional cell carcinomas are strongly positive for both CK7 and CK20; they are GCDFP-15− and they lack signet cells or mucin and may immunostain with uroplakin antibody.

KEY DIAGNOSTIC POINTS

Mammary Paget's Disease
- CK7+, GCDFP-15+, CEA+, CEAD-14 (R-N)

Vulvar Paget's Disease, Primary Adnexal Carcinoma
- CK7+, GCDFP-15+, CEA+/−

Metastatic Colorectal Carcinoma Presenting as Perianal-Vulvar Paget's Disease
- CK7 (N-R), CK 20+, CEA+, GCDFP-15 (N)

Metastatic Transitional Carcinoma Presenting as Perianal-Vulvar Paget's Disease
- CK7+, CK20+, GCDFP-15 (N), CEA−/+

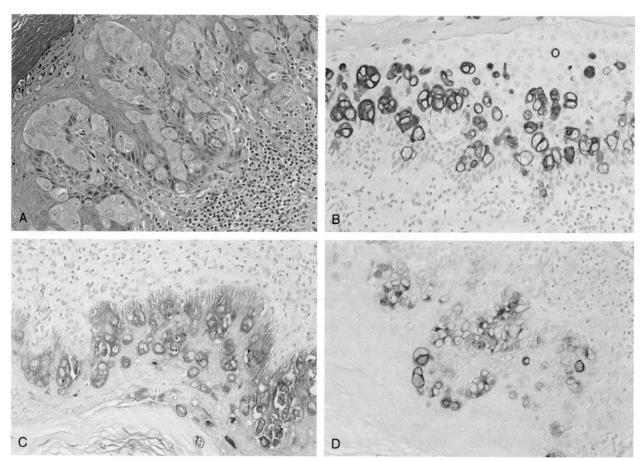

Figure 7–13. A typical case of primary perineal Paget's disease *(A)* is CK7+ *(B)*, CEA+ *(C)*, and GCDFP-15+ *(D)*.

Table 7–11. Useful Diagnostic Antibody Panels

	Antibody		
	Breast	*Versus Lung*	*Versus Liver*
CK7	+	+	−
AE1/AE3	+	+	R-N
CEAD-14	R-N	+	N
GCDFP-15	+/−	N	N
TTF-1	N	+	N
Colon			
CK7	N-R	+	N
CK20	+	N-R	N
TTF-1	N	+	N
Pancreatobiliary			
CK7	+	+	N
CK20	+	N	N
CEA	+	+	N
Prostate			
PSA	+	N	N
PSMA	+	N	N
CEAD-14	N	+	N
pCEA	N	+	+/−c*
Renal Cell			
AE1/AE3	+	+	N-R
CEA	N	+	N
TTF-1	N	+	N
Bladder TCC			
CK7	+	+	N
CK20	+	N	N
Seminoma			
CAM5.2	N-R	+	+
AE1/AE3	N	+	N-R
PLAP	+	N	N
EMA	N	+	−/+
Nonseminoma			
AE1/AE3	+	+	N-R
TTF-1	N	+	N
CK7	+/−	+	N
PLAP	+	N	N
Thyroid			
TTF-1	+	+	N
CEA	N	+	N
Thymus			
CD5	+/−	N	N
TTF-1	N	+	N
CEA	−/+	+	N
Endometrium			
CEAD-14	N	+	N
Vimentin	+/−	−/+	N
AE1/AE3	+	+	N-R
Endocervix			
CEAD-14	N	+	N
AE1/AE3	+	+	N-R
pCEA	+/−	+	+/−c*

Small Cell Carcinoma Lung	*Versus*	*Nonpulmonary Small Cell*	*Versus*	*Merkel Cell*
CK7	−/+	+/−		N
CK20	N	N		+
TTF-1	+	−/+		N
Synaptophysin	+	+		+
Chromogranin	−/+	−/+		+/−
CEA	+/−	+/−		N
NSE	+	+		+

* Canalicular pattern.

GCDFP-15, gross cystic disease fluid protein fraction 15; TTF-1, thyroid transcription factor 1; CEA, carcinoembryonic antigen; PSA, prostate-specific antigen; PSMA, prostate-specific membrane antigen; pCEA, polyclonal carcinoembryonic antigen; PLAP, placenta-like alkaline phosphatase; EMA, epithelial membrane antigen; NSE, neuron-specific enolase.

+, almost always positive; +/−, mostly positive; −/+, mostly negative; R, rare positive cells; N, negative.

Table 7–12. Key Screening Antibodies for Undifferentiated Malignancy

	CAM5.2	Epithelial Membrane Antigen	S-100	Leukocyte Common Antigen	Placenta-Like Alkaline Phosphatase
Carcinoma	+	+	−/+	N	−/+
Melanoma	N	N	+	N	N
Lymphoma	N	N	N	+	N
Nonseminoma	+	N	N	N	+
Germ cell seminoma	R-N	N	N	N	+

SUMMARY

By working closely with the clinician who performs a careful clinical history and assessment, the pathologist should develop a working differential diagnosis based on tumor location or radiologic assessment of the tumor, or both. This information is key to utilizing IHC as a cost-effective tool in patient care. Tables 7–10 to 7–12 summarize useful antibody panels for the diagnostic work-up of MUP.

References

1. Rosai J. Author's response to a letter. Am J Surg Pathol 1999;23:491.
2. Hammar SP. Metastatic adenocarcinoma of unknown primary origin. Hum Pathol 1998;29:1393–1402.
3. Greco F, Hainsworth J. The management of patients with adenocarcinoma of unknown primary site. Semin Oncol 1989;6(Suppl 6):116–122.
4. Haskel CM, Cochran AJ, Barsky SH. Metastasis of unknown origin. Curr Probl Cancer 1988;12:5–58.
5. Krementz ET, Cerise EJ, Foster DS, et al. Metastases of undetermined source. Curr Probl Cancer 1979;4:4–37.
6. Schapira DV, Jerrett AR. The need to consider survival, outcome, and expense when evaluating and treating patients with unknown primary carcinoma. Arch Intern Med 1995;155:2050–2054.
7. Putti T, Win K, Choi Y, et al. Cost effectiveness of immunohistochemistry in surgical pathology. Am J Clin Pathol 1998;110:512A.
8. Steckel RJ, Kagan AR. Metastatic tumors of unknown origin. Cancer 1991;67:1242–1244.
9. Kagan AR, Steckel RJ. The limited role of radiologic imaging in patients with unknown primary tumor. Semin Oncol 1991;18:170–173.
10. Jonk A, Kroon BB, Rumke P, et al. Lymph node metastasis from melanoma with unknown primary site. Br J Surg 1990;77:665–666.
11. Le-Chevalier T, Cvitkivic E, Caille P, et al. Early metastatic cancer of unknown primary origin at presentation: A clinical study of 302 consecutive autopsy patients. Arch Intern Med 1988;148:2035–2039.
12. Kirsten F, Chi CH, Leary JA, et al. Metastatic adeno or undifferentiated carcinoma from an unknown primary site—natural history and guidelines for identification of treatable subsets. Q J Med 1987;62:143–161.
13. Van der Gaast A, Verwei J, Plantane AS, et al. The value of immunocytochemistry in patients with poorly differentiated adenocarcinomas and undifferentiated carcinomas of unknown primary. J Cancer Res Clin Oncol 1996;122:181–185.
14. Greco FA, Hainsworth JD. Poorly differentiated carcinoma or adenocarcinoma of unknown primary site: Long term results with cisplatin based chemotherapy. Semin Oncol 1994;21:77–82.
15. Greco FA, Hainsworth JD. The management of patients with adenocarcinoma and poorly differentiated carcinoma of unknown primary site. Semin Oncol 1989;16:116–122.
16. Matthews P, Ellis IO. Use of immunocytochemistry in a diagnosis of metastatic carcinoma. Ann Med 1996;28:38–44.
17. Mackay B, Ordonez NG. Pathologic evaluation of neoplasms with unknown primary tumor site. Semin Oncol 1993;20:206–228.
18. Osteen RT, Kopf G, Wilson RE. In pursuit of the unknown primary. Am J Surg 1978;135:494.
19. Ayoub JP, Hess KR, Abbruzzese MC, et al. Unknown primary tumors metastatic to liver. J Clin Oncol 1998;16:2105–2112.
20. Guthrie THJ. Treatable carcinoma of unknown origin. Am J Med 1989;298:74–78.
21. Hainsworth JD, Greco FA. Managing carcinomas of unknown primary site. Oncology (Williston Park). 1988;2:439–524.
22. Lenzi R, Hess KR, Abbruzzese MC, et al. Poorly differentiated carcinoma and poorly differentiated adenocarcinoma of unknown origin: Favorable subsets of patients with unknown-primary carcinoma. J Clin Oncol 1997;15:2056–2066.
23. Perchalski JE, Hall KL, Dewar MA. Metastasis of unknown origin. Prim Care 1992;19:747–757.
24. Haskell CM, Cochran AJ, Barski SH, et al. Current problems in cancer. Cancer 1988;2:5–58.
25. Jakobsen JH, Johanssen J, Jurgensen KE. Neck lymph node metastases from an unknown primary tumor. Ugeskr Laeger 1991;153:428–430.
26. Hainsworth JD, Greco FA. Poorly differentiated carcinoma and poorly differentiated adenocarcinoma of unknown primary tumor site. Semin Oncol 1993;20:279–286.
27. Hainsworth JD, Wright EP, Johnson DH, et al. Poorly differentiated carcinoma of unknown primary site: Clinical usefulness of immunoperoxidase staining. J Clin Oncol 1991;9:1931–1938.
28. Huebner G, Tamme C, Schouber C, et al. Prognostically different subgroups in patients with carcinoma of unknown primary. J Chemother Infect Dis Malig 1989;1:816.
29. Kambhu SA, Kelsen DP, Fiore J, et al. Metastatic adenocarcinomas of unknown primary site: Prognostic variables and treatment results. Am J Clin Oncol 1990;13:55–60.
30. Gil GM, Vadell NC, Fabregat X, et al. Yield of diagnostic tests in neoplasms of unknown origin: A retrospective study. Rev Clin Esp 1990;186:252–258.
31. Romeu J, Texido A, Rosell R, et al. Carcinoma of unknown origin: Diagnostic study of 48 cases and its clinical yield. Med Clin (Barc) 1989;92:201–206.
32. Renshaw AA, Pinkus GS, Corson JM. CD34 and AE1/AE3 diagnostic discriminates in a distinction of solitary fibrous tumor of the pleura from sarcomatoid mesothelioma. Appl Immunohistochem 1994;2:94–102.
33. Cho KR, Epstein JI. Metastatic prostatic carcinoma to supradiaphragmatic lymph nodes: A clinicopathologic and immunohistochemical study. Am J Surg Pathol 1987;11:457–463.
34. Nguyen C, Shenouda G, Black MJ, et al. Metastatic squamous cell carcinoma to cervical lymph nodes from unknown primary mucosal sites. Head Neck 1994;16:58–63.

35. Willis D, Brown PW, Roger A. Adenocarcinoma from an unknown primary presenting in women with an axillary mass. Clin Oncol (R Coll Radiol) 1990;2:189–192.
36. Ringenberg QS, Doll DC, Loy TS, et al. Malignant ascites of unknown origin. Cancer 1989;64:753–755.
37. Sears D, Hajdu SI. The cytologic diagnosis of malignant neoplasms in pleura and peritoneal effusions. Acta Cytol 1987;31:85–97.
38. Rougraff BT, Kneisl JS, Simon MA. Skeletal metastases of unknown origin: A prospective study of a diagnostic strategy J Bone Joint Surg Am 1993;75:1276–1281.
39. Pisharodi LR, Lavoie R, Bedrossian CW. Differential diagnostic dilemmas in malignant fine needle aspirates of liver: A practical approach to final diagnosis. Diagn Cytopathol 1995;12:364–371.
40. Perry A, Parisi JE, Kurtin PJ. Metastatic adenocarcinoma to the brain: An immunohistochemical approach. Hum Pathol 1997;28:938–943.
41. Perry A, White C. Colon biopsies of metastatic neoplasms in central nervous system: The surgical pathologist's prospective. Brain Pathol 1994;4:435.
42. Debevec M. Management of patients with brain metastases of unknown origin. Neoplasma 1990;37:601–606.
43. Merchutt MP. Brain metastases from undiagnosed systemic neoplasms. Arch Intern Med 1989;149:1076–1080.
44. Nussbaum ES, Djalilian A, Cho KH, et al. Brain metastases: Histology, multiplicity, surgery and survival. Cancer 1996;15:1781–1788.
45. Nguyen LN, Maor MH, Oswald MJ. Brain metastases as the only manifestation of an undetected primary tumor. Cancer 1998;15:2181–2184.
46. Lagerwaard FJ, Levendag PC, Nowak PJ, et al. Identification of prognostic factors in patients with brain metastases: A review of 1292 patients. Int J Radiat Oncol Biol Phys 1999;1:793–803.
47. Martelli G, Pilotti S, Lepara P, et al. Fine needle aspiration cytology and superficial lymph nodes: Analysis of 266 cases. Eur J Surg Oncol 1989;15:13–16.
48. Lai CR, Pan CC, Tsay SH. Contribution of immunocytochemistry in routine diagnostic cytology. Diagn Cytopathol 1996;14:221–225.
49. DiBonito L, Falconieri G, Colautti I, et al. The positive peritoneal effusion: A retrospective study of cytopathologic diagnoses with autopsy confirmation. Acta Cytol 1993;37:483–488.
50. Bedrossian CW. Special stains: The old and the new: The impact of immunocytochemistry in effusion cytology. Diagn Cytopathol 1998;18:141–149.
51. Longatto FA, Bisi H, Alves VA, et al. Adenocarcinoma in females detected in serous effusions: Cytomorphologic aspects and immunocytochemical reactivity to cytokeratins 7 and 20. Acta Cytol 1997;41:961–971.
52. Lidang JM, Johansen P. Immunocytochemical staining of serous effusions: An additional method in the routine cytology practice? Cytopathology 1994;5:93–103.
53. Bonnefoi H, Smith IE. How should cancer presenting as a malignant pleural effusion be managed? Br J Cancer 1996;74:832–835.
54. Ascoli V, Taccogna S, Scalzo CC, et al. Utility of cytokeratin 20 in identifying the origin of metastatic carcinomas and effusions. Diagn Cytopathol 1995;12:303–308.
55. Moll R. Cytokeratins in the histological diagnosis of malignant tumors. Int J Biol Markers 1994;9:63–69.
56. Miettinin M. Keratin immunohistochemistry: Update of applications and pitfalls. Pathol Annu 1993;1:113–143.
57. Quinlan RA, Schiller DL, Hatzfeld M, et al. Patterns of expression and organization of cytokeratin intermediate filaments. Ann NY Acad Sci 1985;455:282–306.
58. Moll R, Franke WW, Schiller DL, et al. The catalog of human cytokeratins: Patterns of expression in normal epithelia, tumors and cultured cells. Cell 1982;31:11–24.
59. Schaafsma HE, Ramaekers FCS. Cytokeratin subtyping in normal and neoplastic epithelium: Basic principles in diagnostic applications. Pathol Annu 1994;29(Part 1):21–62.
60. Rosenberg M, Fuchs E, LeBeau M, et al. Three epidermal and one simple epithelial type II keratin genes mapped to
61. Rosenberg M, Chaudhury A, Shows TB, et al. A group of type I keratin genes on human chromosome 17: Characterization and expression. Mol Cell Biol 1988;8:722–726.
62. Romano V, Bosco P, Rocchi M, et al. Chromosomal assignments of human type I and type II cytokeratin genes to different chromosomes. Cytogenet Cell Genet 1988;48:148–153.
63. Franke WW, Schmidt E, Schiller DL, et al. Differentiation related patterns of expression of proteins of intermediate size in tissues and cultured cells. Cold Spring Harbor Symp Quant Biol 1982;46:431–445.
64. Wang MP, Zee S, Zarbo RJ, et al. Coordinate expression of cytokeratin 7 and 20 defines unique subsets of carcinomas. Appl Immunohistochem 1995;3:99–107.
65. Stasik PC, Purkis PE, Laigh IN, et al. Keratin 19: Predicted amino acid sequence and broad tissue distribution suggest evolution from keratinocyte keratins. J Invest Dermatol 1989;92:707.
66. Bartek J, Bartkoba J, Taylor-Papadimitriou J, et al. Differential expression of keratin 19 in normal human epithelial tissues revealed by monospecific monoclonal antibodies. Histochem J 1986;18:656.
67. Van Niekerk CC, Jap PHK, Ramakers FCS, et al. Immunohistochemical demonstration of keratin 7 in routinely fixed paraffin embedded human tissues. J Pathol 1991;165:145–152.
68. Ramakers F, Van Niekerk C, Poels L, et al. Use of monoclonal antibodies to keratin 7 and the differential diagnosis of adenocarcinomas. Am J Pathol 1990;136:641–655.
69. Loy TS, Calaluce RD. Utility of cytokeratin immunostaining in separating pulmonary adenocarcinomas from colonic adenocarcinomas. Am J Clin Pathol 1994;102:764–767.
70. Van de Molengraft FJJM, Van Niekerk CC, Jap PHK, et al. OV-TL 12/30 (keratin 7 antibody) is a marker of glandular differentiation in lung cancer. Histopathology 1993;22:35–38.
71. Prayson RA, Hart WR, Petras RE. Pseudomyxoma peritonei: A clinicopathologic study of 19 cases with emphasis on site of origin and nature of associated ovarian tumors. Am J Surg Pathol 1994;18:591–603.
72. Ronnett BM, Shmookler BM, Diener-West M, et al. Immunohistochemical evidence supporting the appendiceal origin of pseudomyxoma peritonei in women. Int J Gyn Pathol 1997;16:1–9.
73. Ronnett BM, Kurman RJ, Shmookler BM, et al. The morphologic spectrum of ovarian metastases of appendiceal adenocarcinomas: A clinicopathologic and immunohistochemical analysis of tumors often misinterpreted as primary ovarian tumors or metastatic tumors. Am J Surg Pathol 1997;21:1144–1155.
74. Loy TS, Calaluce RD, Keeney GL. Cytokeratin immunostaining in differentiating primary ovarian carcinoma from metastatic colonic adenocarcinoma. Mod Pathol 1996;9:1040–1044.
75. Guerrieri C, Franlund B, Boeryd B. Expression of cytokeratin 7 in simultaneous mucinous tumors of the ovary and appendix. Mod Pathol 1995;8:573–576.
76. Berezowski K, Stastny J, Kornstein MJ. Cytokeratin 7 and 20 and carcinoembryonic antigen in ovarian and colonic carcinoma. Mod Pathol 1996;9:426–429.
77. Ueda G, Sawada M, Ogawa H, et al. Immunohistochemical study of cytokeratin 7 for the differential diagnosis of adenocarcinomas in the ovary. Gynecol Oncol 1993;51:219–223.
78. Ramakers F, Huysmans A, Schaart G, et al. Tissue distribution of keratin 7 as monitored by a monoclonal antibody. Exp Cell Res 1987;170:235–249.
79. Osborne M, VanLessen G, Weber K, et al. Methods in laboratory investigation: Differential diagnosis of gastrointestinal carcinomas by using monoclonal antibody specific for individual keratin polypeptides. Lab Invest 1986;55:497.
80. Miettinen M, Fetsch JF. Keratin 7 reactivity in endothelial

cells: A potential pitfall in diagnostic immunohistochemistry. Appl Immunohistochem 1997;5:229–233.

81. VanEyken P, Sciot R, Brock B, et al. Abundant expression of cytokeratin 7 in fibrolamellar carcinoma of the liver. Histopathology 1990;17:101–106.

82. Moll R, Schiller DL, Franke WW. Identification of protein IT of the intestinal cytoskeleton as a novel type I cytokeratin with unusual properties and expression patterns. J Cell Biol 1990;111:567.

83. Miettinen M. Keratin 20: Immunohistochemical marker for gastrointestinal, urothelial and Merkel cell carcinomas. Mod Pathol 1995;8:384–388.

84. Moll R, Zimbelmann R, Goldschmidt MD, et al. The human gene in coding cytokeratin 20 and its expression during fetal development and in gastrointestinal carcinomas. Differentiation 1993;53:75–93.

85. Moll R, Lowe A, Laufer J, et al. Cytokeratin 20 in human carcinomas: A new histodiagnostic marker detected by monoclonal antibodies. Am J Pathol 1992;140:427–447.

86. Tot T. Adenocarcinomas metastatic to the liver: The value of cytokeratins 20 and 7 in the search for unknown primary tumors. Cancer 1999;85:171–177.

87. Delgado Y, Melamed J, Feiner H. Expression of cytokeratins 7 and 20 in 87 breast cancers. Am J Clin Pathol 1998; 110:517A.

88. Fischer HP, Altmannsberger M, Wilber K, et al. Keratin polypeptides in malignant epithelial liver tumors: Differential diagnosis and histogenetic aspects. Am J Pathol 1987;127:530.

89. VanEyken P, Sciot R, Paterson A, et al. Cytokeratin expression in hepatocellular carcinoma: An immunohistochemical study. Hum Pathol 1988;19:562.

90. Kim M-K, Park CK. Variable cytokeratin 7/20 profiles in carcinomas involving the liver. Appl Immunohistochem Mol Morphol 1999;7:52–57.

91. Makhlouf HR, Ishak KG, Goodman ZD. Epithelioid hemangioendothelioma of the liver: A clinicopathologic study of 137 cases. Cancer 1999;85:562–582.

92. Nandedkar MA, Palazzo J, Abbondanzo SL, et al. CD45 (leukocyte common antigen) immunoreactivity in metastatic undifferentiated and neuroendocrine carcinoma: A potential diagnostic pitfall. Mod Pathol 1998;11:1204–1210.

93. Millward C, Weidner N. CD 30 (Ber-H2) expression in non-hemopoietic tumors. Appl Immunohistochem 1998;6: 164–168.

94. Gown AM, Vogel AM. Anti-intermediate filament monoclonal antibodies: Tissue specific tools in tumor diagnosis. Surv Synth Pathol 1984;3:369–385.

95. Gown AM, Vogel AM. Monoclonal antibodies to human intermediate filament proteins. II: Distribution of filament proteins in normal human tissues. Am J Pathol 1984;114: 309–321.

96. Gown AM, Vogel AM. Monoclonal antibodies to human intermediate filament proteins. III: Analysis of tumors. Am J Clin Pathol 1985;84:413–424.

97. Santeusanio G, D'Alfonso V, Lafrte E, et al. Antibodies to cytokeratin 14 specifically identify oncocytes (Hürthle cells) in thyroid lesions and tumors. Appl Immunohistochem 1997;5:223–228.

98. Cover J, Oates J, Edwards C. Anti-cytokeratin 5-6: A positive marker for epithelioid mesothelioma. Histopathology 1997;31:140–143.

99. Gotzos V, Fogt P, Celio MR. The calcium binding protein calretinin is a selective marker for malignant pleural mesotheliomas of the epithelial type. Pathol Res Pract 1996;192:137–147.

100. Ordonez NG. Value of cytokeratin 5/6 immunostaining in distinguishing epithelial mesothelioma of the pleura from lung adenocarcinoma. Am J Surg Pathol 1998;22:1215–1221.

101. Argani P, Rosai J. Hyperplastic mesothelial cells in lymph nodes: Report of 6 cases of a benign process that can simulate metastatic involvement by mesothelioma or carcinoma. Hum Pathol 1998;29:339–346.

102. Miettinen M. Keratin subsets in spindle cell sarcomas: Keratins are widespread but synovial sarcoma contains a distinctive keratin polypeptide pattern and desmoplakins. Am J Pathol 1991;138:505–513.

103. Miettinen M. Keratin immunohistochemistry: Update of applications and pitfalls. Pathol Annu 1993;28:113–143.

104. Miettinen M. Immunoreactivity for cytokeratin and epithelial membrane antigen in leiomyosarcomas. Arch Pathol Lab Med 1988;112:637–640.

105. Litzky LA, Brooks JJ. Cytokeratin immunoreactivity in malignant fibrous histiocytoma and spindle cell tumors: Comparison between frozen and paraffin embedded tissues. Mod Pathol 1992;5:30–34.

106. Rosenberg AE, O'Connell JX, Dickerson GR, et al. Expression of epithelial markers in malignant fibrous histiocytoma of the musculoskeletal system: An immunohistochemical and electron microscopic study. Hum Pathol 1993;24:284–293.

107. Hazelbag HM, Mooi WJ, Fleuren GJ, et al. Chain specific keratin profile of epithelioid soft tissue sarcomas: An immunohistochemical study on synovial sarcoma and epithelioid sarcoma. Appl Immunohistochem 1996;4:176–183.

108. Alobeid B, Brooks JJ, Zhang PJ. Cytokeratin subset immunoreactivity in sarcomas using a large panel of cytokeratin subset antibodies. Appl Immunohistochem 1998;6:154–157.

109. Zarbo RJ, Gown AM, Nagel RB, et al. Anomalous cytokeratin expression in malignant melanoma: One and two dimensional Western blot analysis and immunohistochemical survey of 100 melanomas. Mod Pathol 1990;3:494–501.

110. Traweek ST, Liu J, Battifora H. Keratin gene expression in non-epithelial tissues: Detection with polymerase chain reaction. Am J Pathol 1993;142:1111–1118.

111. Swanson PE. Heffalumps, jagulars and cheshire cats. Am J Clin Pathol 1991;95:S2–S7.

112. Alobeid B, Brooks JJ, Zhang PJ. Aberrant cytokeratin subset immunoreactivity in sarcomas using a large panel of cytokeratin subset antibodies. Appl Immunohistochem 1998;6:154–157.

113. Rizeq MN, Van De Rijn M, Hendrickson MR, et al. A comparative immunohistochemical study of uterine smooth muscle neoplasms with emphasis on the epithelioid variant. Hum Pathol 1994;25:671–677.

114. Brown DC, Theaker JM, Banks PM, et al. Cytokeratin expression in smooth muscle and smooth muscle tumors. Histopathology 1987;11:477.

115. Miettinen M, Rapola J. Immunohistochemical spectrum of rhabdomyosarcoma and rhabdomyosarcoma-like tumors: Expression of cytokeratin and the 68kD neurofilament protein. Am J Surg Pathol 1989;13:120–126.

116. Hirose T, Kudo E, Hasegawa T, et al. Expression of intermediate filaments in malignant fibrous histiocytomas. Hum Pathol 1989;20:871–877.

117. Jones HJ, Anthony PP. Metastatic prostatic carcinoma presenting as left-sided cervical lymphadenopathy: A series of 11 cases. Histopathology 1992;21:149–154.

118. Fletcher CD, Beham A, Bekir S, et al. Epithelioid angiosarcoma of deep soft tissue: A distinctive tumor readily mistaken for an epithelial neoplasm. Am J Surg Pathol 1991; 15:915–922.

119. Eusebi V, Carangiu ML, Dina R, et al. Keratin positive epithelioid angiosarcoma of thyroid: A report of four cases. Am J Surg Pathol 1990;14:737.

120. Meis-Kindblom JM, Kindblom LG. Angiosarcoma of soft tissue: A study of 80 cases. Am J Surg Pathol 1998;22: 683–697.

121. Kwaspen FH, Smedts FM, Broos A, et al. Reproducible and highly sensitive detection of the broad spectrum epithelial marker keratin 19 in routine cancer diagnosis. Histopathology 1997;31:503–516.

122. McCluggage WG, Clarke R, Toner PG. Cutaneous epithelioid angiosarcoma exhibiting cytokeratin positivity. Histopathology 1995;27:291–294.

123. Jochum W, Schroder S, Risti B, et al. Cytokeratin positive angiosarcoma of the adrenal gland. Pathologe 1994;15:181–186.

124. Goldblum JR, Weiss TW. Epithelioid angiosarcoma of the pulmonary artery. Hum Pathol 1995;26:1275–1277.

125. Hasegawa T, Fujii Y, Seki K, et al. Epithelioid angiosarcoma of bone. Hum Pathol 1997;28:985–989.

126. Gown AM, Boyd H, Chang Y, et al. Smooth muscle cells can express cytokeratins of simple epithelium: Immunocytochemical and biochemical studies in vitro and in vivo. Am J Pathol 1988;132:223.

127. Knapp AC, Franke WW. Spontaneous losses of control of cytokeratin gene expression in transformed nonepithelial human cells occurring at different levels of regulation. Cell 1989;59:67.

128. Frisman DM, McCarthy WF, Schleiff P, et al. Immunocytochemistry in the differential diagnosis of effusions: Use of logistic regression to select the panel of antibodies to distinguish adenocarcinomas from mesothelial proliferations. Mod Pathol 1993;6:179–184.

129. Ordonez NG, Tornos C. Malignant peripheral nerve sheath tumor of the pleura with epithelial and rhabdomyoblastic differentiation: Report of a case clinically simulating mesothelioma. Am J Surg Pathol 1997;21:1395–1398.

130. Banks DR, Jansen JF, Oberle E, et al. Cytokeratin positivity in fine needle aspirates of melanomas and sarcomas. Diagn Cytopathol 1995;12:230–233.

131. Rosai J, Pinkus GS. Immunohistochemical demonstration of epithelial differentiation in adamantinoma of the tibia. Am J Surg Pathol 1982;6:427.

132. Heikinheimo K, Persson S, Kindblom L-G, et al. Expression of different cytokeratin subclasses in human chordoma. J Pathol 1991;164:145.

133. Gerharz CD, Moll R, Meister P, et al. Cytoskeletal heterogeneity of an epithelioid sarcoma with expression of vimentin, cytokeratins and neurofilaments. Am J Surg Pathol 1990;14:274.

134. Battifora H, ed. Diagnostic Uses of Antibodies to Keratins: A Review and Immunohistochemical Comparison of 7 Monoclonal and 3 Polyclonal Antibodies. Philadelphia: Field and Wood, 1988.

135. Smith KJ, Skelton HG, 3rd, Morgan AM, et al. Spindle cell neoplasms coexpressing cytokeratin and vimentin. J Cutan Pathol 1992;19:286–293.

136. Mooi WJ, Deenik W, Peterse JL, et al. Keratin immunoreactivity in melanoma of soft parts (clear cell sarcoma). Histopathology 1995;27:61–65.

137. Ben-Izhak A, Stark P, Lebi R, et al. Epithelial markers in malignant melanoma: A study of primary lesions and their metastases. Am J Dermatopathol 1994;16:241–246.

138. Gatter KC, Ralfkliaer E, Skinner JM, et al. An immunocytochemical study of malignant melanoma and its differential diagnosis from other malignant tumors. J Clin Pathol 1985;38:1353–1357.

139. Miettinin M, Franssila K. Immunohistochemical spectrum of malignant melanoma: The common presence of keratin. Lab Invest 1989;61:623–629.

140. Cosgrove M, Fitzgibbons P, Scherrod A, et al. Intermediate filament expression in astrocytic neoplasms. Am J Surg Pathol 1989;13:144–145.

141. Krihl VK, Yang HY, Moskal JR, et al. Keratin expression in astrocytomas: An immunofluorescence and biochemical reassessment. Virchows Arch 1997;431:139–147.

142. Bacchi C, Zarbo RJ, Jiang JJ, et al. Do glioma cells express cytokeratin? Appl Immunohistochem 1995;3:45–53.

143. Probst-Cousin S, Villagran-Lillo R, Lahl R, et al. Secretory meningioma: Clinical, histologic, and immunohistochemical findings in 31 cases. Cancer 1997;79:2003–2015.

144. Meis J, Ordonez NG, Bruner JM. Meningiomas: An immunohistochemical study of 50 cases. Arch Pathol Lab Med 1986;110:934.

145. Artleich A, Schmidt D. Immunohistochemical profile of meningiomas and their histologic subtypes. Hum Pathol 1990;21:843.

146. Radley MG, DiSant'agnese PA, Eskin TA, et al. Epithelial differentiation in meningiomas: An immunohistochemical, histochemical and ultrastructural study—with review of the literature. Am J Clin Pathol 1989;92:26–31.

147. Gould VE, Bloom KJ, Franke WW, et al. Increased numbers of cytokeratin positive interstitial reticulum cells in reactive, inflammatory and neoplastic lymphadenopathies: Hyperplasia or induced expression? Virchows Arch 1995;425:617–629.

148. Lasota J, Hyjek E, Koo CH, et al. Cytokeratin positive large cell lymphomas of B-cell lineage: A study of five phenotypically unusual cases verified by polymerase chain reaction. Am J Surg Pathol 1996;20:346–354.

149. Cho J, Gong C, Choe G, et al. Extrafollicular reticulum cells in pathologic lymph nodes. J Korean Med Sci 1994;9:9–15.

150. Zoltowska A. Immunohistochemical comparative investigations of lymphoid tissue in reactive processes, myasthenic thymuses and Hodgkin's disease. Arch Immunol Ther Exp 1995;43:15–22.

151. Ramaekers F, Haag D, Rap P, et al. Immunochemical demonstration of keratin and vimentin in cytologic aspirates. Acta Cytol 1984;28:385–392.

152. Iuzzolino P, Bontempini L, Doglioni C, et al. Keratin immunoreactivity in extrafollicular reticular cells of the lymph node. Am J Clin Pathol 1989;91:239–240.

153. Franke WW, Moll R. Cytoskeletal components of lymphoid organs. I: Synthesis of cytokeratins 8 and 18 and desmin in subpopulations of extrafollicular reticulum cells of human lymph nodes, tonsils and spleen. Differentiation 1987;36:145–163.

154. Doglioni C, Dell'Orto P, Zanetti G, et al. Cytokeratin immunoreactive cells of lymph nodes and spleen in normal and pathologic conditions. Virchows Arch (A) 1990;416:479–490.

155. Carbone A, Manconi R, Poletti A, et al. Heterogeneous immunostaining patterns of follicular dendritic reticulum cells in human lymphoid tissue with selected antibodies reactive with different cell lineages. Hum Pathol 1988;19:51–56.

156. Battifora H, Kapinski M. The influence of protease digestion and duration of fixation on the immunostaining of keratins: A comparison of formalin and ethanol fixation. J Histochem Cytochem 1986;34:1095–1099.

157. Frierson HF, Bellafiore FJ, Gaffey MJ, et al. Cytokeratin in anaplastic large cell lymphoma. Mod Pathol 1994;7:317–321.

158. Kolarik J, Rejthar A, Lauerova L, et al. Monoclonal antibodies against individual cytokeratins in the detection of metastatic spread. Int J Cancer 1988;3:50.

159. Petruch UR, Homy H-P, Keiserling E. Frequent expression of hemopoietic and nonhemopoietic antigens by neoplastic plasma cells: An immunohistochemical study using formalin-fixed paraffin embedded tissue. Histopathology 1992;20:35.

160. Watherspoon AC, Norton AJ, Isaacson PG. Immunoreactive cytokeratins in plasmacytomas. Histopathology 1989;14:141.

161. Gastmann C, Altmannsberger M, Osborne M, et al. Cytokeratin expression and vimentin content in large cell anaplastic lymphomas and other non-Hodgkin's lymphomas. Am J Pathol 1991;138:1413.

162. Delsol G, AlSaati T, Gatter KC, et al. Coexpression of epithelial membrane antigen (EMA), Ki-1 and interleukin-2 receptor by anaplastic large cell lymphomas. Am J Pathol 1988;130:59.

163. Miettinin M. Immunostaining of intermediate filament proteins in paraffin sections: Evaluation of optimal protease treatment to improve the immunoreactivity. Pathol Res Pract 1989;184:431–435.

164. Battifora H: Assessment of antigen damage in immunohistochemistry: The vimentin internal control. Am J Clin Pathol 1991;96:669–671.

165. Ramakers FCS, Haag D, Kant A, et al. Co-expression of keratin and vimentin-type intermediate filaments in human metastatic carcinoma cells. Proc Natl Acad Sci USA 1983;80:2618–2622.

166. McNutt MA, Bolen JW, Gown AM, et al. Co-expression of intermediate filaments in human epithelial neoplasms. Ultrastruct Pathol 1985;9:31–43.

167. Geisinger KR, Dabbs DJ, Marshall RB. Malignant mixed mullerian tumors and ultrastructural and immunohistochemical analysis with histogenetic considerations. Cancer 1987;59:1781–1790.

168. Dabbs DJ, Geisinger K, Norris HT. Intermediate filaments in endometrial and endocervical carcinoma: The diagnos-

tic utility of vimentin patterns. Am J Surg Pathol 1986;10:568–576.

169. Dabbs DJ, Sturtz K, Zaino RJ. The immunohistochemical discrimination of endometrioid adenocarcinoma. Hum Pathol 1996;27:172–177.

170. Pritchard DG, Todd CW, Eghan ML. Chemistry of carcinoembryonic antigen. Methods Cancer Res 1978;14:55–85.

171. Buchegger F, Schreyer M, Correl S, et al. Monoclonal antibodies identify a CEA cross-reacting antigen of 95 KD (MCA-95) distinct in antigenicity and tissue distribution from the previously described MCA 55 KD. Int J Cancer 1984;33:643–649.

172. Nach J, Pusztaszeri G. Carcinoembryonic antigen: Demonstration of a partial identity between CEA and a normal glycoprotein. Immunochemistry 1972;9:1031–1033.

173. Svenberg T. Carcinoembryonic antigen-like substances of human bile: Isolation and partial characterization. Int J Cancer 1976;17:588–596.

174. Nagora H, Tsusumi Y, Watanabe K, et al. Immunohistochemistry of carcinoembryonic antigen, secretory component and lysozyme in benign and malignant common bile duct tissues. Virchows Arch (Pathol Anat) 1984;403:271–280.

175. Pavelic ZP, Petrelli NJ, Herrera L, et al. D-14 monoclonal antibody to carcinoembryonic antigen: Immunohistochemical analysis of formalin-fixed, paraffin embedded human colorectal carcinoma, tumors of non-colorectal origin and normal tissues. J Cancer Res Clin Oncol 1990;116:51–56.

176. Pavelic ZP, Pavelic L, Pavelic K, et al. Utility of anti-carcinoembryonic antigen monoclonal antibodies for differentiating ovarian adenocarcinomas from gastrointestinal metastasis to the ovary. Gynecol Oncol 1991;40:112–117.

177. Fabian C, Dabbs DJ. The immunohistochemical discrimination of metastatic breast carcinoma in lung. Breast J 1997;3:135–141.

178. Maeda T, Kajiyama K, Adachi E, et al. The expression of cytokeratin 7, 19 and 20 in primary and metastatic carcinomas of the liver. Mod Pathol 1996;9:901–909.

179. Osborne M, VanLessen G, Weber K, et al. Differential diagnosis of gastrointestinal carcinomas by using monoclonal antibodies specific for individual keratin polypeptides. Lab Invest 1986;55:497–504.

180. Ferrandez-Izquierdo A, Llombart-Bosch A. Immunohistochemical characterization of 130 cases of primary hepatic carcinomas. Pathol Res Pract 1987;182:783–791.

181. Chedid A, Chejfec G, Eichorst M, et al. Antigenic markers of hepatocellular carcinoma. Cancer 1990;65:84–87.

182. Ronnett BM, Kurman R, Zahn CM, et al. Pseudomyxoma peritonei in women: A clinicopathologic analysis of 30 cases with emphasis on site of origin, prognosis and relationship to ovarian mucinous tumors of low malignant potential. Hum Pathol 1995;26:509–524.

183. Wick MR, Siegal GP. Monoclonal antibodies to carcinoembryonic antigen in diagnostic immunohistochemistry. In: Wick MR, Siegal GP, eds. Monoclonal Antibodies in Diagnostic Immunohistochemistry. New York: Marcel Dekker, 1988.

184. Sheahan K, O'Brian MJ, Burke D, et al. Differential reactivities of carcinoembryonic antigen and CEA-related monoclonal and polyclonal antibodies in common epithelial malignancies. Am J Clin Pathol 1990;94:157–164.

185. Ma CK, Zarbo RJ, Frierson HF, et al. Comparative immunohistochemical study of primary and metastatic carcinomas of the liver. Am J Clin Pathol 1993;99:551–557.

186. Balaton A, Nehama-Sibony M, Gotheil C, et al. Distinction between hepatocellular carcinoma, cholangiocarcinoma and metastatic carcinoma based on immunohistochemical staining for carcinoembryonic antigen and for cytokeratin 19 on paraffin sections. J Pathol 1988;156:305–310.

187. Gottschalk-Sabag S, Ron N, Glick T. Use of CD-34 and factor VIII to diagnose hepatocellular carcinoma on fine needle aspirates. Acta Cytol 1998;42:691–696.

188. Cui S, Hanno H, Sakata A, et al. Enhanced CD-34 expression of sinusoid-like vascular endothelial cells in hepatocellular carcinoma. Pathol Int 1996;46:751–756.

189. Wennerberg AE, Nalesnik MA, Coleman WB. Hepatocyte paraffin 1: A monoclonal antibody that reacts with hepatocytes and can be used for differential diagnosis of hepatic tumors. Am J Pathol 1993;143:1050–1056.

190. Sinard J, Macleay LJ, Melamed J. Hepatoid adenocarcinoma in the urinary bladder: Unusual localization of a newly recognized tumor type. Cancer 1994;73:1919–1925.

191. Ishikura H, Fukasawa Y, Ogasawara K, et al. An AFP-producing gastric carcinoma with features of hepatic differentiation: A case report. Cancer 1985;56:840–848.

192. Hilkens J, Buijs F, Hilgers J, et al. Monoclonal antibodies against human milk-fat globule membrane detecting differentiation antigens of the mammary gland and its tumors. Int J Cancer 1984;34:197–206.

193. McGuckin MA, Walsh MD, Hohn BG, et al. Prognostic significance of MUC1 epithelial mucin expression in breast cancer. Hum Pathol 1996;26:432–439.

194. Zoretsky JZ, Weiss M, Tsafaty I, et al. Expression of genes coding of PS2, C-erB2 estrogen receptor and the H23 breast tumor associated antigen: A comparative analysis in breast cancer. FEBS Lett 1990;265:46–50.

195. Hilkens J, Ligtenberg MJL, Vos HL, et al. Cell membrane associated mucins and their adhesion property. Trends Biochem Sci 1992;17:359–363.

196. Pinkus GS, Etheridge CL, O'Connor EM. Are keratin proteins a better tumor marker than epithelial membrane antigen? A comparative immunohistochemical study of various paraffin-embedded neoplasms using monoclonal and polyclonal antibodies. Am J Clin Pathol 1986;85:269–277.

197. Gatter KC, Alcock C, Heryet A, et al. The clinical importance of analyzing tumors of uncertain origin by immunohistological techniques. Lancet 1985;1:1302–1305.

198. Wick MR, Swanson PE, eds. Immunohistochemical Findings in Tumors of the Skin. New York: Marcel Dekker, 1989.

199. Hilkens J, Buijs F. Biosynthesis of NAM-6, an epithelial sialomucin. J Biol Chem 1988;263:4215–4222.

200. Hilkens J, Buijs F, Ligtenberg M. Complexity of MAM-6, an epithelial sialomucin associated with carcinomas. Cancer Res 1989;49:786–793.

201. Gendler S, Taylor-Papadimitriou J, Duhig T, et al. Immunogenic region of a human polymorphic epithelial mucin expressed by carcinomas is made up of tandem repeats. J Biol Chem 1988;263:12820–12823.

202. Hayes DF, Zurawski VR, Kufe DW. Comparison of circulating CA15-3 and carcinoembryonic antigen levels in patients with breast cancer. J Clin Oncol 1986;4:1532–1550.

203. Kufe D, Inghirami G, Abe M, et al. Differential reactivity of a novel monoclonal antibody (DF3) with human malignant vs benign breast tumors. Hybridoma 1984;3:223–232.

204. Peterson JA, Zava DT, Duwe AK, et al. Biochemical and histological characterization of antigens preferentially expressed on the surface and cytoplasm of breast carcinoma cells identified by monoclonal antibodies against a human milk fat globule. Hybridoma 1990;9:221–235.

205. Peterson JA, Couto JR, Taylor M, et al. Selection of tumor-specific epitopes on target antigens for radioimmunotherapy. Cancer Res 1995;55:5847S–5851S.

206. Swanson P, ed. Monoclonal Antibodies to Human Milk Fat Globule Proteins. New York: Marcel Dekker, 1988.

207. Al-Naffussi A, Carder PJ. Monoclonal antibodies in the cytodiagnosis of serous effusions. Cytopathology 1990;1:119–128.

208. Leong A-Y, Parkinson R, Milios J. "Thick" cell membranes revealed by immunocytochemical staining: A clue to the diagnosis of mesothelioma. Diagn Cytopathol 1990;6:9–13.

209. Singh HK, Silverman JF, Burns L, et al. Significance of epithelial membrane antigen in the workup of problematic serous effusions. Diagn Cytopathol 1995;13:3–7.

210. Delsol G, Gatter KC, Stein H, et al. Human lymphoid cells express epithelial membrane antigen. Lancet 1984;2:1124–1129.

211. Chittal SM, Delsol G. The interface between Hogkin's disease and anaplastic large cell lymphoma. Cancer Surv 1997;30:87–105.

212. Stein H, Hansmann M-L, Lennert K, et al. Reed-Sternberg and Hodgkin's cells in lymphocyte predominant Hodgkin's

disease of nodular subtype contain J-chain. Am J Clin Pathol 1986;86:292–297.

213. Chittal SM, Caveriviere P, Schwarting R, et al. Monoclonal antibodies in the diagnosis of Hodgkin's disease: The search for a rational panel. Am J Surg Pathol 1988;12:9–21.

214. Gatter KC, Abdulaziz Z, Beverly P, et al. Use of monoclonal antibodies for the histopathological diagnosis of human malignancy. J Clin Pathol 1982;35:1253–1267.

215. Sarkar AB, Akagi T, Yoshino T, et al. Expression of vimentin and epithelial membrane antigen in malignant lymphomas. Acta Pathol Jpn 1990;40:581–587.

216. Hall PA, D'Ardenne J, Stansfeld AG. Paraffin section of immunohistochemistry. I: Non-Hodgkin's lymphoma. Histopathology 1988;13:149–160.

217. Strickler JG, Weiss LM, Copenhaver CM, et al. Monoclonal antibodies reactive in routinely processed tissue sections of malignant lymphoma, with emphasis on T-cell lymphomas. Hum Pathol 1987;18:808–814.

218. Fujimoto J, Hata J, Ishii E, et al. Ki1 lymphomas in childhood: Immunohistochemical analysis and the significance of epithelial membrane antigen (EMA) as a new marker. Virchows Arch A Pathol Anat Histopathol 1988;412:307–314.

219. Al Saati T, Caveriviere P, Gorguet B, et al. Epithelial antigen in hemopoietic neoplasms. [letter] Hum Pathol 1986;17:533–534.

220. Leocini L, Del Vecchio MT, Kraft R, et al. Hodgkin's disease and CD30 positive anaplastic large cell lymphomas—a continuous spectrum of malignant disorders. Am J Pathol 1990;137:1047–1057.

221. Carbone A, Gloghini A, Volpe R. Paraffin section immunohistochemistry in the diagnosis of Hodgkin's disease and anaplastic large cell (CD30+) lymphomas. Virchows Arch A Pathol Anat Histopathol 1992;420:527–532.

222. Piris M, Brown DC, Gatter KC, et al. CD30 expression in non-Hodgkin's lymphoma. Histopathology 1990;17:211–218.

223. Chott A, Kasere K, Augustin I, et al. Ki-1 positive large cell lymphoma: A clinicopathologic study of 41 cases. Am J Surg Pathol 1990;14:439–448.

224. Pilieri S, Bocchia M, Baroni CD, et al. Anaplastic large cell lymphoma (CD30+/Ki-1+): Results of a prospective clinicopathologic study of 69 cases. Br J Haematol 1994;86:513–523.

225. Shek TWH, Yuen ST, Luk ISC, et al. Germ cell tumor as a diagnostic pitfall of metastatic carcinoma. J Clin Pathol 1996;49:223–225.

226. Giwercman A, Marks A, Bailey D, et al. M2A—a monoclonal antibody as a marker for carcinoma in-situ germ cells of the human adult testis. Acta Pathol Microbiol Immunol Scand (A) 1988;96:667–670.

227. Jacobson GK, Norgaard-Pedersen D. Placental alkaline phosphatase in testicular germ cell tumors and carcinoma in situ of the testis: An immunohistochemical study. Acta Pathol Microbiol Immunol Scand (A) 1984;92:323–329.

228. Giwercman A, Andrews PW, Jorgensen M. et al. Immunohistochemical expression of embryonal marker TRA-1-60 in carcinoma in-situ and germ cell tumors of the testis. Cancer 1993;72:1308–1314.

229. Fogel M, Lifschitz-Nercer B, Moll R. Heterogeneity of intermediate filament expression in human testicular seminomas. Differentiation 1990;45:242–249.

230. Burke AP, Mostofi FK. Placental alkaline phosphatase immunohistochemistry of intratubular malignant germ cells and associated testicular germ cell tumors. Hum Pathol 1988;19:663–670.

231. Cummings OW, Ulbright TM, Eble JM, et al. Spermatocytic seminoma: An immunohistochemical study. Hum Pathol 1994;25:54–59.

232. Niehans GA, Nanibel JC, Copland GT, et al. Immunohistochemistry of germ cell and trophoblastic neoplasms. Cancer 1988;62:1113–1123.

233. Nanibel JC, Jessuran J, Wick MR, et al. Placental alkaline phosphatase immunoreactivity in testicular germ cell tumors. Am J Surg Pathol 1987;11:21–29.

234. Uchiba T, Shimoda T, Miyata H, et al. Immunoperoxidase study of alkaline phosphatase in testicular tumors. Cancer 1981;48:1455–1462.

235. Hustin J, Collettee J, Franchimont P. Immunohistochemical demonstration of placental alkaline phosphatase in various states of testicular development and in germ cell tumors. Int J Androl 1987;10:29–35.

236. Wick MR, Swanson PE, Manivel JC. Placental-like alkaline phosphatase reactivity in human tumors: An immunohistochemical study of 520 cases. Hum Pathol 1987;18:946–954.

237. Bailey D, Marks A, Stratis M, et al. Immunohistochemical staining of germ cell tumors and intratubular malignant germ cells of the testis using antibody to placental alkaline phosphatase and a monoclonal antiseminoma antibody. Mod Pathol 1991;4:167–171.

238. Lles RK, Ind TE, Chard T. Production of placenta-like alkaline phosphatase and PLAP-like material in epithelial germ cell and non-germ cell tumors in vitro. Br J Cancer 1994;69:274–278.

239. Watanabe H, Tokuyama H, Ohta H, et al. Expression of placental alkaline phosphatase in gastric and colorectal cancers: An immunohistochemical study using the prepared monoclonal antibody. Cancer 1990;66:2575–2582.

240. Mostofi FK, Sesterhenn RA, David CJJ. Immunopathology of germ cell tumors of the testis. Semin Diagn Pathol 1987;4:320–341.

241. Jacobsen GK, Jacobsen M. Alpha-fetoprotein (AFP) and human chorionic gonadotropin in testicular germ cell tumors: A prospective immunohistochemical study. Acta Pathol Microbiol Immunol Scand (A) 1983;91:165–176.

242. Eglen DE, Ulbright T. The differential diagnosis of yolk sac tumor and seminoma: Usefulness of cytokeratin, alpha-fetoprotein and alpha-1-antitrypsin immunoperoxidase reactions. Am J Clin Pathol 1987;88:328–332.

243. Devouassoux-Shisheboran M, Schammel DP, Tavassoli FA. Ovarian hepatoid yolk sac tumors: Morphological, immunohistochemical and ultrastructural features. Histopathology 1999;34:462–469.

244. Wiedemann MB, Kuhn C, Schwechheimer K, et al. Synaptophysin identified by metastases of neuroendocrine tumors by immunocytochemistry and immunoblotting. Am J Clin Pathol 1987;88:560–569.

245. Wilson BS, Lloyd RV. Detection of chromogranin in neuroendocrine cells with a monoclonal antibody. Am J Pathol 1984;115:458–468.

246. Lloyd RV, Wilson BS. Specific endocrine marker defined by a monoclonal antibody. Science 1983;222:628–630.

247. DeStephano DV, Lloyd RV, Pike AM, et al. Pituitary adenomas: An immunohistochemical study of hormone production and chromogranin localization. Am J Pathol 1984;116:464–472.

248. Lloyd RV, Mervak T, Schmidt K, et al. Immunohistochemical detection of chromogranin and neuron-specific enolase in pancreatic endocrine neoplasms. Am J Surg Pathol 1984;8:607–614.

249. Wick MR, Siegal GP, eds. Monoclonal Antibodies to Chromogranin: Characterization and Comparison with Other Neuroendocrine Markers. New York: Marcel Dekker, 1988.

250. Wiedemann B, Franke WW. Identification and localization of synaptophysin, an integral membrane glycoprotein of MW 38,000 characteristic of presynaptic vesicles. Cell 1985;41:1017–1028.

251. Thomas L, Hartung K, Langosch D, et al. Identification of synaptophysin as a hexomeric channel protein of the synaptic vesicle membrane. Science 1988;242:1050–1053.

252. Staren ED, Gould VE, Warren WH, et al. Neuroendocrine carcinomas of the colon and rectum: A clinicopathologic evaluation. Surgery 1988;104:1080–1089.

253. Piehl MR, Gould VE, Warren WH, et al. Immunohistochemical identification of exocrine and neuroendocrine subsets of large cell carcinomas. Pathol Res Pract 1988;183:675–682.

254. Guinee DG Jr, Fishback MF, Koss MN, et al. The spectrum of immunohistochemical staining of small cell lung carci-

noma and specimens from transbronchial and open lung biopsies. Am J Clin Pathol 1994;102:406–414.

255. Kayser K, Schmid W, Ebert W, et al. Expression of neuro-endocrine markers (neuron specific enolase, synaptophysin and bombesin) in carcinoma of the lung. Pathol Res Pract 1988;183:412–417.

256. Abel T, Balch CM. The differentiation antigen of human NK and K-cells identified by a monoclonal antibody (HNK-1). J Immunol 1981;127:1024–1029.

257. Mechtersheimer G. Towards the phenotyping of soft tissue tumors by cell surface molecules. Virchows Arch A Pathol Anat Histopathol 1991;419:7–28.

258. Baylon SB, Jackson RD, Goodwin G, et al. Neuroendo-crine-related biochemistry in the spectrum of human lung cancers. Exp Lung Res 1982;3:209–223.

259. Caillaud JM, Benjelloun S, Bosq J, et al. HNK-1 defined antigen detected in paraffin embedded neuroectodermal tumors and those derived from cells of the amine precursor uptake and decarboxylation system. Cancer Res 1984;44:4432–4439.

260. Shioda Y, Nagura H, Tsutsumi Y, et al. Distribution of Leu-7 (HNK-1) antigen in human digestive organs: An immunohistochemical study with monoclonal antibody. Histochem J 1984;16:843–854.

261. Cole SP, Mirski A, McGarry RC, et al. Differential expression of the Leu-7 antigen on human lung tumor cells. Cancer Res 1985;45:4285–4290.

262. Battifora H, Silva E. The use of antikeratin antibodies in the immunohistochemical distinction between neuroendocrine (Merkel cell) carcinoma of the skin, lymphoma and oat cell carcinoma. Cancer 1986;58:1040–1046.

263. Osborne M, Dirk T, Kaser H, et al. Immunohistochemical localization of neurofilaments and neuron-specific enolase in 29 cases of neuroblastoma. Am J Pathol 1986;122:437–442.

264. Tsokos M, Linnoila RI, Chandra RS, et al. Neuron-specific enolase in the diagnosis of neuroblastoma and other small round cell tumors in children. Hum Pathol 1984;15:575–584.

265. Vinores SA, Bonnin JN, Rubenstein LJ, et al. Immunohisto-chemical demonstration of neuron specific enolase in neoplasms of the CNS and other tumors. Arch Pathol Lab Med 1984;108:536–540.

266. Jiang C, Tan Y, Li E. Histopathological and immunohisto-chemical studies on medullary thyroid carcinoma. Chung Hua Ping Li Hsueh Tsa Chih 1996;25:332–335.

267. Kargi A, Yorukoglu A, Aktas S. Neuroendocrine differenti-ation in non-neuroendocrine thyroid carcinoma. Thyroid 1996;6:207–210.

268. Kovacs CS, Mase RM, Kovacs K, et al. Thyroid medullary carcinoma with thyroglobulin immunoreactivity in sporadic multiple endocrine neoplasia type 2-B. Cancer 1994;74:928–932.

269. Ruck P, Horny HP, Greschniok A, et al. Non-specific im-munostaining of blast cells of acute leukemia by antibodies against non-hemopoietic antigens. Hematol Pathol 1995;9:39–56.

270. DiLoreto C, Pglisi F, DiLauro V, et al. Immunocytochemi-cal expression of tissue specific transcription factor-1 in lung carcinoma. J Clin Pathol 1997;50:30–32.

271. DiLoreto C, Pglisi F, DiLauro V, et al. TTF-1 protein expression in pleural malignant mesotheliomas and adeno-carcinomas of the lung. Cancer Lett 1998;124:73–78.

272. Fabbro D, DiLoreto C, Stamerra O, et al. TTF-1 gene expression and human lung tumors. Eur J Cancer 1996;32A:512–517.

273. Bejarno PA, Baughman RP, Biddinger PW, et al. Surfactant proteins and thyroid transcription factor 1 in pulmonary and breast carcinomas. Mod Pathol 1996;9:445–452.

274. Lazzaro D, Price M, DeFelice M, DiLauro R. The transcrip-tion factor TTF-1 is expressed at the onset of thyroid and lung morphogenesis and in restricted regions of the fetal brain. Development 1991;113:1093–1104.

275. Stahlman MT, Gray ME, Whitsett JA. Expression of thy-roid transcription factor-1 (TTF-1) and fetal and neo-natal human lung. J Histochem Cytochem 1996;44:673–678.

276. Anwar F, Schmidt RA. Thyroid transcription factor-1 (TTF-1) distinguishes mesothelioma from pulmonary ade-nocarcinoma. Lab Invest 1997;79:181A.

277. Guazzi S, Price M, DeFelice M, et al. Thyroid nuclear factor 1 (TTF-1) contains a homeodomain and displays a novel DNA binding specificity. Endo J 1990;9:3631–3639.

278. Khoor A, Whitsett JA, Stahlman MT, et al. Utility of sur-factant protein B precursor and thyroid transcription fac-tor-1 in differentiating adenocarcinoma from malignant mesothelioma. Hum Pathol 1999;30:695–700.

279. Folpe AL, Gown AM, Lamps LW, et al. Thyroid transcrip-tion factor-1 immunohistochemical evaluation of pulmo-nary neuroendocrine tumors. Mod Pathol 1999;12:5–8.

280. Holzinger A, Dingle S, Bejarano PA, et al. Monoclonal antibody to thyroid transcription factor-1: Production, characterization and usefulness in tumor diagnosis. Hy-bridoma 1996;15:49–53.

281. Tan J, Sidhu G, Greco A, et al. Villin, cytokeratin 7 and cytokeratin 20 expression in pulmonary adenocarcinoma with ultrastructural evidence of microvilli with rootlets. Hum Pathol 1998;29:390–396.

282. Nambu Y, Iannettoni MD, Orringer MB, et al. Unique ex-pression patterns and alterations in the intestinal protein villin in primary and metastatic pulmonary adenocarcino-mas. Mol Carcinog 1998;23:233–242.

283. Sharma S, Tan J, Sidhu G, et al. Lung adenocarcinomas metastatic to the brain with and without ultrastructural evidence of rootlets: An electron microscopic and immunohistochemical study using cytokeratins 7 and 20 and villin. Ultrastruct Pathol 1998;22:385–391.

284. Bacchi CE, Gown AM. Distribution and pattern of expres-sion of villin, a gastrointestinal-associated cytoskeletal protein in human carcinomas: A study employing paraffin-embedded tissue. Lab Invest 1991;64:418–424.

285. Lowe FC, Trauzzi SJ. Prostatic acid phosphatase in 1993: Its limited clinical utility. Urol Clin North Am 1993;20:589–596.

286. Komoshida S, Tsutsumi Y. Extraprostatic localization of prostatic acid phosphatase and prostate specific antigen: Distribution in cloacogenic glandular epithelium and sex dependent expression. Hum Pathol 1990;21:1108–1115.

287. Kote RJ, Taylor CR. Prostate, Bladder, and Kidney. Phila-delphia: WB Saunders, 1994.

288. Frazier HA, Humphrey PA, Burchette JL, et al. Immunore-active prostate specific antigen in male periurethral glands. J Urol 1992;147:246–250.

289. Elgamaol A, van de Voorde W, van Poppel W, et al. Im-munohistochemical localization of prostate-specific mark-ers within the accessory periurethral glands of Calper, Lat-tre and Morgagni. Urology 1994;434:84–90.

290. Nowels K, Kent E, Ranshl K. Prostate specific antigen and acid phosphatase-reactive cells in cystitis cystica and glan-dularis. Arch Pathol Lab Med 1988;112:734–738.

291. Golz R, Shubert GE. Prostate specific antigen: Immunore-activity in urachal remnants. J Urol 1989;141:1480–1484.

292. Van Krieken JH. Prostate marker immunoreactivity in sali-vary gland neoplasms—a rare pitfall in immunohisto-chemistry. Am J Surg Pathol 1993;17:410–414.

293. Alanen KA, Kuopio T, Koskinen PJ, et al. Immunohisto-chemical labeling for prostate specific antigen in non-pros-tatic tissues. Pathol Res Pract 1996;192:233–237.

294. Bostwick DG. Prostate specific antigen: Current role in di-agnostic pathology of prostate cancer. Am J Clin Pathol 1994;102(Suppl):S31–S37.

295. Kuriyama J, Wang M, Lee CL, et al. Multiple marker evalu-ation in human prostate cancer with use of tissue specific antigens. J Natl Cancer Inst 1982;68:99–105.

296. Nadji J, Tabei SZ, Castro A, et al. Prostatic origin of tu-mors: An immunohistochemical study. Am J Clin Pathol 1980;73:735–739.

297. Millar EA, Sharma MK, Lessells AM. Ductal (endome-trioid) adenocarcinoma of the prostate: A clinicopathologic study of 16 cases. Histopathology 1996;29:11–19.

298. Lee SS. Endometrioid adenocarcinoma of the prostate: A clinicopathologic and immunohistochemical study. J Surg Oncol 1994;55:235–238.

299. Leong FJ, Leong AS, Swift J. Signet ring carcinoma of the prostate. Pathol Res Pract 1996;192:1232–1238.

300. Kremer S, Farnham RJ, Glen JF, et al. Comparative morphology of primary and secondary deposits of prostatic adenocarcinoma. Cancer 1981;38:271–273.

301. Bovenberg SA, Vanderzvet CJJ, Vanderkrast T, et al. Prostate specific antigen expression in prostate cancer and its metastasis. J Urol Pathol 1993;1:55–62.

302. Estabon JN, Battifora H. Tumor immunophenotype: Comparison between primary neoplasm and its metastases. Mod Pathol 1990;3:192–196.

303. Bodey B, Birdie B, Kaiser H. Immunocytochemical detection of prostate specific antigen expression in human primary and metastatic melanomas. Anticancer Res 1997;17:2343–2346.

304. Horoszewicz JS, Kawinski E, Murphy GP. Monoclonal antibodies to a new antigenic marker in epithelial prostatic cells and serum prostatic cancer patients. Anticancer Res 1987;7:927–936.

305. Wright GLJ, Haley C, Beckett NO, et al. Expression of prostate-specific membrane antigen in normal, benign and malignant tissues. Urol Oncol 1995;1:18–28.

306. Silver DA, Pellicer I, Fair WR, et al. Prostate-specific membrane antigen expression in normal and malignant human tissues. Clin Cancer Res 1997;3:81–85.

307. Murphy GP, Elgamal A-A, Su SL, et al. Current evaluation of the tissue localization and diagnostic utility of prostate specific membrane antigen. Cancer 1998;83:2259–2269.

308. Bostwick DG, Pacelli A, Blute M, et al. Prostate specific membrane antigen expression in prostatic intraepithelial neoplasia and adenocarcinoma: A study of 184 cases. Cancer 1998;82:2256–2261.

309. Murphy GP, Barren RJ, Erickson SJ, et al. Evaluation and comparison of two new prostate carcinoma markers: Free-prostate specific antigen and prostate specific membrane antigen. 1996;78:809–818.

310. Troyer JK, Beckett ML, White GLJ. Location of prostate-specific membrane antigen in the LNCaP prostate carcinoma cell line. Prostate 1997;30:232–242.

311. Murphy GP, Teno WT, Holmes EH, et al. Measurement of prostate-specific membrane antigen in the serum with a new antibody. Prostate 1996;28:266–271.

312. Moll R, Wu X, Lin JH, et al. Uroplakins, specific membrane proteins of urothelial umbrella cells, as histologic markers of metastatic transitional cell carcinoma. Am J Pathol 1995; 147:1383–1397.

313. Wu RL, Osman I, Wu XR, et al. Uroplakin II gene is expressed in transitional cell carcinoma but not in Bilharzial bladder squamous cell carcinoma: Alternative pathways of bladder epithelial differentiation and tumor formation. Cancer Res 1998;58:1291–1297.

314. Pearlman WH, Giueriguian JD, Sawyer ME. A specific progesterone-binding component of human breast cyst fluid. J Biol Chem 1973;248:5736–5741.

315. Haagensen DE Jr, Mazoujian G, Holder WD Jr, et al. Evaluation of a breast cyst fluid protein detectable in the plasma of breast carcinoma patients. Ann Surg 1977;185:279–285.

316. Murphy LC, Lee-Wing M, Goldenberg GJ, et al. Expression of the gene encoding a prolactin-inducible protein by human breast cancers in vivo. Cancer Res 1987;47:4160–4164.

317. Eusebi V, Magalhaes F, Azzopardi JG. Pleomorphic lobular carcinoma of the breast: An aggressive tumor showing apocrine differentiation. Hum Pathol 1992;23:655-662.

318. Mazoujian G, Parish TH, Haagensen DEJ. Immunoperoxidase location of GCDFP-15 with mouse monoclonal antibodies versus rabbit antiserum. J Histochem Cytochem 1988;36:377–382.

319. Losi L, Lorenzini RL, Eusebi V, et al. Aprocrine differentiation in invasive carcinoma of the breast: Comparison of monoclonal and polyclonal gross cystic disease fluid protein-15 antibodies with prolactin-inducible protein mRNA gene expression. Appl Immunohistochem 1995;3:91–98.

320. Mazoujian G, Pinkus GS, David S, et al. Immunohistochemistry of a breast gross cystic disease fluid protein (GCDFP-15): A marker of apocrine epithelium and breast carcinomas with apocrine features. Am J Pathol 1983;110:105–112.

321. Mazoujian G, Margolis R. Immunohistochemistry of gross cystic disease fluid protein (GCDFP-15) in 65 benign sweat gland tumors of the skin. Am J Dermatopathol 1988;10:28–35.

322. Swanson PE, Pettinato G, Lillemoe TJ, et al. Gross cystic disease fluid protein-15 in salivary gland tumors. Arch Pathol Lab Med 1991;115:158–163.

323. Viacava P, Naccarato AG, Bevilacqua G. Spectrum of GCDFP-15 expression in human fetal and adult normal tissues. Virchows Arch 1998;432:255–260.

324. Wick MR, Lillemoe TJ, Copland GT, et al. Gross cystic disease fluid protein-15 as a marker for breast cancer: Immunohistochemical analysis of 690 human neoplasms and comparison with alpha-lactalbumin. Hum Pathol 1989;20:281–287.

325. Raab S, Berg SC, Swanson PE, et al. Adenocarcinoma in lung in patients with breast cancer: A prospective analysis of the discriminatory value of immunohistology. Am J Clin Pathol 1993;100:27–35.

326. Kufmann O, Deidesheimer T, Muehlenberg M, et al. Immunohistochemical differentiation of metastatic breast carcinomas from metastatic adenocarcinomas of other common sites. Histopathology 1996;29:233–240.

327. Busam KJ, Jungbluth AA. Melan-A, a new melanocytic differentiation marker. Adv Anat Pathol 1996;6:12–18.

328. Jungbluth AA, Busam KJ, Gerald WL, et al. A103: An anti–melan-A monoclonal antibody for the detection of malignant melanoma in paraffin-embedded tissues. Am J Surg Pathol 1998;22:595–602.

329. Busam KJ, Iverson K, Coplin KA, et al. Immunoreactivity for A103, an antibody to melan-A (Mart-1) in adrenal cortical and other steroid tumors. Am J Surg Pathol 1998;1:57.

330. Renshaw AA, Granter SR. A comparison of A103 and inhibin reactivity in adrenal cortical tumors: Distinction from hepatocellular carcinoma and renal tumors. Mod Pathol 1998;3:1160–1164.

331. Hofbauer GF, Kamarashev J, Geertsen R. Melan-A/MART-1 immunoreactivity in formalin-fixed paraffin-embedded primary and metastatic melanoma: Frequency and distribution. Melanoma Res 1998;8:337–343.

332. Arber DA, Weiss LM. CD5: A review. Appl Immunohistochem 1995;3:1–22.

333. Hishima T, Fukayama M, Fujisawa M, et al. CD5 expression in thymic carcinoma. Am J Pathol 1994;145:268–275.

334. Dorfman DM, Shahsafaei A, Chan JKC. Thymic carcinomas, but not thymomas and carcinomas of other sites, show CD5 immunoreactivity. Am J Surg Pathol 1997;21:936–940.

335. Berezowski K, Grimes MM, Gal A, et al. CD5 immunoreactivity of epithelial cells in thymic carcinoma and CASTLE using paraffin-embedded tissue. Am J Clin Pathol 1996;106:483–486.

336. Kornstein MJ, Rosai J. CD5 labeling of thymic carcinomas and other non-lymphoid neoplasms. Am J Clin Pathol 1998;109:722–726.

337. Tateyama H, Eimoto T, Tada T, et al. Immunoreactivity of a new CD5 antibody with normal epithelium and malignant tumors including thymic carcinoma. Am J Clin Pathol 1999;111:235–242.

338. Kuo TT, Chan JK. Thymic carcinoma arising in thymoma is associated with alterations in immunohistochemical profile. Am J Surg Pathol 1998;22:1474–1481.

339. Suster S, Moran CA. Spindle cell thymic carcinoma: Clinicopathologic and immunohistochemical study of a distinctive variant of primary thymic epithelial neoplasm. Am J Surg Pathol 1999;23:691–700.

340. Wick MR, Loy T, Mills SE, et al. Malignant epithelioid pleural mesothelioma versus peripheral pulmonary adenocarcinoma: A histochemical, ultrastructural and immunohistologic study of 103 cases. Hum Pathol 1990;21:759–766.

341. Johnston WW. Applications of monoclonal antibodies in

clinical cytology as exemplified by studies with monoclonal antibody B72.3. Acta Cytol 1987;31:537–566.

342. Johnson VG, Schlom J, Paterson AJ, et al. Analysis of a human tumor-associated glycoprotein (TAG-72) identified by monoclonal antibody B72.3. Cancer Res 1986;46:850–857.

343. Ordonez NG. The immunohistochemical diagnosis of mesothelioma: Differentiation of mesothelioma and lung adenocarcinoma. Am J Surg Pathol 1989;13:276–291.

344. Garcia-Prats MD, Ballestin C, Sotelo T, et al. A comparative evaluation of immunohistochemical markers for the differential diagnosis of malignant pleural tumors. Histopathology 1998;32:462–472.

345. Riera JR, Astengo-Osuna C, Longmate JA, et al. The immunohistochemical diagnostic panel for epithelial mesothelioma: A re-evaluation after heat induced epitope retrieval. Am J Surg Pathol 1997;21:1409–1419.

346. Szpak CA, Johnston WW, Roggli V, et al. The diagnostic distinction between malignant mesothelioma of the pleura and adenocarcinoma of the lung as defined by a monoclonal antibody (B72.3). Am J Pathol 1986;122:252–260.

347. Sheibani K, Battifora H, Burke JS. Antigenic phenotype of malignant mesotheliomas and pulmonary adenocarcinomas: An immunohistologic analysis demonstrating the value of Leu M1 antigen. Am J Pathol 1986;123:212–219.

348. Brown RW, Clark GM, Tandon AK, et al. Multiple-marker immunohistochemical phenotypes distinguishing malignant pleural mesothelioma from pulmonary adenocarcinoma. Hum Pathol 1993;24:347–354.

349. McCaughey WT, Colby TV, Battifora H, et al. Diagnosis of diffuse malignant mesothelioma: Experience of a US/Canadian mesothelioma panel. Mod Pathol 1991;4:342–353.

350. Wirth PR, Legier J, Wright GL Jr. Immunohistochemical evaluation of seven antibodies for differentiation of pleural mesothelioma from lung adenocarcinoma. Cancer 1991;67:655–662.

351. Leers MP, Aarts MM, Theunissen PH: E-Cadherin and calretinin: A useful combination of immunochemical markers for differentiation between mesothelioma and metastatic adenocarcinoma. Histopathology 1998;32:209–216.

352. Jordon D, Jagirdar J, Kaneko M. Blood group antigens, Lewis x and Lewis y, in the diagnostic discrimination of malignant mesothelioma versus adenocarcinoma. Am J Pathol 1989;135:931–937.

353. Gaffey MJ, Mills SE, Swanson PE, et al. Immunoreactivity for Ber-EP4 in adenocarcinomas, adenomatoid tumors and malignant mesotheliomas. Am J Surg Pathol 1992;16:593–599.

354. Sheibani K, Shin SS, Kezirian J, et al. Ber-EP4 antibody as a discriminant in a differential diagnosis of malignant mesothelioma versus adenocarcinoma. Am J Surg Pathol 1991;15:779–784.

355. Ordonez NG. Value of the Ber-EP4 antibody in differentiating epithelial pleural mesothelioma from adenocarcinoma: The MD Anderson experience and a critical review of the literature. Am J Clin Pathol 1998;109:85–89.

356. Ruitenbeek T, Gouw AS, Poppema S. Immunocytology of body cavity fluids: MOC-31, a monoclonal antibody discriminating between mesothelial and epithelial cells. Arch Pathol Lab Med 1994;118:265–269.

357. Delahaye M, Hoogsteden HC, Vanderkwast TH. Immunocytochemistry of malignant mesothelioma: OV632 as a marker of malignant mesothelioma. J Pathol 1991;165:137–143.

358. Edwards C, Oates J. OV632 and MOC31 in a diagnosis of mesothelioma and adenocarcinoma: An assessment of their use in formalin-fixed and paraffin wax embedded material. J Clin Pathol 1995;48:626–630.

359. Sosolik RC, McGaughey VR, DeYoung BR. Anti-MOC-31: A potential addition to the pulmonary adenocarcinoma vs. mesothelioma immunohistochemistry panel. Mod Pathol 1997;10:716–719.

360. Ordonez NG. Value of the MOC-31 monoclonal antibody in differentiating epithelial pleural mesothelioma from lung adenocarcinoma. Hum Pathol 1998;29:166–169.

361. Andressen C, Blumcke I, Celio MR. Calcium binding proteins: Selective markers of nerve cells. Cell Tissue Res 1993;271:181–208.

362. Doglioni C, Tos AP, Laurino L, et al. Calretinin: A novel immunocytochemical marker for mesothelioma. Am J Surg Pathol 1996;20:1037–1046.

363. Ordonez NG. Value of calretinin immunostaining in differentiating epithelial mesothelioma from lung adenocarcinoma. Mod Pathol 1998;11:929–933.

364. Ordonez NG. Value of antibodies 44-3A6 SM3 HBME-1 and thrombomodulin in differentiating epithelial pleural mesothelioma from lung adenocarcinoma: A comparative study with other commonly used antibodies. Am J Surg Pathol 1997;21:1399–1408.

365. Ordonez NG. Value of thrombomodulin immunostaining in a diagnosis of mesothelioma. Histopathology 1997;31:25–30.

366. Deamant FT, Pombo MT, Battifora H. Estrogen receptor immunohistochemistry as a predictor of site of origin in metastatic breast cancer. Appl Immunohistochem 1993;1:188–192.

367. Bacchi CE, Garcia RL, Gown AM. Immunolocalization of estrogen and progesterone receptors in neuroendocrine tumors of the lung, skin, gastrointestinal and female genital tracts. Appl Immunohistochem 1997;5:17–22.

368. Cagle PT, Mody DR, Schwartz MR. Estrogen and progesterone receptors in bronchogenic carcinoma. Cancer Res 1990;50:632–635.

369. Su JM, Shu HK, Chang H, et al. Expression of estrogen and progesterone receptors in non-small cell lung cancer: Immunohistochemical study. Anticancer Res 1996;16:3803–3806.

370. Kaiser U, Hofmann J, Schilli M, et al. Steroid hormone receptors in cell lines and tumor biopsies of human lung cancer. Int J Cancer 1996;67:357–364.

371. Beattie CW, Hansen NW, Thomas PA. Steroid receptors in human lung cancer. Cancer Res 1985;45:4206–4214.

372. Vargas SO, Leslie KO, Vacek PM, et al. Estrogen receptor related protein P29 in primary non-small cell carcinoma: Pathologic and prognostic correlations. Cancer 1998;82:1495–1500.

373. Ashikari R, Park K, Huvos AG, et al. Paget's disease of the breast. Cancer 1970;26:680–685.

374. Kister SJ, Haagensen CD. Paget's disease of the breast. Am J Surg 1977;119:606–609.

375. Salvadori BG, Saccozzi R. Analysis of 100 cases of Paget's disease of the breast. Tumori 1976;62:529–536.

376. Lundquist K, Kohler S, Rouse RV. Intraepidermal cytokeratin 7 expression is not restricted to Paget cells but is also seen in Toker cells and Merkel cells. Am J Surg Pathol 1999;23:212–219.

377. Tani EM, Skoog L. Immunocytochemical detection of estrogen receptors in mammary Paget cells. Acta Cytol 1988;23:825–828.

378. Meissner K, Riviere A, Haupt G, et al. Study of neu-protein expression in mammary Paget's disease with and without underlying breast carcinoma and in extramammary Paget's disease. Am J Pathol 1990;137:1305–1309.

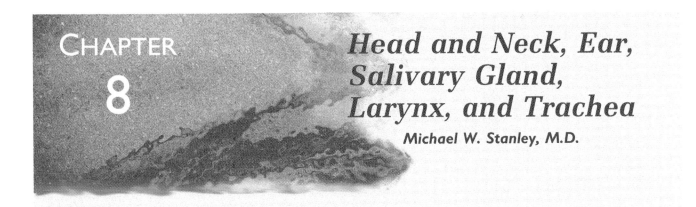

CHAPTER 8

Head and Neck, Ear, Salivary Gland, Larynx, and Trachea

Michael W. Stanley, M.D.

MASSES THAT ARE NOT UNIQUE TO THE HEAD AND NECK

Many types of tumors that are seen more commonly in other sites are occasionally seen in the head and neck. They are discussed in detail in other chapters but are summarized here in Table 8–1. The major exception is the family of squamous epithelial lesions, as these hold a position of preeminence in head and neck pathology in terms of the number of patients affected. In some instances, identification of a specific malignancy in various head and neck sites will lead at once to a search for a primary lesion that is more likely to be seated elsewhere. Many of these are relatively common types of carcinoma, some of which can be immunohistochemically addressed with considerable diagnostic success, as discussed in Chapter 7. This scenario almost always heralds a high-stage malignancy that may leave the patient with severely limited treatment options.

Immunostains for cytokeratin 7 (CK7) and CK20 are useful when evaluating metastatic adenocarcinomas, as seen in Figure 8–1. The pattern of metastatic adenocarcinoma seen (CK7+ and CK20−) suggests possible origin in the lung, breast, ovary (nonmucinous), or endometrium. This contrasts with the reverse pattern, which is typical of colonic adenocarcinomas.

Immunohistochemistry is a sensitive way to detect metastatic deposits. This has been applied to searching for even the most minimal disease in sentinel lymph nodes (Fig. 8–2). This procedure was initially used for staging malignant melanomas but is now more commonly used in the evaluation of breast carcinoma. The clinical significance of detecting micrometastases is not yet clear.

Other lesions pose diagnostic difficulties that may be addressed with only limited success using immunostains. They are discussed in the sections that follow. Attention is given to problems that remain difficult after the most thorough evaluation. Experience has led me to conclude that cases that are difficult by fine needle aspiration (FNA) are also difficult at the time of frozen section, often generating the same differential diagnostic considerations on both occasions.[1] I now extend that observation to include various head and neck masses encountered at the surgical bench.

SQUAMOUS EPITHELIAL PROLIFERATIONS AND NASOPHARYNGEAL CARCINOMA

Included in the category of squamous epithelial proliferations and nasopharyngeal carcinoma are intraepithelial preneoplasia and invasive squamous cell carcinomas with various degrees of differentiation. With the exception of the salivary glands, in which primary squamous cell carcinoma is a rarity, virtually all head and neck mucosal sites host these processes. In their classic form, they usually pose little diagnostic difficulty. However, a number of variations can lead to problems, as summarized in Table 8–2.

The most common difficulties are of fundamental clinical significance and involve distinctions between benign epithelium and low-grade malignancies or between in situ and invasive carcinomas. Immunohistochemistry has little to offer in resolving questions about lesions that consist of differentiated squamous cells and thus does nothing to help in these situations.

When one must make an assessment of possible invasion, the traditional methods of surgical pathology—including deeper levels, looking at the contour of cell nests, inspecting the stroma for reactive alterations, and finally requesting repeat biopsy—are the mainstay of diagnosis. In some instances, another clinical manifestation of the disease can resolve questions about invasion. In my experience, this is most commonly accomplished when a cervical lymph node suitable for FNA is discovered.

There is investigational work to suggest that we may soon be able to address questions about invasion by looking at various tissue components that are altered as a part of the invasion process. Immu-

Table 8–1. Masses That Are Not Unique to the Head and Neck but May Be Encountered Occasionally

Nasopharynx, paranasal sinuses, and nasal cavity	Salivary gland–type masses
	Central nervous system and meningeal neoplasms
	Malignant melanoma
	Paraganglioma
	Various soft tissue tumors
	Metastatic malignancies
	Hematopoietic neoplasms
Salivary glands	Amyloidosis
	Various uncommon soft tissue or bone tumors
	Paraganglioma
	Small cell anaplastic carcinoma
	Metastatic malignancies
	Hematopoietic neoplasms
Larynx and trachea	Amyloidosis
	Salivary gland–type masses
	Malignant melanoma
	Various uncommon soft tissue or bone tumors
	Paraganglioma
	Small cell anaplastic carcinoma
	Metastatic malignancies
	Hematopoietic neoplasms
Ear	Amyloidosis
	Gouty tophi
	Various primarily cutaneous lesions
	Salivary gland–type masses
	Malignant melanoma
	Various uncommon soft tissue or bone tumors
	Paraganglioma
	Meningioma
	Metastatic malignancies
	Hematopoietic neoplasms

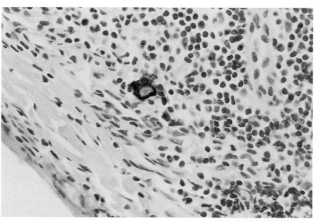

Figure 8–2. A "sentinel" cervical lymph node containing a single HMB-45+ cell representing minimal metastatic malignant melanoma. The cell stains strongly, but its nucleus and large nucleolus are visible through the brown reaction product. (×400)

nohistochemical assessment of basement membrane integrity (staining for laminin, type IV collagen, and proteoglycans) has been diagnostically disappointing.[2] Studying cutaneous squamous cell carcinomas and their precursors (actinic keratoses), Tsukifuji and colleagues reported differences in distributions of metalloproteinase-1 (MMP-1), MMP-2, and MMP-3.[3] Their investigation employed in situ hybridization for mRNAs but suggested that immunohistochemical methods should be studied in this context. Davidson and coworkers studied squamous cell carcinomas of the uterine cervix and high-grade cervical intraepithelial neoplasias and found increased expression of MMP-9 in both epithelial and stromal cells. This work looked at both the protein (immunohistochemistry) and its mRNA (in situ hybridization). Of particular note is their suggestion that strong stromal cell expression of MMP-9 mRNA characterizes some invasive carcinomas.[4]

Acantholytic ("adenoid") squamous cell carcinomas arise most often in head and neck cutaneous sites in elderly individuals, but they can be encountered as mucosa-based primary tumors or as metastatic deposits.[5–7] Tumor cell desquamation into the centers of rounded cell nests imparts a pseudoglandular appearance that may be recapitulated in FNA material. When cytoplasmic evidence of squamous differentiation is detected, these tumors are often mistaken for adenosquamous carci-

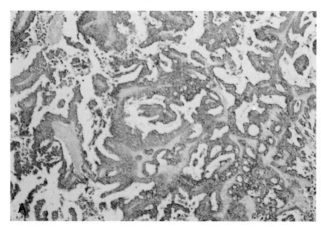
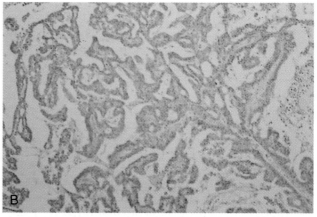

Figure 8–1. A metastatic adenocarcinoma from a pulmonary carcinoma that was undetected at the time of presentation. This metastatic deposit is positive for CK7 *(A)* and negative for CK20 *(B)*. (×400).

Table 8–2. Diagnostic Problems in Squamous Proliferations of the Head and Neck

Type of Squamous Lesion	Mistaken Lesion	Approach to Diagnostic Resolution
Inverted nasal papilloma	Invasive squamous cell carcinoma	Routine histologic methods only
Pseudoepitheliomatous hyperplasia	Invasive squamous cell carcinoma	Routine histologic methods only
In situ squamous cell carcinoma	Invasive squamous cell carcinoma	Routine histologic methods only
Acantholytic squamous cell carcinoma	Adenocarcinoma*	Mucin stains, CK20, LeuM1, Electron microscopy
Verrucous carcinoma	Benign mucosal hyperplasia	Routine histologic methods only
Spindle cell carcinoma	Sarcoma or malignant melanoma	Cytokeratins, electron microscopy
Basaloid squamous cell carcinoma	Adenoid cystic carcinoma	34βE12, electron microscopy
Poorly differentiated nasopharyngeal carcinoma	Malignant lymphoma	Cytokeratin, CD45, epithelial membrane antigen

* Markers that may be more organ-specific include prostate-specific antigen, hormone receptor proteins, gross cystic disease fluid protein-15, CA 125, and CA 19.9, but they are infrequently helpful in carcinomas involving the head and neck.

noma, mucoepidermoid carcinoma (MEC) or, in the skin, various adnexal neoplasms. Evidence of mucin production with mucicarmine or periodic acid–Schiff (PAS) stains is not present. Immunohistochemical and ultrastructural evidence of glandular differentiation is similarly absent. Immunostains for CK20 have found considerable utility in evaluation of carcinomas from the colon and other gastrointestinal sites.[8–10] These stains are negative in squamous cell carcinomas, suggesting that this stain may be useful when acantholytic squamous cell carcinoma might be mistaken for metastatic adenocarcinoma.

Spindle cell squamous carcinoma may be monophasic or biphasic with respect to the presence of an identifiable epithelioid component.[11–17] Furthermore, some of the latter may show only minimal or very focal epithelioid differentiation. Rarely, spindle cell carcinoma may be mixed with other variants of squamous cell carcinoma.[13] Many examples show positive immunohistochemical staining for epithelial markers (CK and epithelial membrane antigen [EMA]), but this may be very focal. The need for broad spectrum anti-CK cocktails has been emphasized.[11, 14] Furthermore, positive staining for vimentin neither excludes a diagnosis of carcinoma nor confirms a suspicion of sarcoma. It is also prudent to include spindle cell malignant melanoma in the differential diagnosis and to address this possibility with immunostains (S-100 protein, HMB-45 and MART-1). In the most difficult cases, performing electron microscopy to search for tonofilaments and rudimentary desmosomes can be diagnostic. In each of the larger series, there remains a residuum of spindle cell squamous carcinomas that show no evidence of epithelial differentiation by either immunohistochemistry or electron microscopy.[11, 12]

Basaloid squamous cell carcinoma occurs in a wide variety of upper aerodigestive tract sites, as well as in the bronchi, vulva, and anus.[18–22] It often presents with high-stage disease and follows an aggressive course. Keys to the diagnosis include foci of conventional squamous differentiation and associated surface epithelial dysplasia. CK stains are usually positive, with 34βE12 marking all cases

in the series of Banks and coworkers, and AE1/AE3 and CAM5.2 marking 80% of 40 tumors.[18] Some cases may show limited immunoreactivity for S-100 protein, EMA, Leu7, and smooth muscle actin.[18, 19, 21] Markers of malignant melanoma (S-100 protein and HMB-45) and most markers of neuroendocrine differentiation (chromogranin, synaptophysin, and neurofibrillary protein) are generally negative.

In cytologic samples, basaloid squamous cell carcinoma is most often mistaken for small cell undifferentiated carcinoma,[23, 24] prompting Banks and coworkers to suggest that this diagnosis be considered when one evaluates metastatic deposits in a patient with an upper aerodigestive tract mass.

Adenoid cystic carcinoma (ACC) is another "small blue cell" tumor that must be distinguished from basaloid squamous cell carcinoma.[25–27] The solid or anaplastic type of ACC can be especially problematic. Ultrastructural features of glandular differentiation in the former contrast with squamous differentiation in the latter.[19, 27] After examining a large number of epithelial and neuroendocrine markers, Morice and Ferreiro noted that the most reliable differential immunohistochemical finding was staining of most basaloid squamous cell carcinomas (22 of 23) with 34βE12, a marker of high molecular weight CK.[25] Small cell undifferentiated carcinomas and ACCs were negative.

Nasopharyngeal carcinoma often presents with a cervical lymph node metastasis in the face of a primary tumor that can be difficult to identify. Immunohistochemistry can be used to add confidence to the diagnosis, as illustrated in Figure 8–3.

MASSES OF THE NASAL CAVITY, PARANASAL SINUSES, AND NASOPHARYNX

Sinonasal Carcinoma

Sinonasal carcinomas are a diverse group of epithelial malignancies that are united by a common set of locations and a tendency to present at an advanced local stage with bone destruction. The

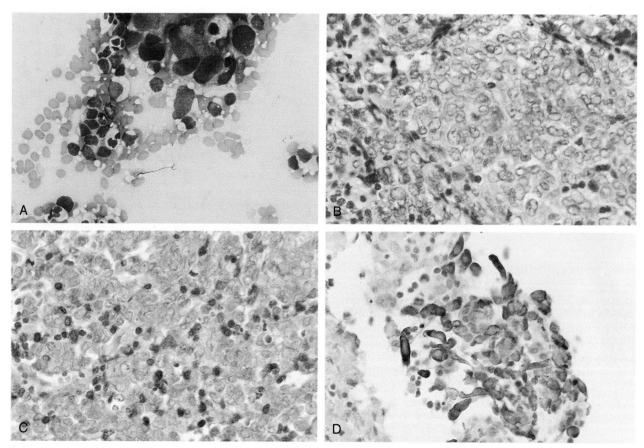

Figure 8–3. Evaluation of nasopharyngeal carcinoma that has presented as a cervical lymph node metastasis. *A,* Fine needle aspiration initially suggests the diagnosis by showing a combination of unremarkable lymphoid cells and cohesive clusters of malignant epithelioid cells. (Diff-Quik stain, ×400) *B,* Histologically, the tumor consists of undifferentiated cells that appear epithelial because they occur in nests. Lymphocytes are scattered through the background. (H&E, ×400) *C,* Immunostaining with the lymphocyte marker CD45 shows the lymphocytes and confirms that the large undifferentiated cells are not hematopoietic in nature. (×400) *D,* Staining with a cocktail of anticytokeratin monoclonal antibodies confirms the epithelial nature of the tumor cells. (×400)

histologic types include all the squamous cell carcinoma variants previously discussed, as well as adenocarcinoma and the very aggressive undifferentiated or anaplastic carcinoma. The designation *adenocarcinoma* is reserved for tumors that do not have features of any specific salivary gland carcinoma. The previously discussed immunohistochemical observations apply to these neoplasms.

Wick and coworkers emphasized application of an antibody panel with markers of epithelial (CK, EMA), melanocytic (S-100 protein, HMB-45), and neuroendocrine differentiation (synaptophysin) to distinguish undifferentiated carcinoma, malignant melanoma, and olfactory neuroblastoma, respectively.[28]

Nasopharyngeal Angiofibroma

A clinicopathologically distinctive lesion, nasopharyngeal angiofibroma rarely requires special tests for accurate diagnosis, and immunohistochemistry has little to offer. The stroma can vary

from loose to dense and is inhabited by cells that stain only for vimentin.[29] The biology of this lesion was elucidated by Hwang and coworkers when they applied immunohistochemistry to demonstrate androgen receptors in 18 of 24 cases.[30] Two had progesterone receptors, and none showed estrogen receptor proteins. The potential therapeutic implications of these observations remain incompletely investigated.

Olfactory Neuroblastoma (Esthesioneuroblastoma)

The neuroblastic nature of olfactory neuroblastoma is manifested by proliferation of small, uniform cells that tend to be arranged in small nests. These collections are separated by neurofibrillary tangles. Homer-Wright rosettes may be seen, but ganglion cell differentiation is rarely encountered.[31, 32] Cervical lymph node metastases have been described in FNA studies.[33]

Diagnostic difficulties occur when the small cells

are mistaken for malignant lymphoma, leukemia, rhabdomyosarcoma, undifferentiated sinonasal carcinoma, or malignant melanoma. The relationship between olfactory neuroblastoma and the Ewing's sarcoma group of neoplasms, as well as the potential therapeutic implications of these nosologic distinctions, remains incompletely evaluated.[32, 34] These issues will undoubtedly be addressed with increasing sophistication using molecular diagnostic techniques. In some instances, the characteristic histopathologic features described above are altered by compartmentalizing sclerosis or vascular proliferation, leading to further diagnostic difficulty.

Ultrastructural features of neural differentiation are present in virtually all cases and include dense core neurosecretory granules and microtubule-contained cell processes. In keeping with this picture, most examples are immunohistochemically positive with neural markers (synaptophysin, chromogranin). Epithelial markers (CKs, EMA) are usually negative, as are studies for bcl-2 and p53 overexpression.[35] Scattered cells may show positive staining for S-100 protein or glial fibrillary acidic protein (GFAP).[36]

MASSES OF THE LARYNX AND TRACHEA

As noted in Table 8–1, numerous lesions that are more common in other sites can occur in the larynx and trachea; all are addressed in detail in other chapters. The most common set of lesions in the larynx and trachea includes squamous cell carcinoma, with its variants and precursors. These were discussed previously, and special diagnostic issues were summarized in Table 8–2.

MASSES INVOLVING THE EXTERNAL, MIDDLE, AND INNER EAR

External Ear

A wide variety of lesions that may be seen in the ear is summarized in Table 8–1. All are uncommon, with the exception of squamous cell carcinoma and basal cell carcinoma. Each of these lesions affects mostly the skin of the external ear but may be encountered in the external auditory canal.

Adenomas[37, 38] and adenocarcinomas[39–42] of the external auditory canal are usually considered related to ceruminous glands. Unfortunately, the terms *ceruminoma, ceruminous adenoma,* and *ceruminous carcinoma* have been applied to several diverse lesions, with highly variable clinical significance. These include apparently true cerumen gland masses, dermal eccrine cylindroma, syringocystadenoma papilliferum, and ACC of the salivary gland type.

The distinction between adenomas and adenocarcinomas in the external auditory canal can be difficult, as many of the malignant lesions are well differentiated and manifest their nature only in local recurrences rather than in metastases. Ulceration, invasion, pleomorphism, and mitotic figures are histopathologic clues to malignancy. Extramammary Paget's disease in association with ceruminous adenocarcinoma is rare.[41]

The immunohistochemistry of these tumors has not been described. Cankar and Crowley noted the presence of a myoepithelial layer in ceruminous adenomas but not in the adenocarcinomas.[42] Whether or not immunohistochemical reagents targeted to this cell layer would be diagnostically useful remains to be investigated.

It is also important to distinguish between dermal eccrine cylindroma and the much more ominous ACC of the external auditory canal or skin.[43] Immunohistochemistry is of little utility in this regard.

Internal and Middle Ear

Middle ear adenoma (MEA) and carcinoid tumor of the middle ear probably represent the same entity with differing levels of neuroendocrine differentiation, although some authors continue to regard them as separate entities. The growth pattern features solid, glandular, or trabecular areas, without appreciable necrosis, nuclear atypia, or mitotic activity. Various degrees of mucin production and ultrastructural evidence of neurosecretory granules have been described. Lysozyme can be demonstrated immunohistochemically in most cases and is also present in the normal middle ear mucosa.[44–48]

The most important differential diagnostic consideration in the middle ear is between MEA and adenocarcinoma; the two have been confused. Each has also been mistaken for carcinoma arising in the external ear or in the salivary glands and extending to involve the middle ear secondarily. Carcinomas that arise primarily in the middle ear are locally aggressive, with bone invasion not usually seen in MEA.[49] The diagnosis rests on the prominent papillary architecture of the carcinomas, in contrast to the adenomas, which lack this feature. It has been suggested that papillary middle ear carcinoma may represent a major visceral manifestation of von Hippel-Lindau disease.[50]

SALIVARY GLAND MASSES

The salivary glands host an extraordinarily diverse array of neoplasms. Most are proliferations of ductal and myoepithelial cells in various combinations; acinar cells participate infrequently. Interpretation of histologic material is further complicated by the fact that a variety of secondary alterations is common to several different entities. They include clear cell change, cystic change, oncocytic cytologic features, sebaceous differentiation, and prominent lymphoid stroma, as summarized in Table 8–3. Furthermore, many of these entities are uncommon so that most individuals' experience with a specific type of tumor may be very limited.

Pleomorphic Adenoma

The immunohistochemical features of pleomorphic adenoma (PA) have been investigated extensively, as summarized in Table 8–4.[51–59] S-100 protein can be expressed in both the epithelial and myoepithelial compartments, leading us to expect considerable overlap between its decoration of PA and other tumor types. Furthermore, much of the S-100 labeling observed in non-neoplastic salivary gland tissue is apparently related to a rich plexus of nerve fibers rather than to myoepithelial cells.[52]

Staining for GFAP has been localized to the myoepithelial cells that appear to be the most undifferentiated ultrastructurally, in a pattern similar to neoplastic cartilage.[55] This marker has proved diagnostically useful in both histopathologic[53] and in FNA cytologic studies.[56] The majority of pleo-

Table 8–4. Immunohistochemistry of Pleomorphic Adenoma

Ductal cells	Cytokeratins
	Epithelial membrane antigen
	Lysozyme
	Lactoferrin
	GCDFP-15
	CEA
	Alpha-1-antitrypsin
	Alpha-1-antichymotrypsin
	Prostatic acid phosphatase
	Prostate-specific antigen
Myoepithelial cells	Cytokeratins
	Actins
	S-100 protein
	Fibronectin
	GFAP

GCDFP-15, gross cystic disease fluid protein-15; CEA, carcinoembryonic antigen; GFAP, glial fibrillary acidic protein.

morphic adenomas are positive, whereas normal salivary gland tissue, chronic sialoadenitis, basal cell adenomas, ACC, and low-grade MEC give negative results. This finding seems limited in its diagnostic utility, since examples of PA with well-developed chondromyxoid stroma pose the least diagnostic difficulty and are not likely to be mistaken for any of the negatively staining entities listed earlier. The particular utility of this marker in the differential diagnosis with polymorphous low-grade adenocarcinoma is discussed subsequently.

Despite having studied a small number of cases, van Krieken warns that salivary gland PA and some carcinomas may show immunoreactivity for prostatic acid phosphatase and prostate-specific antigen (PSA).[51] This has obvious clinical implications for male patients who present with adenocarcinoma of unknown primary site. Felix and coworkers noted that a loss of immunohistochemically demonstrable type IV collagen around tumor cell nests may indicate a proclivity for metastatic behavior in carcinoma ex-PA.[59]

Differential diagnostic problems can occur when most of a PA consists of spindled myoepithelial cells, especially when nuclear palisading occurs; neurilemmoma and leiomyoma are the most likely considerations.[58] Takeda and Shimono studied two such cases and found the spindle cells to be uniformly negative for markers of smooth muscle differentiation (desmin, muscle-specific actin [HHF-35], alpha smooth muscle actin, and myoglobin).

Table 8–3. Secondary Alteration Common to Various Salivary Gland Neoplasms

Clear cell change	Oncocytic tumors
	Myoepithelioma
	Acinic cell carcinoma
	Mucoepidermoid carcinoma
	Epithelial-myoepithelial carcinoma
	Adenocarcinoma
	Clear cell carcinoma
Oncocytic cytology	Pleomorphic adenoma
	Myoepithelioma
	Warthin's tumor
	Oncocytic tumors
	Mucoepidermoid carcinoma
	Acinic cell carcinoma
	"Oncocytoid" adenocarcinoma
Cystic change	Non-neoplastic duct obstructive lesions
	Pleomorphic adenoma
	Basal cell adenomas
	Warthin's tumor
	Mucoepidermoid carcinoma
	Acinic cell carcinoma
Lymphoid stroma	Non-neoplastic duct obstructive lesions
	Warthin's tumor
	Lymphoepithelial cyst
	Lymphoepithelial lesion
	Oncocytic tumors
	Acinic cell carcinoma
	Mucoepidermoid carcinoma
Sebaceous differentiation	Sebaceous neoplasms
	Pleomorphic adenoma
	Basal cell adenoma
	Warthin's tumor
	Mucoepidermoid carcinoma

Myoepithelioma and Malignant Myoepithelioma

Myoepithelioma and malignant myoepithelioma are uncommon entities that probably represent the extreme end of the PA morphologic spectrum, in which the entire lesion is overgrown by myoepithelial cells. Both tumors have the same clinical features.[60, 61] The cells may be spindled, clear, oncocytoid, or plasmacytoid. Preservation of the entity is useful in that it directs the differential diagnostic thinking along lines that may help to avoid mistaking these benign lesions for a variety of other spindle cell or epithelioid neoplasms. Both the spindle cell type and the plasmacytoid lesions show positive immunostaining for vimentin, CKs, S-100 protein, and GFAP, but only the spindle cell type demonstrates smooth muscle actin and muscle-specific actin.[62]

Malignant myoepithelioma features invasive growth and mitotic figures, in addition to the immunohistochemical profile noted previously.[63–65] Michal and coworkers suggested that clear cell change in concert with a myoepithelial immunoprofile distinguishes clear cell malignant myoepithelioma from hyalinizing clear cell carcinoma (CCC), which lacks these markers.[65]

Warthin's Tumor

Diagnostic difficulty is rarely presented by Warthin's tumor. In some instances, partial infarction with markedly atypical squamous metaplasia may suggest squamous cell carcinoma, but this is a more serious source of diagnostic difficulty in FNA than in examination of excised tumors. The previous comments regarding squamous lesions apply to this problem. The epithelial cells show a duct cell–like immunophenotype (positive for CKs, carcinoembryonic antigen [CEA], and S-100 protein), whereas the lymphocytic component features both T cells and polyclonal B cells.[66, 67]

Basal Cell Adenoma and Adenocarcinoma

These architecturally diverse lesions are distinguished from PA by the absence of chondromyxoid stroma as reflected by negative staining for GFAP. In the small numbers of cases studied to date, variable positivity of the epithelial cells for CEA, EMA, actin, CKs, vimentin, and S-100 protein have been described.[68–70]

This tumor's lack of spindle cell or plasmacytoid features points away from myoepithelioma. The distinction from basal cell adenocarcinoma is based on a lack of infiltration in the benign lesions, since both entities usually show bland cytologic features. Some adenomas have a minor cylindromatous-appearing component but lack the infiltration and perineural invasion typical of ACC. Prasad and coworkers noted that three novel smooth muscle–specific proteins (alpha smooth muscle actin, smooth muscle myosin heavy chains, and calponin) can be demonstrated immunohistochemically in ACC but not in basal cell adenomas (specifically the canalicular type).[71] If confirmed and extended, this observation might be diagnosti-

cally useful in the often difficult differential diagnosis. Those who encounter this sometimes insoluble dilemma in FNA would especially welcome such a test.

Oncocytoma and Malignant Oncocytoma

Oncocytoma and dominant masses of nodular oncocytic hyperplasia occasionally come to surgical excision. One example with a positive immunostain for PSA was clinically difficult to distinguish from metastatic prostatic carcinoma.[72] Malignant oncocytoma is extremely rare. Infiltrative growth indicates malignancy. Confirmation of oncocytic differentiation, preferably by electron microscopy, distinguishes this tumor from adenocarcinoma with "oncocytoid" cytoplasmic features. A single case with widespread metastases has been described as immunohistochemically positive for alpha-1 antitrypsin, alpha-1-antichymotrypsin, lactoferrin, and CEA, but negative for S-100 protein and muscle-specific actin (HHF-35).[73]

Mucoepidermoid Carcinoma

One problem in evaluating the literature describing MEC is that some investigators do not sort their findings according to tumor grade with sufficient rigor so that the significance of some observations is difficult to ascertain. The most common diagnostic maneuver directed toward MEC is the mucicarmine stain. A positive reaction helps to exclude other types of carcinoma, especially the family of squamous lesions that was previously discussed.

Earlier studies found limited CK expression in MEC,[74] but later investigations with more contemporary reagents have provided more information.[75] Specifically, Loyola and coworkers noted staining patterns summarized in Table 8–5.[75] This information is of limited diagnostic utility but suggests a histogenetic relationship to certain parts of the salivary gland duct system. These authors noted muscle-specific actin only in stromal cells and heterogeneous vimentin staining in a minority of cases.

Studying 25 MECs of diverse grades and sites of origin, Cho and coworkers described immunohistochemically detectable c-erb-B2 in 36%, with a tendency for overexpression to be seen in higher grade neoplasms.[76] Whether this has any prognostic significance greater than that derived from tumor grade and size remains unclear.

Acinic Cell Carcinoma

Diagnostic difficulties can arise because of the architectural diversity of acinic cell carcinoma. Solid, microcystic, follicular, and papillary-cystic

Table 8–5. Intermediate Filament Staining in Mucoepidermoid Carcinoma

Cytokeratin	Squamous Basal and Parabasal Cells	Luminal Columnar Cells	Intermediate Cells	Mucinous Cells
7	−	+	+	+
8	−	+	+	+
18	−	+	+	+
19	−	+	+	−
14	−	−	+	+
13	−	−	+	−

patterns lead to consideration of MEC and metastatic thyroid carcinoma. Clear cell change expands the differential diagnosis, and one must consider primary CCC, metastatic renal cell carcinoma, and myoepithelial neoplasms. If the cells show characteristic PAS-positive cytoplasmic granules, or if these zymogen granules can be demonstrated by electron microscopy, the diagnosis is secure. Other cases are more difficult. Amylase immunohistochemistry has been suggested by some as a diagnostic tool,[77, 78] but other investigators have not found this useful.[79] The microcystic pattern may rarely suggest metastatic thyroid carcinoma; thyroglobulin immunostains are useful in this setting. Neuroendocrine differentiation is rare.[80]

Adenoid Cystic Carcinoma

ACC is a complex neoplasm that contains both luminal (ductal) and abluminal (myoepithelial) cells, which show differing immunohistochemical profiles.[81–85] The extracellular spheres and cylinders mark as basement membrane material with immunostains against laminin, type IV collagen, heparan sulfate proteoglycans, and entactin.[81, 85] Cheng and coworkers also noted these materials to be distributed through the tumor stroma and around nests of neoplastic cells.[81]

The luminal cells show glandular epithelial-type markers, including CEA, EMA, and CKs. The myoepithelial cells demonstrate positivity for vimentin and muscle-specific actin and show variable staining for CKs.[82–85] Published descriptions of staining for S-100 protein in both luminal and myoepithelial cells are inconsistent.

Ozono and coworkers identified progesterone receptors, estradiol, and progesterone in ACCs, suggesting that this neoplasm might be a target tissue for estrogen.[86] However, an immunohistochemical search for estrogen receptor protein was negative when applied to paraffin-embedded sections.[87]

Polymorphous Low-Grade Adenocarcinoma

Several investigators have reported some combination of positive epithelial markers in virtually all cases of polymorphous low-grade adenocarcinoma (PLGA) examined (CK, EMA, CEA).[88–90] Results with S-100 and muscle-specific actin have been more variable.

This histologically variable neoplasm is most often confused with PA. The most useful differential diagnostic immunostain appears to be GFAP, although only a relatively small number of cases has been evaluated.[91, 92] The results of applying this stain to PA and PLGA are summarized in Table 8–6. Gnepp and coworkers noted diffuse staining of PLGA for EMA and CKs and suggested that this might be useful in distinguishing this tumor from ACC, in which more restricted staining with a luminal pattern is expected.[90]

Epithelial Myoepithelial Carcinoma

Epithelial myoepithelial carcinoma (EMC) is a distinctive neoplasm that features tubular structures with an inner layer of ductal cells and an outer layer of clear cells. The few cases that have been evaluated in immunohistochemical terms show ductal differentiation in the inner cells (CK) and myoepithelial features in the clear cells (S-100 protein, vimentin, muscle-specific actin).[93–95] Although both ductal and myoepithelial cells are prominent in many salivary gland lesions, most

Table 8–6. Comparative Immunostaining for Glial Fibrillary Acidic Protein in Pleomorphic Adenomas and Polymorphous Low-Grade Adenocarcinoma

Tumor	Reference	Glial Fibrillary Acidic Protein Cases Studied	Glial Fibrillary Acidic Protein Distribution
Polymorphous low-grade adenocarcinoma	91	0/7	
	92	2/14	Epithelial and very focal
Pleomorphic adenoma	91	11/11	
	92	14/15	All staining confined to stromal cells

differential diagnostic problems with EMC can be avoided if the biphasic cell arrangement and marked myoepithelial cell clearing are noted carefully.

Clear Cell Carcinoma

As noted in Table 8–4, clear cell change can be a feature of many salivary gland neoplasms. However, a small group of tumors show this feature diffusely and lack histologic foci that point toward the other entities. Such cases are usually rich in collagenous stroma and were formerly designated *hyalinizing CCC.* Examples studied to date show positive staining for CKs and variable reactions for vimentin, GFAP, and S-100 protein.[96–98]

Salivary Duct Carcinoma

Salivary duct carcinoma (SDC) is operatively defined as a carcinoma that shows a strong histologic resemblance to ductal carcinoma of the breast. Many are of high nuclear grade with prominent, comedo-like necrosis, but a low-grade form of this tumor has also been described.[99] The epithelial phenotype of the cells is virtually always manifested by positive immunostains for CK and EMA.[99–103] A majority of cases also shows c-erb-B2 overexpression,[104] as well as positive staining for gross cystic disease fluid protein-15 (GCDFP-15),[103, 105] alpha-lactalbumin,[103] and B72.3.[101] Results obtained with immunostains for S-100 protein have been contradictory.[99, 102]

The histologic similarity of SDC to breast carcinoma has led several investigators to search immunohistochemically for evidence of hormone receptors. Estrogen receptor protein was identified in only 1 of 67 tumors,[103, 105–107] whereas progesterone receptors were found in only 3 of 41 cases.[105–107] In the series of Kapadia and Barnes, 11 of 12 tumors were positive for androgen receptors.[105] The possible therapeutic implications of these data remain to be investigated.

Wick and coworkers have used the term *morphologic mimicry* to unite histologically identical ductal carcinomas of the breast, salivary glands, and sweat glands.[107] They noted relative differences in immunoprofiles as follows: less frequent expression of GCDFP-15 in the cutaneous carcinomas, a low rate of CEA detection in breast carcinomas, and an absence of estrogen receptors in SDC. However, they also pointed out the limited clinical utility of these observations in evaluating a patient with disseminated disease.

Undifferentiated Small Cell Carcinoma

Previously, a morphologic distinction was made between neuroendocrine and ductal small cell carcinomas based on the presence or absence of ul-

trastructurally demonstrable dense core granules. In an immunohistochemical study of 11 cases, Gnepp and Wick found expression of at least 1 neuroendocrine marker in each neoplasm (synaptophysin, chromogranin, neuron-specific enolase, and Leu7).[108] These authors conclude that all such tumors are neuroendocrine.

Chan and colleagues studied a large number of small cell carcinomas from a variety of sites and compared their immunostaining for CK20 with that of 34 Merkel cell carcinomas. Most Merkel cell carcinomas (33 of 34) and several salivary gland small cell carcinomas (3 of 5) were positive, whereas only 2 of 48 cases from other sites showed this marker.[109]

Large Cell Undifferentiated Carcinoma

Large cell undifferentiated carcinomas are uncommon salivary gland neoplasms for which the differential diagnosis includes malignant melanoma, poorly differentiated adenocarcinoma or squamous cell carcinoma, metastatic malignancy of various types, large cell malignant lymphoma, and anaplastic lymphoma. The evaluation of such neoplasms is discussed in other chapters.

References

1. Stanley M. Head and neck cytology. In: Silverberg SG, DeLellis RA, Frable W, eds. Principles and Practice of Surgical Pathology and Cytopathology, vol. 1. 3rd ed. New York: Churchill Livingstone, 1997:1007–1008.
2. Kumagai S, Kojima S, Imai K, et al. Immunohistologic distribution of basement membrane in oral squamous cell carcinoma. Head Neck 1994;16:51–57.
3. Tsukifuji R, Tagawa K, Hatamochi A, et al. Expression of matrix metalloproteinase-1, -2 and -3 in squamous cell carcinoma and actinic keratosis. Br J Cancer 1999;80:1087–1091.
4. Davidson B, Goldberg I, Kopolovic J, et al. Expression of matrix metalloproteinase-9 in squamous cell carcinoma of the uterine cervix—clinicopathologic study using immunohistochemistry and mRNA in situ hybridization. Gynecol Oncol 1999;72:380–386.
5. Nappi O, Pettinato G, Wick MR. Adenoid (acantholytic) squamous cell carcinoma of the skin. J Cutan Pathol 1989;16:114–121.
6. Hertenstein JC. Pathologic quiz case 1: Acantholytic squamous cell carcinoma. Arch Otolaryngol Head Neck Surg 1986;112:780–782.
7. Dodd LG. Fine-needle aspiration cytology of adenoid (acantholytic) squamous-cell carcinoma. Diagn Cytopathol 1995;12:168–172.
8. Moll R, Lowe A, Laufer J, et al. Cytokeratin 20 in human carcinomas: A new, histodiagnostic marker detected by monoclonal antibodies. Am J Pathol 1992;140:427–447.
9. Ascoli V, Taccogna S, Scalzo CC, et al. Utility of cytokeratin 20 in identifying the origin of metastatic carcinomas in effusions. Diagn Cytopathol 1995;12:303–308.
10. Tan J, Sidhu G, Greco MA, et al. Villin, cytokeratin 7 and cytokeratin 20 expression in pulmonary adenocarcinoma with ultrastructural evidence of microvilli with rootlets. Hum Pathol 1998;29:390–396.
11. Zarbo RJ, Crissman JD, Venkat H, et al. Spindle-cell carcinoma of the upper aerodigestive tract mucosa: An immunohistochemical and ultrastructural study of 18 biphasic

tumors and comparison with seven monophasic tumors. Am J Surg Pathol 1986;10:741–753.

12. Ellis GL, Langloss JM, Heffner DK, et al. Spindle-cell carcinoma of the aerodigestive tract: An immunohistochemical analysis of 21 cases. Am J Surg Pathol 1987;11:335–342.

13. Muller S, Barnes L. Basaloid squamous cell carcinoma of the head and neck with a spindle cell component: An unusual histologic variant. Arch Pathol Lab Med 1995;119:181–182.

14. Takata T, Ito H, Ogawa I, Miyauchi M, et al. Spindle cell squamous carcinoma of the oral region: An immunohistochemical and ultrastructural study on the histogenesis and differential diagnosis with a clinicopathologic analysis of six cases. Virchows Arch A Pathol Anat Histopathol 1991:419:177–182.

15. Leonardi E, Dalri P, Pusiol T, et al. Spindle-cell carcinoma of head and neck region: A clinicopathologic and immunohistochemical study of eight cases. J Otorhinolaryngol 1986;48:275–281.

16. Recher G. Spindle cell squamous carcinoma of the larynx: Clinico-pathological study of seven cases. J Laryngol Otol 1985;99:871–879.

17. Leventon GS, Evans HL: Sarcomatoid squamous cell carcinoma of the mucous membranes of the head and neck: A clinicopathologic study of 20 cases. Cancer 1981;48:994–1003.

18. Banks ER, Frierson HF Jr, Mills SE, et al. Basaloid squamous cell carcinoma of the head and neck: A clinicopathologic and immunohistochemical study of 40 cases. Am J Surg Pathol 1992;16:939–946.

19. Sarbia M, Verreet P, Bittinger F, et al. Basaloid squamous cell carcinoma of the esophagus: Diagnosis and prognosis. Cancer 1997;79:1871–1878.

20. Ferlito A, Altavilla G, Rinaldo A, et al. Basaloid squamous cell carcinoma of the larynx and hypopharynx. Ann Otorhinolaryngol 1997;10:1024–1035.

21. Wieneke JA, Thompson LD, Wenig BM. Basaloid squamous cell carcinoma of the sinonasal tract. Cancer 1999;85:841–854.

22. Altavilla G, Mannara GM, Rinaldo A, et al. Basaloid squamous cell carcinoma of the oral cavity and oropharynx. J Otorhinolaryngol 1999;61:169–173.

23. Vesoulis Z. Metastatic laryngeal basaloid squamous cell carcinoma simulating primary small cell carcinoma of the lung on fine needle aspiration lung biopsy. Acta Cytol 1998;42:783–787.

24. Banks ER, Frierson HF Jr, Covell J. Fine needle aspiration cytologic findings in metastatic basaloid squamous cell carcinoma of the head and neck. Acta Cytol 1992;36:126–131.

25. Morice WG, Ferreiro JA. Distinction of basaloid squamous cell carcinoma from adenoid cystic and small cell undifferentiated carcinoma by immunohistochemistry. Hum Pathol 1998;29:609–612.

26. Klijanienko J, el-Naggar A, Ponzio-Prion A, et al. Basaloid squamous cell carcinoma of the head and neck: Immunohistochemical comparison with adenoid cystic carcinoma and squamous cell carcinoma. Arch Otolaryngol 1993;119:887–890.

27. Hewan-Lowe K, Dardick I. Ultrastructural distinction of basaloid squamous carcinoma and adenoid cystic carcinoma. Ultrastruct Pathol 1995;19:371–381.

28. Wick MR, Stanley SJ, Swanson PE: Immunohistochemical diagnosis of sinonasal melanoma, carcinoma and neuroblastoma with monoclonal antibodies HMB-45 and anti-synaptophysin. Arch Pathol Lab Med 1988;112:616–620.

29. Beham A, Fletcher CD, Kainz J, et al. Nasopharyngeal angiofibroma: An immunohistochemical study of 32 cases. Virchows Arch A Pathol Anat Histopathol 1993;423:281–285.

30. Hwang HC, Mills SE, Patterson K, et al. Expression of androgen receptors in nasopharyngeal angiofibroma: An immunohistochemical study of 24 cases. Mod Pathol 1998;11:1122–1126.

31. Taraszewska A, Czorniuk-Silwa A, Dambska M. Olfactory neuroblastoma (esthesioneuroblastoma): Histologic and im-munohistochemical study. Folia Neuropathol 1998;36:81–86.

32. Argani P, Perez-Ordonez B, Xiao H, et al. Olfactory neuroblastoma is not related to the Ewing family of tumors: Absence of EWS/FL11 gene fusion and MIC2 expression. Am J Surg Pathol 1998;22:391–398.

33. Collins BT, Cramer HM, Hearn SA. Fine needle aspiration of metastatic olfactory neuroblastoma. Acta Cytol 1997:41:802–810.

34. Devaney K, Wenig BM, Abbondanzo SL. Olfactory neuroblastoma and other round cell lesions of the sinonasal region. Mod Pathol 1996;9:658–663.

35. Hirose T, Scheithauer BW, Lopes MB, et al. Olfactory neuroblastoma: An immunohistochemical, ultrastructural and flow cytometric study. Cancer 1995;76:4–19.

36. Taxy JB, Bharani NK, Mills SE, et al. The spectrum of olfactory neural tumors: A light microscopic, immunohistochemical and ultrastructural analysis. Am J Surg Pathol 1986;10:687–695.

37. Moss R, Labay G, Mehta N. Ceruminoma revisited. Am J Otol 1987;8:485–488.

38. Mills RG, Douglas-Jones T, Williams RG. Ceruminoma—a defunct diagnosis. J Laryngol Otol 1998;109:180–188.

39. Michel RG, Woodard BH, Shelburne JD, et al. Ceruminous gland adenocarcinoma: A light and electron microscopic study. Cancer 1978;8:541–543.

40. Nadasdy T, Kemeny E, Molnar G, et al. Adenocarcinoma of ceruminous glands: Ultrastructural, immunohistochemical and lectin histochemical studies. Acta Morphol Hung 1991;39:157–165.

41. Fligiel Z, Kaneko M. Extramammary Paget's disease of the external ear in association with ceruminous gland carcinoma: A case report. Cancer 1975;36:1072–1076.

42. Cankar V, Crowley H. Tumors of the ceruminous glands. Arch Otolaryngol Cancer 1964;17:67–75.

43. Wolf BA, Gluckman JL, Wirman JA. Benign dermal cylindroma of the external auditory canal: A clinicopathologic report. Am J Otolaryngol 1985;6:35–38.

44. Ribe A, Fernandez PL, Ostertag H, et al. Middle-ear adenoma (MEA): A report of two cases, one with prominent aplasmacytoid features. Histopathology 1997;30:359–364.

45. Arnold B, Zietz C, Muller-Hocker J, et al. Adenoma of the middle ear mucosa. Eur Arch Otorhinolaryngol 1996;253:65–68.

46. Hardingham M. Adenoma of the middle ear. Arch Otolaryngol Head Neck Surg 1995;121:342–344.

47. Stanley MW, Horwitz CA, Levinson RM, et al. Carcinoid tumors of the middle ear. Am J Clin Pathol 1987;87:592–600.

48. Mills SE, Fechner RE. Middle ear adenoma: A cytologically uniform neoplasm displaying a variety of architectural patterns. Am J Surg Pathol 1984;8:677–685.

49. Gaffey MJ, Mills SE, Fechner RE, et al. Aggressive papillary middle ear tumor: A clinicopathologic entity distinct from middle ear adenoma. Am J Surg Pathol 1988;12:790–797.

50. Gaffey MJ, Mills SE, Boyd JC. Aggressive papillary tumor of middle ear/temporal bone and adnexal papillary cystadenoma: Manifestations of von Hippel-Lindau disease. Am J Surg Pathol 1994;18:1254–1260.

51. van Krieken JH. Prostate marker immunoreactivity in salivary gland neoplasms: A rare pitfall in immunohistochemistry. Am J Surg Pathol 1993;17:410–414.

52. Dardick I, Stratis M, Parks WR, et al. S-100 protein antibodies do not label normal salivary gland myoepithelium: Histogenetic implications for salivary gland tumors. Am J Pathol 1991;138:619–658.

53. Nishimura T, Furukawa M, Kawahara E, et al. Differential diagnosis of pleomorphic adenoma by immunohistochemical means. J Laryngol Otol 1991:105:1057–1060.

54. Hirano T, Kashiwado I, Suzuki I, et al. Immunohistopathological properties of pleomorphic adenoma in salivary gland. J Nippon Med School 1990;57:172–179.

55. Anderson C, Knibbs DR, Abbott SJ, et al. Glial fibrillary acidic protein expression in pleomorphic adenoma of salivary gland: An immunoelectron microscopic study. Ultrastruct Pathol 1990;14:263–271.

56. Ostrzega N, Cheng L, Layfield L. Glial fibrillary acidic protein immunoreactivity in fine-needle aspiration of salivary gland lesions: A useful adjunct for the differential diagnosis of salivary gland neoplasms. Diagn Cytopathol 1989;5:145–149.

57. Takahashi H, Tsuda N, Tezuka F, et al. Immunohistochemical localization of carcinoembryonic antigen in carcinoma in pleomorphic adenoma of salivary gland: Use in the diagnosis of benign and malignant lesions. Tohoku J Exp Med 1986;149:329–340.

58. Takeda Y, Shimono M. Pleomorphic adenoma with nuclear palisading arrangement of modified myoepithelial cells: Histopathologic and immunohistochemical study. Bull Tokyo Dent Coll 1999;40:27–34.

59. Felix A, Rosa JC, Fonseca I, et al. Laminin and collagen IV in pleomorphic adenoma and carcinoma ex-pleomorphic adenoma: An immunohistochemical study. Hum Pathol 1999;30:964–969.

60. Simpson RH, Jones H, Beasley P. Benign myoepithelioma of the salivary glands: A true entity? Histopathology 1995;27:1–9.

61. Skalova A, Michal M, Ryska A, et al. Oncocytic myoepithelioma and pleomorphic adenoma of the salivary glands. Virchows Arch 1999;434:537–546.

62. Franquemont DW, Mills SE. Plasmacytoid monomorphic adenoma of salivary glands: Absence of myogenous differentiation and comparison to spindle cell myoepithelioma. Am J Surg Pathol 1993;17:146–153.

63. Sierra DA, Alamillos FJ, Lopez-Beltran A, et al. Malignant myoepithelioma of the salivary glands: Clinicopathological and immunohistochemical features. Br J Oral Maxillofac Surg 1999;37:64–66.

64. Nagao T, Sugano I, Ishida Y, et al. Salivary gland malignant myoepithelioma: A clinicopathologic and immunohistochemical study of ten cases. Cancer 1998;83:1292–1299.

65. Michal M, Skalova A, Simpson RH, et al. Clear cell malignant myoepithelioma of the salivary glands. Histopathology 1996;2:309–315.

66. Ohmori T, Uraga N, Tabei R. Warthin's tumor as a hamartomatous dysplastic lesion: A histochemical and immunohistochemical study. Histol Histopathol 1991;6:559–565.

67. Segami N, Fukuda M, Manabe T. Immunohistological study of the epithelial components of Warthin's tumor. Int J Oral Maxillofac Surg 1989;18:133–137.

68. Ferreiro JA: Immunocytochemistry of basal cell adenoma of the major salivary glands. Histopathology 1994;24:539–542.

69. Ogawa I, Nikai H, Takata T, et al. The cellular composition of basal cell adenoma of the parotid gland: An immunohistochemical analysis. Oral Surg Oral Med Oral Pathol 1990;70:619–626.

70. Hamano H, Abiko Y, Hashimoto S, et al. Immunohistochemical study of basal cell adenoma in the parotid gland. Bull Tokyo Dent Coll 1990;31:23–31.

71. Prasad AR, Savera AT, Gown AM, et al. The myoepithelial phenotype in 135 benign and malignant salivary gland tumors other than pleomorphic adenoma. Arch Pathol Lab Med 1999;123:801–806.

72. Holmes GF, Eisele DW, Rosenthal D, et al. PSA immunoreactivity in a parotid oncocytoma: A diagnostic pitfall in discriminating primary neoplasms from metastatic prostate cancer. Diagn Cytopathol 1998;19:221–225.

73. Sugimoto T, Wakizono S, Uemura T, et al. Malignant oncocytoma of the parotid gland: A case report with an immunohistochemical and ultrastructural study. J Laryngol Otol 1993;107:69–74.

74. Huang JW, Mori M, Yamada K, et al. Mucoepidermoid carcinoma of the salivary glands: Immunohistochemical distribution of intermediate filament proteins, involucrin and secretory proteins. Anticancer Res 1992;12:811–820.

75. Loyola AM, de Sousa SO, Araujo NS, et al. Study of minor salivary gland mucoepidermoid carcinoma differentiation used on immunohistochemical expression of cytokeratins, vimentin and muscle-specific actin. Oral Oncol 1998;34:112–118.

76. Cho KJ, Kim JY, Lee SS, et al. Mucoepidermoid carcinoma

of the salivary gland: A clinico-pathologic and immunohistochemical study for c-erbB-2 oncoprotein. J Korean Med Sci 1997;12:499–504.

77. Ordonez NG, Batsakis JG. Acinic cell carcinoma of the nasal cavity: Electron-optic and immunohistochemical observations. J Laryngol Otol 1986;100:345–349.

78. Utsunomiya T, Yamamoto H, Kuyama K, et al. Acinic cell carcinoma of the palate: Case report and immunohistochemical observation. Arch Otolaryngol 1999:125:1025–1028.

79. Egan M, Crocker J, Nar P. Localization of salivary amylase and epithelial membrane antigen in salivary gland tumors by means of immunoperoxidase and immunogold-silver techniques. J Laryngol Otol 1988;102:242–247.

80. Ito K, Kakudo K, Mori I, et al. Neuroendocrine differentiation in a case of acinic cell carcinoma of the parotid gland. Acta Pathol Japonica 1990;40:279–287.

81. Cheng J, Saku T, Okabe H, et al. Basement membranes in adenoid cystic carcinoma: An immunohistochemical study. Cancer 1992;6:2631–2640.

82. Gunhan O, Evren G, Demiriz M, et al. Expression of S-100 protein, epithelial membrane antigen, carcinoembryonic antigen and alpha fetoprotein in normal salivary glands and primary salivary gland tumors. J Nihon Univ School Dent 1992;34:240–248.

83. Chomette G, Auriol M, Vaillant JM, et al. Heterogeneity and co-expression of intermediate filament proteins in adenoid cystic carcinoma of salivary glands. Pathol Biol 1991;39:110–116.

84. Bergman R, Lichtig C, Moscona RA, et al. A comparative immunohistochemical study of adenoid cystic carcinoma of the skin and salivary glands. Am J Dermatopathol 1991;13:162–168.

85. Chen JC, Gnepp DR, Bedrossian CW. Adenoid cystic carcinoma of the salivary glands: An immunohistochemical analysis. Oral Surg Oral Med Oral Pathol 1988;65:316–326.

86. Ozono S, Onozuka M, Ito Y. Immunohistochemical localization of estradiol, progesterone, and progesterone receptor in human salivary glands and salivary adenoid cystic carcinomas. Cell Struct Funct 1992;17:169–175.

87. Miller AS, Hartman GG, Chen SY, et al. Estrogen receptor assay in polymorphous low-grade adenocarcinoma and adenoid cystic carcinoma of salivary gland origin: An immunohistochemical study. Oral Surg Oral Med Oral Pathol 1994;77:36–40.

88. Araujo V, Sousa S, Jaeger M, et al. Characterization of the cellular component of polymorphous low grade adenocarcinoma by immunohistochemistry and electron microscopy. Oral Oncol 1999;35:164–172.

89. Perez-Ordonez B, Linkov I, Huvos AG. Polymorphous low grade adenocarcinoma of minor salivary glands: A study of 17 cases with emphasis on cell differentiation. Histopathology 1998;32:521–529.

90. Gnepp DR, Chen JC, Warren C. Polymorphous low grade adenocarcinoma of minor salivary glands: An immunohistochemical and clinicopathologic study. Am J Surg Pathol 1988;12:461–468.

91. Anderson C, Krutchkoff D, Pedersen C, et al. Polymorphous low grade adenocarcinoma of minor salivary glands: A clinicopathologic and comparative immunohistochemical study. Mod Pathol 1990;3:76–82.

92. Gnepp DR, el-Mofty S. Polymorphous low grade adenocarcinoma: Glial fibrillary acidic protein staining in the differential diagnosis with cellular mixed tumors. Oral Surg Oral Med Oral Pathol 1997;83:691–695.

93. Fonseca I, Soares J. Epithelial-myoepithelial carcinoma of the salivary glands: A study of 22 cases. Virchows Arch 1993;422:389–396.

94. Tralongo V, Daniele E. Epithelial-myoepithelial carcinoma of the salivary glands: A review of the literature. Anticancer Res 1998;18:603–608.

95. Shuangshoti S, Lutigaviboon V, Kasantikul V. Epithelial-myoepithelial carcinoma of parotid gland: A case report with immunohistochemical and ultrastructural studies. J Med Assoc Thai 1998;81:712–716.

96. Simpson RH, Sarsfield PT, Babajews AV. Clear cell carci-

noma of minor salivary glands. Histopathology 1990;17:433–438.

97. Milchgrub S, Gnepp DR, Vuitch F, et al. Hyalinizing clear cell carcinoma of salivary gland. Am J Surg Pathol 1994;18:240–241.

98. Shrestha P, Yang LT, Liu BL, et al. Clear cell carcinoma of salivary glands: Immunohistochemical evaluation of clear tumor cells. Anticancer Res 1994;14:825–836.

99. Delgado R, Klimstra D, Albores-Saavedra J. Low grade SDC: A distinctive variant with a low grade histology and a predominant intraductal growth pattern. Cancer 1996;78:958–967.

100. Delgado R, Vuitch F, Albores-Saavedra J. Salivary duct carcinoma. Cancer 1993;72:1503–1512.

101. Drandwein MS, Jagirdar J, Patil J, et al. Salivary duct carcinoma (cribriform salivary carcinoma of excretory ducts): A clinicopathologic and immunohistochemical study of 12 cases. Cancer 1990;65:2307–2314.

102. Yoshihara T, Shino A, Ishii T, Kawakami M. Ultrastructural and immunohistochemical study of salivary duct carcinoma of the parotid gland. Ultrastruct Pathol 1994;18:553–558.

103. Lewis JE, McKinney BC, Weiland LH, et al. Salivary duct carcinoma: Clinicopathologic and immunohistochemical review of 26 cases. Cancer 1996;77:223–230.

104. Martinez-Barba E, Cortes-Guardiola JA, Minguela-Puras A, et al. Salivary duct carcinoma: Clinicopathologic and immunohistochemical studies. J Craniomaxillofac Surg 1997;25:328–334.

105. Kapadia SB, Barnes L. Expression of androgen receptor, gross cystic disease fluid protein, and CD 44 in salivary duct carcinoma. Mod Pathol 1998;11:1033–1038.

106. Barnes L, Rao U, Contis L, et al. Salivary duct carcinoma. Part II: Immunohistochemical evaluation of 13 cases for estrogen and progesterone receptors, cathepsin D, and c-erbB-2 protein. Oral Med Oral Surg Oral Pathol 1994;78:74–80.

107. Wick MR, Ockner DM, Mills SE, et al. Homologous carcinomas of the breasts, skin, and salivary glands: A histologic and immunohistochemical comparison of ductal mammary carcinoma, ductal sweat gland carcinoma, and salivary duct carcinoma. Am J Clin Pathol 1998;109:75–84.

108. Gnepp DR, Wick MR. Small cell carcinoma of the major salivary glands: An immunohistochemical study. Cancer 1990;66:185–192.

109. Chan JK, Suster S, Wenig BM, et al. Cytokeratin 20 immunoreactivity distinguishes Merkel cell (primary cutaneous neuroendocrine carcinomas) and salivary gland small cell carcinomas from small cell carcinomas of various sites. Am J Surg Pathol 1997;21:226–234.

CHAPTER 9

Diagnostic Immunohistochemistry of Endocrine Tumors

Ronald A. DeLellis, M.D. and
Sandra J. Shin, M.D.

The application of immunohistochemical methods has had a profound impact on the understanding of the normal endocrine system and its changes in a wide variety of disease states. In particular, these methods have led to the development of a series of functional classifications of endocrine tumors that have supplemented and, in some cases, supplanted traditional morphologic classifications.[1] The use of immunohistochemistry has been critical for the recognition of new tumor entities, the identification of sites of origin of metastatic tumors, and prognostic assessments, based on patterns of hormone expression and the presence of a variety of other markers. Immunohistochemical methods have played a key role in the identification of precursors of endocrine tumors and in elucidating the steps in the hyperplasia-neoplasia sequence. The purpose of this chapter is to review the major classes of immunohistochemical markers currently used in the assessment of endocrine tumors and to review the diagnostic applications of these methods for endocrine tumors of specific sites.

IMMUNOHISTOCHEMICAL MARKERS OF ENDOCRINE TUMORS

Hormones

An important approach to the diagnosis and classification of endocrine tumors relies on the demonstration of their hormonal content.[1, 2] This can be accomplished by the use of antibodies directed against the mature hormones and hormone precursors. An additional approach involves the use of in situ hybridization (hybridization histochemistry) for the demonstration of specific hormonal messenger RNAs (mRNAs). The latter approach is discussed in detail in several reviews.[3, 4] Virtually all classes of hormones (small peptides, large polypeptide hormones, steroids, amines) and hormone receptors can be visualized in immuno-

histochemical formats.[2, 5] With the advent of microwave-based antigen retrieval methods, the vast majority of these products can be demonstrated in formalin-fixed, paraffin-embedded samples. With few exceptions, however, hormonal products cannot be used as lineage-specific markers.[6] For example, somatostatin is present in the D cells of the pancreatic islets, gastrointestinal and bronchopulmonary endocrine cells, thymic endocrine cells, and thyroid C cells. Therefore, the presence of immunoreactive somatostatin by itself does not provide evidence of the site of origin of a metastatic lesion. The discussion of individual hormones is addressed in sections on specific endocrine cell types and their corresponding tumors.

Enzymes

Enzymes that are active in the biosynthesis and processing of hormones are important markers of endocrine cells.[6] Immunoreactivity for aromatic L-amino acid decarboxylase, for example, is widely distributed in neuroendocrine cells.[7] Tyrosine hydroxylase, dopamine β-hydroxylase, phenylethanolamine N-methyl transferase, in contrast, have a narrower tissue distribution and are confined to known sites of catecholamine biosynthesis.[8] Immunolocalization of these enzymes permits catecholamine synthesizing abilities to be deduced from paraffin sections. The presence of immunoreactive enzyme, however, does not necessarily imply that the enzyme is present in a functional form.[6]

A variety of endopeptidases and carboxypeptidases that are required for the formation of biologically active peptides from precursor molecules are present in the secretory granules of neuroendocrine cells. They include the prohormone convertases PC1/PC3 and PC2 and carboxypeptidases H and E.[9, 10] The proconvertases are widely distributed in neuroendocrine cells and their corresponding tumors, whereas other types of endocrine cells (thyroid follicular cells, parathyroid chief cells, adrenal cortical cells, and testis) are negative.[10] Neu-

209

roendocrine cells with a neural phenotype (e.g., adrenal medullary cells, Merkel cells) contain a predominance of PC2, whereas epithelial neuroendocrine cells contain a predominance of PC3. With the exception of parathyroid cells, the presence of PC2 and PC3 correlates with the presence of chromogranins and secretogranins. PC2 and PC1/PC3 are present in normal pituitaries and in pituitary adenomas, with adrenocorticotropic hormone (ACTH)-producing adenomas containing a predominance of PC1/PC3, and other adenomas expressing a predominance of PC2.[9] Both peptidylglycine alpha-amidating monooxygenase and peptidylamidoglycolate lyase are present in neuroendocrine secretory granules.[11] These enzymes are responsible for the alpha-amidation of the C-terminal regions of peptide hormones. This function is critical for biologic activity of the peptides.

Neuron-specific enolase (NSE) is an additional enzyme that has been studied extensively in neuroendocrine cells.[12] This enzyme is the most acidic isoenzyme of the glycolytic enzyme enolase and is present both in neurons and in neuroendocrine cells.[12] The enolases are products of three genetic loci that have been designated alpha, beta, and gamma. Non-neuronal enolase (alpha-alpha) is present in fetal tissues of different types, glial cells, and many non-neuroendocrine tissues in the adult. Muscle enolase is of the beta-beta type, whereas the neuronal form of enolase has been designated gamma-gamma. Hybrid enolases are present in megakaryocytes and a variety of other cell types. NSE (gamma-gamma) replaces non-neuronal enolase during the migration and differentiation of neurons, and the appearance of this isoenzyme heralds the formation of synapses and electrical excitability. Although many earlier studies used NSE as a specific marker of neuroendocrine cells, more recent studies have indicated that the specificity of this marker using polyclonal antisera is low.[13, 14] Seshi and coworkers reported a high degree of specificity with monoclonal antibodies to the gamma-gamma form of NSE.[15] Some of the monoclonal antibodies to NSE react predominantly with nerve fibers, whereas others react with the perikaryon exclusively or with the perikaryon and associated nerve fibers. In contrast to the polyclonal antisera, monoclonal antibodies stain neuronal cells in a more selective fashion. Some monoclonal antibodies to NSE also react with adrenal medullary cells and subsets of pancreatic endocrine cells.

The protein gene product 9.5 (PGP9.5) is a ubiquitin carboxyterminal hydrolase that plays a role in the catalytic degradation of abnormal denatured proteins.[16-18] PGP9.5 is present in neurons and nerve fibers and in a variety of neuroendocrine cells, with the possible exception of those in the normal gastrointestinal tract. In contrast, carcinoid tumors and a variety of other neuroendocrine tumors contain PGP9.5. The patterns of staining for NSE and PGP9.5 are generally similar in that posi-

tive cells show diffuse cytoplasmic reactivity that is unrelated to the type of hormone produced or the degree of cellular differentiation.[19] Comparative studies, however, have demonstrated that some neuroendocrine tumors may be positive for PGP9.5 and negative for NSE, whereas others may be positive for NSE and negative for PGP9.5. Antibodies to PGP9.5 are particularly useful for the demonstration of neurons and cells with neuronal differentiation.

Histaminase (diamine oxidase) has been used as marker for some neuroendocrine cells and their tumors. This enzyme is present in high concentrations in medullary thyroid carcinomas but is not detectable in C-cell hyperplasia.[20] Small cell carcinomas of the lung and other neuroendocrine neoplasms are variably positive for histaminase. High serum levels of histaminase also occur in pregnancy, and immunohistochemical studies have revealed the presence of this enzyme in decidual cells.

Enzymes of the biosynthetic pathway of steroid hormones can also be demonstrated effectively in immunohistochemical formats. Among the enzymes that have been localized are $P450_{scc}$ (cholesterol side chain cleavage), 3β-hydroxysteroid dehydrogenase, 21-hydroxylase, 17α-hydroxylase, and 11β-hydroxylase.[21-23] To date, however, there have not been extensive studies evaluating antibodies to these enzymes as diagnostic reagents.

Chromogranins, Secretogranins, and Other Granule Proteins

The chromogranins and secretogranins represent the major constituents of neuroendocrine secretory granules.[24-28] Three major chromogranin proteins have been identified and categorized and have been designated chromogranin A, chromogranin B, and secretogranin II. The chromogranin and secretogranin proteins contain multiple dibasic residues that are sites for endogenous proteolytic processing to smaller peptides. These proteins are widely distributed in neurons and neuroendocrine cells. Many neuroendocrine cells contain all three granins, whereas others show distinctive patterns of distribution. For example, the pancreatic beta cells contain only chromogranin A, whereas pituitary lactotrophs and somatotrophs contain a predominance of chromogranin B.

Tissue-specific patterns and ratios of the chromogranin to secretogranin proteins are typically maintained in neuroendocrine tumors. For example, chromogranin A is the major granin expressed by gastric carcinoids and serotonin-producing carcinoids of the appendix and ileum. In contrast, strong immunoreactivity for chromogranin B and secretogranin II is typical of rectal carcinoids and small cell carcinomas and of prolactinomas, which lack chromogranin A.[29, 30] Numerous chromogranin A fragments, including chromostatin, pancreastatin, parastatin, and vasostatin, have also been identified.

HISL-19 and PHE5 are monoclonal antibodies that have also been used in studies of neuroendocrine tumors.[19, 31–33] HISL-19 was produced against human islet cells and reacts with proteins that are distinct from chromogranin A and B and secretogranin II. In normal islets, glucagon cells are more reactive than other islet cell types. Reactivity for HISL-19 is present both in Golgi regions and in secretory granules.[19, 33] This antibody also stains a variety of other neuroendocrine cell types and their corresponding tumors.[33] PHE5 was produced against human pheochromocytomas and reacts with a protein that is distinct from chromogranin A.[32] This antibody also reacts with a variety of normal and neoplastic neuroendocrine cells.

Synaptophysin and Other Synaptic Vesicle Proteins

Synaptophysin is a calcium-binding glycoprotein (38,000 kd), which is the most abundant integral membrane protein constituent of synaptic vesicles of neurons.[34] It is also present in a wide spectrum of neuroendocrine cells and in many of their corresponding tumors. Typically, synaptophysin reactivity is present in a punctate pattern in synaptic regions of neurons and is present diffusely throughout the cytoplasm of neuroendocrine cells. Ultrastructurally, synaptophysin is present in microvesicles, whereas chromogranin is present in secretory granules.[35] These differences suggest that chromogranins and synaptophysin may be complementary generic neuroendocrine markers. Synaptophysin immunoreactivity, however, is not specific to neuroendocrine cells because it is also present in adrenal cortical cells.[36] Synaptic vesicle protein 2 (SV2) is present in the nervous system and in a wide variety of neuroendocrine cells. Portela-Gomes and coworkers demonstrated that it is a sensitive marker for neuroendocrine tumors of all types, particularly hindgut carcinoids.[36a]

CD57

The CD57 antigen is present on subsets of T cells and natural killer cells.[37–39] Antibodies to CD57 also react with Schwann cells, oligodendroglial cells, and a variety of neuroendocrine cells of both neural and epithelial types. Additionally, CD57 positivity is present in prostatic, renal, and cortical thymic epithelial cells. Antibodies to CD57 react with varying proportions of neural tumors, including schwannomas, neurofibromas, neuromas, and granular cell tumors. Among endocrine tumors, CD57 has been used most commonly as a marker for neuroendocrine tumors. For example, CD57 is present in 100% of pheochromocytomas, 85% of extra-adrenal paragangliomas, 50% of

small cell bronchogenic carcinomas, and 85% of carcinoids of diverse origins. However, CD57 is not restricted in its distribution to neuroendocrine tumors, since reactivity is present in more than 95% of papillary thyroid carcinomas and approximately 70% of follicular carcinomas.[40] Nonendocrine tumors that are frequently CD57+ include prostatic carcinomas, thymomas, and a variety of small, round, blue cell tumors. These results indicate that the use of CD57 antibodies alone is unreliable for the specific identification of neuroendocrine tumors.

Neural Cell Adhesion Molecule (CD56)

The neural cell adhesion molecules (NCAMs) comprise a family of glycoproteins that play critical roles in cell binding, migration, and differentiation.[41] The NCAM family includes three principal moieties that are generated from alternative splicing of RNA from a gene that is a member of the immunoglobulin supergene family. The molecules are modified post-translationally by phosphorylation, glycosylation, and sulfation. The homophilic binding properties of NCAMs are modulated by the differential expression of polysialic acid. Although initial studies indicated that NCAM was restricted in its distribution to the nervous system, more recent studies indicate a wider distribution, including the adrenal medulla and cortex (zona glomerulosa), cardiac muscle, thyroid follicular epithelium, proximal renal tubular epithelium, hepatocytes, gastric parietal cells, and islets of Langerhans. Among tumors, both follicular and papillary thyroid carcinomas as well as renal cell carcinomas and hepatocellular carcinomas are NCAM+.[42] The Leu7 antigen, recognized by the HNK-1 monoclonal antibody, has now been identified as a carbohydrate epitope present on NCAM and a number of other adhesion molecules. Most neuroendocrine cells and tumors with neurosecretory granules contain both NCAM mRNA and NCAM protein.[43] Antibodies to a long chain form of polysialic acid (polySia) found on NCAM have been used in studies of normal and neoplastic C cells and neuroendocrine tumors of the lung.[44, 45]

Intermediate Filaments

With the exception of steroid-synthesizing cells, cytokeratins are the major intermediate filaments of endocrine cells. The cytokeratins are members of the intermediate filament (10 nm) superfamily of cytoskeletal proteins.[46] They differ from other cytoskeletal filaments on the basis of size and other physical and chemical properties. Microfilaments (5 to 15 nm) contain actin, whereas the 25-nm microtubules contain tubulin. Other types of intermediate filaments that are present in endocrine cells and their supporting elements include vimentin, glial fibrillary acidic protein (GFAP), and the neurofilament proteins. The cytokeratins are the largest and most complex group of intermediate filaments and include a family of at least 30 proteins with molecular weights ranging from 40 to 68 kd. The type II keratins are basic and include eight epithelial proteins (CK1 to CK8). The type II keratins are more acidic and include 11 epithelial keratins that are designated CK9 to CK20. Pairs of basic and acidic keratins are expressed differentially in epithelial cells at different stages of development and differentiation. They can be identified immunohistochemically using pancytokeratin antibodies that react with epitopes on multiple different molecular weight cytokeratin proteins or with chain-specific monoclonal antibodies that recognize one specific cytokeratin type. The cytokeratins are distributed in tissue-specific patterns, and primary tumors tend to recapitulate the cytokeratin profiles of the cells from which they are derived.[47-49] In some cases, cytokeratin expression patterns tend to be simple, whereas in other cases, complex patterns of cytokeratin expression are apparent. Vimentin (57 kd) is also expressed together with cytokeratins in many normal and neoplastic endocrine cell types. In steroid-producing cells, vimentin is the major intermediate filament protein.

The neurofilaments are composed of heteropolymers of three different subunits with molecular weights of 70, 170, and 195 kd, corresponding to low (L), medium (M), and high (H) molecular weight subunits.[50] All three neurofilament subunits are phosphorylated in proportion to the molecular weight of each subunit. The neurofilaments represent the major intermediate filaments of mature and developing neurons, paraganglionic cells, and certain normal neuroendocrine cells. These intermediate filaments are expressed in tumors with evidence of neuronal differentiation and are also present to varying degrees in neuroendocrine tumors of epithelial type, which also express cytokeratins. Normal epithelial neuroendocrine type cells (pancreatic islets, Merkel cells) most commonly lack neurofilament immunoreactivity, whereas their corresponding neoplasms are commonly positive for this marker. Moreover, the pattern of staining in a dot-like area corresponding to the Golgi region is typical of neuroendocrine neoplasms. The studies of Perez and coworkers have suggested that the differential expression of neurofilament subtypes is related to tumor site.[51] Glial fibrillary acidic protein (GFAP) (50 kd) is the major intermediate filament type of fibrous and protoplasmic astrocytes. GFAP is also present in nonmyelinated Schwann cells, supporting cells of the anterior pituitary and paraganglia, and in a variety of carcinomas. Immunoreactive GFAP is also present in mixed tumors of the skin and salivary glands, nerve sheath tumors, and chordomas.

Transcription Factors

Transcription factors are proteins that bind to regulatory elements in the promoter and enhancer regions of DNA and stimulate or inhibit gene expression and protein synthesis.[52] Transcription factors may be tissue-specific or may be present in a variety of different tissue types. Many of the so-called tissue-specific transcription factors, however, are not restricted to a single tissue type. For example, thyroid transcription factor-1 (TTF-1) is present both in thyroid follicular cells and in lung, whereas the adrenal 4 site/steroidogenic factor (ad4BP/SF-1) is present in steroid-producing cells and in certain anterior pituitary cell types. The pituitary transcription factor, Pit-1, is present in certain cells of the adenohypophysis and is also present in the placenta. Immunohistochemical applications of the transcription factor localization are discussed in subsequent sections.

TUMORS OF SPECIFIC SITES

Adenohypophysis

The cell types of the adenohypophysis were categorized originally on the basis of their reactivities with hematoxylin and eosin as acidophils, basophils, and chromophobes. With more sophisticated histochemical staining sequences, the three cell types were subdivided further. For example, acidophils were further differentiated into the orange G-positive prolactin-positive cells and the erythrosin-positive growth hormone–producing cells. The subsequent development of immunohistochemical methods allowed the distinction of cell types based on their specific hormones.[53] The major cell types and their corresponding products include somatotrophs (growth hormone), lactotrophs (prolactin), mammosomatotrophs (growth hormone, prolactin), thyrotrophs (thyroid-stimulating hormone), corticotrophs (adrenocorticotropin, beta-endorphin, melanocyte-stimulating hormone), and gonadotrophs (follicle-stimulating hormone, luteinizing hormone). The somatotrophs are present predominantly in the lateral wings and account for approximately 50% of the cells of the adenohypophysis. Lactotrophs predominate at the posterolateral edges of the gland and account for 15 to 25% of the cells. The corticotrophs are present primarily in the central mucoid wedge and account for 15 to 20% of the cells. Thyrotrophs account for 5% of the cells and are located in the anteromedial regions of the gland. The gonadotrophs compose approximately 5% of the cell populations and are scattered throughout the anterior lobe.

In addition to the hormone-producing cells, a second cell population is also present (folliculostellate cells) in the normal gland.[54] The latter cells have a dendritic shape and typically encircle the hormone-positive cells. The folliculostellate cells

Table 9–1. Immunohistochemistry of Pituitary Adenomas

Tumor Type	Hormones	Transcription Factors and Receptors	Cytokeratins
Densely granulated somato-troph adenoma	Growth hormone, alpha subunit	Pit-1	Perinuclear staining for CAM5.2
Sparsely granulated somato-troph adenoma with fibrous bodies	Growth hormone (faint, focal, juxtanuclear), alpha subunit (weak)	Pit-1	Globular positivity for CAM5.2
Mammosomatotroph adenoma	Growth hormone (strong), prolactin (weak)	Pit-1, focal estrogen receptor positivity	Perinuclear staining for CAM5.2 with foci of globular staining
Sparsely granulated lacto-troph adenoma	Prolactin (juxtanuclear), alpha subunit (focal)	Pit-1, focal estrogen receptor positivity	
Densely granulated lacto-troph adenoma	Prolactin (diffuse positivity)		
Acidophil stem cell adenoma	Prolactin (diffuse), growth hormone (scant)		
Thyrotroph adenoma	Beta–Thyroid-stimulating hormone and alpha subunit		
Densely granulated cortico-troph adenoma	Adrenocorticotropin and beta-endorphin		Strong and diffuse staining for CAM5.2 with perinuclear accentuation
Sparsely granulated cortico-troph adenoma	Adrenocorticotropin (weak)		Strong cytoplasmic staining for CAM5.2
Crooke cell adenoma	Adrenocorticotropin (weak, peripheral)		Abundant staining for CAM5.2
Gonadotroph adenoma	Alpha subunit, beta–follicle-stimulating hormone, beta-luteinizing hormone	SF-1	
Null cell adenoma and onco-cytoma	Alpha subunit, beta–follicle-stimulating hormone, beta-luteinizing hormone	SF-1	

are positive for S-100 protein and are variably positive for GFAP.

Pituitary adenomas are currently classified according to their content of specific hormones as summarized in Table 9–1 (Figs. 9–1 and 9–2). The tumors also have distinctive patterns of reactivity with antibodies to transcription factors and cytokeratins. Ninety-four percent contain CK8, but in approximately half of these cases, the staining is focal and is present in the form of perinuclear dots. Approximately 50% of adenomas exhibit keratin immunoreactivity with the AE1/AE3 keratin antibody, whereas 6% and 9% are reactive with CKs 19 and 7, respectively.[48] These tumors are also typically positive for generic neuroendocrine markers, including chromogranin (100%), synaptophysin (91%), and NSE (89%).[30, 48–55] Immunoreactivity for the monoclonal antibody HBME-1 (produced against mesothelioma cells) has been found in approximately 25% of pituitary adenomas, predominantly in the extracellular matrix.[48] p53 has been demonstrated in one of four (25%)

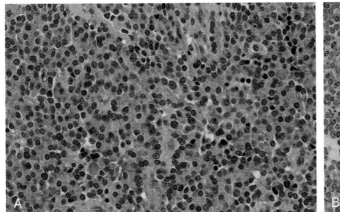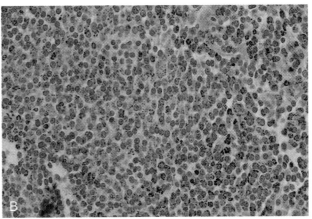

Figure 9–1. A, Pituitary adenoma. (H&E) *B,* Immunoperoxidase stain for prolactin. The cells show weak granular cytoplasmic positivity (sparsely granulated prolactinoma).

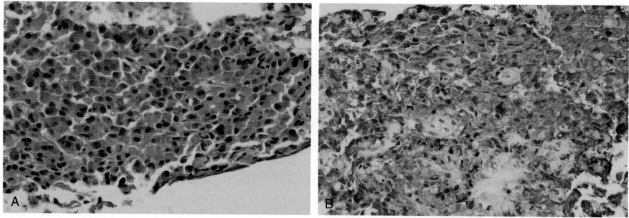

Figure 9–2. A, Pituitary adenoma. (H&E) *B*, Immunoperoxidase stain for growth hormone. All the cells contain immunoreactive growth hormone.

pituitary adenomas, whereas MIC2 and bcl-2 are absent.[56] In contrast to their presence in the normal anterior pituitary, S-100 protein–positive folliculostellate cells are absent from pituitary adenomas.[56]

Pineal Gland

Most primary tumors of the pineal gland originate from pineocytes, which represent modified neurons similar to retinal photoreceptor cells.[57] The remaining tumors of this organ include tumors of germ cell origin and those of glial origin. Pineocytomas are typically positive for NSE, synaptophysin, neurofilament proteins, tau protein, and microtubule-associated protein-2 (MAP2) (Fig. 9–3).[57–59] GFAP and S-100 protein have been found in 75% and 83% of cases, respectively. S antigen, a protein localized in photoreceptor cells, has been demonstrated in 28% of pineocytomas and 50% of pineoblastomas.[60, 61] In contrast to germ cell tumors, pineocytomas are negative for placental alka-

line phosphatase, human chorionic gonadotropin (hCG), and alpha-fetoprotein.[57]

Thyroid Gland

The epithelial components of the thyroid gland include follicular cells and C cells. Follicular cells contain thyroglobulin (TGB), thyroxine (T_4), and triiodothyronine (T_3) which can be demonstrated in frozen sections and in formalin-fixed, paraffin-embedded sections, whereas the major product of the C cell is calcitonin.

Follicular Cells and Their Neoplasms

TGB is a 660-kd glycoprotein with a sedimentation constant of 19S. Iodoproteins of higher and lower sedimentation constants have also been localized immunohistochemically.[62] There is considerable variation in TGB staining intensity in normal glands. The cuboidal to columnar cells of

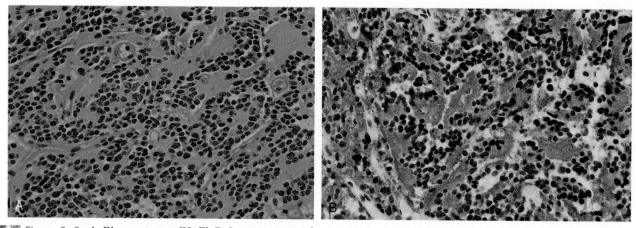

Figure 9–3. A, Pineocytoma. (H&E) *B*, Immunoperoxidase stain for synaptophysin. The cell processes show strong reactivity for synaptophysin.

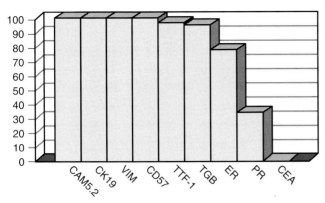

Figure 9–4. Distribution of markers in papillary thyroid carcinoma. CK19, cytokeratin 19; VIM, vimentin; TTF-1, thyroid transcription factor-1; TGB, thyroglobulin; ER, estrogen receptor; PR, progesterone receptor; CEA, carcinoembryonic antigen.

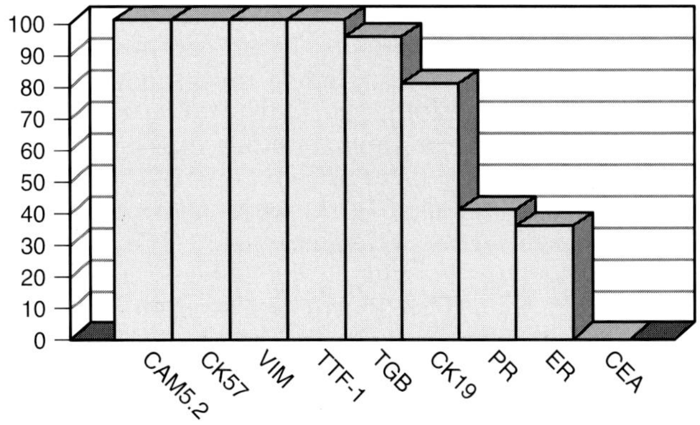

Figure 9–5. Distribution of markers in follicular thyroid carcinoma. CK19, cytokeratin 19; VIM, vimentin; TTF-1, thyroid transcription factor-1; TGB, thyroglobulin; ER, estrogen receptor; PR, progesterone receptor; CEA, carcinoembryonic antigen.

the normal gland consistently exhibit greater degrees of TGB immunoreactivity than the flattened (atrophic) cells of follicles that are distended with colloid. Variation in the staining of colloid is also apparent. Hyperplastic cells are typically strongly stained for TGB, whereas cells lining involuted follicles are weakly reactive or negative. Follicular cells both in Graves' disease and the hyperplastic phase of Hashimoto's disease are moderately to strongly positive for TGB.

Follicular adenomas are positive for TGB but also show considerable variability in staining intensity based on the functional status of the component cells.[62] Hyperfunctional adenomas exhibit strong positivity for TGB, whereas the cells of macrofollicular adenomas show considerably less reactivity and may be negative. Normofollicular adenomas show moderate immunoreactivity for TGB, whereas adenomas with a more solid structure contain smaller amounts of TGB in the component cells. The hyalinizing trabecular adenomas are typically positive for TGB and may also exhibit positivity for some neuroendocrine markers, including chromogranin A and hormonal peptides (neurotensin, endorphins).[63] It has been observed that hyalinizing trabecular adenomas demonstrate plasma membrane patterns of staining with the monoclonal antibody MIB-1.[63a]

The frequency of TGB positivity in thyroid carcinomas is dependent on the degree of differentiation and the histologic subtype. Generally, poorly differentiated carcinomas contain less TGB than do better differentiated tumors. The levels of TGB mRNA are also correspondingly lower in poorly differentiated than in well-differentiated thyroid carcinomas.[64] TGB immunoreactivity is present in more than 95% of papillary and follicular carcinomas (Figs. 9–4 to 9–6.) Since TGB is also expressed in metastatic lesions, stains for this marker are particularly valuable in establishing the origins of metastatic tumors. Immunoreactivity for TGB in differentiated follicular and papillary tumors is

generally present in a patchy distribution. Although some cells exhibit diffuse and uniform staining, others show focal apical or basal positivity. Some tumor cells may be completely unreactive and for this reason, the absence of TGB in a small biopsy sample does not exclude the possibility of a thyroid origin in a metastatic site. Rarely, TGB immunoreactivity as demonstrated with monoclonal antibodies and polyclonal antisera has been reported in nonthyroid malignancies.[65]

Poorly differentiated thyroid carcinomas of the insular type are usually TGB+ both in the colloid and in the component tumor cells, although the extent of cellular staining is generally weak and focal.[66] Undifferentiated (anaplastic) thyroid carcinomas are most commonly negative for TGB. In the series reported by Ordonez and coworkers, 5 of 32 (15.6%) cases of anaplastic carcinoma exhibited TGB immunoreactivity in a small number of cells using both monoclonal antibodies and polyclonal antisera.[67] In this series, positivity was present in 3

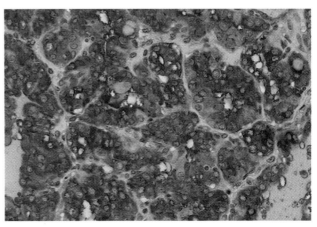

Figure 9–6. Papillary thyroid carcinoma. The cells in this well-differentiated tumor reveal uniform reactivity for thyroglobulin. (Immunoperoxidase stain for thyroglobulin)

of 8 giant cell, 1 of 4 spindle cell, 0 of 6 squamoid, and 0 of 13 mixed variants. Examination of serial sections in these cases failed to reveal evidence of entrapped normal follicular cells or foci of differentiated thyroid carcinoma. Other authors, however, have failed to demonstrate any TGB immunoreactivity in anaplastic carcinomas except in foci of residual differentiated carcinoma.[68]

Antibodies to T_3 and T_4 have been used less extensively than TGB in studies of thyroid carcinoma. Kawaoi and coworkers reported T_4 positivity in 95% of papillary carcinomas and 54% of follicular carcinomas but in no cases of anaplastic thyroid carcinoma. T_3 was present in 66% of papillary carcinomas, 81% of follicular carcinomas, and 45% of anaplastic carcinomas.[69] The significance of T_3 staining in the absence of T_4 immunoreactivity, however, is unknown.

There is an extensive body of literature on the distribution of intermediate filaments in normal and neoplastic follicular cells (Table 9–2).[70–79] Broad spectrum keratin antibodies (AE1/AE3, CAM5.2) react with normal and hyperplastic follicular cells, follicular cells in chronic thyroiditis, and all tumor types. Antibodies to high molecular weight keratins (plantar callus), in contrast, have been reported to react with some follicular cells in 8% of normal thyroids, 44% of hyperplastic glands, and all cases of thyroiditis. High molecular weight keratins were present in 100% of papillary carcinomas, 6% of follicular carcinomas, and 20% of anaplastic carcinomas in one study.[71] These patterns of immunoreactivity with antisera raised against plantar callus, however, have not been adequately explained in terms of keratin subtypes. It has been suggested that this staining most probably results from reactivity with CK19.

Studies reported by Schelfhout and coworkers have demonstrated uniform reactivity for CK19 in 100% of papillary carcinomas (Fig. 9–7).[73] Focal reactivity for CK19 (in <5% of the tumor cells)

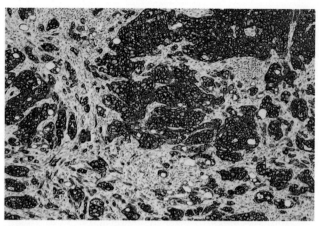

Figure 9–7. Papillary thyroid carcinoma. The tumor cells exhibit intense cytoplasmic staining. (Immunoperoxidase stain for CK19)

was present in 80% of follicular carcinomas and 90% of follicular adenomas, whereas 90% of colloid nodules demonstrated more diffuse positivity in less than 50% of the cells. These data were largely confirmed by Raphael and associates.[74]

More recent studies have demonstrated that normal thyroid strongly expresses the simple epithelial cytokeratins CK7 and CK18 and to a lesser extent CK8 and CK19 but not stratified epithelial cytokeratins.[75] The same patterns of staining were present in lymphocytic thyroiditis, but reactivity for CK19 was more intense. Immunoreactivity for CK7, CK8, CK18, and CK19 was present in both papillary and follicular carcinomas, although the extent and intensity of CK19 staining was greater in papillary carcinomas. However, CK19 was present in all cases of follicular carcinoma at least focally.[75] The stratified epithelial CK5/CK6 and CK13 were present in 27 of 41 (66%) and 14 of 41 (34%) of papillary carcinomas, respectively, but these keratins were absent from other tumor types. Miettinen and associates observed CK19 in all papillary carcinomas and in approximately 50% of follicular carcinomas, whereas CK5/CK6 was present focally in papillary carcinomas.[76] Kragsterman and coworkers concluded that CK19 is of limited value as a marker for routine histopathologic diagnosis but that the presence of this marker should raise the suspicion of papillary carcinoma.[78]

Baloch and coworkers examined a large series of papillary carcinomas of both usual types and follicular variants for a spectrum of cytokeratins, including CK5/CK6/CK18, CK18, CK10/CK13, CK20, CK17, and CK19.[77] In this series, all cases of papillary carcinoma, including the follicular variant, were positive for CK19 (Fig. 9–8). The follicular variants showed strong immunoreactivity in areas with nuclear features of papillary carcinoma, whereas the remaining areas showed moderate to strong staining. Similar but less intense patterns of staining were observed for CK17 and CK20. Normal thyroid parenchyma immediately adjacent to

Table 9–2. Cytokeratin Distribution in Papillary Carcinomas and Follicular Tumors*

Cytokeratin Type	Papillary (%)	Follicular (%)
8	100	100
18	100	100
7	100	100
19	98*	84*
1, 5, 10, 11/14	97	22
5, 6	68	8
17	40	15
13	30	0
20	26	12
14	11	10
4	2.4	0

* Although CK19 is present in both papillary carcinomas and follicular tumors, the extent of staining is consistently higher in papillary carcinomas.

Data based on studies reported by Schelfhout,[73] Raphael,[74] Fonseca,[75] Miettinen,[76] Baloch,[77] Kragsterman,[78] and Liberman and their coworkers.[79]

the follicular variants was also positive, whereas normal thyroid tissue adjacent to the usual variants was negative. Follicular adenomas, follicular carcinomas, and hyperplastic nodules were negative for CK19. The reasons for the discrepancies in CK19 immunoreactivity in follicular tumors between this and other series is unknown.

There is considerable controversy with respect to the presence of CK19 in hyalinizing trabecular tumors of the thyroid. Fonseca and coworkers reported CK19 in all cases of hyalinizing trabecular adenomas and suggested that this tumor represented a peculiar encapsulated variant of papillary carcinoma.[78a] Hirokawa and colleagues, in contrast, found no or minimal CK19 in their series of cases.[78b]

Liberman and Weidner studied the distribution of high molecular weight cytokeratins as demonstrable with the monoclonal antibody 34βE12 (CK1, CK5, CK10, and CK14) and antibodies to involucrin, a structural protein of the stratum corneum, in a series of papillary and follicular carcinomas.[79] Antibodies to high molecular weight cytokeratins reacted with 91% of papillary carcinomas, including the follicular variant, and 20% of follicular neoplasms (adenomas and carcinomas). In general, the staining pattern in papillary carcinomas was strong and patchy, whereas follicular neoplasms stained weakly. Involucrin was positive in 72.5% of papillary carcinomas and 29% of follicular tumors. It has been suggested that the pattern of staining with 34βE12 might be best explained by the presence of an epitope on CK1 or by an epitope that is not recognized by other monoclonal antibodies to CK5, CK10, and CK14.[79]

Cytokeratins are demonstrable in 70 to 75% of anaplastic carcinomas using antibodies AE1/AE3, 34βH11, and CAM5.2, whereas approximately 30% exhibit reactivity with 34βE12 (Fig. 9–9).[67, 68] Poorly differentiated carcinomas exhibit positivity in 100% of cases with broad spectrum cytokeratin antibodies.[66]

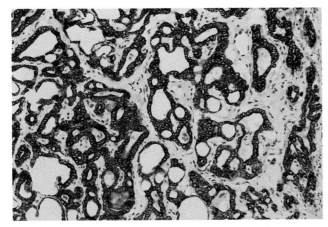

Figure 9–8. Papillary thyroid carcinoma, follicular variant. The tumor cells exhibit intense and uniform cytoplasmic staining. (Immunoperoxidase stain for CK19)

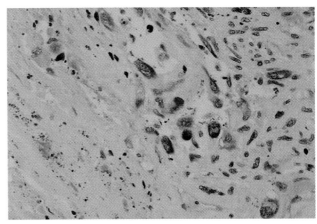

Figure 9–9. Anaplastic (undifferentiated) thyroid carcinoma. Individual tumor cells reveal cytoplasmic staining. (Immunoperoxidase stain for broad spectrum cytokeratins)

Vimentin is coexpressed with cytokeratins in the vast majority of normal and neoplastic thyroids.[71] In the series of Miettinen and colleagues, follicular and papillary tumors expressed vimentin in more than 50% of the tumor cells. Immunoreactivity for vimentin was generally present in the basal portions of the cells in contrast to the more diffuse cytoplasmic reactivity for cytokeratins. Vimentin immunoreactivity has been reported in 94% of anaplastic thyroid carcinomas.

Carcinoembryonic antigen (CEA) is generally absent from nonmedullary thyroid carcinomas. Using six different monoclonal CEA antibodies, Dasovic-Knezevic and colleagues found that 10 papillary, 10 follicular, and 8 anaplastic carcinomas were negative for CEA.[80] Ordonez and coworkers, in contrast, reported CEA immunoreactivity in 9% of anaplastic thyroid carcinomas using a monoclonal antibody.[67] CD15 is present in approximately 30% of papillary carcinomas.[81] The studies of Schroder and associates indicate that the expression of CD15 is more likely to occur in tumors at advanced stages.[81] Thus, CD15 has been considered a prognostic marker for these tumors. Ghali and coworkers reported strong positive staining for CD57 in 100% of papillary and follicular carcinomas, whereas focal positive staining was present in 25% of colloidal goiters and 21% of follicular adenomas.[40] Other authors, however, have questioned the specificity of CD57 as a marker of malignancy in thyroid tumors.[82, 83] The monoclonal antibody HBME-1 has been assessed for its efficacy in differentiating benign and malignant lesions both in aspirates (direct smears and cell blocks) and in tissue sections.[84] Miettinen and Kerkkainen demonstrated positivity for this marker in 100% of papillary and follicular carcinomas but in only 30% of follicular adenomas in histologic sections.[84a] In aspirated material, HBME-1 was detected in five of seven (72%) papillary carcinomas, one of one follicular carcinoma, and one of one anaplastic carcinoma.[84]

In contrast, there was no staining of five follicular adenomas hyperplastic nodules, three Hurthle cell adenomas, one case of chronic thyroiditis and one case of nodular goiter. In tissue sections, HBME-1 was present in 13 of 13 (100%) carcinomas and in 3 of 5 follicular adenomas with hyperplastic nodules, 1 of 3 cases of chronic thyroiditis, 11 cases of chronic thyroiditis, and 0 of 1 case of nodular goiter. In benign lesions, the staining was focal in contrast to the more uniform reactivity of the malignant tumors. These findings have suggested that positive staining for HBME-1 can be a valuable adjunct in the cytologic diagnosis of thyroid malignancies. However, a positive finding does not guarantee the diagnosis of malignancy.

CA 15-3 and CA 19-9 are variably expressed in thyroid follicular tumors. Both follicular and papillary carcinomas reveal positivity in 100% of cases for CA 15-3, whereas CA 19-9 is present in 70% of papillary tumors but in no follicular carcinomas.[85] CA 125 immunoreactivity has been reported in approximately 40% of papillary carcinomas.[65] The distribution of mucin-related antigens has also been analyzed in thyroid tumors.[86] These studies have demonstrated that MUC1 plays a key role in the glycosylation features of well-differentiated thyroid carcinomas. However, there are no consistent differences between papillary and follicular carcinomas with respect to the expression of mucins.

S-100 protein has also been studied in neoplastic lesions of the thyroid gland. McLaren and Cossar reported positivity in 100% of papillary carcinomas, 75% of follicular carcinomas, 37.5% of follicular adenomas, and 28.5% of papillary hyperplasias.[87]

The distribution of p53 has been examined in cases of thyroid carcinoma. In the series reported by Soares and coworkers, p53 was absent from 14 cases of goiter and adenoma and from 12 cases of papillary carcinoma. p53 was present in 20% of follicular carcinomas (predominantly of the widely invasive type), 16% of poorly differentiated carci-

nomas, and 67% of undifferentiated carcinomas.[88] In the series reported by Holm and Nesland, 6 of 32 (19%) papillary carcinomas, 5 of 29 (17%) follicular carcinomas, and 18 of 24 (75%) undifferentiated carcinomas were p53+. In contrast, the RB gene product was present in all thyroid carcinomas.[89]

The *ret* oncogene protein has been demonstrated by immunohistochemistry both in papillary carcinomas and in a subset of hyalinizing trabecular adenomas.[89a–c] However, additional studies are required to ascertain the sensitivity and specificity of *ret* antibodies in immunohistochemical formats for the specific identification of papillary carcinomas.[89d]

Steroid receptors are variably expressed in thyroid tumors. Bur and associates reported estrogen receptor positivity in 8 of 39 (21%) papillary carcinomas, 0 of 5 follicular tumors (three adenomas and two carcinomas), and 0 of 15 Hurthle cell tumors.[90] Progesterone receptor positivity was present in 13 of 39 (33%) papillary carcinomas, 2 of 5 (40%) follicular tumors (one third were adenomas and one half were carcinomas), and 8 of 15 (53%) Hurthle cell tumors. There was no significant correlation between gender, age, or pathologic findings associated with aggressive behavior and the estrogen/progesterone receptor status of the tumors.

Antibodies to mitochondrial antigens are of value in the identification of thyroid tumors with oncocytic (Hurthle cell) features.[91] Positive cells typically exhibit intense cytoplasmic positivity corresponding to the distribution of mitochondria (Fig. 9–10).

TTF-1 is a homeodomain-containing transcription factor that is expressed in the thyroid, diencephalon, and lung. TTF-1 regulates the expression of thyroperoxidase and TGB genes in the thyroid. In the lung, TTF-1 plays an important role in the specific expression of surfactant proteins A, B, and C and Clara cell secretory protein. TTF-1 immunoreactivity has been reported in 96% of papillary, 100% of follicular, 20% of Hurthle cell, 100% of insular, and 90% of medullary carcinomas (Fig. 9–11).[92] Eighty-two percent of metastatic thyroid car-

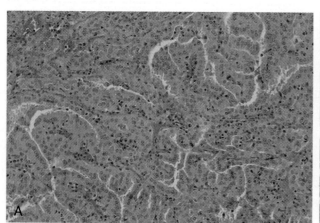
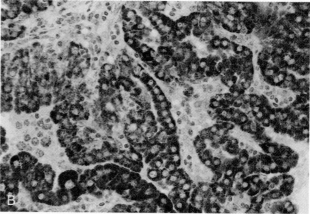

▌ *Figure 9–10. A,* Papillary thyroid carcinoma, oncocytic type. (H&E) *B,* Immunoperoxidase stain for mitochondria using the antibody MITO-113. Tumor cells exhibit intense granular cytoplasmic staining.

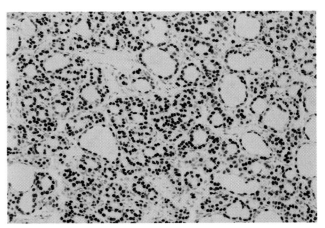

Figure 9–11. Well-differentiated follicular thyroid carcinoma. The tumor cells reveal nuclear positivity. (Immunoperoxidase stain for thyroid transcription factor-1)

cinomas were positive, whereas all anaplastic carcinomas studied to date were negative for TTF-1. In the lung, this marker has been reported in 72.5% of adenocarcinomas, 10% of squamous carcinomas, 26% of large cell carcinomas, 75% of large cell neuroendocrine carcinomas, 30.5% of typical carcinoids, 100% of atypical carcinoids, 94% of small cell carcinomas, and 100% of alveolar adenomas. In contrast, only 2 of 286 adenocarcinomas of nonpulmonary and nonthyroid types exhibited TTF-1 immunoreactivity. In their study of thyroid and pulmonary carcinomas, Kaufmann and Dietel demonstrated reactivity for surfactant protein A in three of seven thyroid carcinomas in a focal pattern.[93] Byrd-Gloster and coworkers reported that TTF-1 is useful in the distinction of pulmonary small cell carcinomas from Merkel cell carcinomas.[94] In their study, 97% of small cell bronchogenic carcinomas were TTF-1+, whereas none of 21 Merkel cell tumors exhibited positivity. However, TTF-1 has been reported in some nonpulmonary small cell carcinomas, including those arising in the prostate, urinary bladder, and uterine cervix.[95]

KEY DIAGNOSTIC POINTS OF THYROID CARCINOMAS

- Poorly differentiated carcinomas contain less TGB than do better differentiated tumors
- TGB is present in more than 95% of papillary and follicular carcinomas
- Anaplastic thyroid carcinomas are mostly TGB−
- The vast majority of papillary carcinomas are CK19+; however, CK19 is also present in other thyroid tumor types.
- 34βE12 clone (keratin 903, high molecular weight keratin) is positive in more than 90% of papillary carcinomas

- Low molecular weight and broad spectrum keratins are present in up to 75% of anaplastic carcinomas
- Vimentin is coexpressed regularly in thyroid carcinomas
- CEA is absent in follicular-papillary carcinomas but positive in medullary carcinoma and certain metastatic carcinomas to thyroid
- TTF-1 is positive in 96% of papillary, 100% of follicular, 20% of Hurthle cell, and 90% of medullary carcinomas; anaplastic carcinomas are essentially negative for TTF-1

C Cells and Medullary Thyroid Carcinoma

C cells, the second major endocrine cell population of the thyroid gland, are the primary sites of synthesis and storage of calcitonin. These cells also synthesize a variety of other regulatory products, including somatostatin and gastrin-releasing peptide, and amines.[96, 97] They can be distinguished from the follicular cells on the basis of their content of calcitonin and the presence of generic neuroendocrine markers, including NSE, chromogranin A, and synaptophysin.

C cells in normal glands have an exclusive intrafollicular topography and are concentrated at the junctions of the upper and middle thirds of the lobes.[96] In patients with multiple endocrine neoplasia, type 2 (MEN2), C-cell hyperplasia has been recognized as the precursor of medullary thyroid carcinoma. Detailed immunohistochemical studies have shown that C-cell hyperplasia is characterized by increased numbers of C-cells within the follicles in the same regions of the gland where C cells normally predominate (Fig. 9–12). These relationships are maintained in areas of more advanced C-cell hyperplasia, where C cells often

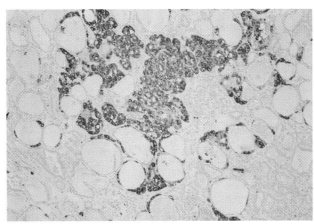

Figure 9–12. C-cell hyperplasia from a patient with multiple endocrine neoplasia, type 2A. Hyperplastic C cells surround individual follicles and in some areas replace follicles. (Immunoperoxidase stain for calcitonin)

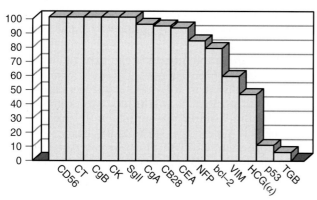

Figure 9–13. Distribution of markers in medullary thyroid carcinoma. CT, calcitonin; CgB, chromogranin B; CK, cytokeratin; SgII, secretogranin II; CgA, chromogranin A; CB28, calbindin D_{28k}; CEA, carcinoembryonic antigen; NFP, neurofilament protein; VIM, vimentin; HCG(α), human chorionic gonadotropin alpha; TGB, thyroglobulin.

completely encircle and displace the follicular epithelium centrally. Nodular hyperplasia is characterized by the complete obliteration of the follicular space by proliferating C cells. The earliest phases of medullary carcinoma are characterized by invasion of C cells through the follicular basement membrane. In addition to its occurrence in patients with MEN2, C-cell hyperplasia may occur in patients with hypercalcemia or hypergastrinemia and around follicular or papillary neoplasms. This type of C-cell hyperplasia has been termed *secondary hyperplasia* in contrast to the hyperplasia occurring in patients with MEN2 (primary or "neoplastic" hyperplasia).[98]

Medullary thyroid carcinomas are positive for calcitonin in more than 95% of cases (Figs. 9–13 and 9–14).[97, 99, 100] In rare cases that are negative for calcitonin peptide, calcitonin mRNA may be demonstrated by in situ hybridization.[101] Rarely, small cell carcinomas resembling oat cell carcinomas may occur and have been reported to be nega-

tive for calcitonin peptide and the corresponding mRNA.[102] Several studies have suggested that the patterns of calcitonin staining in these tumors may have prognostic significance and that tumors with low levels of calcitonin may behave more aggressively. Franc and coworkers have demonstrated in univariate analyses that patients with tumors containing fewer than 50% calcitonin immunoreactive cells had less favorable survival patterns than did patients whose tumors contained more than 50% immunoreactive cells.[103] In multivariate analyses, the five parameters that were significantly associated with a lower survival included necrosis (p = .001), squamous foci (p = .002), age greater than 45 years (p = .004), presence of oxyphils (p = .025), and less than 50% calcitonin immunoreactive cells (p = .04). In addition to calcitonin, normal and neoplastic C cells contain the calcitonin gene-related peptide (CGRP).[104] CGRP results from alternate splicing of the primary transcript of the calcitonin gene. The normal thyroid expresses calcitonin predominantly, whereas CGRP is found primarily in the central and peripheral nervous system. In medullary carcinomas, calcitonin and CGRP are produced in a concordant manner.[105]

A variety of other peptides have been demonstrated by immunohistochemistry, and their presence has been confirmed by correlative radioimmunoassays of tumor extracts. Somatostatin and gastrin-releasing peptide are found commonly in medullary thyroid carcinomas.[106, 107] Scopsi and coworkers used antisera raised against four different regions of the prosomatostatin molecule and demonstrated positive staining in 100% (33 of 33) of cases.[106] Most, but not all, of the somatostatin-positive cells were also positive for calcitonin. Somatostatin immunoreactive cells are generally present singly or in small groups, representing less than 5% of the entire tumor cell population. The somatostatin-positive cells have a dendritic shape with branching cell processes extending between adjacent tumor cells. Gastrin-releasing peptide is present in approximately 30% of medullary carci-

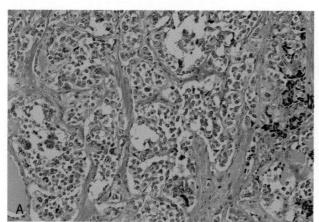
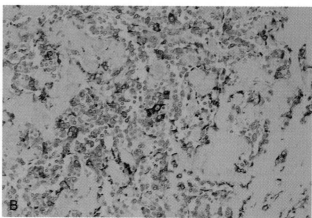

Figure 9–14. A, Medullary thyroid carcinoma. (H&E) *B,* This tumor exhibits considerable variation in staining intensity in different cells. (Immunoperoxidase stain for calcitonin)

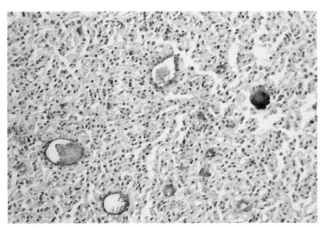

Figure 9–15. Medullary thyroid carcinoma. Thyroglobulin-positive follicles are entrapped within the tumor. (Immunoperoxidase stain for thyroglobulin)

nomas.[107] Other peptide products that are present in these tumors include ACTH and other pro-opiomelanocortin peptides, neurotensin, substance P, and vasoactive intestinal peptide (VIP).[99] The alpha chain of hCG has been demonstrated in 46% (17 of 37) of cases.[108]

Both catecholamines and serotonin are present in medullary thyroid carcinomas. Uribe and coworkers demonstrated serotonin immunoreactivity in 70% (14 of 20) of cases.[100] Serotonin immunoreactivity in these tumors is generally present in cells with a dendritic morphology, similar to that of the somatostatin-positive cells.

TGB may occur in medullary thyroid carcinoma as entrapped follicles, single follicular cells, or extracellular deposits (Fig. 9–15). This phenomenon is most likely to occur at the junction of the tumor and the adjacent thyroid parenchyma or along vascular septa. In one series, TGB immunoreactivity was present in approximately 60% of primary thyroid tumors but in no case of metastatic medullary thyroid carcinoma.[109] True mixed tumors with C-cell and follicular features have also been reported. These tumors are composed of cells that contain calcitonin or other peptides and TGB.[110, 111] The existence of such tumors may explain the rare cases of medullary thyroid carcinoma that have the capacity for radioactive iodine uptake.

The proposed origin of tumors with mixed medullary and follicular features has been controversial. Volante and coworkers have proposed an origin from two different progenitors.[112] According to their hypothesis, neoplastic transformation of C cells leads to the development of medullary thyroid carcinoma with entrapped normal follicles. Stimulation of the entrapped follicular cells results in hyperplasia and ultimately follicular (or papillary) neoplasia (hostage hypothesis). Neoplastic C cells and follicular cells would have the capacity to metastasize and could explain the presence of both components in distant sites.

Medullary carcinomas are typically positive for the entire battery of generic neuroendocrine markers, including NSE, the chromogranin proteins, synaptophysin, and histaminase.[96, 99] Since NSE is also expressed in a variety of non–C-cell neoplasms, it should never be used as the sole marker to distinguish medullary carcinomas from other thyroid tumor types. In addition to chromogranin A, medullary carcinomas also consistently express chromogranin B and secretogranin II.[113] The calcium-binding protein calbindin-D_{28K}, which is also regarded as a general neuroendocrine marker, has been found in 95% (18 of 19) of medullary carcinomas.[114]

Polysialic acid of NCAM is consistently expressed in medullary carcinomas. Komminoth and coworkers demonstrated that 100% (33 of 33) of medullary carcinomas were positive, whereas other thyroid tumor types were consistently negative.[105] Strong polySia immunoreactivity occurs in all cases of primary C-cell hyperplasia, whereas normal C cells and C cells in cases of secondary C-cell hyperplasia were negative in most cases.

Bcl-2 immunoreactivity is present in 79% (26 of 33) of cases of medullary carcinoma.[115] In the study reported by Viale and associates, lack of bcl-2 immunoreactivity correlated significantly with shorter survival ($p = .0001$).[115] In multivariate analyses, lack of bcl-2 was an independent predictor of poor prognosis. Viale and colleagues also demonstrated that p53 immunoreactivity was present in 12% (4 of 33) of medullary carcinomas.[115] Holm and Nesland reported p53 immunoreactivity in 13% (6 of 46) of medullary carcinomas.[89]

CEA as detected by both monoclonal antibodies and polyclonal antisera is present in the vast majority of medullary carcinomas.[116] Monoclonal antibodies that are specific to CEA react with approximately 75% of cases of medullary carcinoma but not with other tumor types.[117] Antibodies that react with epitopes present on CEA and the nonspecific cross-reacting antigens react with almost 90% of medullary carcinomas but also give positive reactions with other thyroid tumor types. Several groups have demonstrated that some medullary thyroid carcinomas may lose their ability to synthesize and secrete calcitonin while maintaining their capacity for CEA production and that such tumors may have an aggressive course.[118] Franc and coworkers demonstrated that patients with medullary carcinomas containing more than 50% CEA-positive cells and less than 50% calcitonin-positive cells had a poorer prognosis compared with other groups.[103]

Medullary carcinomas are typically positive for low molecular weight cytokeratins. Vimentin immunoreactivity is present in approximately 60% of cases, whereas neurofilament proteins have been reported in 85% (10 of 12) cases.[119] Normal C cells have been reported to lack neurofilament proteins but are typically positive for low molecular weight cytokeratins and are variably positive for vimentin.

KEY DIAGNOSTIC POINTS OF MEDULLARY THYROID CARCINOMA

- Normal C cells have intrafollicular topography and immunostain with calcitonin
- Ninety-five percent of medullary carcinomas are positive for calcitonin. Other peptides may also be present
- True mixed C-cell and follicular tumors are rare
- Generic neuroendocrine markers are typically positive in medullary carcinoma and include NSE, synaptophysin, chromogranins A and B, and secretogranin II

Parathyroid Glands

Immunohistochemical analysis of parathyroid hormone (PTH) has proved difficult because of both the lack of suitable antibodies and the low level of hormone storage within the chief cells.[120] Antigen retrieval methods, however, have greatly facilitated the localization of PTH in formalin-fixed, paraffin-embedded sections (Fig. 9–16).[121] Both PTH and chromogranin A are demonstrable in the vast majority of normal, hyperplastic, and neoplastic parathyroid glands. In normal glands, chief cells stain more intensely for PTH and chromogranin A than do oncocytes. Hyperplastic glands generally stain less intensely than do normal glands. The intensity of staining for PTH and chromogranin A is less intense in adenomas than in normal and hyperplastic glands. Generally, however, staining of the rim of adjacent normal parathyroid is more intense than that of the adenomas.[121] A similar pattern of reactivity has been observed in in situ hybridization preparations with probes to parathyroid mRNA.[122] In a single case of parathyroid carcinoma, Tomita reported positive staining for PTH but no significant reaction for chromogranin A.[121] Patterns of PTH reactivity generally correspond to the levels of extractable PTH, with the highest levels being present in normal glands and the lowest in adenomatous glands.[123] In addition to PTH, PTH-related protein has also been demonstrated by immunohistochemistry.[124]

Schmid and coworkers reported that 14% (12 of 86) of hyperplastic parathyroid glands demonstrated focal reactivity for chromogranin B and that in 10 of 12 of these cases calcitonin was colocalized with chromogranin B.[125] CGRP was found in a small proportion of the calcitonin cells in 4 of 10 of the cases. These observations were confirmed by the demonstration of mRNAs for calcitonin and CGRP. The results of this study indicate that calcitonin and CGRP may be synthesized and stored in hyperplastic parathyroid chief cells.

CD4 immunoreactivity using the anti-Leu3a and OKT4D antibodies has been demonstrated both in normal and abnormal parathyroid glands.[126] Positive staining was restricted to chief cells, whereas oncocytic cells were nonreactive. Normal, hyperplastic, and neoplastic cells demonstrated positive staining primarily on cell surfaces. In contrast, parathyroid carcinomas demonstrated primarily cytoplasmic staining. Although the functional significance of CD4-like immunoreactivity is unknown, this moiety may play a role in calcium-regulated PTH release.

The distribution of cyclin D1 has also been examined in normal and neoplastic parathyroid tissue.[127] In normal glands, cyclin D1 was present in 6% of cases. In contrast cyclin D1 was present in 10 of 11 (91%) parathyroid carcinomas, 11 of 38 (39%) parathyroid adenomas, and 11 of 18 (61%) hyperplastic parathyroid glands. These studies confirm the high frequency of cyclin D1 expression in adenomas and carcinomas, but they also indicate that high levels of expression may also occur in cases of hyperplasia.[127]

The distinction between parathyroid adenomas and carcinomas is, on occasion, extremely difficult. Several studies have used MIB-1 to aid in the differential diagnosis. Abbona and coworkers re-

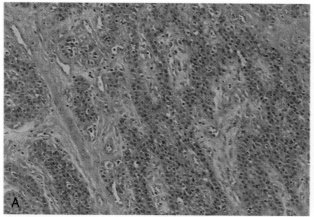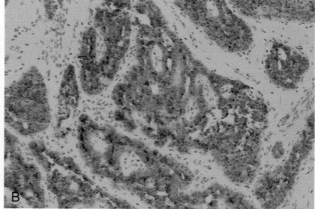

Figure 9–16. *A*, Intrathyroidal parathyroid adenoma. *B*, The chief cells exhibit strong cytoplasmic reactivity. (Immunoperoxidase stain for parathyroid hormone)

ported a significant difference between carcinomas (aggressive and nonaggressive) and adenomas with respect to MIB-1 scores.[128] There were no significant differences, however, between nonaggressive carcinomas and adenomas. Conversely, mitotic rates and MIB-1 scores of clinically aggressive carcinomas were significantly higher than in adenomas. Vargas and coworkers reported that an MIB-1 fraction in excess of 40 positive signals per 1000 cells correlated strongly with malignancy.[129] p27 (Kip 1) has also been examined in parathyroid hyperplasia, adenoma, and carcinoma.[130] The p27 labeling index was 56.8 ± 3.4 for adenomas and 13.9 ± 2.6 for carcinomas, whereas the MIB-1 labeling index was significantly higher in carcinomas than in adenomas. These findings suggest that both p27 and MIB-1 may be helpful when used together for the distinction of parathyroid adenomas and carcinomas.

Another approach to the distinction of parathyroid adenomas and carcinomas involves the use of antibodies to the retinoblastoma (RB) protein. Cryns and coworkers reported the absence of RB protein in a small series of carcinomas, whereas this protein was present in adenomas.[131] However, Vargas and coworkers demonstrated positive staining for RB in 100% of adenomas and 80% of carcinomas.[129] More recently, Farnebo and coworkers also demonstrated the lack of utility of RB immunoreactivity for the distinction of adenomas and carcinomas.[132]

p53 has also been examined in normal, hyperplastic, and neoplastic parathyroid tissues. In the study reported by Kayath and colleagues, p53 was present in 36% (10 of 28) of adenomas, 42% (5 of 12) of cases of primary hyperplasia, 72% (13 of 18) of cases of diffuse hyperplasia, 44% (17 of 39) of cases of nodular hyperplasia, and 40% (2 of 5) of adenomas.[133] These results indicate that the analysis of p53 by immunohistochemistry is not useful in the distinction of the various proliferative states of the parathyroid.

The intermediate filament profiles of normal and neoplastic parathyroid tissue have been studied by Miettinen and associates.[134] Both normal and adenomatous parathyroid glands contain CK8, CK18, and CK19. Vimentin was restricted to stromal cells. The chief cells of normal parathyroid gland were negative for neurofilament proteins, but 33% of adenomas contained some neurofilament-positive cells that also stained positively for cytokeratins.

Adrenal Gland

ADRENAL CORTEX

Markers that have been used for the identification of adrenal cortical cells include steroidogenic enzymes, the monoclonal antibody D11, Ad4BP, A103 (melan A), and inhibin A (Fig. 9–17). Studies reported by Sasano and coworkers demon-

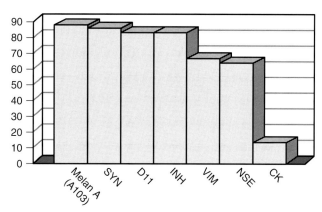

Figure 9–17. Distribution of markers in adrenal cortical carcinoma. SYN, synaptophysin; INH, inhibin; VIM, vimentin; NSE, neuron-specific enolase; CK, cytokeratin.

strated strong staining for $P450_{17\alpha}$ in the fasciculata and reticularis zones of patients with Cushing's disease.[21-23] Cortical adenomas associated with cortisol overproduction demonstrated strong staining for this enzyme, whereas the adjacent zona reticularis showed weak staining, consistent with suppression of the normal gland.

The monoclonal antibody D11 recognizes several 59kd proteins capable of binding apolipoprotein E.[135, 136] Approximately 80% of adrenal cortical tumors show positive nuclear staining for D11; however, 100% of hepatocellular carcinomas, 60% of lung carcinomas and occasional renal carcinomas have been reported to show cytoplasmic staining for this marker.[137] The nuclear adrenal 4 binding protein (Ad4BP) which is also known as steroid factor (SF)-1 is a transcription factor that regulates steroidogenic cytochrome P450 gene expression. Ad4BP has been reported in 100% of adrenal cortical carcinomas while no cases of renal cell carcinoma, hepatocellular carcinoma or other tumor types (including pheochromocytoma) exhibited positivity.[138]

The monoclonal antibody A103 (melan A) has been used primarily for the identification of malignant melanoma (Fig. 9–18; see also Fig. 9–17). This antibody cross-reacts with an epitope which is present in steroid-producing cells, including those of the adrenal cortex.[139] Busam and coworkers reported A103 immunoreactivity in 100% of adrenal cortical carcinomas but in no cases of renal cell carcinoma, hepatocellular carcinoma, pheochromocytoma, or other types of epithelial tumors.[139] In a smaller series, Renshaw and Granter reported positive staining in two of four adrenal cortical carcinomas.[140] A103 is also of considerable use in the evaluation of cytologic specimens from adrenal aspirates.[141]

The inhibin A antibody is also useful for the identification of steroid-producing cells.[142] Fetsch and coworkers used this antibody for the identification of adrenal cortical tumors in cytologic prep-

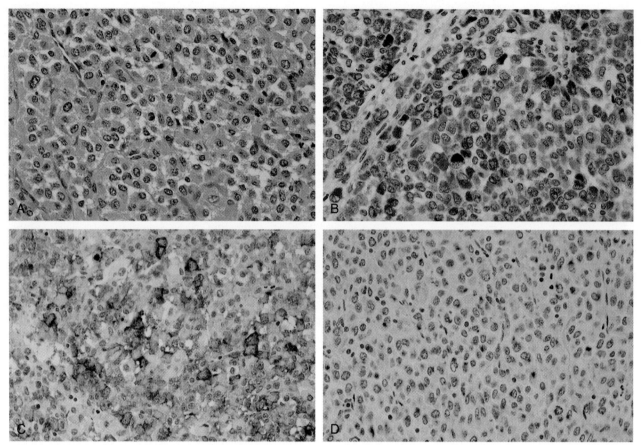

Figure 9–18. *A,* Adrenal cortical carcinoma. (H&E) *B,* The tumor cells exhibit granular cytoplasmic positivity. (Immunoperoxidase stain for melan A [A103]) *C,* The tumor cells show strong cytoplasmic staining. (Immunoperoxidase stain for synaptophysin) *D,* There is focal cytoplasmic staining. (Immunoperoxidase stain for cytokeratins, CAM5.2)

arations.[143] They reported positive staining in 100% of adrenal cortical tumors but in no cases of renal cell carcinoma. Renshaw and Granter demonstrated that inhibin A and A103 are useful in the immunohistochemical identification of adrenal cortical neoplasms and that A103 is marginally more specific and inhibin A slightly more sensitive for the identification of cortical tumors.[140]

Adrenal cortical carcinomas may show evidence of neuroendocrine differentiation, as manifested by immunoreactivity for synaptophysin, neurofilament proteins, and NSE[36, 144] (Fig. 9–18*C*). In contrast to pheochromocytomas, however, adrenal cortical car-

cinomas are typically negative for the chromogranin proteins. In one series, 60% of cortical carcinomas were positive for the low molecular weight neurofilament protein, 80% were positive for synaptophysin, and 60% were positive for NSE.[144] The significance of these findings with respect to the histogenesis of cortical carcinomas is unknown.

The differentiation of adrenal cortical carcinomas from metastatic carcinomas to the adrenal gland may be extremely difficult (Table 9–3). This distinction may be facilitated by studies of the distribution of intermediate filaments, particularly cy-

Table 9–3. Differential Diagnosis of Adrenal Cortical Carcinoma

Tumor Type	A103	Inhibin	Cyto-keratin	Vimentin	S-100	Epithelial Membrane Antigen	Chromo-granin	Synapto-physin	Neuro-filaments	Carcino-embryonic Antigen	Alpha-Fetoprotein
Adrenocortical carcinoma	+	+	−/+	+	+/−	N	N	+/−	+/−	N	N
Pheochromocytoma	N	N	N	+	+	N	+	+	+	N	N
Renal cell carcinoma	N	N	+	+	+/−	+	N	N	N	N	N
Hepatocellular carcinoma	N	N	+	+	+/−	+/−	N	N	N	+	+
Metastatic adenocarcinoma	N	N	+	+	+/−	+	N	N	N	+	N

+, almost always positive; +/−, mostly positive; −/+, mostly negative; N, negative.

tokeratins and vimentin. Normal and neoplastic adrenal cortical cells are typically vimentin-positive but exhibit considerable differences in patterns of cytokeratin immunoreactivity depending on factors such as tissue preparation (fixed versus frozen) and the reactivities of the cytokeratin antibodies.[145, 146] With fresh frozen tissues and with formalin-fixed, paraffin-embedded tissues subjected to microwave antigen retrieval, cytokeratin immunoreactivity may be present focally in up to 60% of adrenal cortical neoplasms, particularly with CAM5.2 (see Fig. 9–18D). The typical intermediate filament profile for cortical carcinomas is, therefore, vimentin-positive with variable weak cytokeratin immunoreactivity.[147, 148] Metastases to the adrenal gland, in contrast, are more likely to exhibit intense cytokeratin staining and are also usually positive for CEA, CD15, and epithelial membrane antigen (EMA), whereas adrenal cortical carcinomas are negative for these markers.

Bcl-2 is typically present in all cell layers of the normal adrenal cortex but is consistently absent from the medulla. Fogt and coworkers demonstrated bcl-2 immunoreactivity in 23 of 23 cortical adenomas and carcinomas but in only 1 of 11 pheochromocytomas.[149] This study suggests that bcl-2 may be helpful in the differential diagnosis of adrenal cortical and medullary tumors.

ADRENAL MEDULLA AND EXTRA-ADRENAL PARAGANGLIA

The major cell types of the adrenal medulla and extra-adrenal paraganglia include the catecholamine-synthesizing cells and the supporting or sustentacular cells.[150, 151] Both catecholamines and catecholamine-synthesizing enzymes have been demonstrated in these cells with immunofluorescent techniques in frozen sections and immunoperoxidase techniques in paraffin-embedded material.[8, 150–152] The catecholamine-synthesizing cells

typically exhibit positivity for a variety of generic neuroendocrine markers and are variably positive for certain peptide hormones. Sustentacular cells, in contrast, are positive for S-100 protein.[150]

The adrenal medullary cells and extra-adrenal paraganglionic cells and their tumors typically exhibit a neurofilament- and vimentin-positive phenotype.[50, 145, 153] The presence of cytokeratin immunoreactivity in these tumors has been controversial. Kimura and coworkers have reported cytokeratin immunoreactivity in 13 of 45 (29%) pheochromocytomas using a broad spectrum cytokeratin antibody.[119] Cytokeratin immunoreactivity was generally sparse, but positive cells were sometimes present in small groups or clusters. In contrast to the cytokeratin positivity in pheochromocytomas, extra-adrenal paragangliomas in Kimura and associates' study were cytokeratin-negative. Other authors, however, have failed to demonstrate cytokeratins in pheochromocytomas and extra-adrenal paragangliomas. Chetty and colleagues examined 18 extra-adrenal paragangliomas and 7 pheochromocytomas for cytokeratins using the antibodies AE1/AE3, CAM5.2, and 34βE12 after microwave antigen retrieval.[154] Reactivity with AE1/AE3 and CAM5.2 was present in three extra-adrenal paragangliomas (cauda equina, intravagal, and orbital). None of the pheochromocytomas was positive. Other epithelial markers, such as EMA, are typically negative in pheochromocytomas and paragangliomas.

NSE is present in virtually all pheochromocytomas and paragangliomas.[150, 155] Synaptophysin is present in 100% of cases, whereas chromogranin A is expressed in more than 95%.[150, 155, 156] Generally, chromogranin immunoreactivity is more intense in normal than in neoplastic cells of paraganglionic tissue (Fig. 9–19A). Chromogranin immunoreactivity appears in a distinctive granular pattern, whereas NSE immunoreactivity appears diffusely within the cytoplasm. Synaptophysin immunoreactivity is present in 100% of cases. Another generic

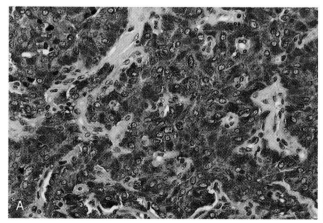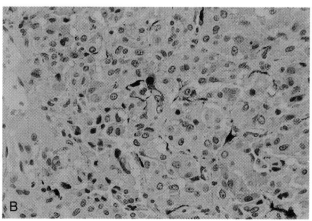

Figure 9–19. A, Adrenal pheochromocytoma. The tumor cells exhibit intense cytoplasmic staining. (Immunoperoxidase stain for chromogranin A) B, Positivity is restricted to the sustentacular cells. (Immunoperoxidase stain for S-100 protein)

neuroendocrine marker that has been analyzed in these tumors is PGP9.5, which is present in approximately 80% of reported cases.[157] S-100 protein is present only in the sustentacular cells (see Fig. 9–19*B*).

In the normal adrenal gland, CD56 is present in the medulla and the zona glomerulosa.[42] Pheochromocytomas are typically strongly positive. Komminoth and associates used a monoclonal antibody that binds specifically to a long chain form of polysialic acid (polySia) found on NCAM and demonstrated staining restricted to the medulla of normal human glands.[36] One hundred percent of pheochromocytomas were diffusely polySia-positive, whereas 8 of 28 (28%) cortical carcinomas exhibited focal positivity.

In addition to catecholamines, serotonin immunoreactivity has been demonstrated in approximately 80% of pheochromocytomas.[155] Both pheochromocytomas and extra-adrenal paragangliomas may also contain peptide hormones, including neuropeptide Y (64%), substance P (36%), calcitonin (21%), and leu- and met-enkephalin (70%).[155, 157] Several studies indicated that determination of circulating levels of neuropeptide Y may be useful in the diagnosis and monitoring of patients with these tumors. Hellman and coworkers demonstrated that neuropeptide Y mRNA is present in all benign pheochromocytomas but in only 30% of malignant pheochromocytomas.[157a]

Although alpha inhibin is considered to be a specific marker for cortical neoplasms, Pelkey and coworkers reported immunoreactivity in 2 of 19 pheochromocytomas.[142]

Clarke and coworkers used a variety of markers to aid in the distinction of benign and malignant pheochromocytomas.[158] In their study, an MIB-1 labeling index of greater than 3% yielded a specificity of 100% and a sensitivity of 50% for predicting malignant behavior in these tumors. As indicated in prior studies, S-100 positivity had a significant

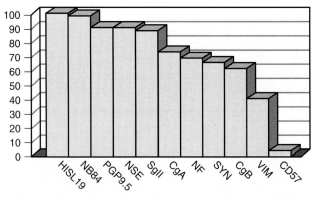

Figure 9–20. Distribution of markers in neuroblastoma. PGP9.5, protein gene product 9.5; NSE, neuron-specific enolase; SgII, secretogranin II; CgA, chromogranin A; NF, neurofilament; SYN, synaptophysin; CgB, chromogranin B; VIM, vimentin.

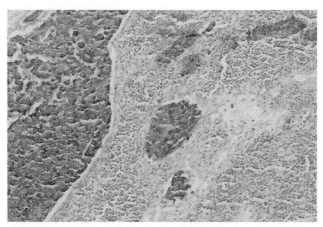

Figure 9–21. Metastatic neuroblastoma involving a lymph node. Positive staining is restricted to the tumor cells. (Immunoperoxidase stain for neuron-specific enolase)

(p = .02) but nonlinear association with benign tumors and the absence of S-100 correlated with greater tumor weight. Cathepsin B, cathepsin D, and type IV collagenase were present in both benign and malignant tumors, as were c-met, bcl-2, and basic fibroblast growth factor.

Neuroblastomas are small, round, blue cell tumors that may arise in the adrenal gland as well as in a variety of extra-adrenal sites. The differential diagnosis is wide and includes rhabdomyosarcoma, Ewing's sarcoma–primitive neuroectodermal tumor (ES-PNET), medulloblastoma, small cell osteosarcoma, lymphoblastic lymphoma, blastematous Wilms' tumor, and small cell desmoplastic tumor. Numerous markers have been used for the diagnosis of neuroblastomas, including neuroendocrine markers, cytoskeletal proteins, catecholamine-synthesizing enzymes, and neuroblastoma-"specific" antibodies[159–165] (Fig. 9–20). Many of these markers lack specificity or sensitivity, or both, as individual reagents and must be used as panels.

NSE is present in 85 to 100% of cases of neuroblastoma, and a similarly high level of positivity has been reported for PGP9.5 (Fig. 9–21).[163] However, both of neuroblastoma these markers may also be present in other small, round, blue cell tumors. Wirnsberger and colleagues reported that among antibodies directed against chromogranins and related proteins, HISL-19 was present in 100%, followed by chromogranin A (52%) and chromogranin A and B (45%) (Fig. 9–22*A*).[163] Neurofilament protein was present in 80% and was localized primarily in cell processes or nerve fibers, whereas synaptophysin was present in 75% of cases. Dopamine β-hydroxylase was present in 75% of cases. In general, reactivity for these markers was greater in well differentiated than in poorly differentiated neuroblastomas.[163] Among peptide hormones, VIP was present in 30% and

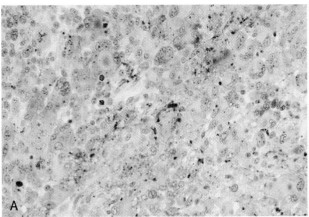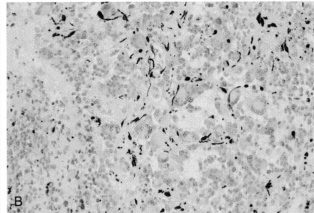

Figure 9–22. A, Extra-adrenal neuroblastoma. There is a distinct granular positivity in areas of process formation. (Immunoperoxidase stain for chromogranin A) *B,* Extra-adrenal neuroblastoma. Positivity is restricted to the sustentacular (stromal) cells. (Immunoperoxidase stain for S-100 protein)

neuropeptide Y was present in 10%. CD57 was not found in any neuroblastoma but was demonstrable in seven of seven ganglioneuromas.[163] Microtubule-associated protein-1 (MAP1) and MAP2 and beta-tubulin are present in 100% of cases, but the number of cases studied to date has been small.[164, 165] S-100 protein is restricted in its distribution to the sustentacular (stromal) cells (see Fig. 9–22*B*).

CD99 is a useful marker for the distinction of neuroblastomas from other small, round, blue cell tumors.[166–170] More than 100 cases of neuroblastoma have now been studied for CD99, and all have been negative. In contrast, nearly 100% of cases of ES-PNET are CD99-positive. Anti–β_2-microglobulin is another marker that is negative in neuroblastoma but positive in approximately 75% of ES-PNET.[171]

Worthy of note is an immunohistochemical marker, NB84, that is a monoclonal antibody raised to neuroblastoma cells.[171] Miettinen and co-workers studied 22 cases of undifferentiated neuroblastomas and 83 cases of differentiated neuroblastomas (total of 105 cases) and found that 21 of 22 (95.5%) of the former and all (83 of 83; 100%) of the latter (total 104 of 105; 99%) showed immunoreactivity for NB84.[172] In addition, 4 of 5 (80%) of ES-PNETs and 3 of 3 (100%) of desmoplastic small, round cell tumors also showed positive staining. In contrast, 7 of 39 (17.9%) of ES and 1 of 14 (7.1%) cases of blastematous Wilms' tumors were NB84-positive. Alveolar and embryonal rhabdomyosarcomas, lymphoblastic lymphomas, and pulmonary small cell carcinomas were negative.[172] However, Folpe and coworkers reported NB84 immunoreactivity in 3 of 13 rhabdomyosarcomas, 10 of 11 medulloblastomas, 1 of 9 esthesioneuroblastomas, and 2 of 3 small cell osteosarcomas.[173] A panel of antibodies including NB84, CD99, cytokeratins, lymphoid, and muscle-specific markers should be used in rendering a diagnosis of neuroblastoma.

KEY DIAGNOSTIC POINTS OF THE ADRENAL CORTEX

- Typically positive for vimentin and inconsistent, weak or focal keratin immunostaining in formalin fixed tissues
- Metastases to adrenal gland are almost always strongly, diffusely keratin-positive, and are usually positive for CEA, EMA, and CD15
- Nuclear staining for D11 in 80% of cortical tumors, but cytoplasmic staining in hepatoma, lung carcinoma, and some renal carcinomas
- Ad4BP decorates 100% of cortical carcinomas but has no reactivity with renal cell carcinoma, hepatoma, or pheochromocytoma
- A103 immunostains 100% of adrenal cortical tumors but is negative in other carcinomas
- Inhibin A immunostains 100% of adrenal cortical tumors
- Adrenal cortical carcinomas may immunostain with synaptophysin, NSE, or neuro-filaments but are typically chromogranin-negative. Chromogranin is useful to distinguish adrenal cortical carcinomas (all chromogranin-negative) useful to distinguish from pheochromocytomas (majority chromogranin-positive)

Gastrointestinal Endocrine Cells

The carcinoid tumors of the gastrointestinal tract have been divided into three major groups based on their origins from foregut, midgut, and hindgut derivatives. There is a strong correlation between their sites of origin and the distribution patterns of peptide hormones and amines. For example, serotonin is present in 89% of midgut carcinoids, 30% of foregut carcinoids, and 12.5% of hindgut carcinoids (Table 9–4).[174]

Carcinoid tumors are typically positive for cyto-

Table 9–4. Hormonal Profiles of Gastrointestinal Carcinoids			
Product	**Foregut (%+)**	**Midgut (%+)**	**Hindgut (%+)**
Serotonin	30	89	13
Somatostatin	80	4	63
Substance P	10	41	0
Pancreatic polypeptide	0	0	88
Glucagon	10	0	50
Calcitonin	0	11	0
Adrenocorticotropic hormone	20	4	0
Gastrin	30	0	0

keratins, with 100% exhibiting positivity for CAM5.2 and 80% exhibiting positivity with other pancytokeratin antibodies.[175, 176] Thirty-eight percent are positive for CK20.[177] Approximately 25% are positive for vimentin, and neurofilament proteins are present in a variable proportion. Carcinoid tumors are positive for a wide variety of generic neuroendocrine markers. NSE is present in nearly 80% of cases, whereas PGP9.5 is present in approximately 90%.[16] The reactivity of other neuroendocrine markers differs according to the site of origin.[178] Synaptophysin is present in 100% of carcinoids at all sites. Chromogranin A is present in 88 to 100% of foregut, 100% of midgut, and 24 to 40% of hindgut carcinoids (Figs. 9–23 and 9–24). Chromogranin B, in contrast, is present in 100% of hindgut carcinoids.[29, 179] Peptidylglycine alpha-amidating enzyme has been reported in 14% of gastric carcinoids, 100% of ileal carcinoids, and 100% of rectal carcinoids.[179] NCAM is present in 76% of foregut, 58% of midgut, and 20% of hindgut carcinoids. Antibodies to NCAM stain both tumor cells and sustentacular elements.[179] The S-100 protein is present in 41% of foregut carcinoids and 50% of midgut and hindgut tumors. The pattern of staining for S-100 is generally similar to that observed for NCAM, with reactivities present in both tumor cells and sustentacular elements.

CEA is present in approximately 40% of carcinoids with polyclonal antisera or monoclonal antibodies, whereas CD15 is present in 30% of these tumors.[180–182] The monoclonal antibody CA15.3, which identifies both carbohydrate and peptide determinants (MUC1-type mucin), reacts with 75% of carcinoids, whereas CA 19.9, which reacts with sialylated Lewis antigen, is negative.[85]

Prostatic acid phosphatase (PAP) may be present in some carcinoid tumors. In a study of 33 carcinoids of foregut, midgut, and hindgut origins, PAP was present in five of five hindgut tumors, whereas other carcinoids were negative.[183] Prostate-specific antigen, in contrast, is typically negative in these tumors. The alpha chain of hCG is also present to varying extents in carcinoid tumors. Heitz and co-workers reported staining for the alpha chain in 46% of foregut, 25% of hindgut, but in none of 35 midgut carcinoids.[108] Calbindin, a 28,000-kd calcium-binding protein has been localized to subpopulations of central and peripheral nervous system neurons, distal tubular cells of the kidney, and enteric neuroendocrine cells. Immunohistochemical studies have demonstrated that calbindin is present in a small number of neuroendocrine cells, predominantly in the appendix and small intestine, and in 100% of midgut and foregut (gastric) carcinoids.[114] In contrast, calbindin immunoreactivity was absent from a single case of rectal carcinoid.

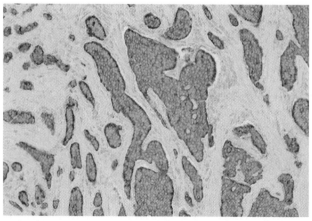

Figure 9–23. Ileal carcinoid tumor. Positive staining is restricted to the nests of tumor cells. (Immunoperoxidase stain for chromogranin A)

Pancreatic Endocrine Cells

Cytokeratin immunoreactivity using broad spectrum antibodies is present in normal pancreatic endocrine cells and in approximately 90% of pancreatic endocrine tumors, whereas CK20 is present in 12.5% of cases (Fig. 9–25).[47, 51, 119, 177, 184] There is variable reactivity for vimentin with approximately 25% of cases showing convincing cytoplasmic staining. Neurofilament immunoreactivity has been reported in 50% of cases. Immunoreactivity for NSE and synaptophysin is present in all normal pancreatic endocrine cells and in virtually all pancreatic endocrine tumors.[185] Chromogranin A is present in approximately 75% of all pancreatic endocrine tumors. Generally, the extent of chromogranin immunoreactivity correlates with the degree of granularity as noted in sections stained for pep-

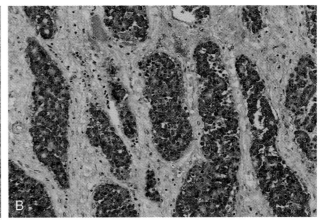

Figure 9–24. A, Metastatic carcinoid involving the liver. The tumor cells show strong cytoplasmic staining. (Immunoperoxidase stain for chromogranin A) *B,* Metastatic carcinoid involving the liver. The tumor cells are strongly positive. (Immunoperoxidase stain for serotonin)

tide hormones.[185] Calbindin has been reported in two of two pancreatic insulinomas.[114] MIC2 (CD99) has been reported in two of five pancreatic endocrine tumors.[168]

The normal islets of Langerhans contain four major cell types.[186] The insulin-producing beta cells compose 60 to 70% of the cells in the main part of the pancreas and 20 to 30% of the cells in the posterior head of the gland. The glucagon-producing alpha cells compose 15 to 20% of the cells in the main portion of the gland and less than 5% of the cells in the posterior head. The delta cells, which produce somatostatin represent 5 to 10% of the cells in the main portion of the gland and approximately 5% of the islet cell population in the posterior portion of the gland. Pancreatic polypeptide (PP) cells represent 70% of the islet cells in the posterior gland and 2 to 5% of the cells in the remaining islets. Approximately 10% of pan-

creatic endocrine cells are present in extrainsular sites, where they are distributed among ductal cells or paraductular acinar cells. Occasional serotonin-producing cells are present in large ducts and are the most likely cell of origin of true carcinoid tumor of the pancreas.

Insulinomas are typically positive for insulin and proinsulin, including cases that are negative by standard histochemical stains.[186, 187] Approximately 50% of insulinomas are multihormonal and may contain cells that are positive for glucagon, somatostatin, PP, gastrin, ACTH, or calcitonin. There is often considerable variation in the staining intensity for insulin, with those cells containing abundant granules ultrastructurally giving the most intense immunoreactivity. Glucagonomas are identified on the basis of reactivity for the corresponding peptide. Both glicentin and glucagon-like peptides are typically present as well. Glucagonomas may also contain peptides unrelated to proglucagon, including somatostatin and insulin.

Somatostatinomas are identified on the basis of their reactivity with antibodies to somatostatin.[186] These tumors may also contain calcitonin, ACTH, and gastrin. Tumors of identical morphology and immunohistochemical profiles also occur within the duodenum. PP-producing tumors are generally classified among nonfunctional tumors, although rarely these tumors may be associated with the syndrome of watery diarrhea, hypokalemia, and achlorhydria (WDHA). In addition to their content of PP, these tumors may contain scattered cells containing other hormonal peptides.

Gastrinomas are characterized by varying degrees of immunoreactivity for gastrin; however, some of these tumors may be nonreactive (Fig. 9–26).[186] In the latter instance, antibodies to different regions of the N- and C-terminal portions of the gastrin molecule may be positive. Some gastrinomas that may be entirely negative for gastrin may give positive signals for gastrin mRNA in in situ hybridization formats.[188] Gastrinomas, similar to other pan-

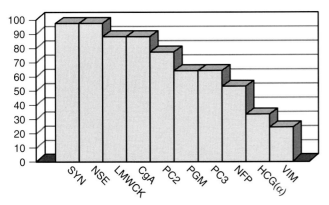

Figure 9–25. Distribution of markers in pancreatic endocrine tumors. SYN, synaptophysin; NSE, neuron-specific enolase; LMWCK, low molecular weight cytokeratin; CgA, chromogranin A; PC2, proconvertase 2; PGM, peptidylglycine alpha-amidating enzyme; PC3, proconvertase 3; NFP, neurofilament protein; HCG(α), human chorionic gonadotropin alpha; VIM, vimentin.

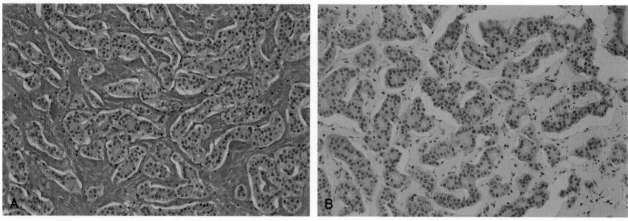

Figure 9–26. A, Pancreatic gastrinoma. (H&E) *B,* The tumor cells show weak cytoplasmic staining. (Immunoperoxidase stain for gastrin)

creatic endocrine tumors, may contain scattered cells positive for glucagon, PP, insulin, somatostatin, serotonin, or ACTH.[189] Gastrinomas may also occur in a variety of extrapancreatic sites, including the duodenum.[186]

VIP-producing tumors have been associated with the syndrome of WDHA. In a series of 28 cases of WDHA studied by Solcia and colleagues, VIP was present in 87% and peptide histidine methionine was present in 57% of cases. Growth hormone–releasing hormone and PP were present in 50% and 53% of cases, respectively.[190] In addition to pancreatic endocrine tumors, ganglioneuromas and ganglioneuroblastomas have been associated with the syndrome of WDHA.

Rare examples of true carcinoid (endocrine cell) tumors may occur within the pancreas, and these tumors contain immunoreactive serotonin. Other tumors occurring as primary pancreatic endocrine tumors may produce growth hormone–releasing hormone associated with acromegaly, ACTH-producing tumors associated with Cushing's syndrome, and PTH or PTH-like peptide tumors associated with hypercalcemia.

Nonfunctional pancreatic endocrine tumors may contain scattered cells positive for a variety of hormones, most commonly PP and glucagon (Fig. 9–27).

The alpha chain of hCG has been regarded as a marker of malignancy in pancreatic endocrine tumors and occurs in approximately 70% of cases (Fig. 9–28).[191] More recent studies, however, have demonstrated immunoreactivity for this marker in benign endocrine pancreatic tumors.[192] Progesterone receptor protein is also demonstrable in pancreatic endocrine tumors.[193]

Pulmonary Endocrine Cells

The neuroendocrine cells of the lung are present as single cells and as small cell clusters that have been termed *neuroepithelial bodies.*[194] These bod-

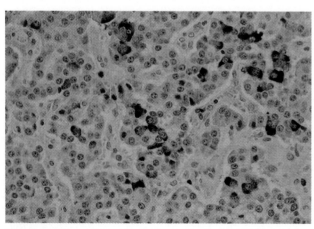

Figure 9–27. Nonfunctional pancreatic endocrine tumor. A few scattered tumor cells are positive. (Immunoperoxidase stain for pancreatic polypeptide)

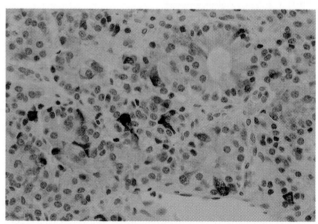

Figure 9–28. Nonfunctional pancreatic endocrine tumor. A few scattered cells are positive. (Immunoperoxidase stain for the alpha chain of human chorionic gonadotropin)

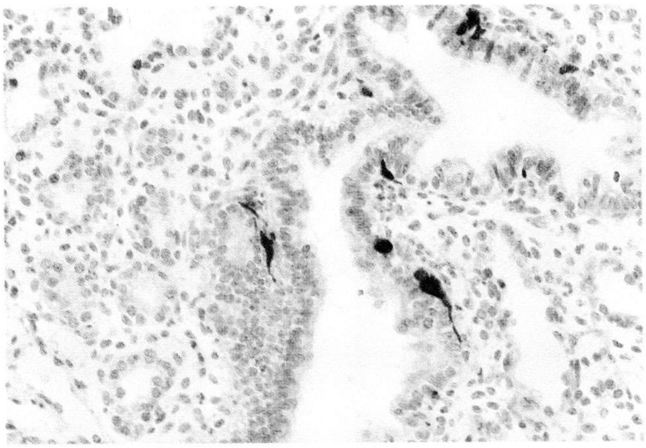

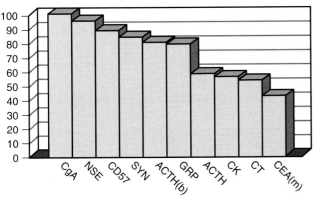

Figure 9–29. Fetal lung. Immunoreactive hormone is present in single cells. (Immunoperoxidase stain for gastrin-releasing peptide)

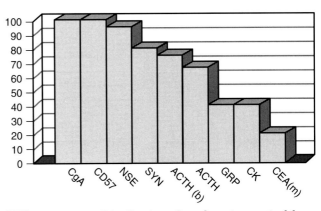

Figure 9–31. Distribution of markers in atypical lung carcinoid. CgA, chromogranin A; NSE, neuron-specific enolase; SYN, synaptophysin; ACTH (b), big adrenocorticotropic hormone; GRP, gastrin-releasing peptide; CK, cytokeratin; CEA(m), monoclonal carcinoembryonic antigen.

ies may have a chemoreceptor function, whereas the single neuroendocrine cells may act as paracrine elements. A variety of regulatory products including serotonin, gastrin-releasing peptide, and calcitonin are present both in single neuroendocrine cells and within neuroepithelial bodies, whereas leu-enkephalin is present only in single neuroendocrine cells (Fig. 9–29).[194] The pulmonary neuroendocrine cells may undergo a series of hyperplastic changes in response to irritation or after exposure to carcinogens. Generally, hyperplastic neuroendocrine cells retain the patterns of expression of regulatory products characteristic of their normal counterparts. More severe forms of hyperplasia and dysplasia are accompanied by the production of ectopic products, including VIP and different molecular forms of ACTH.

Neuroendocrine tumors of the lung include four major entities that can be distinguished on the basis of morphology and immunohistochemical characteristics.[195] The tumor types include typical car-

cinoids (Fig. 9–30), atypical carcinoids (Fig. 9–31), small cell carcinomas (Fig. 9–32), and large cell neuroendocrine carcinomas (Fig. 9–33). Approximately 85% of these tumors are reactive with antibodies to low molecular weight cytokeratins.[195, 196] In the series reported by Travis and associates, reactivity with broad spectrum keratin antibodies (AE1/AE3) was seen, with positive staining in 56% of typical carcinoids, 40% of atypical carcinoids, and 100% of small cell carcinomas and large cell neuroendocrine carcinomas.[195] Eighty-two percent of small cell carcinomas are negative for CK7 and CK20.[49]

NSE is present in more than 95% of pulmonary neuroendocrine tumors of all types.[195] Chromogranin A is present in 100% of typical and atypical carcinoids, in 80% of large cell neuroendocrine carcinomas, and in up to 50% of small cell carcinomas, depending on the antigen retrieval method

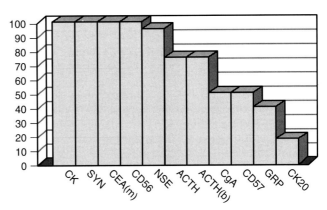

Figure 9–30. Distribution of markers in typical lung carcinoid. CgA, chromogranin A; NSE, neuron-specific enolase; SYN, synaptophysin; ACTH (b), big adrenocorticotropic hormone; GRP, gastrin-releasing peptide; CK, cytokeratin; CT, calcitonin; CEA(m), monoclonal carcinoembryonic antigen.

Figure 9–32. Distribution of markers in small cell carcinoma. CK, cytokeratin; SYN, synaptophysin; CEA(m), monoclonal carcinoembryonic antigen; NSE, neuron-specific enolase; ACTH (b), big adrenocorticotropic hormone; CgA, chromogranin A; GRP, gastrin-releasing peptide.

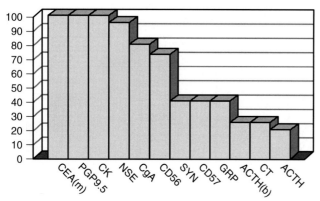

Figure 9–33. Distribution of markers in large cell neuroendocrine carcinoma. CEA(m), monoclonal carcinoembryonic antigen; PGP, protein gene product 9.5; CK, cytokeratin; NSE, neuron-specific enolase; CgA, chromogranin A; SYN, synaptophysin; GRP, gastrin releasing peptide; ACTH (b), big adrenocorticotropic hormone; CT, calcitonin.

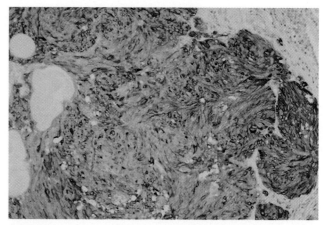

Figure 9–34. Pulmonary tumorlet. The lesional cells are strongly positive. (Immunoperoxidase stain for Leu7)

and sensitivity of the detection method. Synaptophysin is present in 84% of typical carcinoids, 80% of atypical carcinoids, 40% of large cell neuroendocrine carcinomas, and 100% of small cell carcinomas. Leu7 immunoreactivity is present in 89% of typical carcinoids, 100% of atypical carcinoids, and 40% and 50% of large cell neuroendocrine carcinomas and small cell carcinomas, respectively. Pulmonary tumorlets are also positive for Leu7 (Fig. 9–34). CEA (monoclonal) is present in 100% of large cell neuroendocrine carcinomas and small cell carcinomas, 42% of typical carcinoids, and 20% of atypical carcinoids. These tumors also contain a variety of different peptides. Jiang and colleagues[197] also studied large cell neuroendocrine carcinomas and confirmed the findings of Travis and coworkers.[195] In addition, Jiang and coworkers reported positivity for PGP9.5 in 100% of the cases and positivity for TuJ1 (neuron-specific class III beta-tubulin) in 82%. NCAM positivity was present in 73%.[197]

Endocrine Tumors in Other Sites

CERVIX

Carcinoids, small cell carcinomas, and large cell neuroendocrine carcinomas have been reported as primary cervical tumors.[198–200] All the small cell cervical carcinomas studied to date have been cytokeratin-positive, and 92% have been positive for EMA. Reactivity for CEA with polyclonal antisera has been reported in 77%. With respect to neuroendocrine markers, NSE is present in 95%, synaptophysin in 46%, chromogranin A in 43%, and CD57 in 37% (Fig. 9–35). These tumors may also contain peptide and amine hormones, including serotonin (31%), ACTH (23%), and somatostatin (8%). Stoler and associates demonstrated human papillomavirus 18 (HPV18) in 78% of small cell

cervical carcinomas with neuroendocrine differentiation.[201] Chromogranin A immunoreactivity has been reported in all large cell neuroendocrine cervical carcinomas.[200] Synaptophysin staining was positive in 66% of cases, whereas NSE was positive in 50%. Occasional serotonin-positive cells were present in 50% of cases, whereas somatostatin-positive cells were present in 37%. Seventy-five percent of cases contained CEA, as demonstrated with a monoclonal antibody.

PROSTATE

Normal prostatic epithelium contains subpopulations of neuroendocrine cells, which can be identified on the basis of their content of NSE, chromogranin, peptide hormones, and serotonin.[202–204] Prostatic neoplasms with neuroendocrine differentiation include carcinoids, small cell carcinomas, and "usual" adenocarcinomas with subpopulations of neuroendocrine cells (Fig. 9–36). Neuroendo-

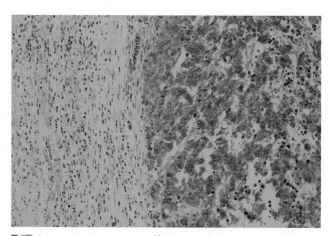

Figure 9–35. Large cell (neuroendocrine) carcinoma of the cervix. Positivity is confined to the tumor cells. (Immunoperoxidase stain for neuron-specific enolase)

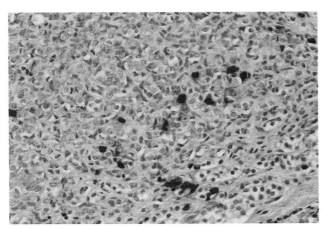

Figure 9–36. Metastatic prostatic adenocarcinoma with neuroendocrine cells. A few scattered cells are positive. (Immunoperoxidase stain for chromogranin A, aminoethylcarbazole as chromogen)

crine differentiation in prostatic carcinomas may be more important in androgen-independent tumors and metastatic tumors than in hormone-sensitive and locally recurrent tumors.[203] Scattered neuroendocrine cells have been demonstrated in up to 88% of cases of high-grade prostatic intraepithelial neoplasia.[205] The highest percentage of cases are immunoreactive for serotonin (73%), NSE (67%), chromogranin (62%), and hCG (30%). In carcinomas of the prostate, 54% contain serotonin, 46% are positive for NSE, 65% are positive for chromogranin, and 22% are positive for hCG. Somatostatin, calcitonin, and ACTH were present in less than 5% of cases.[205] Schmid and coworkers demonstrated that the pattern of chromogranin distribution is correlated with tumor grade.[204] Grade I tumors show positive reactions for chromogranins A and B and secretogranin II, with colocalization of all three products in the majority of neuroendocrine cells. In grade II and grade III tumors, in contrast, chromogranin B is the predominant granin.

SKIN

Merkel cell (neuroendocrine) carcinoma of the skin is an uncommon entity that was first described by Toker as trabecular carcinoma.[206] These tumors are uniformly positive with broad spectrum cytokeratin antibodies and stain positively for CK20 in 97% of cases, with a dot-like pattern of positivity (Fig. 9–37).[177, 207] Other small cell tumors exhibiting CK20 positivity include bronchogenic small cell carcinomas (0.03%), small cell cervical carcinomas (9%), and small cell carcinomas of salivary gland origin (60%). Seventy-eight percent of Merkel cell carcinomas are positive for EMA.[208]

Virtually all Merkel cell carcinomas are positive for NSE.[209] Chromogranins B and A are found in

100% and 72% of the tumors, respectively. Secretoneunin, which is derived from secretogranin II, is present in 22% of cases, whereas synaptophysin is present in 39%.[210] CD99 may be positive in Merkel cell tumors. In the series reported by Nicholson and associates, 12 of 30 cases (40%) were positive for CD99.[211] In nine cases that were consistent with Merkel cell carcinoma clinically, CD99 was positive, whereas CK20 was negative.

BREAST

Neuroendocrine tumors of the breast include carcinoids and neuroendocrine carcinomas of small cell type (Fig. 9–38A).[212–214] Small cell carcinomas are typically positive for cytokeratins, including AE1/AE3 (91%), CAM5.2 (82%), CK7 (78%), and CK19 (78%), whereas stains for CK20 have been reported as negative.[215] Among neuroendocrine markers, NSE is present in 90%, whereas synaptophysin and chromogranin have been reported in 56% and 41%, respectively (see Fig. 9–38B). CD56 and CD57 have been noted in 78% and 43% of cases, respectively. Immunoreactivity for calcitonin has been reported in 27%, whereas stains for gastrin-releasing peptide and serotonin have been reported in 39% and 14% of cases, respectively. Estrogen receptor positivity has been reported in 54%, and progesterone receptor positivity has been reported in 45%. Stains for bcl-2 are consistently positive, but stains for HER-2/neu are negative.[215]

THYMUS

Thymic neuroendocrine tumors include carcinoids, atypical carcinoids, and small cell carcinomas. Thymic small cell carcinomas are typically positive for cytokeratins using the antibodies AE1/AE3 and CAM5.2.[216–218] In general, cytokeratin immunoreactivity is most intense in well-differentiated areas of these tumors, whereas less-differen-

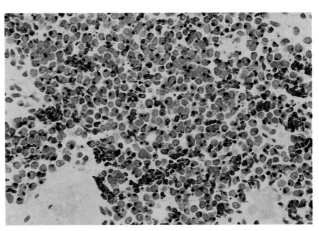

Figure 9–37. Merkel cell carcinoma. The tumor cells show a dot-like pattern of staining. (Immunoperoxidase stain for CK20)

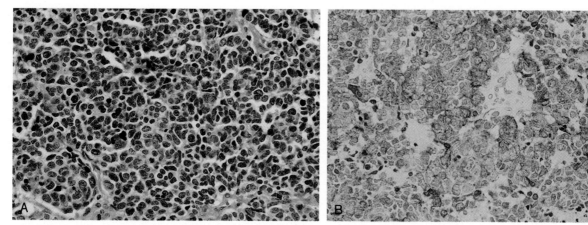

Figure 9–38. *A,* Small cell (neuroendocrine) carcinoma of the breast. (H&E) *B,* Immunoperoxidase stain for chromogranin A. The tumor cells show moderately intense cytoplasmic staining.

tiated areas are sometimes cytokeratin-negative.[217] Among generic neuroendocrine markers, NSE is present in 93%, synaptophysin in 78%, and chromogranin A in 63%. These tumors are also variably positive for peptide and amine hormones, including cholecystokinin (100%), alpha hCG (100%), neurotensin (60%), somatostatin (58%), beta hCG (37.5%), ACTH (34%), CGRP (25%), calcitonin (18%), and serotonin (12.5%).[216–218]

ACKNOWLEDGEMENTS

The authors wish to acknowledge the assistance of Dr. Dennis Frisman's website, ImmunoHisto-Query, for many of the data provided in the bar graphs.

The authors also thank Ms. Madellyn Brito for her help in the preparation of this manuscript.

References

1. DeLellis RA, Wolfe HJ. Contributions of immunohisto-chemical and molecular biological techniques to endocrine pathology. J Histochem Cytochem 1987;35:1347–1351.
2. DeLellis RA. Endocrine tumors. In: Colvin RB, Bhan AK, McCluskey RT, eds. Diagnostic Immunopathology. New York: Raven Press, 1995:551–578.
3. DeLellis RA, Wolfe HJ. Analysis of gene expression in endocrine cells. In: Fenoglio-Preiser CM, Williman CL, eds. Molecular Diagnostics in Pathology. Baltimore: Williams & Wilkins, 1991:299–323.
4. Lloyd RV, Jin L, Kulig E, Fields K. Molecular approaches for the analysis of chromogranins and secretogranins. Diagn Mol Pathol 1992;1:2–15.
5. Portela-Gomes GM, Stridsberg M, Grimelius L, et al. Expression of five different somatostatin receptor subtypes in endocrine cells of the pancreas. Appl Immunohistochem 2000;8:126–132.
6. DeLellis RA, Tischler AS. The dispersed neuroendocrine cell system. In: Kovacs K, Asa SL, eds. Functional Endocrine Pathology. Oxford, Blackwell Science, 1998:529–549.
7. Lauweryns JM, Van Ranst L. Immunocytochemical localization of aromatic L-amino acid decarboxylase in human, rat and mouse bronchopulmonary and gastrointestinal endocrine cells. J Histochem Cytochem 1988;36:1181–1186.
8. Lloyd RV, Sisson JC, Shapiro B, Verhofstad AA. Immuno-histochemical localization of epinephrine, norepinephrine, catecholamine-synthesizing enzymes and chromogranin in neuroendocrine cells and tumors. Am J Pathol 1986;125:45–54.
9. Lloyd RV, Jin L, Qian X, et al. Analysis of the chromo-granin A post-translational cleavage product pancreastatin and the prohormone convertases PC2 and PC3 in normal and neoplastic human pituitaries. Am J Pathol 1995;146:1188–1198.
10. Scopsi L, Gullo M, Rilke F, et al. Proprotein convertases (PC1/PC3 and PC2) in normal and neoplastic tissues: Their use as markers of neuroendocrine differentiation. J Clin Endocrinol Metab 1995;80:294–301.
11. Scopsi L, Lee R, Gullo M, et al. Peptidylglycine, α amidating monooxygenase in neuroendocrine tumors: Its identification, characterization, quantification and relation to the grade of morphologic differentiation, amidated peptide content and granin immunocytochemistry. Appl Immunohistochem 1998;6:120–132.
12. Schmechel D, Marangos PJ, Brightman M. Neurone-specific enolase is a molecular marker for peripheral and central neuroendocrine cells. Nature 1978;276:834–836.
13. Haimoto H, Takahashi Y, Koshikawa T, et al. Immunohis-tochemical localization of gamma enolase in normal human tissues other than nervous and neuroendocrine tissue. Lab Invest 1985;52:257–263.
14. Schmechel DE. Gamma submit of the glycolytic enzyme enolase: Nonspecific or neuron specific? Lab Invest 1985;52:239–242.
15. Seshi B, True L, Carter D, Rosai J. Immunohistochemical characterization of a set of monoclonal antibodies to human neuron-specific enolase. Am J Pathol 1988;131:258–269.
16. Rode J, Dhillon AP, Doran JF, et al. PGP 9.5, a new marker for human neuroendocrine tumors. Histopathology 1985;9:147–158.
17. Li GL, Farooque M, Holtz A, Olsson Y. Expression of the ubiquitin carboxyl-terminal hydrolase PGP 9.5 in axons following spinal cord compression trauma. APMIS 1997;105:384–390.
18. Wilson PO, Barber PC, Hamid QA, et al. The immunolo-calization of protein gene product 9.5 using rabbit poly-clonal and mouse monoclonal antibodies. Br J Exp Pathol 1988;69:91–104.
19. Bordi C, Pilato FP, D'Adda T. Comparative study of several neuroendocrine markers in pancreatic endocrine tumors. Virchows Arch A Pathol Anat Histopathol 1988;413:387–398.
20. Mendelsohn G. Histaminase localization in medullary thyroid carcinoma and small cell lung carcinoma. In: DeLellis RA, ed. Diagnostic Immunohistochemistry. New York: Masson, 1981:299–312.

21. Sasano H, Mason JI, Sasano N. Immunohistochemical analysis of cytochrome P450 17 alpha in human adrenocortical disorders. Hum Pathol 1989;20:113–117.
22. Sasano H, Okamoto M, Sasano N. Immunohistochemical study of cytochrome P-450 11B hydroxylase in human adrenal cortex with mineralo- and glucocorticoid excess. Virchows Arch A Pathol Anat Histopathol 1988;413:313–318.
23. Sasano H, Okamoto M, Mason JI, et al. Immunohistochemical studies of steroidogenic enzymes (aromatase, 17 alpha-hydroxylase and cholesterol side chain cleavage cytochrome P450) in sex cord stromal tumors of the ovary. Hum Pathol 20:1989;452–457.
24. Lloyd RV, Wilson BS. Specific endocrine tissue marker defined by a monoclonal antibody. Science 1983;222:628–630.
25. O'Connor DT, Burton D, Deftos LJ. Chromogranin A: Immunohistology reveals its universal occurrence in normal polypeptide hormone producing endocrine glands. Life Sci 1983;33:1657–1663.
26. Wilson BS, Lloyd RV. Detection of chromogranin in neuroendocrine cells with a monoclonal antibody. Am J Pathol 1984;115:458–468.
27. Hagn C, Schmid KW, Fischer-Colbrie R, Winkler H. Chromogranin A, B, and C in human adrenal medulla and endocrine tissues. Lab Invest 1986;55:405–411.
28. Huttner WB, Gerdes H-H, Rosa P. Chromogranins/secretogranins—widespread constituents of the secretory granule matrix in endocrine cells and neurons. In: Langley K, Gratzl M, eds. Markers for Neural and Endocrine Cells: Molecular and Cell Biology. Weinhein, VCH, 1991.
29. Fahrenkamp AG, Wibbeke C, Winde G. Immunohistochemical distribution of chromogranins A and B and secretogranin II in neuroendocrine tumors of the gastrointestinal tract. Virchows Arch 1995;426:361–367.
30. Schmid KW, Kroll M, Hittmair A, et al. Chromogranin A and B in adenomas of the pituitary: An immunohistochemical study of 42 cases. Am J Surg Pathol 1991;15:1072–1077.
31. Buffa R, Pelagi M, Siccardi AG, et al. Identification of the endocrine cells detected by the monoclonal antibody HISL-19 in human tissues. Basic Appl Histochem 1990;34:259–268.
32. Riddel K, Tippens D, Gown AM. PHE5: A new monoclonal antibody to a unique neuroendocrine granule protein. Lab Invest 1987;56:64A.
33. Krisch K, Horvat G, Krisch I, et al. Immunochemical characterization of a novel secretory protein (defined by monoclonal antibody HISL-19) of peptide hormone producing cells which is distinct from chromogranin A, B and C. Lab Invest 1988;58:411–420.
34. Gould VE, Lee I, Wiedenmann B, et al. Synaptophysin: A novel marker for neurons, certain neuroendocrine cells and their neoplasms. Hum Pathol 1986;17:979–983.
35. Navone F, Jahn R, Di Gioia G, et al. Protein p38: An integral membrane protein specific for small vesicles of neurons and neuroendocrine cells. J Cell Biol 1986;103:2511–2527.
36. Komminoth P, Roth J, Schroder S, et al. Overlapping expression of immunohistochemical markers and synaptophysin mRNA in pheochromocytomas and adrenocortical carcinomas: Implications for the differential diagnosis of adrenal gland tumors. Lab Invest 1995;72:424–431.
36a. Portela-Gomes GM, Lukinius GM, Grinelius L. Synaptic vesicle protein 2: A new neuroendocrine cell marker. Am J Pathol 2000;157:1299–1309.
37. Arber DA, Weirs LM. CD57: A review. Appl Immunohistochem 1995;3:137–152.
38. McGarry RC, Helfand SL, Quarles RH, Roder JC. Recognition of the myelin associated glycoprotein by the monoclonal antibody HNK-1. Nature 1983;306:376–378.
39. Tischler AS, Mobtaker H, Mann K, et al. Anti-lymphocyte antibody Leu 7 (HNK-1) recognizes a constituent of neuroendocrine granule matrix. J Histochem Cytochem 1986;34:1213–1216.
40. Ghali VS, Jimenez EJS, Garcia RL. Distribution of Leu 7

41. antigen (HNK-1) in thyroid tumors: Its usefulness as a diagnostic marker for follicular and papillary carcinomas. Hum Pathol 1992;23:21–25.
41. Langley K, Gratzl M. Neural cell adhesion molecule (NCAM) in neural and endocrine cells. In Langley K, Gratzl M, eds. Markers for Neural and Endocrine Cells: Molecular and Cell Biology. Diagnostic Applications. Weinheim VCH, 1991:133–177.
42. Shipley WR, Hammer RD, Lennington WJ, Macon WR. Paraffin immunohistochemical detection of CD56, a useful marker for neural cell adhesion molecule in normal and neoplastic fixed tissues. Appl Immunohistochem 1997;5:87–93.
43. Jin L, Hemperly JJ, Lloyd RV. Expression of neural cell adhesion molecule in normal and neoplastic human neuroendocrine tissues. Am J Pathol 1991;138:961–969.
44. Komminoth P, Roth J, Saremaslani P, et al. Polysialic acid of the neural cell adhesion molecule in the human thyroid: A marker for medullary thyroid carcinoma and primary C-cell hyperplasia: An immunohistochemical study on 79 thyroid lesions. Am J Surg Pathol 1994;18:399–411.
45. Komminoth P, Roth J, Lackie PM, et al. Polysialic acid of the neural cell adhesion molecule distinguishes small cell lung carcinoma from carcinoids. Am J Pathol 1991;139:297–304.
46. Fuchs E, Weber K. Intermediate filaments: Structure, dynamics, function and disease. Ann Rev Biochem 1994;63:345–382.
47. Hoefler H, Denk H, Lackinger E, et al. Immunocytochemical demonstration of intermediate filament cytoskeleton proteins in human endocrine tissues and (neuro-) endocrine tumors. Virchows Arch A Pathol Anat Histopathol 1986;409:609–626.
48. O'Hara BJ, Paetau A, Miettinen M. Keratin subsets and monoclonal antibody to HBME-1 in chordoma: Immunohistochemical differential diagnosis between tumors simulating chordoma. Hum Pathol 1998;29:119–126.
49. Wang NP, Zee S, Zarbo RJ, et al. Coordinate expression of cytokeratins 7 and 20 defines unique subsets of carcinomas. Appl Immunohistochem 1995;3:99–107.
50. Trojanowski JQ, Lee VM, Schlaepfer WW. An immunohistochemical study of human central and peripheral nervous system tumors, using monoclonal antibodies against neurofilaments and glial filaments. Hum Pathol 1984;15:248–257.
51. Perez MA, Saul SH, Trojanowski JQ. Neurofilament and chromogranin expression in normal and neoplastic neuroendocrine cells of the human gastrointestinal tract and pancreas. Cancer 1990;65:1219–1227.
52. Kulig E, Lloyd RV. Transcription factors and endocrine disease. Endocr Pathol 1996;1:245–250.
53. Asa SL. Atlas of Tumor Pathology: Tumors of the Pituitary Gland. Washington, D.C.: Armed Forces Institute of Pathology, 1998.
54. Girod C, Trouillar J, Dubois MP. Immunocytochemical localization of S100 protein in stellate cells (folliculo-stellate cells) of the anterior lobe of the normal human pituitary. Cell Tissue Res 1985;241:505–511.
55. Lloyd RV, Cano M, Rosa P, et al. Distribution of chromogranin A and secretogranin I (chromogranin B) in neuroendocrine cells and tumors. Am J Pathol 1988;130:296–304.
56. Devaney K, Wenig BM, Abbondanzo SL. Olfactory neuroblastoma and other round cell lesions of the sinonasal region. Mod Pathol 1996;9:658–663.
57. Burger PC, Scheithauer BW. Atlas of Tumor Pathology: Tumors of the Central Nervous System. Third Series. Washington, D.C.: Armed Forces Institute of Pathology, 1994.
58. Coca S, Vaquero J, Escandon J, et al. Immunohistochemical characterization of pineocytomas. Clin Neuropathol 1992;11:298–303.
59. Hayashi K, Hoshida Y, Horie Y, et al. Immunohistochemical study on the distribution of α and β subunits of S100 protein in brain tumors. Acta Neuropathol (Berl) 1991;81:657–663.

60. Korf HW, Klein DC, Zigler JS, et al. S-antigen-like immunoreactivity in a human pineocytoma. Acta Neuropathol (Berl) 1986;69:165–167.
61. Perentes E, Rubinstein LJ, Herman MM, et al. S-antigen immunoreactivity in human pineal glands and pineal parenchymal tumors: A monoclonal antibody study. Acta Neuropathol (Berl) 1986;71:224–227.
62. Bocker W, Dralle H, Dorn G. Thyroglobulin: An immunohistochemical marker in thyroid disease. In: DeLellis RA, ed. Diagnostic Immunohistochemistry. New York: Masson, 1981:37–60.
63. Sambade C, Franssila K, Cameselle-Teijeiro J, et al. Hyalinizing trabecular adenoma: A misnomer for a peculiar tumor of the thyroid gland. Endocr Pathol 1991;2:83–91.
63a. Hirokawa M, Carney JA. Cell membrane and cytoplasmic staining for MIB-1 in hyalinizing trabecular adenoma of the thyroid. Am J Surg Pathol 2000;24:575–578.
64. Berge-Lefranc JL, Cartouzou G, DeMicco C, et al. Quantification of thyroglobulin messenger RNA by in-situ hybridization in differentiated thyroid cancers: Difference between well-differentiated and moderately differentiated histologic types. Cancer 1985;56:345–350.
65. Keen CE, Szakacs S, Okon E, et al. CA125 and thyroglobulin staining in papillary carcinomas of thyroid and ovarian origin is not entirely specific for site of origin. Histopathology 1999;34:113–117.
66. Carcangiu ML, Zampi G, Rosai J. Poorly differentiated ("insular") thyroid carcinoma: A reinterpretation of Langhans' "wuchernde Struma." Am J Surg Pathol 1984;8:655–668.
67. Ordonez NG, El-Naggar AK, Hickey RC, Samaan NA. Anaplastic thyroid carcinoma: Immunocytochemical study of 32 cases. Am J Clin Pathol 1991;96:15–24.
68. Carcangiu ML, Steeper T, Zampi G, Rosai J. Anaplastic thyroid cancer: A study of 70 cases. Am J Clin Pathol 1985;83:135–158.
69. Kawaoi A, Okano T, Nemoto N, et al. Simultaneous detection of thyroglobulin, (T_g) thyroxine (T_4) and tri-iodothyronine (T_3) in nontoxic thyroid tumors by the immunoperoxidase method. Am J Pathol 1982;108:39–49.
70. Henzen-Logmans SC, Mullink H, Ramaekers FC, et al. Expression of cytokeratins and vimentin in epithelial cells of normal and pathologic thyroid tissue. Virchows Arch A Pathol Anat Histopathol 1987;410:347–354.
71. Miettinen M, Franssila K, Lehto V-P, et al. Expression of intermediate filament proteins in thyroid gland and thyroid tumors. Lab Invest 1984;50:262–270.
72. Viale G, Dell'Orto P, Coggi G, Gambacorta M. Co-expression of cytokeratins and vimentin in normal and diseased thyroid glands: Lack of diagnostic utility of vimentin immunostaining. Am J Surg Pathol 1989;13:1034–1040.
73. Schelfhout LJDM, van Muijen GN, Fleuren GJ. Expression of keratin 19 distinguishes papillary thyroid carcinoma from follicular carcinomas and follicular adenoma. Am J Clin Pathol 1989;92:654–658.
74. Raphael SJ, McKeown-Eyssen G, Asa SL. High molecular weight cytokeratin and cytokeratin 19 in the diagnosis of thyroid tumors. Mod Pathol 1994;7:295–300.
75. Fonseca E, Nesland JM, Hoie J, Sobrinho-Simoes M. Pattern of expression of intermediate cytokeratin filaments in the thyroid gland: An immunohistochemical study of simple and stratified epithelial-type cytokeratins. Virchows Arch 1997;430:239–245.
76. Miettinen M, Kovatich AJ, Karkkainen P. Keratin subsets in papillary and follicular thyroid lesions: A paraffin section analysis with diagnostic implications. Virchows Arch 1997;431:407–413.
77. Baloch ZW, Abraham S, Roberts S, LiVolsi VA. Differential expression of cytokeratins in follicular variant of papillary carcinoma: An immunohistochemical study and its diagnostic utility. Hum Pathol 1999;30:1166–1171.
78. Kragsterman B, Grimelius L, Wallin G, et al. Cytokeratin 19 expression in papillary thyroid carcinoma. Appl Immunohistochem 1999;7:181–185.
78a. Fonseca E, Nesland J, Sobrinho-Simoes M. Expression of stratified epithelial cytokeratins in hyalinizing trabecular adenoma supports their relationship with papillary carcinoma of the thyroid. Histopathology 1997;31:330–335.
78b. Hirokawa M, Carney JA, Ohtsuki Y. Hyalinizing trabecular adenoma and papillary carcinoma of the thyroid express different cytokeratin patterns. Am J Surg Pathol 2000;24:877–881.
79. Liberman E, Weidner N. Papillary and follicular neoplasms of the thyroid gland: Differential immunohistochemical staining with high molecular weight keratin and involucrin. Appl Immunohistochem 2000;8:42–48.
80. Dasovic-Knezevic M, Bormer O, Holm R, et al. Carcinoembryonic antigen in medullary thyroid carcinoma: An immunohistochemical study applying six novel monoclonal antibodies. Mod Pathol 1989;2:610–617.
81. Schroder S, Schwarz W, Rehpenning W, et al. Prognostic significance of Leu M1 immunostaining in papillary carcinomas of the thyroid gland. Virchows Arch A Pathol Anat Histopathol 1987;411:435–439.
82. Loy TS, Darkow GV, Spollen LE, Diaz-Arias AA. Immunostaining for Leu 7 in the diagnosis of thyroid carcinoma. Arch Pathol Lab Med 1994;118:172–174.
83. Ostrowski ML, Brown RW, Wheeler TM, et al. Leu 7 immunoreactivity in cytologic specimens of thyroid lesions with an emphasis on follicular neoplasms. Diagn Cytopathol 1995;12:297–302.
84. Sack MJ, Astengo-Osuna C, Lin BT, et al. HBME-1 immunostaining in thyroid fine needle aspirations: A useful marker in the diagnosis of carcinoma. Mod Pathol 1997;10:668–674.
84a. Miettinen M, Karkkainen P. Differential HBME-1 reactivity in benign vs. malignant thyroid tissue is helpful in the diagnosis of thyroid tumors. [abstract] Mod Pathol 1996;5:50A.
85. Gatalica Z, Miettinen M. Distribution of carcinoma antigens CA19-9 and CA15-3: An immunohistochemical study of 400 tumors. Appl Immunohistochem 1994;2:205–211.
86. Alves P, Soares P, Fonseca E, Sobrinho-Simoes M. Papillary thyroid carcinoma overexpresses fully and underglycosylated mucins together with native and sialylated simple mucin antigens and histo-blood group antigens. Endocrine Pathol 1999;10:315–324.
87. McLaren KM, Cossar DW. The immunohistochemical localization of S-100 in the diagnosis of papillary carcinoma of the thyroid. Hum Pathol 1996;27:633–636.
88. Soares P, Cameselle-Teijeiro J, Sobrinho-Simoes M. Immunohistochemical detection of p53 in differentiated, poorly differentiated and undifferentiated carcinomas of the thyroid. Histopathology 1994;24:205–210.
89. Holm R, Nesland JM. Retinoblastoma and p53 tumor suppressor gene protein expression in carcinomas of the thyroid gland. J Pathol 1994;172:267–272.
89a. Tallini G, Santoro M, Helie M, et al. RET/PTC oncogene activation defines a subset of papillary thyroid carcinomas lacking evidence of progression to poorly differentiated or undifferentiated tumor phenotypes. Clin Cancer Res 1998;4:287–294.
89b. Papotti M, Volante M, Guiliano A, et al. RET/PTC activation in hyalinizing trabecular tumors of the thyroid. Am J Surg Pathol 2000;24:1615–1621.
89c. Cheung CC, Boerner SL, MacMillan CM, et al. Hyalinizing trabecular tumor of the thyroid: A variant of papillary carcinoma proved by molecular genetics. Am J Surg Pathol 2000;24:1622–1626.
89d. LiVolsi VA. Hyalinizing trabecular tumor of the thyroid: Adenoma, carcinoma, or neoplasm of uncertain malignant potential? Am J Surg Pathol 2000;24:1683–1684.
90. Bur M, Shiraki W, Masood S. Estrogen and progesterone receptor detection in neoplastic and non-neoplastic thyroid tissue. Mod Pathol 1993;6:469–472.
91. Papotti M, Gugliotta P, Forte G, Bussolati G. Immunocytochemical identification of oxyphilic mitochondrion rich cells. Appl Immunohistochem 1994;2:261–267.
92. Ordonez NG. Thyroid transcription factor 1 is a marker of

lung and thyroid carcinomas. Adv Anat Pathol 2000;7: 123–127.

93. Kaufmann O, Dietel M. Thyroid transcription factor-1 is the superior immunohistochemical marker for pulmonary adenocarcinomas and large cell carcinomas compared to surfactant proteins A and B. Histopathology 2000;36:8–16.

94. Byrd-Gloster AL, Khoor A, Glass LF, et al. Differential expression of thyroid transcription factor-1 in small cell lung carcinoma and Merkel cell tumor. Hum Pathol 2000; 31:58–62.

95. Agoff SN, Lamps LW, Philip AT, et al. Thyroid transcription factor-1 is expressed in extrapulmonary small cell carcinomas but not in other extrapulmonary neuroendocrine tumors. Mod Pathol 2000;13:238–242.

96. DeLellis RA, Wolfe HJ. The pathology of the human calcitonin (C) cell. Pathol Annu 1981;16:25–52.

97. Sikri KL, Varndell IM, Hamid QA, et al. Medullary carcinoma of the thyroid: An immunocytochemical and histochemical study of 25 cases using 8 separate markers. Cancer 1985;56:2481–2491.

98. Perry A, Molberg K, Albores-Saavedra J. Physiologic versus neoplastic C-cell hyperplasia of the thyroid: Separation of distinct histologic and biologic entities. Cancer 1996;77:750–756.

99. Holm R, Sobrinho-Simoes M, Nesland JM, et al. Medullary carcinoma of the thyroid gland: An immunocytochemical study. Ultrastruct Pathol 1985;8:25–41.

100. Uribe M, Fenoglio-Preiser CM, Grimes M, Feind C. Medullary carcinoma of the thyroid gland: Clinical, pathological and immunohistochemical features with a review of the literature. Am J Surg Pathol 1985;9:577–594.

101. Zajac JD, Penschow J, Mason T, et al. Identification of calcitonin and calcitonin gene related peptide messenger RNA in medullary thyroid carcinoma by hybridization histochemistry. J Clin Endocrinol Metab 1986;62:1037–1043.

102. Eusebi V, Damiani S, Riva C, et al. Calcitonin free oat cell carcinoma of the thyroid gland. Virchows Arch A Pathol Anat Histopathol 1990;417:267–271.

103. Franc B, Rosenberg-Bourgin M, Caillou B, et al. Medullary thyroid carcinoma: Search for histological predictors of survival (109 proband case analysis). Hum Pathol 1998;29: 1078–1084.

104. Steenbergh PH, Hoppener JW, Zandberg J, et al. Calcitonin gene related peptide coding sequence is conserved in the human genome and is expressed in medullary thyroid carcinoma. J Clin Endocrinol Metab 1984;59:358–360.

105. Komminoth P, Roth J, Saremaslani P, et al. Polysialic acid of the neural cell adhesion molecule in the human thyroid: A marker for medullary thyroid carcinoma and primary C-cell hyperplasia: An immunohistochemical study on 79 thyroid lesions. Am J Surg Pathol 1994;18:399–411.

106. Scopsi L, Ferrari C, Pilotti S, et al. Immunocytochemical localization and identification of prosomatostatin gene products in medullary carcinoma of human thyroid gland. Hum Pathol 1990;21:820–830.

107. Sunday ME, Wolfe HJ, Roos BA, et al. Gastrin releasing peptide gene expression in developing, hyperplastic and neoplastic thyroid C-cells. Endocrinology 1988;122:1551–1558.

108. Heitz PU, von Herbay G, Kloppel G, et al. The expression of subunits of human chorionic gonadotropin (hCG) by nontrophoblastic, nonendocrine and endocrine tumors. Am J Clin Pathol 1987;88:467–472.

109. DeLellis RA, Moore FM, Wolfe HJ. Thyroglobulin immunoreactivity in human medullary thyroid carcinoma. Lab Invest 1983;48:20A.

110. Holm R, Sobrinho-Simoes M, Nesland JM, Johannessen JV. Concurrent production of calcitonin and thyroglobulin by the same neoplastic cells. Ultrastruct Pathol 1986;10: 241–248.

111. Ljungberg O, Bondeson L, Bondeson AG. Differentiated thyroid carcinoma, intermediate type: A new tumor entity with features of follicular and parafollicular cell carcinomas. Hum Pathol 1984;15:218–228.

112. Volante M, Papotti M, Roth J, et al. Mixed medullary fol-

licular thyroid carcinoma: Molecular evidence for a dual origin of tumor components. Am J Pathol 1999;155:1499–1509.

113. Schmid KW, Fischer-Colbrie R, Hagn C, et al. Chromogranin A and B and secretogranin II in medullary carcinomas of the thyroid. Am J Surg Pathol 1987;11:551–556.

114. Katsetos CD, Jami MM, Krishna L, et al. Novel immunohistochemical localization of 28000 molecular weight (Mr) calcium binding protein (Calbindin-D$_{28k}$) in enterochromaffin cells of the human appendix and neuroendocrine tumors (carcinoids and small cell carcinomas) of the midgut and foregut. Arch Pathol Lab Med 1994;118:633–639.

115. Viale G, Roncalli M, Grimelius L, et al. Prognostic value of bcl-2 immunoreactivity in medullary thyroid carcinoma. Hum Pathol 1995;26:945–950.

116. DeLellis RA, Rule AH, Spiler I, et al. Calcitonin and carcinoembryonic antigen as tumor markers in medullary thyroid carcinoma. Am J Clin Pathol 1978;70:587–594.

117. Schroder S, Kloppel G. Carcinoembryonic antigen and non-specific cross reacting antigen in thyroid cancer: An immunocytochemical study using polyclonal and monoclonal antibodies. Am J Surg Pathol 1987;11:100–108.

118. Mendelsohn G, Wills SA Jr, Baylin SB. Relationship of tissue carcinoembryonic antigen and calcitonin to tumor virulence in medullary thyroid carcinoma: An immunohistochemical study in early, localized and virulent disseminated stages of disease. Cancer 1984;54:657–662.

119. Kimura N, Nakazato Y, Nagura H, Sasano N. Expression of intermediate filaments in neuroendocrine tumors. Arch Pathol Lab Med 1990;114:506–510.

120. Futrell JM, Roth SI, Su SP, et al. Immunocytochemical localization of parathyroid hormone in bovine parathyroid glands and human parathyroid adenomas. Am J Pathol 1979;94:615–622.

121. Tomita T. Immunocytochemical staining patterns for parathyroid hormone and chromogranin in parathyroid hyperplasia, adenoma and carcinoma. Endocr Pathol 1999;10: 145–156.

122. Stork PJ, Herteaux C, Frazier R, et al. Expression and distribution of parathyroid hormone and parathyroid hormone messenger RNA in pathological conditions of the parathyroid gland. Lab Invest 1992;61:169–174.

123. Weber CJ, Russell J, Chryssochoos JT, et al. Parathyroid hormone content distinguishes true normal parathyroids from parathyroids of patients with primary hyperparathyroidism. World J Surg 1996;20:1010–1015.

124. Danks JA, Ebeling PR, Hayman J, et al. Parathyroid hormone related protein: Immunohistochemical localization in cancers and in normal skin. J Bone Miner Res 1989;4: 273–278.

125. Schmid KW, Morgan JM, Baumert M, et al. Calcitonin and calcitonin gene related peptide mRNA detection in a population of hyperplastic parathyroid cells, also expressing chromogranin B. Lab Invest 1995;73:90–95.

126. Hellman P, Karlsson-Parra A, Klareskog L, et al. Expression and function of a CD4 like molecule in parathyroid tissue. Surgery 1996;120:985–992.

127. Vasef MA, Brynes RK, Sturm M, et al. Expression of cyclin D1 in parathyroid carcinomas, adenomas and hyperplasias: A paraffin immunohistochemical study. Mod Pathol 1999;12:412–416.

128. Abbona GC, Papotti M, Gasparri G, Bussolati G. Proliferative activity in parathyroid tumors as detected by Ki-67 immunostaining. Hum Pathol 1995;26:135–138.

129. Vargas MP, Vargas HI, Kleiner DE, Merino MJ. The role of prognostic markers (MIB-1, RB, bcl-2) in the diagnosis of parathyroid tumors. Mod Pathol 1997;10:12–17.

130. Erickson LA, Jin L, Wollan P, et al. Parathyroid hyperplasia, adenomas, and carcinomas: Differential expression of p27 Kip 1 protein. Am J Surg Pathol 1999;23:288–295.

131. Cryns VL, Thor A, Xu H-J, et al. Loss of the retinoblastoma tumor suppressor gene in parathyroid carcinoma. N Engl J Med 1994;330:757–761.

132. Farnebo F, Auer G, Farnebo LO, et al. Evaluation of retinoblastoma and ki-67 immunostaining as diagnostic markers

of benign and malignant parathyroid disease. World J Surg 1999;23:68–74.

133. Kayath MJ, Martin LC, Vieira JG, et al. A comparative study of p53 immunoexpression in parathyroid hyperplasias secondary to uremia, primary hyperplasias, adenomas and carcinomas. Eur J Endocrinol 1998;139:78–83.

134. Miettinen M, Clark R, Lehto VP, et al. Intermediate filament proteins in parathyroid glands and parathyroid adenomas. Arch Pathol Lab Med 1985;109:986–989.

135. Schroder S, Niendorf A, Achilles E, et al. Immunocytochemical differential diagnosis of adrenocortical neoplasms using the monoclonal antibody D11. Virchows Arch A Pathol Anat Histopathol 1990;417:89–96.

136. Schroder S, Padberg BC, Achilles E, et al. Immunocytochemistry in adrenocortical tumors: A clinicopathological study of 72 neoplasms. Virchows Arch A Pathol Anat Histopathol 1992;420:65–70.

137. Tartour E, Caillou B, Tenenbaum F, et al. Immunohistochemical study of adrenocortical carcinoma: Predictive value of the D11 monoclonal antibody. Cancer 1993;72:3296–3303.

138. Sasano H, Shizawa S, Suzuki T, et al. Transcription factor adrenal 4 binding protein as a marker of adrenocortical malignancy. Hum Pathol 1995;26:1154–1156.

139. Busam KJ, Iversen K, Coplan KA, et al. Immunoreactivity for A103, an antibody to melan-A (Mart-1) in adrenocortical and other steroid tumors. Am J Surg Pathol 1998;22:57–63.

140. Renshaw AA, Granter SR. A comparison of A103 and inhibin reactivity in adrenal cortical tumors: Distinction from hepatocellular carcinoma and renal tumors. Mod Pathol 1998;11:1160–1164.

141. Shin SJ, Hoda RS, Ying L, DeLellis RA. Diagnostic utility of the monoclonal antibody A103 in fine-needle aspiration biopsies of the adrenal. Am J Clin Pathol 2000;113:295–302.

142. Pelkey TJ, Frierson HF, Mills SE, Stoler MH. The α submit of inhibin in adrenal cortical neoplasia. Mod Pathol 1998;11:516–524.

143. Fetsch PA, Powers CN, Zakowski M, et al. Anti-alpha inhibin: Marker of choice for the consistent distinction between adrenocortical carcinoma (ACC) and renal cell carcinoma (RCC) in fine needle aspirations (FNA). Cancer 1999;87:168–172.

144. Miettinen M. Neuroendocrine differentiation in adrenocortical carcinoma: New immunohistochemical findings supported by electron microscopy. Lab Invest 1992;66:169–174.

145. Miettinen M, Lehto V-P, Virtanen I. Immunofluorescence microscopic evaluation of the intermediate filament expression of the adrenal cortex and medulla and their tumors. Am J Pathol 1985;118:360–366.

146. Gaffey MJ, Traweek ST, Mills SE, et al. Cytokeratin expression in adrenocortical neoplasia: An immunohistochemical and biochemical study with implications for the differential diagnosis of adrenocortical, hepatocellular and renal cell carcinoma. Hum Pathol 1992;23:144–153.

147. Wick MR, Cherwitz DL, McGlennen RC, Dehner LP. Adrenocortical carcinoma: An immunohistochemical comparison with renal cell carcinoma. Am J Pathol 1986;122:343–352.

148. Cote RJ, Cardon-Cardo C, Reuter VE, Rosen PP. Immunopathology of adrenal and renal cortical tumors: Coordinated change in antigen expression is associated with neoplastic conversion in the adrenal cortex. Am J Pathol 1990;136:1077–1084.

149. Fogt F, Vortmeyer AO, Poremba C, et al. Bcl-2 expression in normal adrenal glands and in adrenal neoplasms. Mod Pathol 1998;11:716–720.

150. Lloyd RV, Shapiro B, Sisson JC, et al. An immunohistochemical study of pheochromocytomas. Arch Pathol Lab Med 1984;108:541–544.

151. Lloyd RV, Blaivas M, Wilson BS. Distribution of chromogranin and S100 protein in normal and abnormal adrenal

medullary tissues. Arch Pathol Lab Med 1985;109:633–635.

152. Verhofstad AAJ, Steinbusch HWM, Joosten JWJ, et al. Immunocytochemical localization of nonadrenaline, adrenaline and serotonin. In: Polak JM, Van Noordens S, eds. Immunohistochemistry: Practical Applications in Pathology and Biology. Bristol, England: Wright-PSG, 1983:143–168.

153. Trojanowski JQ, Lee VM. Expression of neurofilament antigens by normal and neoplastic human adrenal chromaffin cells. N Engl J Med 1985;313:101–104.

154. Chetty R, Pillay P, Jaichand V. Cytokeratin expression in adrenal pheochromocytoma and extra-adrenal paragangliomas. J Clin Pathol 1998;51:477–478.

155. Grignon DJ, Ro JY, Mackay B, et al. Paraganglioma of the urinary bladder: Immunohistochemical, ultrastructural and DNA flow cytometric studies. Hum Pathol 1991;22:1162–1169.

156. Johnson TL, Zarbo RJ, Lloyd RV, Crissman JD. Paragangliomas of the head and neck: Immunohistochemical neuroendocrine and intermediate filament typing. Mod Pathol 1988;1:216–223.

157. Salim SA, Milroy C, Rode J, et al. Immunocytochemical characterization of neuroendocrine tumors of the larynx. Histopathology 1993;23:69–73.

157a. Helman LJ, Cohen PS, Averbuch SD, et al. Neuropeptide Y expression distinguishes malignant from benign pheochromocytoma. J Clin Oncol 1989;7:720–725, 1989.

158. Clarke MR, Weyant RJ, Watson CG, Carty SE. Prognostic markers in pheochromocytoma. Hum Pathol 1998;29:522–526.

159. Triche TJ, Askin F. Neuroblastoma and the differential diagnosis of small-, round-, blue-cell tumors. Hum Pathol 1983;14:569–595.

160. Hachitanda Y, Tsuneyoshi M, Enjoji M. An ultrastructural and immunohistochemical evaluation of cytodifferentiation in neuroblastic tumors. Mod Pathol 1989;2:13–19.

161. Pagani A, Forni M, Tonini GP, et al. Expression of members of the chromogranin family in primary neuroblastomas. Diagn Mol Pathol 1992;1:16–24.

162. Carter RL, Al-sams SZ, Corbett RP, et al. A comparative study of immunohistochemical staining for neuron-specific enolase, protein gene product 9.5 and s-100 in neuroblastoma, Ewing's sarcoma and other round cell tumors in children. Histopathology 1990;16:461–467.

163. Wirnsberger GH, Becker H, Ziervogel K, et al. Diagnostic immunohistochemistry of neuroblastic tumors. Am J Surg Pathol 1992;16:49–57.

164. Franquemont DW, Mills SE, Lack EE. Immunohistochemical detection of neuroblastomatous foci in composite adrenal pheochromocytoma-neuroblastoma. Am J Clin Pathol 1994;102:163–170.

165. Argani P, Erlandson RA, Rosai J. Thymic neuroblastoma in adults: Report of three cases with special emphasis on its association with the syndrome of inappropriate secretion of antidiuretic hormone. Am J Clin Pathol 1997;108:537–543.

166. Fellinger EJ, Garin-Chesa P, Triche TJ, et al. Immunohistochemical analysis of Ewing's sarcoma cell surface antigen p30/32 MIC2. Am J Pathol 1991;39:317–325.

167. Stevenson AJ, Chatten J, Bertoni F, et al. CD99 (p30/32mic2) neuroectodermal/Ewing's sarcoma antigen as an immunohistochemical marker: Review of more than 600 tumors and the literature experience. Appl Immunohistochem 1994;2:231–240.

168. Weidner N, Tjoe J. Immunohistochemical profile of monoclonal antibody O13: Antibody that recognizes glycoprotein p 30/32mic2 and is useful in diagnosing Ewing's sarcoma and peripheral neuroepithelioma. Am J Surg Pathol 1994;18:486–494.

169. Scotlandi K, Serra M, Manara MC, et al. Immunostaining of the p30/32mic2 antigen and molecular detection of EWS rearrangements for the diagnosis of Ewing's sarcoma and peripheral neuroectodermal tumor. Hum Pathol 1996;27:408–416.

170. Hess E, Cohen C, DeRose PB, et al. Nonspecificity of p30/32mic2 immunolocalization with the 013 monoclonal antibody in the diagnosis of Ewing's sarcoma: Application of an algorithmic immunohistochemical analysis. Appl Immunohistochem 1997;5:94–103.

171. Pappo AS, Douglass ED, Meyer WH, et al. Use of HBA 71 and anti-B2-microglobulin to distinguish peripheral neuroepithelioma from neuroblastoma. Hum Pathol 1993;24:880–885.

172. Miettinen M, Chatten J, Paetau A, et al. Monoclonal antibody NB84 in the differential diagnosis of neuroblastoma and other small round cell tumors. Am J Surg Pathol 1998;22:327–332.

173. Folpe AL, Patterson K, Gown AM. Antineuroblastoma antibody NB-84 also identifies a significant subset of other small blue round cell tumors. Appl Immunohistochem 1997;5:239–245.

174. Dayal Y. Endocrine cells of the gut and their neoplasms. In: Norris HT, ed. Pathology of the Colon, Small Intestine and Anus. New York: Churchill Livingstone, 1991:305–366.

175. Moll R, Franke WW. Cytoskeletal differences between human neuroendocrine tumors: A cytoskeletal protein of molecular weight 46000 distinguishes cutaneous from pulmonary neuroendocrine tumors. Differentiation 1985;30:165–175.

176. Burke AP, Sobin LH, Federspiel BH, Shekitka KM. Appendiceal carcinoids: Correlation of histology and immunohistochemistry. Mod Pathol 1989;2:630–637.

177. Miettinen M. Keratin 20: Immunohistochemical marker for gastrointestinal, urothelial, and Merkel cell carcinomas. Mod Pathol 1995;8:384–388.

178. Al-Khafaji B, Noffsinger AE, Miller MA, et al. Immunohistologic analysis of gastrointestinal and pulmonary carcinoid tumors. Hum Pathol 1998;29:992–999.

179. Kimura N, Pilichowska M, Okamoto H, et al. Immunohistochemical expression of chromogranins A and B, prohormone convertases 2 and 3, and amidating enzyme in carcinoid tumors and pancreatic endocrine tumors. Mod Pathol 2000;13:140–146.

180. Thomas RM, Baybick JH, Elsayed AM, Sobin LH. Gastric carcinoids: An immunohistochemical and clinicopathologic study of 104 patients. Cancer 1994;73:2053–2058.

181. Machlouf HR, Burke AP, Sobin LH. Carcinoid tumors of the ampulla of Vater: A comparison with duodenal carcinoid tumors. Cancer 1999;85:1241–1249.

182. Sheibani K, Battifora H, Burke JS, Rappaport H. Leu-M1 antigen in human neoplasms: An immunohistologic study of 400 cases. Am J Surg Pathol 1986;10:227–236.

183. Azumi N, Traweek ST, Battifora H. Prostatic acid phosphatase in carcinoid tumors: Immunohistochemical and immunoblot studies. Am J Surg Pathol 1991;15:785–790.

184. Shah IA, Schlageter M-O, Netto D. Immunoreactivity of neurofilament proteins in neuroendocrine neoplasms. Mod Pathol 1991;4:215–219.

185. Chejfec G, Falkmer S, Grimelius L, et al. Synaptophysin: A new marker for pancreatic neuroendocrine tumors. Am J Surg Pathol 1987;11:241–247.

186. Solcia E, Capella C, Kloppel G. Atlas of Tumor Pathology: Tumors of the Pancreas. Washington, D.C.: Armed Forces Institute of Pathology, 1997.

187. Heitz PU, Kasper M, Polak JM, Kloppel G. Pancreatic endocrine tumors: Immunocytochemical analysis of 125 tumors. Hum Pathol 1982;13:263–271.

188. Perkins PL, McLeod MK, Jin L, et al. Analysis of gastrinomas by immunohistochemistry and in-situ hybridization histochemistry. Diagn Mol Pathol 1992;1:155–164.

189. Le Bodic M-F, Heyman M-F, Lecomete M, et al. Immunohistochemical study of 100 pancreatic tumors in 28 patients with multiple endocrine neoplasia type I. Am J Surg Pathol 1996;20:1378–1384.

190. Solcia E, Capella C, Riva C, et al. The morphology and neuroendocrine profile of pancreatic epithelial VIPomas and extrapancreatic, VIP producing neurogenic tumors. Ann NY Acad Sci 1988;527:508–517.

191. Heitz PU, Kasper M, Kloppel G, et al. Glycoprotein-hormone alpha-chain production by pancreatic endocrine tumors: A specific marker for malignancy: Immunocytochemical analysis of tumors of 155 patients. Cancer 1983;51:277–282.

192. Graeme-Cook F, Nardi G, Compton CC. Immunocytochemical staining for human chorionic gonadotropin subunits does not predict malignancy in insulinomas. Am J Clin Pathol 1990;93:273–276.

193. Viale G, Doglioni C, Gambacorta M, et al. Progesterone receptor immunoreactivity in pancreatic endocrine tumors: An immunocytochemical study of 156 neuroendocrine tumors of the pancreas, gastrointestinal and respiratory tracts and skin. Cancer 1992;70:2268–2277.

194. Gould VE, Linnoila RI, Memoli VA, Warren WH. Neuroendocrine components of the bronchopulmonary tract: Hyperplasias, dysplasias and neoplasias. Lab Invest 1983;49:519–537.

195. Travis WD, Linnoila ID, Tsokos MG, et al. Neuroendocrine tumors of the lung with proposed criteria for large cell neuroendocrine carcinoma: An ultrastructural, immunohistochemical and flow cytometric study of 35 cases. Am J Surg Pathol 1991;15:529–553.

196. Blobel GA, Gould VE, Moll R, et al. Co-expression of neuroendocrine markers and epithelial cytoskeletal proteins in bronchopulmonary neuroendocrine neoplasms. Lab Invest 1985;52:39–51.

197. Jiang S-X, Kameya T, Shoji M, et al. Large cell neuroendocrine carcinoma of the lung: A histological and immunohistochemical study of 22 cases. Am J Surg Pathol 1998;22:526–537.

198. Gersell DJ, Mazoujian G, Mutch DG, Rudloff MA. Small cell undifferentiated carcinoma of the cervix: A clinicopathologic, ultrastructural and immunocytochemical study of 15 cases. Am J Surg Pathol 1988;12:684–698.

199. Abeler VM, Holm R, Nesland JM, Kjorstad KE. Small cell carcinoma of the cervix: A clinicopathologic study of 26 patients. Cancer 1994;73:672–677.

200. Gilks CB, Young RH, Gersell DJ, Clement PB. Large cell neuroendocrine carcinoma of the uterine cervix: A clinicopathologic study of 12 cases. Am J Surg Pathol 1997;21:905–914.

201. Stoler MH, Mills SE, Gersell DJ, Walker AN. Small cell neuroendocrine carcinoma of the cervix: A human papillomavirus 18 associated cancer. Am J Surg Pathol 1991;15:28–32.

202. diSant'Agnese PA, de Mesy Jensen KL, Churukian CJ, et al. Human prostatic endocrine-paracrine (APUD) cells: Distributional analysis with a comparison of serotonin and neuron specific enolase immunoreactivity and silver stains. Arch Pathol Lab Med 1985;109:607–612.

203. diSant'Agnese PA. Neuroendocrine differentiation in prostatic carcinoma: An update. Prostate (Suppl) 1998;8:74–79.

204. Schmid KW, Helpap B, Totsch M, et al. Immunohistochemical localization of chromogranins A and B and secretogranin II in normal, hyperplastic and neoplastic prostate. Histopathology 1994;24:233–239.

205. Bostwick DG, Dousa MK, Crawford BG, Wollan PC. Neuroendocrine differentiation in prostatic intraepithelial neoplasia and adenocarcinoma. Am J Surg Pathol 1994;18:1240–1246.

206. Gould VE, Moll R, Moll I, et al. Neuroendocrine (Merkel) cells of the skin: Hyperplasias, dysplasias and neoplasms. Lab Invest 1985;52:334–353.

207. Chan JKC, Suster S, Wenig BM, et al. Cytokeratin 20 immunoreactivity distinguishes Merkel cell (primary cutaneous neuroendocrine) carcinomas and salivary gland small cell carcinomas from small cell carcinomas of various sites. Am J Surg Pathol 1997;21:226–234.

208. Drijkoningen M, de Wolf-Peeters C, van Limbergen E, Desmet V. Merkel cell tumor of the skin: An immunohistochemical study. Hum Pathol 1986;17:301–307.

209. Sibley RK, Dahl D. Primary neuroendocrine (Merkel cell?) carcinoma of the skin. II: An immunohistochemical study of 21 cases. Am J Surg Pathol 1985;9:109–116.

210. Brinkschmidt C, Stolze P, Fahrenkamp AG, et al. Immuno-histochemical demonstration of chromogranin A, chromo-granin B and secretoneunin in Merkel cell carcinoma of the skin: An immunohistochemical study suggesting two types of Merkel cell carcinoma. Appl Immunohistochem 1995;3: 37–44.
211. Nicholson SA, McDermott MB, Swanson PE, Wick MR. CD99 and cytokeratin 20 in small cell and basaloid tumors of the skin. Appl Immunohistochem Mol Morphol 2000;8: 37–41.
212. Maluf HM, Koerner FC. Carcinomas of the breast with endocrine differentiation: A review. Virchows Arch 1994; 425:449–457.
213. Papotti M, Gherardi G, Eusebi V, et al. Primary oat cell (neuroendocrine) carcinoma of the breast: Report of four cases. Virchows Arch A Pathol Anat Histopathol 1992;420: 103–108.
214. Francois A, Chatikhine VA, Chevallier B, et al. Neuroen-docrine primary small cell carcinoma of the breast: Report of a case and review of the literature. Am J Clin Oncol 1995;18:133–138.
215. Shin SJ, DeLellis RA, Ying BA, Rosen PP. Small cell carci-noma of the breast: A clinico-pathological and immunohis-tochemical study of 9 patients. Am J Surg Pathol 2000;24: 1231–1238.
216. Klemm KM, Moran CA. Primary neuroendocrine carci-noma of the thymus. Semin Diagn Pathol 1999;16:32–41.
217. Moran CA, Suster S. Thymic neuroendocrine carcinomas with combined features ranging from well-differentiated (carcinoid) to small cell carcinoma: A clinicopathologic and immunohistochemical study of 11 cases. Am J Clin Pathol 2000;113:345–350.
218. De Montpreville VT, Macchiarini P, Dulmet E. Thymic neuroendocrine carcinoma (carcinoid): A clinicopathologic study of fourteen cases. J Thorac Cardiovasc Surg 1996; 111:134–141.

CHAPTER 10

Immunohistology of the Mediastinum

Mark R. Wick, M.D.

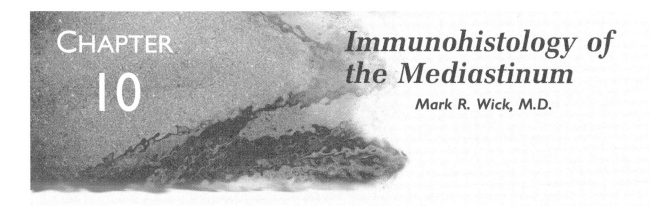

The mediastinum is a relatively confined anatomic site, but it is capable of harboring a wide variety of pathologic processes, both non-neoplastic and neoplastic. These include proliferations of somatic epithelial, lymphoid, mesenchymal, and germ cell types. Surgical pathology of mediastinal disorders is made all the more challenging by the fact that small biopsies—taken either by mediastinoscopy or closed needle biopsy—have become routine as the primary method of diagnosis.[1-6] Therefore, one is often faced with the need to perform numerous immunostaining procedures on such material in order to obtain a meaningful diagnosis in the absence of much morphologic detail. This chapter presents a synopsis of immunohistologic information as applied to that specific context. There is no attempt to be "encyclopedic" in regard to the scope of pathologic entities that may arise in the mediastinum or the panoply of immunoreactants that have been assessed in them. Rather, emphasis is placed on practical differential diagnosis and the role that immunohistology plays in that process.

SPECIFIC IMMUNOREACTANTS OF INTEREST IN MEDIASTINAL LESIONS

There are few cellular proliferations of the mediastinum—neoplastic or otherwise—that are unique to it, and therefore the spectrum of immunoreactants of interest in this topographic region overlaps significantly with that considered in the other chapters of this book. Hence, the biochemical attributes of intermediate filament subtypes, various membrane glycoproteins synthesized by epithelial and hematopoietic cells, and cytoplasmic differentiation-related proteins are not recounted here. The reader is referred to primary discussions of carcinomas, hematolymphoid lesions, specific mesenchymal proliferations, and so on elsewhere in this text. However, a few remarks are made here about reactants that appear to be restricted to mediastinal

disorders or are elaborated in a singular fashion in those diseases.

Thymic "Hormones." Several "hormonal" proteins are apparently synthesized by epithelial cells of the thymus, and these are thought to have distant effects on the development or function of the immunologic system. Such moieties include thymopoietin, thymic humoral factor, thymosin, facteur thymique serique, thymic factor "X," thymic plasma recirculating factor, thymotoxin, thymulin, and thymin.[7] Among them, only thymosin has been evaluated immunohistochemically in human neoplasms, primarily in thymomas, with reactivity being observed in greater than 80% of cases.[8] Nevertheless, there have been no systematic studies of the differential diagnostic utility (or lack thereof) of thymic "hormones," and their practical role in the surgical pathology laboratory is consequently unknown.

Keratin Subclasses. As in many other organs, keratin subsets have been analyzed in the normal thymus and in tumors deriving from it.[9, 10] In particular, cytokeratins (CK) 7, 13, and 18 appear to be expressed in this spectrum of tissues. CK13 is restricted to epithelial cells of the thymic medulla but is shared by thymomas of all types.[9] Indeed, CK7 and CK18 likewise appear to be preferentially seen in neoplastic proliferations of this gland.[9, 10]

ALGORITHMIC IMMUNOHISTOCHEMISTRY OF MEDIASTINAL DISEASE

Perhaps in reaction to the overwhelming number of antibodies that one may now apply to diagnostic questions in surgical pathology, "shotgun" approaches to immunohistology have become so common as to cause concern. Worry over medicolegal liabilities also may prompt one to "empty the reservoir" of reagents in the evaluation of difficult cases. Nonetheless, published experience with well-characterized procedures and antibodies has made this temptation unnecessary. Indeed, a sufficient body of data on reagent specificity and sensitivity is now available so that one may codify it by means of integration into algorithms.

Adjunctive algorithmic diagnosis has several benefits. It provides reproducible strategies for the resolution of recurring problems in histopathology, gives one a prescribed sequence in which the results of predefined antibody-mediated stains may be interpreted, and compensates for the reality that no single reagent is likely to provide a definitive answer in any given case. The last of these three points is an important one, because it has been fashionable (but largely noncontextual and fatuous in the author's opinion) to embrace the practice of "antibody bashing" with regard to the specificity of individual reagents.

There are several caveats that must be heeded before immunohistochemical algorithms can be safely and effectively applied. They include the following:

1. The user (pathologist) must control the processing of all tissues in his or her own laboratory under stringent conditions. If specimen fixation times or conditions vary wildly, so will antibody reactivity patterns.
2. The user (*not* the manufacturer or distributor) must determine the optimal dilutions of all antibody reagents personally. Simple acceptance of commercial recommendations is unwise; published scientific papers on such reagents are more helpful in giving one practical information on this point.
3. The user must accrue data on the spectra of reactivity for all antibodies, over a broad group of pathologic conditions or neoplasms, as processed and studied in his or her own laboratory. Failing the feasibility of this approach, the pathologist must adopt *exactly* the same method of fixation, processing, and staining that is used in published investigations providing the desired information.
4. Algorithms must be based on formal statistical analyses of specificity, sensitivity, and Bayesian predictive values, as applied to predefined differential diagnostic problems. This approach allows for the determination of "relative values" for each determinant in well-characterized settings.
5. The sequence of interpretation of a group of immunostains should be governed by their relative statistical values, moving from most specific to least specific or from highest positive predictive value to lowest.
6. Discrete morphologic categories must be determined for application of the foregoing principles. For example, the author generically classifies all morphologically indeterminate and undifferentiated neoplasms of the mediastinum into one of three major groups—small cell, large polygonal cell, and spindle cell pleomorphic tumors.
7. Immunohistochemical data *must* be applied *only* in the context of thorough morphologic

analysis and well-formulated differential diagnosis. It is and will *always* be true that immunostains are merely diagnostic adjuncts and do not take the place of skill in the interpretation of slides stained with hematoxylin and eosin. A poor histodiagnostician will probably be a worse immunohistochemist! Hence, one must always see to it that clinical information, histologic differential diagnosis, and immunohistologic interpretations fit together in a sensible fashion.
8. Algorithms should be flexible. As new reagents are introduced and suitably characterized, they may be integrated into pre-existing schemes to replace or supplement older antibodies.

Working examples of practical algorithms used in the author's laboratory are presented throughout this chapter. The statistical data used to construct them were gathered over a period of several years using specimens that were fixed routinely in 10% neutral-buffered formalin, primary antibody incubations at 4°C for 16 to 18 hours, the Elite avidin-biotin-peroxidase complex method of immunodetection (Vector Laboratories, Burlingame, CA), and the antibody reagents listed in Table 10–1.

IMMUNOHISTOLOGIC FINDINGS IN SPECIFIC DISEASES OF THE MEDIASTINUM

Cystic Thymoma Versus Cystic Seminoma

In many respects, cystic thymomas are morphologically similar to thymic cysts.[11–13] However, more pertinently, they may also be confused with intrathymic seminomas, which manifest prominent cystic changes.[14, 15] These lesions are usually separated from one another adequately by conventional microscopy, inasmuch as cystic seminoma typically displays a much greater degree of nuclear atypia than does thymoma. However, in small biopsy specimens, this feature may not be clear. The periodic acid–Schiff stain is helpful in delineating the glycogen content that typifies seminomas and may be used to screen for the neoplastic cell aggregates in this particular setting. Similarly, immunostains for placental alkaline phosphatase (PLAP) with a broadly reactive mixture of monoclonal antibodies to keratin are helpful in this setting. Seminomas are uniformly PLAP+ (with a distinct cell membranous pattern of reactivity), but less than 15% will label for keratin.[14–16] Conversely, thymoma is universally keratin-positive and always lacks PLAP.[17, 18]

Differential Diagnosis of Other Thymoma Variants

The favored nosologic scheme for thymomas divides them into several discrete categories based

Table 10–1. Antibodies Used in the Algorithmic Immunohistochemical Analysis of Mediastinal Diseases

Antigen	Antibody (Clone)	Source	Dilution	Antigen	Antibody (Clone)	Source	Dilution
Cytokeratins	AE1	Boehringer-Mannheim	1:100	CD45	PD7/26-2B111	DAKO	1:80
	AE1/AE3	Boehringer-Mannheim	1:150	CD3	Polyclonal	DAKO	1:40
	CAM5.2	Becton-Dickinson	1:150	CD5	CD5/54/B4	Vector	1:4
	MAK6	Triton BioSciences	1:40		4C7	Vector	1:100
CK20	ITKs2O.8	DAKO	1:40	CD43	MT1	BioGenex	1:50
Vimentin	V9	BioGenex	1:2000		DF-T1	DAKO	1:50
Desmin	033	BioGenex	1:2000	CD45RO	UCHL-1	DAKO	1:120
				CD20	L26	DAKO	1:200
Epithelial membrane antigen	E29	DAKO	1:400	"Membrane-bound B-cell antigen"	MB2	BioGenex	1:80
Carcinoembryonic antigen	NG	Boehringer-Mannheim	1:4000	CD74	LN2	BioGenex	1:8
"Epithelial antigen"	BEREP4	DAKO	1:200	CD15	LeuM1	Becton-Dickinson	1:150
Calretinin	Polyclonal	Zymed	1:750	CD30	BerH2	DAKO	1:40
Neuron-specific enolase	Polyclonal	BioGenex	1:450	"Anti-Hodgkin's disease"	BLA.36	DAKO	1:200
Chromogranin A	LK2H1O	Boehringer-Mannheim	1:4000	"Anti–large cell lymphoma"	BNH9	DAKO	1:200
Synaptophysin	SY38	Boehringer-Mannheim	1:40	Lysozyme	Polyclonal	DAKO	1:400
CD57	Leu7	Becton-Dickinson	1:20	Cathepsin B	Polyclonal	ICN Biomed	1:800
S-100 protein	Polyclonal	DAKO	1:300	"Myeloid/Histiocyte Antigen"	MAC387	DAKO	1:800
"Antimelanoma"	HMB-45	BioGenex	1:60	CD68	KP1	DAKO	1:800
Tyrosinase	T311	Novocastra	1:20				
MART-1	A103	BioGenex	1:25	Myeloperoxidase	Polyclonal	DAKO	1:250
Muscle-specific actin	HHF-35	BioGenex	1:400	Ki-67	MIB-1	AMAC	1:200
Alpha-isoform actin	IA4	BioGenex	1:2	PCNA	PC10	Novocastra	1:400
Myogenin	F5D	DAKO	1:10				
MyoD1	AntiMyoD1	DAKO	1:10	p53	DO1	Oncogene Sci	1:160
Placental alkaline phosphatase	Polyclonal	DAKO	1:800		D07	DAKO	1:240
Alpha-fetoprotein	C3	BioGenex	1:40				
CD31	JC/70A	DAKO	1:40				
CD34	Myl 0	DAKO	1:800				

NG, Not given by manufacturer

on cross-sectional microscopic morphology: lymphocyte-predominant (>66% lymphocytes), epithelial-predominant (>66% epithelial cells), mixed lymphoepithelial (34 to 66% epithelial cells), and spindle cell (a subtype of epithelial-predominant thymoma featuring a nearly exclusive composition by fusiform tumor cells).[17, 19–22] However, it must be stated forthrightly that thymoma must be defined as a cytologically bland epithelial neoplasm in order for this system to have clinical usefulness. That utility is not one of prognostication, but rather a cue to the consideration of dissimilar differential diagnostic categories that attend each of the four major histologic categories outlined earlier. Salient diagnostic problems that are specific to these tumor subgroups are presented further on. The distinction between thymoma and primary thymic carcinoma (which may, occasionally, arise in transition *from* thymoma) will be considered later in this discussion.

Lymphocyte-Predominant Thymoma Versus Lymphoid Hyperplasia. In patients with myasthenia gravis, one is asked to distinguish between true thymic hyperplasia[23] and thymoma in surgical specimens. In general, thymoma does not manifest the presence of internal lymphoid follicles, although the latter do occur rarely. In that circumstance, immunostaining for keratin reveals a finely arborizing network of interconnecting epithelial cell processes between the lymphocytes in thymoma (Fig. 10–1), which is not seen in lymphoid hyperplasia.[18, 19, 24]

Lymphocyte-Predominant Thymoma Versus Lymphoma. The imitation of lymphoblastic lymphoma (LL) by selected lymphocyte-rich thymomas is enhanced by the peculiar features of infiltrating lymphocytes in some of the latter tumors; these may show convoluted nuclear contours, increased nucleocytoplasmic ratios, and brisk mitotic activity,[19] as typically seen in LL. Moreover, the immunophenotypes of the lymphocytes in thymomas and those of LL cells are remarkably similar. Both populations are typically labeled for CD1, CD2, CD3, CD99 (MIC2),[25–27] and bcl-2,[27–29] as well as

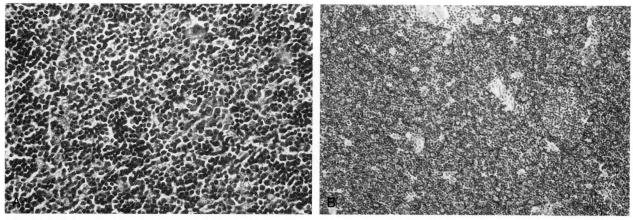

Figure 10–1. Keratin in lymphocyte-predominant thymoma *(A).* Note the delicately "interlocking" pattern of reactivity *(B).*

terminal deoxynucleotidyl transferase.[26, 27, 30–35] Consequently, immunohistochemical distinctions between these neoplasms must be made with extreme caution.

The most helpful immunostain in this differential diagnosis—and one that the author, through regrettable mistakes, has made routine—is an assessment of keratin reactivity. The elaborately interconnecting epithelial cells of lymphocyte predominant thymoma, which are not seen in LL, are distinctive. This *pattern* is essential to differential diagnosis, because LL and other lymphomas of thymus may demonstrate entrapped non-neoplastic thymic epithelial cells that are visible (but widely separated and noninterconnecting) on keratin immunostains.[5, 36]

Predominantly Epithelial Spindle Cell Thymoma Versus Fibrous Histiocytoma and Hemangiopericytoma. Predominantly epithelial thymomas that are constituted by spindle cells may be difficult to separate diagnostically from fibrous histiocytomas or hemangiopericytomas by conventional histologic study.[19] Immunohistochemistry is a more discerning method toward that end, particularly when only small biopsy specimens are available for analysis. Pseudomesenchymal thymomas are univer-

sally positive for keratin and lack vimentin,[18] whereas fibrous histiocytomas and hemangiopericytomas show the opposite of that pattern.[37] In addition, hemangiopericytomas commonly demonstrate reactivity for CD34 (Fig. 10–2),[38] whereas the latter determinant is not expected in thymomas.

Benign Peripheral Nerve Sheath Tumors and Ganglioneuromas

The overwhelming majority of neoplasms encountered in the posterior mediastinum are neurogenic in nature.[39–41] As such, they often show morphologic similarities to one another, thereby presenting diagnostic difficulties. Specifically, Schwann cell neoplasms (peripheral nerve sheath tumors) are usually subdivided into neurofibromas and neurilemomas (schwannomas), because of their differing associations with von Recklinghausen's disease and risk of malignant transformation.[41–44] They also must be separated from ganglioneuromas.[40, 45] All these proliferations are reactive for vimentin and S-100 protein in a uniform manner. In fact, S-100 negativity should cast

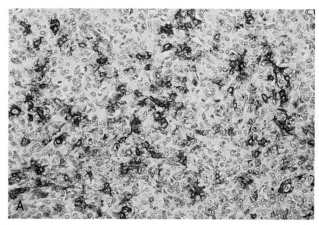
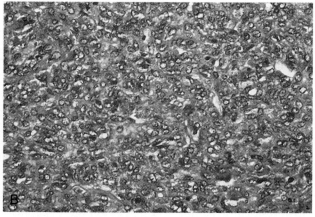

Figure 10–2. CD34 positivity *(A)* in true hemangiopericytoma *(B)* of the mediastinum.

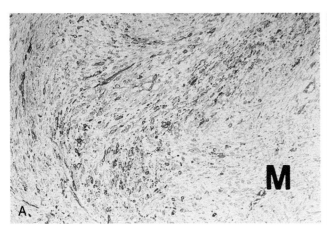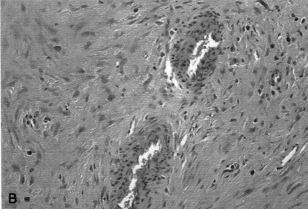

🔖 *Figure 10–3.* Muscle-specific actin (M) *(A)* is present in the proliferating cells of this mediastinal desmoid-type fibromatosis *(B).*

serious doubt on any of the three diagnoses under discussion. Synaptophysin, a synaptic vesicle–related protein that is typical of neuronal and neuroendocrine lesions,[46] is a helpful determinant for the labeling of ganglion cells (which may be focal or widely scattered) in ganglioneuromas.

Fibrogenic and Myofibroblastic Proliferations

Four cytologically bland spindle cell proliferations of the mediastinum may be mistaken for one another histologically, namely, solitary fibrous tumor,[47–49] desmoid-type fibromatosis, sclerosing mediastinitis, and inflammatory myofibroblastic tumor (inflammatory pseudotumor). The immunophenotype of solitary fibrous tumor[49–51] features reactivity for vimentin and CD34, with a lack of keratin, epithelial membrane antigen (EMA), S-100 protein, desmin, and actin.

In contrast, fibromatoses and inflammatory pseudotumors show a mixture of cells labeling for vimentin and muscle-specific actin or alpha isoform actin, with or without desmin (Fig. 10–3).[52–54] The distinction between the latter two lesions must therefore be made on the basis of morphologic features alone. Sclerosing mediastinitis (SM) is composed of spindle cells that are reactive only for vimentin. However, an important caution must be remembered in reference to lesions thought to be SM: Selected malignant lymphomas (especially "obliterative total sclerosis" Hodgkin's disease[14, 55]), metastatic carcinomas, or desmoplastic mesotheliomas may engender a densely fibrotic response in the mediastinal soft tissue or lymph node groups. The actual tumor cells in such cases are consequently sparse and may be surprisingly bland cytologically. Accordingly, they may be overlooked, leading to diagnostic mistakes (Fig. 10–4).[56–58] Thus, stains for keratin, CD15, CD20, CD30, and CD45 should be routine in the assessment of putative cases of SM.

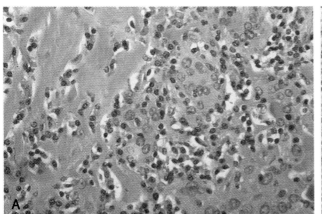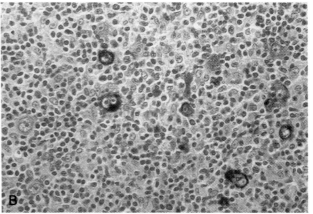

🔖 *Figure 10–4. A,* This dense fibroinflammatory mass in the mediastinum has the appearance of a "tumefactive fibroinflammatory lesion" (fibrosing mediastinitis). However, biopsy of an adjacent lymph node *(B)* demonstrated classic Reed-Sternberg cells (labeled for CD30), establishing a diagnosis of the "total obliterative" nodular sclerosing subtype of Hodgkin's disease.

Table 10–2. Immunoreactants Used in the Differential Diagnosis of Small Cell Indeterminate and Undifferentiated Neoplasms of the Mediastinum

Keratin (monoclonal mixture)
Epithelial membrane antigen
Vimentin
Desmin
Muscle-specific actin
MyoD1
Myogenin
Neuron-specific enolase
Synaptophysin
Chromogranin A
CD15
CD45
CD99 (MIC2 protein)
Ber-EP4
S-100 protein
HMB-45
MART-1
Tyrosinase

Malignant Small Cell Mediastinal Neoplasms (Tables 10–2 and 10–3; Figs. 10–5 to 10–8)

Mediastinal Small Cell Neuroendocrine Carcinoma (Grade III Neuroendocrine Carcinoma, Small Cell Type). Nearly all small cell neuroendocrine carcinomas (SCNCs) involving the mediastinum are metastatic,[59] usually from tumors of the lungs or esophagus. Immunophenotypically, SCNC commonly demonstrates perinuclear punctate labeling for keratin (Fig. 10–9),[18] which is a specific marker of neuroendocrine lineage in a small cell neoplasm. Less frequently, it will show reactivity for one of several neuroendocrine markers such as chromogranin, synaptophysin, CD57, or specific

neuropeptides.[60–65] There are currently no reliable discriminants to distinguish between primary (thymic) and secondary mediastinal SCNCs.

Basaloid Squamous Cell Carcinoma of the Mediastinum. Basaloid squamous cell carcinoma (BSCC) also may be either a primary thymic tumor[64–66] or a mediastinal metastasis from a primary neoplasm of the oropharynx, hypopharynx, larynx, esophagus, lungs, or anorectal region.[67] Keratin is universally present in basaloid squamous cell carcinoma, with a diffuse cytoplasmic pattern of labeling; EMA reactivity also may be observed.[19, 67] Neuroendocrine determinants are, in the author's experience, consistently absent.

Neuroblastoma of the Mediastinum. Characteristically, neuroblastoma (NBL) is a disease of young children,[41, 68] and it is usually located in the posterior mediastinum in these patients.[69, 70] Nonetheless, rare examples of this tumor or its congeners have also been reported in the anterior mediastinum in adults.[71, 72] The immunoprofile of NBL includes variable reactivity for vimentin and neurofilament protein; a proportion of cases lack both of these proteins.[73] Neural features are reflected by positivity for CD57 and synaptophysin (Fig. 10–10).[40] NBLs are universally devoid of markers of myogenous differentiation (desmin, actin, MyoD1, myogenin), a hematolymphoid lineage (CD45), and epithelial character (keratin, EMA).[50, 71]

Mediastinal Primitive Neuroectodermal Tumor. The primitive neuroectodermal tumor (PNET) may rarely occur in the mediastinum, in either the anterior or posterior compartment.[74] The immunophenotype of PNET is similar to that of NBL, but the former of these lesions shows more uniform reactivity for vimentin and only occasionally is labeled for neurofilament protein.[37] Moreover, the CD99 (p30/32 [MIC2]) and MB2 antigens and β_2-micro-

Table 10–3. Percentages of Immunoreactivity for Selected Markers in Malignant Small Cell Tumors of the Mediastinum with Indeterminate or Undifferentiated Histologic Features

Tumor	KER	EMA	VIM	DES	MSA	MYOD1	MYOGN	S100	HMB45	TYR	MART1	NSE	SYN	CGA	BEREP4	CD45	CD15	CD99
PNET/ES	10	0	87	1	3	3	3	10	0	0	0	91	74	0	70	0	0	81
RMS	0	0	91	93	97	91	92	7	0	0	0	37	0	0	0	0	0	20
LL/TAL	0*	0	23	0	0	0	0	10	0	0	0	11	0	0	0	90/78	85/52	10
SCMM	1	3	100	0	0	0	0	97	50	86	87	70	0	0	0	0	0	7
PNBL	0	0	56	0	0	0	0	37	0	0	0	99	65	71	0	0	0	0
MSCSCC	100	83	35	0	0	0	0	52	0	0	0	50	4	0	60	0	0	0
MSCADCA	100	99	12	0	0	0	0	5	0	0	0	44	15	0	92	0	69	0
SCNC	99	73	0	0	0	0	0	0	0	0	0	70	35	40	100	0	18	20
SCUS	0	0	100	0	0	0	0	0	0	0	0	10	0	0	0	0	0	0

* Unless otherwise indicated, the given percentage of reactivity applies to both tumor entities.
KER, keratin (mixture of monoclonal antibodies); EMA, epithelial membrane antigen; VIM, vimentin; DES, desmin; MSA, muscle-specific actin; MYOGN, myogenin; S-100, S100 protein; TYR, tyrosinase; NSE, neuron-specific (gamma dimer) enolase; SYN, synaptophysin; CGA, chromogranin A; PNET, primitive neuroectodermal tumor; ES, Ewing's sarcoma; RMS, rhabdomyosarcoma; LL, lymphoblastic lymphoma; TAL, tumefactive acute myelogenous leukemia; SCMM, small cell malignant melanoma; PNBL, peripheral neuroblastoma; MSCSCC, metastatic small cell squamous cell carcinoma; MSCADCA, metastatic small cell adenocarcinoma; SCNC, small cell neuroendocrine carcinoma; SCUS, small cell undifferentiated sarcoma.
Data from Frisman D. Immunoquery. Available at http://www.immunoquery.com, and the author's experience.

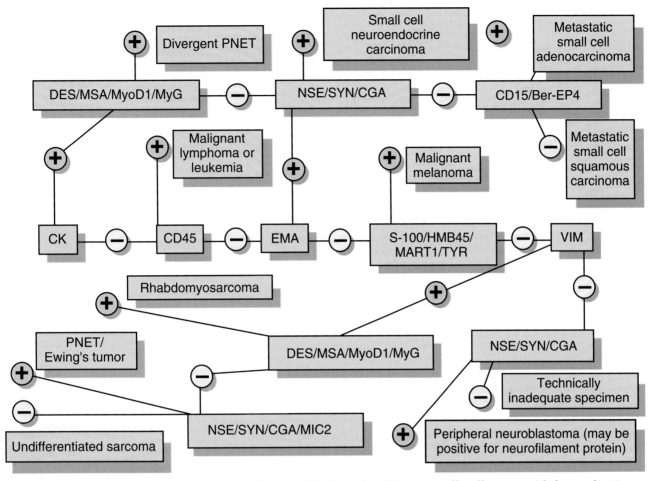

Figure 10–5. Algorithm for immunohistologic evaluation of malignant small cell tumors of the mediastinum. PNET, primitive neuroectodermal tumor; DES, desmin; MyG, myogenin; NSE, neuron-specific enolase; SYN, synaptophysin; CGA, chromogranin A; CK, cytokeratin; EMA, epithelial membrane antigen; TYR, tyrosinase; VIM, vimentin; MSA, muscle-specific actin.

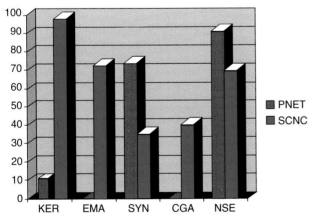

Figure 10–6. Bar graph showing markers of interest in the differential diagnosis of primitive neuroectodermal tumor (PNET) small versus cell neuroendocrine carcinoma (SCNC) of the mediastinum. KER, keratin; EMA, epithelial membrane antigen; SYN, synaptophysin; CGA, chromogranin A; NSE, neuron-specific enolase.

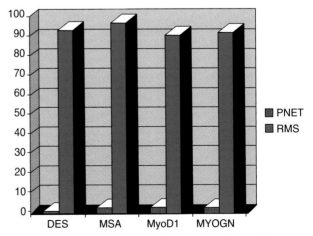

Figure 10–7. Bar graph showing markers of interest in the differential diagnosis of primitive neuroectodermal tumor (PNET) versus rhabdomyosarcoma (RMS) of the mediastinum. DES, desmin; MSA, muscle-specific actin; MYOGN, myogenin.

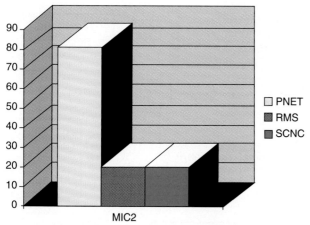

Figure 10–8. Bar graph showing relative rates of positivity for CD99 (MIC2) in primitive neuroectodermal tumor (PNET) versus rhabdomyosarcoma (RMS) versus small cell neuroendocrine carcinoma of the mediastinum (SCNC).

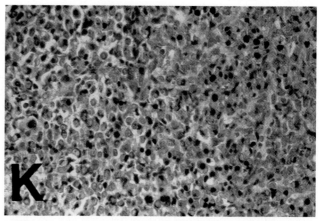

Figure 10–9. Characteristic perinuclear "dots" of immunoreactivity for keratin (K) are evident in this small cell neuroendocrine carcinoma of the mediastinum.

globulin are consistently seen in PNET but not in NBL (Fig. 10–11).[75–77] Synaptophysin and CD57 are detectable in most cases of PNET as well, and examples of this tumor with "divergent" differentiation will also demonstrate focal reactivity for keratin, desmin, and actin.[37, 78] Such lesions also have been termed *desmoplastic small cell tumor of the peritoneum, rhabdomyosarcoma-like small cell tumors of soft tissue,* and *ectomesenchymomas,* among other designations. In some instances, it may be difficult to distinguish between a "solid" alveolar rhabdomyosarcoma (see further on) that is MIC2+ and a PNET with divergent rhabdomyoblastic differentiation, especially if synaptophysin is absent. In such cases, one may have to rely on cytogenetic evaluations, seeking the characteristic t(2;13) or t(1;13) chromosomal translocations of alveolar rhabdomyosarcoma or the t(11;22) translocation of PNET.

Rhabdomyosarcoma of the Mediastinum. Rhabdomyosarcoma of the mediastinum is observed al-

most exclusively in children and adolescents,[40, 79, 80] and may demonstrate embryonal or alveolar architectural features. Nearly all rhabdomyosarcomas express desmin (Fig. 10–12) and muscle-specific actin, together with vimentin. Myoglobin is observed only in large maturing rhabdomyoblasts and is therefore not a particularly useful marker of rhabdomyosarcoma in its purely small cell form. Synaptophysin is lacking in rhabdomyosarcoma, but some cases do demonstrate labeling for CD57 or MIC2.[37, 50, 76, 77, 81] The specificity of desmin and actin for the diagnosis of rhabdomyosarcoma could be challenged, because these determinants may also be seen in smooth muscle neoplasms. Despite that truism, this argument seems superfluous to the author because a small cell variant of leiomyosarcoma does not exist. In any event, nuclear proteins that are apparently restricted to striated muscle—namely, MyoD1 and myogenin[81, 82]—can be applied to the differential diagnosis in question.

Small Cell Malignant Lymphomas of the Mediastinum. Several small cell non-Hodgkin's lym-

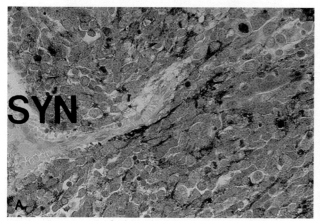

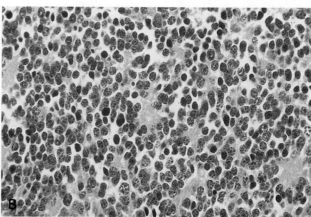

Figure 10–10. Diffuse reactivity for synaptophysin (SYN) *(A)* in mediastinal neuroblastoma *(B).*

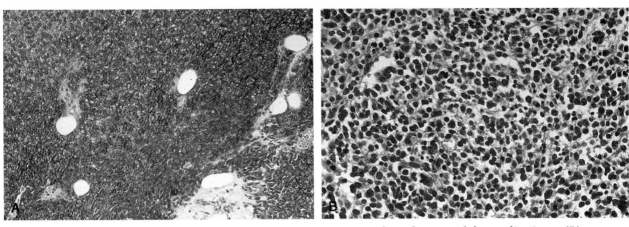

Figure 10–11. Labeling for CD99 (MIC2) *(A)* in primitive neuroectodermal tumor of the mediastinum *(B).*

phomas (SCNHLs) may be observed in the mediastinum as primary lesions. These include LL[83–85] (see earlier), small noncleaved cell (Burkitt's–non-Burkitt's) lymphoma,[86, 87] and lymphomas of the mucosa-associated lymphoid tissue (MALTomas).[88, 89]

Immunohistochemical analysis is helpful in separating these tumor types diagnostically. They usually express the CD45 (leukocyte common) antigen, although uncommon examples of LL lack that marker. LL also is commonly labeled with CD43 reagents (L60, Leu22, MT-1); CD99 antibodies such as HBA-71, O13, or 12E7; and antibodies to bcl-2 protein and TDT (Fig. 10–13).[27] Small noncleaved cell lymphoma expresses CD20, with or without bcl-2 protein.[27] In MALTomas, reactivity for CD10 and CD20 is evident, but CD43, CD99, bcl-2, and TDT are absent[89–92]; CD5 is variably present, but keratin, CD57, synaptophysin, desmin, actin, MyoD1, and myogenin are not detectable in any of these three small cell non-Hodgkin's lymphomas. Roughly 50% are positive for vimentin.[93]

Other Small Cell Mediastinal Neoplasms. In addition to those small cell tumors presented in the foregoing sections, others of a metastatic nature also may involve the mediastinum. These include small cell osteosarcoma and Ewing's sarcoma of bone, as well as small cell malignant melanoma. Except for the last of these possibilities, the primary lesion in such cases is typically obvious, and there is no question of whether the intrathoracic neoplasm might have arisen there. Nonetheless, melanomas are certainly capable of producing distant metastasis in the absence of an obvious primary source. Furthermore, they may assume the guise of a small cell neoplasm, closely resembling SCNC.[94] Immunohistochemical characteristics of small cell melanomas include uniform labeling for S-100 protein, tyrosinase, MART-1, and the HMB-45 antigen,[94, 95] none of which is expected in other small cell neoplasms of the mediastinum.

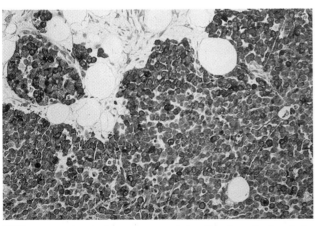

Figure 10–12. Immunoreactivity for desmin in rhabdomyosarcoma of the mediastinum.

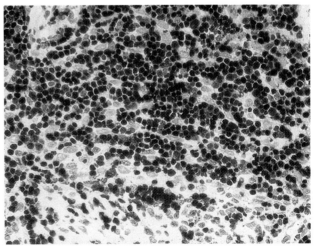

Figure 10–13. Nuclear labeling for terminal deoxynucleotidyl transferase in lymphoblastic lymphoma of the thymus.

Table 10–4. Immunoreactants Used in the Differential Diagnosis of Large Cell Indeterminate and Undifferentiated Neoplasms of the Mediastinum

Keratin (monoclonal mixture)
Vimentin
Synaptophysin
Chromogranin A
CD15
CD30
CD45
Placenta-like alkaline phosphatase
Carcinoembryonic antigen
Ber-EP4
Calretinin
S-100 protein
HMB-45
Tyrosinase
MART-1

Large Polygonal Cell Neoplasms of the Mediastinum (Tables 10–4 and 10–5; Figs. 10–14 to 10–18)

Primary Thymic Carcinomas. Although primary thymic carcinoma (PTC) is an "exciting" diagnosis because of its rarity, it should be remembered that most neoplasms thought to be that entity ultimately prove to represent metastases. Immunohistochemical analysis of PTCs reveals uniform labeling for keratin, and many cases also express EMA. Carcinoembryonic antigen, secretory component, and the TAG-72 antigen are variably seen as well, especially in tumors that show partial or uniform glandular differentiation.[96] However, vimentin is characteristically undetectable in greater than 95% of polygonal cell PTC variants.[18, 97]

Several reports have been made on the expression of CD5 by the epithelial cells of thymic carcinoma but not those of conventional thymoma (Fig. 10–19).[97–100] This statement must be qualified in part, because *atypical* epithelial-predominant thymomas—that is, those in which there is evidence of cytologic atypia that is insufficient for an outright diagnosis of malignancy[17, 21, 39]—also show CD5 positivity in 40% of cases.[99]

Some variability exists in the literature concerning mutant p53 protein as another potential discriminant between thymoma and thymic carcinoma.[101–103] In general, however, it can be stated that immunostains performed with the DO1 and DO3 antibodies against mutant p53 are much more likely to yield positive results in PTC than in conventional thymoma. Hence, this determinant could serve as an adjunct in making the diagnostic distinction between those two entities. Similar claims have been made for Mcl-1 protein[104] and the Fas antigen,[105] but data on those reactants in thymic neoplasms are scarce.

Table 10–5. Percentages of Immunoreactivity for Selected Markers in Malignant Large Polygonal Cell Tumors of the Mediastinum with Indeterminate or Undifferentiated Histologic Features

Tumor	KER	CEA	VIM	CALRET	PLAP	S-100	HMB-45	TYR	MART-1	SYN	CGA	BER-EP4	CD45	CD15	CD30
PTADCA	100	70	5	67	0	0	0	0	0	40	20	70	0	65	0
MADCA	100	75	12	10	10	10	0	0	0	3	5	90	0	70	0
PNEC	100	40	20	0	0	6	0	0	0	80	90	90	0	85	0
MNEC	100	62	20	0	0	10	0	0	0	80	75	90	0	20	0
LCL/TAL	0*	0/50	65	0	0	3	0	0	0	0	0	0	99/85	3/85	23/3
ALCL	0	0	100	0	0	10	0	0	0	0	0	0	90	13	99
SYNHD	0	0	50	0	0	0	0	0	0	0	0	0	6	90	90
MELAN	1	0	100	0	0	97	50	86	90	0	0	0	0	0	0
SEMIN	12	0	70	0	93	0	0	0	0	0	0	0	0	0	3
EMBCA	100	0	17	0	90	0	0	0	0	0	0	0	0	0	80
YST	100	0	50	0	50	0	0	0	0	0	0	0	0	0	20
EPSARCS†	V	0	100	V	0	V	0	0	0	0	0	V	0	0	0
PSCC	100	40	5	0	0	3	0	0	0	40	20	50	0	20	0
MSCC	100	50	30	33	10	10	0	0	0	20	3	50	0	20	0
LELCT	100	0	50	0	0	0	0	0	0	40	20	10	0	0	0
MESOTH	100	0	54	90	3	7	0	0	0	0	2	10	0	1	0
PARAGANG	2	0	40	0	0	40	0	0	0	100	100	0	0	0	0

* Unless otherwise indicated, the given percentage of reactivity applies to both tumor entities.

† Epithelioid synovial sarcoma is reactive for keratin in 100% of cases and Ber-EP4 in 90% of cases. Epithelioid malignant peripheral nerve sheath tumor is reactive for S-100 protein in 80% of cases.

KER, keratin (mixture of monoclonal antibodies); CEA, carcinoembryonic antigen; VIM, vimentin; CALRET, calretinin; PLAP, placental alkaline phosphatase; S-100, S-100 protein; TYR, tyrosinase; SYN, synaptophysin; CGA, chromogranin A; PTADCA, primary thymic adenocarcinoma; MADCA, metastatic adenocarcinoma; PNEC, primary neuroendocrine carcinoma; MNEC, metastatic neuroendocrine carcinoma; LCL, large cell lymphoma; TAL, tumefactive acute myelogenous leukemia; ALCL, anaplastic large cell lymphoma; SYNHD, syncytial Hodgkin's disease; MELAN, malignant melanoma; SEMIN, seminoma; EMBCA, embryonal carcinoma; YST, yolk sac tumor; EPSARCS, sarcomas with epithelioid features; PSCC, primary thymic squamous cell carcinoma; MSCC, metastatic squamous cell carcinoma; LELCT, lymphoepithelioma-like carcinoma of the thymus; MESOTH, mesothelioma; PARAGANG, malignant paraganglioma.

Data from Frisman D. Immunoquery. Available at http://www.immunoquery.com, and the author's experience.

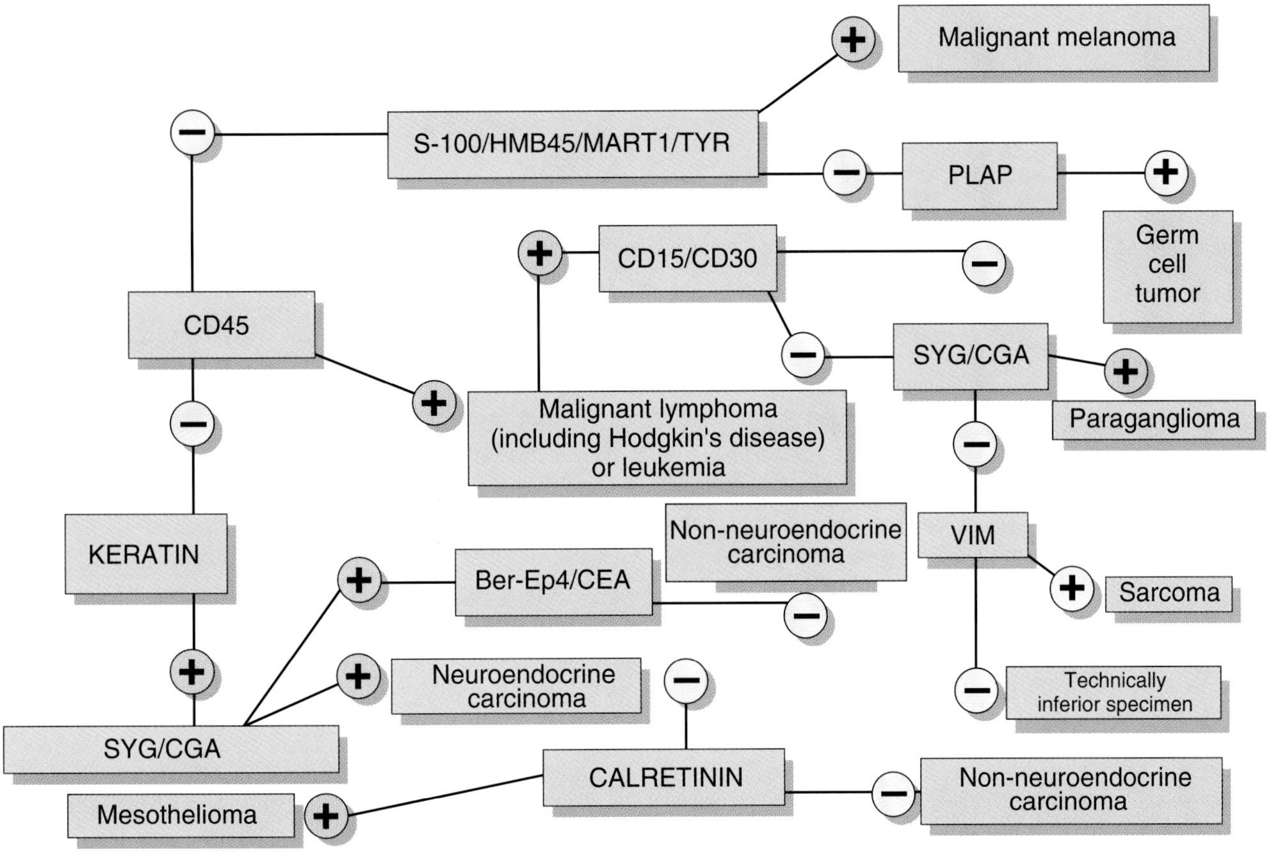

Malignant melanoma
S-100/HMB45/MART1/TYR
PLAP
Germ cell tumor
CD15/CD30
CD45
SYG/CGA
Paraganglioma
Malignant lymphoma (including Hodgkin's disease) or leukemia
Non-neuroendocrine carcinoma
VIM
KERATIN
Ber-Ep4/CEA
Sarcoma
Neuroendocrine carcinoma
Technically inferior specimen
SYG/CGA
CALRETININ
Non-neuroendocrine carcinoma
Mesothelioma

Figure 10–14. Algorithm for immunohistologic evaluation of malignant large polygonal cell tumors of the mediastinum. TYR, tyrosinase; PLAP, placenta-like alkaline phosphatase; SYN, synaptophysin; CGA, chromogranin A; CEA, carcinoembryonic antigen; VIM, vimentin.

90
80
70
60
50
40
30
20
10
0
CALRET
CEA
BeRep 4
Carcinoma
Mesothelioma

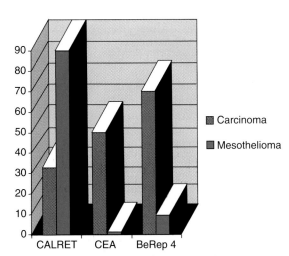

Figure 10–15. Bar graph showing markers of interest in the differential diagnosis of carcinoma versus mesothelioma. CALRET, calretinin; CEA, carcinoembryonic antigen.

90
80
70
60
50
40
30
20
10
0
BerEP4
CEA
S-100
SYN
CGA
ADCA
NEC

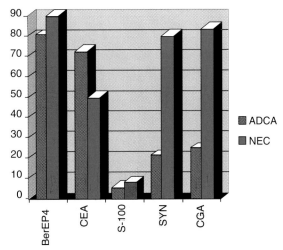

Figure 10–16. Bar graph showing markers of interest in the differential diagnosis between poorly differentiated adenocarcinoma (ADCA) and neuroendocrine carcinoma (NEC) of the mediastinum. CEA, carcinoembryonic antigen; SYN, synaptophysin; CGA, chromogranin A.

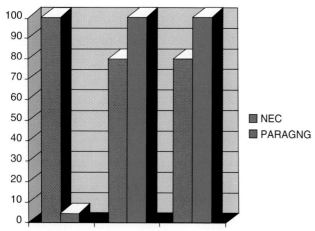

Figure 10–17. Bar graph showing relative reactivity patterns for neuroendocrine carcinoma (NEC) and malignant paraganglioma (PARAGNG) of the mediastinum. KER, keratin; SYN, synaptophysin; CGA, chromogranin A.

Other primary malignant tumors of the thymic region, such as germ cell tumors and lymphomas, are CD5−, and that statement is also said to be applicable to the majority of metastatic mediastinal carcinomas from other organs.[98–100] Future studies are necessary to determine whether such observations withstand the test of time. Conversely, it has been found that MIC2+ lymphocytes are lacking in *both* PTCs and metastatic carcinomas in the thymic region, indicating that CD99 has no role in making the distinction between those neoplasms.[25]

Another facet of PTCs that should be mentioned is their capacity for "occult" neuroendocrine differentiation. Even though there may be no overt morphologic evidence of neuroendocrine features

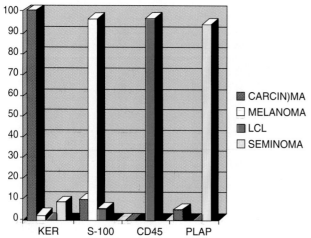

Figure 10–18. Bar graph depicting markers of interest in the differential diagnosis of carcinoma versus metastatic melanoma versus large cell non-Hodgkin's lymphoma (LCL) versus seminoma of the mediastinum. KER, keratin; PLAP, placental alkaline phosphatase.

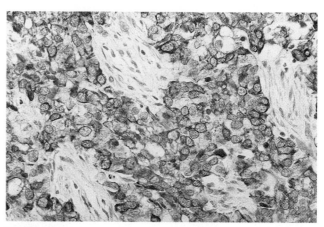

Figure 10–19. Diffuse immunoreactivity for CD5 *(A)* in primary thymic carcinoma *(B).*

in such lesions, immunoreactivity may be observed for synaptophysin, chromogranin A, or CD57 (Fig. 10–20).[106] The biologic significance of those findings is currently uncertain, but they are *not* sufficiently compelling to change the diagnostic classification of these tumors to that of outright "neuroendocrine carcinoma."

Parathyroid Carcinoma of the Mediastinum. Parathyroid carcinomas (PACs) may be seen intrathymically or in the soft tissue of the anterosuperior mediastinum. Its resemblance to thymic neuroendocrine carcinoma is considerable in some cases, and paraganglioma also enters into the differential diagnosis.[107–109] The diagnosis of these lesions is typically straightforward clinically, because of the striking levels of hypercalcemia with which they are associated. Nevertheless, nonsecretory PACs may require immunohistologic evaluation for definitive diagnosis. This can be accomplished through documenting the intracellular presence of parathyroid hormone, which is restricted to parathyroid lesions among the contextual diagnostic possibilities (Fig. 10–21).[110] Otherwise, the immunophenotypes of PAC and other neuroendocrine carcinomas are largely superimposable.[109]

Malignant Mediastinal Germ Cell Tumors. Pure or mixed mediastinal germ cell tumors with seminomatous, embryonal carcinomatous, endodermal sinus tumor, and choriocarcinomatous elements all have the potential to arise in the mediastinum or involve it metastatically.[15, 16, 111–115] Immunohistology is often indispensable in the characterization of such neoplasms, especially in limited tissue samples. The typical phenotype of seminoma is that of a keratin-negative and EMA− tumor with uniform, cell membrane−based reactivity for PLAP (Fig. 10–22).[16, 116] Approximately 10 to 15% of such lesions, however, will indeed demonstrate limited labeling for keratin proteins.[16] Embryonal carcinomas and yolk sac carcinomas differ from the latter description in their acquisition of in-

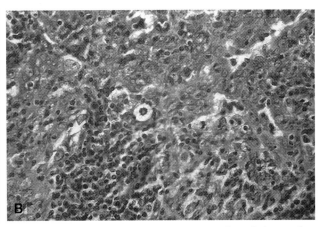

Figure 10–20. "Occult" labeling for synaptophysin (S) *(A)* in a primary thymic carcinoma that did not have neuroendocrine characteristics by conventional morphologic study *(B)*.

tense, diffuse keratin positivity and potential labeling for alpha fetoprotein (AFP).[16, 114, 117] In addition, embryonal carcinoma paradoxically manifests the presence of CD30 (Fig. 10–23),[118] which is typically conceptualized as a hematopoietic determinant. Choriocarcinoma is also globally keratin-reactive, but that neoplasm is further typified by the immunohistologic presence of EMA and β-human chorionic gonadotropin.[16, 119]

Mediastinal "Carcinoid Tumor" (Neuroendocrine Carcinoma, Grades I and II). Immunohistochemically, neuroendocrine carcinomas of the thymus show reproducible positivity for keratin, neuron-specific (gamma dimeric) enolase, synaptophysin, CD57, and chromogranin A.[18, 120–123] Furthermore, even those lesions that have not produced a clinical endocrinopathy can show, at an intracellular level, the presence of specific neuropeptides.[124–126]

Mediastinal Paragangliomas. Intrathoracic paragangliomas may arise in either the anterior mediastinal compartment, in association with the aorticopulmonary root, or in a paravertebral location.[123, 127, 128] The neural nature of paragangliomas

is reflected by their lack of labeling for keratin and EMA. They instead express neurofilament protein, with or without vimentin, similar to NBL.[123] Stains for S-100 protein can be used to label sustentacular cells that surround cellular nests in paragangliomas (Fig. 10–24),[129] and the tumor cells themselves often contain one of the enkephalin peptides.[130]

Mediastinal Large Cell Non-Hodgkin's Lymphoma (Table 10–6; Fig. 10–25). After Hodgkin's disease, large cell non-Hodgkin's lymphoma (LCNHL) is the next most common primary malignancy of the mediastinum.[93] Immunohistology reveals crisp cell membranous reactivity for CD45 in virtually all LCNHLs.[36, 93, 131–134] However, rare examples of "Ki-1+" (CD30+) (large cell anaplastic) lymphoma have been reported at this site,[135] some of which have, in fact, been CD45−. Therefore, it is prudent to evaluate the possible presence of CD30 in the assessment of possible LCNHLs; in the context of simultaneous keratin negativity, that marker is specific for a diagnosis of lymphoma.[93] The belief that most mediastinal LCNHLs show B-cell differentiation is supported by reactivity for

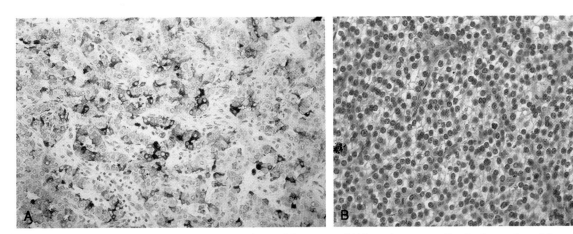

Figure 10–21. Immunoreactivity for parathyroid hormone *(A)* in primary mediastinal parathyroid carcinoma *(B)*.

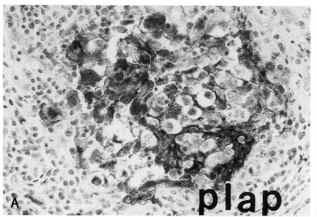
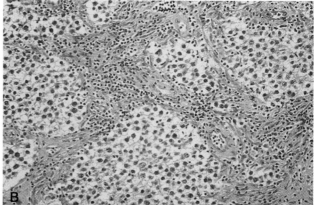

Figure 10–22. Membrane-based immunolabeling for placental alkaline phosphatase (plap) *(A)* in primary mediastinal seminoma *(B)*.

CD20 in most instances (Fig. 10–26),[133, 134, 136] including those with anaplastic features.[135] Only exceptional LCNHLs with T-cell or "true histiocytic" differentiation have been reported in the mediastinum.[93]

"Syncytial" Mediastinal Hodgkin's Disease. Hodgkin's lymphoma (HL) is the most common cytologically malignant mediastinal neoplasm.[93] Although it is felt to arise in the thymus or perithymic lymph nodes in the thorax, this lesion also may involve other contiguous structures by direct extension.[137–139] Most examples of HL are recognizable without the need for immunohistologic assays, but one of its variants, "syncytial" HL, in which mononuclear Reed-Sternberg cells are arranged in sheets, may closely simulate the appearance of a carcinoma or LCNHL.[140] The typical immunophenotype of the Reed-Sternberg cells of HL is that of CD45 negativity, in contrast to its presence in almost all cases of LCNHL.[18, 93] Conversely, Reed-Sternberg cells in syncytial HL coexpress CD15 and CD30 (Fig. 10–27). CD15 is not seen in most LCNHLs, enabling the distinction between these tumor types.[93] Nonetheless, it must be acknowledged that there is a potential overlap between HL and selected examples of CD30+ LCNHL. This makes cytogenetic studies—particularly those for abnormalities at the 5q35 locus, which typify "Ki-1+" large cell lymphomas[141, 142]—a wise inclusion in this context. In reference to its distinction from carcinomas in the mediastinum, syncytial HL uniformly lacks keratin,[18, 93, 140] unlike malignant epithelial neoplasms.

Other Mediastinal Hematopoietic Tumors. Two other hematopoietic neoplasms that may present in the mediastinum are represented by granulocytic sarcoma (extramedullary myelogenous leukemia)[143, 144] and extraosseous plasmacytoma.[145, 146] Immunoreactivity for CD13, CD15, CD33, CD68, and myeloperoxidase is expected in granulocytic sarcoma but not in LCNHL (Fig. 10–28).[147–149] Extraosseous plasmacytoma of the mediastinum can potentially imitate the microscopic appearance of

Figure 10–23. Diffuse positivity for CD30 in thymic embryonal carcinoma.

Table 10–6. Immunoreactants Used in the Differential Diagnosis of Hematopoietic Diseases of the Mediastinum

Keratin
HMB-45
MART-1
Tyrosinase
Placenta-like alkaline phosphatase
CD3
CD15
CD20
CD30
CD43
CD45
CD45RO
CD68
CD74
MB2
BLA.36
BNH9
Cathepsin-B
Lysozyme
Myeloperoxidase

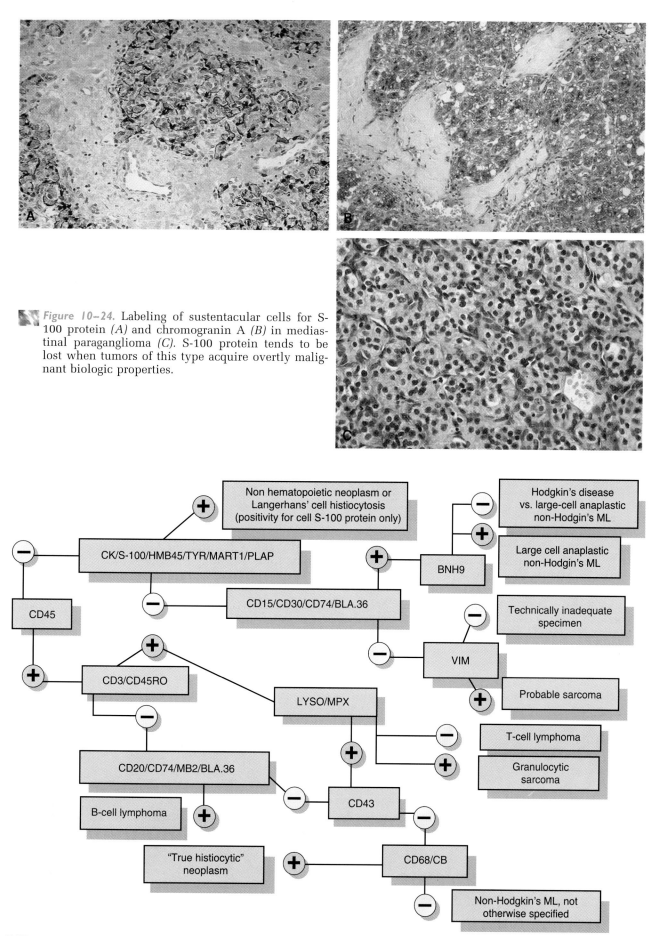

Figure 10–24. Labeling of sustentacular cells for S-100 protein *(A)* and chromogranin A *(B)* in mediastinal paraganglioma *(C).* S-100 protein tends to be lost when tumors of this type acquire overtly malignant biologic properties.

Figure 10–25. Algorithm for immunohistologic evaluation of hematopoietic neoplasms of the mediastinum. ML, malignant lymphoma; TYR, tyrosinase; PLAP, placenta-like alkaline phosphatase; VIM, vimentin; LYSO/MPX, lysozyme/myeloperoxidase; CB, cathepsin B.

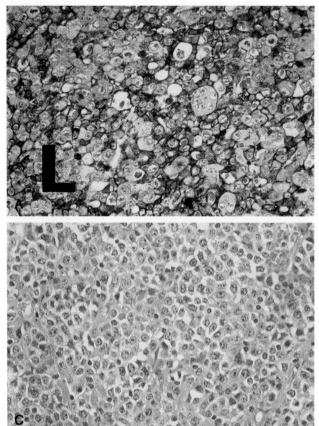

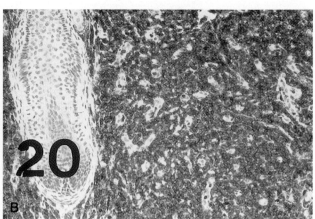

Figure 10–26. Immunoreactivity for CD45 (leukocyte common antigen [L]). *(A)* and CD20 (20) *(B)* in primary large-cell lymphoma of the thymic region *(C)*. L, leukocyte common antigen.

neuroendocrine neoplasms and large cell lymphomas.[145, 146] Extraosseous plasmacytoma of the mediastinum is reactive for light chain immunoglobulins (Fig. 10–29) and CD38 but not for keratin, chromogranin A, or synaptophysin.[150] A special diagnostic trap attending this tumor is its potential to express an EMA-like substance;[151] for the unwary, this result may appear to support a mistaken interpretation of neuroendocrine neoplasia.

Malignant Epithelioid Mesothelioma of the Mediastinum. Although malignant mesotheliomas are usually regarded as tumors of the peripheral pleurae or the peritoneum, they also can be seen in the mediastinum, where they likely take origin from the hilar reflections of the pleural surfaces. The immunophenotype of mesothelioma features intense keratin reactivity in all its histologic variants, including the purely epithelioid form; the same is

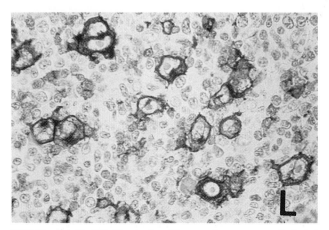

Figure 10–27. Typical cell, membranous, and Golgi zone labeling for CD15 in the Reed-Sternberg cells of mediastinal Hodgkin's disease. L, LeuM1.

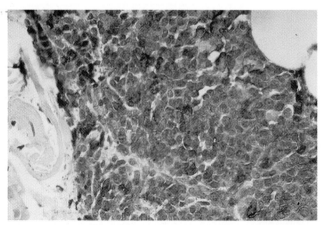

Figure 10–28. Diffuse cytoplasmic reactivity for myeloperoxidase in granulocytic sarcoma of the mediastinum.

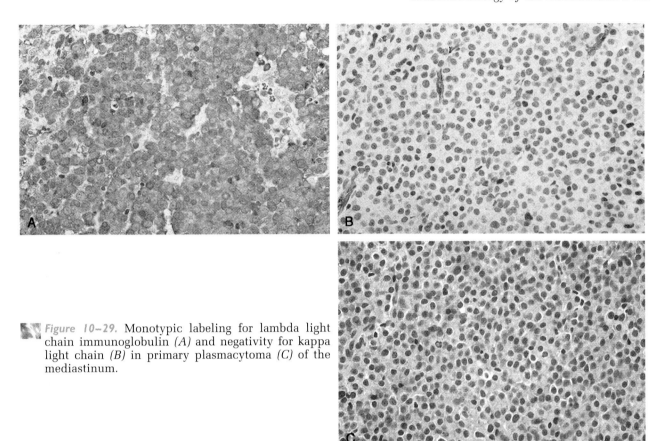

Figure 10-29. Monotypic labeling for lambda light chain immunoglobulin *(A)* and negativity for kappa light chain *(B)* in primary plasmacytoma *(C)* of the mediastinum.

true of calretinin.[152] Vimentin coexpression also may be seen in roughly 50% of mesothelioma cases, and there is also heterogeneous (and not entirely specific) labeling for determinants such as HBME-1[153] and thrombomodulin.[154] Specialized markers of adenocarcinomatous differentiation, including carcinoembryonic antigen, CD15, thyroid transcription factor-1, blood group (e.g., A,B,H, and Lewis) antigens, and the TAG-72 antigen (recognized by antibody B72.3), are absent in mesotheliomas.[155-157]

Metastatic Mediastinal Carcinoma and Melanoma. As stated earlier in this discussion, most nonhematopoietic malignancies of the mediastinum should be presumed metastatic until proved otherwise. Immunohistologic analysis is only variably productive in establishing a site of origin for secondary carcinomas in this location. If determinants are found that are unassociated with PTCs, such as thyroglobulin, prostate-specific antigen, S-100 protein, PLAP, CA19-9 (an enteric carcinoma marker), or CA 125 (a serosal and müllerian tract marker),[158] it is likely that the lesion being studied is, in all likelihood, a metastasis. Conversely, the presence of coexpression of keratin and CD5 would, at least tentatively, appear to support a thymic origin for such a neoplasm.[100]

Mediastinal implants of an amelanotic malignant melanoma rarely represent the initial manifestation of that tumor[159] in the face of no detectable cutaneous or mucosal disease. In that scenario, the differential diagnosis would also include primary or metastatic somatic carcinomas, malignant germ cell tumors, and lymphomas. Immunohistochemical studies show that metastatic large cell melanomas of the mediastinum are devoid of keratin, EMA, PLAP, CD15, CD30, and CD45. Instead, they react with antibodies to vimentin, S-100 protein, tyrosinase, and the MART-1 and HMB-45 antigens.[95, 158, 160]

Mixed Small Cell and Large Cell Malignancies

Mixed Large Cell and Small Cell Non-Hodgkin's Lymphoma (MNHL). There is still some controversy about the definition of MNHL, as it is distinguished from LCNHL. The author uses the rather arbitrary criterion that no more than 30% large cells should be seen in mixed non-Hodgkin's lymphomas. The immunoprofile of MNHL separates it from other malignant mixed cell neoplasms of the mediastinum. It includes reactivity for CD45 in all lesional cells, as well as positivity for CD20 in B-cell tumors or CD3, CD43, or CD45RO in T-cell neoplasms.[161] Keratin is universally absent.

Mixed Cellularity Hodgkin's Disease. Mixed cellularity Hodgkin's disease is superficially similar histologically to MNHL; however, the former of those lesions fails to show labeling for CD45 in the

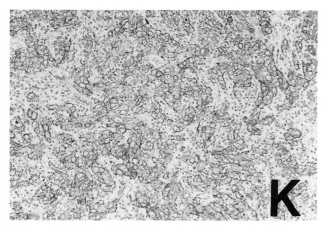

Figure 10–30. Delicately "interlocking" reactivity for keratin (K) in primary lymphoepithelioma-like carcinoma of the thymus.

large tumor cells (Reed-Sternberg cells). Moreover, they also lack CD3, CD20, CD43, and CD45RO but express CD15, with or without CD30, with a distinctive Golgi zone and cell membranous staining pattern.[93, 140, 162] EMA may be observed in some cases of mixed cellularity Hodgkin's disease, but keratin is consistently absent.[162]

Lymphoepithelioma-Like Carcinoma. Lymphoepithelioma-like carcinoma of the thymus features an admixture of large epithelioid cells and small lymphocytes, in likeness to the image of classic nasopharyngeal carcinoma. All cases of lymphoepithelioma-like carcinoma are immunoreactive for keratin (Fig. 10–30) and EMA. Conversely, the large tumor cells are devoid of PLAP, CD3, CD15, CD20, CD30, CD43, CD45, and CD45RO.[18, 65]

Malignant Spindle Cell Mediastinal Tumors (Figs. 10–31 to 10–33; Tables 10–7 and 10–8)

Sarcomatoid Thymic Carcinoma. Comparatively few examples of sarcomatoid thymic carcinoma (STC) have been reported.[65, 163–165] Microscopically, this lesion is characterized by fascicles of fusiform and pleomorphic tumor cells, with little internal organization. Some cases, however, contain limited foci in which cohesive epithelioid cell nests are admixed with spindle cell elements.[66] Biphasic STCs with "carcinoid" elements have also been documented.[166] Snover and colleagues[66] reported an example of STC with focally well-defined rhabdomyogenic differentiation, complete with cyto-

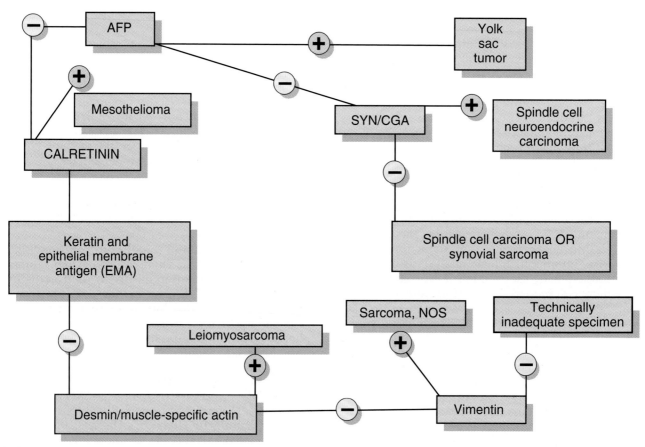

Figure 10–31. Algorithm for immunohistologic evaluation of malignant spindle cell tumors of the mediastinum. AFP, alpha fetoprotein; SYN, synaptophysin; CGA, chromogranin A; NOS, not otherwise specified.

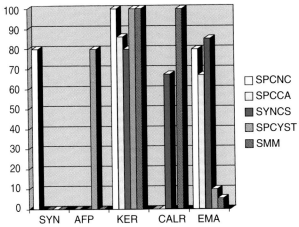

Figure 10–32. Bar graph depicting markers of interest in the differential diagnosis of malignant epithelial spindle cell tumors of the mediastinum. SPCNC, spindle cell neuroendocrine carcinoma; SPCCA, spindle cell carcinoma; SYNSC, synovial sarcoma; SPCYST, spindle cell yolk sac tumor; SMM, sarcomatoid malignant mesothelioma; SYN, synaptophysin; AFP, alpha fetoprotein; KER, keratin, CALR, calretinin; EMA, epithelial membrane antigen.

Table 10–7. Immunoreactants Used in the Differential Diagnosis of Spindle Cell Indeterminate and Undifferentiated Neoplasms of the Mediastinum

Keratin (monoclonal mixture)
Epithelial membrane antigen
Calretinin
Vimentin
Desmin
Muscle-specific actin
Alpha-fetoprotein
Synaptophysin
Chromogranin A

plasmic cross-striations. Some observers may choose to label such lesions as "carcinosarcomas,"[167] but it is the author's opinion that they are basically epithelial in nature, that is, metaplastic or sarcomatoid carcinomas.[168]

Immunohistochemically, the fusiform and pleomorphic cells of STCs express vimentin. Labeling for keratin and EMA is also seen, but it may be quite focal (Fig. 10–34).[19, 168] This finding opens the door to the possibility that a small biopsy specimen could fail to demonstrate any epithelial

markers because of sampling artifact. Tumors showing divergent components, such as myogenic elements, may additionally exhibit immunoreactivity for desmin, actin, myoglobin, MyoD1, or myogenin.[65, 66] Obviously, those potential results underscore the difficulty of establishing a firm diagnosis of STC with limited tissue samples.

An especially troublesome differential diagnosis is the separation of primary mediastinal synovial sarcoma and PTC, because their clinical, electron microscopic, and immunophenotypic features are similar. The demonstration of t(X;18) chromosomal translocations in synovial sarcoma—by fluorescence in situ hybridization or traditional cytogenetic analyses—has now made that tumor consistently identifiable.[169]

Another potential pitfall in the diagnosis of STC is the existence of thymomas that incite the proliferation of an exuberant but reactive spindle cell stroma.[170] This phenomenon produces a biphasic morphologic image and also yields a mutually exclusive immunophenotype in the two lesional components with respect to keratin and vimentin labeling. Hence, the superficial resemblance to "carcinosarcoma" is great, and only through attention to the cytologic blandness of the lesion can diagnostic errors be avoided.

Spindle Cell Carcinoid Tumor of the Thymus. The existence of a spindle cell variant of thymic carcinoid was first documented in 1976 by Levine and Rosai,[171] but it appears to be a very rare tumor subtype, with only a limited number of additional examples having been identified.[172] For all practical purposes, the immunoprofile of this neoplastic variant is identical to that of polygonal cell neuroendocrine carcinomas of the mediastinum, as documented earlier.

Sarcomatoid Mediastinal Malignant Mesothelioma. Aside from its exclusive composition by fusiform and pleomorphic tumor cells, sarcomatoid mediastinal mesothelioma also is dissimilar from its epithelioid or biphasic counterparts in its ultrastructural and immunohistologic features. These closely approximate the specialized pathologic attributes of sarcomatoid carcinoma, as described earlier. They differ from those of the latter entity only in the fact that sarcomatoid mesothelioma is

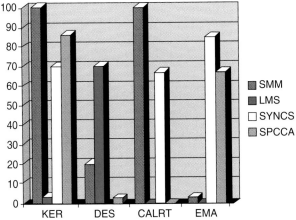

Figure 10–33. Bar graph showing pertinent markers in the differential diagnosis of leiomyosarcoma (LMS) versus malignant epithelial spindle-cell tumors (SPCCA) of the mediastinum. SMM, sarcomatoid malignant mesothelioma; SYNSC, synovial sarcoma; KER, keratin; DES, desmin; CALRT, calretinin; EMA, epithelial membrane antigen.

Table 10–8. Percentages of Immunoreactivity for Selected Markers in Malignant Small Cell Tumors of the Mediastinum with Indeterminate or Undifferentiated Histologic Features

Tumor	KER	EMA	VIM	CALRET	DES	MSA	AFP	SYN	CGA
MESOTH	100	3	86	100	20	90	0	0	0
SCYST	100	10	50	0	0	0	80	0	0
LMS	3	0	89	0	70	90	0	0	0
SPCCA	86	67	96	0	3	10	0	0	0
SYNSC	80	85	100	67	0	0	0	0	0
SPCNC	100	80	3	0	0	10	0	80	75
FS/MFH	1	1	100	0	0	0	0	0	0

KER, keratin (mixture of monoclonal antibodies); EMA, epithelial membrane antigen; VIM, vimentin; CALRET, calretinin; DES, desmin; MSA, muscle-specific actin; AFP, alpha-fetoprotein; SYN, synaptophysin; CGA, chromogranin A; MESOTH, mesothelioma; SCYST, spindle cell yolk sac tumor; LMS, leiomyosarcoma; SPCCA, spindle cell carcinoma (either primary or metastatic); SYNSC, synovial sarcoma; SPCNC, spindle cell neuroendocrine carcinoma; FS, fibrosarcoma; MFH, malignant fibrous histiocytoma.
Data from Frisman D. Immunoquery. Available at http://www.immunoquery.com, and the author's experience.

reactive for calretinin, whereas carcinomas are not.[152]

Sarcomatoid Thymic Yolk Sac Tumor. A peculiar variant of primary mediastinal yolk sac tumor (MYST) has been documented by Moran and Suster.[173] Even though it features a predominance of spindle cells, and as such may be confused with the other neoplastic entities cited in this section, sarcomatoid MYST is identical immunohistologically to "conventional" endodermal sinus tumor (see earlier). Reactivity for keratin and AFP is expected in spindle cell MYST. The second of these markers reproducibly excludes the diagnostic possibility of STC, which lacks AFP.[163–165, 173]

Mediastinal Leiomyosarcoma. Moran and associates[174] have reported the existence of primary mediastinal leiomyosarcomas, which may be observed either in the anterior or posterior compartments. These spindle cell malignancies are uniformly immunoreactive for desmin (Fig. 10–35), muscle-specific actin, or alpha isoform actin, and vimentin may also be present in them. Conversely, EMA, keratin, MyoD1, myoglobin, my-

ogenin, and S-100 protein are absent in leiomyosarcomas.[37]

"Prognostic" Markers in Mediastinal Neoplasms

Attempts have been made at prognosticating the behavior of thymoma through immunohistologic semiquantitation of tumoral proliferative rates with antiproliferating cell nuclear antigen (PCNA) and Ki-67,[175–177] and detection of aberrant expression of bcl-2, Fas, or p53 gene products by immunostaining or blotting methods.[28, 29, 102, 105, 178] In general, these methods have produced no consistently reproducible results. Comparable statements apply to the immunohistologic evaluation of E-cadherin expression.[179, 180] Similarly, there are at present no "molecular" markers of prognosis for other mediastinal neoplasms. Thus, it is the author's belief that currently this aspect of contextual immunohistochemical analysis is beyond the standard practice of surgical pathology.

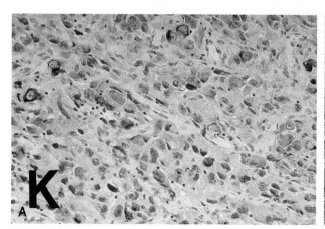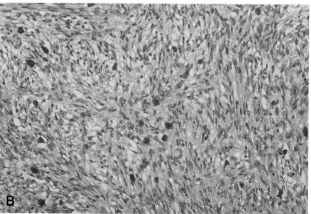

Figure 10–34. Focal immunolabeling for keratin (K) *(A)* in primary sarcomatoid carcinoma of the thymus *(B)*.

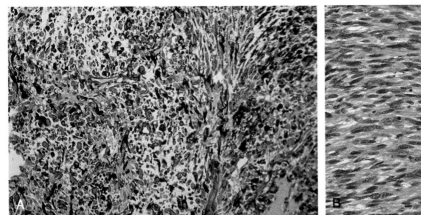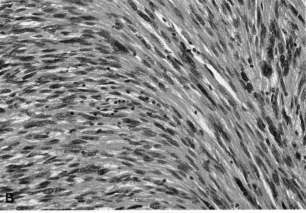

Figure 10–35. Immunoreactivity for desmin *(A)* in mediastinal leiomyosarcoma *(B).*

References

1. Sterrett G, Whitaker D, Shilkin KB, et al. The fine needle aspiration cytology of mediastinal lesions. Cancer 1983;51:127–135.
2. Gherardi G, Marveggio C, Placidi A. Neuroendocrine carcinoma of the thymus: Aspiration biopsy, immunocytochemistry, and clinicopathologic correlates. Diagn Cytopathol 1995;35:158–164.
3. Heilo A. Tumors in the mediastinum: Ultrasound-guided histologic core-needle biopsy. Radiology 1993;189:143–146.
4. Powers CN, Silverman JF, Geisinger KR, et al. Fine needle aspiration biopsy of the mediastinum: A multi-institutional analysis. Am J Clin Pathol 1996;105:168–173.
5. Yu GH, Salhany KE, Gokaslan ST, et al. Thymic epithelial cells as a diagnostic pitfall in the fine needle aspiration diagnosis of primary mediastinal lymphoma. Diagn Cytopathol 1997;16:460–465.
6. Shin HJ, Katz RL. Thymic neoplasia as represented by fine needle aspiration biopsy of anterior mediastinal masses: A practical approach to the differential diagnosis. Acta Cytol 1998;42:855–864.
7. Wick MR, Rosai J. The endocrine thymus. In: Kovacs K, Asa SL, eds. Functional Endocrine Pathology, 2nd ed. Oxford, England, Blackwell, 1998:869–894.
8. Hirokawa K, Utsuyama M, Moriizumi E, et al. Immunohistochemical studies in human thymomas: Localization of thymosin and various cell markers. Virchows Arch B Cell Pathol 1988;55:371–380.
9. Fukai I, Masaoka A, Hashimoto T, et al. Cytokeratins in normal thymus and thymic epithelial tumors. Cancer 1993;71:99–105.
10. Fukai I, Masaoka A, Hashimoto T, et al. Differential diagnosis of thymic carcinoma and lung carcinoma with the use of antibodies to cytokeratins. J Thorac Cardiovasc Surg 1995;110:1670–1675.
11. Wick MR. Mediastinal cysts and intrathoracic thyroid tumors. Semin Diagn Pathol 1990;7:285–294.
12. Sabiston D, Scott HW. Primary neoplasms and cysts of the mediastinum. Ann Surg 1961;136:777–797.
13. LeRoux BT, Kallichurum S, Shama DM. Mediastinal cysts and tumors. Curr Probl Surg 1984;21:1–77.
14. Suster S, Moran CA: Malignant thymic neoplasms that may mimic benign conditions. Semin Diagn Pathol 1995;12:98–10.
15. Moran CA, Suster S: Mediastinal seminomas with prominent cystic changes: A clinicopathologic study of 10 cases. Am J Surg Pathol 1995;25:1047–1053.
16. Niehans GA, Manivel JC, Copland GT, et al. Immunohistochemistry of germ cell and trophoblastic neoplasms. Cancer 1988;62:1113–1123.
17. Suster S, Moran CA. Primary thymic epithelial neoplasms: Spectrum of differentiation and histological features. Semin Diagn Pathol 1999;16:2–17.
18. Wick MR, Simpson RW, Niehans GA, et al. Anterior mediastinal tumors: A clinicopathologic study of 100 cases, with emphasis on immunohistochemical analysis. Prog Surg Pathol 1990;11:79–119.
19. Wick MR, Rosai J. Epithelial tumors. In: Givel JC, ed. Surgery of the Thymus. Berlin: Springer-Verlag, 1990;79–107.
20. Walker AN, Mills SE, Fechner RE. Thymomas and thymic carcinomas. Semin Diagn Pathol 1990;7:250–265.
21. Lewis JE, Wick MR, Scheithauer BW, et al. Thymoma: A clinicopathologic review. Cancer 1987;60:2727–2743.
22. Rosai J, Sobin LH, Caillaud JM, et al. WHO Classification of Thymic Tumors. Geneva, Switzerland, World Health Organization, 1999:1–25.
23. Rice HE, Flake AW, Hori T, et al. Massive thymic hyperplasia: Characterization of a rare mediastinal mass. J Pediatr Surg 1994;29:1561–1564.
24. Battifora H, Sun TT, Bahu RM, et al. The use of antikeratin antiserum as a diagnostic tool: Thymoma versus lymphoma. Hum Pathol 1980;11:635–641.
25. Chan JKC, Tsang WY, Seneviratne S, et al. The MIC2 antibody O13: Practical application for the study of thymic epithelial tumors. Am J Surg Pathol 1995;19:1115–1123.
26. Robertson PB, Neiman RS, Worapongpaiboon S, et al. O13 (CD99) positivity in hematologic proliferations correlates with TdT positivity. Mod Pathol 1997;10:277–282.
27. Soslow RA, Bhargava V, Warnke RA: MIC2, TdT, bcl-2, and CD34 expression in paraffin-embedded high-grade lymphoma/acute lymphoblastic leukemia distinguishes between distinct clinicopathologic entities. Hum Pathol 1997;28:1158–1165.
28. Brocheriou I, Carnot F, Briere J: Immunohistochemical detection of bcl-2 protein in thymoma. Histopathology 1995;27:251–255.
29. Chen FF, Yan JJ, Jin YT, et al. Detection of bcl-2 and p53 in thymoma: Expression of bcl-2 as a reliable marker of tumor aggressiveness. Hum Pathol 1996;27:1089–1092.
30. Chan WC, Zaatari GS, Tabei S, et al. Thymoma: An immunohistochemical study. Am J Clin Pathol 1984;82:160–166.
31. Knowles DM II. Lymphoid cell markers: Their distribution and usefulness in the immunopathologic analysis of lymphoid neoplasms. Am J Surg Pathol 1985;9(Suppl):85–108.
32. Weiss LM, Bindl JM, Picozzi VJ, et al. Lymphoblastic lymphoma: An immunophenotypic study of 26 cases with comparison to T-cell acute lymphoblastic leukemia. Blood 1986;67:474–478.
33. Picker LJ, Weiss LM, Medeiros LJ, et al. Immunophenotypic criteria for the diagnosis of non-Hodgkin's lymphoma. Am J Pathol 1987;128:181–201.
34. Berrih-Aknin S, Safar D, Cohen-Kaminsky S. Analysis of lymphocyte phenotype in human thymomas. Adv Exp Med Biol 1988;237:369–374.

35. Ito M, Taki T, Mihaye M, et al. Lymphocyte subsets in human thymoma studied with monoclonal antibodies. Cancer 1988;61:284–287.
36. Perrone T, Frizzera G, Rosai J. Mediastinal diffuse large-cell lymphoma with sclerosis: A clinicopathologic study of 60 cases. Am J Surg Pathol 1986;10:176–191.
37. Wick MR, Swanson PE, Manivel JC. Immunohistochemical analysis of soft tissue sarcomas: Comparisons with electron microscopy. Appl Pathol 1988;6:169–196.
38. Nappi O, Ritter JH, Pettinato G, et al. Hemangiopericytoma: Histopathological pattern or clinicopathologic entity? Semin Diagn Pathol 1995;12:221–232.
39. Shimosato Y, Mukai K. Tumors of the Mediastinum. In: Rosai J, ed. Atlas of Tumor Pathology, Series 3, Fascicle 21. Washington, D.C., Armed Forces Institute of Pathology, 1997:33–273.
40. Swanson PE. Soft tissue neoplasms of the mediastinum. Semin Diagn Pathol 1991;8:14–34.
41. Marchevsky AM: Mediastinal tumors of peripheral nervous system origin. Semin Diagn Pathol 1999;16:65–78.
42. Chaves-Espinosa JI, Chaves-Fernandez JA, Hoyer OH, et al. Endothoracic neurogenic neoplasms: Analysis of 30 cases. Rev Interamer Radiol 1980;5:49–54.
43. Gale AW, Jelihovsky T, Grant AF, et al. Neurogenic tumors of the mediastinum. Ann Thorac Surg 1974;17:434–443.
44. Davidson KG, Walbaum PR, McCormack RJM. Intrathoracic neural tumors. Thorax 1978;33:359–367.
45. Young DG. Thoracic neuroblastoma/ganglioneuroma. J Pediatr Surg 1983;18:37–41.
46. Gould VE, Wiedenmann B, Lee I, et al. Synaptophysin expression in neuroendocrine neoplasms as determined by immunocytochemistry. Am J Pathol 1987;126:243–257.
47. Witkin GB, Rosai J. Solitary fibrous tumor of the mediastinum: A report of 14 cases. Am J Surg Pathol 1989;13:547–557.
48. Balassiano M, Reichert N, Rosenman Y, et al. Localized fibrous mesothelioma of the mediastinum devoid of pleural connections. Postgrad Med J 1989;65:788–790.
49. Hanau CA, Miettinen M: Solitary fibrous tumor: Histological and immunohistochemical spectrum of benign and malignant variants presenting at different sites. Hum Pathol 1995;26:440–449.
50. Wick MR, Manivel JC, Swanson PE. Contributions of immunohistochemistry to the diagnosis of soft tissue tumors. Prog Surg Pathol 1988;8:197–249.
51. England DM, Hochholzer L, McCarthy MJ. Localized benign and malignant fibrous tumors of the pleura: A clinicopathologic review of 223 cases. Am J Surg Pathol 1989;13:640–658.
52. Swanson PE, Wick MR. Immunohistochemical diagnosis of soft tissue tumors. In: Colvin R, Bhan A, McCluskey R, eds. Diagnostic Immunopathology, 2nd ed. New York: Raven Press, 1995:599–632.
53. Dines DE, Payne WS, Bernatz PE, et al. Mediastinal granulomas and fibrosing mediastinitis. Chest 1979;75:320–324.
54. Coffin CM, Watterson J, Priest JR, et al. Extrapulmonary inflammatory myofibroblastic tumor (inflammatory pseudotumor): A clinicopathologic and immunohistochemical study of 84 cases. Am J Surg Pathol 1995;19:859–872.
55. Lukes RJ, Butler JJ, Hicks EB: Natural history of Hodgkin's disease as related to its pathologic picture. Cancer 1966;19:317–344.
56. Matsubara O, Mark EJ, Ritter JH: Pseudoneoplastic lesions of the lungs, pleural surfaces, and mediastinum. In: Wick MR, Humphrey PA, Ritter JH, eds. Pathology of Pseudoneoplastic Lesions. Philadelphia, Lippincott-Raven, 1997:97–129.
57. Crotty TB, Colby TV, Gay PC, et al. Desmoplastic malignant mesothelioma masquerading as sclerosing mediastinitis: A diagnostic dilemma. Hum Pathol 1992;23:79–82.
58. Ritter JH, Humphrey PA, Wick MR. Malignant neoplasms capable of simulating inflammatory (myofibroblastic) pseudotumors and tumefactive fibroinflammatory lesions: Pseudopseudotumors. Semin Diagn Pathol 1998;15:111–132.
59. Rosai J, Levine GD, Weber WR, et al. Carcinoid tumors and oat cell carcinomas of the thymus. Pathol Annu 1976;11:201–226.
60. Wick MR, Rosai J. Neuroendocrine neoplasms of the thymus. Pathol Res Pract 1988;183:188–199.
61. Kuo TT, Chang JP, Lin FJ, et al. Thymic carcinomas: Histopathological varieties and immunohistochemical study. Am J Surg Pathol 1990;14:24–34.
62. Truong LD, Mody DR, Cagle PT, et al. Thymic carcinoma: A clinicopathologic study of 13 cases. Am J Surg Pathol 1990;14:151–166.
63. Shimizu J, Hayashi Y, Morita K, et al. Primary thymic carcinoma: A clinicopathological and immunohistochemical study. J Surg Oncol 1994;56:159–164.
64. Suster S, Rosai J. Thymic carcinoma: A clinicopathologic study of 60 cases. Cancer 1991;67:1025–1032.
65. Ritter JH, Wick MR. Primary carcinomas of the thymus gland. Semin Diagn Pathol 1999;16:18–31.
66. Snover DC, Levine GD, Rosai J. Thymic carcinomas: Five distinctive histological variants. Am J Surg Pathol 1982;6:451–470.
67. Iezzoni JC, Nass LB. Thymic basaloid carcinoma: A case report and review of the literature. Mod Pathol 1996;9:21–25.
68. DeLorimier AA, Bragg KU, Linden G. Neuroblastoma in childhood. Am J Dis Child 1969;118:441–450.
69. Salter JE Jr, Gibson D, Ordonez NG, et al. Neuroblastoma of the anterior mediastinum in an 80 year old woman. Ultrastruct Pathol 1995;19:305–310.
70. Hachitanda Y, Hata J. Stage IVS neuroblastoma: A clinical, histological, and biological analysis of 45 cases. Hum Pathol 1996;27:1135–1138.
71. Argani P, Erlandson RA, Rosai J. Thymic neuroblastoma in adults: Report of three cases with special emphasis on its association with the syndrome of inappropriate secretion of antidiuretic hormone. Am J Clin Pathol 1997;108:537–543.
72. Asada Y, Marutsuka K, Mitsukawa T, et.al. Ganglioneuroblastoma of the thymus: An adult case with the syndrome of inappropriate secretion of antidiuretic hormone. Hum Pathol 1996;27:506–509.
73. Wirnsberger GH, Becker H, Ziervogel K, et al. Diagnostic immunohistochemistry of neuroblastic tumors. Am J Surg Pathol 1992;16:49–57.
74. Dehner LP. Peripheral and central primitive neuroectodermal tumors: A nosologic concept seeking a consensus. Arch Pathol Lab Med 1986;110:997–1005.
75. Fellinger EJ, Garin-Chesa P, Su SL, et al. Biochemical and genetic characterization of the HBA71 Ewing's sarcoma cell surface antigen. Cancer Res 1991;51:336–340.
76. Dehner LP. Primitive neuroectodermal tumor and Ewing's sarcoma. Am J Surg Pathol 1993;17:1–13.
77. Leong ASY, Wick MR, Swanson PE. Immunohistology and Electron Microscopy of Anaplastic and Pleomorphic Tumors. Cambridge, UK: Cambridge Press, 1997:109–208.
78. Parham DM, Dias P, Kelly DR, et al. Desmin-positivity in primitive neuroectodermal tumors of childhood. Am J Surg Pathol 1992;16:483–492.
79. Pachter MR, Lattes R. Mesenchymal tumors of the mediastinum. I: Tumors of fibrous tissue, adipose tissue, smooth muscle, and striated muscle. Cancer 1963;16:74–94.
80. Suster S, Moran CA, Koss MN. Rhabdomyosarcomas of the anterior mediastinum: Report of four cases unassociated with germ cell, teratomatous, or thymic carcinomatous components. Hum Pathol 1994;25:349–356.
81. Tsokos M. The diagnosis and classification of childhood rhabdomyosarcoma. Semin Diagn Pathol 1994;11:26–38.
82. Cui S, Hano H, Harada T, et al. Evaluation of new monoclonal anti-MyoD1 and anti-myogenin antibodies for the diagnosis of rhabdomyosarcoma. Pathol Int 1999;49:62–68.
83. Nathwani BN, Kim H, Rappaport H. Malignant lymphoma, lymphoblastic. Cancer 1976;38:964–983.
84. Nathwani BN, Diamond LW, Winberg CD, et al. Lymphoblastic lymphoma: A clinicopathologic study of 95 patients. Cancer 1981;48:2347–2357.

85. Shikano T, Arioka H, Kobayashi R, et al. Acute lympho-blastic leukemia and non-Hodgkin's lymphoma with medi-astinal mass—a study of 23 children; different disorders or different stages? Leuk Lymphoma 1994;13:161–167.

86. Trump DL, Mann RB. Diffuse large cell and undifferen-tiated lymphomas with prominent mediastinal involve-ment: A poor prognostic subset of patients with non-Hodg-kin's lymphoma. Cancer 1982;50:277–282.

87. Majolino I, Marceno R, Magrin S, et al. Burkitt's cell leu-kemia with mediastinal mass and unusually good progno-sis. Haematologica 1983;68:287–288.

88. Isaacson PG, Chan JKC, Tang C, et al. Low-grade B-cell lymphoma of mucosa-associated lymphoid tissue arising in the thymus: A thymic lymphoma mimicking myoepi-thelial sialadenitis. Am J Surg Pathol 1990;14:342–351.

89. Takagi N, Nakamura S, Yamamoto K, et al. Malignant lym-phoma of mucosa-associated lymphoid tissue arising in the thymus of a patient with Sjogren's syndrome: A mor-phologic, phenotypic, and genotypic study. Cancer 1992;69:1347–1355.

90. Ozdemirli M, Fanburg-Smith JC, Hartmann DP, et al. Pre-cursor B-lymphoblastic lymphoma presenting as a solitary bone tumor and mimicking Ewing's sarcoma: A report of four cases and review of the literature. Am J Surg Pathol 1998;22:795–804.

91. Zukerberg LR, Medeiros LJ, Ferry JA, et al. Diffuse low-grade B-cell lymphomas: Four clinically distinct subtypes defined by a combination of morphologic and immuno-phenotypic features. Am J Clin Pathol 1993;100:373–385.

92. Banks PM, Isaacson PG: MALT lymphomas in 1997. Am J Clin Pathol 1999;111(Suppl 1):S75–S83.

93. Strickler JG, Kurtin PJ. Mediastinal lymphoma. Semin Diagn Pathol 1991;8:2–13.

94. Nakhleh RE, Wick MR, Rocamora A, et al. Morphologic diversity in malignant melanomas. Am J Clin Pathol 1990;93:731–740.

95. Fetsch PA, Marincola FM, Abati A. The new melanoma markers: MART-1 and Melan-A. Am J Surg Pathol 1999;23:607–610.

96. Matsuno Y, Mukai K, Noguchi M, et al. Histochemical and immunohistochemical evidence of glandular differentia-tion in thymic carcinomas. Acta Pathol Jpn 1989;39:433–438.

97. Kuo TT, Chan JKC. Thymic carcinoma arising in thymoma is associated with alterations in immunohistochemical profile. Am J Surg Pathol 1998;22:1474–1481.

98. Berezowski K, Grimes MM, Gal A, et al. CD5 immunoreac-tivity of epithelial cells in thymic carcinoma and CASTLE using paraffin-embedded tissue. Am J Clin Pathol 1996;106:483–486.

99. Hishima T, Fukayama M, Fujisawa M, et al. CD5 expres-sion in thymic carcinoma. Am J Pathol 1994;145:268–275.

100. Kornstein MJ, Rosai J. CD5 labeling of thymic carcinomas and other non-lymphoid neoplasms. Am J Clin Pathol 1998;109:722–726.

101. Tateyama H, Eimoto T, Tada T, et al. p53 protein expres-sion and p53 gene mutation in thymic epithelial tumors: An immunohistochemical and DNA sequencing study. Am J Clin Pathol 1995;104:375–381.

102. Stefanaki K, Rontogianni D, Kouvidou CH, et al. Expres-sion of p53, mdm2, p21/waf1, and bcl-2 proteins in thy-momas. Histopathology 1997;30:549–555.

103. Weirich G, Schneider P, Fellbaum C, et al. p53 alterations in thymic epithelial tumors. Virchows Arch A 1997;431:17–23.

104. Chen FF, Yan JJ, Chang KC, et al. Immunohistochemical localization of Mcl-1 and bcl-2 proteins in thymic epithe-lial tumors. Histopathology 1996;29:541–547.

105. Tateyama H, Eimoto T, Tada T, et al. Apoptosis, bcl-2 protein, and Fas antigen in thymic epithelial tumors. Mod Pathol 1997;10:983–991.

106. Lauriola L, Erlandson RA, Rosai J. Neuroendocrine differ-entiation is a common feature of thymic carcinoma. Am J Surg Pathol 1998;22:1059–1066.

107. Clark OH. Mediastinal parathyroid tumors. Arch Surg 1988;123:1096–1100.

108. Nathaniels EK, Nathaniels AM, Wang CA. Mediastinal para-thyroid tumors: A clinical and pathological study of 84 cases. Ann Surg 1970;171:165–170.

109. Murphy MN, Glennon PG, Diocee MS, et al. Nonsecretory parathyroid carcinoma of the mediastinum. Cancer 1986;58:2468–2476.

110. Ordonez NG, Ibanez ML, Samaan NA, Hickey RC. Immu-noperoxidase study of uncommon parathyroid tumors. Am J Surg Pathol 1983;7:535–542.

111. Dehner LP. Germ cell tumors of the mediastinum. Semin Diagn Pathol 1990;7:266–284.

112. Wick MR, Ritter JH, Humphrey PA, et al. Clear cell neo-plasms of the endocrine system and thymus. Semin Diagn Pathol 1997;14:183–202.

113. Knapp RH, Hurt RD, Payne WS, et al. Malignant germ cell tumors of the mediastinum. J Thorac Cardiovasc Surg 1985;89:82–89.

114. Truong LD, Harris L, Mattioli C, et al. Endodermal sinus tumor of the mediastinum: A report of seven cases and review of the literature. Cancer 1986;58:730–739.

115. Weidner N. Germ cell tumors of the mediastinum. Semin Diagn Pathol 1999;16:42–50.

116. Moran CA, Suster S, Przygodzki RM, et al. Primary germ cell tumors of the mediastinum. II: Mediastinal semino-mas—a clinicopathologic and immunohistochemical study of 120 cases. Cancer 1997;80:691–698.

117. Moran CA, Suster S. Hepatoid yolk sac tumors of the mediastinum: A clinicopathologic and immunohistologic study of four cases. Am J Surg Pathol 1997;21:1210–1214.

118. Suster S, Moran CA, Dominguez-Malagon, et al. Germ cell tumors of the mediastinum and testis: A comparative im-munohistochemical study of 120 cases. Hum Pathol 1998;29:737–742.

119. Moran CA, Suster S. Primary mediastinal choriocarcino-mas: A clinicopathologic and immunohistochemical study of eight cases. Am J Surg Pathol 1997;21:1007–1012.

120. Klemm KM, Moran CA. Primary neuroendocrine carcino-mas of the thymus. Semin Diagn Pathol 1999;16:32–41.

121. DeMontpreville VT, Macchiarini P, Dulmet E. Thymic neuroendocrine carcinoma (carcinoid): A clinicopathologic study of fourteen cases. J Thorac Cardiovasc Surg 1996;111:134–141.

122. Caceres W, Baldizon C, Sanchez J. Carcinoid tumor of the thymus: A unique neoplasm of the mediastinum. Am J Clin Oncol 1998;21:82–83.

123. Wick MR, Rosai J. Neuroendocrine neoplasms of the medi-astinum. Semin Diagn Pathol 1991;8:35–51.

124. Valli M, Fabris GA, Dewar A, et al. Atypical carcinoid tumor of the thymus: A study of eight cases. Histopathol-ogy 1994;24:371–375.

125. Wick MR, Scheithauer BW. Thymic carcinoid: A histo-logic, immunohistochemical, and ultrastructural study of 12 cases. Cancer 1984;53:475–484.

126. Herbst WM, Kumner W, Hofmann W, et al. Carcinoid tu-mors of the thymus: An immunohistochemical study. Can-cer 1987;60:2465–2470.

127. Odze R, Begin LR. Malignant paraganglioma of the poste-rior mediastinum. Cancer 1990;65:564–569.

128. Olson JL, Salyer WR. Mediastinal paraganglioma (aortic body tumor): A report of four cases, and a review of the literature. Cancer 1978;41:2405–2412.

129. Schroder HD, Johannsen L. Demonstration of S100 protein in sustentacular cells of phaeochromocytomas and para-gangliomas. Histopathology 1986;10:1023–1033.

130. DeLellis RA, Tischler AS, Lee AK, et al. Leu-enkephalin-like immunoreactivity in proliferative lesions of the hu-man adrenal medulla and extra-adrenal paraganglia. Am J Surg Pathol 1983;7:29–37.

131. Lamarre L, Jacobson JO, Aisenberg AC, et al. Primary large cell lymphoma of the mediastinum: A histologic and im-munophenotypic study of 29 cases. Am J Surg Pathol 1989;13:730–739.

132. Suster S. Primary large-cell lymphomas of the mediasti-num. Semin Diagn Pathol 1999;16:51–64.

133. Davis RE, Dorfman RF, Warnke RA. Primary large-cell

lymphoma of the thymus: A diffuse B-cell neoplasm presenting as primary mediastinal lymphoma. Hum Pathol 1990;21:1262–1268.

134. Al-Sharabati M, Chittal S, Duga-Neulat, et al. Primary anterior mediastinal B-cell lymphoma: A clinicopathologic and immunohistochemical study of 16 cases. Cancer 1991; 67:2579–2587.

135. Suster S, Moran CA. Pleomorphic large cell lymphomas of the mediastinum. Am J Surg Pathol 1996;20:224–232.

136. Addis BJ, Isaacson PG. Large-cell lymphoma of the mediastinum: A B-cell tumor of probable thymic origin. Histopathology 1986;10:379–390.

137. Fechner RE. Hodgkin's disease of the thymus. Cancer 1969;23:16–23.

138. Katz A, Lattes R. Granulomatous thymoma or Hodgkin's disease of thymus? A clinical and histologic study and a re-evaluation. Cancer 1969;23:1–15.

139. Lazzarino M, Orlandi E, Paulli M, et al. Treatment outcome and prognostic factors for primary mediastinal (thymic) B-cell lymphoma: A multicenter study of 106 patients. J Clin Oncol 1997;15:1646–1653.

140. Strickler JG, Michie SA, Warnke RA, et al. The "syncytial variant" of nodular sclerosing Hodgkin's disease. Am J Surg Pathol 1986;10:470–477.

141. Frizzera G: The distinction of Hodgkin's disease from anaplastic large cell lymphoma. Semin Diagn Pathol 1992;9: 291–296.

142. Menestrina F, Chilosi M, Scarpa A. Nodular lymphocyte predominant Hodgkin's disease and anaplastic large cell (CD30+) lymphoma: Distinct entities or nonspecific patterns? Semin Diagn Pathol 1995;12:256–269.

143. Kubonishi I, Ohtsuki Y, Machida K, et al. Granulocytic sarcoma as a mediastinal mass. Am J Clin Pathol 1984;83: 730–734.

144. Chubachi A, Miura I, Takahashi N, et al. Acute myelogenous leukemia associated with a mediastinal tumor. Leuk Lymphoma 1993;12:143–146.

145. Niwa K, Tanaka T, Mori H, et al. Extramedullary plasmacytoma of the mediastinum. Jpn J Clin Oncol 1987;17:95–100.

146. Miyazaki T, Kohno S, Sakamoto A, et al. A rare case of extramedullary plasmacytoma in the mediastinum. Intern Med 1992;31:1363–1365.

147. Meis JM, Butler JJ, Osborne BM, et al. Granulocytic sarcoma in nonleukemic patients. Cancer 1986;58:2697–2709.

148. Quintanilla-Martinez L, Zukerberg LR, Ferry JA, et al. Extramedullary tumors of lymphoid or myeloid blasts: The role of immunohistology in diagnosis and classification. Am J Clin Pathol 1995;104:431–443.

149. Goldstein NS, Ritter JH, Argenyi ZB, et al. Granulocytic sarcoma: Potential diagnostic clues from immunostaining patterns seen with anti-lymphoid antibodies. Int J Surg Pathol 1995;2:199–206.

150. Tong AW, Lee JC, Stone MJ. Characterization of a monoclonal antibody having selective reactivity with normal and neoplastic plasma cells. Blood 1987;69:238–245.

151. Petruch UR, Horny HP, Kaiserling E. Frequent expression of haematopoietic and non-haematopoietic antigens by neoplastic plasma cells: An immunohistochemical study using formalin-fixed, paraffin-embedded tissue. Histopathology 1992;20:35–40.

152. Ordonez NG. Role of immunohistochemistry in differentiating epithelial mesothelioma from adenocarcinoma: Review and update. Am J Clin Pathol 1999;112:75–89.

153. Kennedy AD, King G, Kerr KM. HBME-1 and antithrombomodulin in the differential diagnosis of malignant mesothelioma of pleura. J Clin Pathol 1997;50:859–862.

154. Ordonez NG. Value of thrombomodulin immunostaining in the diagnosis of mesothelioma. Histopathology 1997;31: 25–30.

155. Wick MR, Loy T, Mills SE, et al. Malignant epithelioid pleural mesothelioma versus peripheral pulmonary adenocarcinoma: A histochemical, ultrastructural, and immunohistologic study of 103 cases. Hum Pathol 1990;21:759–766.

156. Riera JR, Astengo-Osuna C, Longmate JA, et al. The immunohistochemical diagnostic panel for epithelial mesothelioma: A reevaluation after heat-induced epitope retrieval. Am J Surg Pathol 1997;21:1409–1419.

157. Khoor A, Whitsett JA, Stahlman MT, et al. Utility of surfactant protein B precursor and thyroid transcription factor 1 in differentiating adenocarcinoma of the lung from malignant mesothelioma. Hum Pathol 1999;30:695–700.

158. Wick MR. Immunohistochemistry in the diagnosis of "solid" malignant tumors. In: Jennette JC, ed. Immunohistology in Diagnostic Pathology. Boca Raton: CRC Press, 1989:161–191.

159. Feldman L, Kricun ME. Malignant melanoma presenting as a mediastinal mass. JAMA 1979;241:396–397.

160. Kaufmann O, Koch S, Burghardt J, et al. Tyrosinase, melan-A, and KBA62 as markers for the immunohistochemical identification of metastatic amelanotic melanomas on paraffin sections. Mod Pathol 1998;11:740–746.

161. Andrade RE, Wick MR, Frizzera G, Gajl-Peczalska KJ. Immunophenotyping of hematopoietic malignancies in paraffin sections. Hum Pathol 1988;19:394–402.

162. Said JW: The immunohistochemistry of Hodgkins disease. Semin Diagn Pathol 1992;9:265–271.

163. Suster S, Moran CA. Spindle cell thymic carcinoma: A clinicopathologic and immunohistochemical study of a distinctive variant of primary thymic epithelial neoplasm. Am J Surg Pathol 1999;23:691–700.

164. Suster S, Moran CA. Thymic carcinoma: Spectrum of differentiation and histologic types. Pathology 1998;30:111–122.

165. Moran CA, Suster S. Primary thymic carcinomas. Pathology (Phila) 1996;4:141–153.

166. Kuo TT. Carcinoid tumor of the thymus with divergent sarcomatoid differentiation: Report of a case with histogenetic considerations. Hum Pathol 1994;25:319–323.

167. Suarez-Vilela D, Salas-Valien JS, Gonzalez-Moran MA, et al. Thymic carcinosarcoma associated with a spindle cell thymoma: An immunohistochemical study. Histopathology 1992;21:263–268.

168. Wick MR, Swanson PE. Carcinosarcomas—current perspectives and a historical review of nosological concepts. Semin Diagn Pathol 1993;10:118–127.

169. DeLeeuw B, Suijkerbuijk RF, Olde-Weghuis D, et al. Distinct Xp11.2 breakpoint regions in synovial sarcoma revealed by metaphase and interphase FISH: Relationship to histologic subtypes. Cancer Genet Cytogenet 1994;73:89–94.

170. Suster S, Moran CA, Chan JKC. Thymoma with pseudosarcomatous stroma: Report of an unusual histologic variant of thymic epithelial neoplasm that may simulate carcinosarcoma. Am J Surg Pathol 1997;21:1316–1323.

171. Levine GD, Rosai J. A spindle-cell variant of thymic carcinoid tumor: A clinical, histologic, and fine structural study with emphasis on its distinction from spindle-cell thymoma. Arch Pathol Lab Med 1976;100:293–300.

172. Moran CA, Suster S. Spindle-cell neuroendocrine carcinomas of the thymus (spindle-cell thymic carcinoid): A clinicopathologic and immunohistochemical study of seven cases. Mod Pathol 1999;12:587–591.

173. Moran CA, Suster S. Yolk sac tumors of the mediastinum with prominent spindle cell features: A clinicopathologic study of three cases. Am J Surg Pathol 1997;21:1173–1177.

174. Moran CA, Suster S, Perino G, et al. Malignant smooth muscle tumors presenting as mediastinal soft tissue masses: A clinicopathologic study of 10 cases. Cancer 1994;74:2251–2260.

175. Yang WI, Efird JT, Quintanilla-Martinez L, et al. Cell kinetic study of thymic epithelial tumors using PCNA (PC10) and Ki-67 (MIB-1) antibodies. Hum Pathol 1996;27: 70–76.

176. Pan CC, Ho DM, Chen WY, et al. Ki-67 labelling index correlates with stage and histology but not significantly with prognosis in thymoma. Histopathology 1998;33:453–458.

177. Yang WI, Efird JT, Quintanilla-Martinez L, et al. Cell ki-

netic study of thymic epithelial tumors using PCNA (PC10) and Ki-67 (MIB-1) antibodies. Hum Pathol 1996;27: 70–76.

178. Tateyama H, Eimoto T, Tada T, et al. Apoptosis, bcl-2 protein, and fas antigen in thymic epithelial tumors. Mod Pathol 1997;10:983–991.

179. Yang WI, Yang KM, Hong SW, et al. E-cadherin expression in thymomas. Yonsei Med J 1998;39:37–44.

180. Pan CC, Ho DM, Chen WY, et al. Expression of E-cadherin and alpha- and beta-catenins in thymoma. J Pathol 1998; 184:207–211.

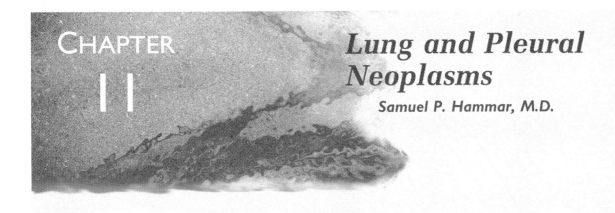

CHAPTER 11

Lung and Pleural Neoplasms

Samuel P. Hammar, M.D.

Immunohistochemistry is an effective, commonly used, adjuvant technique in diagnosing primary and metastatic neoplasms of the lung and pleura. Because of its relative ease of use and specificity, immunohistochemistry has largely replaced mucin histochemistry and electron microscopy in diagnosing pulmonary and pleural neoplasms. In some instances, electron microscopy is diagnostically superior to immunohistochemistry, and cases occur in which neither immunohistochemistry nor electron microscopy is specific for a given neoplasm.

Most primary lung cancers are capable of being diagnosed by histologic criteria alone, although as lung neoplasms become more poorly differentiated and as clinical situations become more complicated, immunohistochemical techniques are often used to confirm or eliminate a pathologic diagnosis. In addition, many neoplasms of different primary origins are morphologically similar to primary lung and pleural neoplasms, and immunohistochemistry is an effective way to distinguish them.

PRIMARY LUNG NEOPLASMS

A wide variety of primary neoplasms occur in the lung. Four major types make up 85 to 90% of primary lung neoplasms: adenocarcinoma, squamous cell carcinoma, small cell carcinoma, and large cell undifferentiated carcinoma.[1] Adenocarcinoma is currently the most frequently diagnosed primary lung cancer in the United States[2, 3] and usually occurs in a subpleural location, although occasionally it is central or intrabronchial. Squamous carcinoma is the second most common primary lung cancer and occurs predominantly in a central distribution arising from mainstem and segmental bronchi. Approximately 10% of primary pulmonary squamous cell carcinomas occur in the periphery of the lung. Small cell lung cancers occur in the central region of the lung arising from neuroendocrine cells in the mainstem bronchi and lobar bronchi, although up to 10% of small cell lung cancers occur in the periphery of the lung.

Large cell undifferentiated carcinomas potentially occur in any location in the lung and make up approximately 8 to 10% of primary lung cancers.

Several antibodies are useful in confirming or eliminating primary lung cancers; those used are dependent on the type of neoplasm suspected and the clinical situation encountered. A list of the antibodies commonly used in detecting, confirming, or eliminating primary lung carcinomas (excluding neuroendocrine carcinomas, which will be discussed later) is presented in Table 11–1.

ANTIBODIES

Keratins are a family of polypeptides that have been separated according to molecular weight and isoelectric point (acidic or basic). Twenty molecular species exist and have been catalogued by Moll and colleagues.[4, 5] CK7 is expressed in many pulmonary epithelial cells, although it is found in a variety of other epithelial cells and in a variety of nonpulmonary carcinomas.[6] When used diagnostically, CK7 is often used with CK20 and nonkeratin antibodies in diagnosing and classifying glandular neoplasms. Most primary pulmonary carcinomas contain several molecular species of keratins, with the exception of small cell carcinoma, which contains low molecular weight keratin.

Vimentin is a 58-kd intermediate filament found predominantly in mesenchymal cells. However, vimentin is expressed in most spindle cell carcinomas[7] and is reported by some to be expressed in a relatively high percentage of pulmonary adenocarcinomas.[8]

A variety of epithelial cell markers (carcinoembryonic antigen [CEA], human milk fat globule protein-2 [HMFG-2], epithelial membrane antigen [EMA], LeuM1 [CD15], B72.3, and BerEP4) is expressed in primary lung carcinomas, predominantly pulmonary adenocarcinomas. Most are nonspecific and have been used in distinguishing epithelial mesothelioma from pulmonary and nonpulmonary adenocarcinoma (see later) and in eval-

Table 11–1. Antibodies Commonly Used to Evaluate Potential Lung Neoplasms (Excluding Neuroendocrine Lung Neoplasms)

Antibody Directed Against	Clone	Characteristics of Antigen	Immunogen	Manufacturer	Dilution	Type of Antigen Retrieval
Keratin	AE1/AE3	AE1—acidic subfamily 40, 48, 50; 56.5 kd AE3—basic subfamily—52, 56, 58, 59, 64, 65–67 kd	Human epidermal keratin	DAKO	1:200	HIER
Keratin	CAM5.2	CK 8, CK 18	Colorectal carcinoma cell line	Becton-Dickinson	1:100	HIER
Keratin	MAK6	CK 8, CK14–CK 16, CK 18, CK 19	Extracellular antigen from MCF-tissue culture and from human sole epidermis	Zymed	1:100	HIER
Keratin	35βH11	CK 8—54 kd	Hep3B hepatocellular carcinoma line	DAKO	1:50	HIER
Keratin	34βE12	Keratins—Moll numbers 1, 5, 10, and 14	Human stratum corneum keratin	DAKO	1:100	HIER
CK5/CK6	D5/16B4	Intermediate filament CK5/CK6 and to slight degree CK 4	Purified CK5	Biocare Medical	1:100	HIER
CK7	OV-TL 12/30	Moll CK 7—54 kd	OTN 11 ovarian carcinoma line	DAKO	1:100	HIER
CK20	K_s20.8	Moll CK 20	Cytoskeletal protein from human duodenal mucosa	DAKO	1:50	HIER
Vimentin	Vim 3B4	Intermediate filament—57 kd	Vimentin from bovine eye lens	DAKO	1:100	HIER
Epithelial membrane antigen (EMA)	E29	Glycoprotein—250–400 kd	Delipidated extract of human milk fat	DAKO	1:100	HIER
Human milk fat globule protein-2 (HMFG-2)	115D8	MAM-6 mucus glycoprotein—>400 kd	Purified human milk fat globule protein	BioGenex	1:25	HIER
Polyclonal carcinoembryonic antigen (pCEA)	—	Antibody recognizes CEA and CEA-like proteins, including nonspecific cross-reacting substance and biliary glycoprotein	Human CEA isolated from metastatic colonic adenocarcinoma	DAKO	1:16,000	HIER
CD15 (LeuM1)	C3D-1	3-fucosyl-N-acetyllactosamine	Purified neutrophils from normal human peripheral blood	DAKO	1:20	HIER
Tumor-associated glycoprotein	B72.3	Glycoprotein in a variety of adenocarcinomas	Membrane-enriched fraction of metastatic breast carcinoma	BioGenex	1:100	HIER
Human epithelial antigen	Ber-EP4	Glycoproteins of 34 and 49 kd on surface and in cytoplasm of all epithelial cells except squamous epithelium, hepatocytes, and parietal cells	MCF-7 cell line	DAKO	1:100	HIER
Thyroid transcription factor-1 (TTF-1)	8G7G3/1	40-kd member of NKx2 family of homeodomain transcription factors	Rat TTF-1 recombinant protein	Biocare Medical	1:200	HIER
S-100 protein	—	S-100 protein A and B	S-100 protein isolated from cow brain	DAKO	1:300	HIER

HIER, heat-induced epitope retrieval.

uating metastatic adenocarcinoma of unknown primary origin[9] (see Chapter 7).

Thyroid transcription factor-1 (TTF-1), a 38- to 40-kd transcription factor member of NKx2 family of homeodomain transcription factors, is expressed in thyroid and pulmonary epithelial cells.[10, 11] TTF-1 binds to and activates the promoters for Clara cell secretory protein and surfactant proteins A, B, and C.[12, 13] As reported in the literature and as observed by me, TTF-1 is expressed in the nuclei of 60 to 75% of pulmonary adenocarcinomas[14–17] and in most small cell lung cancers, atypical carcinoids, large cell neuroendocrine carcinomas, and approximately 35% of typical carcinoids.[18]

The immunohistogram of common lung carcinomas is shown in Figure 11–1.

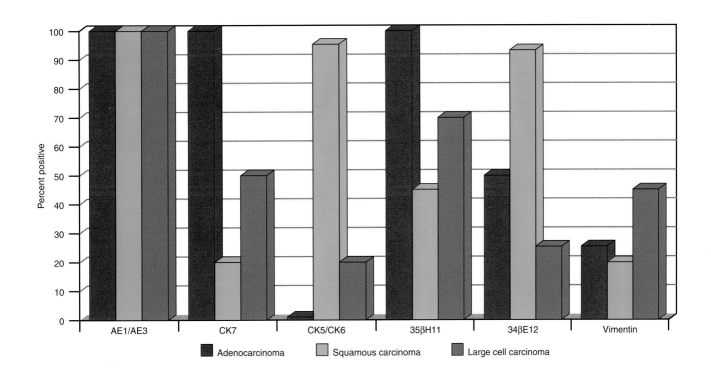

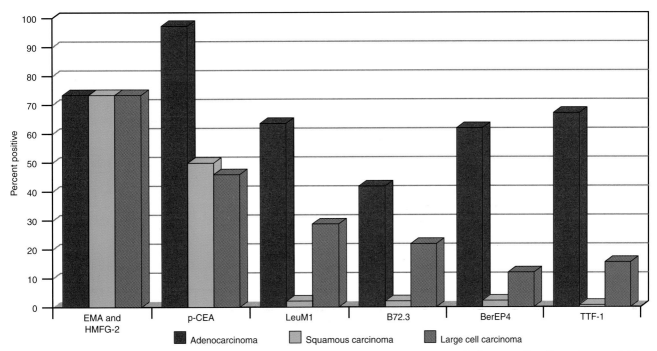

Figure 11–1. Immunohistogram of common primary pulmonary carcinomas, excluding small cell carcinoma. EMA, epithelial membrane antigen; pCEA, polyclonal carcinoembryonic antigen; TTF-1, thyroid transcription factor-1.

NEUROENDOCRINE LUNG NEOPLASMS

Small cell carcinoma is the most common neuroendocrine neoplasm of the lung.[19, 20] The previously described subtypes (lymphocyte-like, intermediate–polygonal-fusiform) are currently lumped together as small cell carcinoma.[21] The entity referred to as a *large cell–small cell carcinoma* has been eliminated.

Other primary neuroendocrine neoplasms of the lung include typical carcinoid, atypical carcinoid, and large cell neuroendocrine carcinoma. There has been significant confusion concerning the entity "atypical carcinoid," with several different names applied to the entity. The designation *atypical carcinoid* was used by Arrigoni and colleagues[22] to describe a neuroendocrine lung neoplasm that differed from typical carcinoid. Atypical carcinoid has been referred to as *malignant carcinoid,*[23] *well-differentiated neuroendocrine carcinoma,*[24] *peripheral small cell carcinoma of lung resembling carcinoid tumor,*[25] and *Kulchitzky cell carcinoma II.*[26]

The current World Health Organization (WHO) International Histological Typing of Lung and Pleural Tumors[27] describes atypical carcinoid as a tumor with neuroendocrine morphology with between 2 and 10 mitoses/10 high power fields (2 mm^2) or with foci of punctate necrosis, or both.

The existence of large cell neuroendocrine carcinoma of the lung was suggested by Gould and Chejfec[28] in 1978, and further described by Hammond and Sause[29] in 1985, Neal and colleagues[30] in 1986, and Barbareschi and associates[31] in 1989. It is not certain whether the neoplasms described by McDowell and colleagues[32] in 1981 were large cell neuroendocrine carcinomas or non–small cell lung carcinomas showing neuroendocrine differentiation.

Travis and associates[33] reported 35 neuroendocrine lung neoplasms in 1991, including 5 large cell neuroendocrine lung neoplasms. Their criteria for diagnosing a neoplasm as a large cell neuroendocrine carcinoma included (1) a tumor with a neuroendocrine appearance by light microscopy that included an organoid, trabecular, palisading, or rosette pattern; (2) large cells with most cells greater than the nuclear diameter of three small resting lymphocytes, a low nuclear to cytoplasmic ratio, polygonal-shaped cells, finely granular eosinophilic cytoplasm with an eosinophilic hue, coarse nuclear chromatin, and frequent nucleoli; (3) a mitotic rate greater than 10 mitoses per 10 high power fields; (4) necrosis; and (5) neuroendocrine features by immunohistochemistry or electron microscopy, or both.

In 1989, I found that there is a wide spectrum of differentiation of neuroendocrine lung neoplasms, and some do not fit into a well-defined category.[34]

Antibodies Used To Detect Neuroendocrine Lung Neoplasms

Neuroendocrine cells occur in many organs and tissues in the body and are part of the "diffuse neuroendocrine system" as described by Pearse[35] and the "dispersed neuroendocrine system" described by Gould and DeLellis.[36] Not surprisingly, neuroendocrine cells and neoplasms formed by cells exhibiting neuroendocrine differentiation show similar immunohistochemical features. They contain a variety of biogenic amines, peptide hormones, and neurotransmitters that can be identified biochemically or immunohistochemically.[37] Immunohistochemical markers are useful in showing neuroendocrine differentiation by a neoplasm but are not necessarily specific. The antibodies commonly used in demonstrating neuroendocrine differentiation are shown in Table 11–2.

Table 11–2. Antibodies Commonly Used in Identifying Neuroendocrine Lung Neoplasms

Antibody Directed Against	Clone	Characteristic of Antigen	Immunogen	Manufacturer	Dilution	Type of Antigen Retrieval
Synaptophysin	—	38-kd membrane component of synaptic vesicles	Synthetic human synaptophysin coupled to ovalbumin	DAKO	1:100	HIER
Chromogranin A	DAK-A3	439 amino acid protein encoded on chromosome 14 residing in neuroendocrine granules	C-terminal 20-kd fragment of chromogranin-A	DAKO	1:100	HIER
Neuro-specific enolase (NSE)	—	46-kd gamma-gamma isoenzyme of enolase	NSE isolated from human brain	DAKO	1:400	HIER
Leu7 CD57	NK-1	110-kd human myeloid cell–associated surface glycoprotein	Antigen from human natural killer cells	BioGenex	1:20	HIER
Neural cell adhesion molecule (NCAM)	UJ13A	125-kd sialoglycoprotein	16-week-old fetal human brain homogenates	DAKO	1:20	HIER

HIER, heat-induced epitope retrieval.

Synaptophysin is a 38-kd glycoprotein component of pre-synaptic vesicles isolated from bovine neurons.[38, 39] In my opinion, it is the most sensitive and most specific screening antibody for neuroendocrine neoplasms. As discussed further on, synaptophysin has occasionally been observed in non-neuroendocrine, non–small cell lung carcinomas.

Chromogranins are a family of acidic proteins containing high concentrations of glutamic acid located in the matrix of neuroendocrine granules in normal and neoplastic neuroendocrine cells.[40, 41] Chromogranin A was discovered by Banks and Helle[42] in 1965 in adrenal medullary cells. Antibodies against chromogranin A are the most specific marker of normal and neoplastic neuroendocrine cells. Expression in a given neoplasm correlates with the number of cytoplasmic neuroendocrine granules that can be evaluated ultrastructurally.

Neuron-specific enolase catalyzes the interconversion of 2-phosphoglycerate and phosphoenolpyruvate in the glycolytic pathway. Enolases are dimers composed of three subunits (alpha, beta, and gamma). Neuron-specific enolase contains a high concentration of gamma enolase and is usually present in high concentrations in neurons and neuroendocrine cells. Unfortunately, neuron-specific enolase is not neuron- or neuroendocrine cell–specific. Neuron-specific enolase has been identified in a wide variety of non-neuron, non-neuroendocrine cells, including smooth muscle cells, myoepithelial cells, renal epithelial cells, plasma cells, and megakaryocytes.[43, 44] Neuron-specific enolase is not uncommonly referred to as *non-specific enolase.* Despite its low specificity, it is a highly sensitive marker for neoplastic neuroendocrine cells.

Other neuroendocrine markers that are occasionally used to identify normal neuroendocrine lung cells and neoplastic neuroendocrine cells include neurofilaments,[45] neural cell adhesion molecules (NCAMs),[46, 47] and Leu7.[48] The most frequent neuropeptides, neuroamines, and hormones found in neuroendocrine lung neoplasms are listed in Table 11–3. TTF-1 is found in a high percentage of small cell carcinomas, atypical carcinoids, and large cell neuroendocrine carcinomas, but in less than 50% of typical carcinoids.

The antibodies I use in evaluating a neoplasm for neuroendocrine differentiation include low molecular weight keratin, high molecular weight keratin, synaptophysin, chromogranin A, TTF-1, and leukocyte common antigen. It should be remembered that CEA is occasionally expressed in neuroendocrine lung neoplasms,[49] and neuron-specific enolase is expressed in nearly all such neoplasms.

An immunohistogram showing the characteristic immunohistochemical staining reactions in neuroendocrine lung neoplasms is shown in Figure 11–2.

Small cell carcinomas, which make up about 20 to 25% of all primary lung cancers, show immunostaining for low molecular weight keratins (CAM5.2, 35βH11); no immunostaining for high molecular weight keratin; immunostaining for synaptophysin, neuron-specific enolase, and CEA (Fig. 11–3); variable staining for chromogranin A; and frequent nuclear immunostaining for TTF-1 (Fig. 11–4). The pattern of staining for low molecular weight keratin and chromogranin is usually punctate (Figs. 11–5 and 11–6). In my experience, most small cell carcinomas do not express chromogranin A, although the expression is dependent on how many neuroendocrine granules are in the cytoplasm of the neoplastic cells. When studied by electron microscopy, there are occasional small cell carcinomas whose tumor cells contain a moderate number of neuroendocrine granules (Fig. 11–7).

Typical carcinoids, atypical carcinoids, and large cell neuroendocrine carcinomas characteristically express low and high molecular weight keratin, synaptophysin, and chromogranin A. Immunohistochemical tests are helpful in identifying these neoplasms as neuroendocrine but are not helpful in separating specific neoplasms from one another. Chromogranin A shows the greatest staining intensity in typical carcinoids (Fig. 11–8), which correlates with relatively frequent cytoplasmic neuroendocrine granules.

RARE PRIMARY LUNG NEOPLASMS

A variety of rare primary neoplasms occur in the lung that are occasionally encountered by pathologists and may cause diagnostic confusion. None is frequent. Examples include sarcomatoid carcinoma (carcinosarcoma, spindle cell carcinoma), pulmonary blastoma, malignant hemangioendothelioma (intravascular bronchioloalveolar tumor), sarcoma, lymphoma, pulmonary Langerhans' cell granulomatosis, Kaposi's sarcoma, clear cell neoplasm (sugar tumor), rhabdoid tumor, sclerosing hemangioma, and inflammatory pseudotumor.[50]

Table 11–3. Neuropeptides, Neuroamines and Hormones Frequently Found in Neuroendocrine Lung Neoplasms

Bombesin
Calcitonin
Adrenocorticotropic hormone (ACTH)
Leu-enkephalin
Gastrin
Somatostatin
Vasoactive intestinal polypeptide
Neurotensin
Arginine vasopressin
Serotonin

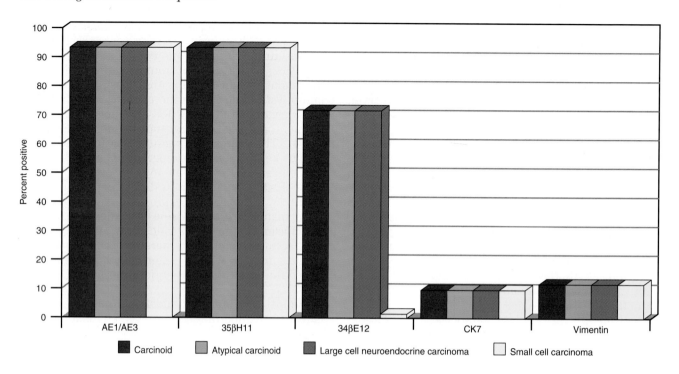

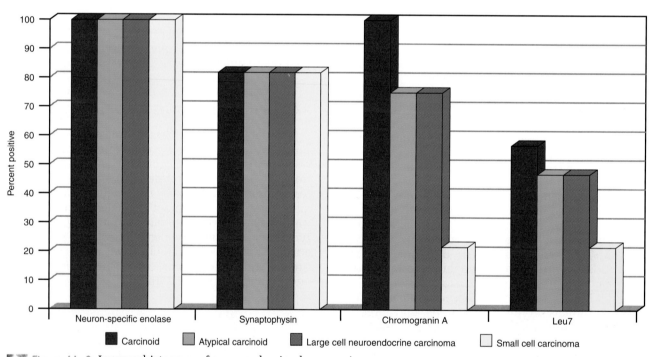

Figure 11–2. Immunohistogram of neuroendocrine lung carcinomas.

Sarcomatoid carcinoma, also referred to as *carcinosarcoma, spindle cell carcinoma, blastoma,* and *teratocarcinoma,* is a neoplasm of epithelial derivation that shows variable differentiation. This neoplasm has been reviewed conceptually by Wick and Swanson.[51] Several studies have evaluated sarcomatoid carcinoma by immunohistochemistry using keratin antibodies or electron microscopy, or both, and concluded that the spindle cell component of the neoplasm was of epithelial deriva-

tion.[52–56] In most instances, the spindle cells coexpress keratin and vimentin (Figs. 11–9 and 11–10), or occasionally keratin and other intermediate filaments such as desmin or actin.

Pleomorphic carcinoma, as defined by Fishback and colleagues,[57] is a neoplasm that occurs predominantly in older individuals and is composed predominantly of spindle cells and large pleomorphic giant cells. In 78 cases, the authors found foci of squamous differentiation in 8% of cases, large

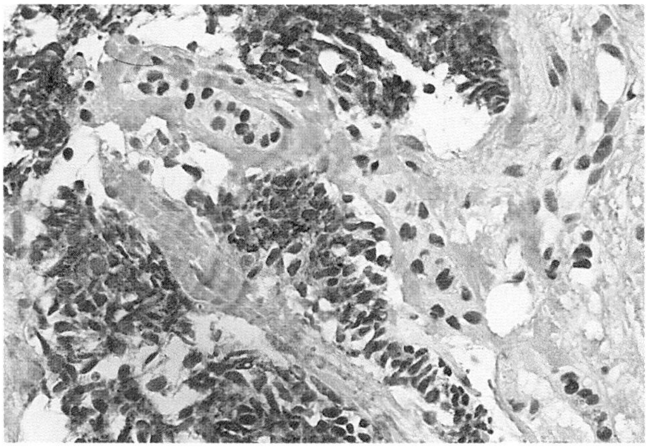

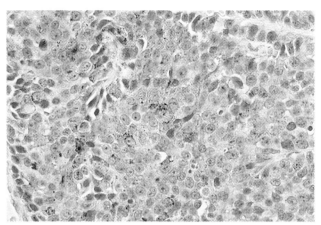

Figure 11–3. Many small cell lung carcinomas express carcinoembryonic antigen. (×400)

Figure 11–6. As shown in this photograph, the immunostaining pattern for chromogranin A in this small cell lung carcinoma is punctate. (×400)

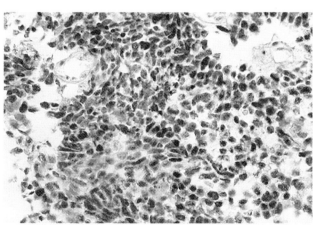

Figure 11–4. This small cell carcinoma of lung shows intense nuclear immunostaining for thyroid transcription factor-1. (×400)

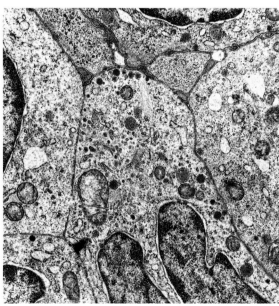

Figure 11–7. In this small cell carcinoma, the neoplastic cells contain a moderate number of cytoplasmic dense core neuroendocrine granules. (×16,000)

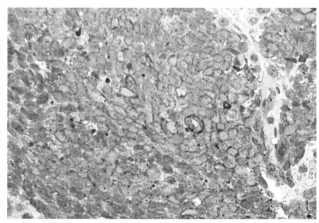

Figure 11–5. Most small cell carcinomas of lung show punctate immunostaining for low molecular weight keratin. (×400)

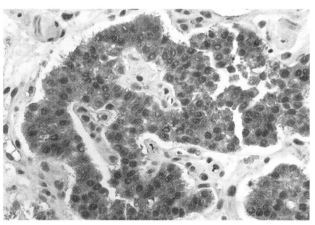

Figure 11–8. This typical carcinoid shows intense cytoplasmic immunostaining for chromogranin A. (×400)

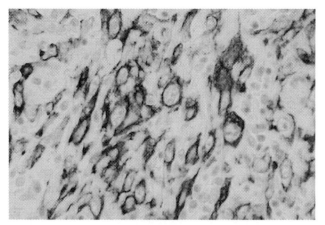

Figure 11–9. This region of sarcomatoid carcinoma showed immunostains of the spindle cells for low molecular weight keratin. (×400)

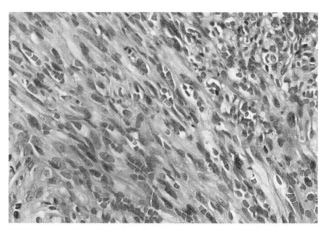

Figure 11–11. The neoplastic cells in Kaposi's sarcoma are spindle-shaped and are in a lymphatic distribution. (×400)

cell undifferentiated carcinoma in 25% of cases, and adenocarcinoma in 45% of cases. The remaining 22% of the neoplasms were composed of neoplastic spindle cells and giant cells. The spindle cells usually express only vimentin. The immunostaining pattern of the epithelial component of the neoplasm will depend on what type of differentiation it shows.

Pulmonary blastomas are usually composed of an epithelial component that forms glandular structures often resembling endometrial glands or fetal glands and a spindle cell component. The epithelial tumor cells occasionally form squamous morulae. As reported by Koss and associates[58] and Yousem and coworkers,[59] these neoplasms differentiate in divergent ways and occasionally show neuroendocrine differentiation. The epithelial cells forming glands immunostain for keratin, CEA, and EMA. The spindle cells express vimentin and, depending on the differentiation of the sarcomatoid component, desmin, actin, and S-100 protein.

Those that contain neuroendocrine elements show markers of neuroendocrine cells.

Primary sarcomas of the lung are rare and occur in various forms. The immunophenotype of the neoplastic cells forming such neoplasms is essentially identical to sarcomas that occur in soft tissue and other organs (see Chapter 3).

With the advent of the acquired immunodeficiency syndrome (AIDS), Kaposi's sarcoma is more frequent and, in most cases, is a metastatic neoplasm in the lung.[60–69] Kaposi's sarcoma follows lymphatic pathways in the lung and often involves lymph nodes. The neoplastic cells are spindle-shaped (Fig. 11–11) and immunostain for vimentin and endothelial cell markers such as CD31 (Fig. 11–12).

Malignant hemangioendothelioma, also referred to as *intravascular bronchioloalveolar tumor,* usually occurs in relatively young women, is bilateral, and takes the form of multiple small nodules that fill alveolar spaces and undergo degeneration, necrosis, and calcification.[50] This neoplasm was ini-

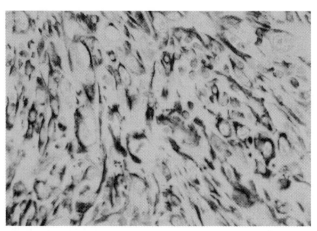

Figure 11–10. Same neoplasm as shown in Figure 11–9. Neoplastic spindle cells show intense immunostaining for vimentin. (×400)

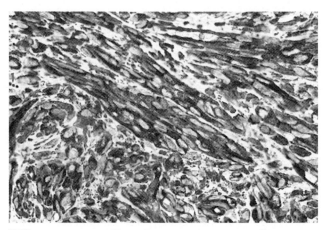

Figure 11–12. Kaposi's sarcoma tumor cells express vascular markers such as CD31. (×400)

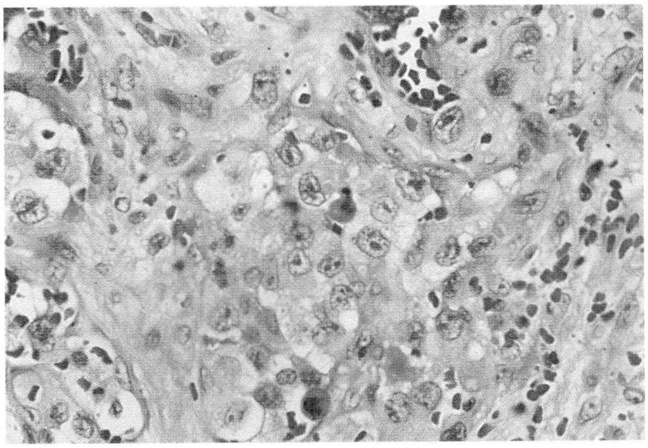

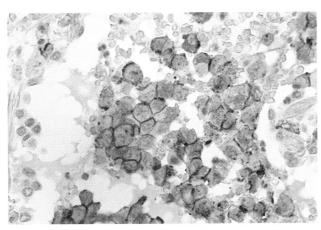

Figure 11–13. In this malignant epithelioid hemangioendothelioma, the neoplastic cells have an epithelial appearance and can be confused with carcinomas. (×400)

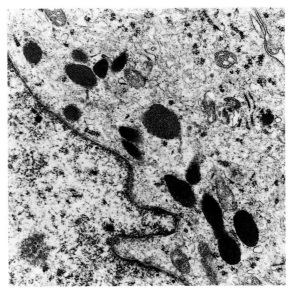

Figure 11–15. In this case, the neoplastic epithelioid hemangioendothelioma cells contained cytoplasmic Weibel-Palade bodies. (×20,000)

tially thought to be of alveolar cell origin. Histologically, the tumor cells are round or polygonal and have an epithelial appearance (Fig. 11–13). They characteristically express endothelial markers such as CD31, CD34, and factor VIII antigen and immunostain for vimentin. Rarely, these neoplasms express keratin (Fig. 11–14). Ultrastructurally, the neoplastic cells often contain Weibel-Palade bodies, which are pathognomonic markers of endothelial cells (Fig. 11–15). Primary angiocarcinomas are rare and can be dedifferentiated without forming obvious vascular channels. The neoplastic cells usually show the same immunohistochemical profile as malignant hemangioendotheliomas.

The lung shows a wide spectrum of primary lymphoproliferative disorders.[70] These are similar to those seen in lymph nodes, and the same immunohistochemical markers apply (see Chapters 4 and 5). Lymphomatoid granulomatosis (LYG) is the most unique primary lymphoma of the lung. Origi-

nally described as an angiocentric and angiodestructive process involving primarily pulmonary veins,[71] it was uncertain if the process represented a primary vasculitis or a neoplasm. LYG is often included in the spectrum of angiocentric immunoproliferative lesions[72] and is composed of a variegated lymphoid infiltrate including mature lymphocytes, plasma cells, and large, highly atypical lymphoid cells (Fig. 11–16). Most of the lymphoid cells mark immunohistochemically as T lymphocytes. As reported by Guinee and associates,[73] the large atypical cells, which are considered to be the neoplastic cells in LYG, show immunostaining for the B lymphocyte marker CD20 (Fig. 11–17). These cells also contain the Epstein-Barr virus genome.

Pulmonary Langerhans cell granulomatosis is another process of hematopoietic cell origin that is of

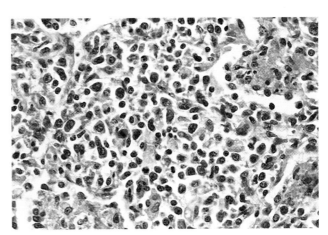

Figure 11–14. Occasional neoplastic epithelioid hemangioendothelioma cells show cytoplasmic immunostaining for keratin. (×400)

Figure 11–16. Lymphomatoid granulomatosis is composed of a variegated lymphoid infiltrate. (×100)

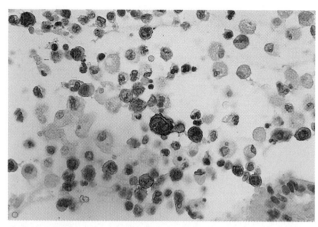

Figure 11–17. The large atypical cells in lymphomatoid granulomatosis express the B cell antigen CD20. (×400)

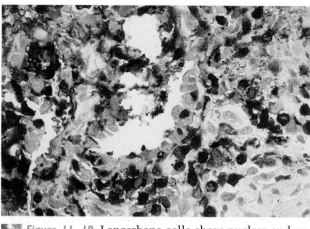

Figure 11–19. Langerhans cells show nuclear and cytoplasmic immunostaining for S-100 protein. (×400)

uncertain neoplastic potential; it occurs as a primary process in the lungs of cigarette smokers predominantly and can cause diagnostic confusion.[74] Also referred to as *pulmonary histiocytosis X* and *pulmonary eosinophilic granuloma,* pulmonary Langerhans cell granulomatosis can present with fever, chills, weight loss, and multiple pulmonary nodules that can be confused with metastatic neoplasm. The pulmonary nodules are composed of Langerhans cells admixed with varying numbers of lymphocytes, plasma cells, eosinophils, neutrophils, and cigarette smoker's macrophages. Langerhans cells are smaller than mature alveolar macrophages and have extensively convoluted nuclei (Fig. 11–18). They immunostain for CD1 and calcium-binding S-100 protein (Fig. 11–19).

Clear cell neoplasms of the lung occur as unencapsulated discrete nodules and are often referred to as *sugar tumors.*[75] Histologically, they are most frequently composed of cells that are relatively uniform in size, shape, and nuclear appearance (Fig. 11–20), although they can be more pleomorphic (Fig. 11–21). The neoplastic cells characteristically contain large amounts of glycogen in their cytoplasm that is ultrastructurally membrane bound. There has been considerable controversy over the cell of origin of this neoplasm. The current hypothesis is that this tumor is derived from a perivascular epithelioid cell similar to that seen in angiomyolipomas of the kidney.[76] The neoplastic cells show immunostaining for vimentin and express HMB-45 and S-100 protein relatively frequently (Fig. 11–22). In some cases, the neoplastic cells express neuron-specific enolase, Leu7, synaptophysin, and HMB-50. They are keratin-negative. As described by Gaffey and coworkers,[77] some neoplastic cells contain melanosomes (Fig. 11–23), as demonstrated ultrastructurally.

Lymphangioleiomyomatosis is a rare, proliferative, but non-neoplastic pulmonary condition and

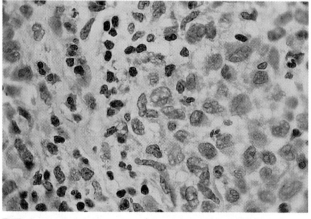

Figure 11–18. Portion of a nodule of pulmonary Langerhans cell granulomatosis. Langerhans cells are smaller than mature alveolar macrophages and have highly convoluted nuclei and a small amount of pale cytoplasm. Note the associated inflammatory cells. (×400)

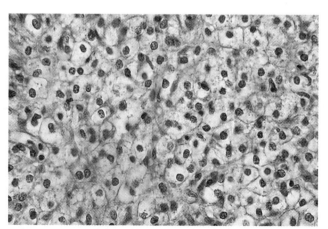

Figure 11–20. This clear cell tumor of lung is composed of relatively uniform cells. The clear cytoplasm is due to glycogen. (×400)

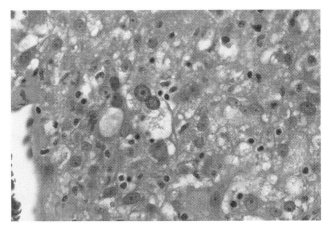

Figure 11–21. This clear cell tumor of lung is composed of significantly more pleomorphic cells than those seen in Figure 11–20. (×400)

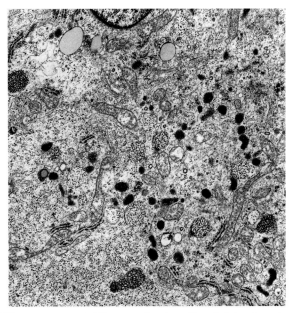

Figure 11–23. The neoplastic cells of this clear lung neoplasm contain melanosomes. (×16,000)

is mentioned briefly because the proliferative cells in this condition express HMB-45.[78, 79] This disease affects women of reproductive age and is characterized by proliferation of atypical smooth cells surrounding lymphatics and blood vessels with cystic space formation. These cells may express actin, vimentin, estrogen receptor protein, progesterone receptor protein, and HMB-45. Patients with lymphangioleiomyomatosis frequently have renal angiomyolipomas.

Sclerosing hemangioma is one of the most extensively studied rare pulmonary neoplasms and usually occurs as a round to oval solitary subpleural mass,[80, 81] the majority of which occur in relatively young women.[82] Most sclerosing hemangiomas are histologically variegated, showing cellular areas, various-sized spaces occasionally containing blood, sclerosis, and papillary structures. In the solid cellular regions, the neoplastic cells are round, oval, and slightly spindle-shaped (Fig. 11–24). The spaces are usually lined by cuboidal or columnar cells that appear morphologically as epithelial cells

and are often different from adjacent tumor cells. Most sclerosing hemangiomas contain varying types and numbers of inflammatory cells, especially mast cells. There have been several immunohistochemical studies of sclerosing hemangiomas. These have been reviewed by Dail.[50] Positive and negative immunohistochemical reactions of the neoplastic cells in the solid areas are contrasted with positive and negative immunohistochemical reactions reported for the lining cells in Table 11–4. In a case I evaluated, the lining cells and tumor cells in solid areas showed intense immunostaining for EMA (Fig. 11–25) and moderately intense cytoplasmic immunostaining for vimentin. Occasional lining cells showed low-intensity immunostaining for ker-

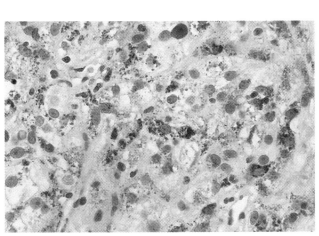

Figure 11–22. The neoplastic cells of this clear cell tumor express HMB-45. (×400)

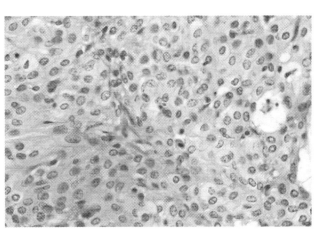

Figure 11–24. In the solid region of this sclerosing hemangioma, the majority of the neoplastic cells are round, oval, and occasionally slightly spindle-shaped. (×400)

Table 11–4. Reported Immunohistochemical Findings in Sclerosing Hemangiomas of Lung

Cells in Solid Regions of Tumor		Cells Lining Spaces in Tumor	
Positive Reactions	*Negative Reactions*	*Positive Reactions*	*Negative Reactions*
Vimentin	Keratin	Keratin	Vimentin
EMA	S-100 protein	Vimentin	S-100 protein
Keratin (rare)		EMA	
		Surfactant apo- protein	
		Clara cell antigen	
		CEA	

EMA, epithelial membrane antigen; CEA, carcinoembryonic antigen.

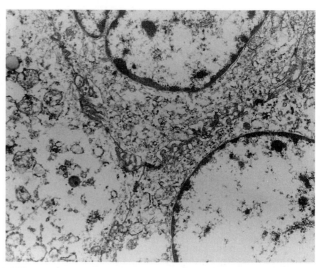

Figure 11–26. Ultrastructurally, the central cells of sclerosing hemangioendotheliomas exhibit epithelioid features with short microvillus processes and small intercellular junctions. (×10,000)

atin. The lining cells and neoplastic cells in solid areas showed no immunostaining for actin, desmin, S-100 protein, HMB-45, CD31, and factor VIII antigen. Ultrastructurally, the neoplastic cells in solid areas had "epithelioid" features, with a short microvillus process and small intercellular junctions (Fig. 11–26).

Malignant rhabdoid tumors of the kidney were described in 1978 by Beckwith and Palmer[83] as highly malignant tumors of infants and children initially thought to represent a variant of Wilms' tumor. Similar neoplasms were described in extra-renal sites and in adults.[84–97] Those that resemble rhabdoid tumors in the kidney but occur in non-renal sites are designated pseudorhabdoid tumors. They have a diverse immunohistochemical phenotype,[84–97] although the majority express vimentin, and many coexpress vimentin and keratin.

Six cases of lung tumors with rhabdoid morphology were described by Cavazza and associates[98] in 1996. These neoplasms were composed predominantly of large, round cells with ovoid nuclei, large nucleoli, and large eosinophilic globular inclusions that compressed the nucleus toward one side of the cell (Fig. 11–27). These six primary

rhabdoid tumors of lung were evaluated immunohistochemically, with 17 antibodies in five cases and 18 antibodies in one case. The rhabdoid component of the tumor immunostained for vimentin in all cases, the intensity of staining usually being high. The cytoplasmic eosinophilic inclusions showed immunostaining for EMA and neuron-specific enolase in five of six cases, chromogranin and broad spectrum keratin in three of six cases, CAM5.2 keratin in two of six cases, neurofilament in two of six cases, and Leu7 and gliofibrillary acidic protein in one of six cases. Synaptophysin was focally positive in three of six cases and CD34 in one of six cases, but did not stain the globular inclusions. Diffuse granular cytoplasmic immunostaining for myoglobulin was observed in one case. The neoplastic cells showed no immunostaining for factor VIII antigen, actin, desmin, S-100 protein, HMB-45, and light-chain immunoglobulin

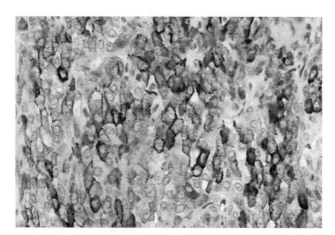

Figure 11–25. This sclerosing hemangioma is composed of cells that show relatively intense immunostaining for epithelial membrane antigen. (×400)

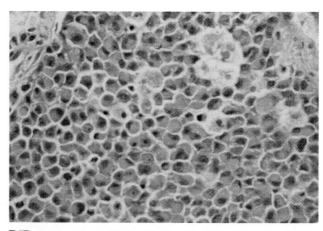

Figure 11–27. This primary rhabdoid tumor of lung is composed of large cells with large, globular eosinophilic inclusions. (×400)

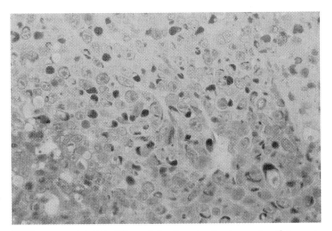

Figure 11-28. The globular inclusions in this primary rhabdoid tumor of the lung show intense immunostaining for vimentin. (×200)

(evaluated in one case). In my experience with six cases, five showed immunostaining for vimentin (Fig. 11–28), and one showed coexpression of vimentin and keratin.

Inflammatory pseudotumors of lung, also referred to as *plasma cell granulomas of lung,* represent less than 1% of all lung tumors.[99] Most occur in persons younger than 40 years old, and 15% arise in persons 1 to 10 years of age.[100, 101] They cause symptoms and signs of cough, chest pain, dyspnea, hemoptysis, clubbing, and fever. Radiographically, they are usually circumscribed but may be irregularly shaped. Pathologically, they are yellowish white and well-circumscribed and can infiltrate normal lung tissue, causing its destruction. Histologically, they are composed of mature plasma cells, macrophages, including multinucleated histiocytic giant cells, lymphocytes, mast cells, neutrophils and spindle-shaped cells. The differential pathologic diagnoses usually include sclerosing hemangioma, malignant fibrous histiocytoma, malignant plasmacytoma and reactive lymphoid proliferation. Immunohistochemically, the plasma cells show polyclonal expression of light-chain immunoglobulin. The spindle cells usually stain as myofibroblasts expressing vimentin and actin, with rare cases in which the spindle cells express keratin. These tumors can be invasive and resemble low-grade sarcomas.[102, 103] Expression of tumor suppressor gene product p53 has been reported helpful in differentiating sarcoma from inflammatory pseudotumor,[104] although this finding has been controversial in differentiating other inflammatory conditions from neoplasms, for example, fibrosing pleuritis versus desmoplastic mesotheliomas. Cytogenetic clonal changes have been reported in inflammatory pseudotumor of lung.[105]

VARIABILITIES AND PITFALLS

Squamous cell carcinomas of lung can show a variety of histologic forms and can be poorly differentiated. Small cell squamous carcinomas of the lung can be confused with small cell neuroendocrine carcinomas. These two neoplasms are contrasted in Table 11–5. The main difference is that small cell squamous carcinomas do not express neuroendocrine markers and usually express high molecular weight keratin and show no immunostaining for TTF-1, whereas small cell neuroendocrine carcinomas typically express neuroendocrine markers, do not show immunostaining for high molecular weight keratin, show punctate immunostaining for low molecular weight keratin, and express TTF-1 in a high percentage of cases.

Squamous carcinomas frequently show spindle cell features. The neoplastic spindle squamous cells often coexpress keratin and vimentin. Some spindle cell squamous carcinomas express predominantly vimentin and relatively small amounts of keratin.

Basaloid carcinoma is a relatively rare lung neoplasm[106] that may be confused with neuroendocrine carcinoma. They are frequently composed of nests of relatively undifferentiated cells with extensive necrosis and palisading of the peripheral cell layer (Fig. 11–29). They may show squamous

Table 11–5. Immunohistochemical Features of Small Cell Squamous Carcinoma of Lung and Small Cell Neuroendocrine Carcinoma of Lung

Type of Neoplasm	Low Molecular Weight Keratin	High Molecular Weight Keratin	CK5/CK6	CK7	CK20	Synaptophysin	Chromogranin A	Thyroid Transcription Factor-1
Small cell squamous cancer	−/+	+/−	+/−	N	R	N	N	N
Small cell neuroendocrine cancer	+*	N	N	R	R	+	−/+†	+

*Pattern of staining is usually punctate using antibody 35βH11.
†Pattern of staining is usually punctate.
+, almost always diffuse, strong positivity; +/−, variable staining, mostly positive; −/+, variable staining, mostly negative; R, rare cells positive; N, almost always negative.

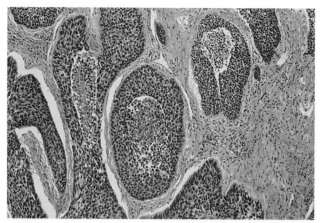

Figure 11–29. This basaloid carcinoma is composed of undifferentiated, relatively small cells and often resembles primary neuroendocrine carcinomas. (×200)

and glandular differentiation, although the degree of this differentiation is usually poorly developed. The glandular component is often composed of small cells. Basaloid carcinoma can be confused with small cell carcinoma, atypical carcinoid, and large cell neuroendocrine carcinoma. Basaloid carcinomas usually express low and high molecular weight keratin and do not express neuroendocrine markers. Basaloid carcinoma is contrasted with small cell carcinoma, atypical carcinoid, and large cell neuroendocrine carcinoma in Table 11–6.

Pulmonary adenocarcinomas are currently the most common primary lung cancer[2, 3] and show a wide range of differentiation. In most cases, pulmonary adenocarcinomas show more than one histologic pattern. Several mucinous forms of primary pulmonary carcinomas exist, including a cystic mucinous form and signet ring adenocarcinoma.

Histologically, it is often impossible to differentiate a primary mucinous pulmonary adenocarcinoma from a metastatic adenocarcinoma from the gastrointestinal (GI) tract, such as the colon. Ultrastructurally, it is also usually impossible to differentiate these neoplasms with respect to their site of origin. The immunohistochemical profile of pulmonary adenocarcinoma is contrasted with metastatic colonic adenocarcinoma in Table 11–7. In general, primary pulmonary adenocarcinoma typically expresses CK7 and TTF-1 and does not express CK20. Metastatic colonic adenocarcinoma expresses CK20 and shows no expression of CK7 or TTF-1. As stated previously, TTF-1 is the best antibody for differentiating primary pulmonary adenocarcinomas from adenocarcinomas of other sites. Approximately 60 to 75% of primary pulmonary adenocarcinomas express TTF-1.

A few primary pulmonary adenocarcinomas may show low intensity immunostaining for S-100 protein.[107] However, it is more common in primary pulmonary adenocarcinomas, especially nonmucinous bronchioloalveolar cell carcinomas, to see S-100 protein–positive dendritic cells admixed with the neoplastic cells (Fig. 11–30).[108] These S-100 protein–positive cells represent Langerhans cells (Fig. 11–31). It has been suggested that these adenocarcinomas secrete a factor that is chemotactic for the Langerhans cells.[109] Langerhans cells, however, can be seen in a wide variety of neoplasms and non-neoplastic conditions.[110]

Antibodies against surfactants are not commercially available in the United States but have been evaluated in diagnosing pulmonary adenocarcinomas. Nonmucinous bronchioloalveolar cell carcinomas not infrequently show intranuclear inclusions that are periodic acid–Schiff (PAS)–diastase positive (Fig. 11–32).[111–114] The intranuclear PAS-positive inclusions immunostain for the apoprotein portion of surfactant (Fig. 11–33). When examined

Table 11–6. Immunohistochemical Features of Basaloid Carcinoma of Lung Compared with Small Cell Carcinoma, Atypical Carcinoid, and Large Cell Neuroendocrine Carcinoma of Lung

Type of Tumor	Low Molecular Weight Keratin	High Molecular Weight Keratin	CK7	CK20	CK5/ CK6	Synaptophysin	Chromogranin A	Carcinoembryonic Antigen	Thyroid Transcription Factor-1
Basaloid carcinoma	+/−	+/−	−/+	R	+/−	N	N	−/+	−/+
Small cell carcinoma	+	N	R	N	N	+	−/+	+/−	+/−
Atypical carcinoid	+/−	+/−	R	N	N	+/−	+	−/+	+/−
Large cell neuroendocrine carcinoma	+/−	+/−	R	N	N	+/−	+	−/+	+/−

+, almost always diffuse, strong, positive staining; +/−, variable staining, mostly positive; −/+, variable staining, mostly negative; R, rare cells positive; N, almost always negative.

Table 11–7. Immunohistochemical Features of Primary Mucinous Pulmonary Adenocarcinomas Contrasted with Metastatic Colonic Adenocarcinomas

	Antibody Directed Against					
Type of Neoplasm	CK7	CK20	CK5/CK6	Carcinoembryonic Antigen	Surfactant Apoprotein-A	Thyroid Transcription Factor-1
Primary pulmonary mucinous tumors	+/−	N	N	+	R	+/−
Metastatic colonic mucin-producing adenocarcinoma	N	+/−	N	+	N	N

+, almost always diffuse, strong positivity; +/−, variable staining, mostly positive; −/+, variable staining, mostly negative; R, rare cells positive; N, almost always negative.

ultrastructurally, these intranuclear inclusions consist of 45-nm-diameter tubules that attach to the inner nuclear membrane (Fig. 11–34).

Surfactant antibodies are not 100% specific for surfactant-producing pulmonary adenocarcinomas. Bejarano and colleagues[14] used immunohistochemical markers to distinguish between primary non–small cell lung carcinoma and metastatic breast carcinoma. They studied 57 primary non–small cell lung cancers, including 46 adenocarcinomas and 51 adenocarcinomas of the breast. They found surfactant protein A, surfactant protein B, and TTF-1 in 49%, 53%, and 63% of non–small cell pulmonary carcinomas, respectively, and 54%, 63%, and 76% of primary pulmonary adenocarcinomas, respectively. Squamous cell lung carcinomas rarely stained with these antibodies. Fifty-one breast carcinomas showed no immunostaining for TTF-1 and surfactant B, although four breast cancers immunostained for surfactant A.

The lung is the site of numerous metastatic neoplasms, and pathologists must be acutely aware of this.[115, 116] Metastatic neoplasms to lung are more common than primary tumors. The problem with differentiating primary from metastatic lung neoplasms is compounded by the frequently similar histologic appearances of the primary and metastatic lung neoplasms. Adenocarcinomas as a group present the greatest challenge to differentiating primary from metastatic lesions. Metastatic tumors to the lung always have to be considered when making a diagnosis of primary lung cancer, even when considering solitary pulmonary nodules.

As discussed by me[9] and others,[117] antibodies against CK7 and CK20 are helpful in distinguishing primary from metastatic carcinoma, although they are not specific. Many GI tract cancers, a few renal cell carcinomas, gynecologic neoplasms, and bladder neoplasms express CK7. TTF-1 is the most specific antibody in identifying pulmonary adenocarcinoma but is negative in about 25 to 40% of cases.

Carcinomas of breast frequently metastasize to pleura and lung, often many years after the initial

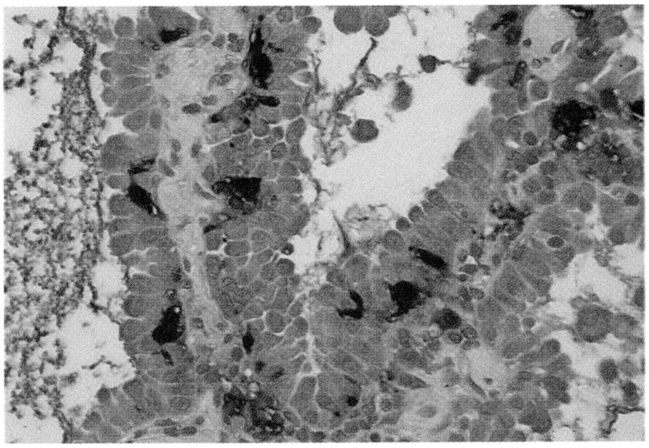

Figure 11–30. This nonmucinous bronchioloalveolar cell carcinoma shows numerous S-100 protein–positive dendritic cells admixed with the tumor cells. (×400)

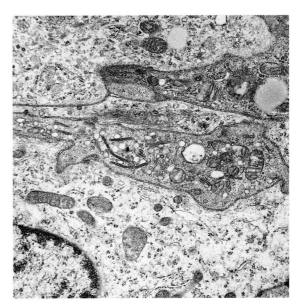

Figure 11–31. Ultrastructurally, the S-100 protein–positive cells represent Langerhans cells. These cells are antigen presenting-processing macrophages that contain peculiar cytoplasmic organelles referred to as *Langerhans cell granules* or *Birbeck granules.* (×20,000)

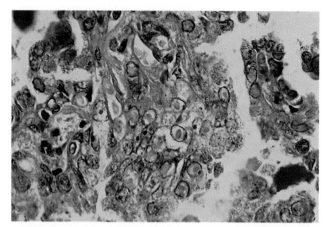

Figure 11–32. This nonmucinous bronchioloalveolar cell carcinoma shows intranuclear periodic acid–Schiff (PAS)-positive inclusions. (×400)

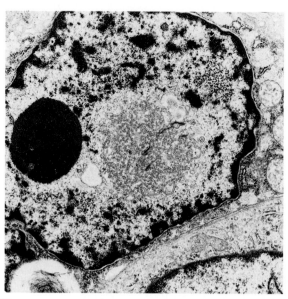

Figure 11–34. Ultrastructurally, the intranuclear inclusions are composed of 45-nm-diameter tubules that connect to the inner nuclear membrane. (×20,000)

diagnosis. Ollayos and associates[118] evaluated the sensitivity of estrogen receptor protein by immunohistochemistry in known cases of adenocarcinoma of colon, pancreas, and lung. Forty-three colonic adenocarcinomas and 18 pancreatic adenocarcinomas showed no nuclear immunostaining for estrogen receptor proteins, whereas 3 of 42 primary pulmonary adenocarcinomas immunostained for estrogen receptor protein.

Canver and colleagues[119] studied sex hormone receptor expression by immunohistochemistry in 64 non–small cell lung cancers. Specimens were stated to have been acetone-fixed. They found no immunostaining for sex hormone receptors in normal lung. However, 62 of 64 non–small cell lung carcinomas showed nuclear immunostaining for estrogen receptor protein. Immunostaining for progesterone receptor protein was negative in 50 cases (78%) and weakly positive in 14 cases (22%).

Bacchi and coworkers[120] reported expression of nuclear estrogen and progesterone receptor pro-

teins in a few pulmonary carcinoids and small cell carcinomas.

I have not observed estrogen or progesterone receptors by immunohistochemistry in 50 primary non–small cell lung cancers using heat epitope antigen retrieval. A few cases of small cell carcinoma have shown nuclear estrogen and progesterone receptor protein expression (Fig. 11–35).

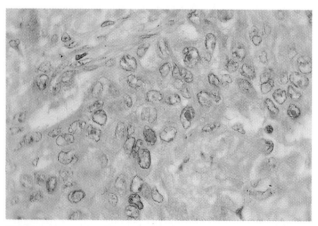

Figure 11–33. The intranuclear inclusions in nonmucinous bronchioloalveolar cell carcinomas immunostain for the apoprotein portion of surfactant A. (×400)

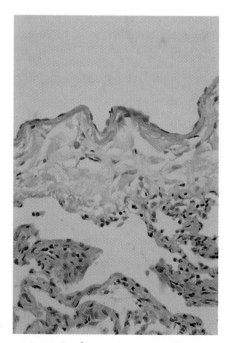

Figure 11–35. In the resting state, the normal pleura is composed of a slightly flattened layer of mesothelial cells with underlying spindle cells, collagen, and elastic tissue. (×200)

The immunophenotype of large cell undifferentiated neoplasms of lung is unpredictable. Most such neoplasms are carcinomas and coexpress keratin and vimentin. Some express only vimentin. There are large cell neoplasms that look like carcinomas but, in fact, are not. Another area of potential confusion is related to observations that non-neuroendocrine, non–small cell carcinomas as determined by histologic appearances express neuroendocrine markers by immunohistochemistry.

Lymphoepithelioma-like carcinoma may occur as a primary lung cancer composed of large anaplastic cells and may be confused with lymphomas and other neoplasms.[121] Most express low and high molecular weight keratins and show ultrastructural features of epithelial differentiation, including desmosomes and intracellular tonofilaments.

Giant cell carcinomas of lung are a subtype of large cell undifferentiated carcinoma composed of at least 40% of cells greater than 40 μm in diameter.[122] They usually coexpress keratin and vimentin. They must be differentiated from metastatic sarcomas and melanomas. Some show cytoplasmic immunostaining for CEA.

Some large cell anaplastic lymphomas have an epithelioid appearance and show immunostaining for keratin.[123] Most Ki-1 (CD30)–positive anaplastic lymphomas express EMA.[124] Some large cell anaplastic lymphomas have ultrastructural features suggesting epithelial differentiation.[125]

As known by most surgical pathologists, malignant melanomas may show significant variability in differentiation. Nearly all show immunostaining for S-100 protein and vimentin, and approximately 50% immunostain for human melanoma black-45 antigen. Rare melanomas immunostain for keratin,[126] which can cause diagnostic confusion.

A list of large cell undifferentiated neoplasms and their immunophenotypes is shown in Table 11–8.

The mediastinum contains a variety of neoplasms, including those of germ cell origin. It can occasionally be difficult to determine if a neoplasm is primary in the lung invading the mediastinum or primary in the mediastinum invading the lung. In addition, thymic carcinomas may show significant variability in differentiation, including cases that show germ cell differentiation. This problem can be compounded because primary lung cancers have been reported to express germ cell markers. Yoshimoto and colleagues[127] reported a case of a poorly differentiated mucin-producing primary pulmonary neoplasm whose tumor cells showed immunostaining for CEA, alpha-fetoprotein, and human chorionic gonadotropin. Autopsy tissue showed these substances in different tumor cells, which the authors interpreted to suggest that the lung cancer consisted of at least three clones of cancer cells with different phenotypes. Kuida and colleagues[128] found human chorionic gonadotropin

expression in 4 of 11 primary lung cancers. The application of TTF-1 would potentially help clarify some cases with respect to a primary mediastinal or pulmonary origin of the neoplasm.

Non–small cell primary lung neoplasms may show neuroendocrine differentiation. This can cause confusion if the neoplasm being evaluated is considered histologically to have features suggestive of a non-neuroendocrine tumor. Visscher and associates[129] evaluated 56 poorly differentiated non–small cell primary lung neoplasms with monoclonal antibodies directed against chromogranin A, synaptophysin, S-100 protein, keratin, vimentin, and neurofilament antigen. These investigators stated that these neoplasms showed no histologic features of neuroendocrine differentiation. Using frozen, unfixed tissue sections, 5 of 17 (29%) large cell undifferentiated carcinomas and 4 of 19 (21%) adenocarcinomas showed immunostaining for chromogranin A or synaptophysin. Diffuse intense immunostaining for synaptophysin was observed in two large cell undifferentiated carcinomas and one poorly differentiated adenocarcinoma. One of 20 (5%) poorly differentiated squamous carcinomas expressed synaptophysin. Ten of 17 (58.8%) large cell undifferentiated carcinomas and 10 of 19 (52.6%) poorly differentiated adenocarcinomas expressed vimentin or neurofilament antigen. The authors concluded that immunohistologic evidence of neuroendocrine differentiation was observed in a significant number of large cell undifferentiated carcinomas and poorly differentiated adenocarcinomas and was accompanied by heterogeneous intermediate filament expression. I have not evaluated neurofilament expression in undifferentiated or poorly differentiated primary lung carcinomas, but more than half of such neoplasms coexpress keratin and vimentin, even if they do not show neuroendocrine differentiation by immunohistochemistry.

Linnoila and colleagues[130] evaluated 113 surgically resected primary lung neoplasms with antibodies against chromogranin A, Leu7, neuron-specific enolase, serotonin, bombesin, calcitonin, adrenocorticotropic hormone (ACTH), vasopressin, neurotensin, CEA, keratin, vimentin, and neurofilament using formalin-fixed, paraffin-embedded sections. They observed that the majority of carcinoids and small cell carcinomas expressed multiple neuroendocrine markers in a high percentage of tumor cells and that approximately 50% of non–small cell lung carcinomas contained subpopulations of tumor cells expressing neuroendocrine markers. They found occasional non–small cell lung carcinomas that showed immunostaining patterns indistinguishable from small cell carcinoma. They found neuroendocrine markers to be expressed more frequently in large cell undifferentiated carcinomas and in adenocarcinomas than in squamous carcinomas.

Mooi and associates[131] evaluated 11 resected primary lung neoplasms classified as large cell carci-

284

Table 11–8. Immunohistochemical Features of Various Types of Large Cell Undifferentiated Neoplasms of Lung

Type of Neoplasm	AE1/AE3	Low Molecular Weight Keratin	High Molecular Weight Keratin	CK7	CK20	Vimentin	Epithelial Membrane Antigen	Carcinoembryonic Antigen	S-100 Protein	HMB-45	CD30	CD20	Neuron-Specific Enolase	Synaptophysin	Chromogranin A
Large cell undifferentiated carcinoma of lung	+	+	+/−	+/−	N	−/+	+/−	−/+	R	N	N	N	−/+	R	R
Giant cell carcinoma of lung	+	+	+/−	+/−	N	−/+	+/−	−/+	R	N	N	N	−/+	R	R
Lymphoepithelioma–like carcinoma of lung	+/−	−/+	+/−	−/+	N	−/+	−/+	−/+	R	N	N	N	R	R	R
Large cell neuroendocrine carcinoma	+/−	+/−	+/−	−/+	N	−/+	−/+	−/+	R	N	N	N	+	+	+/−
Malignant melanoma	R	R	R	R	N	+	R	R	−/+	+/−	R	N	−/+	R	R
Anaplastic lymphoma	R	R	R	N	N	+/−	+/−	R	R	N	+/−	+/−	R	N	N

+, almost always diffuse, strong positivity; +/−, variable staining, mostly positive; −/+, variable staining, mostly negative; R, rare cells positive; N, almost always negative.

noma or squamous cell carcinoma but showing some microscopic resemblance to bronchial carcinoid and small cell carcinoma. All cases were neuron-specific enolase− and protein gene product 9.5−positive, which the authors stated indicated neuroendocrine differentiation. Bombesin and chromogranin were positive in two cases each and C-terminal peptide was expressed in five cases. In six of seven cases evaluated by electron microscopy, dense core neuroendocrine granules were observed. Based on the published photographs of the neoplasms, one might argue that the neoplasms reported represented mixed neuroendocrine−nonneuroendocrine tumors.

Wick and colleagues[132] compared 12 large cell carcinomas of lung showing neuroendocrine differentiation with 15 large cell pulmonary neoplasms showing no neuroendocrine differentiation. From the data presented, the large cell neoplasms showing neuroendocrine differentiation would have been classified by Travis and colleagues'[33] criteria as large cell neuroendocrine carcinomas and not as large cell undifferentiated carcinomas showing focal neuroendocrine differentiation. Of interest and potential importance, the large cell neoplasms with neuroendocrine differentiation had a significantly worse prognosis than did those that did not show neuroendocrine differentiation. The authors suggested that because immunohistochemistry and electron microscopy were necessary to diagnose such neoplasms, they were probably underdiagnosed. Some medical oncologists suggest that all large cell carcinomas of lung be evaluated for neuroendocrine differentiation because of differences in chemotherapeutic treatment. This may or may not be appropriate based on a study discussed further on.

Loy and colleagues[133] evaluated 66 neoplasms that had been examined ultrastructurally with a battery of neuroendocrine markers, including neuron-specific enolase, chromogranin A, Leu7, and synaptophysin, and with a non-neuroendocrine marker B72.3. They studied 11 small cell carcinomas, 4 low-grade neuroendocrine carcinomas (? atypical carcinoids), 2 large cell carcinomas with neuroendocrine differentiation (? large cell neuroendocrine carcinomas), 26 adenocarcinomas, 10 squamous cell carcinomas, and 11 large cell undifferentiated carcinomas. Four of 10 squamous carcinomas, 3 of 26 adenocarcinomas, and 1 of 11 large cell undifferentiated carcinomas showed immunostaining for chromogranin A. Zero of 10 squamous carcinomas, 4 of 26 adenocarcinomas, and 0 of 11 large cell undifferentiated carcinomas showed immunostaining for Leu7. Six of 10 squamous carcinomas, 15 of 26 adenocarcinomas, and 7 of 11 large cell undifferentiated carcinomas showed immunostaining for neuron-specific enolase. Six of 10 squamous carcinomas, 16 of 26 adenocarcinomas, and 7 of 11 large cell undifferentiated carcinomas showed immunostaining for synaptophysin. Overall, 34 of 47 (79%) carcinomas without neuroendocrine features

expressed at least one neuroendocrine immunohistochemical marker. Nineteen of 19 (100%) neuroendocrine carcinomas expressed at least one neuroendocrine marker.

Schleusener and coworkers[134] evaluated 107 patients with stage III A, stage III B, and stage IV non−small cell lung carcinomas (62 adenocarcinomas, 22 squamous cell carcinomas, 18 large cell carcinomas, 5 adenosquamous carcinomas) immunohistochemically with antibodies against keratin, synaptophysin, Leu7, and chromogranin A. Keratin was used as a control and was positive in 99.1% of cases. Thirty-five percent of adenocarcinomas, 41% of squamous cell carcinomas, and 33% of large cell carcinomas expressed at least one neuroendocrine marker. Somewhat surprising was the finding of increased survival in patients whose tumors expressed one or more neuroendocrine markers; however, there was no correlation between neuroendocrine markers and response to chemotherapy.

The bottom line for pathologists is that lung neoplasms that are not classified by histologic criteria as being neuroendocrine neoplasms may express neuroendocrine markers by immunohistochemistry. A summary of these studies showing the frequency of expression of chromogranin A, synaptophysin, neuron-specific enolase, and Leu7 is shown in Figure 11−36.

PLEURAL NEOPLASMS

Neoplasms of the pleura are relatively common, and more metastatic tumors than primary tumors involve the pleura.[116, 135] The differentiation of primary from metastatic pleural neoplasms is an area that has received extensive attention in the discipline of immunohistochemistry. In part, this has been due to an emergence of a marked increase in the understanding of the biology of serosal membranes and the pathology-pathobiology of mesotheliomas.

The celomic cavity develops relatively early in embryogenesis and gives rise to the pleural, peritoneal, and pericardial cavities by partitioning membranes that divide this cavity.[136] Mesotheliomas arise from the serosal tissue of the body cavities. Except for a cohort of insulators studied by Selikoff and colleagues,[137] pleural mesotheliomas account for approximately 90% of all mesotheliomas.

Pleural mesotheliomas show a wide range of histologic differentiation, although they can be divided into four major subtypes: (1) epithelial, (2) sarcomatoid (fibrous, sarcomatous), (3) biphasic, and (4) desmoplastic (a variant of a sarcomatoid mesothelioma).

Immunohistochemistry is the predominant technique used for diagnosing mesotheliomas accurately and differentiating them from primary lung cancers that invade the pleura and from primary lung cancers and neoplasms outside the chest cav-

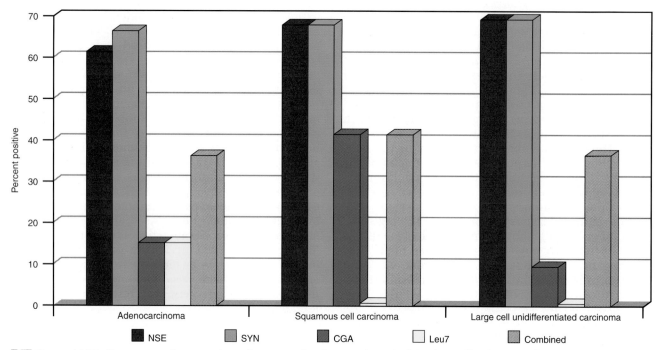

Figure 11-36. Summary of expression of neuroendocrine markers in histologically diagnosed non-neuroendocrine neoplasms. NSE, neuron-specific enolase; SYN, synaptophysin; CGA, chromogranin A.

ity that metastasize to pleura. The four major histologic types of pleural mesothelioma represent a marked oversimplification. For example, there are several different subtypes of epithelial mesotheliomas, including tubulopapillary, histiocytoid, glandular, microcystic, adenoidcystic, signet ring, solid, small cell, large cell, and mesotheliomas composed of relatively pleomorphic large cells. A well-differentiated papillary form of mesothelioma exists primarily in the peritoneal cavity and rarely in the pleural cavity, and it is important to recognize because unlike other mesotheliomas it is usually clinically benign or has a low malignant potential.[138] In addition, serosal membranes are extremely reactive tissues and show a variety of changes when injured, which can be misinterpreted as malignant.[139] Immunohistochemistry is usually not helpful diagnostically in differentiating atypical reactive pleural processes from malignant ones, but it is helpful in identifying the cells in these processes as either epithelial mesothelial cells or pleural spindle cells.

The biology and morphology of the normal pleura has been studied extensively. In the resting state, the pleura is composed of a layer of relatively flattened epithelial mesothelial cells that are separated from the underlying connective tissue components by a basement membrane (see Fig. 11–35). The sub–basement membrane cells are spindle-shaped and are associated with elastic tissue and collagen that is best seen in elastic tissue–stained sections (see Fig. 11–35). Epithelial mesothelial cells and pleural spindle cells show a marked reaction to injury and an increase in number and size (Fig. 11–37). The pleural spindle cells are interesting in that,

by immunohistochemistry, they express keratin, vimentin, actin, and calretinin (Fig. 11–38), and ultrastructurally they have the appearance of myofibroblasts (Fig. 11–39). In 1986, my colleagues and I[140] extensively studied the pleura and its reaction to injury and related the histologic, immunohistochemical, and ultrastructural features of mesotheliomas to the reactive pleural cells. Although doubted by some, there is evidence that epithelial mesothelial cells are derived from a proliferation of sub–basement membrane spindle cells that differentiate into epithelial-mesothelial cells. We named these cells *multipotential-subserosal cells.*

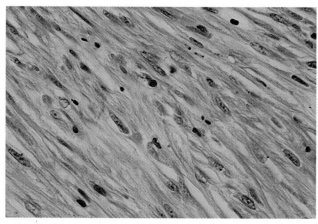

Figure 11–37. When injured, the pleura shows hypertrophy and hyperplasia of lining mesothelial cells and a proliferation of underlying spindle cells that have features of myofibroblasts. (×200)

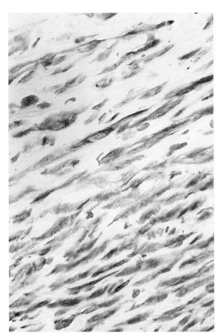

Figure 11–38. The proliferating myofibroblasts of the pleura immunostain keratin, vimentin, actin, and calretinin. (×400)

A variety of antibodies have been used to understand and help diagnose mesotheliomas. They can be divided into three main categories: (1) antibodies that are relatively specific for mesothelial cells and mesotheliomas, which when positive serve as a positive marker for mesotheliomas; (2) antibodies that show no reaction for mesothelial cells or mesotheliomas and when negative serve as a negative marker for mesotheliomas; and (3) other antibodies that may react with mesothelial cells and mesotheliomas but are relatively nonspecific.

As stated, mesotheliomas show a variety of histologic patterns and exhibit a wide range of differentiation. The selection of a panel of antibodies to evaluate a suspected mesothelioma varies depending on the type of differentiation the suspected mesothelioma shows.

The antibodies that are frequently used in diagnosing suspected mesotheliomas are listed and characterized in Table 11–9.

POSITIVE MARKERS

Keratins are found in nearly 100% of mesotheliomas. Keratin antibodies are used primarily to identify neoplastic mesothelial cells, to determine invasion in suspected mesotheliomas, to diagnose sarcomatoid mesotheliomas, and to differentiate sarcomatoid mesothelioma from sarcoma, localized fibrous tumors of the pleura, and other neoplasms that are usually keratin-negative. Low and high molecular weight keratins are detectable in most mesotheliomas, especially low molecular weight cytokeratins (CAM5.2, 35βH11). I use AE1/AE3

keratin as a screening antibody. Cytokeratin expression in mesotheliomas has been reviewed by Henderson and colleagues[141] and Ordonez.[142]

In 1985, Blobel and associates[143] reported that normal and neoplastic mesothelial cells express CK7, CK8, CK18, and CK19, which were cytokeratins typically seen in simple epithelial cells and adenocarcinomas. They found some epithelial mesotheliomas contained CK4, CK16, CK14, and CK17. In a previous publication,[144] they reported that adenocarcinomas contained CK7, CK8, CK18, and CK19 and that squamous carcinomas showed a more complex cytokeratin pattern containing simple epithelial cytokeratins (CK7, CK8, CK18, and CK19) and stratified epithelium-type keratins, specifically CK5/CK6. In 1989, Moll and coworkers[145] used antibody AE14 to demonstrate CK5 reactivity in 12 of 13 epithelial-biphasic mesotheliomas but in 0 of 21 pulmonary adenocarcinomas. They concluded that CK5 was a helpful marker to distinguish between pulmonary adenocarcinomas and epithelial-biphasic mesotheliomas. The AE14 antibody, unfortunately, did not work in paraffin-embedded tissue and it wasn't until 1997 that Clover and colleagues,[146] using commercial monoclonal antibody D5/16B4 that reacted with CK5 and CK6 in formalin-fixed, paraffin-embedded tissue, obtained reactivity in 23 of 23 (100%) epithelial mesotheliomas. Reactivity was observed in 5 of 27 (18.5%) pulmonary adenocarcinomas. In four of five (80%) pulmonary adenocarcinomas, the reactivity was described as being weak or equivocal. In one, it was described as being patchy. Ordonez and colleagues,[142] using the same antibody as did Clover and associates,[146] found positive staining in 40 of 40 (100%) epithelial mesotheliomas, 15 of 15 (100%) squamous carcinomas of lung, and in 0 of

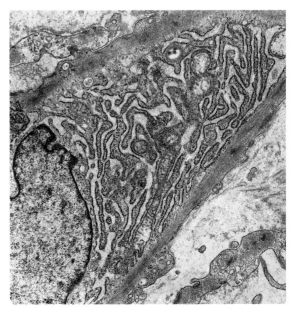

Figure 11–39. The proliferating spindle cells have ultrastructural features of myofibroblasts. (×20,000)

Table 11–9. Antibodies Used to Confirm, Eliminate, or Classify Suspected Mesotheliomas

Antibody Directed Against	Clone	Characteristics of Antigens Recognized	Immunogen	Manufacturer	Dilution	Type of Antigen Retrieval
Keratin	AE1/AE3	Keratins—Moll numbers 1–5, 6, 8, 9, 10, 14–16, 18	Human epidermal keratin	DAKO	1:200	HIER
Keratin	MAK-6	Keratins—Moll numbers 8, 14–16, 18, and 19	Extracellular antigen from MCF-tissue culture and from human sole epidermis	Zymed	1:100	HIER
Keratin	CAM5.2	Keratins—Moll numbers 8, 18	Colorectal carcinoma cell line	Becton-Dickinson	1:100	HIER
Keratin	35βH11	Keratin—Moll number 8	Hep3B hepatocellular carcinoma cell line	DAKO	1:50	HIER
Keratin CK5/CK6	34βE12	Keratins—Moll numbers 1, 5, 10, and 14	Human stratum corneum keratin	DAKO	1:100	HIER
	D5/16B4	Keratins—Moll numbers 5, 6, and to a slight degree 4	Purified CK5	Biocare Medical	1:100	HIER
CK7	OV-TL 12/30	Keratin—Moll number 7	OTN 11 ovarian carcinoma cell line	DAKO	1:100	HIER
CK20	$K_s20.8$	Keratin—Moll number 20	Villi of human duodenal mucosa	DAKO	1:50	HIER
Vimentin	Vim3B4	Intermediate filament—57 kd	Vimentin from bovine eye lens	DAKO	1:100	HIER
Alpha actin	1A4	Alpha smooth muscle isoform of actin	N-terminal decapeptide of human alpha smooth muscle actin	DAKO	1:100	HIER
Muscle-specific actin	HHF-35	42-kd protein in preparations of purified skeletal muscle actin and extracts of aorta, uterus, diaphragm, and heart	SDS extracted protein fraction of human myocardium	DAKO	1:400	HIER
Desmin	D33	53-kd intermediate filament in muscle cells, recognizing 18-kd rod piece of molecule	Desmin purified from porcine stomach	DAKO	1:80	HIER
Calretinin	—	29-kd calcium-binding protein	Human recombinant calretinin	Zymed	1:50	HIER
Mesothelioma antigen	HBME-1	Antigen present in membrane of mesothelial cells	Suspension of human mesothelial cells from malignant epithelial mesothelioma	DAKO	1:500	HIER
Thrombomodulin	1009	Transmembrane glycoprotein of 75-kd molecular weight containing 6 repeated domains homologous with epidermal growth factor	Recombinant thrombomodulin	DAKO	1:50	HIER
Epithelial membrane antigen (EMA)	E29	250- to 400-kd glycoprotein of milk fat globule protein family	Delipidated extract of human milk fat	DAKO	1:100	HIER
Human milk fat globule protein-2 (HMFG-2)	115D8	MAM-6 mucus glycoprotein of >400 kd in glycocalyx of epithelial cells	Purified human milk fat globule protein	BioGenex	1:25	HIER
N-Cadherin	389	Transmembrane glycoprotein involved in calcium-dependent cell adhesion	Intracellular domain of chicken N-cadherin	Zymed	1:100	HIER
Polyclonal carcinoembryonic antigen (pCEA)	—	CEA and CEA-like proteins including nonspecific cross-reacting substance and biliary glycoprotein	Human CEA isolated from metastatic colonic adenocarcinoma	DAKO	1:16,000	HIER
CD15 (LeuM1)	C3D-1	3-fucosyl-N-acetyllactosamine	Purified neutrophils from normal human peripheral blood	DAKO	1:20	HIER
Tumor associated glycoprotein	B72.3	Tumor-associated glycoprotein of wide variety of human adenocarcinomas	Membrane-enriched fraction of metastatic breast carcinoma	BioGenex	1:100	HIER
Human epithelial antigen	Ber-EP4	34- and 49-kd glycoproteins on the surface and in cytoplasm of most epithelial cells, except squamous epithelium, hepatocytes and parietal cells	MCF-7 cell line	DAKO	1:100	HIER

Antigen	Clone	Description	Immunogen/source	Vendor	Dilution	
Thyroglobulin	—	Thyroglobulin	Thyroglobulin from human thyroid glands	DAKO	1:16,000	HIER
Thyroid transcription factor-1 (TTF-1)	8G7C3/1	40-kd member of NKx2 family of homeodomain transcription factors	Rat TTF-1 recombinant protein	Biocare Medical	1:200	HIER
Prostate-specific antigen (PSA)	ER-PR8	33-kd prostate-specific antigen	Purified human prostate-specific antigen	DAKO	1:100	HIER
Prostatic acid phosphatase (PAP)	PASE/4LJ	52-kd human prostatic acid phosphatase	Purified prostatic acid phosphatase from human seminal plasma	DAKO	1:16,000	HIER
Human epithelial-related antigen	MOC-31	40-kd transmembrane glycoprotein present on most normal and malignant epithelial cells	Neuraminidase-treated cells from small cell carcinoma cell line	DAKO	1:50	HIER
Lewis Y antigen	BG8-F3	Difucosylated tetrasaccharide found on type 2 blood group oligosaccharide	SK-LU-3 lung cancer cell line	Signet	1:40	HIER
E-cadherin	4A2C7	Transmembrane glycoprotein in calcium-dependent cell adhesion	Recombinant protein of human E-cadherin	Zymed	1:100	HIER
Gross cystic disease fluid protein-15 (BRST-2)	D6	Pathologic secretion of breast composed of several glycoproteins including 15-kd monomer protein	Gross cystic disease fluid protein-15	Signet	1:50	HIER
Estrogen receptor protein	1D5	66-kd protein member of nuclear hormone receptor that acts as ligand-activated transcription factors	Human recombinant estrogen receptor protein	Biocare Medical	1:200	HIER
c-erb-B2 oncoprotein	—	190-kd protein product of c-erb-B2 proto-oncogene	Synthetic human c-erb-B2 oncoprotein peptide	DAKO	1:500	HIER
Human leukocyte antigen CD45	DAKO-LCA	Five or more high molecular weight glycoproteins on the surface of the majority of human leukocytes	Human peripheral blood lymphocytes maintained in T-cell growth factor	DAKO	1:200	HIER
CD20 human B-lymphocyte antigen	L26	33-kd nonglycosylated membrane-spanning protein	Human tonsil B lymphocyte	DAKO	1:800	HIER
CD3 human T-lymphocyte antigen	—	Intracytoplasmic portion of CD3 antigen	Synthetic human CD3 peptide	DAKO	1:100	HIER
CD30 Ki-1 antigen	Ber-H2	120-kd transmembrane glycoprotein	Co cell line cells	DAKO	1:20	HIER
bcl-2 oncoprotein	124	25-kd integral protein localized in mitochondria that inhibits apoptosis	Synthetic peptide sequence amino acids 41–54 of bcl-2 protein	DAKO	1:20	HIER
Neuron-specific enolase	—	Gamma subunit of enolase	Neuron-specific enolase isolated from human brain	DAKO	1:400	HIER
Chromogranin A	DAK-A3	Member of secretogranin-chromogranin class of proteins in secretory granules of endocrine and neuron cells	C-terminal 20-kd fragment of chromogranin A	DAKO	1:100	HIER
Synaptophysin	—	38-kd membrane component of neuron synaptic vesicles	Synthetic human synaptophysin peptide coupled to ovalbumin	DAKO	1:100	HIER
S-100 protein	—	S-100 protein A and B	S-100 protein isolated from cow brain	DAKO	1:3000	HIER
Melanoma antigen	HMB-45	Neuraminidase-sensitive oligosaccharide side chain of glycoconjugate in immature melanosomes	Extract of pigmented melanoma metastases from lymph nodes	DAKO	1:200	HIER
CD34	My10	105- to 120-kd single-chain transmembrane glycoprotein associated with human hematopoietic progenitor cells	CD34 antigen	Becton-Dickinson	1:50	HIER
CD31	JC/70A	100-kd glycoprotein in endothelial cells and 130-kd glycoprotein in platelets	Membrane preparation of spleen from patient with hairy cell leukemia	DAKO	1:40	HIER
Factor VIII antigen	—	Human von Willebrand factor	von Willebrand factor isolated from human plasma	DAKO	1:2000	HIER

HIER, heat-induced epitope retrieval.

30 pulmonary adenocarcinomas. Focal or weak reactivity was noted in 14 of 93 (15.1%) nonpulmonary adenocarcinomas, specifically 10 of 30 (33.3%) ovarian adenocarcinomas, 2 of 10 (20%) endometrial adenocarcinomas, 1 of 18 (5.6%) breast carcinomas, 1 of 7 (14.3%) thyroid carcinomas, 0 of 10 renal carcinomas, 0 of 10 colonic adenocarcinomas, and 0 of 8 prostatic adenocarcinomas. Cytokeratin profiles of epithelial mesothelioma, pulmonary adenocarcinoma, and squamous cell carcinoma of lung are contrasted in Table 11–10.

Kahn and colleagues[147] reported a difference in the pattern of keratin distribution in benign and malignant mesothelial cells compared with adenocarcinomas. They observed that in mesothelial cells, the keratin filaments were in a perinuclear or peripheral distribution, whereas in adenocarcinomas they showed an arborizing pattern. Kahn and colleagues'[147] report was followed by a more extensive study[148] in which 10 adenocarcinomas, 10 carcinoids, and 4 mesotheliomas were evaluated for keratin intermediate filament distribution using three monoclonal and three polyclonal antibodies against keratin. When they allowed the diaminobenzidine color reaction to proceed for less than 2 minutes, they observed a web-like pattern of reactivity in adenocarcinomas, a punctate crescentic pattern in carcinoids, and a perinuclear staining pattern in mesotheliomas. Although the perinuclear distribution of keratin intermediate filaments is common in epithelial mesotheliomas, it is not seen in all cases, and some pulmonary adenocarcinomas show a perinuclear distribution of keratin. I do not use the "distribution pattern" of keratin diagnostically.

Although 100% of epithelial mesotheliomas express keratin, the percentage of sarcomatoid mesotheliomas reported in the literature to express keratin is variable. Montag and associates[149] detected keratins in 16 of 16 (100%) sarcomatoid mesotheliomas, findings identical to Battifora,[150] who observed keratins in 100% of more than 20 sarcomatoid mesotheliomas examined. In contrast, some investigations have failed to detect keratin in more than 40% of sarcomatoid mesotheliomas.[151-158] The US-Canadian Mesothelioma Panel recognizes cases of keratin-negative sarcomatoid mesothelioma. In my experience with large samples of well-fixed autopsy tissue, keratin expression in sarcomatoid mesotheliomas can be highly variable. Some regions of a sarcomatoid mesothelioma can show intense immunostaining for keratin, and other regions of the same tumor show no keratin staining. This has been observed with "broad spectrum" keratin antibodies (AE1/AE3) and with antibodies against low molecular weight keratin (35βH11, CAM5.2).

Vimentin is a 58-kd intermediate filament found predominantly in cells of mesenchymal derivation. Although initially touted in the late 1970s and early 1980s as being useful in separating carcinomas from sarcomas, vimentin is currently observed in normal epithelial cells and in a variety of carcinomas.[159-162] In my experience, vimentin is expressed in all sarcomatoid mesotheliomas—usually intensely—and in most poorly differentiated and transitional mesotheliomas. Churg[163] reported vimentin expression in two alcohol-fixed epithelial mesotheliomas, one of which was a tubulopapillary variant. Jasani and colleagues[164] observed vimentin expression in 75% of 44 malignant mesotheliomas of all histologic types. However, 46% of 24 pulmonary adenocarcinomas also demonstrated vimentin by immunohistochemical analysis. Mullink and associates[165] found it more common for epithelial mesotheliomas than for pulmonary adenocarcinomas to coexpress keratin and vimentin. I have observed 30 to 45% of epithelial mesotheliomas to coexpress keratin and vimentin.

In my opinion, antibody against calretinin is the most specific and reproducible positive marker of epithelial mesothelioma. Calretinin is a calcium-binding protein similar to S-100 protein.[166, 167] It has a molecular weight of 29 kd and is found in the central and peripheral nervous system and in a wide spectrum of non-neural cells, including steroid-producing cells of ovaries and testes, fat cells, renal tubular epithelial cells, eccrine glands, thymic epithelial cells, and mesothelial cells. Gotzos and coworkers[168] found calretinin immunostaining in 7 of 7 (100%) epithelial mesotheliomas and in the epithelial component of 15 of 15 (100%) biphasic mesotheliomas. They found no immunostaining in sarcomatoid components of biphasic mesotheliomas or in a single case of sarcomatoid mesothelioma. The four lung adenocarcinomas evaluated showed no immunostaining for calretinin. Doglioni and associates[169] found calretinin immunostaining in 44 of 44 (100%) epithelial mesotheliomas and focal staining in 28 of 294 (9.5%) adenocarcinomas of various origins. Doglioni and colleagues[169] found positive staining in three of three (100%) sarcomatoid mesotheliomas and in the sarcomatoid component of five biphasic mesotheliomas. Studying cells in serous fluids, Barberis and associates[170] found immunostaining for calretinin in 8 of 8 (100%) epithelial mesotheliomas and low-intensity immunostaining in 3 of 13 (23.1%) adenocarcinomas. Leers and colleagues[171] observed calretinin immunostaining in 20 of 20 (100%) epithelial mesotheliomas and weak immunostaining in 1 of 21 (4.8%) adenocarcinomas.

Ordonez[172] compared two commercially available calretinin antibodies. He found calretinin immunostaining in 8 of 38 (21.1%) epithelial mesotheliomas and focal, generally weak immunostaining in 14 of 155 (9%) adenocarcinomas of various types using a calretinin antibody obtained from Zymed Laboratories (South San Francisco, CA). In contrast, 28 of 38 (73.1%) epithelial mesotheliomas and 6 of 155 (3.8%) adenocarcinomas showed immunostaining for calretinin using a calretinin antibody from CHEMICON International (Temecula, CA). In my experience using a calretinin antibody

Table 11-10. Cytokeratin Profiles of Epithelial Mesothelioma, Pulmonary Adenocarcinoma, and Squamous Cell Carcinoma of Lung

Type of Neoplasm	Cytokeratin Moll Number, Molecular Weight, and Isoelectric pH																			
	1 68 kd 7.8	2 65.5 kd 7.8	3 63 kd 7.5	4 59 kd 7.3	5 58 kd 7.4	6 56 kd 7.8	7 54 kd 6.0	8 52.5 kd 6.1	9 64 kd 5.4	10 56.5 kd 5.3	11 56 kd 5.3	12 55 kd 4.9	13 54 kd 5.1	14 50 kd 5.3	15 50 kd 4.9	16 48 kd 5.1	17 46 kd 5.1	18 45 kd 5.7	19 40 kd 5.2	20 46 kd 5.2
Primary pulmonary adenocarcinoma	N	N	N	N	N	N	+/-	+/-	N	N	N	N	N	N	N	N	N	+/-	+/-	R
Epithelial mesothelioma	N	N	N	N	+/-	+/-	+/-	+/-	N	N	N	N	N	+/-	N	N	+/-	+/-	+/-	R
Primary pulmonary squamous cell carcinoma	N	N	N	+/-	+/-	+/-	R	-/+	N	N	N	N	N	+/-	-/+	-/+	+/-	-/+	+/-	R

+, almost always diffuse, strong positivity; +/-, variable staining, mostly positive; -/+, variable staining, mostly negative; R, rare cells positive; N, almost always negative.

from Biocare (Walnut Creek, CA), 198 of 210 (94%) epithelial mesotheliomas showed immunostaining for calretinin. As with S-100 protein, the immunostaining pattern for calretinin is in a cytoplasmic and nuclear distribution (Fig. 11–40). It should be noted that reactive, multipotential subserosal spindle cells express calretinin.

The use of the ME1 antibody was initially reported by O'Hara and colleagues[173] in 1990. ME1 is a monoclonal antibody generated from the mesothelial cell line SPC111 and reacted with normal mesothelial cells and malignant epithelial mesotheliomas. This antibody was useful only on frozen section tissue and showed immunostaining of 40 of 40 (100%) epithelial mesotheliomas. Nineteen well and moderately differentiated primary pulmonary adenocarcinomas failed to stain with the ME1 antibody, but one poorly differentiated pulmonary adenocarcinoma showed intense immunostaining. As reviewed by Sheibani and colleagues,[174] Battifora produced an ME1 monoclonal antibody designated HBME-1 that worked in paraffin-embedded, formalin-fixed tissue. As reported by these authors, this antibody showed immunostaining of a relatively high percentage of epithelial mesotheliomas in a cell membrane distribution (Fig. 11–41). In my experience, the intensity of this reaction varies from one case to another. DAKO Product Specification Sheet states that 17 of 19 (89.5) epithelial mesotheliomas showed immunostaining for HBME-1, but the antibody also reacted with 19 of 50 (38%) adenocarcinomas. The specification sheet suggested using the antibody at a dilution of 1:100. In my experience, the antibody should be used at a much greater dilution (1:7500 in our laboratory). Henderson and coworkers[141] use HBME-1 antibody in a dilution between 1:5000 and 1:15,000. They found that when lower dilutions were used, the cytoplasm of many mesotheliomas stained and that a significant number of adenocarcinomas showed cytoplasmic immunostaining. These findings indi-

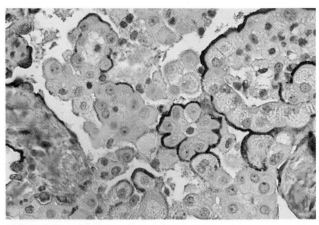

Figure 11–41. Most well to moderately well differentiated epithelial mesotheliomas show thick cell membrane immunostaining for HBME-1. (×400)

cate that HBME-1 should be used at a high dilution to be effective for differentiating epithelial mesotheliomas from other neoplasms. I have not found HBME-1 to be useful in diagnosing sarcomatoid mesotheliomas and have rarely found it to immunostain adenocarcinomas. This antibody reacts with respiratory epithelium and occasionally shows cell membrane staining of primary pulmonary squamous cell carcinomas.

EMA and human milk fat globule protein-2 (HMFG-2) are glycoproteins of high molecular weight (250 to 400 kd) and are known as human milk fat globule proteins. These glycoproteins are in milk fat and in a variety of normal and neoplastic epithelial cells. Antibodies against EMA and HMFG-2 are of use in diagnosing epithelial mesotheliomas in that the majority of epithelial mesotheliomas show immunostaining in a cell membrane distribution. This is different from most adenocarcinomas and other carcinomas, which usually show cytoplasmic immunostaining. My colleagues and I[175] detected EMA in 50 of 64 (78.1%) epithelial mesotheliomas, in 37 of 60 (61.7%) adenocarcinomas, and in 8 of 19 (42%) squamous cell carcinomas. Walz and Koch[176] demonstrated EMA expression in 33 of 44 epithelial mesotheliomas. Wick and associates[177] found immunostaining in 43 of 51 (84%) epithelial mesotheliomas. As stated, antigen is concentrated in the cell membrane and, in most well to moderately well differentiated epithelial mesotheliomas, produces a "thick" reaction (Fig. 11–42) because of the extensive microvillus surface of epithelial mesotheliomas. Henderson and colleagues[178] demonstrated strong cell surface EMA staining in epithelial mesotheliomas and found immunostaining in a surface distribution in some lymphoid cells. It is my experience that most reactive (benign) epithelial mesothelial cells show no immunostaining for EMA or HMFG-2. I have found relatively intense EMA and HMFG-2 cell membrane staining in cases of nonmucinous bronchioloalveolar cell

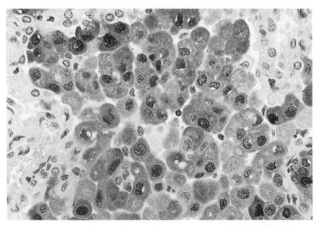

Figure 11–40. Most well and moderately well differentiated epithelial mesotheliomas and a few sarcomatoid mesotheliomas show cytoplasmic and nuclear immunostaining for calretinin. (×400)

carcinomas and in some renal papillary adenocarcinomas.

Thrombomodulin is a plasma membrane–related glycoprotein that has anticoagulant activity. Thrombomodulin antigen is found in several cell types, including mesangial cells, synovial cells, mesothelial cells, endothelial cells, megakaryocytes, and some squamous epithelial cells. Fink and coworkers[179] demonstrated immunostaining for thrombomodulin in eight epithelial mesotheliomas and two mesothelial cell lines. The cell lines were shown by in situ hybridization to possess messenger RNA for thrombomodulin. In contrast, 14 of 15 (93.3%) adenocarcinomas were negative for thrombomodulin, and one showed focal positivity. Collins and coworkers[180] found thrombomodulin expression in 31 of 31 (100%) epithelial mesotheliomas and 4 of 48 (8.3%) pulmonary adenocarcinomas. In contrast, Brown and colleagues[181] observed only 60% of epithelial and biphasic mesotheliomas to express thrombomodulin, whereas 58% of pulmonary adenocarcinomas showed positivity. Ascoli and colleagues[182] identified thrombomodulin in 33 of 33 (100%) epithelial mesotheliomas, in reactive mesothelial cells in 35 effusions, and in 57 of 145 (39.3%) carcinomas in effusions. They reported a different immunohistochemical pattern of staining in benign reactive mesothelial cells, malignant epithelial mesotheliomas, and carcinomas. In benign reactive mesothelial cells, thin linear staining was observed. Thick membrane staining was seen in malignant epithelial mesotheliomas, and cytoplasmic staining was observed in cases of carcinoma.

Cadherins are a family of adhesion proteins important in sorting cells into specialized tissues during morphogenesis.[183, 184] Included in the cadherin family are epithelial (E) cadherin, nerve (N) cadherin, retina (R) cadherin, osteoblast (OB) cadherin, and placental (P) cadherin. N-cadherin is a 135,000-kd protein found in nerve cells, developing muscle cells, and mesothelial cells.[185] Peralta-

Soler and colleagues,[186] using 13A9 anti–N-cadherin monoclonal antibody on frozen sections, observed strong immunoreactivity in 19 of 19 (100%) epithelial mesotheliomas and focal weak reactivity in 3 of 16 (18.8%) pulmonary adenocarcinomas. Using antigen retrieval methodology on paraffin-embedded tissue sections, Han and coworkers[187] reported 12 of 13 (92.3%) epithelial mesotheliomas to be positive for N-cadherin and 1 of 14 (7.1%) pulmonary adenocarcinomas to be positive.

Wilms' tumor suppressor gene resides on the 11p13 chromosome whose inactivation causes susceptibility to Wilms' tumor. This gene is found predominantly in tissues of mesodermal origin. Using frozen tissue sections, Amin and associates[188] observed nuclear immunostaining in 20 of 21 (95.2%) malignant mesotheliomas and in 0 of 26 nonmesothelioma tumors involving lung, including 20 primary non–small cell lung carcinomas. Kumar-Singh and associates,[189] using an antibody adaptable to formalin-fixed, paraffin-embedded tissue, found positive staining of Wilms' tumor suppressor gene products in 39 of 42 (92.9%) mesotheliomas, 2 of 2 (100%) papillary carcinomas of ovary, and 1 of 1 (100%) renal cell carcinoma. Twelve adenocarcinomas of lung, four squamous cell carcinomas of lung, eight metastatic breast adenocarcinomas, and three metastatic adenocarcinomas from colon did not express the Wilms' tumor suppressor gene products. This antibody is potentially useful in diagnosing mesotheliomas and has become commercially available. Using molecular biology techniques, WT1 transcripts were found in 23 of 26 (88.5%) mesothelioma cell lines, in 5 of 8 (62.5%) human malignant mesotheliomas, but in no non–small cell lung cancer cell lines or in a few biopsy specimens.[190]

NEGATIVE MARKERS

Of all antibodies used as exclusionary antibodies for diagnosing epithelial mesothelioma, polyclonal CEA has been used most frequently.

Carcinoembryonic antigen (CEA) is a glycoprotein of approximately 200 kd containing approximately 50% carbohydrate.[191–194] It is referred to as a family[195] and is coded by 29 genes, 18 of which are expressed: 7 belong to the CEA subgroup and 11 belong to the pregnancy-specific subgroup.

Often referred to as an oncofetal antigen, CEA is expressed in normal adult tissues and in a variety of epithelial neoplasms. The CEA subgroup includes biliary glycoprotein and nonspecific cross-reacting substance. The antibody I use is polyclonal and the immunogen is CEA isolated from hepatic metastases of a colonic adenocarcinoma. The antibody reacts with nonspecific cross-reacting substance and biliary glycoprotein. Nonspecific cross-reacting substance is present in granulocytes and monocytes, and biliary glycoprotein is ex-

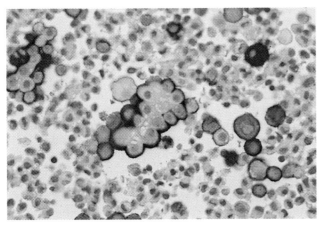

Figure 11–42. Most well to moderately well differentiated epithelial mesotheliomas show thick cell membrane staining for epithelial membrane antigen. (×400)

pressed by a large number of normal epithelial cells and by granulocytes, lymphocytes, and possibly endothelial cells. Therefore, it is likely that there is built-in positive control staining in most tissue sections.

CEA is negative in most epithelial mesotheliomas.[196-198] In contrast, it is found in a high percentage (85 to 100%) of pulmonary adenocarcinomas. Henderson and colleagues[178] analyzed data from 21 separate reports evaluating 598 cases of diffuse malignant mesothelioma and found 58 cases (9.7%) reported to express CEA. In the majority of cases in which a positive reaction was observed, it was usually focal and weak. In the same analysis, 359 of 404 (88.9%) pulmonary adenocarcinomas expressed CEA. I have observed CEA-positive staining in mesotheliomas only rarely, and it has occurred predominantly in those epithelial mesotheliomas that were "mucin"-positive, which correlated with those producing large quantities of hyaluronic acid or proteoglycan. In my experience, polyclonal CEA is the best negative marker of mesothelioma.

LeuM1 is a monoclonal antibody against the membrane-related trisaccharide fucosyl-*N*-acetyl-lactosamine on myelomonocytic cells, where the epitope is also known as CD15 or X-hapten. LeuM1 is found in Reed-Sternberg cells in some cases of Hodgkin's lymphoma. In 1985, Sheibani and Battifora[199] reported LeuM1 in a metastatic, poorly differentiated pulmonary adenocarcinoma. In 1986, Sheibani and colleagues[200] performed immunohistochemical analyses on 400 malignant neoplasms and found LeuM1 immunostaining in 105 of 179 (58.7%) adenocarcinomas and 0 of 18 epithelial mesotheliomas. They subsequently studied 50 primary pulmonary adenocarcinomas and 28 pleural epithelial mesotheliomas, finding expression in 47 of 50 (94%) pulmonary adenocarcinomas and 0 of 28 epithelial mesotheliomas.[201] In another study, Sheibani and associates[202] reported no immunostaining for LeuM1 in 127 cases of malignant mesothelioma. Wick and colleagues[177] identified LeuM1 in 52 of 52 (100%) pulmonary adenocarcinomas and 0 of 51 epithelial mesotheliomas. In contrast, Otis and associates[203] observed immunostaining in only 50% of pulmonary adenocarcinomas and reported LeuM1 expression in epithelial mesotheliomas. Battifora and McCaughey[138] observed focal LeuM1 expression in epithelial mesotheliomas. I have observed several LeuM1-positive epithelial mesotheliomas, the staining usually being focal. In contrast to what has been reported in the literature and despite using heat-induced antigen retrieval, I have observed a positive reaction in only approximately 50% of primary pulmonary adenocarcinomas.

B72.3 is an antibody that recognizes a high molecular weight glycoprotein complex, tumor-associated glycoprotein 72 (TAG-72), derived from a membrane-enriched fraction of human metastatic breast carcinoma. Szpak and coworkers[204] and Or-

donez[205] reported positive immunostaining in 38 of 45 (84.4%) adenocarcinomas of lung compared with 1 of 38 (2.6%) epithelial mesotheliomas. Wick and associates[177] reported that 43 of 52 (82.6%) pulmonary adenocarcinomas expressed B72.3, whereas all 51 epithelial mesotheliomas were negative. In an evaluation of peritoneal mesotheliomas and serous papillary adenocarcinomas of the peritoneum, Bollinger and coworkers[206] reported 43 of 46 (93.4%) serous papillary carcinomas positive for B72.3, whereas 8 epithelial mesotheliomas were negative. Ordonez[142] tabulated the reported literature, finding 69 of 684 (10.1%) epithelial mesotheliomas to show immunostaining for B72.3 (0 to 48% of cases) and 578 of 607 (95.2%) adenocarcinomas to show positivity (47 to 100%). When positive for B72.3, epithelial mesotheliomas usually show only a small percentage of cells to be positive. However, Henderson and associates[141] reported more extensive expression of B72.3 in the cytoplasm of epithelial mesotheliomas and described one case of intracytoplasmic crescentic staining that correlated ultrastructurally with intracytoplasmic glycogen.

BerEP4 is a monoclonal antibody that recognizes the protein moiety of two glycopolypeptides (34- and 39-kd) on human epithelial cells. Latza and colleagues[207] observed BerEP4 reactivity in 142 of 144 (98.6%) adenocarcinomas from various sites and in 0 of 14 epithelial mesotheliomas. Sheibani and associates[208] observed BerEP4 immunoreactivity in 1 of 115 (0.86%) epithelial mesotheliomas and 72 of 83 (86.7%) adenocarcinomas at various sites. Eight of 25 breast carcinomas and 3 renal cell carcinomas studied were negative for BerEP4. Gaffey and colleagues[209] found different results. They reported 103 of 120 (83%) adenocarcinomas to be positive. Ten of 49 (20%) epithelial mesotheliomas were also reactive, as were 2 of 9 (22%) adenomatoid tumors. Gaffey and colleagues[210] reported one epithelial mesothelioma to be diffusely positive. Staining for BerEP4 was usually in a cell membrane distribution. A possible explanation for the difference in these results is that Sheibani and associates[208] used protease type 14 predigestion before BerEP4 staining, whereas Souhami and associates[211] used 0.4% pepsin predigestion for 30 minutes before staining. My colleagues and I currently use heat-induced epitope retrieval and observe approximately 20% of epithelial mesotheliomas to show predominantly low-intensity cell membrane staining. Ordonez[142] listed published studies of BerEP4 reactivity in epithelial mesotheliomas and adenocarcinomas of various types. Seventy-six of 611 (12.4%) epithelial mesotheliomas (0 to 88%) and 940 of 1399 (67.2%) adenocarcinomas (35 to 100%) immunostained for BerEP4.

MOC31 is a monoclonal antibody that reacts with a 38-kd epithelial-associated transmembrane glycoprotein of small cell lung carcinoma known as epithelial glycoprotein-2.[210, 211] MOC31 activity was reported by DeLeij and colleagues[212] in all pulmonary carcinomas, including 28 of 28 (100%) adenocarcinomas. Normal mesothelial cells and neoplastic epithelial mesothelial cells did not react with the antibody. In 1991, Delahaye and associates[213] studied cytologic preparations of serous fluid and found positive MOC31 staining in 2 of 24 (8.3%) epithelial mesotheliomas and in 18 of 31 (58.1%) adenocarcinomas of various origins. Ruitenbeek and coworkers[210] found MOC31 reactivity in 62 of 63 (98.4%) adenocarcinomas and in 0 of 5 epithelial mesotheliomas. Ordonez[214] reported intense MOC31 reactivity in 40 of 40 (100%) pulmonary adenocarcinomas, 11 of 11 (100%) colon adenocarcinomas, 20 of 21 (95.2%) ovarian adenocarcinomas, 9 of 10 (90%) breast adenocarcinomas, and 5 of 13 (38.5%) kidney adenocarcinomas. MOC31 reactivity was seen in 2 of 38 (5.3%) epithelial mesotheliomas, although the degree of staining was usually focal, involving less than 10% of cells. Ordonez[142] listed published studies of MOC31 reactivity in epithelial mesotheliomas and various types of adenocarcinomas. Immunostaining was found in 307 of 333 (92.2%) adenocarcinomas (58 to 100%) and 23 of 158 (14.6%) epithelial mesotheliomas (0 to 88%).

Monoclonal antibody BG8 reacts with SK-LU-3 lung cancer cells that recognize the blood group antigen Lewis[y]. Jordon and colleagues[215] reported reactivity in 18 of 18 (100%) pulmonary adenocarcinomas and in 7 of 30 (23.3%) epithelial mesotheliomas. Reactivity in mesotheliomas was usually focal and limited to a few cells, whereas reactivity in pulmonary adenocarcinomas was usually strong and diffuse. Riera and colleagues[216] evaluated BG8 antibody and found expression in 114 of 123 (92.7%) pulmonary adenocarcinomas and 5 of 57 (8.8%) epithelial mesotheliomas. The staining in epithelial mesotheliomas was usually focal and weak.

E-cadherin (epithelial cadherin) is a 120-kd cell adhesion molecule expressed in epithelial cells.[217, 218] Loss of E-cadherin expression is associated with a higher degree of invasiveness and an increase in malignant potential in several carcinomas, including lung cancers.[219] Peralta-Soler and associates[186] reported intense immunostaining for E-cadherin in 16 of 16 (100%) pulmonary adenocarcinomas and 8 of 19 (42.1%) epithelial mesotheliomas, with the staining usually involving only a few cells. Using formalin-fixed, heat-induced epitope antigen retrieval, 13 of 14 (92.9%) pulmonary carcinomas were positive for E-cadherin and 0 of 13 epithelial mesotheliomas were reactive. Leers and colleagues[220] reported positive reactivity in 20 of 21 (95.2%) adenocarcinomas of various origin and in 3 of 20 (15%) epithelial mesotheliomas. Ordonez,[142] using the commercially available 5H9 anti–E-cadherin antibody on sections of formalin-fixed, paraffin-embedded tissue, found reactivity in 15 of 18 (83.3%) pulmonary adenocarcinomas and 0 of 17 epithelial mesotheliomas. When Ordonez used anti–E-cadherin monoclonal antibody clone 36

(Transduction Laboratory, Lexington, KY), strong reactivity was seen in 6 of 6 (100%) epithelial mesotheliomas. It would, therefore, appear that caution must be exercised when using this antibody and that the 5H9 anti–E-cadherin antibody would be the appropriate one to use.

Blood group–related antigen expression has been used to evaluate epithelial mesotheliomas and pulmonary adenocarcinomas. Wick and colleagues[177] found ABH isoantigen expression in 35 of 52 (67.3%) adenocarcinomas and in 0 of 51 epithelial mesotheliomas. Kawai and coworkers[221] evaluated 20 epithelial, 3 biphasic, and 6 sarcomatous mesotheliomas, 5 reactive mesothelial cell lesions, and 38 well-differentiated pulmonary adenocarcinomas using ABH blood group–related antigen (BGRA-g) antibody and *Helix pomotia* agglutinin (HPAgg). The reactive mesothelial lesions and the mesotheliomas showed no expression for BGRA-g or HPAgg, irrespective of the blood group type. Positive staining for A, B, or H blood group–related antigen was seen in 40 (83%) adenocarcinomas in compatible blood group–type patients. A positive reaction for HPAgg was seen in 16 of 17 (94.1%) cases of blood type A and in all blood type AB patients. Positive staining for HPAgg was observed in 4 of 5 (80%) blood group type B patients and in 4 of 12 (33.3%) with blood group type O.

Riera and coworkers[216] used heat-induced epitope retrieval to study 268 paraffin-embedded, formalin-fixed tumors, including 57 epithelial mesotheliomas and 211 adenocarcinomas of various origin. After statistical analysis, they found that CEA, BerEP4, and BG8 were the best discriminators between adenocarcinoma and epithelial mesothelioma within the entire panel and that the mesothelioma-associated antibodies HBME-1, calretinin, and thrombomodulin were less sensitive and less specific, although they were found useful in certain cases. They observed all adenocarcinomas and mesotheliomas to show intense immunohistochemical staining for keratin with no discernible difference in staining pattern between adenocarcinoma and mesothelioma. Forty-six of 57 (81.5%) mesotheliomas and 66 of 211 (31.2%) adenocarcinomas expressed vimentin. The intensity and distribution of vimentin staining was greater in mesotheliomas than in adenocarcinomas. CEA immunoreactivity was observed in 175 of 211 (82.9%) adenocarcinomas and in no mesotheliomas. Ovarian and breast adenocarcinomas showed 44.8% and 79.3% positive staining, respectively. Focal immunostaining for BerEP4 was observed in 63.7% of adenocarcinomas and in no mesotheliomas. BG8 reactivity was observed in 88.6% of adenocarcinomas and 5 of 57 (8.7%) mesotheliomas, with the neoplastic cells in mesotheliomas staining only focally positive and with less intensity. B72.3 immunostaining was observed in 170 of 211 (80.5%) adenocarcinomas and 2 of 57 (3.5%) mesotheliomas. In the mesotheliomas, immunostaining for B72.3 was focal but intense. Granular cytoplasmic staining for LeuM1 was found in 159 of 211 (75.3%) adenocarcinomas and 104 of 123 (84.5%) pulmonary adenocarcinomas. Two of 57 (3.5%) mesotheliomas showed predominantly focal membrane staining for LeuM1. Diffuse, moderately intense cytoplasmic staining was observed for BerEP4 in 180 of 211 (85.3%) adenocarcinomas and 16 of 57 (28.1%) mesotheliomas. Most adenocarcinomas were stated to show cytoplasmic reactivity. In contrast, 33 of 57 (57.8%) epithelial mesotheliomas showed cell membrane staining usually without cytoplasmic staining. In several cases, a thick pattern of membrane staining was observed, similar to that found with HBME-1.

Concerning mesothelial-related antigens, 28 of 57 (49.1%) epithelial mesotheliomas immunostained for thrombomodulin compared with 13 of 211 (6.1%) adenocarcinomas, 7 of which were pulmonary adenocarcinomas. HBME-1 immunoreactivity was observed in 45 of 57 (78.9%) epithelial mesotheliomas, usually in a circumferentially thick or moderately thick distribution, and in 83 of 211 (39.3%) adenocarcinomas, usually in a thin pattern restricted to the apical region. A thick membrane pattern was observed in 19 of 211 (9%) adenocarcinomas but usually in an apical distribution. Twenty-four of 57 (42.1%) epithelial mesotheliomas showed immunostaining for calretinin; it was cytoplasmic, finely granular, and diffuse in 22 cases and focal in 2 cases, whereas 13 of 211 (6.1%) adenocarcinomas showed weak or moderate staining.

The sensitivity and specificity of the adenocarcinoma and mesothelioma markers observed by Riera and colleagues[216] are shown in Tables 11–11 and 11–12, respectively.

The study by Riera and associates[216] provides a great deal of practical information. In their study, the HBME-1 antibody was used in a dilution of 1:40, which is in contrast to what I use (1:7500) and what Henderson[141] uses (1:5000 to 1:15,000). I have also found a much higher positive staining reaction for calretinin (approximately 95%) in epithelial mesothelioma.

MISCELLANEOUS ANTIBODIES

Expression of p53 tumor suppressor gene products has been evaluated as a method of discriminating between mesothelioma and reactive mesothelial hyperplasia.[222, 223] Ramael and associates[223] evaluated 40 cases of non-neoplastic reactive pleural mesothelial proliferative lesions and 36 epithelial mesotheliomas for p53 tumor suppressor gene product. Using DO-7 and CM-1 antibodies, nuclear immunolabeling for p53 was observed in 25% of mesotheliomas. No reactivity was observed using antibody PAb240. There was no significant difference in reactivity for the p53 tumor suppressor gene product among histologic subtypes of mesothelioma. Mayall and associates[222] evaluated p53 gene product expression using DO-7 and CM-1 antibodies in pepsin predigested tissue sections and found positive reactions in 10 of 16 (62.5%) epithelial mesotheliomas, 9 of 19 (47.4%) biphasic mesotheliomas, 2 of 12 (16.7%) sarcomatoid mesotheliomas, and 0 of 20 reactive mesothelial cell proliferations. These investigators found no difference in p53 gene product expression in asbestos-induced mesotheliomas than in those mesotheliomas that were not caused by asbestos, suggesting that asbestos was not the cause of p53 gene mutation.[224]

Using formalin-fixed, paraffin-embedded tissue sections, Hurlimann[225] reported immunohistochemical desmin expression in 9 of 16 (56.3%) mesotheliomas (8 epithelial and 1 biphasic). Staining was described as being focal or found only in rare tumor cells. Cases showed positive reactivity more frequently with heat-induced epitope retrieval.

Table 11–11. Sensitivity and Specificity of Immunohistochemical Tests Used to Evaluate Adenocarcinomas*

Scoring	1 Sensitivity	1 Specificity	2 Sensitivity	2 Specificity	3 Sensitivity	3 Specificity
CEA-I	83	100	79	100	75	100
CEA-D			75	100	64	100
BG8-I	89	91	82	91	50	96
BG8-D			75	100	42	100
BerEp4-I	64	100	64	100	39	100
BerEp4-D			55	100	29	100
B72.3-I	81	96	77	96	68	96
B72.3-D			50	98	19	98
LeuM1-I	75	96	71	96	55	96
LeuM1-D			55	100	33	100
HMFG-2-CI	85	72	64	79	19	89
HMFG-2-CD		72	73	77	40	89

*Heat induced epitope retrieval (HIER) used when appropriate.
Values are percentages.
I, intensity of staining; D, distribution of staining.
From Riera JR, Astengo-Osuna C, Longmate JA, et al. The immunohistochemical diagnostic panel for epithelial mesothelioma: A re-evaluation after heat-induced epitope retrieval. Am J Surg Pathol 1997;21:1409–1419.

Table 11–12. Sensitivity and Specificity of Immunohistochemical Tests Used to Evaluate Mesotheliomas*

Scoring	1		2		3	
	Sensitivity	*Specificity*	*Sensitivity*	*Specificity*	*Sensitivity*	*Specificity*
Calretinin-I	42	94	31	96	8	100
Calretinin-D	49	94	39	97	16	98
Thrombomodulin-I	49	94	46	95	35	97
Thrombomodulin-D	49	94	32	96	32	96
HBME-1-I†	79	61	74	72	53	91
HBME-1-D†	79	61	65	73	39	89

*HIER (heat-induced epitope retrieval) used when appropriate.
†Only membrane staining interpreted.
I, intensity of staining; D, distribution of staining.
From Riera JR, Astengo-Osuna C, Longmate JA, et al. The immunohistochemical diagnostic panel for epithelial mesothelioma: A re-evaluation after heat-induced epitope retrieval. Am J Surg Pathol 1997;21:1409–1419.

Four of 16 (25%) mesotheliomas (3 epithelial and 1 biphasic) expressed neuron-specific enolase, 5 of 16 (31.3%) immunostained for chromogranin (4 epithelial, 1 biphasic), and 5 of 16 (31.3%) mesotheliomas (all epithelial) were positive for S-100 protein. Only rare tumor cells expressed these neuroepithelial markers.

Azumi and associates[226] used immunohistochemical techniques to study 33 mesotheliomas (32 pleural, 1 peritoneal, 18 epithelial, 10 biphasic, 4 sarcomatoid, 1 desmoplastic) and 37 adenocarcinomas for hyaluronate. Three of 37 (8.1%) adenocarcinomas and all mesotheliomas immunostained for hyaluronate. The location of the staining reaction in the mesotheliomas was membranous in 30 cases, cytoplasmic in 21 cases, and membranous and cytoplasmic in 19 cases. The staining reaction in mesotheliomas was classified as moderate or greater in 27 of 33 (81.8%) cases. The authors concluded that the demonstration of hyaluronate should be considered an important adjunct to be used with other immunohistochemical tests and electron microscopy in diagnosing epithelial mesotheliomas.

Hyaluronan detection in pleural fluid has been advocated as a method of diagnosing mesothelioma.[227] Among 13 patients with pleural fluid hyaluronan concentrations greater than 225 mg/L, no other diagnosis but mesothelioma was noted. The specificity for mesothelioma was 96%, with a cutoff level of 75 mg/L hyaluronan and 100% with a cutoff level of 225 mg/L hyaluronan.

Martensson and associates[228] evaluated hyaluronan in pleural fluid from 19 men with mesothelioma. Tumor volume was estimated on transilluminated computed tomography (CT) with a digital planimeter. An elevated (7100 mg/L) concentration of hyaluronan was found in the pleural fluid in 13 of 19 (68.4%) patients. A positive correlation was found between the initial concentration of hyaluronan in the serum and the concentration of hyaluronan in the pleural fluid. Increasing concentration of circulating hyaluronan correlated positively with an increasing tumor volume in the hyaluronan-producing mesotheliomas, but not in the non–hyaluronan-producing mesotheliomas.

Thylen and associates[229] evaluated the immunohistochemical differences between hyaluronan- and non–hyaluronan-producing malignant mesothelioma and found a significantly higher reactivity to EMA, a higher reactivity to CAM5.2 keratin, and a lower reactivity to vimentin in the hyaluronan-producing epithelial mesotheliomas. All tumors were stated to be negative for CEA. My experience is different from that of Thylen and colleagues[229] in that the mesotheliomas that produce excess amounts of hyaluronic acid or proteoglycans, or both, are more likely to be mucin-positive and to express the "negative markers" of epithelial mesothelioma, such as CEA, LeuM1 and B72.3.

CA 125 is a glycoprotein identified in the cell membrane in coelomic epithelium during embryogenesis and in neoplasms of the female genital tract.[230–233] The antibody to detect CA 125 in histologic sections, OC-125, was initially thought to work only in frozen tissue sections but was adapted to work in formalin-fixed paraffin-embedded sections using enzymatic digestion[234] or heat-induced epitope retrieval.

It soon became apparent that OC-125 reactivity was not restricted to the gynecologic tract. OC-125 reactivity was observed in breast neoplasms,[235] lung neoplasms, and neoplasms of the pleura and peritoneal linings.[238, 239]

The second-generation antibody against CA 125,[236, 237] M-11, is stated to show greater intensity staining than OC-125.[240] M-11 reactivity was demonstrated in mesothelial linings of spontaneous abortion specimens of 6 to 14 weeks' gestation.[241]

I have observed several cases of low-intensity immunostaining of epithelial mesotheliomas for OC-125.

In rare instances, unusual substances have been demonstrated immunohistochemically in mesotheliomas. Okamato and associates[242] reported two neoplasms consistent with primary pleural mesotheliomas that contained anaplastic tumor giant cells with human chorionic gonadotropin, as demonstrated by immunohistochemistry.

McAuley and colleagues[243] evaluated a patient with malignant mesothelioma who had hypercalcemia and an elevated serum concentration of parathyroid-like hormone. They evaluated nine epithelial mesotheliomas for parathyroid-like peptide and found abundant immunopositive cells in eight of nine cases. They also observed parathyroid-like peptide immunoreactivity in normal and reactive epithelial mesothelial cells.

Tateyama and colleagues[244] reported CD5 expression in thymic carcinoma and atypical thymoma and in 9 of 13 (69.2%) mesotheliomas (5 epithelial, 3 biphasic, 1 sarcomatoid). All CD5+ mesotheliomas showed intense intracytoplasmic staining. Eight of 13 (61.5%) pulmonary adenocarcinomas showed low to moderately intense and predominantly cell membrane staining for CD5.

DIAGNOSTIC CONSIDERATIONS

I use a battery of antibodies for evaluating mesothelial proliferative lesions, including reactive and neoplastic processes. Keratin antibodies generally are not used to differentiate mesothelioma from another neoplasm or from a reactive process but to identify the extent of a neoplastic or reactive mesothelial cell process. The antibodies I used to differentiate a well or moderately well differentiated epithelial mesothelioma from a pulmonary adenocarcinoma or nonpulmonary adenocarcinoma include AE1/AE3 cytokeratin, CK7, CK20, CK5/CK6, vimentin, EMA, human milk fat globule protein-2, HBME-1, calretinin, CEA, LeuM1, B72.3, BerEP4, and TTF-1.

The immunohistogram of a well to moderately well differentiated epithelial mesothelioma is shown in Fig. 11–43. A comparison of the immunohistochemical profile of well to moderately well

differentiated epithelial mesothelioma and pulmonary adenocarcinoma is shown in Table 11–13.

Sarcomatoid mesotheliomas characteristically express keratin, usually low molecular weight keratin, vimentin, and frequently muscle-specific/alpha actins. A relatively small percentage (10 to 15%) of sarcomatoid mesotheliomas express calretinin and infrequently CK5/CK6. In my experience, sarcomatoid mesotheliomas, and tumors they may be confused with, do not express the negative markers used to diagnose a well or moderately well differentiated epithelial mesothelioma, such as CEA, LeuM1, B72.3, BerEP4, and BG8. Therefore, I would not include those antibodies in a "screen" of a malignant spindle cell proliferative lesion of the pleura. The immunohistogram of a sarcomatoid mesothelioma is shown in Figure 11–44. The most important immunohistochemical finding in sarcomatoid mesothelioma is coexpression of keratin and vimentin.

Metastatic tumors to the pleura are more common than primary neoplasms. It is imperative that metastases be considered a possibility for any tumor involving the pleura that is being evaluated by immunohistochemistry. In this context, it is important to know clinical information concerning the patient, which may have an influence on the immunohistochemical tests performed. However, the pathologic diagnosis is based on objective findings and not on the clinical history.

Metastatic tumors of unknown primary origin are discussed in Chapter 7 and may involve the pleura. My colleagues and I and others have shown that the most cost-effective way of evaluating a suspected metastatic tumor of unknown primary origin is by pathologic techniques.[245, 246] The

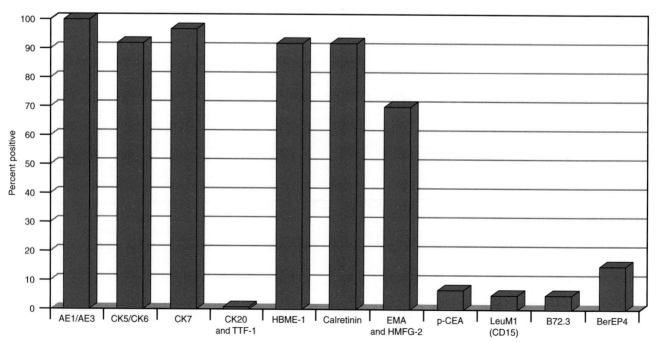

Figure 11–43. Immunohistogram of a well to moderately well differentiated epithelial mesothelioma. EMA, epithelial membrane antigen.

Table 11–13. Comparison of the Immunohistochemical Profile of Well to Moderately Well Differentiated Epithelial Mesothelioma and Well to Moderately Well Differentiated Pulmonary Adenocarcinoma

			Antibody Directed Against											
Type of Neoplasm	AE1/AE3	Low Molecular Weight Keratin	High Molecular Weight Keratin	CK7	CK5/CK6	Carcinoembryonic Antigen	CD15/LeuM1	B72.3	BerEp4	Thyroid Transcription Factor-1	Calretinin	HBME-1	Epithelial Membrane Antigen	Human Milk Fat Globule Protein-2
Well to moderately well differentiated epithelial mesothelioma	+	+	+	+	+/-	R	R	R	-/+	N	+/-	+/-*	+/-	+/-*
Well to moderately well differentiated pulmonary adenocarcinoma	+	+	+/-	+	R	+	+/-	+/-	+/-	+/-	R	R	+/-†	+/-†

*Cell membrane distribution.

†Cytoplasmic distribution.

+, almost always diffuse, strong positivity; +/-, variable staining, mostly positive; -/+, variable staining, mostly negative; R, rare cells positive; N, almost always negative.

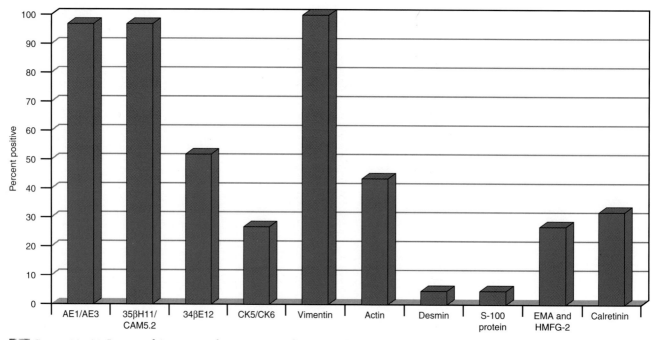

Figure 11–44. Immunohistogram of a sarcomatoid mesothelioma. EMA, epithelial membrane antigen.

histologic appearance of the tumor dictates the antibody selection in such neoplasms. It is important that pathologists recognize the extensive histologic spectrum of mesotheliomas so that uncommon histologic types of mesothelioma are not misdiagnosed as metastatic neoplasms. In cases of suspected pleural mesothelioma, clinical information may be helpful by demonstrating radiographically that a tumor is encasing the lung and by providing evidence that a neoplasm is not identified in other organs or tissues. It must be remembered that localized malignant mesotheliomas occur[247] and that mesotheliomas may be diffuse but beyond the resolution of current radiographic techniques, such as CT and magnetic resonance imaging.

UNCOMMON AND RARE PRIMARY PLEURAL NEOPLASMS

Solitary Fibrous Tumors of the Pleura

Solitary localized fibrous tumors of the pleura are uncommon neoplasms that are thought to arise from subpleural connective tissue cells.[248–250] They occur as neoplasms in the subvisceral-subpleural zone of the lung, within the pleural space attached to the pleura (usually the visceral pleura) by a small pedicle, or in a subparietal pleural location. Such neoplasms may become extremely large and may be associated with unusual clinical situations such as hypoglycemia. Histologically, these neoplasms are composed of spindle cells with varying degrees of cellularity and various amounts of extracellular collagenous tissue. Identifying these neoplasms as malignant can be difficult, with malig-

nant criteria including more than four mitoses per 10 high power fields, hemorrhage, necrosis, and invasion into lung and chest wall.[250] One hundred percent express vimentin, and they are uniformly negative for keratin. About 75 to 80% express CD34,[251, 252] and a slightly greater percentage express the antiapoptosis substance BCL-2.[253] Rare localized fibrous tumors of the pleura express actin.[250] Localized fibrous tumors of the pleura are contrasted to sarcomatoid mesotheliomas and sarcomas (Table 11–14).

Pseudomesotheliomatous Carcinomas of the Lung

Rare primary neoplasms of lung grow in a distribution characteristic of mesothelioma. Five such neoplasms were described by Babolini and Blasi in 1956.[254] Six examples were reported by Harwood and colleagues[255] in 1976; they introduced the term *pseudomesotheliomatous carcinoma*. In 1992, Koss and associates[256] reported on 30 cases of pseudomesotheliomatous adenocarcinoma of lung, 15 of which were from a review of published literature and 15 from the files of the Armed Forces Institute of Pathology. Hartman and Schutze[257] reported 72 cases and designated these neoplasms *mesothelioma-like tumors of the pleura*. A report by Koss and colleagues[258] described 29 cases of pseudomesotheliomatous adenocarcinoma of lung. My colleagues and I[258] reported 17 cases of pseudomesotheliomatous carcinoma of lung in abstract form and are currently preparing a report on 100 cases.

These neoplasms macroscopically look identical

Table 11–14. Comparison of the Immunohistochemical Features of Localized Fibrous Tumors of the Pleura, Sarcomatoid Mesothelioma, and Soft Tissue Sarcomas

Type of Neoplasm	AE1/AE3	Low Molecular Weight Keratin	High Molecular Weight Keratin	CK7	Vimentin	Actin	Desmin	S-100 Protein	CD31
Sarcomatoid mesothelioma	+/−	+/−	−/+	+/−	+	−/+	R	R	N
Localized fibrous tumor of pleura	N	N	N	N	+	−/+	N	N	N
Soft tissue sarcoma	N	N	N	N	+	+/−*	+/−*	+/−*	+/−*

*Positivity depends on type of soft tissue sarcoma.
+, almost always diffuse, strong positivity; +/−, variable staining, mostly positive; −/+, variable staining, mostly negative; R, rare cells positive; N, almost always negative.

to mesothelioma (Fig. 11–45). As reported by Koss and colleagues,[256, 258] and in my[259] experience, the majority of these neoplasms are adenocarcinomas, with the most common histologic subtype being what we refer to as a *tubulodesmoplastic pseudomesotheliomatous adenocarcinoma* (Fig. 11–46). Pseudomesotheliomatous pulmonary adenocarcinomas are usually mucin-positive and express the immunohistochemical markers of a pulmonary adenocarcinoma. Occasionally, these neoplasms show squamous and small cell neuroendocrine differentiation. Some are large cell undifferentiated carcinomas and some may be poorly differentiated and difficult to differentiate from a poorly differentiated mesothelioma. The poorly differentiated neoplasms usually coexpress keratin and vimentin and

may not express specific carcinoma or mesothelioma markers and may be impossible to differentiate from mesothelioma. Koss and associates[256, 258] reported two biphasic variants and my colleagues and I[259] observed one.

The immunohistochemical profile of a pseudomesotheliomatous adenocarcinoma of the lung is the same as a primary pulmonary adenocarcinoma. As reported by my colleagues and myself[259] and Koss and associates,[256, 258] a significant percentage of these neoplasms occur in individuals who were exposed to asbestos and who have elevated concentrations of asbestos in their lung tissue.

Pseudomesotheliomatous Epithelioid Hemangioendothelioma

Rare neoplasms composed of endothelial cells resemble mesotheliomas and are referred to as pseudomesotheliomatous epithelioid hemangioendothelioma or as epithelioid hemangioendothelioma mimicking mesothelioma.[260, 261] The case I contributed to in the Lin series[261] was that of a 50-

Figure 11–45. Macroscopically, pseudomesotheliomatous adenocarcinomas of lung look like diffuse malignant mesotheliomas.

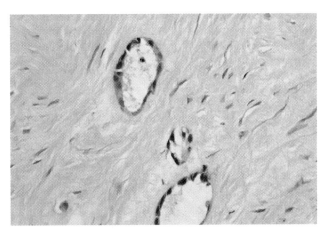

Figure 11–46. The most common histologic appearance of pseudomesotheliomatous adenocarcinoma is a tubulodesmoplastic pattern. (×400)

year-old man who had a potential history of exposure to asbestos while working at a hardware store at age 20 and presented with a right pleural effusion and a tumor encasing the right lung. The initial biopsy was diagnosed by the "treating" pathologist as adenocarcinoma and by another pathologist as an epithelial mesothelioma. The case was referred to me; the pattern of immunoreactivity was confusing in that the neoplastic cells expressed low molecular weight (35βH11) (Fig. 11–47) and high molecular weight keratin (34βE12), vimentin, CD31, factor VIII antigen, and CD34. Ultrastructurally, the neoplastic cells resembled endothelial cells and contained Weibel-Palade bodies in their cytoplasm. The neoplastic cells expressed endothelial cell markers. Keratin expression in epithelioid hemangioendothelioma has been described.[262]

Calcifying Fibrous Pseudotumor of the Pleura

Calcifying fibrous pseudotumor of the pleura is a newly recognized fibrous soft tissue tumor of the pleura that occurs predominantly in younger individuals and presents as a pleural mass radiographically.[263] Patients with this neoplasm usually present with chest pain or cough, or both, and vague chest discomfort. The tumor consists of circumscribed but unencapsulated masses of dense hyalinized collagenous tissue interspersed with a lymphoplasmacytic infiltrate and calcium deposits, many of which have the appearance of psammoma bodies. I have seen three such lesions, and the spindle cells show immunostaining for vimentin and no immunostaining for keratin, alpha actin, desmin, S-100 protein, CD34, and BCL-2.

Primary Desmoid Tumors of the Pleura

These tumors resemble desmoid tumors in other locations and show infiltration of the adjacent fat skeletal muscle by plump spindle cells.[264] Immunohistochemically, the neoplastic spindle cells show immunostaining for vimentin, desmin, smooth muscle actin, and muscle-specific actin. They are negative for S-100 protein and keratin. Ultrastructurally, the neoplastic cells resemble myofibroblasts.

Primary Pleural Thymomas

Thymomas may occur in the pleura and can be confused with mesothelioma.[265–268] They may be

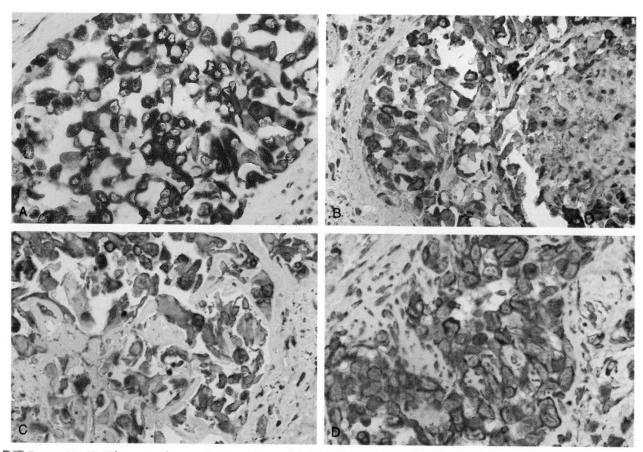

Figure 11–47. This pseudomesotheliomatous epithelioid hemangioendothelioma was initially diagnosed as an adenocarcinoma and then as an epithelial mesothelioma. In this case, the neoplastic cells expressed keratin *(A)* as well as endothelial cell markers CD31 *(B)*, CD34 *(C)*, and factor VIII antigen *(D)*. (×400)

confused with a sarcomatoid mesothelioma with a heavy lymphoid infiltrate or with a lymphohistiocytoid mesothelioma. The cases presented by Moran and colleagues[265] showed no radiographic evidence of a mediastinal tumor, and six cases showed histologic features of a "mixed" (lymphocyte-epithelial) thymoma. The neoplastic thymic epithelial cells express keratin.

Synovial Sarcomas

Synovial sarcomas may occur as primary neoplasms in the pleura and be confused histologically with biphasic and sarcomatoid mesotheliomas.[269] The neoplastic epithelial cells express keratin and show glandular differentiation. The cells forming the glandular structures frequently express CEA and BerEP4 and are positive for neutral mucins, these findings being absent in most epithelial mesotheliomas. Ultrastructurally, the neoplastic epithelial cells in a synovial sarcoma are different from epithelial mesotheliomas having short microvilli and showing glycocalyceal bodies.[270] Monophasic synovial sarcomas could be difficult, if not impossible, to differentiate from sarcomatoid mesotheliomas, although a monophasic variant involving the pleura has not been reported.

Pleuropulmonary Blastoma

Pleuropulmonary blastomas are rare neoplasms that occur predominantly in infants and children and involve the lung or pleura, or both.[271, 272] Rare cases occur in adults.[273] The neoplasm is frequently cystic, with the cysts lined by benign metaplastic epithelium that can be ciliated. The malignant component is composed of differentiated or anaplastic sarcomatous elements, or both, and includes fibrosarcoma, chondrosarcoma, embryonal rhabdomyosarcoma, and mixtures of these elements. The immunohistologic findings are dependent on what type of sarcomatous differentiation occurs.

VARIABILITIES AND PITFALLS

A predominant pitfall of accurately diagnosing mesothelioma is a failure of pathologists to recognize the many histologic patterns that epithelial and sarcomatoid mesotheliomas show. Most immunohistochemical literature discussing mesothelioma concerns epithelial mesothelioma, specifically well and moderately well differentiated epithelial mesotheliomas. Most antibodies used to differentiate mesothelioma from adenocarcinoma discuss tumors that are well or moderately well differentiated. As mesotheliomas become more poorly differentiated, many relatively specific positive markers such as HBME-1, calretinin, and CK5/CK6 fail to stain. Poorly differentiated mesotheliomas characteristically express low molecular weight keratin and occasionally high molecular weight

keratin and vimentin. An absolute diagnosis of such mesotheliomas may be impossible, and the diagnosis may have to state that the histologic and immunohistologic findings are consistent with a poorly differentiated mesothelioma. The "clinical" (diffuse) distribution of a pleural neoplasm can help support the diagnosis.

As reported by Henderson and coworkers[139] and the US-Canadian Mesothelioma Panel,[274] non-neoplastic reactive proliferative pleural lesions may closely simulate mesothelioma. This may be the most difficult area of "diagnostic pleural pathology." Most difficult is differentiating fibrosing pleuritis from desmoplastic mesothelioma and superficially invasive epithelial mesotheliomas from reactive mesothelial proliferations. In my experience, neoplastic epithelial mesothelial cells show cell membrane staining for EMA and human milk fat globule protein-2, whereas reactive non-neoplastic epithelial mesothelial cells usually do not express these antigens.

Unusual and uncommon types of mesothelioma should be mentioned because they can cause diagnostic confusion. Mucin-positive epithelial mesotheliomas are not uncommon. Between 1% and 5% of all moderately well to well differentiated epithelial mesotheliomas show mucicarmine or PAS-diastase staining, or both (see Fig. 11–48). I have extensively described patterns of mucin staining.[275] It is mucin-positive epithelial mesotheliomas that most frequently express immunohistochemical markers that are negative in most epithelial mesotheliomas and that are usually positive in pulmonary adenocarcinomas (CEA, LeuM1, B72.3, BerEP4) (see Fig. 11–42). Mucin-positive epithelial mesotheliomas express calretinin and HBME-1 and show cell membrane staining for EMA and human milk fat globule protein-2. Ultrastructurally, mucin-positive epithelial mesotheliomas frequently contain crystalloid material (Fig. 11–49) in intracellular neolumens, in glandular spaces formed by neoplastic cells, or in the extra-

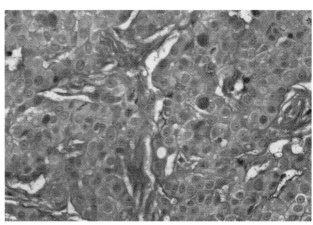

Figure 11–48. This mucin-positive epithelial mesothelioma shows intracellular mucicarmine staining. This reaction can result in an incorrect diagnosis of a mucin-producing adenocarcinoma. (×400)

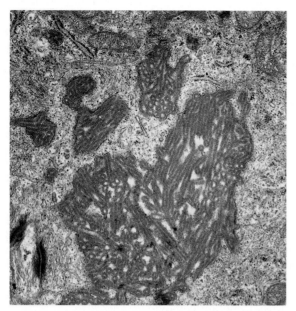

Figure 11–49. In this mucin-positive epithelial meso-thelioma, crystalloid material is located in glandular spaces formed by the neoplastic cells and in intra-cellular neolumens.

cellular space. Some of this crystalloid material is unique to epithelial mesotheliomas.

Some mesotheliomas are composed of small cells and may be confused with small cell lung carcinoma.[276] Mayall and associates[277] reported neuron-specific enolase staining in 46 of 48 (96%) mesotheliomas and Leu7 expression in 14 of 20 (70%) mesotheliomas. Unlike that observed by Hurlimann,[225] the mesotheliomas showed no expression of chromogranin A and bombesin. Mayall and coworkers[276] reported 13 cases of small cell mesothelioma in which there were areas of atypical epithelial mesothelioma and 7 cases in which 90% of the neoplastic cells were small cells. Falconieri and colleagues[278] reported four cases of pseudomesotheliomatous small cell carcinoma of lung that could be confused with small cell mesothelioma. I believe that the best way to differentiate pseudomesotheliomatous small cell lung cancer from small cell mesothelioma would be with TTF-1 (positive in 90% of small cell lung cancers, negative in mesothelioma), CEA (positive in approximately 30 to 50% of small cell lung cancers, negative in small cell mesothelioma), and synaptophysin (positive in 90% of small cell lung cancers, negative in most small cell mesotheliomas).

Lymphohistiocytoid mesothelioma[279] is a rare form of sarcomatoid mesothelioma that initially was histologically thought to be a lymphoma. This mesothelioma is composed of large, mostly round cells admixed with numerous inflammatory cells. This neoplasm can be misdiagnosed as a large cell lymphocytic lymphoma. The neoplastic cells characteristically express low molecular weight keratin and occasionally high molecular weight keratin

and vimentin. Most lymphohistiocytoid mesotheliomas are negative for calretinin, HBME-1, and EMA. Ultrastructurally, the neoplastic cells show intercellular junctions and intracellular tonofilaments.

Well-differentiated papillary epithelial mesothelioma can cause diagnostic confusion, often because pathologists are not familiar with this neoplasm.[138, 280] Most cases occur in the peritoneal cavity of young women (20- to 30-year age group), although they have been reported in the pleura.[281] Macroscopically, they present as multiple serosal surface nodules typically involving the omentum, mesentery, and pelvic cavity. The nodules vary from a few millimeters to several centimeters in maximal dimension. Histologically, they show tubulopapillary differentiation and are composed of well-differentiated, relatively uniform cuboidal cells (Fig. 11–50). The neoplasm can be associated with extensive fibrosis, although unequivocal invasion can be difficult to identify. The immunohistochemical pattern is generally that of a "typical" well-differentiated epithelial mesothelioma, and most cases I have seen show cell membrane immunostaining for EMA or human milk fat globule protein-2. These tumors differ from typical epithelial mesotheliomas in that they usually have a good prognosis and do not progress. However, cases occur that progress, invade, and cause death.

Some epithelial mesotheliomas are composed of small cysts formed by uniform cuboidal mesothelial cells and associated numerous blood vessels (Fig. 11–51). This type of mesothelioma may be difficult to differentiate from a vascular neoplasm. The epithelial mesothelial cells may contain intracytoplasmic hemosiderin (Fig. 11–52). The immunophenotype of such neoplasms is identical to that of other epithelial mesotheliomas. The vascular proliferation may be related to an endothelial growth factor produced by neoplastic mesothelial cells.[282]

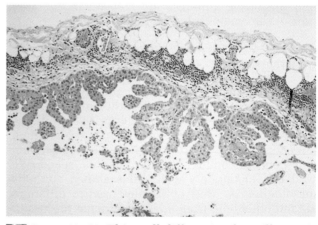

Figure 11–50. This well-differentiated papillary epithelial mesothelioma involving pleura shows papillary differentiation and is composed of relatively small, uniform, cuboidal cells. This type of mesothelioma usually pursues a benign clinical course. (×200)

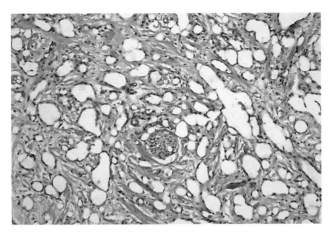

Figure 11-51. This epithelial mesothelioma is composed of small cysts associated with numerous blood vessels. (×200)

Adenomatoid tumors are localized benign mesotheliomas that occur most frequently in the epididymis and cornua of the uterus.[283] These tumors are formed by uniform, small cuboidal cells and can appear invasive. They express keratin and other markers of mesothelial cells and have the characteristic ultrastructural features of mesothelial cells. Adenomatoid tumors have been reported in the pleura.[27]

Hyperplastic mesothelial cells may be found in mediastinal lymph nodes and simulate metastatic epithelial mesothelioma or carcinoma.[284, 285] These atypical mesothelial cells typically occur in nodal sinuses and are most prominent in the subcapsular sinuses. They may be confused with macrophages and, in fact, Ordonez and coworkers[286] have reported that some lesions composed of cells thought to represent reactive mesothelial cells are, in fact, macrophages. The mesothelial cells express the usual positive epithelial mesothelial cell markers and are negative for the antigens that are characteristically negative in epithelial mesothelioma. One

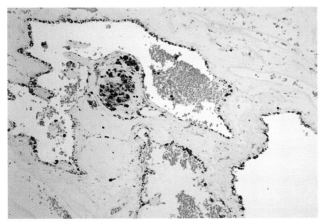

Figure 11-52. The neoplastic mesothelial cells showed abundant intracytoplasmic hemosiderin as demonstrated in this Prussian blue iron-stained section. (×200)

must be aware, however, that epithelial mesotheliomas may be present as metastatic tumors of unknown primary origin in lymph nodes.[287]

Well-differentiated epithelial mesotheliomas and well-differentiated papillary epithelial mesotheliomas need to be differentiated from primary papillary serous carcinomas of the serosa, nearly all of which occur in the peritoneal cavity of women.[288-297] One case has been reported in a man,[298] and rare cases involve the pleural cavity.[141] Histologically, these neoplasms are well differentiated and exhibit a papillary morphology. It is more common to see psammoma bodies in primary papillary carcinomas than in papillary epithelial mesotheliomas, although psammoma bodies are occasionally seen in papillary mesotheliomas, but not in the number seen in primary papillary carcinomas. Primary serosal papillary carcinomas are usually mucicarmine- and PAS-diastase–negative. By immunohistochemistry, the staining pattern can be similar to epithelial mesotheliomas, although Khoury and associates[299] found serous papillary tumors to express one or more of the antigens CEA, LeuM1 (CD15), and TAG-72 (B72.3). In 17 of 20 cases, 7 expressed monoclonal CEA, 6 expressed LeuM1, and 13 were positive for B72.3 when tissue sections were predigested with pepsin. Ultrastructurally, primary papillary serous carcinomas show occasional cilia and outpouchings of straight and relatively short microvilli that are covered by a fuzzy glycocalyx. Sometimes the microvilli are longer and are branched.

Sarcomatoid renal cell carcinomas can metastasize to the pleura in a macroscopic distribution identical to mesothelioma and very closely simulate a sarcomatoid mesothelioma.[300] This tumor can be considered a pseudomesotheliomatous carcinoma but not a primary pulmonary pseudomesotheliomatous carcinoma. The immunostaining pattern of such neoplasms can be identical to a sarcomatoid mesothelioma. The situation can be further complicated because sarcomatoid mesotheliomas can metastasize to the kidney. If an individual is known to have a sarcomatoid renal cell carcinoma and has a spindle cell neoplasm of the pleura, one must strongly consider the possibility of a metastatic sarcomatoid renal cell carcinoma. If the tumor shows a clear cell and a sarcomatoid pattern, metastatic renal cell carcinoma is most likely, although mesotheliomas may show a clear cell pattern.[301]

Malignant melanoma can metastasize to the pleura and simulate mesothelioma. Rare melanomas are keratin-positive[126, 302] and typically express S-100 protein and HMB-45 antigen.

References

1. Hammar SP. Common neoplasms. In: Dail DH, Hammar SP, eds. 2nd ed. Pulmonary Pathology. New York: Springer-Verlag, 1994:1487–1579.

2. Dodds L, Davis S, Polissar L. A population-based study of lung cancer incidence by histological type. J Natl Cancer Inst 1986;76:21–29.

3. Thun MJ, Lally CA, Flannery JT, et al. Cigarette smoking and changes in the histopathology of lung cancer. J Natl Cancer Inst 1997;89:1580–1586.

4. Moll R, Franke WW, Schiller DL, et al. The catalog of human cytokeratins: Patterns of expression in normal epithelia, tumors and cultured cells. Cell 1982;31:11–24.

5. Moll R, Lowe A, Laufer J, et al. Cytokeratin 20 in human carcinomas: A new histodiagnostic marker detected by monoclonal antibodies. Am J Surg Pathol 1992;140:427–447.

6. Ramaekers F, Huysmans A, Schaart G, et al. Tissue distribution of keratin 7 as monitored by a monoclonal antibody. Exp Cell Res 1987;170:235–249.

7. Hammar SP, Hallman KO. Unusual primary lung neoplasms: Spindle cell and undifferentiated carcinomas expressing only vimentin. Ultrastruct Pathol 1990;14:407–422.

8. Upton MP, Hirohashi S, Tome Y, et al. Expression of vimentin in surgically resected adenocarcinomas and large cell carcinomas of lung. Am J Surg Pathol 1986;10:560–567.

9. Hammar SP. Metastatic adenocarcinoma of unknown primary origin. Hum Pathol 1998;29:1393–1402.

10. Guazzi S, Price M, DeFelice M, et al. Thyroid nuclear factor-1 (TTF-1) contains a homeodomain and displays a novel DNA-binding specificity. EMBO J 1990;9:3631–3639.

11. Lazzaro D, Price M, DeFelice M, et al. The transcription factor TTF-1 expressed at the onset of thyroid and lung morphogenesis and in the restricted regions of the foetal brain. Development 1991;113:1093–1094.

12. Bohinski RJ, DiLauro R, Whitsett JA. The lung specific surfactant protein B promoter is a target for thyroid transcription factor-1 and hepatocyte nuclear factor 3, indicating common factors for organ-specific gene expression along the foregut axis. Mol Cell Biol 1994;14:5671–5678.

13. Bohinski RJ, Huffman JA, Whitsett JA, et al. Cis-active elements controlling lung cell–specific expression of human pulmonary surfactant B gene. J Biol Chem 1993;268:11160–11166.

14. Bejarano PA, Baughman RP, Biddinger PW, et al. Surfactant proteins and thyroid transcription factor-1 in pulmonary and breast carcinomas. Mod Pathol 1996;9:445–452.

15. Fabbro D, DiLoreto C, Stamerra O, et al. TTF-1 gene expression in human lung tumors. Eur J Cancer 1996;32A:512–573.

16. DiLoreto C, DiLauro V, Puglisi F, et al. Immunohistochemical expression of tissue specific transcription factor-1 in lung carcinoma. J Clin Pathol 1997;50:30–32.

17. Holzinger A, Dingle S, Bejarano PA, et al. Monoclonal antibody to thyroid transcription factor-1: Production, characterization and usefulness in tumor diagnosis. Hybridoma 1996;15:49–53.

18. Folpe AL, Gown AM, Lamps LW, et al. Thyroid transcription factor-1: Immunohistochemical evaluation in pulmonary neuroendocrine tumors. Mod Pathol 1999;12:5–8.

19. Yesner R. Small cell tumors of the lung. Am J Surg Pathol 1983;7:775–785.

20. Carter D. Small-cell carcinoma of the lung. Am J Surg Pathol 1983;7:787–795.

21. Yesner R. Classification of lung cancer histology. N Engl J Med 1985;312:652–653.

22. Arrigoni MG, Woolner LB, Berantz PE. Atypical carcinoid tumors of the lung. J Thorac Cardiovasc Surg 1972;64:413–421.

23. Leschke H. Über nur regionär bösartige und über krebsig entartete Bronchusadenome bzw: Carcinoide. Virch Arch A Pathol Anat 1956;328:635–657.

24. Warren WH, Memoli VA, Gould VE. Immunohistochemical and ultrastructural analysis of bronchopulmonary neuroendocrine neoplasms. II: Well–differentiated neuroendocrine carcinomas. Ultrastruct Pathol 1984;7:185–199.

25. Mark EJ, Ramirez JF. Peripheral small-cell carcinoma of the lung resembling carcinoid tumor: A clinical and patho-logic study of 14 cases. Arch Pathol Lab Med 1985;109:263–269.

26. Paladugu RR, Benfield JR, Pak HY, et al. Bronchopulmonary Kulchitzky cell carcinomas. Cancer 1985;55:1303–1311.

27. Travis WD, Colby TV, Corrin B, et al. Histological Typing of Lung and Pleural Tumors. New York: Springer-Verlag, 1999.

28. Gould VE, Chejfec G. Ultrastructural and biochemical analysis of pulmonary undifferentiated carcinomas. Hum Pathol 1978;9:377–384.

29. Hammond ME, Sause WT. Large cell neuroendocrine tumors of the lung: Clinical significance and histological definition. Cancer 1985;56:1624–1629.

30. Neal MH, Kosinki R, Cohen P, et al. Atypical endocrine tumors of the lung: A histologic, ultrastructural and clinical study of 19 cases. Hum Pathol 1986;17:1264–1277.

31. Barbareschi M, Mariscotti C, Barberis M, et al. Large cell neuroendocrine carcinoma of the lung. Tumor 1989;75:583–588.

32. McDowell EM, Wilson TS, Trump BF. Atypical endocrine tumors of the lung. Arch Pathol Lab Med 1981;105:20–28.

33. Travis WD, Linnoila I, Tsokos MG, et al. Neuroendocrine tumors of the lung with proposed criteria for large cell neuroendocrine carcinoma: An ultrastructural, immunohistochemical and flow cytometric study of 35 cases. Am J Surg Pathol 1991;15:529–533.

34. Hammar S, Bockus D, Remington F, et al. The unusual spectrum of neuroendocrine lung neoplasms. Ultra Pathol 1989;13:515–560.

35. Pearse AGE. The diffuse neuroendocrine system: An extension of the APUD concept. In: Taylor S, ed. Endocrinology. London: Heinemann, 1972:145–222.

36. Gould VE, DeLellis RA. The neuroendocrine cell system: Its nature, hyperplasias and dysplasias. In: Silverberg SG, ed. Principles and Practice of Surgical Pathology. New York: John Wiley, 1983:1488–1501.

37. Hammar SP, Gould VE. Neuroendocrine neoplasms. In: Azar HA, ed. Pathology of Human Neoplasms: An Atlas of Diagnostic Electron Microscopy and Immunohistochemistry. New York: Raven Press, 1988:333–404.

38. Jahn B, Schibler W, Ouimet C, et al. A 38,000 dalton membrane protein (p38) present in synaptic vesicles. Proc Natl Acad Sci U S A 1985;82:4137–4141.

39. Wiedenmann B, Franke WW. Identification and localization of synaptophysis, an integral membrane glycoprotein of Mr 38,000 characteristic of prosynaptic vesicles. Cell 1985;45:1017–1028.

40. Carmichael SW, Winkler H. The adrenal chromaffin cell. Sci Am 1985;253:40–49.

41. O'Connor DT, Frigon RP. Chromogranin A, the major catecholamine storage vesicle protein. J Biol Chem 1984;259:3237–3247.

42. Banks P, Helle K. The release of protein from the stimulated adrenal medulla. Biochem J 1965;97:40C–41C.

43. Haimoto H, Takahashi V, Koshikawa T, et al. Immunohistochemical localization of gamma enolase in normal human tissues other than nervous and neuroendocrine tissues. Lab Invest 1985;52:257–263.

44. Pahlman S, Esscher T, Nilsson K. Expression of gamma-subunit of enolase, neuron-specific enolase in human non-neuroendocrine tumors and derived cell lines. Lab Invest 1986;54:554–560.

45. Leoncini P, DeMarco EB, Bognoli M, et al. Expression of phosphorylated and non-phosphorylated neurofilament subunits and cytokeratins in neuroendocrine lung tumors. Pathol Res Pract 1989;185:848–855.

46. Komminoth P, Roth J, Lackie PM, et al. Polysialic acid of the neural cell adhesion molecule distinguishes small cell carcinoma from carcinoids. Am J Pathol 1991;139:297–304.

47. Kibbelaar RE, Moolenaar CEC, Michalides RJAM, et al. Expression of the embryonal neural cell adhesion molecule N-CAM in lung carcinoma: Diagnostic usefulness of monoclonal antibody 735 for the distinction between small cell lung cancer and non–small cell lung cancer. J Pathol 1989;159:23–28.

48. Bunn P, Linnoila I, Minna J, et al. Small-cell lung cancer, endocrine cells of the fetal bronchus and other neuroendocrine cells express Leu-7 antigenic determinant present on natural killer cells. Blood 1985;65:764–768.
49. Gibbs AR, Whimster WF. Tumors of the lung and pleura. In: Fletcher CDM, ed. Diagnostic Histopathology of Tumors. Edinburgh: Churchill Livingstone, 1995:127–150.
50. Dail DH. Uncommon neoplasms. In: Dail DH, Hammar SP, eds. Pulmonary Pathology. 2nd ed. New York: Springer-Verlag, 1994:1279–1461.
51. Wick MR, Swanson PE. Carcinosarcomas: Current perspective and a historical review of nosologic concepts. Semin Diagn Pathol 1993;10:118–127.
52. Addis BJ, Corrin B. Pulmonary blastoma, carcinosarcoma and spindle cell carcinoma: An immunohistochemical study of keratin intermediate filaments. J Pathol 1985;147:291–301.
53. Zarbo RJ, Crissman JD, Venkat H, et al. Spindle cell carcinoma of the upper aerodigestive tract mucosa: An immunohistologic and ultrastructural study of 18 biphasic tumors and comparison with seven monophasic spindle cell tumors. Am J Surg Pathol 1986;10:741–753.
54. Humphrey PA, Scroggs MW, Roggli VL, et al. Pulmonary carcinomas with a sarcomatoid element: An immunohistochemical and ultrastructural analysis. Hum Pathol 1988;19:155–165.
55. Colby TV, Bilbao JE, Battifora H, et al. Primary osteosarcoma of the lung: A re-appraisal following immunohistologic study. Arch Pathol Lab Med 1989;113:1147–1150.
56. Nappi O, Glasner SD, Swanson PE, et al. Biphasic and monophasic sarcomatoid carcinomas of the lung: A re-appraisal of "carcinosarcomas" and "spindle cell carcinomas." Am J Clin Pathol 1994;102:331–340.
57. Fishback NF, Travis WD, Moran CA, et al. Pleomorphic (spindle/giant cell) carcinoma of the lung. Cancer 1994;73:2936–2945.
58. Koss MN, Hochholzer L, O'Leary T. Pulmonary blastomas. Cancer 1983;73:265–294.
59. Yousem SA, Wick MR, Randhawa P, et al. Pulmonary blastoma: An immunohistochemical analysis and comparison with fetal lung in its pseudoglandular stage. Am J Clin Pathol 1990;93:167–175.
60. Ognibene FP, Steis RG, Macher AM, et al. Kaposi's sarcoma using pulmonary infiltrates and respiratory failure in the acquired immunodeficiency syndrome. Ann Intern Med 1985;102:471–475.
61. Garay SM, Belenko M, Fazzini E, et al. Pulmonary manifestations of Kaposi's sarcoma. Chest 1987;91:39–43.
62. White DA, Matthay RA. Noninfectious pulmonary complications of infection with the human immunodeficiency virus. Am Rev Respir Dis 1989;140:1763–1787.
63. McLoud TC, Naidich DP. Thoracic disease in the immunocompromised patient. Radiol Clin North Am 1992;30:525–554.
64. Ognibene FP, Shelhamer JH. Kaposi's sarcoma. Clin Chest Med 1988;9:459–465.
65. Heitzman ER. Pulmonary neoplastic lymphoproliferative disease in AIDS: A review. Radiology 1990;177:347–351.
66. Purdy LJ, Colby TV, Yousem SA, et al. Pulmonary Kaposi's sarcoma: Premortem histologic diagnosis. Am J Surg Pathol 1986;10:301–311.
67. Hymes KB, Cheung T, Greene JB, et al. Kaposi's sarcoma in homosexual men: A report of eight cases. Lancet 1981;2:598–600.
68. Kaposi's sarcoma and *Pneumocystis* pneumonia in homosexual men in New York City and California. MMWR 1981;30:305–308.
69. Gottlieb GJ, Ackerman AB. Kaposi's sarcoma: An extensively disseminated form in young homosexual men. Hum Pathol 1982;13:882–892.
70. Colby TV. Lymphoproliferative diseases. In: Dail DH, Hammar SP, Colby TV, eds. Pulmonary Pathology Tumors. New York, Springer-Verlag, 1995:343–368.
71. Liebow AA, Carrington CB, Friedman PJ. Lymphomatoid granulomatosis. Hum Pathol 1972;3:457–558.
72. Jaffe ES. Pulmonary lymphocytic angiitis: A nosologic quandry. Mayo Clin Proc 1988;63:411–415.
73. Guinee D, Jaffe E, Kingma D, et al. Pulmonary lymphomatoid granulomatosis: Evidence for a proliferation of Epstein-Barr virus–infected B lymphocytes with a prominent cell component and vasculitis. Am J Surg Pathol 1994;18:753–764.
74. Hammar SP. Pulmonary histocytosis X (Langerhans) cell granulomatosis. In: Dail DH, Hammar SP, eds. Pulmonary Pathology. 2nd ed. New York: Springer-Verlag, 1994:567–596.
75. Carter D, Patchefsky AS, Mountain CF. Large cell lesions. In: Carter D, Patchefsky AS, eds. Tumors and tumor-like lesions of the lung. Philadelphia: WB Saunders, 1998:271–274.
76. Bonetti F, Pea M, Martigoni G, et al. Clear cell ("sugar tumor") of the lung is a lesion strictly related to angiomyolipoma B the concept of a family of lesions characterized by the presence of the perivascular epithelioid cells (PEC). Pathology 1994;26:230–236.
77. Gaffey M, Mills S, Zarbo R, et al. Clear cell tumor of the lung: Immunohistochemical and ultrastructural evidence of melanogenesis. Am J Surg Pathol 1991;15:644–653.
78. Sullivan EJ. Lymphangioleiomyomatosis: A review. Chest 1998;114:1689–1703.
79. Johnson S. Lymphangioleiomyomatosis: Clinical features, management and basic mechanism. Thorax 1999;54:254–264.
80. Liebow AA, Hubbell DS. Sclerosing hemangioma (histocytoma, xanthoma) of the lung. Cancer 1956;9:53–75.
81. Sogio K, Yokoyama H, Kanedo S, et al. Sclerosing hemangioma of the lung: Radiographic and pathologic study. Ann Thorac Surg 1992;53:295–300.
82. Katzenstein A-LA, Gmelich JT, Carrington CB. Sclerosing hemangioma of the lung: A clinicopathologic study of 51 cases. Am J Surg Pathol 1982;4:343–356.
83. Beckwith JB, Palmer NF. Histopathology and prognosis of Wilms' tumor: Results from the first national Wilms' tumor study. Cancer 1978;55:2850–2853.
84. Small EJ, Gordon GJ, Dahms BB. Malignant rhabdoid tumor of the heart in an infant. Cancer 1985;55:2850–2853.
85. Balaton AJ, Vaury P, Videgrain M. Paravertebral malignant rhabdoid tumor in an adult: A case report of immunocytochemical study. Pathol Res Pract 1987;182:713–718.
86. Harris M, Eyden BP, Joglekar VM. Rhabdoid tumour of the bladder: A histological, ultrastructural and immunohistochemical study. Histopathology 1987;11:1083–1089.
87. Biggs PJ, Garren PD, Posers JM, et al. Malignant rhabdoid tumor of the central nervous system. Hum Pathol 1987;18:332–337.
88. Dervan PA, Cahalane SF, Kneafsey P, et al. Malignant rhabdoid tumor of soft tissue: An ultrastructural and immunohistological study of a pelvic tumour. Histopathology 1987;11:183–190.
89. Parham DM, Peiper S, Robicheaux G, et al. Malignant rhabdoid tumor of the liver: Evidence for epithelial differentiation. Arch Pathol Lab Med 1988;112:61–64.
90. Jakate SM, Mardsen HB, Ingram L. Primary rhabdoid tumour of the brain. Virch Arch A Pathol Anat 1988;412:393–397.
91. Uchida H, Yokoyama S, Nakayama I, Zeze K. An autopsy case of malignant rhabdoid tumor arising from soft parts in the left inguinal region. Acta Pathol Jpn 1988;38:1087–1096.
92. Patron M, Palacious J, Rodriguez–Peralto JL, et al. Malignant rhabdoid tumor of the tongue: A case report with immunohistochemical and ultrastructural findings. Oral Surg Oral Med Oral Pathol 1988;65:67–70.
93. Carter RL, McCarthy KP, al-Sam SZ, et al. Malignant rhabdoid tumour of the bladder with immunohistochemical and ultrastructural evidence suggesting histiocytic origin. Histopathology 1989;14:179–190.
94. Jsujimura T, Wasa A, Kawano K, et al. A case of malignant rhabdoid tumor arising from soft parts of the prepubic region. Acta Pathol Jpn 1989;37:677–682.

95. Cho KR, Rosenshein NB, Epstein JI. Malignant rhabdoid tumor of the kidney and soft tissues: Evidence for a diverse morphological and immunocytochemical phenotype. Arch Pathol Lab Med 1989;113:115–120.

96. Tsokos M, Kouraklis G, Chandra RS, et al. Malignant rhabdoid tumor of the kidney and soft tissues: Evidence for a diverse morphological and immunocytochemical phenotype. Arch Pathol Lab Med 1989;113:115–120.

97. Molenaar WM, DeJong B, Dam-Meiring A, et al. Epithelioid sarcoma or malignant rhabdoid tumor of soft tissue: Epithelioid immunophenotype and rhabdoid karyotype. Hum Pathol 1989;20:347–351.

98. Cavazza A, Colby TV, Tsokos M, et al. Lung tumors with a rhabdoid phenotype. Am J Clin Pathol 1996;105:182–188.

99. Bahadori H, Liebow AA. Plasma cell granuloma of the lung. Cancer 1973;31:191–208.

100. Lane JD, Krohn S, Kolozzi W, Whitehead RE. Plasma cell granuloma of the lung. Dis Chest 1955;27:216–221.

101. Berardi RS, Lee SS, Chen HP, et al. Inflammatory pseudotumors of the lung. Surg Gynecol Obstet 1983;156:89–96.

102. Tang TT, Segura AD, Oechler HW, et al. Inflammatory myofibrohistiocytic proliferation simulating sarcoma in children. Cancer 1990;65:1626–1634.

103. Tan-Liu NS, Matsubara MD, Grillo HC, et al. Invasive fibrous tumor of the tracheobronchial tree: Clinical and pathological study of seven cases. Hum Pathol 1989;20:180–184.

104. Ledet SC, Brown RW, Cagle PT. p53 immunostaining of the differentiation of inflammatory pseudotumor from sarcoma involving the lung. Mod Pathol 1995;8:282–286.

105. Snyder CS, Dell-Aquila M, Haghighi P, et al. Clonal changes in inflammatory pseudotumor of the lung. Cancer 1995;76:1545–1549.

106. Brambill AE. Basaloid carcinoma of the lung. In: Corrin B, ed. Pathology of Lung Tumors. New York: Churchill Livingstone, 1997;71–82.

107. Herrera GA, Turbat–Herrera EA, Lott RL. S100 protein expression by primary and metastatic adenocarcinoma. Am J Clin Pathol 1988;89:168–176.

108. Hammar SP, Bockus D, Remington F, et al. Langerhans' cells and serum precipitating antibodies against fungal antigens in bronchioloalveolar cell carcinomas: Possible association with eosinophilic granuloma. Ultrastruct Pathol 1980;1:19–37.

109. Colasante A, Castrilli G, Aiello FB, et al. Role of cytokines in the distribution of dendritic cells/Langerhans' cell lineage in human primary carcinomas of the lung. Hum Pathol 1995;26:866–872.

110. Hammar SP, Bockus D, Remington F, et al. The widespread distribution of Langerhans' cells in pathologic tissues: An ultrastructural and immunohistochemical study. Hum Pathol 1986;17:894–905.

111. Torikata C, Ishiwata K. Intranuclear tubular structures observed in the cells of alveolar cell carcinomas of the lung. Cancer 1977;40:1194–1201.

112. Singh G, Katyal SL, Torikata C. Carcinoma of type II pneumocytes: Immunodiagnosis of a subtype of bronchioloalveolar carcinoma. Am J Pathol 1981;102:195–208.

113. Singh G, Katyal SL, Torikata C. Carcinoma of type II pneumocytes: PAS staining as a screening test for nuclear inclusions of surfactant-specific apoprotein. Cancer 1982;50:946–948.

114. Ghadially FN, Harawi S, Khan W. Diagnostic ultrastructural markers in alveolar cell carcinoma. J Submicrosc Cytol 1985;17:269–278.

115. Abrams HJ, Spiro R, Goldstein N. Metastases in carcinoma, analysis of 1000 autopsied cases. Cancer 1950;3:74–85.

116. Dail DH. Metastases to and from the lung. In: Dail DH, Hammar SP, Colby TV. Pulmonary Tumors. New York, Springer-Verlag, 1995;369–403.

117. Wang NP, Zee S, Zarbo RJ, et al. Coordinate expression of cytokeratins 7 and 20 defines unique subsets of carcinomas. Appl Immunohist 1995;3:99–107.

118. Ollayos CW, Riordan P, Rushin JM. Estrogen receptor detection in paraffin section of adenocarcinoma of colon, pancreas and lung. Arch Pathol Lab Med 1994;118:630–632.

119. Canver CC, Memoli VA, Vanderveer PL, et al. Sex hormones in non–small cell lung cancer in human beings. J Thorac Cardiovasc Surg 1994;108:153–157.

120. Bacchi CE, Garcia RL, Gown AM. Immunolocalization of estrogen and progesterone receptors in neuroendocrine tumors of lung, skin, gastrointestinal and female genital tracts. Appl Immunohistochem 1997;5:17–22.

121. Butler AE, Colby TV, Weiss L, et al. Lymphoepithelioma-like carcinoma of lung. Am J Surg Pathol 1989;13:632–639.

122. Ginsberg SS, Buzaid AC, Stern H, et al. Giant cell carcinoma of the lung. Cancer 1992;70:606–610.

123. Gustmann C, Altmannsberger M, Osborn M, et al. Cytokeratin expression and vimentin content in large cell anaplastic lymphoma and other non-Hodgkin's lymphoma. Am J Pathol 1991;38:1413–1422.

124. Delsol G, AlSaati T, Gatter KC, et al. Coexpression of epithelial membrane antigen (EMA), Ki-1 and interleukin-2 receptor by anaplastic large cell lymphomas: Diagnostic value in so-called malignant histiocytosis. Am J Pathol 1988;130:59–70.

125. Osborne BM, McKay B, Butler JJ, et al. Large cell lymphoma with microvillus-like projections: An ultrastructural study. Am J Clin Pathol 1983;79:433–450.

126. Bishop PW, Menasce LP, Yates AJ, et al. An immunophenotypic survey of malignant melanomas. Histopathology 1993;23:159–166.

127. Yoshimoto T, Higashino K, Hada T, et al. A primary lung carcinoma producing alpha-fetoprotein, carcinoembryonic antigen and human chorionic gonadotropin. Cancer 1987;60:2744–2750.

128. Kuida CA, Braunstein GD, Shintaku P, et al. Human chorionic gonadotropin expression in lung, breast and renal carcinomas. Arch Pathol Lab Med 1988;112:282–285.

129. Visscher DW, Zarbo RJ, Trojanowski JQ, et al. Neuroendocrine differentiation in poorly differentiated lung carcinomas: A light microscopic and immunohistochemical study. Mod Pathol 1990;3:508–512.

130. Linnoila RI, Mulshine JL, Steinberg SM, et al. Neuroendocrine differentiation in endocrine and nonendocrine lung carcinomas. Am J Clin Pathol 1988;90:641–652.

131. Mooi WJ, Dewar A, Springall D, et al. Non–small cell lung carcinomas with neuroendocrine features: A light microscopic, immunohistochemical and ultrastructural study of 11 cases. Histopathology 1988;13:329–337.

132. Wick MR, Berg LC, Hertz MI. Large cell carcinoma of the lung with neuroendocrine differentiation: a comparison with large cell "undifferentiated" pulmonary tumors. Am J Clin Pathol 1992;97:796–805.

133. Loy TS, Darkow GVD, Quesenberry JT. Immunostaining in the diagnosis of pulmonary neuroendocrine carcinomas: An immunohistochemical study with ultrastructural correlations. Am J Surg Pathol 1995;19:173–182.

134. Schleusener JT, Tazelaar HD, Jung S, et al. Neuroendocrine differentiation is an independent prognostic factor in chemotherapy-treated non–small cell lung carcinoma. Cancer 1996;77:1284–1291.

135. Hammar SP. Pleural diseases. In: Dail DH, Hammar SP, Colby TV, eds. Pulmonary Pathology Tumors. New York, Springer-Verlag, 1995:405–530.

136. Davies J. Human developmental anatomy. New York, Roland Press, 1963:51–52.

137. Selikoff IJ, Seidman H. Asbestos-associated deaths among insulation workers in the United States and Canada, 1967–1987. Ann NY Acad Sci 1991;643:1–14.

138. Battifora H, McCaughey WTE. Tumors of the Serosal Membranes. Washington D.C.: Armed Forces Institute of Pathology, 1995:17–88.

139. Henderson DW, Shilkin KB, Whitaker D. Reactive mesothelial hyperplasia vs. mesothelioma, including mesothelioma in situ: A brief review. Am J Clin Pathol 1998;110:397–404.

140. Bolen JW, Hammar SP, McNutt MA. Reactive and neoplastic serosal tissue: A light-microscopic, ultrastructural and immunocytochemical study. Am J Surg Pathol 1986;10:34–47.

141. Henderson DW, Comin CE, Hammar SP, et al. Malignant mesothelioma of the pleura: Current surgical pathology. In: Corrin B, ed. Pathology of Lung Tumors. New York, Churchill Livingstone, 1997:241−280.

142. Ordonez NG. The immunohistochemical diagnosis of epithelial mesothelioma. Hum Pathol 1999;30:313−323.

143. Blobel GA, Moll R, Franke WW, et al. The intermediate filament cytoskeleton of malignant mesothelioma and its diagnostic significance. Am J Pathol 1985;121:235−247.

144. Blobel GA, Moll R, Franke WW, et al. Cytokeratins in normal lung and lung carcinomas. I: Adenocarcinomas, squamous cell carcinomas and cultured cell lines. Virchows Arch B Cell Pathol 1984;45:407−429.

145. Moll R, Dhovailly D, Sun T-T. Expression of keratin 5 as a distinctive feature of epithelial and biphasic mesotheliomas: An immunohistochemical study using monoclonal antibody AE14. Virchows Arch B Cell Pathol 1989;58:129−145.

146. Clover J, Oates J, Edwards C. Anti-cytokeratin 5/6: A positive marker for epithelial mesothelioma. Histopathology 1997;31:140−143.

147. Kahn HJ, Thorner PS, Yeager H, et al. Immunohistochemical localization of pre-keratin filaments in benign and malignant cells in effusions: Comparison with intermediate filament distribution by electron microscopy. Am J Pathol 1982;109:206−214.

148. Kahn HJ, Thorner PS, Yeger H, et al. Distinct keratin patterns demonstrated by immunoperoxidase staining of adenocarcinomas, carcinoids and mesotheliomas using polyclonal and monoclonal keratin antibodies. Am J Clin Pathol 1986;86:566−574.

149. Montag AG, Pinkus GS, Corson JM. Keratin protein reactivity immunoreactivity of sarcomatoid and mixed types of diffuse malignant mesotheliomas: An immunoperoxidase study of 30 cases. Hum Pathol 1988;19:336−342.

150. Battifora H. The pleura. In: Sternberg SS, ed. Diagnostic surgical pathology. vol. I. New York: Raven Press, 1989: 829−855.

151. Roggli VL, Kolbeck J, Sanfilippo F, et al. Pathology of human mesothelioma: Etiologic and diagnostic considerations. Pathol Annu 1987;22:pt 2:91−131.

152. Al-Izzi M, Thurlow NP, Corrin B. Pleural mesothelioma of connective tissue type, localized fibrous tumour of the pleura and reactive submesothelial hyperplasia: An immunohistochemical comparison. J Pathol 1989;157: 41−44.

153. Blobel GA, Moll R, Franke WW, et al. The intermediate filament cytoskeleton of malignant mesotheliomas and its diagnostic significance. Am J Pathol 1985;121:235−247.

154. Mayall FG, Goddard H, Gibbs AR. Intermediate filament expression in mesotheliomas: Leiomyoid mesotheliomas are not uncommon. Histopathology 1992;21:453−457.

155. Yousem SA, Hochholzer L. Malignant mesotheliomas with osseous and cartilaginous differentiation. Arch Pathol Lab Invest 1987;111:62−66.

156. Wirth PR, Legler J, Wright GL. Immunohistochemical evaluation of seven monoclonal antibodies for differentiation of pleural mesothelioma from lung adenocarcinoma. Cancer 1991;67:655−662.

157. Carter D, Otis CN. Three types of spindle cell tumors of pleura: Fibroma, sarcoma and sarcomatoid mesothelioma. Am J Surg Pathol 1988;12:747−753.

158. Azumi N, Battifora H, Carlson G, et al. Sarcomatous (spindle-cell) mesothelioma of pleura: Immunohistochemical study. Lab Invest 1989;60:4A.

159. McNutt MA, Bolen JW, Gown AM, et al. Coexpression of intermediate filaments in human epithelial neoplasms. Ultrastruct Pathol 1985;9:31−43.

160. Upton MP, Hirohashi S, Tome Y, et al. Expression of vimentin in surgically resected adenocarcinomas and large cell carcinomas of lung. Am J Surg Pathol 1986;10:560−567.

161. Azumi N, Battifora H. The distribution of vimentin and keratin in epithelial and non-epithelial neoplasms: A comprehensive study on formalin and alcohol-fixed tumors. Am J Clin Pathol 1987;88:286−296.

162. Raymond WA, Leong AS-Y. Vimentin B a new prognostic marker in breast carcinoma. J Pathol 1989;158:107−114.

163. Churg A. Immunohistochemical staining for vimentin and keratin in malignant mesothelioma. Am J Surg Pathol 1985;9:360−365.

164. Jasani B, Edwards RE, Thomas ND, et al. The use of vimentin antibodies in the diagnosis of malignant mesothelioma. Virch Arch A Pathol Anat 1985;406:441−448.

165. Mullink H, Henzen-Logmans SC, Alons-van Kordelaan JJM, et al. Simultaneous immunoenzyme staining of vimentin and cytokeratins with monoclonal antibodies as an aid in the differential diagnosis of malignant mesothelioma from pulmonary adenocarcinoma. Virch Arch B Pathol Anat 1986;42:55−65.

166. Andersen C, Blumcke I, Celio MR. Calcium-binding proteins: Selective markers of nerve cells. Cell Tissue Res 1993;271:181−208.

167. Schwaller B, Buchwald P, Blumcke I, et al. Characterization of a polyclonal antiserum against the purified human recombinant calcium binding protein calretinin. Cell Calcium 1993;14:639−648.

168. Gotzos V, Schwaller B, Hertzel N, et al. Expression of the calcium binding protein calretinin in Wi Dr cells and its correlation to their cell cycle. Exp Cell Res 1992;202:292−302.

169. Doglioni C, Dei Tos AP, Laurino L, et al. Calretinin: A novel immunocytochemical marker for mesothelioma. Am J Surg Pathol 1996;20:1037−1046.

170. Barberis MCP, Faleri M, Veronese S, et al. Calretinin: A selective marker of normal and neoplastic mesothelial cells in serous effusions. Acta Cytol 1997;41:1757−1761.

171. Leers MPG, Aarts MMJ, Theunissen PHMH. E-cadherin and calretinin: A useful combination of immunochemical markers for differentiation between mesothelioma and metastatic adenocarcinoma. Histopathology 1998;32:209−216.

172. Ordonez NG. Value of calretinin immunostaining in differentiating epithelial mesothelioma from lung adenocarcinoma. Mod Pathol 1998;10:929−933.

173. O'Hara CJ, Corson JM, Pinkus GS, et al. ME1: A monoclonal antibody that distinguishes epithelial-type mesothelioma from pulmonary adenocarcinoma and extra-pulmonary malignancies. Am J Pathol 1990;136:421−428.

174. Sheibani K, Esteban JM, Bailey A, et al. Immunopathologic and molecular studies as an aid to the diagnosis of malignant mesothelioma. Hum Pathol 1992;23:107−116.

175. Hammar SP, Bolen JW, Bockus D, et al. Ultrastructural and immunohistochemical features of common lung tumors: An overview. Ultrastruct Pathol 1985;9:283−318.

176. Walz R, Koch HK. Malignant pleural mesotheliomas: Some aspects of epidemiology, differential diagnosis and prognosis: Histological and immunohistochemical evaluation and follow-up of mesotheliomas diagnosed from 1964 to January 1985. Pathol Res Pract 1990;186:124−134.

177. Wick MR, Loy T, Mills SE, et al. Malignant epithelioid pleural mesothelioma versus peripheral pulmonary adenocarcinoma: A histochemical, ultrastructural and immunohistologic study of 103 cases. Hum Pathol 1990;21:759−766.

178. Henderson DW, Shilkin KB, Whitaker D, et al. The pathology of mesothelioma, including immunohistology and ultrastructure. In: Henderson DW, Shilkin KB, Langlois SL, Whitaker D, eds. Malignant Mesothelioma. New York: Hemisphere, 1992:69−139.

179. Fink L, Collins CL, Schaefer R, et al. Thrombomodulin expression can be used to differentiate between mesotheliomas and adenocarcinomas. Lab Invest 1992;66:113A.

180. Collins CL, Ordonez NG, Schaefer R, et al. Thrombomodulin expression and pulmonary adenocarcinoma. Am J Pathol 1992;141:827−833.

181. Brown RW, Clark GM, Tandon AK, et al. Multiple-marker immunohistochemical phenotypes distinguishing malignant pleural mesothelioma from pulmonary adenocarcinoma. Hum Pathol 1993;24:347−354.

182. Ascoli V, Scalzo CC, Taccogna S, et al. The diagnostic value of thrombomodulin immunolocalization in serous effusions. Arch Pathol Lab Med 1995;119:1136–1140.

183. Geiger B, Ayalon O. Cadherins. Annu Rev Cell Biol 1992; 8:307–332.

184. Takeichi M. Cadherin cell adhesion receptors as a morphogenetic regulator. Science 1991;251:1451–1455.

185. Hatta K, Takagi S, Fujisawa H, et al. Spatial and temporal expression pattern of N-cadherin cell adhesion molecules correlated with morphogenetic processes of chicken embryos. Dev Biol 1987;120:215–227.

186. Peralta-Soler A, Knudsen KA, Jaurand MC, et al. The differential expression of N-cadherin, E-cadherin distinguished pleural mesotheliomas from lung adenocarcinomas. Hum Pathol 1995;26:1363–1369.

187. Han AC, Peralta-Soler A, Knudsen KA, et al. Differential expression of N-cadherin in pleural mesotheliomas and E-cadherin in lung adenocarcinomas in formalin-fixed, paraffin-embedded tissues. Hum Pathol 1997;28:641–645.

188. Amin KM, Litzky LA, Smythe WR, et al. Wilms' tumor 1 susceptibility (WT1) gene products are selectively expressed in malignant mesothelioma. Am J Pathol 1995;146:344–356.

189. Kumar-Singh S, Segers K, Rodeck O, et al. WT1 mutation in malignant mesothelioma and WT1 immunoreactivity in relation to p53 growth factor expression, cell-type transition and prognosis. J Pathol 1997;181:67–74.

190. Walker C, Rutlen F, Yuan X, et al. Wilms' tumor suppressor gene expression in rat and human mesothelioma. Cancer Res 1994;54:1301–1306.

191. Shivley JE, Beatty JD. CEA-related antigens: Molecular biology and clinical significance. Crit Rev Oncol Hematol 1985;2:355–399.

192. Thompson J, Grunert F, Zimmermann W. Carcinoembryonic antigen gene family: Molecular biology and clinical perspectives. J Clin Lab Anal 1991;5:344–366.

193. Hammarstrom S, Khan WN, Teglund S, et al. The carcinoembryonic antigen family. In: Van Regenmortel MHV, ed. Structure of Antigens. Boca Raton, FL, CRC Press, 1993:341–376.

194. Hammarstrom S, Olsen A, Teglund S, et al. The nature and expression of the human CEA family. In: Stanners C, ed. Cell Adhesion and Clinical Perspectives. Amsterdam: Harwood Academic Publishers, 1997:1–30.

195. Hammarstrom S. The carcinoembryonic antigen (CEA) family: Structures, suggested functions and expression in normal and malignant tissues. Cancer Biol 1999;9:67–81.

196. Wang N-S, Huang S-N, Gold P. Absence of carcinoembryonic antigen–like material in mesothelioma: An immunohistochemical differentiation from other lung cancers. Cancer 1979;44:437–943.

197. Whitaker D, Shilkin KB. Carcinoembryonic antigen in the tissue diagnosis of malignant mesothelioma. Lancet 1981;1:1369–1370.

198. Whitaker D, Sterret GF, Shilkin KB. Detection of tissue CEA-like substance as an aid in the differential diagnosis of malignant mesothelioma. Pathology 1982;14:255–258.

199. Sheibani K, Battifora H. Leu-M1 positivity is not specific for Hodgkin's disease. Am J Clin Pathol 1985;84:682.

200. Sheibani K, Battifora H, Burke JS, et al. Leu-M1 in human neoplasms: An immunohistologic study of 400 cases. Am J Surg Pathol 1986;10:227–236.

201. Sheibani K, Battifora H, Burke J. Antigenic phenotype of malignant mesotheliomas and pulmonary adenocarcinomas: An immunohistologic analysis demonstrating the value of Leu-M1 antigen. Am J Pathol 1986;123:212–219.

202. Sheibani K, Azumi N, Battifora H. Further evidence demonstrating the value of LeuM1 antigen in differential diagnosis of malignant mesothelioma and adenocarcinoma: An immunohistologic evaluation of 395 cases. Lab Invest 1988;58:84A.

203. Otis CN, Carter O, Cole S, et al. Immunohistochemical evaluation of pleural mesothelioma and pulmonary adenocarcinoma. Am J Surg Pathol 1987;11:445–456.

204. Szpak CA, Johnston WW, Roggli V, et al. The diagnostic distinction between malignant mesothelioma and adenocarcinoma of the lung as defined by a monoclonal antibody (B72.3). Am J Pathol 1986;122:252–260.

205. Ordonez NG. The immunohistochemical diagnosis of mesothelioma: Differentiation of mesothelioma and lung adenocarcinoma. Am J Surg Pathol 1989;13:276–291.

206. Bollinger DJ, Wick MR, Dehner LP, et al. Peritoneal malignant mesothelioma versus serous papillary adenocarcinoma: A histochemical and immunohistochemical comparison. Am J Surg Pathol 1989;13:659–670.

207. Latza V, Niedobitek G, Schwarting R, et al. Ber-EP4: New monoclonal antibody which distinguishes epithelia from mesothelia. J Clin Pathol 1990;43:213–219.

208. Sheibani K, Shin SS, Kezirian J, et al. Ber-EP4 antibody as a discriminant in the differential diagnosis of malignant mesothelioma versus adenocarcinoma. Am J Surg Pathol 1991;15:779–784.

209. Gaffey MJ, Mills SE, Swanson PE, et al. Immunoreactivity for Ber-EP4 in adenocarcinomas, adenomatoid tumors and malignant mesotheliomas. Am J Surg Pathol 1992;16:593–599.

210. Riutenbeek T, Gouw ASH, Poppema S. Immunocytology of body cavity fluids: MOC–31, a monoclonal antibody discriminating between mesothelial and epithelial cells. Arch Pathol Lab Med 1994;118:265–269.

211. Souhami RL, Beverly PCL, Bobrow LG. Antigens of small cell lung cancer: First International Workshop. Lancet 1987;2:325–326.

212. DeLeij L, Broers J, Ramaekers F, et al. Monoclonal antibodies in clinical and experimental pathology of lung cancer. In: Roiter DJ, Fleuren GJ, Warner SO, eds. Applications of Monoclonal Antibodies in Tumor Pathology. Dordrecht: Martinus Nijhoff Publishers, 1987:191–210.

213. Delahaye M, Hoogsteden HC, van der Kwast TH. Immunocytochemistry of malignant mesothelioma: OV 632 as a marker of malignant mesothelioma. J Pathol 1991;165:137–143.

214. Ordonez NG. Value of MOC-31 monoclonal antibody in differentiating epithelial pleural mesothelioma from lung adenocarcinoma. Hum Pathol 1998;29:166–169.

215. Jordon D, Jagirdar J, Kaneko M. Blood group antigens Lewis x and Lewis y in the diagnostic discrimination of malignant mesothelioma versus adenocarcinoma. Am J Pathol 1989;135:931–937.

216. Riera JR, Astengo-Osuna C, Longmate JA, et al. The immunohistochemical diagnostic panel for epithelial mesothelioma: A reevaluation after heat-induced epitope retrieval. Am J Surg Pathol 1997;21:1409–1419.

217. Geiger B, Ayalon O. Cadherins. Annu Rev Cell Biol 1992; 8:307–332.

218. Kinsella AR, Green B, Lepts GC, et al. The role of cell-cell adhesion molecule E-cadherin in large bowel tumour cell invasion and metastasis. Br J Cancer 1993;67:904–909.

219. Williams CL, Hayes VY, Hummel AM, et al. Regulation of E-cadherin mediated adhesion by muscarinic acetylcholine receptor in small cell lung carcinoma. J Cell Biol 1993;121:643–654.

220. Leers MPG, Aarts MMJ, Theunissen PTMH. E-cadherin and calretinin: A useful combination of immunochemical markers for differentiation between mesothelioma and metastatic adenocarcinoma. Histopathology 1998;32:209–216.

221. Kawai T, Suzuki M, Torikata C, et al. Expression of blood group–related antigens and Helix pomatia agglutinin in malignant pleural mesothelioma and pulmonary adenocarcinoma. Hum Pathol 1991;22:118–124.

222. Mayall FG, Goddard H, Gibbs AR. p53 immunostaining in the distinction between benign and malignant mesothelial proliferations using formalin-fixed paraffin sections. J Pathol 1992;168:377–381.

223. Ramael M, Lemmens G, Eerdekens C, et al. Immunoreactivity for p53 protein in malignant mesothelioma and nonneoplastic mesothelium. J Pathol 1992;168:371–375.

224. Mayall FG, Goddard H, Gibbs AR. The frequency of p53 immunostaining in asbestos-associated mesotheliomas. Histopathology 1993;22:383–386.

225. Hurlimann J. Desmin and neural marker expression in mesothelial cells and mesotheliomas. Hum Pathol 1994;25: 753–757.
226. Azumi N, Underhill CB, Kagan E, et al. A novel biotinylated probe specific for hyaluronate. Am J Surg Pathol 1992;16:116–121.
227. Thylen A, Wallin J, Martensson G. Hyaluronan in serum as an indicator of progressive disease in hyaluronan-producing malignant mesothelioma. Cancer 1999;86:2000–2005.
228. Martensson G, Thylen A, Lindquist U, et al. The sensitivity of hyaluronan analysis of pleural fluid from patients with malignant mesothelioma and a comparison of different methods. Cancer 1994;73:1406–1410.
229. Thylen A, Levin-Jacobsen AM, Hjerpe A, et al. Immunohistochemical differences between hyaluronan and non-hyaluronan–producing malignant mesothelioma. Eur Respir J 1997;10:404–408.
230. Kabawat SE, Bast RC, Bhan AK, et al. Immunopathologic characterization of a monoclonal antibody that recognizes common surface antigens of human ovarian tumors of serous, endometrioid and clear cell types. Am J Clin Pathol 1983;79:98–104.
231. Kabawat SE, Blast RC, Bhan AK, et al. Tissue distribution of celomic epithelium related antigen recognized by monoclonal antibody OC-125. Int J Gynecol Pathol 1983;2:275–285.
232. Dabbs DJ, Geisinger KR. Selective application of immunohistochemistry in gynecological neoplasms. Pathol Annu 1993;28:pt 1:329–353.
233. Bast RC, Freeney M, Lazarus H, et al. Reactivity of a monoclonal antibody with human ovarian carcinoma. J Clin Invest 1981;68:1331–1337.
234. Koelma IA, Nap M, Rodenburg CJ, et al. The value of tumor marker CA-125 in surgical pathology. Histopathology 1987;11:287–294.
235. Nanbu Y, Fujii S, Konishi I, et al. Immunohistochemical localization of CA-130 in fetal tissue and in normal and neoplastic tissues of the female genital tract. Asia Oceania J Obstet Gynecol 1990;16:379–387.
236. Tamura S, Yamaguchi K, Terada M, et al. Immunohistochemical analysis of CA19-9, SLX and CA–125 in adenoidcystic carcinoma of trachea and bronchus. Nippon Kyobu Shikkan Gakkai Zasshi 1992;3:407–411.
237. Zhou J, Iwasa Y, Konishi I, et al. Papillary serous carcinoma of the peritoneum in women: A clinicopathologic and immunohistochemical study. Cancer 1995;76:429–436.
238. Nouwen EJ, Pollet DE, Eerdekens MW, et al. Immunohistochemical localization of placental alkaline phosphatase, carcinoembryonic antigen and cancer antigen 125 in normal and neoplastic human lung. Cancer Res 1986;46:866–876.
239. Bateman AC, al-Talib RK, Newman T, et al. Immunohistochemical phenotype of malignant mesothelioma: Predictive value of CA-125 and HBME-1 expression. Histopathology 1997;30:49–56.
240. Nap M. Immunohistochemistry of CA-125: Unusual expression in normal tissues, distribution in the human fetus and questions around its application in diagnostic pathology. Int J Biol Markers 1998;13:210–215.
241. O'Brien TJ, Raymond LM, Bannon GA, et al. New monoclonal antibodies identify the glycoprotein carrying the CA-125 epitope. Am J Obstet Gynecol 1991;61:1857–1864.
242. Okamoto H, Matsuno Y, Noguchi M, et al. Malignant pleural mesothelioma producing chorionic gonadotropin: Report of two cases. Am J Surg Pathol 1992;16:969–974.
243. McAuley P, Asa SL, Chiv B, et al. Parathyroid hormone–like peptide in normal and neoplastic mesothelial cells. Cancer 1990;66:1975–1979.
244. Tateyama H, Eimoto T, Tada T, et al. Immunoreactivity of a new CD5 antibody with normal epithelium and malignant tumors including thymic carcinoma. Am J Clin Pathol 1999;111:235–240.

245. Hammar SP, Bockus D, Remington F. Metastatic tumors of unknown origin: An ultrastructural analysis of 265 cases. Ultrastruct Pathol 1987;11:209–250.
246. Gaber AO, Rice P, Eaton C, et al. Metastatic malignant disease of unknown origin. Am J Surg Pathol 1983;145:493–497.
247. Crotty TB, Myers JL, Katzenstein AL, et al. Localized malignant mesothelioma: A clinicopathologic and flow cytometric study. Am J Surg Pathol 1994;18:357–363.
248. Briselli M, Mark EJ, Dickersin GR. Solitary fibrous tumors of the pleura: Eight new cases and review of 360 cases in the literature. Cancer 1981;47:2678–2689.
249. Doucet J, Dardick I, Srigley JR, et al. Localized fibrous tumour of serosal surfaces. Virch Arch A Pathol Anat 1986;409:349–363.
250. England DM, Hochholzer L, McCarthy MJ. Localized benign and malignant fibrous tumors of the pleura: A clinicopathologic review of 223 cases. Am J Surg Pathol 1989;13:640–658.
251. van de Rijn M, Lombard CM, Rouse RV. Expression of CD34 by solitary fibrous tumors of the pleura, mediastinum and lung. Am J Surg Pathol 1994;18:814–820.
252. Flint A, Weiss SW. CD-34 and keratin expression distinguishes solitary fibrous tumor (fibrous mesothelioma) of pleura from desmoplastic mesothelioma. Hum Pathol 1995;26:428–431.
253. Hasegawa T, Matsuno Y, Shimoda T, et al. Frequent expression of bcl-2 protein in solitary fibrous tumors. Jpn J Clin Oncol 1998;28:86–91.
254. Babolini G, Blasi A. The pleural form of primary cancer of the lung. Dis Chest 1956;29:314–323.
255. Harwood TR, Gracey DR, Yokoo H. Pseudomesotheliomatous carcinoma of the lung. Am J Clin Pathol 1976;65:159–167.
256. Koss M, Travis W, Moran C, et al. Pseudomesotheliomatous adenocarcinoma: A reappraisal. Semin Diagn Pathol 1992;9:117–123.
257. Hartman C-A, Schutze H. Mesothelioma-like tumors of the pleura: A review of 72 cases. Cancer Res Clin Oncol 1994;120:331–347.
258. Koss MN, Fleming M, Przygodzki RM, et al. Adenocarcinoma simulating mesothelioma: A clinicopathologic and immunohistochemical study of 29 cases. Ann Diagn Pathol 1998;2:93–102.
259. Robb JA, Hammar SP, Yokoo H. Pseudomesotheliomatous carcinoma of lung. Lab Invest 1993;68:134A.
260. Battifora H. Epithelioid hemangioendothelioma imitating mesothelioma. Appl Immunohistochem 1993;1:220–221.
261. Lin BT-Y, Colby T, Gown AM, et al. Malignant vascular tumors of the serous membranes mimicking mesothelioma: A report of 14 cases. Am J Surg Pathol 1996;20:1431–1439.
262. Gray MH, Rosenberg AE, Dickersin GR, et al. Cytokeratin expression in epithelioid vascular neoplasms. Hum Pathol 1990;21:212–217.
263. Pinkard NB, Wilson RW, Lawless N, et al. Calcifying fibrous pseudotumor of pleura: A report of three cases of a newly described entity involving the pleura. Am J Clin Pathol 1996;105:189–194.
264. Wilson RW, Gallateau-Salle F, Moran CA. Desmoid tumors of the pleura: A clinicopathologic mimic of localized fibrous tumor. Mod Pathol 1999;12:9–14.
265. Moran CA, Travis WD, Rosada-de-Christenson M, et al. Thymomas presenting as pleural tumors: Report of eight cases. Am J Surg Pathol 1992;16:138–144.
266. Payne CB Jr, Morningstar WA, Chester EH. Thymoma of the pleura masquerading as diffuse mesothelioma. Am Rev Respir Dis 1966;94:441–446.
267. Honma K, Shimada K. Metastasizing ectopic thymoma arising in the right thoracic cavity and mimicking diffuse pleural mesothelioma: An autopsy study of a case with review of the literature. Wien Klin Wochenschr 1986;98:14–20.
268. Shih D, Wang J, Tseng H, et al. Primary pleural thymoma. Arch Pathol Lab Med 1997;121:79–82.

269. Gaertner E, Zeren H, Fleming MV, et al. Biphasic synovial sarcomas arising in the pleural cavity: A clinicopathologic study of five cases. Am J Surg Pathol 1996;20:36–45.

270. Ordonez NG, Mahfouz SM, Mackay B. Synovial sarcoma: An immunohistochemical and ultrastructural study. Hum Pathol 1990;21:733–749.

271. Hachitanda Y, Aoyama C, Sato JK, et al. Pleuropulmonary blastoma in childhood: A tumor of divergent differentiation. Am J Surg Pathol 1993;17:382–391.

272. Priest JR, McDermott MB, Bhatia S, et al. Pleuropulmonary blastoma: A clinicopathologic study of 50 cases. Cancer 1997;80:147–161.

273. Hill DA, Sadeghi S, Schultz MZ, et al. Pleuropulmonary blastoma in an adult: An initial case report. Cancer 1999;85:2368–2374.

274. Churg A, Colby TV, Cagle P, et al. The separation of benign and malignant mesothelial proliferations: US-Canadian Mesothelioma Panel. Am J Surg Pathol 2000;24:1183–1200.

275. Hammar SP, Bockus DE, Remington FL, et al. Mucin-positive epithelial mesotheliomas: A histochemical, immunohistochemical and ultrastructural comparison with mucin-producing pulmonary adenocarcinomas. Ultrastruct Pathol 1996;20:293–325.

276. Mayall FG, Gibbs AR. The histology and immunohistochemistry of small cell mesothelioma. Histopathology 1992;20:47–51.

277. Mayall FG, Jasani B, Gibbs AR. Immunohistochemical positivity for neuron specific enolase and Leu 7 in malignant mesotheliomas. J Pathol 1992;165:325–328.

278. Falconieri G, Zanconati F, Bussani R, et al. Small cell carcinoma of lung simulating mesothelioma. Pathol Res Pract 1995;191:1147–1151.

279. Henderson DW, Atwood HD, Constance TJ, et al. Lymphohistiocytoid mesothelioma: A rare lymphomatoid variant of predominantly sarcomatoid mesothelioma. Ultrastruct Pathol 1988;12:367–384.

280. Daya D, McCaughey WTE. Well-differentiated papillary mesothelioma of the peritoneum: A clinicopathologic study of 22 cases. Cancer 1990;65:292–296.

281. Yesner R, Hurwitz A. Localized pleural mesothelioma of epithelial type. J Thorac Surg 1953;26:325–329.

282. Thickett DR, Armstrong L, Millar AB. Vascular endothelial growth factor (VEGF) in inflammatory and malignant pleural effusions. Thorax 1999;54:707–710.

283. Golden A, Ash J. Adenomatoid tumors of genital tract. Am J Pathol 1990;14:63–80.

284. Argani P, Rosai J. Hyperplastic mesothelial cells in lymph nodes: Report of six cases of a benign process that can stimulate metastatic involvement by mesothelioma or carcinoma. Am J Surg Pathol 1998;29:339–346.

285. Brooks JSJ, LiVolsi VA, Pietra GG. Mesothelial cell inclusions in mediastinal lymph nodes mimicking metastatic carcinoma. Am J Clin Pathol 1990;93:741–748.

286. Ordonez NG, Ro JY, Ayal AG. Lesions described as nodular mesothelial hyperplasia are primarily composed of histiocytes. Am J Surg Pathol 1998;22:285–292.

287. Sussman J, Rosai J. Lymph node metastasis as the initial manifestation of malignant mesothelioma: Report of six cases. Am J Surg Pathol 1990;14:819–828.

288. Kannerstein M, Churg J, McCaughey WTE, et al. Papillary tumors of the peritoneum in women: Mesothelioma or papillary carcinoma. Am J Obstet Gynecol 1977;127:306–314.

289. Foyle A, Al-Jabi M, McCaughey WTE. Papillary peritoneal tumors in women. Am J Surg Pathol 1981;5:241–249.

290. Mills SE, Andersen WA, Fechner RE, et al. Serous surface papillary carcinomas: A clinicopathologic study of 10 cases and comparison with stage III-IV ovarian serous carcinoma. Am J Surg Pathol 1988;12:827–834.

291. Bollinger DJ, Wick MR, Dehner LP, et al. Peritoneal malignant mesothelioma versus serous papillary adenocarcinoma: A histochemical and immunohistochemical comparison. Am J Surg Pathol 1989;13:659–670.

292. Raju U, Fine G, Greenwald KA, et al. Primary papillary serous neoplasia of the peritoneum: A clinicopathologic and ultrastructural study of eight cases. Hum Pathol 1989;20:426–436.

293. Bell DA, Scully RE. Benign and borderline serous lesions of the peritoneum in women. Pathol Annu 1989;24:pt 2:1–21.

294. Rutledge ML, Silva EG, McLemore D, et al. Serous surface carcinoma of the ovary and peritoneum: A flow cytometric study. Pathol Annu 1989;24:pt 2:227–235.

295. Bell DA, Scully RE. Serous borderline tumors of the peritoneum. Am J Surg Pathol 1990;14:230–239.

296. Truong LD, Maccato ML, Awalt H, et al. Serous surface carcinoma of the peritoneum: A clinicopathologic study of 22 cases. Hum Pathol 1990;21:99–110.

297. Biscotti CV, Hart WR. Peritoneal serous micropapillomatosis of low malignant potential (serous borderline tumors of the peritoneum): A clinicopathologic study of 17 cases. Am J Surg Pathol 1992;16:467–475.

298. Shah IA, Jayram L, Gani OS, et al. Papillary serous carcinoma of the peritoneum in a man. Cancer 1998;82:860–866.

299. Khoury N, Raju R, Crissman JD, et al. A comparative immunohistochemical study of peritoneal and ovarian tumors, and mesotheliomas. Hum Pathol 1990;21:811–819.

300. Taylor DR, Page W, Huges D, et al. Metastatic renal cell carcinoma mimicking pleural mesothelioma. Thorax 1987;42:901–902.

301. Ordonez NG, Myhre M, Mackay B. Clear cell mesothelioma. Ultrastruct Pathol 1996;20:331–336.

302. Zarbo RJ, Gown AM, Nagle RB, et al. Anomalous cytokeratin expression in malignant melanoma: One- and two-dimensional western blot analysis and immunohistochemical survey of 100 melanomas. Mod Pathol 1990;3:494–501.

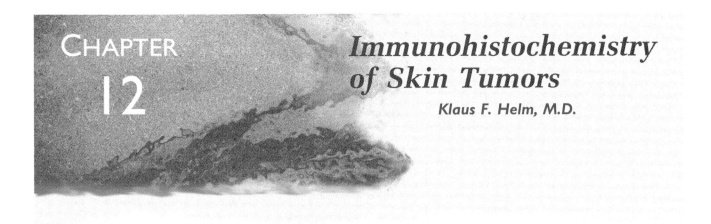

CHAPTER 12

Immunohistochemistry of Skin Tumors

Klaus F. Helm, M.D.

Immunohistochemistry in dermatopathology can be used for diagnosis, prognosis, and research purposes in attempting to understand the pathophysiology of skin diseases. This chapter discusses the use of immunohistochemistry as an adjunctive aid in the diagnosis of a variety of skin tumors.

OVERVIEW OF THE SKIN AND ITS RELEVANT ANTIGENS

The skin is a highly complicated organ, and an in-depth discussion of its components is beyond the scope of this chapter. The following is a brief overview of the skin and some of the relevant antigens used for immunohistochemistry in dermatopathology.

Keratinocytes

Keratinocytes are the building blocks of the epidermis and contain intermediate filaments called *cytokeratins,* which form a cytoskeletal support network. More than 30 different cytokeratin (CK) proteins have been detected. Cytokeratins have been subdivided based both on charge and molecular weight in two-dimensional gel electrophoresis. Cytokeratin filaments are organized in pairs with an acidic cytokeratin paired with a basic cytokeratin. Cytokeratins 1 and 10/11 are markers for differentiated keratinocytes. Cytokeratin 2 paired with cytokeratins 10/11 is found in the palms and soles. Keratinocytes within the basal layers of the epidermis contain cytokeratins 5 and 14/15. In disorders with increased proliferation of the keratinocytes, increased expression of cytokeratins 6 and 16/17 can be detected.[1]

Hair Follicle

The follicular apparatus consists of an external root sheath, which forms a continuum to the over-lying epidermis; an internal root sheath, which forms a canal through which the hair passes; the hair shaft itself, which contains a cuticle, cortex, and occasionally a medulla. Surrounding the hair follicle is a fibroblast-rich connective sheath. At the base of the hair is the hair bulb, which is composed of dermal papilla cells and matrix cells that develop into the internal root sheath and hair follicle. Hair follicles contain approximately 10 unique so-called hard cytokeratins, which differ from epidermal cytokeratins by having a high sulfur content. The keratinocytes within the infundibulum express a cytokeratin profile similar to that of the epidermis. The isthmus expresses CK5/CK6, CK14, CK17, and CK19. The internal root sheath expresses CK4 and CK18.[2] Involucrin, a protein found in the cornified envelope in skin, is expressed by both the infundibulum and isthmus portion of hair follicles. The connective sheath surrounding hair follicles expresses CD34, the human progenitor cell antigen.[3]

Apocrine and Eccrine Glands

Both eccrine and apocrine glands are found in skin. Eccrine glands can be subdivided into three segments: the secretory portion found in deep dermis or fat, the dermal duct, and the intraepidermal duct (acrosyringium). The gland is formed by both clear and dark cells, which are surrounded by a basal lamina and myoepithelial cells. Apocrine glands, like eccrine glands, have three segments: the secretory portion, the intradermal duct, and the intraepidermal duct. On frozen sections, eccrine and apocrine glands exhibit a somewhat different enzyme profile. Eccrine glands contain beta-glucuronidase, succinic dehydrogenase, aminopeptidase, and alkaline phosphatase, whereas apocrine glands contain phosphorylase, alkaline phosphatase, and succinic dehydrogenase.[4, 5] The eccrine and apocrine ducts are identical and cannot be distinguished using morphologic or immunohistochemical techniques. All segments of both eccrine and apocrine glands contain cytokeratins.[6] The intra-epidermal and dermal ducts stain strongly with AE1, an antibody against CK10, CK14/CK15, CK16, and CK19. AE1, CAM5.2 (an antibody against simple cytokeratins 8 and 18), and epithelial membrane antigen (EMA) stain the secretory glands.[6] Eccrine glands exhibit stronger staining with carcinoembryonic antigen (CEA) in contrast to apocrine glands. Conversely, apocrine glands express better staining for gross cystic disease fluid protein-15 (GCDFP-15).[7-9] An antibody, IKH-4, has been described that stains the eccrine but not apocrine secretory coil.[10]

Sebaceous Glands

Sebaceous glands are lipid-secreting glands associated with hair follicles. Using frozen tissue, the presence of lipid can be detected using lipid stains such as oil-red-O. The glands also stain with antibody against EMA,[11] but there are no specific antibodies that will stain sebaceous glands only.

Dermis

The dermis is composed of connective tissue composed of collagen and elastic fibers produced by fibroblasts. Fibroblasts and other mesenchymal cells can be detected easily based on the presence of intermediate filament vimentin. Within the dermis blood vessels, lymphatics, nerves, and dermal appendages can be found (see earlier). Mast cells can also be detected in a perivascular distribution. Studies have also demonstrated a dendritic cell population that has immunologic function within the dermis; these cells are called *dermal dendrocytes*. These dermal dendrocytes, analogous to lymphocytes, express different antigen profiles. Dermal dendrocytes in the papillary dermis and around blood vessels express clotting factor XIIIa, whereas dermal dendrocytes in the reticular and adventitial dermis express the human progenitor cell antigen CD34.[12, 13] As our knowledge of dermal dendrocytes increases, different subtypes will be characterized further.

Epidermal Dendritic-Clear Cells

Within the epidermis, three types of clear and dendritic cells can be detected; namely, melanocytes, Langerhans cells, and Merkel cells. Each of these cells can be involved in both reactive and neoplastic processes. Melanocytes and melanocytic tumors are discussed in great detail in Chapter 6. Langerhans cells are important antigen-processing cells that present antigens to lymphocytes. Langerhans cells express CD1, HLA-DR, HLA-DP, and HLA-DQ surface molecules. Although considered by some scientists to be tissue macrophages, unlike

macrophages, Langerhans cells contain less lysosomal antigens and lack Fc and complement receptors. Using frozen sections, Langerhans cells can be detected using antibody OKT6. In paraffin sections, Langerhans cells stain with S-100 marker, but S-100 also stains melanocytes within the epidermis.[14, 15] Langerhans cells also immunostain with the newly available antibody against CD1.

Merkel cells are unique cells found in the basal epithelial layer and have a yet unclear but probable neural function in the skin. Merkel cells contain neural enzymes such as neuron-specific enolase, chromogranin, and synaptophysin. They also contain neurofilaments and cytokeratin filaments, and stain specifically for CK20.[16, 17]

ANTIBODIES

The principle of immunohistochemistry depends on the fact that different tumors exhibit different immunohistochemical profiles. Successful use of immunohistochemistry requires a knowledge of the specific antibodies available and their staining patterns.[18, 19] Table 12−1 lists commonly used antibodies that can be helpful in diagnosing skin tumors. Since no single antibody is 100% specific or sensitive, a panel of antibodies should always be used for diagnostic purposes.

Epithelial Markers

Ber-EP4

Ber-EP4 is an antiepithelial antibody that binds to a membrane glycoprotein. In normal skin, it stains apocrine, eccrine secretory coil, outer sheath epithelium of vellus follicles, and internal root sheath epithelium of vellus follicles.[20] The epithelium of anagen hair follicles does not stain. A variety of different cutaneous tumors stain for Ber-EP4, including basal cell carcinomas, basaloid foci in nevus sebaceus, trichoepitheliomas, Merkel cell carcinoma, Paget's disease of breast, and mixed tumors.[20-24] Staining for Ber-EP4 can be helpful in differentiating between basal cell carcinomas, which stain strongly and diffusely positive, and squamous cell carcinomas, which exhibit negative staining (Fig. 12−1).[20, 23, 24]

KEY DIAGNOSTIC POINTS OF BerEP4

- It strongly stains basal cell carcinomas, whereas squamous cell carcinomas are negative.
- There are overlapping features between basal cell carcinomas and squamous cell carcinomas in basosquamous cell carcinoma.
- Follicular staining or staining of follicular neoplasms should not be misinterpreted as a basal cell carcinoma.

Table 12–1. Common Antibodies Used in Dermatopathology

Primary Antibody	Catalog No.	Source	City	First Antibody Type	Clone	Pretreatment	Second Ab Method	Staining
Epithelial Tumors								
Ber-EP4	M0804	DAKO	Carpinteria	Mouse	124	Pronase	ABC	Basal cell carcinoma, some adnexal neoplasms
Epithelial membrane antigen	M0613	DAKO	Carpinteria	Mouse	E29	None	ABC	Sebaceous carcinoma, epithelioid sarcoma Will not stain stratified squamous epithelium or squamous cell carcinomas
Cytokeratin (AE1/AE3)	1124161	Boehringer Mannheim	Indianapolis	Mouse	AE1, AE3	Auto/zyme	ABC	All epithelial tumors
Cytokeratin (K903)	C34903	Enzo Diagnostics	Farmingdale	Mouse	34βE12	Antigen retrieval	ABC	Squamous cell carcinomas
Cytokeratin (MAK-6)	28-0001	Zymed	South San Francisco	Mouse	Mono	Pre-digestion with Auto/zyme	ABC	Squamous cell carcinoms
Melanocytic Tumors								
S-100	PU058-UP	BioGenex	San Ramon	Rabbit	Poly	None	ABC	Melanocytes, Langerhans cells chondrocytes, lipocytes
HMB-45	MA-930	Enzo Diagnostics	New York	Mouse	Mono	None	ABC	Activated melanocytes, melanoma, Spitz nevi
Spindle Cell Tumors								
CD31	M0786	DAKO	Carpinteria	Mouse	JC/70A	Pronase	ABC	Blood vessels
CD34 (QBEND/10)	MU236-UC	BioGenex	San Ramon	Mouse	QBEND/10	Microwave	Streptavidin	Blood vessels, dermal dendrocytes
Desmin	MO760	DAKO	Carpinteria	Mouse	D33	None	ABC	Skeletal and smooth muscle
Factor XIIIa	233498	Calbiochem-Novabiochem	San Diego	Rabbit	Poly	None	ABC	Dermal dendrocytes
Muscle-specific actin	O11D	BioGenex	Foster City	Mouse	Mono	None	ABC	Smooth muscle
Glandular Neoplasms								
Cytokeratins: CAM5.2	92-0005	Becton-Dickinson	Triangle Park	Mouse	Cam5.2	Predigestion with Auto/zyme	ABC	Adenocarcinoma, apocrine, and eccrine ducts and neoplasms, some sebaceous carcinomas
CK7	MU255-UC	BioGenex	San Ramon	Mouse	OV-TL 12/30	Antigen retrieval	ABC	Adenocarcinoma
CEA	208M	Biomeda	Foster City	Rabbit	Poly	None	ABC	Adenocarcinoma, eccrine, apocrine ducts
GCDFP-15 (BRST-2)	611-01	Signet	Dedham	Mouse	D6	None	Streptavidin	Apocrine glands

Table continued on following page

315

Table 12–1. Common Antibodies Used in Dermatopathology *Continued*

Primary Antibody	Source	Catalog No.	City	First Antibody Type	Clone	Pretreatment	Second Ab Method	Staining
Small Round Cell Neoplasms								
Neuron-specific enolase	DAKO	MO873	Carpinteria	Mouse	BBS/N C/v1-H14	Antigen retrieval	ABC	Neuroendocrine tumors
Chromogranin	Biomeda	003d	Foster City	Mouse	—	None	ABC	Neuroendocrine tumors
Synaptophysin	BioGenex	MU363-UC	San Ramon	Mouse	Snp88	Antigen retrieval	ABC	Neuroendocrine tumors
CK20	BioGenex	MU315-UC	San Ramon	Mouse	It-KS20.8	Antigen retrieval	ABC	Merkel cell carcinoma
Neurofilaments	Immunotech	0168	Westbrook	Bovine	Pool-3 clones	Predigestion with pronase	ABC	Small cell carcinoma
Histiocytic Markers								
HAM 56	Enzo	MA-935	Farmingdale	Mouse	Mono	None	ABC	Histiocytes, melanophages
CD68	DAKO	MO814	Carpinteria	Mouse	KP-1	Predigestion with auto/zyme	ABC	Histiocytes, giant cells, some atypical fibroxanthomas
MAC387	DAKO	MO747	Carpinteria	Mouse	MAC387	None	ABC	Histiocytes
Proliferating Markers								
MIB-1(Ki-67)	BioGenex	MU297-UC	San Ramon	Mouse	MIB-1	Antigen retrieval	Streptavidin	Proliferating cells
PCNA	DAKO	M879	Carpinteria	Mouse	PC10	Antigen retrieval	ABC	Proliferating cells
Miscellaneous Markers								
CD44	DAKO	A072	Carpinteria	Mouse	Ber-EP4	Predigestion with pronase	ABC	Basal layer of epidermis, basal cell carcinoma, and follicular tumors
BCL-2								

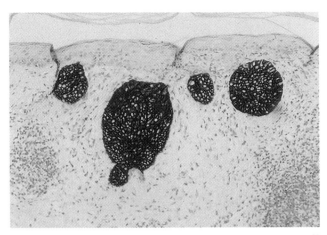

Figure 12–1. Diffuse Ber-EP4 staining of a basal cell carcinoma.

CYTOKERATINS

A wide variety of antibodies against cytokeratins can be found.[25] AE1/AE3 is a cocktail antibody preparation that stains a mixture of high and low molecular weight acidic (AE1) and basic (AE3) cytokeratins. K903 is an antibody that stains only high molecular weight cytokeratins.[1, 5, 10, 14] MAK-6, another antibody cocktail, stains CK8, CK14, CK15, CK16, CK18, and CK19. The epidermis and follicular epithelium contain cytokeratins and stain with these antibodies. A wide variety of antibodies against specific cytokeratins are available, but because many are ineffective on paraffin-embedded, formalin-fixed specimens, they are rarely used in diagnostic skin pathology. The use of CAM5.2 and 35βH11, antibodies against low molecular weight simple cytokeratins, is discussed under the section on Glandular Markers.

Cytokeratin stains have a limited use in diagnosing skin tumors and are useful primarily in confirming the presence of an epithelial neoplasm—namely, a squamous cell carcinoma or adnexal tumor—and exclude a mesenchymal, melanocytic, or hematopoietic tumor. An important caveat in the use of cytokeratin stains is that cytokeratin antibodies may nonspecifically cross-react with other antigens, particularly if too high a concentration is used.

KEY DIAGNOSTIC POINTS OF CYTOKERATINS

- Detection of high molecular weight cytokeratins (K903, AE1/AE3, MAK-6) is helpful in confirming the diagnosis of squamous cell carcinoma.
- Detection of low molecular weight cytokeratins (CAM5.2, 35βH11) is helpful in determining the glandular nature of the tumor, for example, adenocarcinoma, Paget's disease, or extramammary Paget's disease.

- Cytokeratin stains are not useful in distinguishing between metastatic adenocarcinoma and adnexal carcinoma.

Melanocytic Markers (See Chapter 6)

S-100 PROTEIN

S-100 is a protein originally detected in glial cells and was soluble in 100% ammonium sulfate. S-100 protein can be detected in melanocytes, Langerhans cells, dermal dendrocytes, sweat ducts, chondrocytes, and occasionally in lipocytes.[26–32] In the skin, S-100 is primarily used to detect undifferentiated melanocytic neoplasms, or Langerhans cells in Langerhans cell granulomatosis.[31] Rare S-100–negative melanomas do exist.[33]

KEY DIAGNOSTIC POINTS OF S-100

- It is the most sensitive marker for melanocytic tumors.
- S-100 cannot be used to distinguish between benign and malignant melanocytic tumors.
- Staining of Langerhans cells within the epidermis needs to be distinguished from melanocytes.
- S-100 will also stain some dermal dendrocytes.

HMB-45

HMB-45 detects a glycoprotein in premelanosome complex and stains melanoma cells. An important pitfall in the use of HMB-45 is that it also stains activated melanocytes overlying a scar, in benign nevi, and in Spitz nevi.[34–39] Another pitfall in the use of HMB-45 is that frequently the tumor cells in spindle cell–desmoplastic melanoma do not stain.[39]

KEY DIAGNOSTIC POINTS OF HMB-45

- It is a more specific marker for melanoma then is S-100, but it is not as sensitive.
- Activated melanocytes and Spitz nevi stain with this antigen.
- Desmoplastic–spindle cell melanomas are HMB-45–.

Newer Melanocytic Markers

Melanocytes express a variety of different tumor antigens such as MART, MAGE, glycoprotein 100, and tyrosinase.[40, 41] These are discussed in Chapter 6.

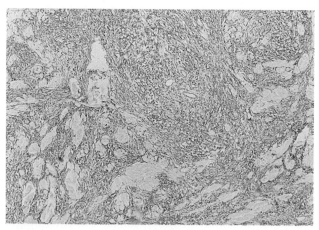

Figure 12–2. Strong staining of a dermatofibrosarcoma protuberans with CD34.

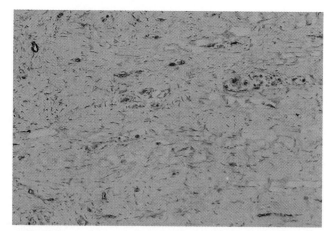

Figure 12–3. Lack of staining of a dermatofibroma for CD34.

Mesenchymal Markers

CD34

The human progenitor cell antigen CD34 is a surface antigen expressed on normal hematopoietic progenitors. In normal skin, CD34 expression can be detected by spindle-shaped cells in perivascular, interstitial, and adventitial connective tissue, and in blood vessels. Staining for CD34 is most helpful in differentiating between dermatofibrosarcoma, which stains strongly positive, and dermatofibromas, which do not stain (Figs. 12–2 and 12–3).[42–47] Some other tumors that express CD34 are lipomas and neurofibromas, angiosarcoma, Kaposi's sarcoma, malignant fibrous histiocytoma, epithelioid sarcoma, giant cell fibroblastoma, pleomorphic fibromas, fibrous papules, and eruptive fibromas.[48–61] There is also decreased staining for CD34 in lesions of scleroderma and morphea.[62] The utility of staining the basal cell carcinomas and trichoepitheliomas for CD34 as a differentiating feature has been debated.[24, 63–66] Reportedly, the stroma surrounding trichoepitheliomas stains with CD34, in contrast to the negative staining of stroma in basal cell carcinomas, but not all investigators have been able to confirm this finding.[24, 66]

KEY DIAGNOSTIC POINTS OF CD34

- CD34 is helpful in distinguishing between dermatofibrosarcoma protuberans (positive) and dermatofibroma (negative).
- It is helpful in distinguishing between persistent or recurrent dermatofibrosarcoma protuberans and scars.
- A diagnostic pitfall is that normal populations of dermal dendrocytes stain with CD34.
- CD34 also stains lipomas, neurofibromas, and other mesenchymal tumors.

FACTOR XIIIA

Factor XIIIa is a protransglutaminase of the final part of the coagulation pathway that stabilizes clot formation by cross-linking fibronectin to collagen. Factor XIIIa is a tetrameric protein consisting of two pairs of subunits (two alpha subunits and two beta subunits).[67, 68] Factor XIIIa can be detected in dendritic connective tissue cells in the dermis and in some macrophages. Antibodies for factor XIIIa label dermatofibromas (Fig. 12–4), fibrous papules of the nose, neurofibromas, juvenile xanthogranulomas, palisading cutaneous fibrous histiocytomas, multicentric reticulohistiocytosis, dermal dendrocytomas, indeterminate cell histiocytomas, some atypical fibroxanthomas, and atypical fibroblasts in radiation dermatitis.[69–77]

KEY DIAGNOSTIC POINTS OF FACTOR XIIIA

- Factor XIIIa stains dermatofibromas, fibrous papules, and neurofibromas.

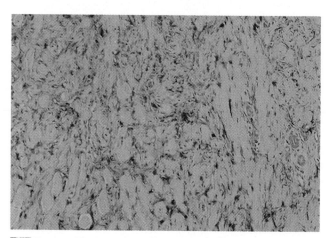

Figure 12–4. Factor XIIIa labeling of a dermatofibroma.

- Increased staining can be seen in stroma of a variety of different tumors such as Kaposi's sarcoma and atypical fibroxanthoma.[70, 78]
- A diagnostic pitfall to avoid is interpreting staining of the tumor's stroma as relevant.

VIMENTIN

Vimentin is a ubiquitous evolutionarily conserved 57-kd intermediate filament expressed during embryonic development. In adults, it is retained in mesenchymal cells, fibroblasts, endothelial cells, macrophages, melanocytes, and lymphocytes. Staining for vimentin is primarily helpful in determining the mesenchymal origin of the tumor. Some carcinomas, and rarely melanomas, express vimentin.[79-81]

KEY DIAGNOSTIC POINTS OF VIMENTIN

- It is a good generalized marker for mesenchymal tumors.
- A diagnostic pitfall is that occasional non-mesenchymal tumors such as carcinomas and melanomas can express vimentin.

INTERMEDIATE FILAMENTS FOR MUSCLE

Actin is a microfilamentous contractile protein found in both striated and smooth muscle cells. Six different actin subtypes have been identified. HHF-35, muscle-specific actin, is an antibody that stains both smooth and skeletal muscle, in contrast to 1A4 or 7GFA1, which stain only smooth muscle. Desmin is a 53-kd cytoplasmic protein found in both striated and smooth muscle cells. Antibodies against actin and desmin are primarily used in dermatopathology to distinguish leiomyosarcoma from other sarcomas.[82] Actin staining has also been reported in dermatofibromas, dermatomyofibromas, proliferative fasciitis, dermatofibrosarcomas, and atypical fibroxanthomas.[46, 77, 83, 84] Other tumors with a muscular component such as glomus tumors (Fig. 12–5), or angiomyolipomas, also exhibit positive immunoreactivity.[85]

KEY DIAGNOSTIC POINTS OF ACTIN AND DESMIN

- They are helpful in confirming origin from muscle in mesenchymal neoplasms.
- Actin staining can be found in some dermatofibromas, dermatomyofibroma, atypical fibroxanthoma, proliferative fasciitis, and dermatofibrosarcoma protuberans.

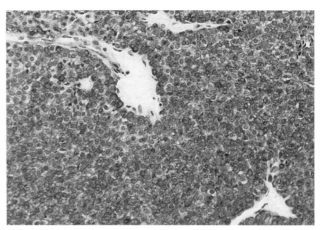

Figure 12–5. Smooth muscle actin staining of a glomus tumor.

Vascular Markers

CD31

CD31, or platelet-endothelial cell adhesion molecule, is a 130-kd glycoprotein found on the surface of platelets, endothelial cells, neutrophils, and monocytes.[86] In one study, CD31 stained 35 of 53 vascular lesions, with one case of Kaposi's sarcoma and one case of angiosarcoma failing to stain.[87] This result was comparable to staining of blood vessels with CD34, but unlike CD34, other nonvascular tumors did not stain with CD31. Therefore, CD31 is a more specific vascular marker.

KEY DIAGNOSTIC POINTS OF CD31

- CD31 is helpful in confirming a vascular origin of tumors.
- It is a more specific vascular marker than CD34 and is more sensitive then *Ulex europaeus I* (UEAI) agglutinin and factor VIII.
- A diagnostic pitfall is that sensitivity for vascular tumors is still only approximately 66%.

ULEX EUROPAEUS I AGGLUTININ

UEAI is a lectin found in endothelial cells. In the skin, UEAI can also be detected in the upper stratum spinosum, in the internal root sheath of hair follicles, and apocrine cells.[88-92] Staining for UEAI agglutinin is not widely performed anymore because staining is technically more difficult, and other more sensitive markers such as CD31 exist. In the study by Sankey and colleagues, all cases of Kaposi's sarcoma failed to stain with UEAI.[93] Staining for UEAI has been used to distinguish between squamous cell carcinomas and trichilemmal carcinomas; since UEAI is expressed in the internal root sheath of hair follicles, stronger staining is seen in trichilemmal carcinomas.[94]

KEY DIAGNOSTIC POINTS OF *ULEX EUROPAEUS I* AGGLUTININ

- Better markers for vascular tumors such as CD31 and CD34 exist.
- UEAI may be helpful in some follicular adnexal tumors because it does stain the internal root sheath of hair follicles.

FACTOR VIII

Factor VIII is a clotting factor found on endothelial cells. Staining for factor VIII can be detected in vascular tumors. Like UEAI agglutinin, the use of factor VIII has decreased because of the existence of more sensitive markers, such as CD34 and CD31. Sankey and coworkers' study of Kaposi's sarcoma showed that the tumors were only weakly positive for factor VIII.[93]

Neuroendocrine Markers

BOMBESIN, CHROMOGRANIN, NEURON-SPECIFIC ENOLASE, SYNAPTOPHYSIN

The markers used to detect neuroendocrine differentiation include synaptophysin, chromogranin, neuron-specific enolase, and bombesin. Chromogranin is a catecholamine carrier protein and a major component of dense-core granules. Neuron-specific enolase is an enzyme of the glycolic pathway. Synaptophysin is a transmembrane glycoprotein of presynaptic vesicles. Bombesin is a tetradecapeptide found in neurons and some endocrine cells. These markers are most helpful in diagnosing small blue cell tumors such as Merkel cell carcinoma. Since none of the antibodies have a 100% sensitivity, usually a panel of antibodies is used to increase the sensitivity.[95–97] Neuron-specific enolase and chromogranin staining has been reported to occur rarely in basal cell carcinomas,[98] and weak staining for neuron-specific enolase can be seen in basaloid squamous cell carcinomas.[99]

KEY DIAGNOSTIC POINTS OF BOMBESIN, CHROMOGRANIN, NEURON-SPECIFIC ENOLASE, AND SYNAPTOPHYSIN

- They are helpful in confirming the diagnosis of Merkel cell carcinoma.
- A panel of antibodies increases sensitivity.
- A diagnostic pitfall is that small cell carcinoma of the lung or other sites will also stain.
- Another diagnostic pitfall is that neuron-specific enolase and chromogranin staining can occur in basal cell carcinomas.

CK20

CK20, which was first described by Moll and colleagues,[114] is expressed in gastric epithelium, urothelium, small intestinal epithelium, and Merkel cells. In the skin, staining for CK20 is used to confirm the diagnosis of Merkel cell carcinoma. Merkel cell carcinomas usually exhibit a characteristic perinuclear dot staining pattern (Fig. 12–6), but occasionally a diffuse cytoplasmic or perinuclear rim pattern can be found. Since approximately 97% of Merkel cell carcinomas stain with CK20, in contrast to 5% of oat cell carcinomas of the lung, the presence or absence of staining provides ancillary data in the attempt to distinguish between metastatic oat cell and primary Merkel cell carcinoma of the skin.[17] However, small cell carcinoma from other sites such as salivary gland, as well as carcinoid tumors, can also stain for CK20.[17, 100] Other skin tumors such as melanoma, squamous cell carcinoma, basal cell carcinoma, and adnexal neoplasms do not express CK20.

KEY DIAGNOSTIC POINTS OF CK20

- CK20 is the most sensitive marker for Merkel cell carcinoma with a perinuclear dot staining pattern.
- A diagnostic pitfall is that rare metastatic oat cell carcinomas can also stain.
- Thyroid-transcription factor-1 (TTF-1) is positive in 95% of pulmonary oat cell cancers and uniformly negative in Merkel cell tumors.

GLIAL FIBRILLARY ACIDIC PROTEIN

Glial fibrillary acidic protein (GFAP) is a 51-kd intermediate filament found in astrocytes, ependymal cells, and oligodendroglia.[101] GFAP staining can be used to distinguish between neural nevi

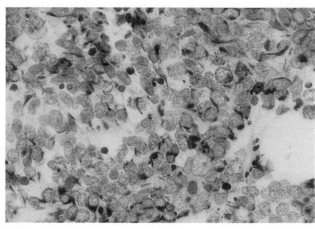

Figure 12–6. Perinuclear dot staining of a Merkel cell carcinoma with CK20.

and neurofibromas.[102] Staining for GFAP is also seen in schwannomas (positive), the periphery of chondroid syringomas, and heterotopic glial nodules.[103–106] A newly reported entity, benign polymorphous mesenchymal tumor (mesenchymal hamartoma) of soft parts, contains garland-shaped structures composed of GFAP+ cells.[107] Staining for GFAP is not present in palisaded encapsulated neuromas.[108, 109]

KEY DIAGNOSTIC POINTS OF GLIAL FIBRILLARY ACIDIC PROTEIN

* GFAP is an intermediate filament found in astrocytes, oligodendroglia, and ependymal cells.
* It can be used to distinguish between neurofibromas and neurotized nevi.
* It is expressed in schwannomas, heterotopic glial nodules, chondroid syringoma, and polymorphous mesenchymal tumor.

NEUROFILAMENTS

Axons of the central and peripheral nervous system contain unique type IV intermediate filaments with molecular weights of 68, 150, and 200 kd. Antibodies against neurofilaments can be used to stain neural tumors.[108, 110, 111] Coexpression of neurofilaments and cytokeratins in a perinuclear dot-like pattern provides strong evidence for neuroendocrine differentiation.[96, 110, 112–114]

KEY DIAGNOSTIC POINTS OF NEUROFILAMENTS

* Neurofilaments stain neural tumors.
* There is a characteristic perinuclear dot staining pattern in Merkel cell carcinoma.

LEU7

Leu7 is an antibody raised against human lymphoid cells and binds to human natural killer-1 (HNK-1) cells. Leu7 is a membrane glycoprotein that can be found on neuroectodermal cells. In the skin, it stains nerves and both apocrine and eccrine glands. Staining for Leu7 is primarily used to identify neural tumors. Its sensitivity varies; in one study, only one of four nerve sheath myxomas stained,[115] whereas staining of the capsule was seen in 10 of 10 palisaded encapsulated neuromas.[108] Leu7, however, can also be expressed by leiomyosarcomas. Loss of expression occurs in anaplastic tumors.[116]

KEY DIAGNOSTIC POINTS OF LEU7

* Leu7 is a neural marker, but sensitivity varies.
* A diagnostic pitfall is that staining has also been reported in leiomyosarcomas.

Glandular Markers

GROSS CYSTIC DISEASE FLUID PROTEIN

Gross cystic disease fluid protein (GCDFP) is a family of proteins with different molecular weights isolated from breast cystic fluid. The most commonly used antibody in diagnostic pathology is BRST-2, which binds to GCDFP-15. In the skin, staining for GCDFP localizes to both apocrine and eccrine gland; therefore, staining should be considered evidence for glandular-ductal differentiation.[117] GCDFP-15 staining appears to be relatively specific for apocrine neoplasms. GCDFP-15 staining can be found in hidradenoma papilliferum, hidrocystoma, syringocystadenoma papilliferum, mixed tumor, mucinous carcinoma, metastatic sweat gland adenocarcinoma, and microcystic adnexal carcinoma.[7–9, 117, 118] Since these neoplasms can be diagnosed using morphologic features, staining for GCDFP-15 is primarily of academic interest. Finally, metastatic breast carcinoma and mammary and extramammary Paget's disease express positive immunoreactivity. GCDFP-15 staining cannot be used to distinguish between a primary malignant adnexal neoplasm and metastatic adenocarcinoma.[119]

KEY DIAGNOSTIC POINTS OF GROSS CYSTIC DISEASE FLUID PROTEIN

* GCDFP is a marker of apocrine differentiation mainly used to help confirm the diagnosis of extramammary Paget's disease or Paget's disease.
* A diagnostic pitfall is that it cannot be used to distinguish between primary malignant adnexal neoplasm and metastatic adenocarcinoma of the breast.

CARCINOEMBRYONIC ANTIGEN

CEA was one of the first markers used in immunohistochemistry and was originally felt to be an oncoprotein specific for colonic carcinoma. Subsequent studies demonstrated other tumors such as lung, pancreas, and breast can also express CEA. Molecular biology and gene cloning studies have demonstrated a CEA gene family, which belongs to the immunoglobulin superfamily. The protein products include the classic 180-kd glycoprotein, a 160-kd biliary glycoprotein, and nonspecific cross-reacting antigens.[120] In the skin, CEA has been considered a marker for sweat gland differentiation,

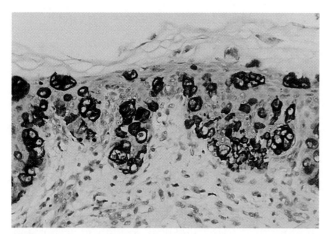

Figure 12–7. Pagetoid cells of extramammary Paget's disease marking with CEA.

but both eccrine and apocrine glands can exhibit some expression. Although staining can be found in ductal foci in sweat gland tumors,[121–129] studies have demonstrated CEA staining in squamous cell carcinomas, seborrheic keratosis, actinic keratosis, Bowen's disease, and warts.[130] CEA staining can also be detected rarely in malignant melanomas.[131] Metze and coworkers demonstrated BGP CEA in sebaceous neoplasms,[120] but Johnson and associates did not find staining for CEA helpful in ocular sebaceous neoplasms.[132] Both monoclonal and polyclonal antibodies against the different glycoproteins can be purchased. In general, there is less cross-reactivity with the monoclonal antibody. As in other markers for glandular tissue, CEA is not helpful in distinguishing between primary adnexal neoplasms and metastatic tumors.[123] Staining for CEA is most beneficial in distinguishing between extramammary Paget's disease and other neoplasms with pagetoid spread.[124, 127, 130, 131, 133–146] (Fig. 12–7).

KEY DIAGNOSTIC POINTS OF CARCINOEMBRYONIC ANTIGEN

- It is a marker for eccrine differentiation but can also stain sebaceous and epithelial neoplasms.
- CEA is most helpful in staining extramammary Paget's disease.

EPITHELIAL MEMBRANE ANTIGEN

EMA is a glycoprotein originally isolated from mammary secretory cells. Three different antibodies—E29, HMFG-1, and HMFG-2—that bind to EMA are available. In the skin, EMA stains eccrine, apocrine, and sebaceous glands. The epidermis normally does not stain. A variety of different adnexal tumors, including trichoepithelioma, microcystic adnexal carcinoma, syringomas, acrospiromas, mixed tumors, poromas, and sweat gland carcinomas,

will stain.[11, 121, 125, 132, 147, 148] Since these tumors can be diagnosed based on morphology, immunoreactivity for EMA is primarily used in staining for extramammary Paget's disease, sebaceous tumors, and epithelioid sarcoma.[11, 137, 141, 145, 149–153] Neuromas, palisaded encapsulated neuroma, and schwannomas exhibit EMA staining in the periphery of the tumors in the areas of the perineurium. Perineuromas also exhibit staining.[48, 50, 109, 115, 154–156] Since epidermis normally does not stain with EMA, EMA is not helpful in diagnosing squamous cell carcinoma, although in a study by Tatemoto and colleagues, 85% of squamous cell carcinomas did stain.[152]

CAM5.2 AND 35βH11

CAM5.2 and 35βH11 are monoclonal antibodies that bind to low molecular weight CK8 and to CK18.[25, 157] In the skin, staining of sweat glands is seen. The epidermis or stratified squamous epithelium do not stain with these antibodies. Tumors that mark with CAM5.2 include Merkel cell carcinoma, metastatic carcinoma, extramammary and mammary Paget's disease, some basal cell carcinomas, and sebaceous carcinomas.[135–137, 139, 153, 158, 159] CAM5.2 staining has also been reported to occur in melanoma of soft parts (clear cell sarcoma).[160] Staining for CAM5.2 is most helpful in diagnosing Paget's disease or extramammary Paget's disease[135] or in confirming the glandular nature of a neoplasm, either primary adnexal or metastatic. By using a panel of antibodies—anti–common leukocyte antigen (anti-LCA), anti-EMA, anti-CK, anti–S-100 protein, and antivimentin—undifferentiated tumors could be classified as mesenchymal, lymphoid, or epithelial in origin in 85.5% of cases.[161]

KEY DIAGNOSTIC POINTS OF CAM5.2 AND 35βH11

- They detect low molecular weight cytokeratin present in most glandular neoplasms.
- A pitfall to avoid is the rare expression of simple cytokeratins in melanomas.

CK7

Antibodies (OV-TL 12/30) to CK7 stain lung, breast, ovary, endometrium, and neuroendocrine tissues. In the skin, staining of basal cell carcinomas and trichoepitheliomas has been reported.[63, 162] Staining for CK7 has been proposed to be a specific and sensitive marker for extramammary and mammary Paget's disease, staining 21 of 22 and 19 of 22 cases, respectively.[163] Normal pale cells, so-called Toker cells, found in nipple epithelium also stain for CK7.[163] The use of CK7 in conjunction with CK20 may be helpful in determining the site of origin of some malignant neoplasms. CK7–

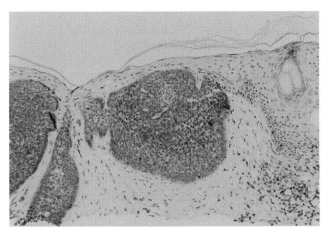

Figure 12–8. BCL-2 staining of a basal cell carcinoma.

staining with CK20 staining is most indicative of tumors of gastrointestinal origin.[164]

KEY DIAGNOSTIC POINTS OF CK7

- CK7 is a helpful marker for Paget's disease and extramammary Paget's disease.
- Toker cells in the nipple also stain.
- When used in a panel with CK20, CK20+ and CK7– staining is indicative of a gastrointestinal origin for the tumor.

Miscellaneous Markers

BCL-2
BCL-2 is an oncoprotein that inhibits apoptosis. In normal skin, the basal cell layer stains for BCL-2. Staining for BCL-2 has been proposed to be beneficial in distinguishing between basal cell carcinomas and trichoepitheliomas.[63, 165] In basal cell carcinomas, the entire tumor lobule stains, whereas in trichoepitheliomas, only the cells in the periphery stain (Figs. 12–8 and 12–9). Not all authors have been able to confirm the utility of these findings.[21, 24] Since BCL-2 does stain basal cell carcinomas, lack of staining can be a useful finding in distinguishing between superficial basal cell carcinomas and actinic keratosis.[166] BCL-2 staining is found in follicular lymphomas, and its utility in distinguishing between reactive versus neoplastic lymphoid infiltrates is being debated.

KEY DIAGNOSTIC POINTS OF BCL-2

- BCL-2 stains the basal cell layer of epidermis.
- It has possible utility in distinguishing between basal cell carcinomas and trichoepitheliomas.
- It has possible utility in distinguishing be-

tween actinic keratosis and basal cell carcinomas.

HISTIOCYTIC MARKERS—HAM 56, MAC387, AND CD68
HAM 56 and MAC387 are monoclonal antibodies against macrophages. A variety of antibodies are available against a 110-kd glycoprotein associated with lysosomes in the CD68 cluster. These include KP-1, Y2/131, Y1/82A, EBM/11, Ki-M6, and Ki-M7. Staining for HAM 56 has been reported useful in distinguishing between melanocytes and melanophages.[167] MAC387 has not been found to be a very specific histiocytic marker, and in one study, MAC387 reacted with 148 soft tissue sarcomas, 29 carcinomas, and 10 melanomas.[168] The most commonly used antibody in dermatopathology is KP-1. Staining for KP-1 is found in rare true histiocytic lymphomas.[169] KP-1 stains xanthogranulomas and the giant cells in some cases of atypical fibroxanthoma and malignant fibrous histiocytoma.[73, 77, 170] Binder reported 18 of 25 cases of malignant fibrous histiocytoma to be positive[171]; however, Smith did not find staining in 12 cases of pleomorphic and myxoid malignant fibrous histiocytomas nor in 9 of 19 cases of an adenomatoid variant.[172] Unfortunately, these findings are not specific, since giant cells in a variety of other entities, including melanoma and dermatofibromas, stain with KP-1.[43, 173] Schwann cells found in granular cell tumors or schwannomas and granular cell dermatofibromas also stain.[174–176]

KEY DIAGNOSTIC POINTS OF HISTIOCYTIC MARKERS

- HAM 56 is helpful in distinguishing between melanocytes and melanophages.
- KP-1 is expressed in some cases of atypical

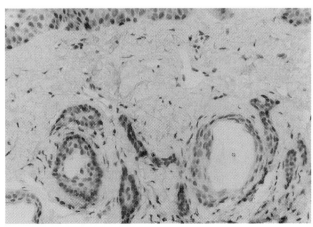

Figure 12–9. Rim pattern with BCL-2 staining of a trichoepithelioma.

fibroxanthoma and malignant fibrous histiocytoma.

- KP-1 is also expressed in juvenile xanthogranuloma, some melanomas, some dermatofibromas, granular cell tumors, and neural tumors.
- MAC387 is not a very specific histiocytic marker.

CD44

CD44 is a cell surface protein involved in cell-to-cell and cell-to-matrix adhesion and lymphocyte-homing activity. CD44 is expressed in epidermal keratinocytes, hair follicles, and sebaceous and eccrine cells.[177, 178] Aberrant CD44 expression has been reported in a variety of tumors, and expression of CD44 has been correlated with more aggressive behavior. Basal cell carcinomas do not exhibit immunolabeling for CD44, in contrast to squamous cell carcinomas and metastatic adenocarcinomas in which almost 100% of cells are labeled.[179] CD44 expression by Merkel cell carcinoma in the skin may correlate with metastatic risk.[180] The data of CD44 expression in melanoma has been somewhat conflicting, and some isoforms of CD44 can be found in normal and atypical nevi.[181]

KEY DIAGNOSTIC POINTS OF CD44

- Expression may be related to progression in some tumors, such as Merkel cell carcinoma, and their ability to metastasize.
- CD44 is expressed by squamous cell carcinomas but not basal cell carcinomas.
- Further studies are needed before the utility of CD44 as a marker can be established.

DIAGNOSTIC DILEMMAS FOR WHICH IMMUNOHISTOCHEMISTRY CAN BE HELPFUL

Pagetoid Cells Within the Epidermis

The diagnosis of tumors presenting with pagetoid spread of cells within the epidermis can be difficult. The histologic differential diagnosis includes melanoma, Paget's disease, extramammary Paget's disease, Bowen's disease, and occasionally sebaceous carcinoma, trichilemmal carcinoma, mycosis fungoides (pagetoid reticulosis), and Langerhans cell granulomatosis.

A recommended panel that is helpful in distinguishing among melanoma, extramammary Paget's disease, and Bowen's disease is given in Table 12−2.

The pagetoid cells in Paget's disease can express low molecular weight cytokeratins (CK7, CK8, and CK18), tumor markers such as CEA, milk fat globule protein (CA 15-3), KA93, oncogenes p53 and c-*erb*-B2/*neu,* and miscellaneous antigens such as EMA and GCDFP-15. The frequency of reported staining with the various antibodies is shown in Figure 12−1. Conversely, the pagetoid cells in melanoma are negative for these markers; they stain with S-100 and HMB-45. In squamous cell carcinoma, the tumor cells are low molecular weight cytokeratin− negative (CAM5.2−) and stain for high molecular weight cytokeratins (K903).

The pagetoid cells in extramammary Paget's disease stain slightly differently and more polymorphous than do those in Paget's disease because the origin of the cells may be more polymorphous. In approximately one third of extramammary Paget's disease cases, there may be an underlying adenocarcinoma from the gastrointestinal or genitourinary tract, in one third of cases, there may be an underlying adnexal carcinoma, and in one third of cases no associated malignancy can be found. These tumors may originate from pluripotential stem cells found in the epidermis. The staining pattern of extramammary Paget's disease reflects the underlying disease. Most cases are CEA+, CAM5.2+, EMA+, and CK7+ (see Fig. 12−7).[134, 135, 182, 183] Cases associated with an underlying colonic adenocarcinoma usually also stain with CK20 and are GCDFP−, whereas primary extramammary Paget's disease with no associated adenocarcinoma is CK20− and GCDFP+.[182, 183, 197]

Occasionally, the tumor cells in both Paget's disease and extramammary Paget's disease can contain melanin and stain with S-100. Therefore, to avoid an erroneous diagnosis of melanoma, a panel of antibodies should always be used because melanomas will be CAM5.2−, CEA−, and EMA−.

Small Cell Carcinoma

The differential diagnosis of malignant tumors composed of small blue cells includes Merkel cell

Table 12−2. Immunohistochemical Profile for Tumors with Pagetoid Spread

	S-100	CK7	HMB-45	CAM5.2	C-*erb*-B2	EMA	K903
Paget's disease; extramammary Paget's disease	−/+	+	N	+	+	+	N
Melanoma	+	N	+	N	N	N	+
Bowen's disease	N	N	N	N	N	N	+

EMA, epithelial membrane antigen; +, almost always positive; −/+, sometimes positive; N, negative.

Table 12–3. Immunohistochemical Profile for Small Cell Carcinoma

	S-100	HMB-45	CK20	Neuron-Specific Enolase	Synaptophysin	Chromogranin	Neurofilament	Leukocyte Common Antigen
Melanoma	+	+	N	N	N	N	N	N
Merkel cell carcinoma	N	N	+	+/−	+/−	+/−	+	N
Lymphoma	N	N	N	N	N	N	N	+
Neuroblastoma	N	N	N	+	+	+/−	+/−	N
Oat cell carcinoma	N	N	N	+/−	+/−	+/−	N	N

+, almost always positive; +/−, mostly positive; N, negative.

carcinoma, melanoma, lymphoma, squamous cell carcinoma, Ewing's sarcoma, and neuroblastoma. Ewing's sarcoma and neuroblastoma rarely occur in the skin. The recommended panel to distinguish between these tumors is listed in Table 12–3. Merkel cells usually express CK20 (see Fig. 12–6) or neuron-specific enolase (Fig. 12–10), synaptophysin, bombesin, chromogranin, and neurofilaments. Of these stains, CK20 is the most sensitive and specific. The majority of melanomas are S-100+ or HMB-45+, and lymphomas express leukocyte common antigen (LCA). Small cell carcinoma of the lung can express neuron-specific enolase, synaptophysin, bombesin, and chromogranin, but generally they do not exhibit the characteristic perinuclear dot staining of Merkel cell carcinoma with CK20 or neurofilaments. Approximately 95% of pulmonary small cell carcinomas are positive with TTF-1.

Spindle Cell Tumors

Table 12–4 shows the expected staining of a variety of malignant spindle cell neoplasms of the skin.

DERMATOFIBROMA VERSUS DERMATOFIBROSARCOMA PROTUBERANS

One of the difficult problems encountered in dermatopathology is distinguishing between an early dermatofibrosarcoma protuberans (DFSP) and a dermatofibroma. Staining for CD34 and factor XIIIa is most helpful, with the majority of DFSP exhibiting strong diffuse staining for CD34 and negativity for factor XIIIa (see Figs. 12–2 and 12–3). In contrast, dermatofibromas are factor XIIIa+ and CD34−. An important pitfall to avoid in the interpretation of the staining pattern is that some normal fibroblasts within the dermis and adventitial dermis stain for CD34, and frequently factor XIIIa+ staining can be found in the stroma of a variety of different neoplasms. Therefore, proper interpretation of the stains requires differentiating among the tumor, normal connective tissue, and tumor stroma. Scars do not stain with CD34, and this fact has been used to help differentiate and find the margins of recurrent DFSP.

Another pitfall to avoid is to consider CD34 staining synonymous with DFSP. Lipomas and neurofibromas stain with CD34, and a variety of rarer CD34-staining tumors include solitary fibrous tumor, CD34+ eruptive fibromas, and congenital CD34+ granular cell dendrocytosis.

ATYPICAL FIBROXANTHOMA VERSUS LEIOMYOSARCOMA, SPINDLE CELL SQUAMOUS CELL CARCINOMA, AND SPINDLE CELL MELANOMA

Malignant spindle cell tumors can be difficult to diagnose based purely on histologic appearance. The differential diagnosis of malignant spindle cell tumors that appear to be arising in proximity to the epidermis includes atypical fibroxanthoma, spindle cell tumors (desmoplastic melanoma), and spindle cell squamous cell carcinoma. Squamous cell carcinomas should express high molecular weight cytokeratins and stain for AE1/AE3, K903,

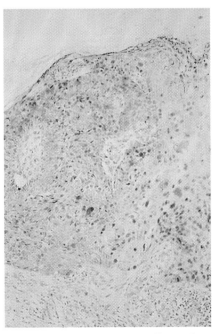

Figure 12–10. Proliferating cell nuclear antigen (PCNA) staining of a squamous cell carcinoma.

Table 12–4. Malignant Spindle Cell Tumors

Tumor	Vimentin	CD34	Factor XIIIa	S-100	Smooth Muscle Actin	Desmin	KP-1	AE1/AE3 (Cytokeratin)
Dermatofibrosarcoma protuberans	+	+	N	N	N	N	N	N
Spindle cell small cell carcinoma	N	N	N	N	N	N	N	+
Spindle cell melanoma	+	N	N	+	N	N	N	N
Atypical fibroxanthoma	+	N	R (stroma)	R (stroma)	N	N	+/− (tumor)	N
Leiomyosarcoma	+	N	N	N	+	+	N	N

+, almost always positive; N, negative; R, rare.

or MAK-6 antibodies. Desmoplastic melanomas are S-100+. There is no single immunostain that universally stains atypical fibroxanthoma. By definition, they should be cytokeratin stain–negative, and in fact some atypical fibroxanthomas may simply be poorly differentiated squamous cell carcinomas that no longer express detectable cytokeratin filaments. The tumor cells in atypical fibroxanthomas may stain with KP-1 (CD68), MAC387, lysozyme, alpha-1-antitrypsin, or alpha-1-antichymotrypsin. The stroma in atypical fibroxanthoma may contain S-100 and factor XIIIa dendritic cells so that interpretation of the staining pattern requires distinguishing between tumor and stroma. The relationship between atypical fibroxanthoma and malignant fibrous histiocytoma is debatable. Whether atypical fibroxanthoma simply represents a smaller superficial version of malignant fibrous histiocytoma is yet to be proved. An antibody against LN2—which stains B cells, Reed-Sternberg cells, and macrophages—was detected in 90% of malignant fibrous histiocytomas in one study, yet 90% of atypical fibroxanthomas were negative or expressed weak staining.

DIAGNOSTIC DILEMMAS FOR WHICH IMMUNOHISTOCHEMISTRY IS OCCASIONALLY USEFUL

Carcinoma Metastatic to the Skin

In the majority of cases, patients with metastasis to the skin have a known primary tumor, and the diagnosis can be made by comparing the histologic features with the metastasis and primary neoplasm. Occasionally, however, skin metastasis may be the presenting feature of the malignancy. An adenocarcinoma on the chest wall of a woman is most likely from an underlying breast cancer. Adenocarcinomas in men most likely arise from the gastrointestinal tract or lung. A dilemma in which immunohistochemistry is useful is distinguishing between pyogenic granulomas and metastatic renal cell carcinoma. In one study of patients with renal cell carcinoma, the skin findings were the first indication of disease in six of nine patients with

metastatic lesions to the skin. Histologically, metastatic renal cell carcinoma can be very vascular and the clear renal cells difficult to see on routine histologic examination. The renal cells stain with antibodies against cytokeratins. Immunohistochemistry with staining for CK20 can also provide some ancillary data to help distinguish between metastatic oat cell carcinoma and Merkel cell carcinoma (see earlier).[17] The expression of CK20 and the lack of expression of CK7 is indicative of a possible colorectal carcinoma.[164] In one study, the combined staining for GCDFP and estrogen protein receptor provided sensitivity, specificity, and positive predictive values of 83%, 91%, and 95%, respectively, in diagnosing metastatic cutaneous breast carcinoma.[119] Conversely, immunohistochemistry is not helpful in distinguishing between primary malignant adnexal neoplasm and metastatic adenocarcinoma. Malignant eccrine and apocrine adnexal neoplasms can resemble metastatic adenocarcinomas to the skin, and like adenocarcinomas they express CEA, GCDFP, and low and high molecular weight cytokeratins.

Vascular Tumors

In the majority of cases, the diagnosis of vascular tumors do not require adjunctive immunohistochemical studies. Occasionally, however, some malignant tumors such as malignant fibrous histiocytoma and giant cell fibroblastoma, have angiomatoid-like areas that can resemble a vascular neoplasm.[59, 87, 172, 184]

DIAGNOSTIC DILEMMAS FOR WHICH IMMUNOHISTOCHEMISTRY IS OF POSSIBLE UTILITY

Basal Cell Carcinoma Versus Adnexal Neoplasms

Basal cell carcinomas can usually be diagnosed based on morphology of basaloid tumor cells with uniform nuclei, inconspicuous nucleoli, and peripheral palisading. However, some adnexal tumors such as trichoepitheliomas and sebaceous epithelimomas or carcinomas can resemble basal cell carcinomas. Trichoepitheliomas histologically resemble basal cell carcinomas because both tumors contain basaloid cells with focal peripheral palisading and a fibrotic stroma. Smoller and colleagues reported that basal cell carcinomas stain diffusely positive with BCL-2, whereas in trichoepitheliomas, only the cells in the periphery of the lobules stain (see Figs. 12–8 and 12–9).[185] In basal cell carcinomas, the tumor stroma is CD34−, whereas the stroma in trichoepitheliomas is focally CD34+. Subsequent studies debated the utility of these stains.[24, 66] Sebaceous neoplasms like basal cell carcinomas can contain immature basaloid staining cells, but unlike basal cell carcinomas, sebocytes with vacuolated scalloped nuclei can be found. Sebaceous neoplasms, unlike basal cell carcinomas, can express EMA.[11, 132, 153] Some sebaceous carcinomas can also express low molecular weight cytokeratins detected with CAM5.2 and GCDFP-15 (BRST-1) antibodies.[153]

Squamous Cell Carcinoma Versus Keratoacanthoma

The relationship between keratoacanthomas and squamous cell carcinomas is controversial.[186] Some pathologists feel that keratoacanthomas are a type of squamous cell carcinoma, and therefore distinguishing between a keratoacanthoma and squamous cell carcinoma is not necessary. Nevertheless, keratoacanthomas may exhibit a unique clinical course and regress spontaneously. If differentiation between a keratoacanthoma and squamous cell carcinoma is necessary, immunohistochemical stains can offer some utility. Keratoacanthomas, unlike squamous cell carcinomas, exhibit a more organized growth pattern when stained for proliferating cells with Ki-67 or proliferating cell nuclear antigen (PCNA).[187–189] In keratoacanthomas, the peripheral cells of the tumor lobules stain, in contrast to a more diffuse, haphazard staining pattern in squamous cell carcinomas (Figs. 12–10 and 12–11).

Melanoma Versus Nevus

Occasionally, immunohistochemical stains can provide ancillary data that are helpful in distinguishing between benign and malignant melanocytic tumors. HMB-45 staining of Spitz nevi demonstrates maturation with staining of the melanocytes within the upper dermis and epidermis, with lack of staining of deeper melanocytes.[35, 190] Staining for proliferating cells can also be helpful in some cases because in melanomas there are a larger number of dermal tumor cells proliferating in contrast to benign nevi.[191–196] Since all the studies demonstrate some overlapping values, the final diagnosis does require synthesis of the entire picture, not just the immunohistochemical results.

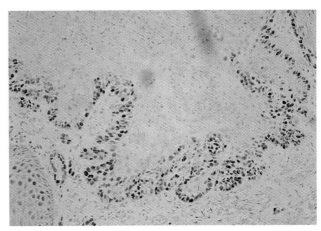

Figure 12–11. Rim pattern of PCNA staining in a keratoacanthoma.

CONCLUSION

The utility of immunohistochemistry continues to evolve. Currently, immunohistochemical stains need to be interpreted in conjunction with pathologic and clinical findings. As new antibodies become available and better data accumulate, the use of immunohistochemistry will become more widespread, not only for diagnosis but also ultimately for prognosis.

References

1. Steinert PM, Freedberg IM. Molecular and cellular biology of cytokeratins. In: Goldsmith LA, ed. Physiology, Biochemistry and Molecular Biology of the Skin. 2nd ed. New York: Oxford University Press 1991:113–147.
2. Gillespie JM. The structural proteins of hair: Isolation, characterization, regulation of biosynthesis. In: Goldsmith LA, ed. Physiology, Biochemistry, Molecular Biology of the Skin. 2nd ed. New York: Oxford University Press, 1991:625–659.
3. Nickoloff BJ. PECAM-1 (CD31) is expressed on proliferating endothelial cells, stromal spindle-shaped cells, dermal dendrocytes in Kaposi's sarcoma. [letter] Arch Dermatol 1993;129:250–251.
4. Lobitz WCJ, Holyoke JB, Brophy D. Histochemical evidence for human eccrine sweat duct activity. Arch Dermatol 1955;172:229–234.
5. Saga K, Morimoto Y. Ultrastructural localization of alkaline phosphatase activity in human eccrine and apocrine sweat glands. J Histochem Cytochem 1995;43:927–932.
6. Watanabe S, Ichikawa E, Takanashi S, Takahashi H. Immunohistochemical localization of cytokeratins in normal eccrine glands, with monoclonal antibodies in routinely processed, formalin-fixed, paraffin-embedded sections. J Am Acad Dermatol 1993;28(2 Pt 1):203–212.
7. Ansai S, Koseki S, Hozumi Y, Kondo S. An immunohistochemical study of lysozyme, CD-15 (Leu M1), gross cystic disease fluid protein-15 in various skin tumors: Assessment of the specificity and sensitivity of markers of apocrine differentiation. Am J Dermatopathol 1995;17:249–255.
8. Mazoujian G. Immunohistochemistry of GCDFP-24 and zinc alpha2 glycoprotein in benign sweat gland tumors. Am J Dermatopathol 1990;12:452–457.
9. Mazoujian G, Margolis R. Immunohistochemistry of gross cystic disease fluid protein (GCDFP-15) in 65 benign sweat

gland tumors of the skin. Am J Dermatopathol 1988;10: 28–35.

10. Ishihara M, Mehregan OR, Hashimoto K, et al. Staining of eccrine and apocrine neoplasms and metastatic adenocarcinoma with IKH-4, a monoclonal antibody specific for the eccrine gland. J Cutan Pathol 1998;25:100–105.

11. Latham JA, Redfern CP, Thody AJ, DeKretser TA. Immunohistochemical markers of human sebaceous gland differentiation. J Histochem Cytochem 1989;37:729–734.

12. Fear JD, Jackson P, Gray C, et al. Localization of factor XIII in human tissue using an immunoperoxidase technique. J Clin Pathol 1984;37:560–563.

13. Nickoloff BJ. The human progenitor cell antigen (CD34) is localized on endothelial cells, dermal dendritic cells, perifollicular cells in formalin-fixed normal skin, on proliferating endothelial cells and stromal spindle-shaped cells in Kaposi's sarcoma. Arch Dermatol 1991;127:523–529.

14. de Fraissinette A, Dezutter-Dambuyant C, Schmitt O, Thivolet J. Ontogeny of Langerhans cells: Phenotypic differentiation from the bone marrow to the skin. Dev Comp Immunol 1990;14:335–346.

15. Schmitt D, Dezutter-Dambuyant C, Brochier J, Thivolet J, et al. Subclustering of CD1 monoclonal antibodies based on the reactivity on human Langerhans cells. Immunol Lett 1986;12:231–235.

16. Drijkoningen M, de Wolf-Peeters C, van Limbergen E, Desmet V. Merkel cell tumor of the skin: An immunohistochemical study. Hum Pathol 1986;17:301–307.

17. Scott MP, Helm KF. Cytokeratin 20: A marker for diagnosing Merkel cell carcinoma. Am J Dermatopathol 1999;21: 16–20.

18. Hudson AR, Smoller BR. Immunohistochemistry in diagnostic dermatopathology. Dermatol Clin 1999;17:667–689.

19. Wallace ML, Smoller BR. Immunohistochemistry in diagnostic dermatopathology. J Am Acad Dermatol 1996;34(2 Pt 1):163–183, quiz 184–186.

20. Latza U, Niedobitek G, Schwarting R, et al. Ber-EP4: New monoclonal antibody which distinguishes epithelia from mesothelial. J Clin Pathol 1990;43:213–219.

21. Barrett TL, Smith KJ, Williams J, et al. Immunohistochemical staining for Ber-EP4, p53, proliferating cell nuclear antigen, Ki-67, bcl-2, CD34, factor XIIIa in nevus sebaceus. Mod Pathol 1999;12:450–455.

22. Jimenez FJ, Burchette JL Jr, Grichnik JM, Hitchcock MG. Ber-EP4 immunoreactivity in normal skin and cutaneous neoplasms. Mod Pathol 1995;8:854–858.

23. Kist D, Perkins W, Christ S, Zachary CB. Anti-human epithelial antigen (Ber-EP4) helps define basal cell carcinoma masked by inflammation. Dermatol Surg 1997;23:1067–1070.

24. Swanson PE, Fitzpatrick MM, Ritter JH, et al. Immunohistologic differential diagnosis of basal cell carcinoma, squamous cell carcinoma, trichoepithelioma in small cutaneous biopsy specimens. J Cutan Pathol 1998;25:153–159.

25. Goddard MJ, Wilson B, Grant JW. Comparison of commercially available cytokeratin antibodies in normal and neoplastic adult epithelial and non-epithelial tissues. J Clin Pathol 1991;44:660–663.

26. Boni R, Burg G, Doguoglu A, et al. Immunohistochemical localization of the Ca2+ binding S100 proteins in normal human skin and melanocytic lesions. Br J Dermatol 1997; 137:39–43.

27. Cochran AJ, Wen DR. S-100 protein as a marker for melanocytic and other tumours. Pathology 1985;17:340–345.

28. Kahn HJ, Marks A, Thom H, Baumal R. Role of antibody to S100 protein in diagnostic pathology. Am J Clin Pathol 1983;79:341–347.

29. Kahn HJ, Baumal R, Marks A. The value of immunohistochemical studies using antibody to S100 protein in dermatopathology. Int J Dermatol 1984;23:38–44.

30. Modlin RL, Rowden G, Taylor CR, Rea TH. Comparison of S-100 and OKT6 antisera in human skin. J Invest Dermatol 1984;83:206–209.

31. Nakajima T, Watanabe S, Sato Y, et al. S-100 protein in Langerhans cells, interdigitating reticulum cells and histiocytosis X cells. Gann 1982;73:429–432.

32. Takahashi K, Isobe T, Ohtsuki Y, et al. Immunohistochemical study on the distribution of alpha and beta subunits of S-100 protein in human neoplasm and normal tissues. Virchows Arch B 1984;45:385–396.

33. Argenyi ZB, Cain C, Bromley C, et al. S-100 protein–negative malignant melanoma: Fact or fiction? A light-microscopic and immunohistochemical study. Am J Dermatopathol 1994;16:233–240.

34. Smoller BR, McNutt NS, Hsu A. HMB-45 recognizes stimulated melanocytes. J Cutan Pathol 1989;16:49–53.

35. Bergman R, Dromi R, Trau H, et al. The pattern of HMB-45 antibody staining in compound Spitz nevi. Am J Dermatopathol 1995;17:542–546.

36. Tronnier M, Wolff HH. UV-irradiated melanocytic nevi simulating melanoma in situ. Am J Dermatopathol 1995; 17:1–6.

37. Colombari R, Bonetti F, Zamboni G, et al. Distribution of melanoma specific antibody (HMB-45) in benign and malignant melanocytic tumours: An immunohistochemical study on paraffin sections. Virchows Arch A Pathol Anat Histopathol 1988;413:17–24.

38. Kanitakis J, Hermier C, Chouvet B, Thivolet J. Reactivity of HMB-45 monoclonal antibody with sweat-gland tumours of the skin. Acta Dermatovenereol 1991;71:426–428.

39. Wick MR, Swanson PE, Rocamora A. Recognition of malignant melanoma by monoclonal antibody HMB-45: An immunohistochemical study of 200 paraffin-embedded cutaneous tumors. J Cutan Pathol 1988;15:201–207.

40. Fetsch PA, Marincola FM, Filie A, et al. Melanoma-associated antigen recognized by T cells (MART-1): The advent of a preferred immunocytochemical antibody for the diagnosis of metastatic malignant melanoma with fine-needle aspiration. Cancer 1999;87:37–42.

41. Bhawan J. Mel-5: A novel antibody for differential diagnosis of epidermal pigmented lesions of the skin in paraffin-embedded sections. Melanoma Res 1997;7:43–48.

42. Abenoza P, Lillemoe T. CD34 and factor XIIIa in the differential diagnosis of dermatofibroma and dermatofibrosarcoma protuberans. [see comments] Am J Dermatopathol 1993;15:429–434.

43. Altman DA, Nickoloff BJ, Fivenson DP. Differential expression of factor XIIIa and CD34 in cutaneous mesenchymal tumors. J Cutan Pathol 1993;20:154–158.

44. Cohen PR, Rapin RP, Farhood AI. Dermatofibroma and dermatofibrosarcoma protuberans: Differential expression of CD34 and factor XIIIa. [letter; comment] Am J Dermatopathol 1994;16:573–574.

45. Goldblum JR, Tuthill RJ. CD34 and factor-XIIIa immunoreactivity in dermatofibrosarcoma protuberans and dermatofibroma. Am J Dermatopathol 1997;19:147–153.

46. Prieto VG, Reed JA, Shea CR. Immunohistochemistry of dermatofibromas and benign fibrous histiocytomas. J Cutan Pathol 1995;22:336–341.

47. Wick MR, Ritter JH, Lind AC, Swanson PE. The pathological distinction between "deep penetrating" dermatofibroma and dermatofibrosarcoma protuberans. Semin Cutan Med Surg 1999;18:91–98.

48. Mentzel T, Dei Tos AP, Fletcher CD. Perineurioma (storiform perineurial fibroma): Clinico-pathological analysis of four cases. Histopathology 1994;25:261–267.

49. Mentzel T, Beham A, Calonje E, et al. Epithelioid hemangioendothelioma of skin and soft tissues: Clinicopathologic and immunohistochemical study of 30 cases. Am J Surg Pathol 1997;21:363–374.

50. Mentzel T. Cutaneous neural neoplasms—an update. Verh Dtsch Ges Pathol 1998;82:309–316.

51. Mentzel T, Partanen TA, Kutzner H. Hobnail hemangioma ("targetoid hemosiderotic hemangioma"): Clinicopathologic and immunohistochemical analysis of 62 cases. J Cutan Pathol 1999;26:279–286.

52. Orchard GE, Zelger B, Jones EW, Jones RR. An immunocytochemical assessment of 19 cases of cutaneous angiosarcoma. Histopathology 1996;28:235–240.

53. Park HR, Park YK. Assessment of diagnostic utility of anti-CD34 in soft tissue tumors. J Korean Med Sci 1995;10: 436–441.

54. Prescott RJ, Banerjee SS, Eyden BP, Haboubi NY. Cutane-

ous epithelioid angiosarcoma: A clinicopathological study of four cases. Histopathology 1994;25:421–429.

55. Pursley HG, Williford PM, Groben PA, White WL. CD34-positive eruptive fibromas. J Cutan Pathol 1998;25:122–125.

56. Quante M, Patel NK, Hill S, et al. Epithelioid hemangioendothelioma presenting in the skin: A clinicopathologic study of eight cases. Am J Dermatopathol 1998;20:541–546.

57. Russell Jones R, Orchard G, Zelger B, Wilson Jones E. Immunostaining for CD31 and CD34 in Kaposi sarcoma. J Clin Pathol 1995;48:1011–1016.

58. Shea CR, Salob S, Reed JA, et al. CD34-reactive fibrous papule of the nose. J Am Acad Dermatol 1996;35(2 Pt 2): 342–345.

59. Silverman JS, Tamsen A. A cutaneous case of giant cell angiofibroma occurring with dermatofibrosarcoma protuberans and showing bimodal CD34+ fibroblastic and FXIIIa+ histiocytic immunophenotype. J Cutan Pathol 1998;25:265–270.

60. Smoller BR, Apfelberg DB. Infantile (juvenile) capillary hemangioma: A tumor of heterogeneous cellular elements. J Cutan Pathol 1993;20:330–336.

61. Stewart M, Smoller BR. Multiple lesions of intravascular papillary endothelial hyperplasia (Masson's lesions). Arch Pathol Lab Med 1994;118:315–316.

62. Skobieranda K, Helm KF. Decreased expression of the human progenitor cell antigen (CD34) in morphea. Am J Dermatopathol 1995;17:471–475.

63. Poniecka AW, Alexis JB. An immunohistochemical study of basal cell carcinoma and trichoepithelioma. Am J Dermatopathol 1999;21:332–336.

64. Kirchmann TT, Prieto VG, Smoller BR. CD34 staining pattern distinguishes basal cell carcinoma from trichoepithelioma. [see comments] Arch Dermatol 1994;130:589–592.

65. Illueca C, Monteagudo C, Revert A, Llombart-Bosch A. Diagnostic value of CD34 immunostaining in desmoplastic trichilemmoma. J Cutan Pathol 1998;25:435–439.

66. Basarab TG, Orchard R. Russell-Jones R. The use of immunostaining for bcl-2 and CD34 and the lectin peanut agglutinin in differentiating between basal cell carcinomas and trichoepitheliomas. Am J Dermatopathol 1998;20:448–452.

67. Cerio R, Griffiths CE, Cooper KD, et al. Characterization of factor XIIIa positive dermal dendritic cells in normal and inflamed skin. Br J Dermatol 1989;121:421–431.

68. Fivenson DP, Nickoloff BJ. Distinctive dendritic cell subsets expressing factor XIIIa, CD1a, CD1b and CD1c in mycosis fungoides and psoriasis. J Cutan Pathol 1995;22:223–228.

69. Moretto JC, Soslow RA, Smoller BR. Atypical cells in radiation dermatitis express factor XIIIa. Am J Dermatopathol 1998;20:370–372.

70. Pierard-Franchimont C, Arrese JE, Nikkels AF, et al. Factor XIIIa–positive dendrocytes and proliferative activity of cutaneous cancers. Virchows Arch 1996;429:43–48.

71. Sidoroff A, Zelger B, Steiner H, Smith N. Indeterminate cell histiocytosis—a clinicopathological entity with features of both X- and non-X histiocytosis. Br J Dermatol 1996;134:525–532.

72. Perrin C, Lacour JP, Michiels JF, et al. Multicentric reticulohistiocytosis: Immunohistological and ultrastructural study: A pathology of dendritic cell lineage. Am J Dermatopathol 1992;14:418–425.

73. Zelger B, Cerio R, Orchard G, et al. Histologic and immunohistochemical study comparing xanthoma disseminatum and histiocytosis X. Arch Dermatol 1992;128:1207–1212.

74. Nickoloff BJ, Wood GS, Chu M, et al. Disseminated dermal dendrocytomas: A new cutaneous fibrohistiocytic proliferative disorder? Am J Surg Pathol 1990;14:867–871.

75. Cerio R, Spaull J, Jones EW. Histiocytoma cutis: A tumour of dermal dendrocytes (dermal dendrocytoma). Br J Dermatol 1989;120:197–206.

76. Helm KF, Helm T, Helm F. Palisading cutaneous fibrous histiocytoma: An immunohistochemical study demonstrating differentiation from dermal dendrocytes. Am J Dermatopathol 1993;15:559–561.

77. Longacre TA, Smoller BR, Rouse RV. Atypical fibroxanthoma: Multiple immunohistologic profiles. Am J Surg Pathol 1993;17:1199–1209.

78. Kumar D, Sanchez RL, Kumar S. Dendrocyte population in cutaneous and extracutaneous Kaposi's sarcoma. Am J Dermatopathol 1992;14:298–303.

79. Miettinen M, Franssila K. Immunohistochemical spectrum of malignant melanoma: The common presence of cytokeratins. Lab Invest 1989;61:623–628.

80. Ben-Izhak O, Stark P, Levy R, et al. Epithelial markers in malignant melanoma: A study of primary lesions and their metastases. Am J Dermatopathol 1994;16:241–246.

81. Caselitz J, Janner M, Breitbart E, et al. Malignant melanomas contain only the vimentin type of intermediate filaments. Virchows Arch A Pathol Anat Histopathol 1983; 400:43–51.

82. Kahn H, Baumal R, From L. Role of immunohistochemistry in the diagnosis of undifferentiated tumors involving the skin. J Am Acad Dermatol 1986;14:1063–1072.

83. Colome MI, Sanchez RL. Dermatomyofibroma: Report of two cases. J Cutan Pathol 1994;21:371–376.

84. LeBoit PE, Barr RJ. Smooth-muscle proliferation in dermatofibromas. Am J Dermatopathol 1994;16:155–160.

85. Herbst WM, Nakayama K, Hornstein OP. Glomus tumours of the skin: An immunohistochemical investigation of the expression of marker proteins. Br J Dermatol 1991;124: 172–176.

86. Fernandez JE, Deaglio S, Donati D, et al. Analysis of the distribution of human CD38 and of its ligand CD31 in normal tissues. J Biol Reg Homeostat Agents 1998;12:81–91.

87. DeYoung BR, Swanson PE, Argenyi ZB, et al. CD31 immunoreactivity in mesenchymal neoplasms of the skin and subcutis: Report of 145 cases and review of putative immunohistologic markers of endothelial differentiation. J Cutan Pathol 1995;22:215–222.

88. Miettinen M, Holthofer H, Lehto VP, et al. *Ulex europaeus I* lectin as a marker for tumors derived from endothelial cells. Am J Clin Pathol 1983;79:32–36.

89. Schaumburg-Lever G. Ultrastructural localization of lectin-binding sites in normal skin. J Invest Dermatol 1990;94: 465–470.

90. Suzuki Y, Hashimoto K, Crissman J, et al. The value of blood group-specific lectin and endothelial associated antibodies in the diagnosis of vascular proliferations. J Cutan Pathol 1986;13:408–419.

91. Cooper PH. Angiosarcomas of the skin. Semin Diagn Pathol 1987;4:2–17.

92. Tsubura A, Fujita Y, Sasaki M, Morii S. Lectin-binding profiles for normal skin appendages and their tumors. J Cutan Pathol 1992;19:483–489.

93. Sankey EA, More L, Dhillon AP. QBEnd/10: A new immunostain for the routine diagnosis of Kaposi's sarcoma. [see comments] J Pathol 1990;161:267–271.

94. Ko T, Muramatsu T, Shirai T. Distribution of lectin UEA-I in trichilemmal carcinoma, squamous cell carcinoma, other epithelial tumors of the skin. J Dermatol 1996;23: 389–393.

95. Perez-Ordonez B, Caruana SM, Huvos AG, Shah JP. Small cell neuroendocrine carcinoma of the nasal cavity and paranasal sinuses. Hum Pathol 1998;29:826–832.

96. Wirnsberger GH, Becker H, Ziervogel K, Hofler H. Diagnostic immunohistochemistry of neuroblastic tumors. Am J Surg Pathol 1992;16:49–57.

97. Erlandson RA, Nesland JM. Tumors of the endocrine/neuroendocrine system: an overview. Ultrastruct Pathol 1994; 18:149–170.

98. George E, Swanson PE, Wick MR. Neuroendocrine differentiation in basal cell carcinoma: An immunohistochemical study. Am J Dermatopathol 1989;11:131–135.

99. Banks ER, Frierson HF Jr, Mills SE. Basaloid squamous cell carcinoma of the head and neck: A clinicopathologic and immunohistochemical study of 40 cases. Am J Surg Pathol 1992;16:939–946.

100. Chan JK, Suster S, Wenig BM, et al. Cytokeratin 20 immunoreactivity distinguishes Merkel cell (primary cutaneous neuroendocrine) carcinomas and salivary gland small cell carcinomas from small cell carcinomas of various sites. Am J Surg Pathol 1997;21:226–234.

101. Onodera K, Takahashi T, Watanabe R, et al. Distribution of

glial fibrillary acidic protein (GFAP) in the intermediate filaments of the cultured cells from a patient with tuberous sclerosis. J Dermatol 1990;17:395–402.

102. Gray MH, Smoller BR, McNutt NS, Hsu A. Neurofibromas and neurotized melanocytic nevi are immunohistochemically distinct neoplasms. Am J Dermatopathol 1990;12:234–241.

103. Argenyi ZB, Balogh K, Goeken JA. Immunohistochemical characterization of chondroid syringomas. Am J Clin Pathol 1988;90:662–669.

104. Argenyi ZB, Goodenberger ME, Strauss JS. Congenital neural hamartoma ("fascicular schwannoma"): A light microscopic, immunohistochemical, ultrastructural study. Am J Dermatopathol 1990;12:283–293.

105. Mori M, Shrestha P, Sakamoto F, et al. Histogenesis and possible mechanism of chondroid changes in mixed tumour of the skin: Immunohistochemical evaluation of bone morphogenetic protein, glycosaminoglycans, cytokeratin, vimentin and neuronal markers. Arch Dermatol Res 1994;286:285–292.

106. Theaker JM, Fletcher CD. Heterotopic glial nodules: A light microscopic and immunohistochemical study. Histopathology 1991;18:255–260.

107. Michal M, Sokol L. Benign polymorphous mesenchymal tumor (mesenchymal hamartoma) of soft parts: Report of two cases. Am J Dermatopathol 1997;19:271–275.

108. Albrecht S, Kahn HJ, From L. Palisaded encapsulated neuroma: An immunohistochemical study. Mod Pathol 1989;2:403–406.

109. Argenyi ZB. Immunohistochemical characterization of palisaded, encapsulated neuroma. J Cutan Pathol 1990;17:329–335.

110. Dreno B, Mousset S, Stalder JF, et al. A study of intermediate filaments (cytokeratin, vimentin, neurofilament) in two cases of Merkel cell tumor. J Cutan Pathol 1985;12:37–45.

111. Kanitakis J, Bourchany D, Faure M, Claudy A. Expression of the intermediate filament peripherin in skin tumors. Eur J Dermatol 1998;8:339–342.

112. Bayrou O, Avril MF, Charpentier P, et al. Primary neuroendocrine carcinoma of the skin: Clinicopathologic study of 18 cases. J Am Acad Dermatol 1991;24(2 Pt 1):198–207.

113. Miettinen M, Lehto VP, Virtanen I, et al. Neuroendocrine carcinoma of the skin (Merkel cell carcinoma): Ultrastructural and immunohistochemical demonstration of neurofilaments. Ultrastruct Pathol 1983;4:219–225.

114. Moll R, Osborn M, Hartschuh W, et al. Variability of expression and arrangement of cytokeratin and neurofilaments in cutaneous neuroendocrine carcinomas (Merkel cell tumors): Immunocytochemical and biochemical analysis of twelve cases. Ultrastruct Pathol 1986;10:473–495.

115. Argenyi ZB, LeBoit PE, Santa Cruz D, et al. Nerve sheath myxoma (neurothekeoma) of the skin: Light microscopic and immunohistochemical reappraisal of the cellular variant. J Cutan Pathol 1993;20: 294–303.

116. Swanson PE, Stanley MW, Scheithauer BW, Wick MR. Primary cutaneous leiomyosarcoma: A histological and immunohistochemical study of 9 cases, with ultrastructural correlation. J Cutan Pathol 1988;15:129–141.

117. Tsubura A, Senzaki H, Sasaki M, et al. Immunohistochemical demonstration of breast-derived and/or carcinoma-associated glycoproteins in normal skin appendages and their tumors. J Cutan Pathol 1992;19:73–79.

118. Komatsu T. An immunohistochemical study of cutaneous tumors using an antibody to the breast cyst fluid protein (GCDFP-15). Nippon Hifuka Gakkai Zasshi 1989;99:991–997.

119. Ormsby AH, Snow JL, Su WP, Goellner JR. Diagnostic immunohistochemistry of cutaneous metastatic breast carcinoma: A statistical analysis of the utility of gross cystic disease fluid protein-15 and estrogen receptor protein. J Am Acad Dermatol 1995;32(5 Pt 1):711–716.

120. Metze D, Soyer HP, Zelger B, et al. Expression of a glycoprotein of the carcinoembryonic antigen family in normal and neoplastic sebaceous glands: Limited role of carcino-

121. Heyderman E, Graham RM, Chapman DV, et al. Epithelial markers in primary skin cancer: An immunoperoxidase study of the distribution of epithelial membrane antigen (EMA) and carcinoembryonic antigen (CEA) in 65 primary skin carcinomas. Histopathology 1984;8:423–434.

122. Maiorana AE, Nigrisoli M, Papotti M. Immunohistochemical markers of sweat gland tumors. J Cutan Pathol 1986;13:187–196.

123. Metze D, Grunert F, Neumaier M, et al. Neoplasms with sweat gland differentiation express various glycoproteins of the carcinoembryonic antigen (CEA) family. J Cutan Pathol 1996;23:1–11.

124. Metze D, Luger TA. Ultrastructural localization of carcinoembryonic antigen (CEA) glycoproteins and epithelial membrane antigen (EMA) in normal and neoplastic sweat glands. J Cutan Pathol 1996;23:518–529.

125. Mohri S, Oh S. An immunohistochemical study of mixed tumor of the skin. J Dermatol 1991;18:414–419.

126. Penneys NS, Nadji M, Ziegels-Weissman J, et al. Carcinoembryonic antigen in sweat-gland carcinomas. Cancer 1982;50:1608–1611.

127. Tamaki K, Furue M, Matsukawa A, et al. Presence and distribution of carcinoembryonic antigen and lectin-binding sites in benign apocrine sweat gland tumours. Br J Dermatol 1985;113:565–571.

128. Tokura Y, Yoshikuni K, Teraki Y, et al. Immunohistochemically detectable duct-like structures in benign and malignant eccrine poromas: CEA and involucrin immunostaining. [see comments] J Dermatol 1989;16:133–141.

129. Wollina U, Castelli E, Rulke D. Immunohistochemistry of eccrine poroma and porocarcinoma—more than acrosyringeal tumors? Recent Results Cancer Res 1995;139:303–316.

130. Egawa K, Honda Y, Ono T, Kuroki M. Immunohistochemical demonstration of carcinoembryonic antigen and related antigens in various cutaneous keratinous neoplasms and verruca vulgaris. Br J Dermatol 1998;139:178–185.

131. Sanders DS, Evans AT, Allen CA, et al. Classification of CEA-related positivity in primary and metastatic malignant melanoma. J Pathol 1994;172:343–348.

132. Johnson JS, Lee JA, Cotton DW, et al. Dimorphic immunohistochemical staining in ocular sebaceous neoplasms: A useful diagnostic aid. Eye 1999;13(Pt 1):104–108.

133. Haneke E. Immunohistochemical detection of carcinoembryonic antigen and protein S-100 in sweat gland tumors. Z Hautkrankheiten 1986;61:32–46.

134. Battles OE, Page DL, Johnson JE. Cytokeratins, CEA, mucin histochemistry in the diagnosis and characterization of extramammary Paget's disease. Am J Clin Pathol 1997;108:6–12.

135. Helm KF, Goellner JR, Peters MS. Immunohistochemical stains in extramammary Paget's disease. Am J Dermatopathol 1992;14:402–407.

136. Hitchcock A, Topham S, Bell J, et al. Routine diagnosis of mammary Paget's disease: A modern approach. Am J Surg Pathol 1992;16:58–61.

137. Jones RR, Spaull J, Gusterson B. The histogenesis of mammary and extramammary Paget's disease. [see comments] Histopathology 1989;14:409–416.

138. Miller LR, McCunniff AJ, Randall ME. An immunohistochemical study of perianal Paget's disease: Possible origins and clinical implications. Cancer 1992;69:2166–2171.

139. Ramachandra S, Gillett CE, Millis RR. A comparative immunohistochemical study of mammary and extramammary Paget's disease and superficial spreading melanoma, with particular emphasis on melanocytic markers. Virchows Arch 1996;429:371–376.

140. Nakamura G, Shikata N, Shoji T, et al. Immunohistochemical study of mammary and extramammary Paget's disease. Anticancer Res 1995;15:467–470.

141. Guarner J, Cohen C, DeRose PB. Histogenesis of extramammary and mammary Paget cells: An immunohistochemical study. Am J Dermatopathol 1989;11:313–318.

142. Mazoujian G, Pinkus GS, Haagensen DE Jr. Extramammary

Paget's disease—evidence for an apocrine origin: An immunoperoxidase study of gross cystic disease fluid protein-15, carcinoembryonic antigen, cytokeratin proteins. Am J Surg Pathol 1984;8:43–50.

143. Cohen C, Guarner J, DeRose PB. Mammary Paget's disease and associated carcinoma: An immunohistochemical study. Arch Pathol Lab Med 1993;117:291–294.

144. Furukawa F, Kashihara M, Miyauchi H, et al. Evaluation of carcinoembryonic antigen in extramammary Paget's disease. J Cutan Pathol 1984;11:558–561.

145. Olson DJ, Fujimura M, Swanson P, Okagaki T. Immunohistochemical features of Paget's disease of the vulva with and without adenocarcinoma. Int J Gynecol Pathol 1991; 10:285–295.

146. Ordonez NG, Awalt H, Mackay B. Mammary and extramammary Paget's disease: An immunocytochemical and ultrastructural study. Cancer 1987;59:1173–1183.

147. Wiley EL, Milchgrub S, Freeman RG, Kim ES. Sweat gland adenomas: Immunohistochemical study with emphasis on myoepithelial differentiation. J Cutan Pathol 1993;20:337–343.

148. Takanashi M, Urabe A, Nakayama J, Hori Y. Distribution of epithelial membrane antigen in eccrine poroma. Dermatologica 1991;183:187–190.

149. Miettinen M, Fanburg-Smith JC, Virolainen M, et al. Epithelioid sarcoma: An immunohistochemical analysis of 112 classical and variant cases and a discussion of the differential diagnosis. Hum Pathol 1999;30:934–942.

150. Daimaru Y, Hashimoto H, Tsuneyoshi M, Enjoji M. Epithelial profile of epithelioid sarcoma: An immunohistochemical analysis of eight cases. Cancer 1987;59:134–141.

151. Arber DA, Kandalaft PL, Mehta P, Battifora H. Vimentin-negative epithelioid sarcoma: The value of an immunohistochemical panel that includes CD34. Am J Surg Pathol 1993;17:302–307.

152. Tatemoto Y, Saka M, Tanimura T, Mori M. Immunohistochemical observations on binding of monoclonal antibody to epithelial membrane antigen in epithelial tumors of the oral cavity and skin. Oral Surg Oral Med Oral Pathol 1987; 64:721–726.

153. Sinard JH. Immunohistochemical distinction of ocular sebaceous carcinoma from basal cell and squamous cell carcinoma. Arch Ophthalmol 1999;117:776–783.

154. Ahn SK, Choi EH, Won JH, Lee SH. Idiopathic solitary neuroma of skin with unusual histologic changes. J Cutan Pathol 1995;22:570–573.

155. Megahed M. Palisaded encapsulated neuroma (solitary circumscribed neuroma): A clinicopathologic and immunohistochemical study. [see comments] Am J Dermatopathol 1994;16:120–125.

156. Zelger BG, Steiner H, Kutzner H, et al. Verocay body–prominent cutaneous schwannoma. [see comments] Am J Dermatopathol 1997;19:242–249.

157. Tsubura A, Okada H, Sasaki M, et al. Immunohistochemical demonstration of cytokeratins 8 and 14 in benign tumours of the skin appendage. Pathol Anat Histopathol 1991; 418:503–507.

158. Smith KJ, Tuur S, Corvette D, et al. Cytokeratin 7 staining in mammary and extramammary Paget's disease. Mod Pathol 1997;10:1069–1074.

159. Prieto VG, Lugo J, McNutt NS. Intermediate- and low-molecular-weight cytokeratin detection with the monoclonal antibody MNF116: An immunohistochemical study on 232 paraffin-embedded cutaneous lesions. J Cutan Pathol 1996;23:234–241.

160. Mooi WJ, Deenik W, Peterse JL, Hogendoorn PC. Keratin immunoreactivity in melanoma of soft parts (clear cell sarcoma). Histopathology 1995;27:61–65.

161. Vege DS, Soman CS, Joshi UA, et al. Undifferentiated tumors: An immunohistochemical analysis on biopsies. J Surg Oncol 1994;57:273–276.

162. Habets JM, Tank B, Vuzevski VD, et al. Immunoelectron microscopic studies on cytokeratins in human basal cell carcinoma. Anticancer Res 1989;9:65–70.

163. Lundquist K, Kohler S, Rouse RV. Intraepidermal cytoker-
atin 7 expression is not restricted to Paget cells but is also seen in Toker cells and Merkel cells. Am J Surg Pathol 1999;23:212–219.

164. Blumenfeld W, Turi GK, Harrison G, et al. Utility of cytokeratin 7 and 20 subset analysis as an aid in the identification of primary site of origin of malignancy in cytologic specimens. Diagn Cytopathol 1999;20:63–66.

165. Smoller BR, Van De Rijn M, Lebrun D, Warnke RA. Bcl-2 expression reliably distinguishes trichoepitheliomas from basal cell carcinomas. Br J Dermatol 1994;131:28–31.

166. Mills AE. Solar keratosis can be distinguished from superficial basal cell carcinoma by expression of bcl-2. Am J Dermatopathol 1997;19:443–445.

167. Fleming MG, Bergfeld WF. A simple immunochemical technique for distinguishing melanocytes and melanophages in paraffin-embedded tissue. J Cutan Pathol 1990;17: 77–81.

168. Loftus B, Loh LC, Curran B, et al. Mac387: Its non-specificity as a tumour marker or marker of histiocytes. [see comments] Histopathology 1991;19:251–255.

169. Copie-Bergman C, Wotherspoon AC, Norton AJ, et al. True histiocytic lymphoma: A morphologic, immunohistochemical, molecular genetic study of 13 cases. Am J Surg Pathol 1998;22:1386–1392.

170. Tomaszewski MM, Lupton GP. Atypical fibroxanthoma: An unusual variant with osteoclast-like giant cells. [see comments] Am J Surg Pathol 1997;21:213–218.

171. Binder SW, Said JW, Shintaku IP, Pinkus GS. A histiocyte-specific marker in the diagnosis of malignant fibrous histiocytoma: Use of monoclonal antibody KP-1 (CD68). [see comments] Am J Clin Pathol 1992;97:759–763.

172. Smith ME, Costa MJ, Weiss SW. Evaluation of CD68 and other histiocytic antigens in angiomatoid malignant fibrous histiocytoma. [see comments] Am J Surg Pathol 1991;15: 757–763.

173. Helm KF. Malignant melanoma masquerading as malignant fibrous histiocytoma. Am J Dermatopathol 1997;19: 473–476.

174. Kaiserling E, Ruck P, Xiao JC. Congenital epulis and granular cell tumor: A histologic and immunohistochemical study. Oral Surg Oral Med Oral Pathol Oral Radiol Endod 1995;80:687–697.

175. Nikkels AF, Arrese Estrada J, Pierard-Franchimont C, Pierard GE. CD68 and factor XIIIa expressions in granular-cell tumor of the skin. Dermatology 1993;186:106–108.

176. Zelger BG, Steiner H, Kutzner H, et al. Granular cell dermatofibroma. Histopathology 1997;31:258–262.

177. Seelentag WK, Gunthert U, Saremaslani P, et al. CD44 standard and variant isoform expression in normal human skin appendages and epidermis. Histochem Cell Biol 1996; 106:283–289.

178. Hale LP, Patel DD, Clark RE, Haynes BF. Distribution of CD44 variant isoforms in human skin: Differential expression in components of benign and malignant epithelia. J Cutan Pathol 1995;22:536–545.

179. Prieto VG, Reed JA, McNutt NS, et al. Differential expression of CD44 in malignant cutaneous epithelial neoplasms. Am J Dermatopathol 1995;17:447–451.

180. Penneys NS, Shapiro S. CD44 expression in Merkel cell carcinoma may correlate with risk of metastasis. J Cutan Pathol 1994;21:22–26.

181. Manten-Horst E, Danen EH, Smit L, et al. Expression of CD44 splice variants in human cutaneous melanoma and melanoma cell lines is related to tumor progression and metastatic potential. Int J Cancer 1995;64:182–188.

182. Goldblum JR, Hart WR. Perianal Paget's disease: A histologic and immunohistochemical study of 11 cases with and without associated rectal adenocarcinoma. Am J Surg Pathol 1998;22:170–179.

183. Goldblum JR, Hart WR. Vulvar Paget's disease: A clinicopathologic and immunohistochemical study of 19 cases. Am J Surg Pathol 1997;21:1178–1187.

184. Nappi O, Wick MR, Pettinato G, et al. Pseudovascular adenoid squamous cell carcinoma of the skin: A neoplasm that may be mistaken for angiosarcoma. Am J Surg Pathol 1992;16:429–438.

185. Smoller BR, Van De Rijn M, Lebrun D, Warnke RA. BCL-2 expression reliably distinguishes trichoepitheliomas from basal cell carcinomas. [see comments] Br J Dermatol 1994; 131:28−31.
186. LeBoit PE. Is keratoacanthoma a variant of squamous cell carcinoma: New insights into an old controversy . . . soon? [editorial; comment] Am J Dermatopathol 1995;17: 319−320.
187. Cain CT, Niemann TH, Argenyi ZB. Keratoacanthoma versus squamous cell carcinoma: An immunohistochemical reappraisal of p53 protein and proliferating cell nuclear antigen expression in keratoacanthoma-like tumors. [see comments] Am J Dermatopathol 1995;17:324−331.
188. Li J, Lee YS. Proliferating cell nuclear antigen (PCNA) expression in pseudoepitheliomatous hyperplasia, keratoacanthoma and squamous cell carcinoma of the skin. Ann Acad Med Singapore 1996;25:526−530.
189. Phillips P, Helm KF. Proliferating cell nuclear antigen distribution in keratoacanthoma and squamous cell carcinoma. J Cutan Pathol 1993;20:424−428.
190. Mirecka JM, Korabiowska A, Schauer A. Comparative distribution of S-100 protein and antigen HMB-45 in various types of melanomas and naevi. Polish J Pathol 1995;46: 167−172.
191. Bjornhagen V, Bonfoco E, Brahme EM, et al. Morphometric, DNA, proliferating cell nuclear antigen measurements in benign melanocytic lesions and cutaneous malignant melanoma. Am J Dermatopathol 1994;16:615−623.
192. Kuwata T, Kitagawa M, Kasuga T. Proliferative activity of primary cutaneous melanocytic tumours. Virchows Arch A Pathol Anat Histopathol 1993;423:359−364.
193. Hofmann-Wellenhof R, Rieger E, Smolle J, Kerl H. Proliferative activity in Spitz's naevi compared with other melanocytic skin lesions. Melanoma Res 1993;3:313−317.
194. Niemann TH, Argenyi ZB. Immunohistochemical study of Spitz nevi and malignant melanoma with use of antibody to proliferating cell nuclear antigen. Am J Dermatopathol 1993; 5:441−445.
195. Tu P, Miyauchi S, Miki Y. Proliferative activities in Spitz nevus compared with melanocytic nevus and malignant melanoma using expression of PCNA/cyclin and mitotic rate. Am J Dermatopathol 1993;15:311−314.
196. Rieger E, Hofmann-Wellenhof R, Soyer HP, et al. Comparison of proliferative activity as assessed by proliferating cell nuclear antigen (PCNA) and Ki-67 monoclonal antibodies in melanocytic skin lesions: A quantitative immunohistochemical study. J Cutan Pathol 1993;20:229−236.
197. Kohler S, Smoller BR. Gross cystic disease fluid protein reactivity in extramammary Paget's disease with and without associated internal malignancy. Am J Dermatopathol 1976;18:118−123.

CHAPTER 13

Immunohistochemistry of the Gastrointestinal Tract, Pancreas, Bile Ducts, Gallbladder, and Liver

Neal S. Goldstein, M.D. and
Jan F. Silverman, M.D.

This chapter is divided into three sections, (1) gastrointestinal (GI) tract, (2) pancreaticobiliary system, which includes the extrahepatic bile ducts and gallbladder, and (3) liver. We have attempted to compile the innumerable immunohistochemical studies that have been applied to these organs into a cogent, useful, and relevant text. Immunohistochemical results depend on standardized methodologies and techniques. In general, studies that have not used antigen retrieval pretreatment and those that have used other, older techniques have been excluded from this discussion.

The three sections are preceded by a general introductory discussion of cytokeratins, their composition within neoplasms, and carcinoembryonic antigen (CEA). We have included this précis because cytokeratin differential response and CEA staining are integral components of the text that follows.

CYTOKERATIN DIFFERENTIAL STAINING

Cytokeratin is an intermediate filament, along with glial fibrillary acidic protein, desmin, vimentin, and neurofilament. "Acidic" and "basic" cytokeratin proteins associate together to form a single cytokeratin filament.[1-3] For instance, cytokeratin 8 (CK8) is usually paired with cytokeratin 18 (CK18), cytokeratin 7 (CK7) is usually paired with cytokeratin 19 (CK19), and cytokeratin 5 (CK5) is usually paired with cytokeratin 14 (CK14). A cytokeratin antibody can bind to an epitope that is found on a unique or selected number of acid or basic proteins constituting a cytokeratin filament and, thus, can help identify subsets of epithelial cells.[4] Alternatively, a cytokeratin antibody can bind to an epitope that is present on most acidic or basic cytokeratin proteins, thus reacting with the cytokeratin filaments that are found in many different types of epithelial cells. The combination of cytokeratins AE1 (acidic) and AE3 (basic), or AE1/AE3, is an example of the latter type of cytokeratin antibody "cocktail," or pankeratin.[5]

Cytokeratins can also be divided into low and high molecular weight groups. Specific antibodies have been developed that bind with cytokeratin epitopes that are generally limited to cytokeratins within each group. Gown[1] gives the examples of cytokeratins 35βH11 and 34βE12 (CK5, CK10, CK11, and CK14), antibodies that are directed to proteins specific for low and high molecular weight cytokeratins. The neoplasms discussed in this chapter can be distinguished on the basis of staining with these two groups of antibodies, as follows:

- Carcinomas that react to (i.e., stain with) both low and high molecular weight cytokeratin antibodies include esophageal and gastric adenocarcinomas, pancreaticobiliary adenocarcinomas, cholangiocarcinomas, breast carcinomas, pulmonary large cell carcinomas and adenocarcinomas, and transitional cell carcinomas.
- Carcinomas that react only to low molecular weight cytokeratin antibodies include colorectal adenocarcinomas, hepatocellular carcinomas, carcinoids, atypical carcinoids, and small cell carcinomas, thymic carcinomas, and prostatic adenocarcinoma.[1]
- Carcinomas that react only to high molecular weight cytokeratin antibodies include esophageal squamous carcinomas and most anal canal nonglandular carcinomas.

Cytokeratin-specific antibodies that are directed toward epitopes expressed in a limited number of epithelial cells can assist in identifying the site of primary or metastatic neoplasm. Antibodies to CK7 and CK20 are the most widely studied and used in this context, especially when used in combination (*CK7/CK20 coordinate staining pattern*). The strength of beliefs about the specificity of these antibodies as reliable markers of the site of origin of a carcinoma varies among authors. Some believe that CK7/CK20 coordinate expression can reliably distinguish among many neoplasms, including those that appear to have a similar histogenesis, such as colorectal adenocarcinoma and ovarian mucinous adenocarcinoma arising in association with an intestinal type mucinous noninvasive neoplasm.[1] It is our view that CK7/CK20 coordinate expression staining patterns can reliably predict the site of a carcinoma when the staining pattern of the two carcinomas in the differential diagnosis have markedly different CK7/CK20 coordinate staining expression. Some carcinomas can display a variety of CK7/CK20 staining patterns, despite having a predominant pattern, thus limiting the diagnostic utility of the two antibodies.

Many studies on CK7/CK20 coordinate expression have been published from different laboratories that have utilized different techniques on specimens that were processed and fixed in different manners. Additionally, the proportion of stained cells that qualifies a neoplasm as showing a "positive reaction" varies from 1 to 50% in studies.[6–9] The latter point cannot be underemphasized, because one of the more frequently cited large studies on CK7/CK20 coordinate staining in numerous neoplasms classified a tumor as showing a positive reaction with either CK7 or CK20 if 1% of the neoplastic cells stained. We believe that the differences in proportion of stained cells used to label a reaction as positive is one major contributor to the sometimes large differences in the distribution of CK7/CK20 staining.

In general, however, with these methodologic issues taken into account, most carcinomas have a predominant staining pattern and show a spectrum of CK7/CK20 coordinate staining. This predominance or spectrum can be extreme or almost minimal. We have attempted to provide ranges of expression of single-antibody and coordinate CK7/CK20 staining in this chapter, and we have included the minority staining patterns in a Differential Diagnosis Panel when they potentially contribute to the distinction between two neoplasms.

CARCINOEMBRYONIC ANTIGEN

Carcinoembryonic antigen (CEA) is a glycoprotein within a glycoprotein superfamily that includes biliary glycoprotein and nonspecific cross-reacting antigen.[10–12] Polyclonal and many monoclonal antibodies identify antigens that are present on many of the glycoproteins within the CEA "family."[1] Neutrophils, which contain nonspecific cross-reacting protein, are frequently positive with polyclonal CEA antibodies and many of the monoclonal CEA antibodies. Tissues that contain extensive necrosis or inflammation stain with CEA antibodies that react with nonspecific cross-reacting protein and produce a staining pattern that appears to contain extensive background, or nonspecific, staining. Similarly, tissues from the pancreaticobiliary system, gallbladder, and liver can appear to have background or nonspecific staining with many CEA antibodies because CEA antibody binds to biliary glycoprotein. In our expe-

rience, these staining effects can be dramatically increased in the presence of marked cholestasis.

Newer monoclonal CEA antibody clones are available that react with epitopes found predominantly on the "true" CEA glycoprotein; their use can significantly reduce the background necrosis and neutrophil staining seen with other monoclonal and polyclonal CEA antibodies.[13]

GASTROINTESTINAL TRACT

Several lesions that have similar morphologies and immunohistochemical profiles throughout the GI tract are covered under general topics, including neuroendocrine lesions and mesenchymal neoplasms; we then discuss site-specific lesions.

Neuroendocrine Cell Lesions

Neuroendocrine cell lesions of the GI tract can be immunohistochemically defined (1) from their staining pattern to a small group of "neuroendocrine"-specific antibodies or (2) from their predominant hormone production. The latter classification has little practical utility. Some neuroendocrine neoplasms express no polypeptides or hormones, whereas others demonstrate a broad spectrum of substances. In addition, the metastases of some carcinoid tumors can express hormones different from those expressed by the primary neoplasm.[14] Serum hormone or neuropeptide determinations have replaced immunohistochemical detection. Although this chapter mentions the predominant hormone or neuropeptide associated with some lesions, this information is not an endorsement for the use of such determinations in diagnostic surgical pathology.

NEUROENDOCRINE-RELATED AND CYTOKERATIN ANTIBODIES

Neuroendocrine cells are immunohistochemically defined by their staining with synaptophysin, chromogranin, protein gene product 9.5 (PGP9.5), and Leu7.[15–29] Synaptophysin is a membrane glycoprotein of presynaptic vesicles. Its expression is independent of chromogranin A.[28, 30] Chromogranin A is a soluble protein within neurosecretory granules.[28, 30] Leu7 (CD57) cross-reacts with an epitope on a protein within neurosecretory granules.[28, 30] Chromogranin and synaptophysin are the most commonly employed antibodies to identify neuroendocrine differentiation. Chromogranin is more specific but less sensitive than synaptophysin.[28] Most non-neoplastic neuroendocrine lesions and low-grade neuroendocrine neoplasms (carcinoids) diffusely and strongly stain with these antibodies in a cytoplasmic distribution that is proportional to the number of intracytoplasmic neurosecretory granules. However, some carcinoids either fail to stain or only weakly stain with chromogranin, a feature that may reflect differences in the type of amines contained within the tumor cell cytoplasm.[31] Use of both antibodies is preferred for this reason.

High-grade neuroendocrine carcinomas contain fewer intracytoplasmic neurosecretory granules, and therefore, fewer numbers of such cells stain, and with less intensity, with chromogranin and synaptophysin. Often, cells from high-grade neuroendocrine carcinomas (small cell carcinoma) show no chromogranin staining despite the use of high-temperature antigen retrieval in buffers with varying acidities. Conversely, CD56 (neural cell adhesion molecule [NCAM]) usually produces stronger positivity in a greater number of high-grade neuroendocrine carcinoma cells than synaptophysin or chromogranin (personal experience).[32, 33]

Neuron-specific enolase (NSE) also stains neuroendocrine cells. We and other authors believe that the low specificity of NSE limits its utility.[34] However, the lack of NSE reaction should cause one to question the presence of neuroendocrine differentiation of a neoplasm (Fig. 13–1).

Carcinoids contain predominantly low molecular weight cytokeratins. They diffusely stain with keratin CAM5.2 and keratin 35βH11 and show little or no positivity with high molecular weight keratins such as 34βE12.[35, 36] In our experience, keratin CAM5.2 produces stronger and more diffuse staining than keratin AE1/AE3.

GI carcinoid neuroendocrine neoplasms stain with villin in approximately 85% of cases.[37] In contrast, pancreatic islet carcinoids do not stain with villin, suggesting that this antibody is useful in distinguishing between these two sites.[37]

NEUROENDOCRINE TUMORS OF THE ESOPHAGUS

Carcinoid tumors rarely occur in the esophagus. Like pulmonary carcinoids, they stain diffusely

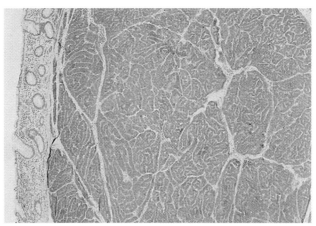

Figure 13–1. Rectal carcinoid showing strong positivity for neuron-specific enolase (NSE), with overlying negative-staining rectal mucosa. The carcinoid tumor was also positive for low molecular weight cytokeratin, chromogranin, and synaptophysin. (Low-power magnification)

and strongly with antibodies to synaptophysin, chromogranin, and CEA (Table 13–1) (personal experience).[38–41]

NEUROENDOCRINE CELL LESIONS OF THE GASTRIC FUNDUS

Enterochromaffin-like (ECL) cells are the predominant neuroendocrine cell of fundic glands. ECL cells can produce histamine and 5-hydroxytryptamine. Immunohistochemically, hyperplastic and neoplastic ECL lesions diffusely and strongly stain with antibodies to chromogranin A and synaptophysin.[16, 42–45]

There are two types of fundic ECL lesions, hypergastrinemia-related and sporadic.[17] Gastrin is a trophic factor for ECL cells.[46] Hypergastrinemia-related fundic ECL lesions include a spectrum of proliferations that range from hyperplasia to dys-

Table 13–1. Antibody Staining of Low-Grade Neuroendocrine Neoplasms (Carcinoid) of the Gastrointestinal Tract

Antibody	Immunostaining	Comments
CEA	−/+	The greater percentage of positivity is among tumors that form glands
EMA	−/+	Colorectal carcinoids are more often positive than gastric or proximal small intestinal carcinoids
Calcitonin	R	In positive carcinoids, distinction with metastatic thyroid medullary can be impossible
S-100 protein	R	Excluding those tumors with positive sustentacular cells
PAP	R	Colorectal carcinoids can occasionally be PAP-positive; uncommon in gastric carcinoids
PSA	N	See text
Chromogranin	+/−	See text
Synaptophysin	+	More sensitive than chromogranin
Alpha inhibin	R	Approximately 10% of carcinoids are positive, with staining in approximately 5% of neoplastic cells (chapter reference 840)
Vimentin	R	Although positivity is uncommon, it is more often seen in colorectal carcinoids than in gastric or proximal small intestine carcinoids

N, negative; R, rare; +/−, more cases positive than negative; −/+, more negative cases than positive.

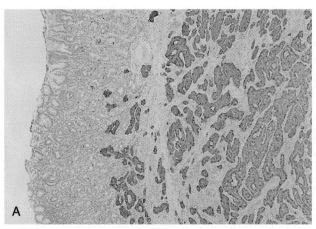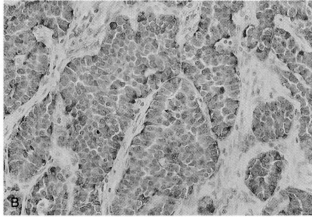

Figure 13–2. *A*, Gastric carcinoid consisting of nests of chromogranin-positive cells in the submucosa, with overlying negative-staining gastric mucosa. (Low-power magnification) *B*, High-power nest of gastric carcinoid demonstrating strong diffuse cytoplasmic-positive staining of the cells for chromogranin. (High-power magnification)

plasia (so-called) and carcinoids. We refer the reader to the major GI pathology textbooks or articles for the characterization of these lesions.[45, 47–51]

Omeprazole is an antireflux medication that acts by blocking hydrogen channels in parietal cells (i.e., it is a proton pump inhibitor). Hypergastrinemia can occur secondary to the hypoacidity induced by long-term omeprazole therapy. ECL cell hyperplasia is thought to occur in response to the hypergastrinemia, in a process similar to that for chronic atrophic gastritis and Zollinger-Ellison syndrome. It is not clear whether immunohistochemically apparent ECL hyperplasia occurs in all patients receiving long-term omeprazole therapy. Nevertheless, gastroenterologists occasionally procure fundic gland biopsy specimens and request an assessment of the degree of ECL cell hyperplasia.[52] In our experience, the number of ECL cells in these specimens appears normal with routine hematoxylin and eosin stain; only by applying chromogranin or synaptophysin can one appreciate mild degrees of ECL cell hyperplasia. Chromogranin and synaptophysin stain ECL cells equally well.

Primary gastrin-producing endocrine cell hyperplasia of the antral mucosa occurs sporadically in patients with peptic ulcer disease or subtypes of *Helicobacter pylori* chronic gastritis and secondarily in patients with severe chronic atrophic gastritis. Chromogranin and synaptophysin can be employed to quantify gastrin-producing endocrine cell hyperplasia, but this method is less desirable than antigastrin antibody serum quantitative measurements.[53, 54]

Fundic ECL carcinoids immunohistochemically stain with chromogranin and synaptophysin antibodies (see Table 13–1)*; most but not all studies demonstrate similar staining patterns with the two

antibodies. One study reported that 3 of 20 carcinoids did not stain with synaptophysin, 3 stained focally, and the other 13 stained diffusely and strongly.[19] In contrast, all of the tumors stained with chromogranin, 2 of which showed focal staining patterns (Fig. 13–2*A*).

NEUROENDOCRINE CELL LESIONS OF THE DUODENUM

Endocrine cell hyperplasia can occur in the duodenum in association with untreated celiac sprue. The cells stain with synaptophysin and chromogranin antibodies.[44, 63, 64]

Duodenal carcinoids frequently immunostain with gastrin antibodies, although other hormones can be expressed and immunohistochemically identified (see Table 13–1). Some duodenal carcinoids produce the Zollinger-Ellison syndrome,[15, 20, 65–68] with most occurring in the bulb. These neoplasms diffusely and strongly stain with chromogranin and synaptophysin.[22, 44]

Carcinoids that are composed predominantly of somatostatin-staining cells also develop in the duodenum, most commonly around the sphincter of Oddi or ampulla of Vater.[69–75] They can mimic adenocarcinomas because of their tubule-forming histology. One study found that only about 50% of these neoplasms immunostain with chromogranin A and diffusely stain with epithelial membrane antigen (EMA), a feature that can increase diagnostic confusion with adenocarcinoma.[15] However, other studies have found the opposite result, reporting that most of the carcinoids diffusely stained with chromogranin.[25, 69] The presence of psammoma bodies in a duodenal neoplasm composed of tubules can suggest the correct diagnosis.[76] A 1999 study concluded that ampullary carcinoids, although geographically close, should be considered an entity distinct from duodenal carcinoids.[29]

---

*References 15, 16, 18, 22, 25, 42, 44, 51, 55–62.

NEUROENDOCRINE CELL LESIONS OF THE JEJUNUM, ILEUM, AND CECUM

Most carcinoid tumors of the jejunum, ileum, and cecum are of the enterochromaffin (EC) cell type and immunostain with antiserotonin and substance P antibodies (see Table 13–1).[77] Serotonin can be released into the blood stream, producing the classic carcinoid syndrome. Approximately 90 to 95% of these tumors diffusely and strongly stain with synaptophysin, chromogranin, and CD57 (Leu7).[25, 77–82] In our experience, synaptophysin, chromogranin, and CD57 (Leu7) usually produce identical staining patterns within a neoplasm; rarely, however, one antibody either is negative or stains significantly fewer cells than the other antibodies.

S-100 protein rarely stains sustentacular cells of occasional carcinoids. The presence of sustentacular cells in approximately 10% of distal bowel carcinoids is interesting in regard to a possible relationship with paragangliomas, but the clinical significance of this finding is unknown.[77, 83] CK7 diffusely stains carcinoids of both the small and large intestine, whereas appendiceal carcinoids are usually nonreactive.[84, 85] Prostatic acid phosphatase (PAP) stains between 20 and 100% of distal small bowel and cecum carcinoids.[53, 77] To verify these reports, we stained five small bowel carcinoids with PAP and prostate-specific antigen (PSA). We found that they stained diffusely and strongly with PAP antibodies but none stained with the PSA antibody, a finding also identical to that reported by other authors.[77] CEA stains approximately 66% of carcinoids from these sites.[77]

NEUROENDOCRINE CARCINOIDS OF THE APPENDIX

Typical non–goblet cell appendiceal carcinoids, unlike jejunal and ileal carcinoids, frequently have S-100 protein–positive sustentacular cells around the solid tumor EC cell nests (see Table 13–1).[86, 87] Tubular carcinoids have been reported to stain less often with chromogranin.[88] It has been our experience, however, that such tumors stain diffusely and strongly with chromogranin and synaptophysin when antigen retrieval is employed. CK7 is negative or focally positive in approximately 10% of neoplasms (see preceding discussion).

Goblet cell carcinoids and mixed adenocarcinoma-carcinoids are discussed in the section on Mixed Epithelial and Endocrine Lesions.

COLON CARCINOIDS

Carcinoids of the colon occur predominantly in two locations, the cecum and proximal-right colon and the distal sigmoid and rectum. Most cecal and proximal-right colon carcinoids are composed of EC cells that stain with antibodies to serotonin, chromogranin, and synaptophysin (see Table 13–1).[89–91] Like jejunal and ileal carcinoids, most proximal-right colon carcinoids lack S-100 protein–staining sustentacular cells.[53] Approximately 12% stain with vimentin.[61]

Sigmoid and rectal carcinoids can stain diffusely and strongly with PAP (see Table 13–1).[92, 93] PSA has been uniformly negative in these tumors. Chromogranin has been reported to stain such cells less often than the 100% staining by synaptophysin, with a reported range of 50 to 80% for chromogranin, depending on the method of detection used. In general, the earlier studies that did not use antigen retrieval methods reported lower percentages of tumors staining with chromogranin.[22, 25, 44, 82, 91–96] In our experience, rectosigmoid carcinoids frequently are chromogranin-negative and synaptophysin-positive. CEA stains approximately 25% of such tumors. Of the positively staining tumors, approximately 70% show focal to patchy positivity of weak to moderate intensity.[92] Vimentin stains approximately 50% of rectal carcinoids.[61, 93, 97]

OTHER NEUROENDOCRINE CELL TUMORS

Intermediate-Grade Neuroendocrine Carcinoma (Atypical Carcinoid)

Intermediate-grade neurocrine carcinomas, or atypical carcinoids, are not well defined in the GI tract, and many authors have included them under the carcinoid designation.[98, 99] These tumors have a unique morphology, retaining to some degree their carcinoid nested pattern and cytology, which is overlaid by necrosis, and overt cytologic atypia. They can also have a single-file infiltrative pattern. In our experience, these tumors strongly and diffusely stain with synaptophysin (monoclonal or polyclonal antibodies), and less often with chromogranin A.

High-Grade Neuroendocrine (Small Cell) Carcinoma

High-grade neuroendocrine (small cell) carcinoma has an aggressive behavior similar to its counterpart in the lung. These neoplasms can arise in any part of the GI tract from the esophagus to the anus.[99–125] Small cell and large cell variants have been described.[118]

The morphology of these tumors is similar to that of small cell carcinoma of the lung. A cautious approach is recommended to making a diagnosis of neuroendocrine carcinoma on the basis of morphology alone, because typical, poorly differentiated adenocarcinoma, especially of the colon, can have a neuroendocrine appearance yet be shown to have no neuroendocrine differentiation by immunohistochemical or electron microscopic techniques (see later discussion of adenocarcinomas with neuroendocrine differentiation). This differ-

Table 13–2. Antibody Staining of High-Grade Neuroendocrine (Small Cell Undifferentiated) Carcinoma of the Gastrointestinal Tract

Antibody	Immunostaining	Comments
Chromogranin	+/−	See text
Synaptophysin	+/−	80% if polyclonal antibody with antigen retrieval is used
		Lower % if monoclonal antibody is used
CEA	N–R	Gastric and duodenal show focal positivity in 10–20% of neoplasms
		Almost never positive in appendiceal, ileal, and colorectal neoplasms
Keratin AE1/AE3	−/+	Frequently weakly positive with no perinuclear dot
Keratin CAM5.2	+/−	Frequently with diffuse cytoplasmic decoration with perinuclear dot accentuation
Keratin 34βE12	N–R	Positive neoplasms usually show only focal, weak staining
EMA	−/+	Frequently weak
Vimentin	R	See text
CK20	N–R	See text
beta hCG	Unknown	Studied only in gastric small cell carcinomas
Neurofilament	R	See text

N, negative; N–R, negative to rare; R, rare; +/−, more positive cases than negative; −/+, more negative cases than positive.

ence is more than semantic, because patients with high-grade neuroendocrine carcinoma are frequently treated with a pulmonary small cell undifferentiated chemoradiation regimen, rather than surgery. The use of NSE is not recommended because of its nonspecificity.

Our immunohistochemical approach to confirming high-grade neuroendocrine carcinomas is to stain them with keratins CAM5.2 and 35βH11, synaptophysin, and chromogranin A (Table 13–2). Some authors have also used CD57(Leu7), with approximately the same results as for chromogranin in regard to sensitivity and specificity.[102, 107, 109, 117, 124]

Gastrointestinal high-grade neuroendocrine carcinomas contain only low molecular weight cytokeratins. In our experience, staining with keratin CAM5.2 or 35βH11 is almost always present. However, staining can be variable; both antibodies can stain, or one antibody will be diffusely and strongly positive while the other is negative. Approximately 50% of high-grade neuroendocrine carcinomas of the GI tract have a perinuclear dot with these antibodies, more often with keratin CAM5.2.[111, 126, 127] Our and other authors' experiences find keratin AE1/AE3 is less specific and usually stains fewer tumor cells with less intensity than keratins CAM5.2 or 35βH11.[102] In addition, we have seen GI high-grade neuroendocrine carcinomas that fail to stain with keratin AE1/AE3 yet strongly immunostain with keratin CAM5.2. This point is important, because some neuroendocrine carcinomas display only keratin CAM5.2 staining and do not immunostain with chromogranin or synaptophysin.

The characteristic perinuclear dot staining pattern seen with keratin CAM5.2 is frequently maintained in crushed or distorted biopsy specimens, whereas chromogranin and synaptophysin staining not infrequently becomes uninterpretable under these conditions. EMA stains in a distribution and intensity similar to keratin AE1/AE3 and is therefore not a preferred antibody.[128] Unlike Merkel cell carcinomas of the skin, high-grade neuroendocrine carcinomas of the GI tract do not stain with CK20,

so this antibody can be used to help distinguish between the two carcinomas.[127]

Villin is not useful in distinguishing the primary site of a high-grade neuroendocrine carcinoma because such a tumor from any site appears to stain diffusely and strongly with this antibody.[37] We have found that vimentin and neurofilament staining are consistently negative and that S-100 stains isolated cells in such tumors. CEA can occasionally stain isolated tumor cells of carcinomas located in the esophagus and stomach,[105] whereas colonic small cell undifferentiated carcinomas almost never stain with CEA.[117, 128] Human chorionic gonadotrophin (hCG) has been reported to diffusely stain gastric high-grade neuroendocrine carcinomas.[110]

Chromogranin A stains 0 to 70% of high-grade neuroendocrine carcinomas.* This spectrum of staining is partially due to technical factors, with studies using antigen retrieval reporting reactivity in close to 70%, and partially to interpretive reasons, with some reports including tumors with rare stained cells as a "positive" result.

Synaptophysin can show greater variations in staining, depending on whether a polyclonal or monoclonal antibody is used. Staining is usually stronger and involves more cells if a polyclonal antibody is used, with positive results reported in 33 to 80% of these tumors.[98, 105, 110, 116–118]

MIXED EPITHELIAL AND ENDOCRINE LESIONS

Mixed Carcinoid-Adenoma and Carcinoid-Adenocarcinoma

Admixtures of typical carcinoid and adenoma or adenocarcinoma within a single neoplasm are uncommon but well documented in all parts of the GI tract.[58, 129–139] Those neoplasms that show no areas of histologic transition between the carcinoid and adenoma or adenocarcinoma have been termed

---

*References 98, 99, 103–105, 108, 110, 116–118, 122.

collision tumors. Some neoplasms show transitions between malignant glands and endocrine cell nests, the so-called adenocarcinoid. The heterogeneity within neoplasms in regard to endocrine cell differentiation sometimes can be extreme. One case report described a gastric tumor with adenocarcinoma, carcinoid, microglandular carcinoid, and neuroendocrine mucinous carcinoma.[140]

Chromogranin and synaptophysin usually diffusely and strongly stain the carcinoid and intermediate-grade neuroendocrine cell carcinoma transition components. CEA rarely stains the nests of endocrine or transition type cells but usually immunostains the glandular component strongly. S-100 protein immunostains sustentacular cells around the endocrine cell nests.[58, 131, 138, 139]

Appendiceal Tubular and Goblet Cell Carcinoids

The goblet cell carcinoid is one of the more common variants of mixed tumors.[28, 88, 130, 131, 141–145] The spectrum of mixed neoplasms includes the tubular carcinoid with occasional goblet cells, the goblet cell carcinoid, and mixed signet ring cell–mucinous adenocarcinoma–carcinoid tumors.[145]

Tubular carcinoids with rare admixed goblet cells stain (carcinoid cells and goblet cells) diffusely and strongly stain with antibodies to cytokeratin, such as keratin AE1/AE3. Unlike typical carcinoids of the appendix, which usually either do not stain or have only focal, weak staining with CEA, tubular carcinoids strongly stain with this antibody.[145] Chromogranin with no antigen retrieval has been reported to stain only 33 to 50% of tumors in a patchy, weak to moderate pattern.[88, 145, 146] In our experience, chromogranin used with heat antigen retrieval, strongly and diffusely stains the endocrine cells and occasional goblet cells of these neoplasms.

Goblet cell carcinoids also diffusely and strongly stain with antibodies to keratin AE1/AE3 and CEA.[141, 145] The admixed endocrine cells stain with chromogranin and synaptophysin.[88, 141, 145] In our experience, consistent staining of the endocrine cell component with chromogranin and synaptophysin is achieved only through the use of heat antigen retrieval and highly sensitive signal detection systems.[147, 148] Synaptophysin produces a stronger and larger intracytoplasmic staining signal than chromogranin. Fewer goblet cells stain with chromogranin and synaptophysin, in the range of 25 to 50% with weak to moderate intensity.

Mixed High-Grade Neuroendocrine Carcinoma and Adenocarcinoma

High-grade neuroendocrine carcinomas (small cell carcinomas) uncommonly arise in conjunction with adenomas, poorly differentiated mucinous adenocarcinoma, or typical glandular adenocarcinoma.[98, 99, 117, 122, 149] Transition zones can be observed between the two regions, but this is not a consistent feature. The previous comments about the immunohistochemistry of pure high-grade neuroendocrine carcinoma apply also to these tumors. The adenocarcinomas stain as typical enteric glandular malignancies with the immunohistochemical phenotype characteristic of each region of the GI tract.

Mesenchymal Lesions

GASTROINTESTINAL STROMAL TUMORS

The immunohistochemistry of GI stromal tumors (GISTs) has produced an extensive body of literature that continues to expand. The results of many of the studies were used to support various authors' opinions about the histogenesis or direction of differentiation of the neoplastic cells, with occasional prognostic implications.

The immunohistochemical phenotype of GIST cells is broad. Depending upon their origin in the GI tract, these tumors can show (1) predominantly smooth muscle differentiation, (2) predominantly neural differentiation, (3) mixed smooth muscle and neural differentiation, or (4) neither smooth muscle nor neural differentiation. Neurogenic differentiation may be entirely schwannian or toward autonomic nerve cells. A GIST can express different antigens within different foci of the same neoplasm. Subtypes or variants of GISTs have been recognized, generating the terms *leiomyoma, neurolemmoma, gastrointestinal autonomic nerve tumor* (GANT), and *plexosarcomas* for these neoplasms.

Despite the intense academic interest in GISTs, we believe that there are no conclusive or definitive associations between the immunohistochemical staining patterns of GISTs and their malignant potential,[150–152] despite some suggestions that most GISTs with prominent autonomic nerve cell differentiation are malignant.[153–155] The location of the GIST has some correlation with the immunostaining pattern. One group noted that small intestine GISTs stain less commonly with CD34 than gastric GISTs.[156] The utility of characterizing the immunohistochemical staining profile of GISTs, aside from academic interest, is in the distinction between GISTs and other lesions.[157]

The frequency of antibodies that have been reported to stain GISTs varies greatly, because many of the early studies used no pretreatment. This discussion is limited to later studies that have used heat or enzyme pretreatment. Following is a compiled list of the more common antibodies that have been applied to GISTs.[150, 151, 154–156, 158–215]

KEY DIAGNOSTIC POINTS

- Vimentin: Diffuse and strong cytoplasmic staining occurs when citrate buffer heat pretreatment (HIER) is used. The significance of this antibody is related to the ability of the neoplastic cells to express immunohistochemically detectable antigens (positive control) rather than to shedding light on the specific histogenesis or direction of differentiation of the neoplasm.

- CD34: Diffuse and strong cytoplasmic staining is seen in approximately 70% of GISTs when HIER is used (Fig. 13–3). The other 30% show patchy, moderate staining. The "neural" differentiated GISTs (schwannian or autonomic nerve) tend to have fewer CD34+ cells with weaker intensity than neoplasms with smooth muscle differentiated GISTs. Neoplasms of the abdominal colon stain infrequently with this antibody. Less than 3% of GISTs show CD34 staining unless heat antigen retrieval pretreatment is used.
- Muscle-specific actin (HHF-35): Diffuse HHF-35 reactivity of moderate intensity occurs in approximately 25% of GISTs when HIER is used; 50% of neoplasms show patchy or focal staining.
- Smooth muscle actin: Approximately 20% of GISTs show diffuse staining with moderate intensity when HIER is used, whereas 25% have patchy, weak staining.
- Desmin: Approximately 10% of neoplasms show diffuse strong staining, whereas 33% show patchy cytoplasmic staining with weak to moderate intensity, when HIER or enzyme pretreatment is used.
- S-100 protein: Approximately 5% of GISTs show more than half of the cells stain (nuclear or cytoplasmic), whereas in 35% of tumors, there is staining only of individual or small clusters of cells, with moderate to strong nuclear and cytoplasmic intensity, when HIER is used.
- Keratin AE1/AE3: Approximately 5% of

GISTs usually show staining of individual cells, with moderate intensity, when HIER is used. Signet ring variants have been uniformly negative.[174]
- Keratin CAM5.2: Approximately 40% of cases stain with individual or small clusters of cells showing positivity, whereas 5% show positivity in a greater number of cells, which would be considered focal positivity. Staining, even when only individual cells are positive, is usually of moderate to strong intensity when HIER is used. Signet ring variants have been uniformly negative.[174]
- Synaptophysin: Approximately 10% of cases stain with synaptophysin, usually as scattered cells with weak to moderate intensity, when HIER is used. GISTs with autonomic nerve cell differentiation are the most common subtype to be synaptophysin-positive. Gastric neoplasms most commonly show staining of the highest number of cells and with the greatest intensity.
- Chromogranin: Approximately 5% of cases stain, usually as scattered cells with weak to moderate intensity, when HIER is used.
- Neurofilament: Staining is seen in approximately 5% of cases, usually as scattered cells with weak to moderate intensity, when HIER is used.
- Glial fibrillary acidic protein (GFAP): Approximately 5% of cases stain, usually as scattered cells with weak to moderate intensity, when HIER is used.
- PGP9.5: One study noted positivity with this antibody in 9 of 10 cases.[216] The clinical application of PGP9.5 remains to be defined.
- BCL-2: One study found that the staining pattern with BCL-2 tends to mirror that with CD34,[159] but another study demonstrated a heterogeneous staining pattern.[217] Given the

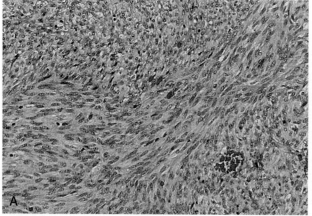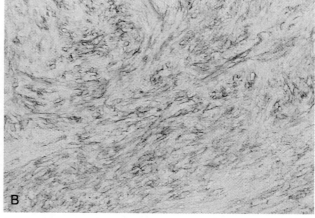

Figure 13–3. *A,* Gastrointestinal stromal tumor (GIST) consisting of interlacing fascicles of uniform, spindle-shaped cells. The GIST measured 7 cm but demonstrated no evidence of significant atypia, increased mitotic activity, or necrosis. The findings were interpreted as GIST of uncertain malignant potential. (Low-power magnification) *B,* The GIST stained positive for CD34, with negative staining for muscle-specific actin and S-100. (Intermediate-power magnification)

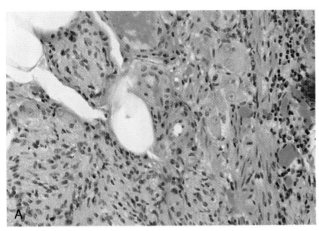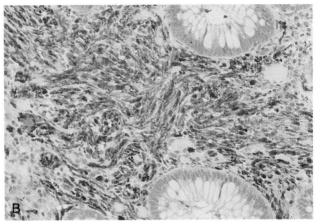

Figure 13–4. *A,* Ganglioneuroma of the sigmoid colon, demonstrating spindle-shaped cells and scattered ganglion cells in the lamina propria. (Low-power magnification) *B,* S-100–positive staining of the Schwann cells of the sigmoid colon ganglioneuroma. (Low-power magnification)

inconsistent staining in GISTs and the positivity in other spindle cell neoplasms, the utility of BCL-2 is low.

* CD117: The c-*kit* proto-oncogene product stains interstitial cells of Cajal, which are involved in the regulation of gut motility (pacemaker cell). This antibody has been found to be expressed in 85% of GISTs, whereas the responses in schwannomas, solitary fibrous tumors, and Kaposi's sarcomas are uniformly negative.[218] Studies have suggested that the majority of GISTs (especially gastric and small intestine), regardless of their degree of smooth muscle or neural differentiation, either are of interstitial cell of Cajal origination or have interstitial cell of Cajal differentiation.[209] As additional studies on this topic are published, CD117 will undoubtedly be found to be a useful antibody in the identification of GISTs. Until then, its utility in daily practice remains to be defined.

When CD34 was noted to stain the majority of GISTs, it became fashionable to characterize a CD34+ spindle cell neoplasm of the abdomen as a GIST. This practice is now questionable with the recognition that CD34 stains many neoplasms, including the solitary fibrous tumors of soft tissue, gastric inflammatory fibroid polyps, and dedifferentiated liposarcoma.[159, 219] A significant minority of GISTs, especially the high-grade sarcomas, express only vimentin.[168]

LEIOMYOMAS

The esophagus and distal colon are sites in which immunohistochemically phenotypic and morphologic leiomyomas and leiomyosarcomas occur. They usually stain diffusely and strongly with desmin and HHF-35, and not with CD34.[188, 189]

NEURAL TUMORS

Ganglioneuroma

Ganglioneuromas and neurofibromas can be seen in the GI tract as isolated lesions, a component of the multiple endocrine neoplasia (MEN) type 2b syndrome, and occasionally as component of von Recklinghausen's disease or other syndromes and complexes. Such tumors most commonly are incidental findings in the colon or appendix. As with the more common non-GI ganglioneuromas, the immunohistochemical staining profile depends on the composition of ganglion and Schwann cells.[220–222] Ganglion cells stain with NSE, synaptophysin, and neurofilament. S-100 protein stains the spindle cell component in the majority of cases and usually the satellite cells around the ganglion cells (Fig. 13–4).

Schwannoma

Schwannoma, representing a neoplasm distinct from GIST, has been reported,[156, 168, 223–226] with most examples described in the stomach. By definition, these neoplasms are CD34– but stain strongly and diffusely with S-100 protein. CD57 and GFAP are usually focally positive. Microscopically, these neoplasms share many features with CD34+ GISTs.

Paraganglioma

There are histologic similarities among paraganglioma-pheochromocytomas that secondarily involve the GI tract (most often from the retroperitoneal regions), carcinoid tumors, and the rare primary GI paraganglioma.[227] Paraganglioma cells stain with antibodies to chromogranin and synaptophysin, and like carcinoid tumors, they can express various polypeptides, such as leu-enkephalin, pancreatic polypeptide, vasoactive intestinal peptide (VIP), adrenocorticotropic hormone (ACTH), calcitonin, and bombesin. Unlike carcinoid tumors of the GI tract, which diffusely and strongly immunostain with keratin AE1/AE3 and CAM5.2 antibodies, paragangliomas almost always (>98% of cases) do not express these keratin antibodies.[227–234]

Gangliocytic Paraganglioma

Gangliocytic paragangliomas arise almost always in the duodenum, most commonly in the periampullary submucosa.[235] These tumors are composed of three cell types, each having its own immunohistochemical profile.[235–242] The proportions of the three cells can vary among tumors. The spindled, nerve sheath type cells that form the stroma and encircling sustentacular cells immunostain with S-100 protein and occasionally with synaptophysin and neurofilament. The ganglion-like cells stain diffusely and strongly with synaptophysin and occasionally with neurofilament.

The endocrine, epithelioid cells that form the paraganglioma-like nests stain with chromogranin in approximately 70% of cases, with a range of staining patterns from scattered to diffusely positive cells. Cytokeratins stain these cells in approximately 50% of cases, with only a minority of cases describing punctate cytoplasmic positivity. PGP9.5 has been reported to diffusely stain the endocrine, epithelioid cells in the few case reports that have utilized this antibody.

Esophageal Lesions and Neoplasms

ACHALASIA

Achalasia is predominantly a medically treated disease. Patients with severe achalasia occasionally require esophagectomy. Immunohistochemically, the absence or decreased number of ganglion cells can be illuminated by S-100 staining of the esophageal wall.[243, 244]

BARRETT'S ESOPHAGUS

Cytokeratins 7 and 20

Ormsby and colleagues[245] have found that the pattern of CK7 and CK20 staining can reliably distinguish between Barrett's esophagus and gastric cardia intestinal metaplasia.[245] In Barrett's esophagus, the entire epithelium of the mucosa stains with CK7, and the surface epithelium stains with CK20 (Fig. 13–5). In contrast, the cells of intestinal metaplasia in the gastric cardia mucosa showed no CK7 staining but strong CK20 staining in the superficial and deep gland compartments. Although the utility of these stains is promising, we believe that the use of these antibodies in this context remains in the research realm until additional studies replicate the reported results.

Villin

Villin is a calcium-regulated, actin-binding protein on the epithelial cell brush border of enterocytes and subsets of renal tubule epithelial cells. Commercial antivillin antibodies are available that work in formalin-fixed, paraffin-embedded tissue. Studies conducted in the late 1990s have reported staining of Barrett's esophagus in 80 to 100% of cases.[246–250] The utility of this finding is unknown, because questions such as the frequency of villin staining of intestinal metaplasia of the cardia in the absence of Barrett's esophagus have not been addressed.

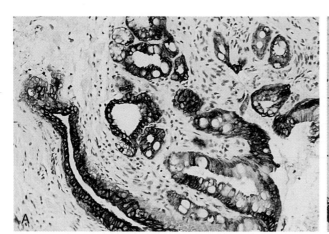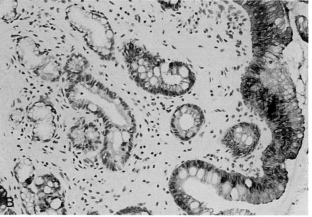

Figure 13–5. *A,* Barrett's esophagus with entire epithelium staining positive with cytokeratin 7 (CK7). (Intermediate-power magnification) *B,* The surface epithelium stains positive for CK20, with negative staining of the underlying mucosa. This pattern is different from that seen in gastric intestinal metaplasia, in which the gastric cardiac mucosa demonstrates a lack of CK7 staining and strong CK20 staining of both the superficial and deep glandular components. (Intermediate-power magnification)

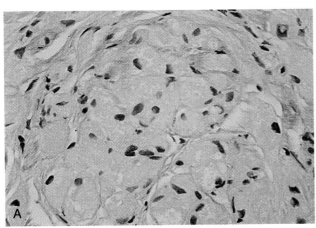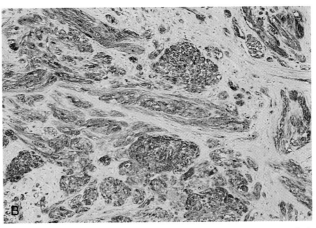

Figure 13–6. *A,* Granular cell tumor consisting of a loose cluster of polygonal-shaped cells with eosinophilic granular cytoplasm. (H&E) *B,* S-100 diffusely stains the granular cells. (Intermediate-power magnification)

p53 Protein

Normal p53 protein has an extremely short half-life and is found in very small quantities inside cells. It cannot be detected in normal cells with the use of immunohistochemistry. The p53 protein from abnormal p53 genes has a longer half-life than normal p53 protein, builds up inside cells, and can be immunohistochemically detected with anti-p53 antibodies. In theory, overexpression of p53, as a surrogate marker for p53 gene mutations, is an immunohistochemical "test" for neoplasia (dysplasia). However, this is not the case in practice, because correlation between staining and gene abnormalities is not precise.[251]

Most but not all studies have found that p53 staining of Barrett's esophagus cell nuclei occurs with rising frequency with increasing grades of dysplasia, and most adenocarcinomas associated with Barrett's esophagus react with p53 antibodies.[252-256] One study found p53 positivity in the nuclei of Barrett's esophagus cells in none of cases in which specimens were negative for dysplasia, in 9% of cases that showed indefinite or low-grade dysplasia, in 55% of cases that showed high-grade dysplasia, and in 87% of cases with adenocarcinoma.[257] Another study found p53 staining in no cases of nondysplastic Barrett's esophagus mucosa and low-grade dysplasia, in 69% of high-grade dysplasias, and in 67% of intramucosal adenocarcinomas.[255]

These findings have led some authors to suggest that positive p53 response is a marker of neoplastic progression and can be used as an adjunct to the histologic evaluation of dysplasia or premalignant lesions in Barrett's esophagus.[257, 258] However, the false-positive and false-negative rates of p53 staining in Barrett's esophagus are not completely defined, and the clinical utility of this test has yet to be determined.[259] In support of the latter opinion, a study found that 4 of 11 nondysplastic specimens, 3 of 10 low-grade dysplastic specimens, 11 of 13 high-grade dysplastic specimens, and 9 of 10 adenocarcinoma specimens were p53+.[260]

In our experience, p53 staining can occur in Barrett's esophagus epithelium that is inflamed or is indeterminate for dysplasia and in some specimens with low-grade dysplasia, but the staining reaction is usually weak and focal in these conditions. The nuclear staining does not always occur in the most atypical cells. In contrast, in high-grade dysplasia, staining usually is strong and restricted to the most atypical-appearing nuclei. In our opinion, p53 staining, when strongly expressed in many nuclei, can be used to help distinguish between reactive cytologic changes and high-grade dysplasia.

PRIMARY ESOPHAGEAL NEOPLASMS

Mesenchymal Neoplasms

Smooth muscle neoplasms and GISTs are discussed in the general section on mesenchymal neoplasms of the GI tract. Most esophageal GISTs demonstrate smooth muscle differentiation consistent with leiomyomas and, rarely, leiomyosarcomas.

Granular Cell Tumors

Granular cell tumors of the esophagus are uncommon but not rare. Immunohistochemically, they stain just like granular cell tumors of other sites. S-100 protein and vimentin stain strongly and diffusely (100%) in almost all tumor cells (Fig. 13–6). Desmin stains rare (<5%) cases in a patchy distribution and with weak intensity. CD57 stains more than 50% of tumor cells with moderate intensity. Keratin CAM5.2 and EMA staining reactions have been consistently negative.[261-263] Earlier studies that used relatively less specific CEA antibodies reported positivity; however, later studies using monoclonal CEA antibodies report either no or rare, individual cell positivity.[264-267]

Squamous Cell Carcinoma

Squamous cell carcinoma is the most common neoplasm of the esophagus, although the incidence of adenocarcinoma is growing. Neoplastic squamous cells contain a preponderance of high molecular weight cytokeratins and usually no, or minimal amounts of, low molecular weight keratins. Accordingly, reactions to the high molecular weight keratin 34βE11 antibody and pankeratin antibody AE1/AE3 are usually positive, whereas responses to the antibodies that stain low or predominantly low molecular weight keratins, such as 35βH11 and CAM5.2, are negative.

Few distinguishing antibodies can be used to separate primary from metastatic squamous cell carcinomas. In the context of a mediastinal mass and the distinction from thymic carcinoma, CD5 has been found to be specific for thymic carcinomas. Care in regard to the specific CD5 antibody clone and to the pH of the antigen retrieval solution used is imperative, because studies have shown relative nonspecificity for thymic carcinoma with some but not all CD5 antibodies and decreased immunoreactivity depending on the pH of the antigen retrieval solution.[268, 269] Poorly differentiated squamous carcinomas diffusely stain with calretinin, making it a useless antibody in the distinction between squamous cell carcinoma and mesothelioma (personal experience).[270]

Following is a list of antibodies and their staining properties of squamous cell carcinoma.

KEY DIAGNOSTIC POINTS

- Keratin CAM5.2: Almost all squamous cell carcinomas strongly stain, most commonly in more than 50% of neoplastic cells.[271] The CK18 component of keratin CAM5.2 accounts for the majority of tumor positivity.[271]
- Keratin AE1/AE3: Almost all squamous cell carcinomas strongly stain in a diffuse cytoplasmic distribution.[272]
- Keratin 35βH11: This antibody does not stain esophageal squamous cell carcinomas.[273]
- Keratin 34βE12: Almost all squamous cell carcinomas strongly stain in a diffuse cytoplasmic distribution with this antibody.[273]
- CK19: Overall, approximately 85 to 100% of esophageal squamous cell carcinomas react positively to CK19.[271, 274] Staining response greatly depends on tumor grade. Approximately 70% of well- and moderately differentiated carcinomas are reactive, most commonly in less than 50% of neoplastic cells. All poorly differentiated squamous cell carcinomas stain with CK19, almost always in more than 50% of neoplastic cells.[271]
- CK20: All neoplasms have demonstrated a negative response to this antibody.[274, 275]
- CK7: From none to 30% of squamous cell carcinomas are reactive with this anti-body.[271, 276] A similar percentage of tumors of all grades are reactive, most commonly in an occasional to rare, single cell or small tumor nest pattern.[3, 271]
- CK7/CK20 coordinate staining: Almost all squamous cell carcinomas are negative to both cytokeratins if a positive result is defined as staining in more than 50% of the neoplastic cells.
- CK5: This antibody, especially the D5/16B4 clone, stains almost all squamous cell carcinomas.[3, 277, 278]
- Involucrin: Almost all squamous cell carcinomas strongly and diffusely stain with involucrin in a cytoplasmic distribution.[274]
- Thrombomodulin: Almost all squamous cell carcinomas strongly stain with thrombomodulin in a diffuse cytoplasmic distribution.[279, 280] In the context of a mediastinal mass or metastatic carcinoma in another location, thrombomodulin cannot be used to distinguish between squamous cell carcinomas and transitional cell carcinomas (TCCs). However, esophageal squamous cell carcinoma cells are CK20−, whereas TCC cells are CK20+.

Differential Diagnoses. Esophageal squamous cell carcinoma does not frequently require immunohistochemical evaluation to distinguish it from other neoplasms. However, several points bear mentioning. Squamous cell carcinomas from all sites of the body have the same or extremely similar immunophenotypes and therefore cannot be distinguished immunohistochemically.[3] Occasionally, it is important to distinguish poorly differentiated squamous cell carcinoma from adenocarcinoma. CK7, CK20, and CK5 are useful in this context.[3] Most squamous cell carcinomas are CK7−, CK20−, and CK5+. Adenocarcinomas of the esophagus, stomach, and lung almost always stain with CK7, CK20, or both, but not with CK5.

Paget's Disease

Rare cases of Paget's disease–like squamous cell carcinoma have been described. The Paget's disease cells stained strongly with keratins CAM5.2 and 35βH11, weakly with keratin AE1/AE3, and not with S-100 protein, gross cystic disease fluid protein-15 (GCDFP-15), EMA, or CEA.[281]

Basaloid Squamous Carcinomas

Basaloid squamous carcinomas are considered variants of squamous cell carcinoma. Most studies have reported diffuse staining with pankeratin; however, several authors have noted either no staining or focal and weak staining of the basaloid carcinoma components with keratins CAM5.2 and AE1/AE3.[282, 283] CK19 reportedly stains the peripheral layer of carcinomatous cells around the basaloid nests of malignant cells.[284] Some authors have shown immunohistochemical and electron microscopic evidence of myoepithelial differentiation within basaloid carcinoma cells, with S-100 and actin positivity of the peripheral cells in tumor nests.[282, 283, 285] This type of divergent differentiation is not surprising, given the poorly differentiated nature of the cells.

High-grade neuroendocrine (small cell) carcinomas can be distinguished from basaloid squamous carcinomas by the latter neoplasm's lack of (1) staining with chromogranin, synaptophysin, and Leu7,[286] and (2) a perinuclear dot pattern of positivity with keratin antibodies.[283] Caution is recommended regarding the reactivity of the neuroendocrine stains, because many high-grade neuroendocrine carcinomas (small cell carcinomas) do not stain with chromogranin and Leu7 antibodies (see Neuroendocrine-Related and Cytokeratin Antibodies).

Poorly differentiated squamous cell carcinoma can be distinguished from basaloid squamous cell carcinoma by diffuse strong staining with BCL-2 in basaloid squamous carcinomas and lack of staining in poorly differentiated squamous cell carcinomas.[287] CEA is usually negative in basaloid squamous carcinomas but is positive in some poorly differentiated squamous cell carcinomas.[282, 288] Most basaloid squamous cell carcinomas diffusely express vimentin,[283] in contrast to only a minority of poorly differentiated squamous cell carcinomas.

Adenocarcinoma

Most of the antibody profiles from the few studies on esophageal adenocarcinomas suggest that the immunophenotypes of adenocarcinomas of the lower esophagus and stomach are highly similar, if not identical.[260, 289–293] The immunohistochemical features of gastric adenocarcinomas are detailed in Table 13–3.

Mucoepidermoid Carcinoma

As defined by some authors, mucoepidermoid carcinoma differs from squamous cell carcinoma with glandular differentiation (adenosquamous) through the presence in mucoepidermoid carcinoma of a diffuse mixture of mucin-secreting cells and squamous cells.[289] The glandular cells of these tumors are strongly CEA+, just like esophageal adenocarcinoma cells.

Adenoid Cystic Carcinoma

The term *adenoid cystic carcinoma* has been applied (1) to neoplasms that are identical in morphology and immunohistochemical staining pattern to salivary gland adenoid cystic carcinomas

Table 13–3. Antibody Staining of Gastric Adenocarcinoma

Antibody	Immunostaining	Comments and References*
Synaptophysin	−/+	See text
Chromogranin	−/+	
Keratin AE1/AE3	+	Diffuse and strong[444, 723]
Keratin 35βH11	+	Diffuse and strong[273, 723, 841]
Keratin CAM5.2	+/−	Diffuse and strong
		The remaining neoplasms show moderate to weak staining[332, 723]
EMA	+	Refs 723, 733
CK7	+/−	See text
CK20	+/−	See text
CK7−/CK20+	−/+	See text
CK7+/CK20+	−/+	
C7+/CK20−	+	
C7−/CK20−	R	
CK17	−/+	See text
CK19	+	Refs 842, 843
KP-1 (CD68)	−/+	See text
CA 19-9	+/−	See text
CEA	+	See text
ER	R	See text
PR	R	See text
BerEP4	+	Refs 332, 554, 555
CD99 (MIC2)	−/+	Ref 844
GCDFP-15	N	See text
CD30	N	Ref 412
CA 125	R	See text
Vimentin	R	See text
AFP	N	Not positive in usual type adenocarcinoma
		Can be positive in clear cell and hepatoid variants
beta hCG	−/+	See text
Calretinin	N	Ref 550
S-100 protein	−/+	See text
B72.3	+	Refs 332, 371, 845
Alpha inhibin	N	Ref 392

*Superscript numbers indicate chapter references.

N, negative; R, rare; +/−, more positive cases than negative; −/+, more negative cases than positive.

and (2) to basaloid squamous carcinomas that form cribriform structures that simulate the high-grade adenoid cystic pattern.[294] Most esophageal "adenoid cystic" carcinomas are basaloid squamous carcinomas[282]; however, occasional true adenoid cystic carcinomas have been reported.[295, 296] True adenoid cystic carcinomas stain diffusely and strongly with keratins CAM5.2 and AE1/AE3. High molecular weight keratin 34βE12 and CEA stain ductal cells, and conversely, S-100, actin, and vimentin stain the basaloid cells.[282, 296]

It has been our experience that pseudo–adenoid cystic basaloid squamous carcinomas usually stain focally and weakly with keratin AE1/AE3 and slightly more diffusely with keratin CAM5.2. Keratin 34βE12 and CEA reactivity are negative or are positive in small clusters or individual cells in a random distribution. S-100 stains only rare cells in a random distribution. Vimentin reactivity is diffusely positive.

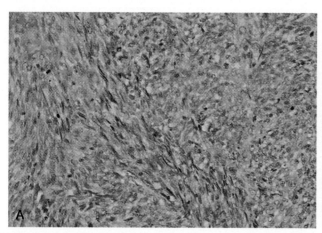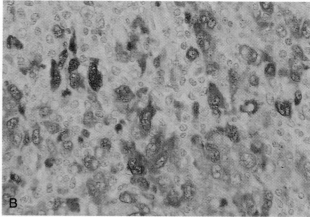

Figure 13–7. A, Poorly differentiated malignancy in the esophagus, having a spindle, sarcomatoid appearance. (Low magnification) *B,* Immunoperoxidase staining demonstrates positivity of the cells for S-100. The tumor cells were also HMB-45+, which is consistent with a primary esophageal malignant melanoma. (High-power magnification)

Carcinomas with Spindle Cell or Mesenchymal Differentiation (Carcinosarcomas)

The esophagus is one of the more common sites of these rare neoplasms. The malignant spindle cell components of the morphologically biphasic neoplasms can express cytokeratin and other epithelial antigens, such as EMA. The number of spindle cells and the intensity which they immunostain with keratin CAM5.2, 35βH11, 34βE12, or AE1/AE3 can markedly vary. Most studies have reported no or only focal staining with these keratin antibodies.[297-302] One study noted that among the small group of neoplasms with keratin-positive spindle cells, AE1/AE3 stained a greater number of spindle cells than CAM5.2 or 35βH11.[303]

Malignant Melanoma

Primary esophageal malignant melanomas are rare.[304, 305] Like their cutaneous counterparts, they stain with vimentin, S-100 protein, HMB-45, MART-1, and tyrosinase (Fig. 13–7).[306]

NEOPLASMS METASTATIC TO THE ESOPHAGUS

The esophagus is occasionally the site of metastatic carcinomas.[307, 308] Most metastatic malignan-cies involving the esophagus manifest late in the clinical course. The following discussion is presented to enable the reader to choose appropriate immunohistochemical panels when there is a question whether an esophageal tumor is a metastasis or a primary neoplasm.

Metastatic lung carcinoma, usually squamous cell carcinoma, is the main neoplasm that can manifest as a primary esophageal carcinoma, which immunohistochemically cannot be distinguished from esophageal squamous cell carcinoma. Metastatic breast carcinoma can rarely occur many years after the primary carcinoma and can simulate a primary esophageal neoplasm (Table 13–4 lists the immunohistochemical differential diagnostic antibodies).[309, 310] An autopsy series revealed the lung, followed by the breast, stomach, and cervix, to be the most common source of metastatic malignancies.[307]

Metastatic hepatocellular carcinomas (HCCs) were reported in esophageal veins in 24% of 55 patients with cirrhosis and carcinoma in one series.[311] Immunohistochemically, HCCs can be distinguished from esophageal adenocarcinomas with the antibody to HepPar 1,[312] which is positive in almost all hepatocellular carcinomas. Polyclonal CEA can also show canalicular staining in HCCs that is not seen in esophageal adenocarcinomas. Caution is needed in the use of polyclonal CEA,

Table 13–4. Gastric Carcinoma Versus Breast Carcinoma

Antibody	Gastric Signet Ring	Breast Lobular	Gastric Intestinal (Glandular)	Breast Ductal
CK7−/CK20+	−/+	N	Not useful	Not useful
ER	N	+/−	N	+/−
GCDFP-15	N	+/−	N	+/−
CK17	Not useful	Not useful	N	+/−
CEA (isomeric, monoclonal)	+	R−N	+	R−N

N, negative; R−N, rare to negative; +/−, more positive cases than negative; −/+, more negative cases than positive.

because both carcinomas can show diffuse cytoplasmic staining. Monoclonal CEA is positive in esophageal adenocarcinomas and negative in HCCs.

Metastatic thyroid carcinoma can be identified with the use of thyroid-stimulating hormone (TSH) and thyroid transcription factor (TTF).[313] TTF can also stain lung adenocarcinomas but is negative in esophageal and gastric adenocarcinomas.

Gastric Neoplasms

ADENOCARCINOMAS OF THE USUAL TYPE

Table 13–3 lists the antibodies and their staining patterns in gastric intestinal and signet ring cell adenocarcinomas, and their relative staining frequencies. In our experience, gastric glandular and signet ring cell adenocarcinomas have the same cytokeratin staining patterns. No consistent differences between glandular and signet ring cell adenocarcinomas have been detected. The two morphologic types, signet ring cell and glandular, appear to represent a spectrum of differentiation, with little differences in cytokeratin immunophenotype.[3, 314]

KEY DIAGNOSTIC POINTS

• Chromogranin and synaptophysin: Glandular-intestinal gastric adenocarcinomas that have no histologic neuroendocrine cell differentiation can show chromogranin positivity within rare neoplastic cells, in the range of one or two positive cells per several malignant glands. Staining of signet ring cell carcinoma can also be positive in up to 70% of cases.[315–320] Other authors have noted a tendency for synaptophysin to show weak staining in some adenocarcinomas.[28] One

study found rare chromogranin-positive cells in 61% of adenocarcinomas that invaded the submucosa, in 21% of adenocarcinomas that extended beyond the submucosa, and in 11% of metastases.[321] The occasional neuroendocrine cell positivity in usual-type adenocarcinoma is so common that the finding should be considered part of the spectrum of a typical immunohistochemical staining profile. Therefore, gastric carcinomas that have no histologic features of neuroendocrine cell differentiation but stain focally with either synaptophysin or chromogranin should not be considered neuroendocrine carcinomas.

• CK7: Approximately 40% of gastric adenocarcinomas are nonreactive. Focal positivity occurs in approximately 10% of neoplasms, and 50% are extensively positive.[276, 322–324]

• CK20: Forty percent of gastric adenocarcinomas are CK20 nonreactive, 20% are focally positive, and 40% are extensively positive (includes intestinal and signet ring cell types).[275, 322, 323, 325, 326]

• CK7/CK20 coordinate staining patterns: Gastric adenocarcinoma is, in our and others' experiences, extremely heterogeneous in its CK7/CK20 coordinate staining patterns.[1] It does not have a predominant pattern; a significant minority of gastric adenocarcinomas stain with each of the four possible CK7/CK20 patterns (Fig. 13–8). This limits the use of CK7/CK20 coordinate staining as part of differential diagnosis antibody panels for gastric adenocarcinoma. Approximately 30% of gastric adenocarcinomas have a CK7+/CK20+ pattern; 40% have a CK7−/CK20+ pattern; 20% have a CK7+/CK20− pattern; and 10% have a CK7−/CK20− pattern.[6, 323]

• CK17: In our experience, essentially all gastric adenocarcinomas, including signet ring cell and glandular types, do not stain with

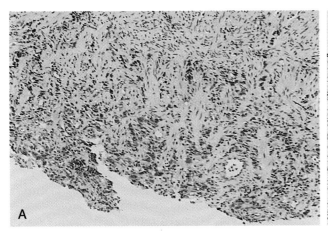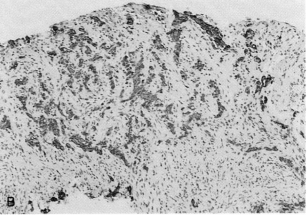

Figure 13–8. A, Gastric carcinoma consisting of nests and cords of malignant cells infiltrating throughout the wall of the stomach. (H&E, low-power magnification) *B,* Positive staining of the poorly differentiated gastric carcinoma for CK20. The CK7 stain was negative, a pattern seen in approximately 40% of gastric carcinomas. (Low-power magnification)

CK17. Occasional neoplasms show rare, singly stained cells. Our results are dissimilar to those of one group of authors who reported that signet ring cell carcinomas stain in approximately 50% of cases.[327] However, intestinal type adenocarcinomas uniformly lack staining.[327]

- KP-1 (CD68): Slightly more than 33% of gastric adenocarcinomas stain with KP-1, in which less than 33% of cells of each neoplasm demonstrated positive staining.[328]
- CA 19-9: Approximately 50 to 70% of adenocarcinomas stain with CA 19-9 in a cytoplasmic or membranous-luminal pattern.[329–331] In one study, more than half of the neoplastic cells stained in 47% of the reactive neoplasms. Approximately 33% of the reactive tumors displayed positivity in one fourth to one half of cells, and another 20% of the tumors had reactivity in less than one fourth of the neoplastic cells.[331] Signet ring cell types stain with slightly greater frequency but equal intensity (personal experience).[325]
- CEA: There is little difference in reactivity between monoclonal and polyclonal antibodies in gastric carcinomas.[332] Polyclonal CEA stains almost all adenocarcinomas, whereas the positivity rate is 98% with the use of a variety of monoclonal antibodies.[290, 319, 333] Monoclonal and polyclonal antibodies become important when CEA is used as part of differential diagnostic panels (see later).
- Estrogen receptor (ER): Studies of ER staining of gastric carcinomas have produced markedly varied results. Some authors, using heat pretreatment and the antibody clone ER1D5, have reported no staining of either the signet ring type or intestinal type adenocarcinomas.[292, 325, 334] Other studies have shown weak reactivity in scattered cells in a minority to a slight majority of carcinomas with the use of a variety of antibodies and pretreatment regimens.[335–344]

A plausible explanation for these varied results comes from a correlative study in which ER messenger RNA (mRNA) was detected in all gastric carcinomas. The results of enzyme immunoassays were positive in all the carcinomas (mean = 1.8 fmol/mg protein), but immunohistochemistry failed to stain the nuclei of the neoplastic cells.[345, 346] Other studies have biochemically confirmed the presence of ER in most gastric carcinomas.[347–349] Rare studies have found ER levels in gastric carcinoma similar to those in breast carcinoma.[350] Identical issues are seen with ER staining of colorectal adenocarcinomas (see Colorectal Adenocarcinomas of the Usual Type for a discussion of these issues).

Immunohistochemically, the number of ER+ cells in gastric carcinomas is almost always well below that seen in ER+ breast carcinomas. In our experience, gastric carcinomas can show faint positivity in up to 10% of neoplastic cell nuclei. Well-differentiated adenocarcinomas show this rare, weakly positive staining pattern more commonly than poorly differentiated neoplasms.[337]

- Progesterone receptor (PR): Some studies report no staining of intestinal or signet ring cell types.[325] However, other studies have shown positivity in 25% of gastric carcinomas.[342, 344] These issues are the same as those already described for ER (see earlier).
- GCDFP-15: No intestinal type adenocarcinomas stain with this antibody,[351, 352] and less than 5% of signet ring adenocarcinomas are focally positive.[325, 353]
- CA 125: Seven percent of gastric adenocarcinomas are reactive to CA 125, usually as single cells or in small, focal areas.[330, 354]
- Vimentin: Responses of glandular and signet ring adenocarcinomas to vimentin are uniformly negative according to some authors[355] or express focal positivity in 33% of tumors according to others.[356] Poorly differentiated carcinomas that have a solid pattern can coexpress vimentin (see section on Spindled, Rhabdoid, and Undifferentiated Carcinomas).
- Alpha-fetoprotein (AFP): So-called yolk sac or hepatoid differentiation occasionally occurs in gastric carcinomas. Usually, AFP+ regions have histologic features of either clear cell, yolk sac, or hepatocellular carcinoma.[357–362] Although all of these neoplasms can be AFP+, one group of authors suggests that gastric adenocarcinoma with hepatoid differentiation has alpha-1-antitrypsin (AAT) staining but yolk sac differentiation is AAT−.[358] Typical signet ring and intestinal adenocarcinomas fail to stain with AFP.[332, 360] In our experience of three cases, gastric adenocarcinoma with hepatoid differentiation shows focal staining with the HepPar 1 antibody, whereas yolk sac differentiation within a gastric carcinoma shows no staining. If confirmed, these results suggest that positive staining with HepPar 1 is useful in distinguishing primary hepatocellular carcinoma (HCC) (HepPar 1 reactive) and metastatic gastric carcinoma with hepatoid differentiation (HepPar 1 nonreactive).
- Beta human chorionic gonadotropin (beta hCG): Fifteen to 30% of typical gastric adenocarcinomas (intestinal and signet ring cell types) stain with beta hCG. These beta hCG–positive neoplasms usually have no features of choriocarcinoma, but gastric choriocarcinoma has rarely been reported.[363, 364]
- S-100 protein: Twenty percent of adenocarcinomas been reported to stain with S-100 protein, with reactivity in less than 25% of cells in the positive cases.[365]

Differential Diagnostic Panels
Breast Lobular Versus Gastric Signet Ring Cell Carcinoma (Table 13–4)

Antibodies: GCDFP-15, ER, CK7, CK20

There can be remarkable histologic similarity between gastric signet ring cell carcinoma and metastatic breast carcinoma.[366, 367] GCDFP-15 is nonreactive in gastric carcinomas and reactive in approximately 50 to 100% of breast lobular carcinomas.[353, 368] GCDFP-15 frequently stains almost 100% of the signet ring cell variant of lobular carcinoma in a perinuclear dot pattern.[353, 369] Although occasional authors have described ER positivity in gastric carcinoma, almost all recent studies have uniformly reported no reactivity.[292, 368] Usually, the majority of lobular carcinoma cells stain with ER.[368]

CK7/CK20 coordinate staining can be used as adjunctive support; approximately 40% of gastric signet ring cell carcinomas show a CK7–/CK20+ pattern, compared with no lobular carcinomas (personal experience) (Fig. 13–9).[6, 367] Other CK7/CK20 staining patterns are noncontributory.

CEA reactivity, specifically the newer monoclonal clones, such as the D14 clone, are diffusely positive in gastric adenocarcinoma and rarely positive in breast lobular carcinoma (personal experience).

Breast Ductal Versus Gastric Intestinal Type Adenocarcinoma (see Table 13–4)

Antibodies: GCDFP-15, ER, CK17, CEA

GCDFP-15 is nonreactive in gastric carcinomas and positive in 33 to 60% of breast ductal carcinomas, most commonly in those showing apocrine features.[325, 368, 370, 371]

Although occasional authors have reported ER positivity in gastric intestinal type carcinoma, most have reported no staining.[292, 368] In contrast, breast ductal carcinomas are positive in approximately 60% of cases.[292, 370, 372–375]

Approximately 50% of breast ductal carcinomas stain with CK17, compared with no reported staining of gastric intestinal type adenocarcinomas.[327] The experiences at William Beaumont Hospital have yielded identical results. Gastric glandular adenocarcinomas are uniformly nonreactive with CK17, compared with patchy to diffuse staining in approximately 50% of breast ductal carcinomas. CK17+ ductal adenocarcinomas are usually poorly differentiated, and the stained cells are usually within the centers of neoplastic nests. We have found that breast lobular carcinomas are uniformly nonreactive with CK17, including the pleomorphic lobular variant.

CEA can be useful in distinguishing between the two neoplasms, depending on the antibody clone. The new monoclonal antibodies, such as the D14 clone, are diffusely reactive in gastric carcinomas, compared with no or focal staining of breast ductal adenocarcinomas (personal experience).

CK7/CK20 coordinate staining is not useful in this situation because of the high percentage of staining of each pattern in gastric carcinoma.[6]

We are aware of laboratories that use S-100 protein and villin as part of this antibody panel, with reactivity by the former antibody as supportive evidence of a breast ductal adenocarcinoma and reactivity by the latter as supportive evidence of a gastric adenocarcinoma.[374, 376–378] We do not use these antibodies in this differential panel because we have found that S-100 protein is not as frequently positive in breast ductal adenocarcinomas as reported in the literature, and we have not as yet investigated the staining patterns of villin in those two neoplasms.

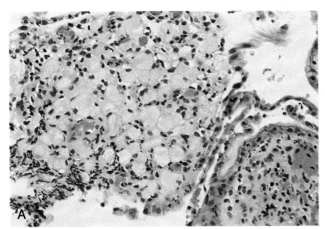 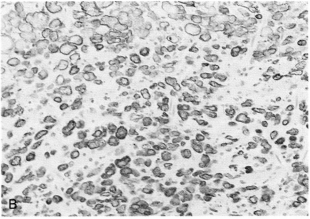

Figure 13–9. A, Signet ring carcinoma in endoscopic biopsy characterized by loose clusters of signet ring cells having large mucin vacuoles with eccentrically placed, atypical nuclei. (H&E, low-power magnification) *B,* Immunoperoxidase stain for CK20 decorates the scattered signet ring cells in the lamina propria, consistent with a gastric carcinoma rather than metastatic lobular carcinoma. Cytokeratin studies can also be of value in differentiating signet ring carcinoma cells from mucinophages, which would not stain for epithelial markers. (Low-power magnification)

Table 13–5. Lung Adenocarcinoma Versus Gastric Glandular Adenocarcinoma

Antibody	Result	
	Gastric Glandular	*Lung*
CK7−/CK20+	−/+	N
TTF	N	+/−

N, negative; +/−, more positive cases than negative; −/+, more negative cases than positive.

Pancreaticobiliary Versus Gastric Intestinal Type Adenocarcinoma

Antibodies: CK17, CA 125

CK17 stains slightly less than 50% of pancreaticobiliary adenocarcinomas, usually in a strong, patchy to diffuse distribution. Gastric intestinal type adenocarcinomas are nonreactive (personal experience).[327]

CA 125 reactivity occurs in more than 50% of pancreaticobiliary adenocarcinomas, compared with almost no staining in gastric carcinomas (see later section on Pancreaticobiliary Ductal Adenocarcinoma). Reactivity in gastric carcinomas almost always consists of staining of less than 10% of cells. Reactivity in greater than 50% of a neoplasm's cells would be strongly supportive of a pancreaticobiliary adenocarcinoma.

CK7 and CK20 do not play a role in the differential because of an extensive overlap in the coordinate staining of the two adenocarcinomas.[6]

Lung Versus Gastric Adenocarcinoma
(Table 13–5)

Antibodies: CK7, CK20, TTF

Cytokeratins 7 and 20 are useful only when a neoplasm expresses the CK7−/CK20+ pattern. Approximately 40% of gastric adenocarcinomas have this pattern, compared with no lung adenocarcinomas. All other CK7/CK20 coordinate staining patterns can be observed in a significant minority of both neoplasms and are therefore not useful.[6, 322–324, 326, 370, 379–381]

TTF stains the majority of pulmonary nonbronchioloalveolar adenocarcinomas and does not stain gastric adenocarcinomas.[379, 382–386]

Prostatic Versus Gastric (Glandular or Signet Ring Cell Type) Adenocarcinoma

Antibodies: PSA, PAP, CEA, CK20

Prostatic signet ring adenocarcinomas stain with PAP or PSA, or both.[387] They either do not stain or show only focal staining with CEA. In contrast, gastric signet ring cell carcinomas stain diffusely and strongly with CEA and do not stain with either PSA or PAP.

CK20 is useful only if it is extensively reactive, because prostate adenocarcinomas almost never show diffuse CK20 positivity. Up to 20% of prostate adenocarcinomas have been reported to show CK20 staining. The staining distribution in these "positive" prostate tumors is almost always extremely focal, with single cell or small groups of glands with positive patterns, compared with diffuse, strong positivity in colon adenocarcinomas.[6, 326]

Müllerian Endometrioid Versus Gastric Intestinal Type Adenocarcinoma (Table 13–6)

Antibodies: CK7, CK20, CA 125

CK7 is a useful initial antibody in this differential diagnosis, because approximately 50% of gastric carcinomas are nonreactive. A negative CK7 reaction supports a diagnosis of gastric adenocarcinoma, as more than 95% of endometrioid adenocarcinomas are CK7+. Approximately 40% of gastric adenocarcinomas express a CK7−/CK20+ pattern, which has not been reported in endometrioid adenocarcinomas. Other patterns of CK7/CK20 coordinate staining are not useful because of the overlap in positivity between the two neoplasms.[6, 322, 323, 326]

CA 125 rarely stains gastric carcinomas; if there is reactivity, this antibody usually stains less than 25% of cells (personal experience).[330] In contrast,

Table 13–6. Müllerian Carcinomas Versus Gastric Glandular Adenocarcinoma

Antibody	Result			
	Gastric Glandular	*Endometrioid*	*Serous Papillary*	*Mucinous*
CK7	−/+	+	Not useful	Not useful
CK7−/CK20+	−/+	N	Not useful	Not useful
CA 125	R	+	+	Not useful
CEA (polyclonal)	+	R	R	Not useful
CK20	−/+	Not useful	N	Not useful

N, negative; R, rare; −/+, more negative cases than positive.

endometrioid adenocarcinomas diffusely and strongly stain with CA 125.[388]

Polyclonal CEA is reactive in the majority of gastric adenocarcinomas, compared with rarely in endometrioid adenocarcinomas, with "positive" endometrioid neoplasms showing reactivity of less than 25% of cells (personal experience).[389]

Müllerian Serous Papillary Versus Gastric Intestinal Type Adenocarcinoma (see Table 13–6)

Antibodies: CK20, CA 125, CEA
CK20 is useful if extensively positive in this differential diagnosis, because only rare müllerian serous papillary carcinomas stain focally, whereas 40% of gastric carcinomas stain extensively. Focal staining with CK20 is not a useful finding because both neoplasms can produce this pattern.[326]

CA 125 stains less than 10% of gastric carcinomas.[330] In our experience, "positive" gastric carcinomas have extremely rare reactive cells. Serous papillary carcinomas diffusely and strongly stain with CA 125.[388]

Polyclonal CEA and monoclonal CEA-D14 clone are reactive in the majority of gastric adenocarcinomas but only very rarely in müllerian serous papillary carcinomas (personal experience).[389]

Müllerian Mucinous Versus Gastric Intestinal Type Adenocarcinoma

No known antibody panels distinguish these two neoplasms.

Adrenal Cortical Carcinomas Versus Gastric Adenocarcinoma

Antibodies: keratin 35βH11, keratin CAM5.2, EMA, alpha inhibin, melan-A
Almost all gastric adenocarcinomas are keratin- and EMA-positive, but less than 5% of adrenal cortical carcinomas stain with the keratins or EMA antibodies. Conversely, responses to inhibin and melan-A have been reported to be positive in most adrenal cortical carcinomas, and in our and others' experiences, these antibodies do not stain gastric adenocarcinomas (personal experience).[390–392]

Pheochromocytoma-Paraganglioma Versus Gastric Adenocarcinoma

Antibodies: keratin AE1/AE3, keratin CAM5.2, EMA, synaptophysin, chromogranin
Gastric adenocarcinomas diffusely and strongly stain with the keratin and EMA antibodies, and rarely stain with synaptophysin and chromogranin.

Conversely, pheochromocytomas-paragangliomas do not, or weakly stain with the keratin or EMA antibodies and diffusely and strongly stain with synaptophysin and chromogranin.[233, 234]

Colon Versus Gastric Adenocarcinoma

See discussion of this topic in later section on neoplasms of the colon.

OTHER GASTRIC NEOPLASMS

Poorly Differentiated and Undifferentiated Carcinomas

Almost all poorly differentiated and undifferentiated carcinomas diffusely express keratin CAM5.2, whereas approximately 10% coexpress vimentin.[393] Rarely, undifferentiated carcinomas and high-grade lymphomas overlap immunohistochemically. There are extremely rare reports of high-grade lymphoma reactivity with keratins AE1/AE3 and CAM5.2 and EMA, and no reactivity with CD45RB (leukocyte common antigen [LCA]).[394, 395] These "keratin-positive" lymphomas do not stain with high molecular weight keratin antibodies. Unfortunately, this feature does not help distinguish between lymphoma and carcinoma, because many poorly differentiated carcinomas also do not stain with high molecular weight keratin antibodies.

We have observed that the "keratin-positive" lymphoma has become an increasingly common differential diagnostic problem with the use of heat antigen retrieval. One of the false-positive reactions that can be produced by the application of too much energy during antigen retrieval are lymphocytes that stain with high and low molecular weight cytokeratin (and S-100) antibodies. A clue that a section has been "over-retrieved" is that the cytokeratin-positive lymphocytes are positive within the nucleus and have a nucleolar accentuation. Molecular genetic techniques or electron microscopy may be needed to establish a diagnosis of lymphoma or carcinoma, respectively.

These cases serve to demonstrate that immunohistochemistry does not always identify the type of neoplasm or sometimes produces spurious staining patterns.[394, 396] However, evaluation of the vast majority of undifferentiated malignancies of the stomach can be resolved with a panel consisting of keratin CAM5.2, LCA, and B-cell and T-cell antibodies (Fig. 13–10).

Rhabdoid Neoplasms

The rhabdoid morphology is not unique to a specific type of neoplasm but rather is a phenotypic expression of poorly differentiated neoplastic

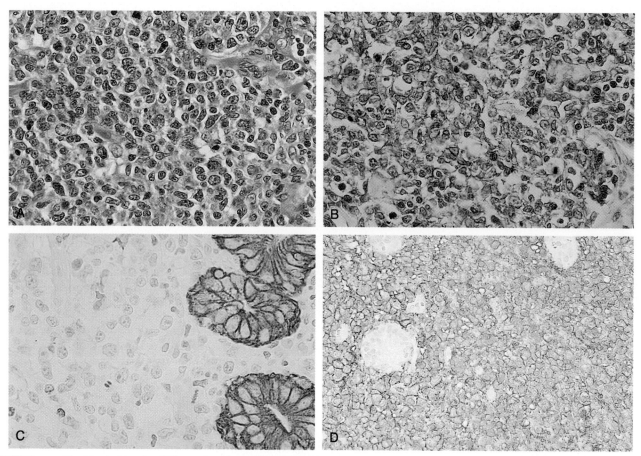

Figure 13–10. A, Poorly differentiated small cell malignancy in the stomach consisting of small malignant cells having high nuclear to cytoplasmic ratios arranged in a dissociative fashion. (Low-power magnification) *B,* Initial impression of gastric non-Hodgkin's lymphoma was confirmed with positive staining of the neoplastic cells for CD20 (L26), a common B-cell marker. (Low-power magnification) *C,* The neoplastic lymphoid cells stain negatively for the low molecular weight cytokeratin CAM5.2, in contrast to the nearby benign gastric mucosa, which shows diffuse cytoplasmic staining. (High-power magnification) *D,* The lymphoma cells show membranous and cytoplasmic staining for CD20. (Intermediate-power magnification)

cells and, frequently, aggressive behavior. Neoplasms that can display the rhabdoid morphology include lymphoma, melanoma, GISTs, and poorly differentiated or undifferentiated carcinomas.[397, 398] In many such neoplasms, including poorly differentiated and undifferentiated carcinomas, vimentin constitutes the intracytoplasmic whorl.[393, 397, 399] Rhabdoid gastric carcinomas only focally stain with EMA and keratins CAM5.2, 34βE12, and 35βH11. The use of several keratin antibodies is recommended because of possible immunostaining with only one antibody. Rhabdoid gastric carcinomas are negative with desmin, actin, and chromogranin.[355]

Spindle Cell Differentiation (Sarcomatoid Carcinoma)

As in the colon and esophagus, spindle cell differentiation has been described in carcinomas of the stomach and intestinal tract. These tumors typically stain only with vimentin, and occasionally with keratin.[400, 401] See the Esophagus section for additional discussion.

Neoplasms of the Small Bowel and Ampulla of Vater

One study has reported that ampulla of Vater adenocarcinomas are immunophenotypically similar to small bowel and colorectal adenocarcinomas, with 60% of neoplasms showing a CK7−/CK20+ pattern and 20% showing a CK7+/CK20+ pattern. However, unlike colon adenocarcinomas, the remaining 20% of neoplasms at the ampulla of Vater had a CK7−/CK20− pattern.[7] These immunophenotypes were also distinct from most pancreaticobiliary ductal adenocarcinomas, of which 65% showed a CK7+/CK20− pattern and the remaining 35% a CK7−/CK20− pattern. Studies using CA 19-9 support a mixed origin for ampullary adenocarcinomas, with some tumors showing a small bowel staining pattern and others a biliary pattern.[402]

Table 13–7. Antibody Staining of Colorectal Adenocarcinoma

Antibody	Immunostaining	Comments and References*
Cytokeratin 35βH11	+	Ref 723
Keratin AE1/AE3	+	Refs 464, 723
Cytokeratin 34βE12	N	Ref 273
Cytokeratin CAM5.2	+	Keratin CAM5.2 stains a greater percentage of poorly differentiated adenocarcinomas than keratin AE1/AE3[464, 723]
EMA	+/−	Refs 723, 733
CK7	R	See text
CK20	+	See text
CK7−/CK20+	+/−	See text
CK7+/CK20+	R	
CK7−/CK20−	R	
CK7+/CK20−	N	
CK17	N	Ref 327
CK19	+	See text
CK5/CK6	N	Ref 278
KP-1 (CD68)	R	Usually less than 10% of cells in each "positive" neoplasm[328]
CA 19-9	+/−	Refs 325, 329–331, 371, 426; see text
CEA	+	See text
ER	N	Focal weak staining in "positive" cases; see text
PR	N	Focal weak staining in "positive" cases; see text
BerEP4	+	Refs 381, 554, 555
Villin	+	See text
GCDFP-15	N	Refs 325, 351, 352, 370, 371
CD30	N	Ref 412; see text
CA 125	R	"Positive" tumors usually show single cells or small focal areas[354, 371]
Vimentin	R	See text
Synaptophysin	R	See text
Chromogranin	−/+	See text
HMB-45	N	See text
Calretinin	R	Refs 270, 550
PLAP	−/+	Usually in a strong, membranous pattern[846]
S-100 protein	−/+	0–25% of colon adenocarcinomas positive In "positive" cases, less than 20% of cells stain[365, 377, 427]
B72.3	+	Usually a diffuse, strong, cytoplasmic pattern[371]
TTF	N	Ref 382 and personal experience
PE-10	N	Ref 438
Thrombomodulin	−/+	See text
Alpha inhibin	R	Approximatelly 5% show strong staining; 75% have weak staining[392]

*Superscript numbers indicate chapter references.
 N, negative; R, rare; +/−, more positive cases than negative; −/+, more negative cases than positive.

Neoplasms of the Colon and Rectum

MEDICAL DISEASES

Hirschsprung's Disease

Immunohistochemical staining of rectal biopsy specimens to assist in the search for ganglion cells can facilitate the diagnosis of Hirschsprung's disease. Ganglion cells stain with NSE and cathepsin D.[403, 404] Satellite cells that surround neurons strongly stain with S-100 protein, producing a visible negative halo effect around the neuron.

COLORECTAL ADENOCARCINOMAS OF THE USUAL TYPE (Table 13–7)

Colorectal adenocarcinoma cells contain low molecular weight keratins CK8, CK18, CK19, and CK20.[1, 3] They typically stain with keratins AE1/AE3, CAM5.2, and 35βH11, and not with 34βH12. Colorectal adenocarcinoma is the prototypical carcinoma that is CK7−/CK20+. Following is a list of antibodies and their staining properties in colorec-

tal adenocarcinoma; Table 13–7 lists the percentage of staining.

KEY DIAGNOSTIC POINTS

- CK7: Approximately 75% of colorectal adenocarcinomas do not stain, 20% show focal (5 to 50%) positivity, and 5% show an extensively (>50%) positive response.[8, 276, 322–324, 405–409] The range of positivity in colorectal adenocarcinomas is 5 to 30%, which may reflect the antibody clone used in the study. Moll[3] reports that the monoclonal antibody OV-TL 12/20 produces the largest span of staining.
- CK20: Approximately 5% of adenocarcinomas do not stain, 3 to 15% show focal positivity, and 85 to 100% are extensively positive.* Staining by CK20 antibodies does not diminish with increasing grade of tumor.[3]

---

*References 8, 275, 322, 323, 325, 326, 405–410.

- CK7/CK20 coordinate staining patterns: It has become "common pathology knowledge" that colorectal adenocarcinomas are CK7–. One should keep in mind, however, that 20% are CK+ to some degree. Approximately 75% of colonic adenocarcinomas show a CK7–/CK20+ pattern, 10 to 20% a CK7+/CK20+ pattern, and 5 to 15% a CK7–/CK20– pattern; none have a CK7+/CK20– pattern (Fig. 13–11).[6, 370, 380, 407, 411]
- CK17: Some authors have reported the response to CK17 to be uniformly negative in all colorectal tumors studied.[327] This statement may be true if "positivity" is defined as staining within the majority of neoplastic cells. CK17 staining has been noted by others, however, to be associated with features of dedifferentiation. CK17 staining in colorectal adenocarcinoma is most common with high-grade tumors and therefore can be seen as single or small groups of cells at the leading edge of a poorly differentiated adenocarcinoma.[3] We have also noticed this feature, with CK17- positive single cells or rare small clusters of cells along the advancing edge of an adenocarcinoma. Overall, we have not encountered a primary colorectal adenocarcinoma in which more than 50% of the neoplastic cells were CK17+.
- CK19: Studies have reported a broad range of CK19 positivity, which limits the use of this antibody in differential staining.
- CD30: We have noted that CD30 frequently stains all grades and types of colon adenocarcinoma in a cytoplasmic granular pattern if extensive blocking of endogenous biotin prior to the application of the CD30 antibody is not performed.[412]
- ER: Approximately zero to 10% of neoplasms are positive with ER with the use of contemporary antibodies, such as the ER1D5 clone and HIER.* Studies using different antibodies and enzyme pretreatment also have reported 0 to 25% positive cases, with most carcinomas showing only focal staining.[292, 342, 372, 415–417] Most but not all immunoassay studies have identified ER in colon adenocarcinomas, usually at low levels.[414, 418–423] These differences may be related in part to technique of ER identification, because ER mRNA has been identified in colorectal adenocarcinomas.[424]
- PR: Zero to 80% of colorectal adenocarcinomas are positive with HIER.[325, 370] The issues regarding the presence and amount of PRs in colorectal adenocarcinoma are the same as those for ERs.[425]
- CA 19-9: In one study, more than half of the neoplastic cells stained in approximately 50% of the "positive" colorectal adenocarcinomas. Approximately 30% of the "positive" tumors displayed positivity in one fourth to one half of cells, and another 20% of the tumors displayed positivity in less than one fourth of the neoplastic cells.[331]
- CEA: Eighty percent to 100% of neoplasms show strong and diffuse staining, depending on the antibody. Most studies report 95 to 100% positivity.[325, 333, 371, 406, 426–429] There are no significant differences in the staining of colorectal adenocarcinomas between monoclonal and polyclonal antibodies.[290] However, in some cases in which CEA is being used as a differential diagnostic antibody, differences between monoclonal and polyclonal antibodies become important (see later).
- Thrombomodulin: Studies have shown marked variation in the positivity of this antibody in colonic adenocarcinomas. One study reported that all colonic adenocarcinomas failed to stain.[430] However, another study of metastatic colon adenocarcinomas in serous effusions reported that 42% of 31 cases showed positive responses.[431]
- Villin: A brush border, microfilament-associated, actin-binding protein, villin is related to rootlet formation.[376, 378] All colon adenocarcinomas are positive for this protein, either in a diffuse or focal cytoplasmic pattern or in a brush border pattern.[376, 378, 405]
- HMB-45: There have been no reports of diffuse cytoplasmic staining of colon adenocarcinoma cells.[432, 433]
- Vimentin: No staining of colon adenocarcinomas (usual type) has been reported.[356, 427].
- Chromogranin and synaptophysin: Typical colon adenocarcinomas that have no histologic neuroendocrine cell differentiation can show chromogranin-positive neoplastic cells, in the range of one or two positive cells per

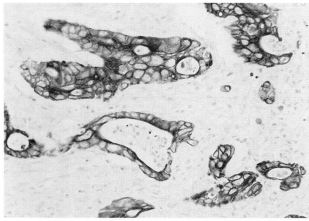

Figure 13–11. Colon carcinoma demonstrating the typical pattern of CK20+ cells. The CK7 stain was negative. (Intermediate-power magnification)

---

*References 292, 325, 338, 370, 371, 413, 414.

Table 13–8. Lung Adenocarcinoma Versus Colorectal Adenocarcinoma

Antibody	Result Colorectal	Lung
CK7–/CK20+	+	N
CK7+/CK20–	N	+/–
CK17	N	+
PE-10	N	+/–
TTF	N	+/–

N, negative; +/–, more positive cases than negative.

Table 13–9. Gastric Adenocarcinoma Versus Colorectal Adenocarcinoma

Antibody	Result Colorectal	Gastric
CK7+/CK20–	N	–/+
CK17	N	–/+

N, negative; –/+, more negative cases than positive.

Colon Versus Gastric Adenocarcinoma (Table 13–9)

Antibodies: CK17, CK7, CK20

The CK17 response is positive in less than 50% of gastric adenocarcinomas, but in "positive" neoplasms, this antibody usually produces a strong and diffuse staining pattern (personal experience). In contrast, colorectal adenocarcinomas either do not stain with CK17 or show extremely focal staining (personal experience).

CK7 and CK20 play a small role in distinguishing the two adenocarcinomas, because only 10 to 20% of gastric adenocarcinomas prominently show the CK7+/CK20– coordinate staining pattern, which is not seen in colorectal adenocarcinomas (Fig. 13–12). The remaining patterns can be seen in both tumors.[6, 326] (For additional references, see discussions of CK7 and CK20 in the Key Diagnostic Points for both gastric and colorectal adenocarcinomas of the usual type.)

Differential Diagnostic Panels

A summary of differential diagnostic antibody panels for various tumors is given here.

Colon Versus Lung Adenocarcinoma (Table 13–8)

Antibodies: CK7, CK20, CK17, PE-10 (pulmonary surfactant apoprotein), TTF

Colon adenocarcinomas usually show the CK7–/CK20+ coordinate staining pattern, a tendency that has not as yet been reported in lung adenocarcinoma. In contrast, lung adenocarcinomas most commonly express the CK7+/CK20– pattern, which has not been reported in colon adenocarcinomas. The CK7+/CK20+ pattern is not helpful because it can be observed in both lung and colorectal adenocarcinomas.[6, 326, 380] In our experience, CK20 staining in lung adenocarcinomas is usually focal. We have not encountered a diffusely CK20+, nonmucinous primary lung adenocarcinoma.

Pulmonary adenocarcinomas are usually extensively CK17+, whereas colorectal adenocarcinomas either do not stain or show extremely focal positivity.[327]

PE-10 has been noted to stain the majority of nonmucinous adenocarcinomas but no colon adenocarcinomas.[438] This antibody had not been commercially released at the time of this writing.

All colon adenocarcinomas have reportedly been negative with TTF, whereas the majority of lung adenocarcinomas are positive.[382, 383]

Colon Versus Pancreaticobiliary and Gallbladder Adenocarcinoma (Table 13–10)

Antibodies: CK7, CK20, CA 125, CK17
Colon, pancreaticobiliary, and gallbladder adeno-

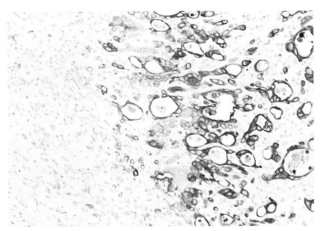

Figure 13–12. Moderately differentiated adenocarcinoma metastatic to the liver and perihepatic lymph nodes. The carcinoma is positive for CK7, with negative staining for CK20, which is more consistent with a gastric primary than a colonic primary.

Table 13–10. Pancreatobiliary Adenocarcinoma Versus Colorectal Adenocarcinoma

	Result	
Antibody	*Colorectal*	*Pancreatobiliary*
CK7−/CK20+	+	R
CK7+/CK20−	N	+/−
CA 125	R	+/−
CK17	N	+

N, negative; R, rare; +/−, more positive cases than negative.

carcinomas frequently metastasize to the liver. Metastatic colon adenocarcinoma occasionally is associated with an intrabiliary growth mimicking cholangiocarcinoma.[439] Only the CK7−/CK20+ and CK7+/CK20− coordinate staining patterns are useful in this context. Colonic adenocarcinomas are usually CK7−/CK20+, compared with none to only 10% of pancreaticobiliary adenocarcinomas. Conversely, approximately 25% (range, 0 to 65%) of pancreaticobiliary adenocarcinomas show a CK7+/CK20− pattern, which is not seen in colorectal adenocarcinomas. There is significant overlap of the other staining patterns in the two neoplasms.[6–8, 275, 276, 322–326, 405, 406, 408, 409]

Approximately 5% of colon adenocarcinomas are positive with CA 125, which is usually in a focal, single-cell pattern, compared with 50% of pancreaticobiliary adenocarcinomas, in which the staining is usually diffuse and strong.[330, 371, 440]

CK17 stains more than 90% of pancreaticobiliary adenocarcinomas, and usually more than 50% of the neoplastic cells. Colon adenocarcinomas do not stain to this extent with this antibody (see earlier discussion).[327]

Colon Versus Intrahepatic Cholangiocarcinoma

Although cholangiocarcinoma is a biliary adenocarcinoma, its immunophenotype is not identical to that of pancreatic and extrahepatic biliary adenocarcinoma. Therefore, a separate Differential Diagnostic Panel is presented in the Liver section.

Table 13–11. Breast Ductal Adenocarcinoma Versus Colorectal Adenocarcinoma

	Result	
Antibody	*Colorectal*	*Breast Ductal*
CK7−/CK20+	+/−	R
CEA	+	R
Villin	+/−	N
CK7+/CK20−	N	+
GCDFP-15	N	+/−
ER	N	+/−

N, negative; R, rare; +/−, more positive cases than negative.

Table 13–12. Müllerian Carcinomas Versus Colorectal Adenocarcinoma of the Usual Type

	Result		
Antibody	*Colorectal*	*Endometrioid*	*Serous Papillary*
CK7−/CK20+	+	N	N
CEA monoclonal	+	R	R
CEA polyclonal	+	−/+	R
Villin	+/−	N	
CK7	R	+	+
CK7+/CK20−	N	+/−	+/−
CA 125	R	+	+
Vimentin	N	+/−	
CD56	N	+/−	
ER	N	+/−	+/−

N, negative; R, rare; +/−, more positive cases than negative; −/+, more negative cases than positive.

Colon Versus Breast Adenocarcinoma (Table 13–11)

Antibodies: CK7, CK20, GCDFP-15, CEA, ER

Unlike colon adenocarcinomas, 80 to 90% of breast carcinomas show the CK7+/CK20− coordinate staining pattern. Conversely, less than 5% of breast ductal carcinomas show the CK7−/CK20+ pattern that is seen in 75% of colorectal adenocarcinomas. The other patterns show significant overlap in the two neoplasms.[6, 8, 322–326, 370, 379, 380, 440]

The GCDFP-15 reaction is positive in 50% of breast carcinomas, most commonly in lobular carcinomas, and is uniformly negative in colon adenocarcinomas.[325, 370, 371, 441]

CEA (polyclonal) staining is positive in 95% of colon adenocarcinomas compared with only 10 to 30% of breast adenocarcinomas.*

Caution is advised with the use of CEA, because CEA+ breast carcinomas usually show strong and diffuse staining.

As noted previously, with the use of contemporary antigen retrieval methods and the 1D5 clone, ER staining has rarely been reported as positive in colon adenocarcinomas, and usually comprises rare, single stained cells. In contrast, breast ductal carcinomas are ER+ in approximately 60% of cases.[292, 370, 372–375]

Colon Versus Müllerian Endometrioid Adenocarcinoma (Table 13–12)

Antibodies: CK7, CK20, CEA, CA 125, vimentin CD56

CK7 staining is a useful initial test because more than 95% of endometrioid adenocarcinomas stain with this antibody but only rare colon adenocarcinomas do so. When CK7 is used in combination

---

*References 32, 371, 373, 428, 429, 440, 442–444.

with CK20, endometrioid adenocarcinomas do not express the typical CK7−/CK20+ pattern seen in 75% of colorectal adenocarcinomas. The CK7+/CK20− coordinate staining pattern is seen in 85% of endometrioid adenocarcinomas but in no colorectal adenocarcinomas. The other patterns overlap sufficiently in the two neoplasms.[6, 8, 322–324, 326, 370, 380, 406, 411, 440, 445, 446]

Monoclonal CEA staining is positive in 95% or more of colon adenocarcinomas, compared with only 5 to 10% of endometrioid adenocarcinomas.* Polyclonal CEA staining is positive in a similar percentage of colon adenocarcinomas. In contrast with monoclonal CEA, we have found, polyclonal CEA stains approximately 33% of endometrioid adenocarcinomas.[428, 429, 440, 444] Lagendijk and associates[441] point out that colon adenocarcinoma usually shows a greater degree of positivity with CEA than with CK7, whereas CK7 staining is expressed to a greater degree than CEA in primary ovarian carcinoma.

CA 125 is positive in 95% of endometrioid adenocarcinomas, compared with only 5% of colon adenocarcinomas.[330, 371, 406, 440]

Vimentin stains 50 to 90% of endometrioid adenocarcinomas, but is positive in less than 5% of colon adenocarcinomas.[356, 409, 427]

CD56 stains rare colon adenocarcinomas in an extremely focal, single cell pattern, compared with approximately 50% of endometrioid adenocarcinomas, in which more than 50% of cells stain.[32, 33]

Colon Versus Müllerian Serous Papillary Adenocarcinoma (see Table 13–12)

Antibodies: CK7, CK20, CEA, CA 125, ER

As with the distinction from endometrioid adenocarcinomas, CK7 is a useful antibody to use initially for serous papillary adenocarcinomas because it stains more than 95% of such neoplasms. No serous carcinomas show the CK7−/CK20+ coordinate staining pattern. Forty to 100% of serous carcinomas show a CK7+/CK20− pattern.[6, 322–324, 326, 406, 411]

Polyclonal CEA staining is positive in 95% of colon adenocarcinomas, compared with less than 10% of serous papillary adenocarcinomas.[371, 388, 389, 406, 448, 449]

CA 125 stains almost all serous papillary adenocarcinomas but only 5% of colorectal adenocarcinomas.[330, 354, 371, 388, 389, 449, 450]

The response to ER is positive in approximately 50% of serous papillary carcinomas, of which approximately 75% stain strongly. Only weak and focal staining is seen in less than 2% of colorectal adenocarcinomas.[292]

Colon Mucinous Versus Ovarian Mucinous Adenocarcinoma (Table 13–13)

Antibodies: CK7, CK20, CEA, vimentin, CA 125

Twenty-five percent of ovarian mucinous adenocarcinomas demonstrate the CK7+/CK20− coordinate staining pattern, which is not seen in colon mucinous adenocarcinomas. The majority of ovarian mucinous adenocarcinomas express a CK7+/CK20+ staining pattern. The CK20 staining is usually focal in ovarian mucinous adenocarcinomas; however, it occasionally can be diffuse (personal experience). Because the CK7+/CK20+ and the other two coordinate staining patterns can be seen in significant numbers of colorectal adenocarcinomas, we believe that the presence of any staining pattern other than CK7+/CK20− is not useful in separating the two neoplasms.[6, 8, 322–324, 326, 370, 380, 406, 409, 411, 440, 445, 451, 452]

CEA is negative in approximately one third of ovarian mucinous adenocarcinomas. When negative, it is a useful finding, because (almost) all colorectal adenocarcinomas do stain with CEA.[409]

CA 125 staining has a similar utility, as it is extensively positive in approximately 60% of ovarian mucinous adenocarcinomas, compared with only focal, weak staining in 15% of colorectal mucinous adenocarcinomas (typical colonic adenocarcinomas stain less frequently and with fewer cells per "positive" neoplasm).[409] We have not observed a diffusely and strongly positive CA 125 staining pattern in mucinous colorectal adenocarcinoma.

Vimentin is useful in positively identifying a minority of ovarian mucinous adenocarcinomas. Approximately 15% of ovarian mucinous adenocarcinomas stain in a strong and diffuse pattern with vimentin, compared with essentially no colorectal mucinous adenocarcinomas.[409] Rare colorectal adenocarcinomas can focally express vimentin.

Colon Adenocarcinoma Versus Transitional Cell Carcinoma

Antibodies: none

CK7 and CK20 do not play a role in this differential diagnosis, because only 10% of transitional

---

Table 13–13. Ovarian Mucinous Adenocarcinoma Versus Colorectal Mucinous Adenocarcinoma

	Result	
Antibody	*Colorectal*	*Ovarian*
CEA	+	R
CA 125	R	+/−
CK7+/CK20−	N	+
Vimentin	R	−/+

N, negative; R, rare; +/−, more positive cases than negative; −/+, more negative cases than positive.

Table 13–14. Renal Cell Carcinoma (RCC) Versus Colorectal Adenocarcinoma

Antibody	Result	
	Colorectal Adenocarcinoma	*RCC*
CK20	+	R–N
CEA	+	N
CA 19-9	+/−	R
Vimentin	R	+/−

R, rare; R–N, rare to negative; +/−, more positive cases than negative; −/+, more negative cases than positive.

cell carcinomas show the characteristically non–colon adenocarcinoma CK7+/CK20− coordinate staining pattern. Ninety percent of transitional cell carcinomas express the CK7+/CK20+ pattern, which can be seen in 10 to 20% of colon adenocarcinomas with a pattern.[6]

Thrombomodulin staining has been uniformly positive in transitional cell carcinomas and negative in colon adenocarcinomas according to some authors[430]; other authors, however, have reported positivity of colon adenocarcinomas in serous effusions.[431] In our experience, colon adenocarcinomas either do not stain or show extremely focal staining with thrombomodulin.

Colon Versus Bladder or Urachal Adenocarcinoma

No known antibody panels reliably distinguish between colon and bladder or urachal adenocarcinomas.[453]

Colon Adenocarcinoma Versus Renal Carcinoma (Table 13–14)

Antibodies: CK20, CEA, CA 19-9, vimentin
The immunohistochemical distinction between colon adenocarcinoma and renal cell carcinoma (RCC) suffers from one major drawback: The identification of RCC is one of exclusion. Except for vimentin, there are no "positive" RCC antibodies.

The CK20 staining response is focally positive in 3 to 15% of colon adenocarcinomas and extensively positive in 85 to 100%.* In contrast, less than 5% of RCCs stain with CK20, and those that do show only rare single cell or focal staining.[6, 326, 370, 410]

CK7 is not useful in this differential diagnosis because both neoplasms almost always fail to stain with it.

CEA stains more than 95% of colon adenocarcinomas with use of a monoclonal CEA, compared with less than 10% of RCCs.[8, 332, 427, 444, 454]

CA 19-9 stains approximately 70 to 90% of

colon adenocarcinomas.[325, 329–331, 371, 426] In contrast, only about 5% of RCCs stain with this antibody.[329, 331]

Vimentin staining, although nonspecific, can be found in RCCs of increasing grade, with Fuhrman grade 4 neoplasms displaying almost 100% vimentin positivity. In contrast, less than 2% of usual type colon adenocarcinomas stain focally with vimentin.[356, 427, 455, 456] Care must be taken in regard to undifferentiated colon carcinomas (see later), because they frequently stain with vimentin.

Colon Versus Prostate Adenocarcinoma (Table 13–15)

Antibodies: PSA, PAP, CA 19-9, CEA, CK20
PSA is positive in 90% of prostate adenocarcinomas and is negative in colorectal carcinomas.[387, 457–461]

PAP is positive in more than 95% of prostate adenocarcinomas and negative in colon adenocarcinomas.[387, 459–461]

CA 19-9 stains approximately 80% of colon adenocarcinomas and less than 10% of prostate adenocarcinomas; the prostate tumors that do stain usually show only focal positivity.[8, 329, 331]

Polyclonal CEA, as noted previously, is positive in a diffuse and strong staining pattern in the vast majority of colon adenocarcinomas, compared with focal positivity in approximately 20% of prostate adenocarcinomas.[460] Therefore, diffuse strong staining is indicative of colorectal adenocarcinoma, and an absence of staining is indicative of prostate adenocarcinoma.

CK20 staining has been reported to be positive in up to 20% of prostate adenocarcinomas. However, the staining pattern in these "positive" prostate tumors is almost always extremely focal, with a single cell positive pattern, compared with diffuse, strong positivity in colon adenocarcinomas.[6, 326]

CK7/CK20 coordinate staining is not useful in distinguishing these neoplasms because of the extensive overlap in staining patterns.[6]

Table 13–15. Prostate Versus Colorectal Adenocarcinoma

Antibody	Result	
	Colorectal	*Prostate*
PSA	N	+
PAP	N	+
CA 19-9	+/−	−/+
CK20	+	−/+
CEA (polyclonal)	+	−/+

N, negative; +/−, more positive cases than negative; −/+, more negative cases than positive.

*References 8, 275, 322, 323, 325, 326, 405, 406, 408, 409.

UNDIFFERENTIATED CARCINOMAS AND NEUROENDOCRINE DIFFERENTIATION

Undifferentiated colon carcinomas consist of solid sheets of large cells with vesicular nuclei and prominent nucleoli. Squamous differentiation is common.[462, 463] Distinction from lymphoma is frequently required. Undifferentiated carcinomas often stain with keratins CAM5.2 and 35βH11 and with the pankeratin antibodies of keratin AE1/AE3 to a lesser degree (personal experience).[464, 465] Squamous cell carcinoma is negative with CEA and keratin CAM5.2 and positive with high molecular weight keratin 34βE12.[462]

Poorly differentiated and undifferentiated carcinomas can have cytologic or architectural features that suggest neuroendocrine differentiation or a high-grade neuroendocrine carcinoma. Approximately 33 to 66% of these carcinomas either have no chromogranin or synaptophysin positivity or display rare positive cells.[28, 116, 436, 466] One study found that approximately 50% of poorly differentiated or undifferentiated neoplasms show admixtures of synaptophysin or chromogranin positive and negative cells; the authors termed these neoplasms *mixed adenocarcinoma-neuroendocrine carcinomas.*[466] In these cases, the synaptophysin or chromogranin positivity is usually localized to regions of cells rather than shown as isolated positive cells distributed throughout the neoplasm.

CD56 staining is also useful in confirming high-grade neuroendocrine cell differentiation.[32] The CEA staining is usually negative in the neuroendocrine cell regions and positive in the non-neuroendocrine carcinoma regions (personal experience).

SIGNET RING CELL ADENOCARCINOMAS

The staining pattern in signet ring cell carcinomas of the colon is identical to that in glandular colon adenocarcinomas (personal experience).[353] Signet ring cell adenocarcinomas are not well-characterized immunohistochemically. Distinction from metastatic gastric signet ring cell carcinoma can be made through the use of the appropriate antibody panel (see earlier Colon Versus Gastric Adenocarcinoma section).

CLEAR CELL ADENOCARCINOMAS

Clear cell adenocarcinomas have the same immunohistochemical phenotype as typical adenocarcinomas, despite the lack of mucin and the presence of glycogen in clear cell adenocarcinomas.[467]

CARCINOMAS WITH SPINDLE CELL DIFFERENTIATION (PLEOMORPHIC CARCINOMA, SARCOMATOID CARCINOMA)

Carcinomas with spindle cell differentiation are uncommon in the colon and small bowel. They can acquire a variety of morphologic patterns, including sheets of loosely cohesive large cell, focal, rhabdoid-appearing cells and spindle (sarcomatoid) cells.[465, 468–474] Keratin staining can be focally positive; therefore, application of several keratin antibodies, such as pankeratin AE1/AE3 and keratins CAM5.2 and 34βE11, is recommended. Keratin positivity has been described in all cases. In our experience, the spindle cell regions are least often positive. Most cases demonstrate diffuse and strong vimentin coexpression. EMA and CA 125 staining can be focally positive. Desmin stains approximately one third of cases, whereas S-100, CEA, HMB-45, chromogranin, synaptophysin, AFP, and LCA have uniformly been negative. Frequently, carcinomas with spindle cell differentiation show histologic and immunohistochemical overlap with high-grade GISTs. Both can coexpress keratin and vimentin and can be focally EMA+, desmin-positive, and CD34−. Electron microscopy has been suggested as the final arbitrating ancillary technique in such cases.[471]

CARCINOMAS WITH RHABDOID CELL DIFFERENTIATION

Carcinomas with rhabdoid cell differentiation have many of the same immunohistochemical features as undifferentiated carcinomas with spindle cell differentiation.[469, 475, 476] The rhabdoid cells usually stain with vimentin and variably stain with keratin. In our experience, rhabdoid carcinoma cells more often stain with keratins CAM5.2 and 35βH11 than with AE1/AE3 or EMA. Transitions between usual type adenocarcinoma, spindle cell regions, and rhabdoid morphologies can be seen.

Adenocarcinomas of the Appendix

Appendiceal neoplasms are derived from the same mucosa as colonic neoplasms and, thus, stain in an identical pattern. Seventy-five percent and 60% of appendiceal cystadenomas and carcinomas are CK7−, respectively[452]; most are CK20+. Neoplastic cells within pseudomyxoma peritonei lesions that are associated with appendiceal neoplasms stain with the same pattern as the appendiceal neoplasms in the majority of cases.[452, 477] Cytokeratin staining patterns have been used as supportive evidence that simultaneous appendiceal mucinous neoplasms and ovarian mucinous borderline neoplasms are derived from the same group of neoplastic cells, which probably originated in the appendix.[452, 478, 479]

Neoplasms of the Anus

NORMAL STRUCTURES

Forty percent of normal anal glands have been noted to stain with antibodies to PSA and PAP.[480]

ANAL TRANSITION ZONE NEOPLASMS

Squamous Cell Carcinoma

Anal squamous cell carcinomas are similar to squamous cell carcinomas of other sites; see the earlier discussion of esophageal squamous cell carcinoma for differential diagnoses.

High molecular weight cytokeratin is the predominant intermediate filament in anal squamous cell carcinomas. Therefore, these neoplasms stain with keratins AE1/AE3 and 34βE12. Most contain little, if any, low molecular weight cytokeratin and do not stain with keratins CAM5.2 and 35βH11.[1, 2] High-grade and spindle cell variants usually show patchy staining with cytokeratin CAM5.2 and vimentin.[481]

Basaloid Cell and Cloacogenic Carcinomas

In general, the squamous cell carcinoma variants basaloid cell carcinoma and cloacogenic carcinoma show keratin staining patterns similar to those of their anal squamous cell counterpart. Comparative immunohistochemical studies have shown that cloacogenic carcinoma has a keratin profile similar to that of the basal layer of the squamous transition zone, and anal glands.[482] We have found that basaloid areas show a greater degree of positivity with cytokeratin 35βH11 than squamous cell carcinomas. Most of these carcinomas show focal to patchy, weak to moderate CEA positivity. A similar staining pattern is seen with B72.3 and BerEP4. The William Beaumont Hospital experience of approximately 20 such neoplasms, demonstrated that these tumors failed to stain with PSA, PAP, GCDFP-15, ER, and PR.

High-grade neuroendocrine (small cell) carcinomas of the rectum can be immunohistochemically distinguished from basaloid cloacogenic carcinomas on the basis of the former's (1) perinuclear dot keratin CAM5.2 staining pattern, (2) immunoreactivity to synaptophysin, chromogranin, and Leu7, and (3) lack of staining to CEA.[128] Although it has been our experience that cloacogenic carcinomas occasionally stain focally and weakly to moderately with synaptophysin, they do not immunostain with antibodies to chromogranin. Unlike high-grade neuroendocrine carcinomas, cloacogenic carcinomas strongly and diffusely stain with CEA, and their staining pattern with keratin CAM5.2 is diffusely cytoplasmic, without a perinuclear dot accentuation.

Anal Paget's Disease

The cell of origin of anal Paget's disease has become an area of great interest. Following is a list of antibodies studied for their utility in the diagnosis of anal Paget's disease.

KEY DIAGNOSTIC POINTS

- Keratin 34βE12: There is no staining of extramammary Paget's cells with 34βE12.[483]

- Keratin AE1/AE3: Staining of 80% of Paget's disease cases with AE1/AE3 has been reported.[484]
- Keratin CAM5.2: All cases of extramammary Paget's disease show diffuse strong staining with CAM5.2.[484–486]
- S-100 protein: No S-100 protein staining of extramammary Paget's disease cells has been reported.[483, 487]
- GCDFP-15: Approximately 33 to 50% of cases stain with GCDFP-15.[483, 484, 487, 488] The staining pattern has varied from focal to diffuse.
- CEA: Almost all cases are positive with CEA. There is strong staining in approximately 75%, and moderate staining in 20%, of extramammary Paget's disease cells.[484–487]
- BerEP4: The response to BerEP4 is negative in 20% of cases of extramammary Paget's disease, and moderate to strong in the remaining 80%.[486]
- CK7: Staining is diffuse and strong in all cases of extramammary or perianal Paget's disease cells, in contrast to the surrounding, normal squamous epithelium, which fails to stain with CK7.[484, 486–489]
- CK20: Focal staining with CK20 is seen in 20 to 50% of cases; the cases that do show staining are almost always associated with rectal adenocarcinoma (see later).[484, 486–489]
- CK7/CK20 coordinate staining pattern: Those cases of perianal Paget's disease that are associated with an underlying colon adenocarcinoma have been noted to be C7+/CK20+, in contrast to those that do not have this association, which are CK7+/CK20−.[487, 488] To state this concept the other way: Of the patients with perianal Paget's disease that are CK7+/CK20+, approximately 90% have had an associated rectal adenocarcinoma.[484, 488] The immunohistochemical profile of perianal Paget's disease cells is identical to the profiles of invasive rectal adenocarcinoma cells.[488, 490] A CK7+/CK20+ pattern can also be seen in cases of perianal Paget's disease associated with transitional cell carcinoma of the bladder.

RARE TUMORS OF THE ANUS

Clear Cell Carcinomas

Clear cell carcinomas occasionally arise in the anus. They have been reported to stain with keratin CAM5.2, CEA, and EMA. AFP, PSA, and PAP have failed to immunostain the tumor cells.[491]

Spindled, Rhabdoid, and Undifferentiated Carcinomas

As in other regions of the GI tract, poorly differentiated carcinomas with spindled (sarcomatoid), rhabdoid, and undifferentiated morphology can occasionally arise in the anus.[492, 493] Immunohistochemical issues regarding these tumors are identical to those discussed in the section on colonic carcinomas with these morphologies.

PANCREAS, EXTRAHEPATIC BILE DUCTS, AND GALLBLADDER

This section discusses the immunohistochemistry of neoplasms of the pancreas, extrahepatic biliary system, and gallbladder. Similar lesions can arise from any of these locations, with the exception of a few carcinomas specific to the pancreas. The immunohistochemical phenotypes of biliary adenocarcinomas of the pancreatic ducts, extrahepatic bile ducts, and the gallbladder are identical. The immunohistochemical studies can be applied to resected specimens as well as needle core biopsy and fine needle aspirate specimens.

CK8 and CK18 are produced by exocrine acinar cells, endocrine islets, and duct cells.[494] CK7 and CK19 are found normally only in ductal cells.[494] CK20 is not found in normal pancreatic cells of any type.[494]

Medical Diseases

Idiopathic chronic pancreatitis accounts for 10 to 40% of all cases of chronic pancreatitis and is the most common condition, second only to alcohol abuse.[495] Patients can have associated autoimmune diseases, to which the term *sclerosing pancreatitis* has been applied. T cells predominate in the inflammatory infiltrate in this condition, a finding similar to the composition of inflammatory infiltrate involving extrahepatic and intrahepatic bile ducts in sclerosing cholangitis.[495]

Neuroendocrine Cell Neoplasms

Neuroendocrine neoplasms of the ampulla of Vater, pancreas, biliary system, and gallbladder include a spectrum of lesions varying from the low-grade carcinoid to the high-grade, small cell carcinoma.[76, 113, 496–514] This group of neoplasms can be immunohistochemically defined by their immunostaining with "neuroendocrine"-specific antibodies or from their predominant hormone production (Table 13–16). The latter form of tumor classification, especially in the pancreas, where numerous hormones and prohormones are produced by the same cell, has limited practical diagnostic utility in the identification of neuroendocrine neoplasms and their distinction from other pancreatic neoplasms[503] but does have prognostic importance. In this context, serum hormone or neuropeptide measurements have replaced mere immunohistochemical detection of these hormones.

In general, almost 100% of neuroendocrine neoplasms stain with antibodies for synaptophysin, and 80% stain with chromogranin, PGP9.5, and

Table 13–16. Antibody Staining of Pancreatobiliary Endocrine Neoplasms

Antibody	Immunostaining	Comments
Synaptophysin	+	Slight, to moderate, decreased staining in high-grade carcinomas
CD57	+	Moderately decreased staining in high-grade carcinomas
CD56	+	Markedly decreased staining in high-grade carcinomas
Chromogranin	+/−	Approximately 80% in low-grade neoplasms
		Markedly decreased staining in high-grade carcinomas
PGP 9.5	+/−	Approximately 80%
		Moderately decreased staining in high-grade carcinomas
Keratin CAM5.2	+/−	Approximately 80%
		Maintains positivity more often in high-grade carcinomas
Keratin AE1/AE3	−/+	Approximately 60%
		Markedly decreased staining in high-grade carcinomas
		High-grade carcinomas usually do not stain
CK19	+/−	Approximately 50% positive in low-grade carcinomas
		Usually negative in high-grade carcinomas
CK7	N–R	Similar staining in carcinomas of all grades
CK20	N–R	Approximately 10%
		Similar staining in carcinomas of all grades
CA 19-9	+/−	Approximatelly 50%
		Markedly decreased staining in high-grade carcinomas
Vimentin	R	Approximately 20%
EMA	R	Approximately 10%
S-100 protein	N	
CEA	−/+	Marked variation, from none to diffuse and strong
		Most studies report no staining
		Low-grade neoplasms stain more often than high-grade neoplasms.

N, negative; N–R, negative to rare; R, rare, +/−, more positive cases than negative; −/+, more negative cases than positive.

CD57 (Leu7).* Higher-grade neoplasms (small cell carcinomas) stain with less intensity and less often with antibodies to synaptophysin and chromogranin, whereas staining with CD56 and CD57 is frequently strong and in a membranous pattern in these neoplasms.[28, 30, 32, 33] Caution is advised in regard to the specificity of neoplasms that stain with CD56 (NCAM [neural cell adhesion molecule]). Not only do carcinoid tumors and small cell carcinomas show positivity; cells from thyroid follicular and papillary adenocarcinomas, hepatocellular carcinomas, and squamous cell carcinomas also can react to this antibody.[32]

Approximately 80% of neuroendocrine neoplasms stain with keratin CAM5.2, and approximately 60% with keratin AE1/AE3. Staining is frequently in a perinuclear dot distribution.[517, 518] These tumors also diffusely and strongly express CK8 and CK18, which are components of keratin CAM5.2. Approximately 50% express CK19. CK7 rarely stains pancreaticobiliary neuroendocrine neoplasms of any grade.[518] CK20 staining is positive in approximately 10% of endocrine neoplasms.[326] CA 19-9 stains approximately 50% of tumors in a focal distribution.[506] Vimentin staining occurs in a focal pattern in approximately 20% of carcinoids.[61, 356, 519]

High-grade pancreatic neuroendocrine carcinomas can stain with calcitonin, a finding that can lead to the false diagnosis of a high-grade thyroid medullary carcinoma, especially in the evaluation of a metastatic lesion.[15, 505, 520]

Neuroendocrine neoplasms of all grades do not stain with EMA or ER. Rare tumors are diffusely positive with CEA, and there has been one report of AFP positivity.[521]

One study reported strong, diffuse S-100 protein positivity within an otherwise typical pancreatic neuroendocrine neoplasm, an extremely rare finding in neuroendocrine tumors.[515] The patient in this report had von Hippel–Lindau (VHL) disease. An association between the S-100 protein positivity and VHL is unknown.

One author found that PR was present in 58% of pancreatic neuroendocrine neoplasms of varying grades, compared with no staining response in non–islet cell tumors.[504] This author recommended the use of PR to discriminate between pancreatic and nonpancreatic neoplasms. We have had no experience with this antibody in this context.

One small study reported that a minority of pancreatic islet cell tumors, unlike small bowel carcinoids, stained with neurofilament.[500]

There is one report of a low-grade neuroendocrine neoplasm that was composed of cells identical to those seen in solid (papillary) and cystic tumors of the pancreas, except that neurosecretory granules were seen on electron microscopy. The neoplasm did not stain with chromogranin or synaptophysin with the use of contemporary immunohistochemical staining techniques.[522]

---

*References 15–29, 503, 507, 509, 510, 515–517.

Mixed Neuroendocrine— Exocrine/Ductal Neoplasms (So-Called Amphicrine Tumors)

Two types of mixed neoplasms have been described. One type consists of a mixed, collision type tumor with immunohistochemically recognizable separate components. The neuroendocrine component varies in these tumors from typical, low-grade carcinoid (islet) to high-grade, small cell carcinoma–like. The glandular component is usually typical ductal adenocarcinoma. Usually, the entire neoplasm expresses keratin CAM5.2. The ductal cells are CEA+, and the neuroendocrine component, is positive with chromogranin, synaptophysin, CD56, and CD57.[523–527]

The second, much less common type consists of an immunohistochemically single neoplasm with neoplastic cells that express exocrine/ductal and neuroendocrine features (*amphicrine tumor*). Cells show homogeneous expression of synaptophysin, CEA, and CA 19-9.[526, 528, 529] Dense core granules are present in cells with exocrine/ductal features. The existence of this neoplasm has been questioned by some authors.[530]

Mixed exocrine/ductal-endocrine neoplasms should be separated from pancreaticobiliary ductal adenocarcinomas, which frequently contain scattered endocrine cells (see later).

Mixed acinic-endocrine neoplasms are discussed later, in the section on Acinic Cell Carcinomas.

Mesenchymal Neoplasms

Mesenchymal neoplasms of the pancreas, gallbladder, and extrahepatic bile ducts are rare. Inflammatory myofibroblastic tumors (IMTs) (inflammatory pseudotumors) and schwannomas are the predominant neoplasms in case reports and studies of small series, admixed with rare leiomyosarcomas and malignant peripheral nerve sheath tumors.[531–536] The immunohistochemistry of these neoplasms is identical to that of IMTs and schwannomas arising elsewhere. IMTs must be distinguished from fibrosing spindle cell pancreatic adenocarcinoma. Cytokeratin antibodies are positive in the latter but do not stain IMTs.

Pancreaticobiliary Ductal Adenocarcinomas

Following is a list of antibodies and their staining patterns in ductal adenocarcinomas from the pancreaticobiliary system (Table 13–17). It appears that the immunohistochemical phenotype of pancreatic ductal adenocarcinomas is identical to that of common bile duct, cystic duct, and gallbladder adenocarcinomas; therefore, they are discussed as a single group of neoplasms.[6, 275, 323, 537, 538] This situation is in contrast with that of cholangiocarcinoma (intrahepatic biliary adenocarcinoma), which

Table 13–17. Antibody Staining of Pancreaticobiliary Ductal Adenocarcinoma

Antibody	Immunostaining	Comments and References
Synaptophysin	−/+	See above text
Chromogranin	−/+	
Keratin AE1/AE3	+	Refs 444, 723
Keratin 35βH11	+	Ref 723
Keratin CAM5.2	+	Refs 518, 545, 723
EMA	+	Refs 444, 545, 546, 623, 723
CK7	+	See text
CK20	+/−	See text
CK7+/CK20−	+/−	See text
CK7+/CK20+	−/+	
CK7−/CK20+	R	
CK7−/CK20−	R	
CK17	+	See text
CK19	+	Ref 7
CA 19-9	+	See text
CEA	+	See text
ER	N	Refs 292, 325, 372
PR	N	Ref 325
BerEP4	+	Refs 332, 554
PAP	N	Ref 847
PSA	N	Refs 458, 847
GCDFP-15	N	Refs 325, 351, 352
CA 125	+/−	See text
Vimentin	N	Refs 325, 356, 518
AFP	N	See text
Calretinin	−/+	See text
S-100 protein	N	Ref 365
B72.3	+	Ref 549
Thrombomodulin	+/−	Approximately 50% of neoplasms[848]
CD56	N	Ref 33
CD57	N	Ref 33
Alpha inhibin	N	Ref 392

N, negative; R, rare; +/−, more positive cases than negative; −/+, more negative cases than positive.

has a slightly different immunophenotype (see section on the Liver). Some studies suggest that ampullary adenocarcinomas have an immunophenotype identical to that of small bowel rather than pancreaticobiliary adenocarcinomas (see GI section for this discussion).[7] A variety of histologic appearances of the neoplasms have been described at all these locations.

Pancreaticobiliary ductal adenocarcinomas in general have a cytokeratin immunophenotype identical to that of normal pancreatic ducts, including positive CK8, CK18, and CK19, and variable CK7 positivity.[3]

KEY DIAGNOSTIC POINTS

- Chromogranin and synaptophysin: Neuroendocrine differentiation in typical ductal adenocarcinomas consists of two types of expression.[528] Scattered flask-shaped neuroendocrine cells that stain with synaptophysin, chromogranin, or Leu7 and are situated at the base of the gland are common, with a prevalence ranging from 80% of papillary adenocarcinomas to 12% of poorly differentiated adenocarcinomas. The second, less com-

mon type, consists of diffuse, homogeneous, and strong synaptophysin reactivity.[528] We do not consider this type of expression to be consistent with a ductal adenocarcinoma; see further discussion in the preceding section on Mixed Neuroendocrine–Exocrine/Ductal Neoplasms.[33]

- CK7: Ductal adenocarcinomas frequently stain in a heterogeneous pattern with CK7. Approximately 90% of pancreaticobiliary adenocarcinomas usually stain diffusely with CK7.[7, 276, 324] One study reported 87% diffuse positivity, and 13% no staining.[323] We have found that if more than 10% staining of neoplastic cells is considered positive, almost 100% of ductal adenocarcinomas are CK7+.

- CK20: CK20 staining has produced markedly different results in pancreaticobiliary adenocarcinomas. In general, approximately 50% show strong positivity. Some pancreaticobiliary ductal adenocarcinomas either do not stain or show focal patchy staining.[7, 275, 325, 326, 539] One study found that only 40% of neoplasms showed 5 to 80% positivity, with none having more than 80% positive cells. Another study found diffuse staining in 22%, focal positivity in 17%, and no staining in 61% of neoplasms.[323]

- CK7/CK20 coordinate staining pattern: The literature contains markedly varied results in regard to CK7/CK20 staining patterns. Two factors probably account for these disparate results: (1) the marked variation of cytokeratin expression by adenocarcinoma cells among different regions of the areas of the same pancreatic ductal adenocarcinoma and (2) the similarly great variation in the percentage of stained cells used to define a "positive" immunoreaction, which ranges from 1 to 50%.

We believe that staining of more than 10% of cells should be considered a "positive" reaction. Most studies report the CK7+/CK20+ staining pattern as the most common, with approximately 60% of tumors showing it (range 25 to 65%).[6, 7, 323] The second most common pattern is the CK7+/CK20− pattern, seen in approximately 25% of neoplasms (range, 0 to 65%). The range of positivity for the CK7−/CK20− pattern is 0 to 35%, and that for the CK7−/CK20+ pattern is 0 to 10%. One report of pseudomyxoma peritonei caused by pancreatic adenocarcinoma noted the neoplasm to be CK7−/CK20+.[540]

- CK17: More than 90% of pancreatic adenocarcinomas express CK17. Approximately half of "positive" tumors contain more than 50% positive cells.[327]

- CK19: Pancreatic adenocarcinomas diffusely and strongly express CK19.[7, 518, 541]

- CA 19-9: Approximately 75 to 95% of pancreatic adenocarcinomas show diffuse strong staining with CA 19-9. Staining is usually of

Table 13–18. Pancreaticobiliary Adenocarcinoma Versus Breast Carcinoma

| Antibody | Result | | |
	Pancreaticobiliary	Breast Lobular	Breast Ductal
ER	N	+/−	+/−
GCDFP-15	N	+/−	+/−
S-100 protein	N	−/+	−/+
CK17	+	N	N
CK20	+/−	R	R

N, negative; R, rare; +/−, more positive cases than negative; −/+, more negative cases than positive.

the apical cytoplasm and membrane, and within the amorphous material inside the lumen of the malignant glands.[329, 331, 537, 538, 542–544]

- CEA: Pancreaticobiliary ductal adenocarcinomas diffusely and strongly stain with polyclonal and monoclonal CEA, including the new isomeric forms.[332, 444, 538, 541, 545, 546] When classified according to anatomic sites within the pancreas and extrahepatic bile ducts, all of the neoplasms have a similar distribution with a predominantly cytoplasmic staining pattern.[537] If a neoplasm does not diffusely and strongly stain with CEA, consideration should be given to a diagnosis of metastasis or acinic or neuroendocrine carcinoma, regardless of the architecture of the neoplasm.[547] CEA stains the cytoplasm, luminal membrane, and amorphous contents within glands in well-differentiated adenocarcinomas. Poorly differentiated carcinomas that merge into anaplastic neoplasms sometimes show focal or no staining. Normal ducts do not stain with CEA.[548] Although immunohistochemistry results should not be used to determine malignancy, one should seriously consider that a lesion may be a pancreaticobiliary adenocarcinoma if it fails to stain with CEA.
- CA 125: Approximately 50% of pancreatic adenocarcinomas show luminal cytoplasmic staining with CA 125.[330] More often there is patchy, individual, or small clusters of positive cells.
- B72.3: Staining usually occurs in 80% of pancreaticobiliary adenocarcinomas, usually in an apical cytoplasmic membrane pattern, and amorphous debris is noted within malignant glands.[544, 549]
- Calretinin: Approximately 20% of pancreaticobiliary adenocarcinomas stain with calretinin.[270, 550]
- AFP: Most AFP+ neoplasms have clear cell, yolk sac–like regions (see Clear Cell and Hepatoid Neoplasms section). As with adenocarcinomas of the stomach, rare cases of pancreaticobiliary adenocarcinomas that have a ductal

morphology are AFP+,[551] but almost all typical ductal carcinomas are AFP−.[332]

Differential Diagnostic Panels
Breast Ductal Versus Pancreatic Carcinoma (Table 13–18)

Antibodies: CK17, GCDFP-15, ER, CK20, S-100
CK17 stains the majority of pancreaticobiliary adenocarcinomas in a strong, diffuse pattern. Conversely, the majority of breast ductal carcinomas do not stain, and those that do show rare positive cells[327] and are usually within the centers of solid high-grade carcinoma nests (personal experience).

CK20 stains approximately 50% of pancreaticobiliary adenocarcinomas, compared with less than 10% of ductal adenocarcinomas.[6, 322, 323, 326]

GCDFP-15 is negative in pancreaticobiliary adenocarcinomas and positive in approximately 50 to 100% of breast lobular carcinomas.[353, 368, 369]

Pancreaticobiliary adenocarcinomas do not stain with ER, whereas many breast carcinomas do.[368]

S-100 protein stains approximately 50% of breast carcinomas, compared with almost no pancreaticobiliary adenocarcinomas.[365, 374]

CK7 and CK20 are not useful in this differential diagnosis because of the complete overlap in the distribution of staining combinations in the two neoplasms.[6]

Prostatic Versus Pancreaticobiliary Adenocarcinoma (Table 13–19)

Antibodies: PSA, PAP, CEA, CK7, CK20, CK19
Prostatic adenocarcinomas stain with PAP and PSA in the majority of cases, compared with an absence of staining in pancreaticobiliary adenocarcinomas.[387]

Prostate adenocarcinomas also either do not stain or very focally stain with CEA; in contrast, pancreaticobiliary adenocarcinomas stain diffusely and strongly with CEA.

A CK7−/CK20− coordinate staining pattern is seen in 60% of prostate adenocarcinomas but not in pancreaticobiliary adenocarcinomas.[6] The other

Table 13–19. Pancreaticobiliary Adenocarcinoma Versus Prostate Adenocarcinoma

| Antibody | Result | |
	Pancreaticobiliary	Prostate
PSA	N	+
PAP	N	+
CK7−/CK20−	N	+/−
CEA	+	−/+
CK17	+	N

+, almost always positive; N, negative; +/−, more positive cases than negative; −/+, more negative cases than positive.

Table 13–20. Pancreaticobiliary Adenocarcinoma Versus Lung Adenocarcinoma

Antibody	Result Pancreaticobiliary	Lung
TTF	N	+
PE-10	N	+
CK20	+/−	R
CA 125	+/−	R

+, almost always positive; N, negative; R, rare; +/−, more positive cases than negative.

patterns significantly overlap in distribution, making them nondiagnostic.

CK17 stains almost all pancreaticobiliary adenocarcinomas; in contrast, there is either no or extremely focal staining in prostate adenocarcinomas.

Lung Versus Pancreaticobiliary Adenocarcinoma (Table 13–20)

Antibodies: TTF, PE-10, CK20, CA 125, CK17

TTF and PE-10 stain lung adenocarcinomas and fail to stain ductal adenocarcinomas.[379, 382, 383, 552, 553]

CA 125 stains approximately 50% of pancreaticobiliary adenocarcinomas in a diffuse pattern; the rare lung adenocarcinomas that are positive usually show patchy staining.

CK20 stains approximately a third of pancreaticobiliary adenocarcinomas in a diffuse pattern, compared with only rare lung adenocarcinomas, which usually show only focal staining.

CK17 stains almost all pancreaticobiliary adenocarcinomas, with approximately half of "positive" neoplasms containing more than 50% positive cells. In contrast, only about 50% of lung adenocarcinomas are positive. Of the "positive" lung adenocarcinomas, approximately 80% show scattered positive or less than 10% positive cells.[327]

CK7/CK20 coordinate staining patterns are not useful in this differential diagnosis because of the overlap in the distribution of patterns.[6]

Pancreaticobiliary Adenocarcinoma Versus Mesothelioma (Table 13–21)

Antibodies: CEA (monoclonal), CA 19-9, BerEP4, CD15, B72.3, CK17, vimentin, calretinin

CEA, CA 19-9, BerEP4, CD15, and B72.3 stain almost all pancreaticobiliary adenocarcinomas but only infrequently stain mesotheliomas.[331, 332, 381, 388, 444, 450, 544, 550, 554–565]

CK17 stains almost all pancreaticobiliary adenocarcinomas, with the majority showing greater than 50% positive cells. In contrast, approximately 80% of pleural mesotheliomas do not stain. Positively responding mesotheliomas show only rare scattered positive cells.[327]

Conversely, vimentin almost never stains pancreaticobiliary adenocarcinomas but does stain at

Table 13–21. Pancreaticobiliary Adenocarcinoma Versus Mesothelioma

Antibody	Result Pancreaticobiliary Adenocarcinoma	Mesothelioma
CEA (monoclonal)	+	R–N
CA 19-9	+	−/+
BerEP4	+	R
B72.3	+	R
CD15	+	R
Calretinin	N	+/−
Vimentin	N	+

+, almost always positive; N, negative; R, rare; R–N, rare to negative; +/−, more positive cases than negative; −/+, more negative cases than positive.

least 70% of mesotheliomas, which usually show diffuse strong staining.[388, 556, 559–561]

Müllerian Endometrioid and Serous Papillary Carcinomas Versus Pancreaticobiliary Adenocarcinoma (Table 13–22)

Antibodies: CEA (monoclonal), ER, S-100 protein, CK17

Isomeric monoclonal CEA stains the majority of pancreaticobiliary adenocarcinomas. Only rarely does it stain endometrioid and serous papillary adenocarcinomas, with "positive" tumors containing less than 25% positive cells (personal experience).[389]

CK17 stains almost all pancreaticobiliary adenocarcinomas, usually in a strong and diffuse pattern. In contrast, endometrioid and serous papillary adenocarcinomas, although frequently positive, usually show staining of only individual, rare cells (personal experience).[327]

ER stains almost all endometrioid and serous papillary adenocarcinomas but no pancreaticobiliary adenocarcinomas.

S-100 protein stains approximately 75% of serous carcinomas and 50% of endometrioid adeno-

Table 13–22. Pancreaticobiliary Adenocarcinoma Versus Müllerian Endometrioid and Serous Papillary Adenocarcinoma

Antibody	Result Pancreaticobiliary	Endometrioid and Serous Papillary
CEA (monoclonal)	+	R
CK20	+/−	R
ER	N	+/−
S-100 protein	N	+/−
Calretinin	N	+/−
Vimentin (endometrioid only)	N	+/−

+, almost always positive; N, negative; R, rare; +/−, more positive cases than negative.

carcinomas, compared with almost no staining of pancreaticobiliary adenocarcinomas.[365, 389]

CA 125 staining is not useful for this differentiation because both neoplasms are positive.[330, 566] Similarly, CK7/CK20 coordinate staining patterns are not useful in separating the two neoplasms because of the extensive overlap of patterns.[6, 326]

Müllerian Mucinous Versus Pancreatic Adenocarcinoma

No known antibody panels distinguish müllerian mucinous from pancreatic adenocarcinoma.

Renal Cell Carcinoma Versus Pancreatic Adenocarcinoma

Antibodies: CA 125, CK7, CK20, B72.3
Pancreatic adenocarcinomas express CA 125 in approximately 50% of cases, whereas renal carcinomas do not stain with this antibody.[330]

Similarly, B72.3 stains almost all pancreaticobiliary adenocarcinomas, but RCCs either do not stain or show only extremely focal staining.[549]

CK7/CK20 coordinate staining is useful if it yields a CK7–/CK20– pattern. Approximately 75% of RCCs stain in this pattern, compared with no pancreaticobiliary adenocarcinomas.[6]

Adenosquamous Carcinoma

Adenosquamous differentiation can be found in a significant minority of poorly differentiated ductal adenocarcinomas.[567] Both regions stain with keratin AE1/AE3. In some studies, the squamous cells did not stain with CEA but the glandular components were diffusely positive. Other studies

reported strong CEA staining of the squamous carcinoma cells.[538, 567, 568]

Both the glandular and squamous cells almost always stain diffusely with keratin CAM5.2 and CK19. In the majority of neoplasms, the squamous cell component has a CA 19-9 staining pattern similar to that of the glandular component.[568] CK5/CK6 staining also occurs in regions of squamous differentiation.[3] Involucrin selectively stains the squamous cell component. Keratin 35βH11 was reported as negative in all cases.[569]

Undifferentiated, Spindled (Sarcomatoid), Pleomorphic, and Giant Cell Carcinomas

Sarcomatoid and pleomorphic are poorly differentiated variants of adenocarcinomas. Spindled (sarcomatoid), pleomorphic giant cell, and poorly differentiated, typical ductal adenocarcinoma are frequently admixed, and squamous differentiation is common. The spindled regions can have the appearance of malignant fibrous histiocytoma or fibrosarcoma. The neoplastic cells of these variants stain to variable extents with keratins AE1/AE3, CAM5.2, 35βH11, and CK7, CK8, CK18, and CK19 (Fig. 13–13).[518, 570–581] The degree to which they stain varies among and within neoplasms. Use of a large battery of keratins is recommended if proof of epithelial differentiation of the spindled (sarcomatoid) regions is needed. EMA and CEA staining are usually negative in the spindled anaplastic areas.[567, 572, 575–577, 582] Admixed benign giant cell tumor areas have the immunophenotype characteristics of giant cell tumor of bone (see later). Typical of all spindled (sarcomatoid) anaplastic carcinomas, the spindle cells strongly and diffusely stain with vimentin.[518, 575–578]

Undifferentiated, spindle cell (sarcomatoid) car-

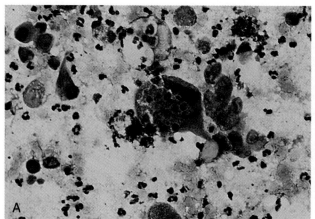
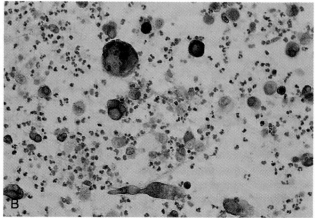

Figure 13–13. A, Fine needle aspiration (FNA) biopsy of pleomorphic giant cell (PGC) carcinoma of the pancreas consisting of pleomorphic malignant cells, including some multinucleated tumor giant cells demonstrating phagocytosis of neutrophils. (Diff-Quik, intermediate-power magnification) B, Positive staining of the malignant cells for broad spectrum cytokeratin (AE1/AE3) in an FNA of PGC of the pancreas. (Low-power magnification)

cinomas that lack glandular or squamous carcinoma differentiation on hematoxylin and eosin staining can appear morphologically similar to malignant melanoma, malignant peripheral nerve sheath tumors, and other spindle-shaped sarcomas that usually originate in the retroperitoneum. Although pancreaticobiliary undifferentiated, spindle cell carcinomas can occasionally show focal S-100 protein positivity, they do not stain with HMB-45, MART-1, or tyrosinase (personal experience).

No immunohistochemical panel can distinguish pancreaticobiliary undifferentiated, spindle cell (sarcomatoid) carcinoma from similar-appearing carcinomas that arise in the lung, thyroid, esophagus, or other locations.

Rhabdoid Carcinomas

Rhabdoid neoplasms have rarely been described in the pancreas. Like their counterparts in the GI tract, they stain with keratin CAM5.2, with vimentin, which highlights the perinuclear whorl, and weakly with EMA.[399, 583]

Mucinous Cystic and Intraductal Papillary Neoplasms

For immunohistochemical purposes, the category mucinous cystic and intraductal papillary neoplasms includes mucinous cystic neoplasms, mucin-hypersecreting neoplasm, mucin-producing tumor, mucinous duct ectasia, duct-ectatic mucinous cystadenoma, and intraductal papillary neoplasms (mucinous and nonmucinous).[584] The epithelial cells of these neoplasms stain strongly and diffusely with cytokeratins AE1/AE3 and CAM5.2, and EMA.[585–590] Approximately 75% stain with CK7 in a diffuse pattern, and 50% with CK20, more often in a focal pattern.[588] These neoplasms stain diffusely with CK18, but unlike ductal adenocarcinomas, which almost always stain diffusely and strongly with CK19, only a small minority of mucinous cystic and intraductal papillary neoplasms are positive.[587]

CEA and CA 19-9 staining has produced variable results. Most studies have reported strong, diffuse CEA and CA 19-9 staining.[575, 585, 590–592] Some studies have reported that most mucinous and intraductal neoplasms stain in a focal distribution with these antibodies (in contrast to ductal adenocarcinomas),[586, 587, 593] and still other studies report marked variation within neoplasms.[588] Some authors have suggested that patchy CEA staining is evidence for precursor lesions of certain cell types.[592] B72.3 stains approximately 33% of these neoplasms.[585] Admixed occasional endocrine cells within the epithelial lining, evidenced by chromogranin or synaptophysin staining, can be found in approximately 10% of tumors in a distribution similar to that seen in ductal adenocarcinomas.[585, 590, 594] S-100 protein and CA 125 do not stain these tumors.[585–587, 589] Mucin-poor cystadenocarcinoma variants are identical in staining pattern to mucin-rich neoplasms.[595] Rare AFP+ tumors have been described.[596]

Ovarian-like stroma can be present immediately around mucinous cystic neoplasms. These regions are frequently positive with vimentin, smooth muscle actin (SMA), and muscle-specific actin (HHF-35). ER has been found in approximately 20 to 80% (mean, approximately 33% of cases).[585, 589, 590, 597] Alpha inhibin and calretinin stain the thecal-like stromal regions in a patchy distribution.[589] The CD34 staining response is negative.[597]

Osteoclast-like giant cells can be rarely found in association with mucinous cystic neoplasms (see later Giant Cell Tumors section).[598, 599]

One group of authors reported a mucinous cystadenocarcinoma that had AFP production, identified through the use of contemporary immunohistochemical techniques.[593]

MUCINOUS CYSTADENOCARCINOMA WITH SPINDLE CELL (SARCOMATOID) DIFFERENTIATION

This subtype of mucinous cystadenocarcinoma has areas of spindle cell (sarcomatoid) differentiation, frequently as a mural nodule within the cystic regions.[575, 600] The spindled areas stain with SMA, ER, and PR.[600] Like many spindle cell (sarcomatoid) carcinomas, these tumors frequently do not stain with keratin or EMA or show focal positivity.[575, 600]

Intraductal Oncocytic Papillary Neoplasm of the Pancreas

One group of authors described 11 cases of a distinctive intraductal papillary oncocytic neoplasm that had a different immunohistochemical staining pattern from that of the mucin-rich and mucin-poor intraductal papillary neoplasms described previously.[584] B72.3 showed diffuse positivity in all cases, with most displaying 75% cell positivity.[584] Unlike the previously described neoplasms, less than 50% of the tumors in this series stained with CEA (monoclonal and polyclonal), predominantly in a membrane pattern. No cells showed cytoplasmic staining. CA 19-9 stained only two of the neoplasms, and the CA 125 staining response was negative in all cases.

Giant Cell Tumors

There are two types of giant cell tumors of the pancreas, (1) osteoclast-like giant cell tumor that can resemble giant cell tumor of bone and (2) pleomorphic giant cell carcinoma.[576, 599]

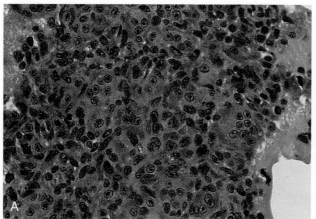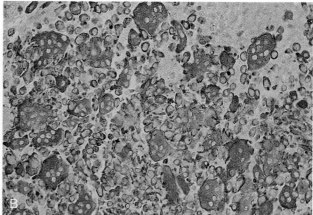

Figure 13–14. A, Osteoclastic giant cell tumor of the pancreas having an appearance similar to that of a giant cell tumor of bone. Sheets of osteoclastic-like giant cells are appreciated in the cell block from the FNA. (H&E, intermediate magnification) *B,* Immunohistochemical stain for vimentin decorates the osteoclastic cells. (Intermediate-power magnification)

Osteoclast-like giant cell tumors have an immunophenotype identical to that of similar-appearing cells in giant cell tumors of bone.[598, 601] The osteoclast-like giant cells that are not overtly malignant stain with CD68, CD45 (LCA), CD71, alpha-1-antichymotrypsin, and vimentin (Fig. 13–14). Most studies demonstrate that these cells do not stain with EMA, cytokeratins, or lysozyme. The mononuclear cells (of varying atypicality) usually are similar in immunophenotype to the osteoclast-like multinucleated cells and do not stain with cytokeratin antibodies.[576, 578, 598, 599, 601–603] Weak EMA positivity of mononuclear cells has been reported in a minority of neoplasms.[598] Many of these neoplasms have coexistent invasive ductal adenocarcinoma, either as a collision type tumor or as intimately admixed single or small clusters of malignant adenocarcinomas cells, and these regions have the characteristic immunophenotype of pancreatic ductal adenocarcinoma (see earlier).

The giant cells in pleomorphic giant cell carcinoma are anaplastic carcinoma cells. Pleomorphic giant cell carcinoma can also be admixed with mixed osteoclast-like giant cell tumor cells.[573]

Acinic Cell Carcinomas (Table 13–23)

Seventy-five percent to 100% of acinic cell carcinomas stain with keratins AE1/AE3 and CAM5.2 and CK7, CK8, CK16, and CK19. CAM5.2 stains a larger percentage of acinic cell carcinoma cells with greater intensity than AE1/AE3.[518, 542, 604–606] One third of the "positive" cases show only focal keratin staining that is frequently weak. The EMA staining response is usually negative or focally positive,[605] but occasional cases have been reported to show diffuse positivity.[604] Ninety percent

of acinic cell carcinomas stain with trypsin and alpha-1-antichymotrypsin.[604, 605, 607] CA 19.9 and B72.3 stain approximately 33% of architecturally solid neoplasms, but infrequently, acinic cell carcinomas have other staining patterns. Approximately 10 to 30% of neoplasms focally and weakly stain with chromogranin and CEA, but most studies report no staining.[542, 605–608] Vimentin is usually negative.[518] AFP staining is usually negative except for rare case reports.[609–611]

Mixed acinic-endocrine neoplasms occasionally have been described.[612, 613] The cells of these neoplasms show both pancreatic acinar cell differentiation, characterized by their staining with antibodies to trypsin, chymotrypsin, and lipase, and endocrine differentiation, characterized by their reaction to chromogranin and synaptophysin. Most cells expressed only one line of differentiation.

Table 13–23. Antibody Staining of Acinic Cell Carcinoma

Antibody	Immuno-staining	Comments
Chromogranin	N–R	See text
Keratin AE1/AE3	+/−	See text
Keratin CAM5.2	+	See text
CK7	+/−	See text
CK19	+/−	See text
Trypsin	+	See text
Chymotrypsin	+	See text
CA 19-9	−/+	Usually solid pattern neoplasms
B72.3	+/−	Usually solid pattern neoplasms
EMA	R	Usually focal and weak (see text)
CEA	N–R	See text
Vimentin	N	See text

+, almost always positive; N, negative; N–R, negative to rare; R, rare; +/−, more positive than negative cases; −/+, more negative cases than positive.

Table 13–24. Antibody Staining of Solid and Cystic (Papillary) Acinic Cell Carcinoma*

Antibody	Immunostaining
Alpha-1-antichymotrypsin	+
A1AT	+
Vimentin	+
CK20	+/−
Keratin AE1/AE3	+/−
Synaptophysin	+/−
Chromogranin	R
ER	R
PR	R
Keratin CAM5.2	R
CK7	R
CK19	R
EMA	N
Calretinin	N
CEA	N
CA 19-9	N
S-100 protein	N
AFP	N

*For comments, see text.
  +, almost always positive; N, negative; R, rare; +/−, more positive cases than negative; −/+, more negative cases than positive.

Solid and Cystic (Papillary) Neoplasms
(Table 13–24)

Neoplastic cells have consistently shown diffuse positivity with alpha-1-antitrypsin (A1AT), alpha-1-antichymotrypsin, and vimentin.[518, 614–617] Keratin AE1/AE3 and CK20 stain a minority of neoplastic cells in an inconsistent fashion.[614, 618, 619] Even fewer neoplasms (5 to 20%) stain with keratins 7, 8, 18, and 19.[518, 615, 617] Synaptophysin staining is diffuse in approximately 33 to 50% of cases (Fig. 13–15).[615, 616] Diffuse chromogranin staining has rarely been reported.[619] ER diffusely stains approximately 20% of cases,[614, 616, 617, 620] and an even smaller percentage of cases

have been reported to stain with PR.[614, 621] The neoplasms do not stain with EMA,[616, 618] calretinin,[550] AFP,[616] CEA, CA 19-9,[607, 614, 616, 619, 622] or S-100 protein.[616–618]

Differentiating Between Microacinar and Solid Neoplasms (Table 13–25)

Solid and microacinar carcinoid neoplasms can be histologically similar to pancreaticobiliary ductal adenocarcinomas, acinic carcinomas, and solid and cystic (papillary) carcinomas.[542, 547, 623, 624] Neuroendocrine carcinomas, unlike any of the other neoplasms in the differential diagnosis, diffusely and strongly stain with the neuroendocrine antibodies synaptophysin, chromogranin, CD56, and CD57. Although solid and cystic (papillary) neoplasms can occasionally show moderately diffuse staining with synaptophysin, they do not stain with chromogranin or the other neuroendocrine markers. Similarly, neuroendocrine neoplasms can be distinguished from ductal adenocarcinomas on the basis of their staining with neuroendocrine markers, which is not seen in ductal adenocarcinomas.

Solid or cystic and papillary carcinoma may be distinguished from pancreaticobiliary ductal adenocarcinoma as follows. CK7, CEA, CA 19-9, EMA, keratin CAM5.2, and CK19 stain ductal adenocarcinomas but not solid and cystic (papillary) neoplasms. Acinic cell carcinomas can be distinguished from solid and cystic (papillary) neoplasms in their positivity to lipase. However, many laboratories do not have this antibody; therefore, a diffuse, strong staining response to vimentin in solid and cystic (papillary) neoplasms is a useful distinguishing feature. Neuroendocrine and ductal carcinomas do not diffusely and strongly stain with vimentin.

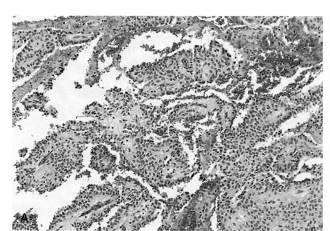 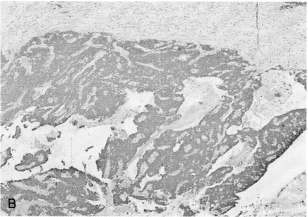

Figure 13–15. *A,* Papillary and cystic neoplasm of the pancreas showing characteristic papillary fronds lined by uniform, mildly atypical cells with associated nearby hemorrhage and necrosis. (Low-power magnification) *B,* Synaptophysin positivity of the neoplastic cells of a papillary and cystic tumor of the pancreas. (Low-power magnification)

Table 13–25. **Immunohistochemical Differential Diagnostic Panel for Microacinar Carcinoma**

Antibody	Result			
	Neuroendocrine	Pancreatobiliary Ductal	Acinic	Solid and Cystic (Papillary)
Synaptophysin	+	−/+	N	+/−
Chromogranin	+	−/+	N	R
CD56	+	N	N	N
CD57	+	N	N	N
Alpha-1-antichymotrypsin	R	R	+	+
Lipase	N	N	+	N
CK7	R	+	−/+	R
CK19	+/−	+	+/−	R
EMA	N	+	R	N
CEA	R	+	N	N
CA 19-9	+/−	+	−/+	N
Vimentin	R	N	N	+

+, almost always positive; N, negative; R, rare; −/+, more positive cases than negative; −/+, more negative cases than positive.

Clear Cell and Hepatoid Neoplasms

Clear cell carcinomas have been described in the pancreas, extrahepatic ducts, and gallbladder.[625, 626] "Clear cell carcinoma" from these regions comprises several immunohistochemically distinct neoplasms, such as (1) typical ductal adenocarcinomas that contain abundant glycogen, (2) yolk sac–like or enteric carcinomas with antibody staining results similar to those described in the stomach, and (3) hepatoid carcinomas. The immunohistochemical profiles of the latter two neoplasms overlap. AFP, alpha inhibin, and many other antibodies, including many lymphoid CD antibodies, can be positive in clear cell carcinomas from any nonrenal site, in our and others' experiences.[627] We have found that most of this staining is due to spurious, endogenous biotin–produced reactions. Appropriate pre-primary antibody slide preparation eliminates most of these reactions. CEA can produce focal staining, compared with the strong and diffuse staining that is seen in ductal adenocarcinomas.[626] Vimentin and neuroendocrine markers are negative.[541, 626]

Clear cell "sugar" tumors can occur in the pancreas. Despite the epithelioid nature of the cells, they do not stain with keratins AE1/AE3 or CAM5.2, chromogranin, or lipase. Like sugar tumors in other organs, they do stain with actin and HMB-45.[628]

Immunohistochemistry is useful in clarifying the subtype of a clear cell neoplasm. Antibodies should be applied to differentiate neuroendocrine differentiation, clear cell carcinoma, "sugar tumor," and GIST.[629]

Serous Cystadenomas (Microcystic Adenomas)

The epithelial cells lining serous cystadenomas stain strongly and diffusely with keratin AE1/AE3 and EMA.[448, 630, 631] Some authors have reported no staining with keratin CAM5.2,[448, 630] but others have noted diffuse positivity.[631] The cyst-lining cells do not stain with CEA, factor VIII, or chromogranin.[448, 630, 632] CA 19-9 staining can be focally present.[632, 633]

Miscellaneous Lesions

Lymphoepithelial cyst of the pancreas is an uncommon entity. The squamous epithelium of the cyst reacts with keratin AE1/AE3, and the adjacent lymphocytes are an admixture of CD3+ T cells and CD20+ B cells.[634]

LIVER

Biotin Blocking of Liver Tissue Specimens

Hepatocytes contain abundant amounts of biotin,[635] which can bind or react with many secondary antibodies that are components of contemporary chromogen systems, producing extensive nonspecific staining that can be falsely interpreted as a positive reaction.[636–640] This effect is more pronounced with the use of antigen retrieval.[641, 642] Unless "blocked," endogenous biotin in hepatocytes produces spurious staining in response to almost every antibody. There also can be a high level of background staining, making interpretation of staining extremely difficult. Lack of recognition of the effect of hepatocyte biotin on immunohistochemistry has produced conflicting staining results and has been the focus of several reports.[635, 640, 641, 643]

Blocking of endogenous hepatocyte biotin is required prior to application of primary antibodies. "Biotin blocks" are readily available from commercial or noncommercial sources. We have found that the efficacy of noncommercial biotin blocks can vary greatly, despite Herculean attempts at quality control, and therefore, we prefer to use biotin blocks from commercial sources.

Liver tissue can also contain greater concentrations of peroxidase than many other tissues, partly because of the numerous erythrocytes, both intact and lysed by procedures, within hepatic sinusoids and other vascular structures. Unless the peroxidase is deactivated prior to application of the primary antibody, extremely high levels of background staining or false-positive antibody reactions frequently occur. We have found that incubating the liver tissues in a low-concentration H_2O_2-methanol solution bath for a longer time than used for other tissues can eliminate this problem.

Immunophenotype of Hepatocellular Constituents

Initial immunohistochemical staining profiles of HCC and cholangiocarcinoma (CC) suggested that these carcinomas had immunophenotypes identical to those of benign hepatocytes and intrahepatic bile duct epithelial cells.[644, 645] Numerous studies examined these issues in detail, with extensive debates regarding the truth of the original findings. With the passage of time, the accumulation of studies, and the development of more sensitive techniques, it has become clear that these "truths" are incorrect. HCCs frequently express some degree of biliary type cytokeratin phenotype. The immunophenotypes of HCC and CC are not identical to those of their benign counterparts. Because of this historical aspect of the immunophenotype of HCC, CC, and mixed HCC-CC, we discuss constituent cells and structures of the liver before delving into the immunophenotypes of primary hepatic carcinomas.

BENIGN HEPATOCYTES

Embryonal hepatocytes contain CK8, CK18, and CK19. CK19 expression disappears by the 10th week of gestation.[646, 647] Mature hepatocytes in the normal liver contain only CK8 and CK18 and therefore stain diffusely and strongly with keratin CAM5.2.[85, 644, 645, 648, 649] Staining with CAM5.2 shows an intensity gradient, with the strongest staining in acinar zone 1 hepatocytes.[648] Additionally, a rim of intensely stained hepatocytes around the terminal hepatic venules and subjacent to subhepatic venules can be seen with keratin CAM5.2.[648] Most hepatocytes stain with keratin 35βH11, which reacts with CK8 only.[390, 650] They do not stain with CK7 (Fig. 13–16),[85, 648] CK19,[85, 312, 390, 648, 651] CK20,[275] keratin 34βE12,[650, 652] or vimentin.[390, 653]

HepPar 1 stains hepatocytes (normal architecture or in cirrhosis) in a diffuse, coarsely granular, cytoplasmic pattern without canalicular accentuation.[312, 654, 655] CD57 (NCAM, Leu19) weakly stains normal hepatocytes.[32] Polyclonal CEA stains the canaliculi of normal hepatocytes in a thin, membranous pattern.[656] Normal hepatocytes do not stain with AFP,

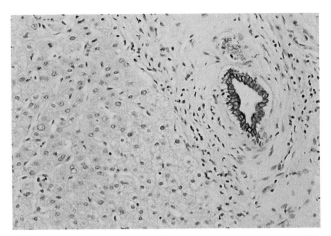

Figure 13–16. Benign liver tissue showing negative staining of the hepatocytes for CK7, with a positive-staining bile duct. (Low-power magnification)

but liver cells constituting cirrhotic nodules occasionally show focal staining.[657, 658]

Hepatocytes, sometimes arranged in a thin encircling rim at the periphery of cirrhotic nodules, can stain with keratin AE1/AE3, CK7, and CK19.[651] Staining with these keratins is thought to represent biliary differentiation.[85] This phenomenon may represent a form of stem cell differentiation similar to the so-called small cell parenchymal reaction seen around the portal tracts in cases of chronic biliary obstruction (see later).

INTRAHEPATIC BILE DUCTS AND PERIBILIARY GLANDS

The epithelial cells of intrahepatic bile ducts stain diffusely and strongly with CK7, CK8, CK18, and CK19 (see Fig. 13–16).[85, 312, 648, 649, 659, 660] They also stain with antibodies AE1/AE3, 35βH11, and 34βE12.[650] Normal bile ducts do not stain with CK20,[275] unlike normal pancreatic ducts, which stain strongly.[275] Normal intrahepatic peribiliary glands show weak reactivity to CA 19-9 and no staining with CEA.[661, 662] One study noted an association between growing intensity of CA 19-9 and CEA staining of the cells within peribiliary glands and increasing degrees of cellular atypia.[661]

STEM CELLS, BILE DUCTULES, AND HEPATOCYTES IN ACUTE AND CHRONIC LIVER DISEASE

Cuboidal hepatocyte-like cells are present in the parenchyma immediately adjacent to portal tracts or within bile ductules at the periphery of portal tracts in cases of chronic biliary obstruction and during the regenerative phase after a episode of fulminant hepatitis.[660] These cells may be a proliferation of stem cells that normally reside in or compose the small ducts that connect bile canaliculi to the canals of Hering.[646, 652, 660, 663–668] Despite their hepatocyte-like or bile duct–like histologic appearance, these cells can show a bile duct immunophenotype or coexpress a bile duct and hepatocyte immunophenotype.[654, 664, 668, 669]

The existence of a hepatic stem cell that can differentiate toward hepatocytes or bile ducts is a useful concept to consider before one deals with the immunophenotype of liver lesions.[663, 665] Differentiation toward the stem cell phenotype in hepatocytes around the periphery of cirrhotic nodules can explain their bile duct–like keratin immunophenotype.[670–672] Similarly, differentiation of malignant hepatocytes toward a stem cell phenotype and secondarily toward bile duct epithelial cells can be used to rationalize the results of many studies reporting a minority of HCCs (especially those that are high-grade) immunostaining with antigens and having a keratin profile that is characteristic of cholangiocarcinoma. The same theory can also explain the reason that a minority of CCs can have the immunohistochemical features of HCCs as well as the existence of mixed HCC-CCs. The stem cell concept has been suggested as the underpinning that partially explains the differing morphologies and immunohistochemical profiles of hepatoblastomas.

SINUSOIDAL ENDOTHELIAL CELLS

The sinusoid endothelial cells in the normal liver differ from the endothelial cells of normal arteries and veins in that most of the former cells do not stain with CD34, factor VIII, CD31, or *Ulex europaeus*.[673–678] Focal staining of some endothelial cells in the vicinity of portal tracts or fibrous septa has been noted in a minority of cases.[676]

Weak to moderate staining with *Ulex*, CD31, and factor VIII and weak patchy staining with CD34, typically of endothelial cells, can be seen in cirrhosis.[676]

Medical Diseases

ALPHA-1-ANTITRYPSIN DEFICIENCY

The hallmark of A1AT deficiency is intracytoplasmic globules that stain with alpha-1-antitrypsin. Staining is most intense and prevalent in periportal or periseptal hepatocytes (Fig. 13–17).[679–681] Intrahepatocyte globules in end-stage hepatic disease of various causes are also A1AT globules, and their appearance usually signifies an unsuspected A1AT abnormality.[681]

MALLORY BODIES

Mallory bodies (MBs) are intracytoplasmic accumulations of keratin filaments or fragments of cytokeratin (Fig. 13–18).[672, 682, 683] The type of cytokeratin filament in MBs is heterogeneous, the major component is high molecular weight fragments and filaments,[12, 682, 684] and they stain with keratin 34βE12. MBs usually strongly and diffusely stain with CK18, one of the reactants of keratin CAM5.2.[672] MBs also occasionally react with CK7 and CK19. We have found that keratin CAM5.2 is suboptimal for identifying MBs, because they are hard to see against the background of normal diffuse cytoplasmic staining seen with this antibody.

HEPATITIS B VIRUS

Immunohistochemical staining of liver tissue for hepatitis B virus (HBV) antigens as a routine component of patient care has been replaced by both serum and liver tissue virus DNA measurements using the polymerase chain reaction (PCR) test and serologic tests for the antigens HBcAg, HBeAg, and HBsAg and their respective antibodies. Staining in selected instances, such as of a specimen from a transplant recipient or to shed light on the mecha-

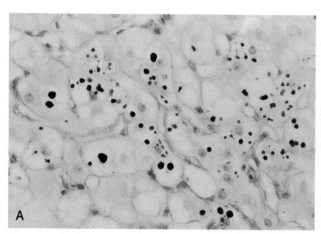 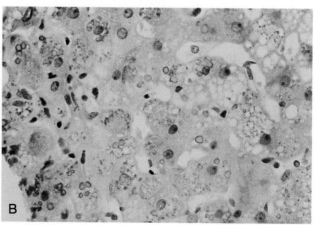

Figure 13–17. A, Periodic acid–Schiff (PAS)-positive D globules in hepatocytes in a biopsy specimen of alpha-1-antitrypsin. (High-power magnification) *B,* Immunoperoxidase stain for alpha-1-antitrypsin demonstrates numerous positive-staining globules in the hepatocytes, showing characteristic peripheral rimming. (Intermediate-power magnification)

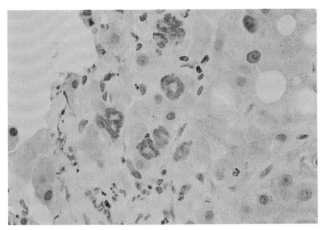

Figure 13–18. Mallory bodies in alcoholic hepatitis staining with broad spectrum cytokeratin (AE1/AE3). (High-power magnification)

nisms of HCC development in HBV-infected patients, is useful.[685] HBsAg (hepatitis B surface antigen) immunolocalization has been noted along the hepatocyte cell membrane, diffusely cytoplasmic, or as an intracytoplasmic inclusion (Fig. 13–19).[686–688] HBcAg (hepatitis B core antigen) staining can be seen as weak cytoplasmic or, more commonly, as strongly nuclear. Staining of nuclei indicates active, complete virus production and is associated with elevated serum HBV DNA levels.[686]

HEPATITIS C VIRUS

Like the use of HBV immunohistochemical staining, the routine use of hepatitis C virus (HCV) immunostaining of liver tissue has yet to be defined.[689] Most of the commercially available antibodies to HCV, an RNA virus, are directed against HCV core polypeptides.[690–697] Diffuse, cytoplasmic staining of hepatocytes has been identified

in approximately 75% of patients with chronic HCV hepatitis (Fig. 13–20).[694] The number of positive cells can vary markedly and does not appear to correlate with liver function test values.[698] Immunohistochemically positive cells can be seen in 70% of reverse transcriptase (RT)-negative/PCR+ cases.[690] Nuclear staining has not been identified. The cells of proliferated bile ductules also occasionally show cytoplasmic staining, a phenomenon thought to be reflective of their origin from hepatocyte cords.[694] HCV+ cells usually show no degenerative changes, a feature that strongly supports the hypothesis that necrosis and its sequelae are immune-mediated rather than the result of direct HCV-induced cytotoxic effects.[694] HCV can also be identified in hepatocytes and malignant lymphoma cells in primary hepatic lymphomas that arise in association with HCV.[699]

PRIMARY SCLEROSING CHOLANGITIS AND PRIMARY BILIARY CIRRHOSIS

Primary sclerosing cholangitis (PSC) and primary biliary cirrhosis (PBC) are different in pathogenesis. Both diseases, however, pose a problem in regard to evaluation of the severity of bile duct loss in liver biopsy specimens.[700] CK7 is useful in this context, because it either strongly stains the nascent bile ducts or, in their absence, leaves a notable lack of staining next to the portal artery. We and others have found this antibody to be helpful for this purpose.[659, 701] It is not helpful in distinguishing between PSC and PBC.

Both PSC and PBC also cause a loss of the peribiliary vascular plexus that normally surrounds medium and large interlobular bile ducts.[702] The pattern of loss is different in the two diseases, a feature that occasionally can be of diagnostic assistance. In PSC, any of the endothelial antibodies (*Ulex*, factor VIII, CD31, or CD34) shows the peri-

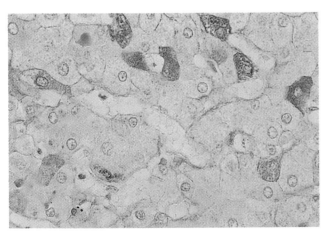

Figure 13–19. Immunoperoxidase stain for hepatitis B surface antigen, revealing scattered cells with characteristic crescent-shaped cytoplasmic staining. (High-power magnification)

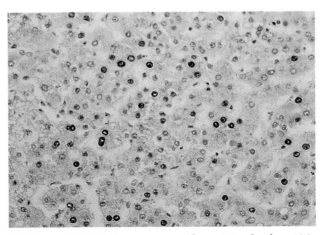

Figure 13–20. Immunoperoxidase stain for hepatitis C antigen showing numerous scattered cells with strong positive nuclear staining. (Low-power magnification)

ductal capillaries to be preserved but pushed away from the duct basement membrane by concentric rings of collagen. In PBC, peribiliary vessels are destroyed by the ductocentric inflammation.[702]

The inflammatory infiltrate in PSC and PBC consists mainly of T lymphocytes that stain with CD3 and CD45RO.[703, 704] In PBC and so-called autoimmune cholangitis, CD4+ and CD8+ T cells are admixed, and CD56+ or CD57+ cells are rare.[703]

Benign Primary Hepatic Lesions

HEPATOCELLULAR ADENOMAS

The hepatocytes that compose adenomas have the immunohistochemical profile of normal, noncirrhotic hepatocytes.[649]

CD34 (QBend-10) has been advocated as an ancillary antibody to distinguish between adenoma and HCC.[705] CD34 does not stain the normal sinusoidal endothelial cells that surround the hepatocyte structures in adenomas, but it does stain the endothelial cells in HCC.[673, 705]

Focal Nodular Hyperplasia

The hepatocytes within the cirrhosis-like nodules composing focal nodular hyperplasia (FNH) stain with CAM5.2 just like normal hepatocytes. Additionally, a variable number of hepatocytes adjacent to fibrous septa stain with CK7 and CK19. Some of the CK7+ cells are continuous with ductular structures within the fibrous septa.[649, 671] These results reflect the ability of hepatocytes to express a biliary (CK7 and CK19) immunophenotype and support the opinion that some bile ductules within fibrous septa of cirrhosis are the result of hepatocyte metaplasia.[649]

Like the staining pattern in cirrhosis, the endothelial cells lining the sinusoids within FNH show moderate to prominent staining with *Ulex* and CD34, and weak staining with factor VIII and CD31.[676] This feature contrasts with the lack of staining of endothelial cells lining the sinuses of normal parenchyma.

BILE DUCT (PERIBILIARY) HAMARTOMAS AND ADENOMAS

The immunophenotypes of the cells forming the bile ducts in bile duct hamartomas and adenomas are identical to those of normal bile ducts, including diffuse CK7 and CK19 positivity.[706, 707]

Malignant Hepatic Lesions

HEPATOBLASTOMAS

Hepatoblastomas can be composed of a wide array of epithelial and mesenchymal cells with different lines of differentiation, including endocrine, melanocytic, and neural.[660, 708] Cells with hepatic differentiation can be divided on the basis of morphologic criteria into embryonal, fetal, small cell, and anaplastic types.[660, 708] It has been suggested that hepatoblastomas are derived from pluripotent stem cells, referred to as *small cells*.[660, 668] This theory is based on the observations that so-called small cells, similar to the cells observed around the portal tracts in chronic obstructive biliary processes, are found in a variety of morphologic cell types of hepatoblastomas. These cells can predominantly express or coexpress hepatocyte or bile duct keratin profiles and other cellular antigens.[660, 668]

Hepatoblastomas stain with many antibodies.[709] Embryonal or fetal type carcinoma cells stain with chromogranin in approximately 50% of cases and with AFP in approximately 75% of carcinomas, and reactions to many clones of low and high molecular weight keratins have been identified in both cell types, including those considered characteristic of biliary differentiation.[710, 711] Unlike HCCs, hepatoblastomas stain with vimentin in approximately 75% of cases.

Almost all of the small round blue cell neoplasms of childhood can involve the liver or tissue near the liver, and occasionally, the distinction between hepatoblastoma and the other neoplasms in this group can be challenging. Cytokeratin is positive in hepatoblastomas and Wilms' tumors. One study compared the staining patterns of hepatoblastomas with those of childhood germ cell neoplasms, primitive neuroendocrine tumors (PNETs), Ewing's sarcomas, rhabdomyosarcomas, neuroblastomas, rhabdoid tumors, lymphomas, and Wilms' tumors through the use of HepPar 1, polyclonal CEA, and monoclonal CEA.[712] All of the fetal hepatoblastomas stained with polyclonal CEA in a canalicular and diffuse pattern, whereas none of the other, nonhepatoblastoma neoplasms had a canalicular staining pattern. Embryonal hepatoblastomas less often stained with polyclonal CEA or had a canalicular staining pattern. HepPar 1 stained all of the hepatoblastomas and none of the nonhepatoblastoma neoplasms. The authors of this study concluded that polyclonal CEA and HepPar 1 are the optimum antibodies for positive distinction of hepatoblastomas from the other, nonhepatoblastoma small round cell neoplasms of childhood.

HEPATOCELLULAR CARCINOMAS OF THE USUAL TYPE

HCC cells predominantly contain the low molecular weight CK8 and CK18 and contain no or minimal amounts of high molecular weight cytokeratins.[85, 649, 713, 714] Accordingly, they stain with the low molecular weight keratin antibody CAM5.2 and either do not stain or show only weak, patchy staining with the high molecular weight cytokeratin antibody 34βH12.[1] We have found that CAM5.2 is the most reliable cytokeratin antibody for HCCs because it stains the highest number of HCC cells of all grades with the strongest intensity. Although keratin 35βH11 is also a low molecular weight cytokeratin antibody, we have found that HCCs of all grades display markedly heterogeneous staining with this antibody. In our experience, keratin 35βH11 stains HCC cells in an inconsistent and unreliable pattern. Additionally, despite the presence of low molecular weight cytokeratins, we and other authors have found that the keratin AE1/AE3 does not stain HCCs in useful numbers or with medium or strong intensity. Most HCCs do not stain with CK7 or CK20, and those that do usually show only focal, weak staining.

The definition of what constitutes biliary differentiation within otherwise typical HCCs and the point at which an HCC becomes a mixed HCC-CC are controversial. Most of this controversy is based on the comparison of keratin subtype expression by malignant hepatocytes with the expression of benign hepatocytes and bile ducts. Keratin antibody AE1/AE3 staining is thought by some authors to be indicative of biliary (cholangiocarcinoma) differentiation.[715] HCC cells that respond positively to keratin AE1/AE3 frequently also do so to CK19, another keratin that is characteristically seen in cholangiocarcinoma.[715] Some authors consider histologically typical HCCs that focally stain with keratin AE1/AE3 or CK19, or both as displaying biliary differentiation.

One study identified biliary differentiation on the basis of keratin AE1/AE3 or CK19 staining in 30% of HCCs.[715] This finding may be of significance because HCCs with biliary differentiation have been shown to be associated with a shorter survival time[715] but are usually also of higher grade. One group of authors believe that HCCs with focal areas that have a histologic resemblance to CC should be considered mixed HCC-CC, on the basis of the finding that these CC-like areas display a CK7/CK19 staining profile similar to that of pure CCs.[716] The same issue affects monoclonal CEA, which is not expressed in well-differentiated HCCs but can focally stain typical, poorly differentiated HCCs.[332]

We cannot dispute the opinion that biliary type keratin expression or monoclonal CEA staining of HCCs is evidence of biliary differentiation within otherwise histologically typical HCC and therefore points to classification as a neoplasm other than pure HCC, such as mixed HCC-CC. However, we prefer to view these results in a different light. Given the evidence for the existence of human hepatic stem cells, the ability of benign hepatocytes to transform into bile ductules, under certain pathologic conditions, that are partially composed of cells displaying hepatocyte and biliary differentiation, and evidence that embryonal hepatocytes express "biliary" type cytokeratins, it is not unexpected to observe this type of keratin (or focal monoclonal CEA) staining in malignant hepatocytes.

We and other authors do not view focal staining with biliary type keratins or monoclonal CEA alone as sufficient criteria to label an otherwise typical HCC as a mixed HCC-CC.[332, 649, 714, 717, 718] We restrict use of the immunohistochemical label *mixed HCC-CC* for neoplasms with cells that stain with the global immunohistochemical profile characteristic of either HCC and CC (see later discussion of mixed HCC-CCs and the differential diagnostic panel for HCC versus CC). These opinions are in keeping with our view of the immunohistochemical profile of all malignancies as presented in other sections of this chapter. There is usually a predominant staining pattern, but a range of staining responses with any antibody is the rule, not the exception.

Some authors have described neuroendocrine differentiation in up to 50% of HCCs.[719, 720] "Neuroendocrine" differentiation in these studies has consisted of a positive response to S-100 or CD57 (Leu7). Chromogranin and synaptophysin are seen in less than 10% of HCCs.[720] Positive staining with the latter two antibodies is usually extremely focal and weak.

KEY DIAGNOSTIC POINTS (Table 13–26)

- Keratin AE1/AE3: AE1/AE3 staining has been reported in approximately 20% of HCCs (range, 5 to 33%).[444, 715, 721, 722] HCC grade influences the percentage of "positive" cases as well as the number of positive cells within a neoplasm. Few well-differentiated HCCs are AE1+/AE3+, compared with approximately 33% of poorly differentiated HCCs.[444] Staining occurs in moderately and poorly differentiated carcinomas as isolated or discrete clusters of HCC cells that form various histologic patterns, including acinar structures.[715] The lack of AE1/AE3 positivity is weak support that a neoplasm is an HCC in the context of an antibody panel that is being used to distinguish one type of carcinoma from HCC. A positive staining response is diagnostically noncontributory in this context.

- Keratin CAM5.2: A positive response to CAM5.2 occurs in 90 to 95% of HCCs.[332, 390, 656, 721, 723–726] Staining can be diffusely cytoplasmic, membranous, or both.[726]

- Keratin 35βH11: Approximately 75% of HCCs (range 70 to 85%) show a positive response to 35βH11. We and others have found that the staining intensity of positive cases is usually weak to moderate, and rarely strong.[390, 650, 651, 723, 727, 728]

- CK7: Overall, approximately 15% (range, 0–25%) of HCCs stain to some extent with CK7.[6, 8, 85, 679, 716, 724] The numbers of cells that stain with CK7 are as follows: 50% of HCCs have no staining, 30% have focal staining, 10 to 20% show staining of less than 50% of

Table 13–26. Antibody Staining of Hepatocellular Carcinoma

Antibody	Immunostaining	Comments and References*
Pankeratin (MAK-6)	+	Refs 390, 721
Keratin AE1/AE3	−/+	See text
Keratin 35βH11	+	See text
Keratin CAM5.2	+	See text
EMA	−/+	See text
CK7	R	See text
CK20	R	See text
CK7+/CK20−	N	See text
CK7+/CK20+	R	
CK7−/CK20+	−/+	
CK7−/CK20−	+	
CK17	N	Ref 327
HepPar 1	+	See text
CK19	R	See text
CA 19-9	N	Refs 8, 329, 331, 651, 679, 718
CEA		
Monoclonal	N–R	See text
Polyclonal	+/−	See text
AFP	+	See text
A1AT	+	See text
BerEP4	R	See text
GCDFP-15	N	Refs 351, 352, 849
CA 125	R	Approximately 10% (range, 0–20%) of HCCs are positive[330]
Vimentin	R	See text
Calretinin	N	Ref 550
S-100 protein	R	Refs 377, 731
B72.3	R	<10% of HCCs are positive (range, 5–20%)[332, 730]
CD56	+	Weak staining of most HCCs[32]
CD57	R	3–15% of HCCs positive[332, 730]
Inhibin	R	See text
Synaptophysin	R	Approximately 5% positive; range, 0–20%[726]
Chromogranin	R	Approximately 5% positive; range 0–15%[719]
PLAP	N	Ref 846
Melan-A (A103)	N	Ref 734

*Superscript numbers indicate chapter references.
  N, negative; N–R, negative to rare; R, rare; +/−, more positive cases than negative; −/+, more negative cases than positive.

cells, and none to 5% of HCCs show greater than 50% staining cells.[8, 716] The significance of CK7 positivity in HCCs has been the subject of debate (see preceding discussion).[649, 714] CK7 positivity is related to the degree of HCC differentiation, poorly differentiated HCCs yielding the highest percentage of "positive" carcinomas.[649, 714, 724]

- CK20: Overall, approximately 20% of HCCs are positive with CK20 (range, 10 to 30%).[6, 8, 312, 326] Staining in many "positive" cases is weak and patchy; HCCs almost never show diffuse strong staining.[275] Approximately 80% of HCCs show no staining with CK20, another 15% show focal staining, and 5% show staining of less than 50% of malignant cells.[8, 312]

- CK7/CK20 coordinate staining pattern: Approximately 75% of HCCs have a CK7−/CK20− staining pattern, 15% have a CK7+/CK20− pattern, 5% have a CK7+/CK20+ pattern, and none has a CK7−/CK20+ pattern.[6]

- CK19: Most studies have reported an overall CK19 positivity rate in HCCs of approximately 10% (range, 0 to 20%).[8, 85, 390, 651, 679, 716, 729] "Positive" tumors usually show only focal staining of malignant hepatocytes.[8, 716] Occasional studies have reported a positivity rate of 30 to 100%,[312, 715, 718, 724] with some studies considering a "positive" tumor as showing staining of more than 5% of the malignant hepatocytes. A relationship between HCC grade and staining with CK19 has been noted by two authors, the highest percentage of "positive" tumors occurring among poorly differentiated HCCs.[718, 724]

- Monoclonal CEA: Almost all studies have reported less than 5% staining of HCCs with monoclonal CEA (range, 0 to 5%), with "positive" cases showing extremely patchy staining.[8, 332, 444, 651, 726, 730] Two studies have reported rates of 10% and 20% positive responses in HCCs.[332, 730] One of these studies found that HCC grade was related to monoclonal CEA positivity, with no staining of well-differentiated HCCs, 8% staining of moderately differentiated HCCs, and 16% staining of poorly differentiated HCCs.[332]

- Polyclonal CEA: In contrast with responses to monoclonal CEA, staining of HCCs with polyclonal CEA is common, with overall positivity in approximately 70% (range, 60 to 95%). Staining occurs in a canalicular pattern or is diffusely cytoplasmic.

A canalicular staining pattern with polyclonal CEA is specific for HCC and has not been observed in other carcinomas (see later Differential Diagnostic Panel). Overall, 40 to 80% of HCCs show a canalicular staining pattern.[332, 651, 656, 718, 726, 729] Canalicular staining by polyclonal CEA is inversely associated with HCC grade; 75% of well-differentiated, 70% of moderately differentiated, and 25 to 50% of poorly differentiated HCCs show this pattern (Fig. 13–21).[332, 444, 726, 729]

Approximately 50% of HCCs show diffuse cytoplasmic staining with polyclonal CEA.[332] Similar to the canalicular staining pattern, diffuse cytoplasmic staining with polyclonal CEA is associated with HCC grade.[726] Less than 5% of well-differentiated and moderately differentiated HCCs and almost 20% of poorly differentiated HCCs show diffuse cytoplasmic staining.[332, 444]

- Vimentin: Most studies report no or minimal staining of HCC cells with vimentin, with a general positivity rate of approximately 5% (range, 0 to 10%).[356, 390, 651, 653, 731] Rare stud-

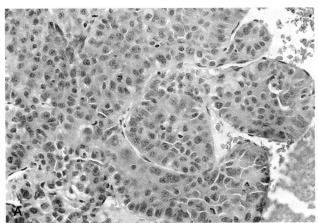 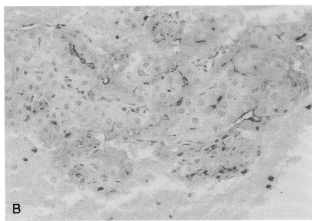

Figure 13–21. *A,* Cell block from an FNA biopsy of a large liver mass showing the characteristic appearance of moderately differentiated hepatocellular carcinoma consisting of thick nests and cords of neoplastic cells with sinusoidal rimming. (H&E, intermediate-power magnification) *B,* Canalicular staining pattern with polyclonal carcinoembryonic antigen (CEA) is typically seen in hepatocellular carcinoma. (Low-power magnification)

ies have noted staining in up to 33% of cases.[390] Vimentin positivity of HCCs occurs almost completely within the high-grade HCC group.[732]

- Factor XIIIa: Markedly variable results with this antibody have been reported. Some studies have noted cytoplasmic staining of the majority of HCCs.[651, 730] One group of authors reported no staining of malignant hepatocytes; rather, they found staining of Kupffer cells within HCCs.[312]
- AFP: AFP staining in HCCs suffers from a lack of sensitivity. Overall, approximately 50% of HCCs stain with AFP, with a reported staining range of 20 to 75%.* Positivity correlates with HCC grade, poorly differentiated neoplasms having only a small percentage (5 to 20%) of "positive" cases.[332, 718, 732]
- HepPar 1: Approximately 80 to 100% of HCCs (range, 40 to 100%) stain with HepPar 1. Staining usually occurs in a moderate to strong and diffuse pattern but occasionally in a focal distribution.[312, 712, 715, 726] Staining consists of numerous, small, intracytoplasmic vesicles.[726] The distribution of staining does not correlate with HCC grade.[312]
- A1AT: Approximately 50% of HCCs stain with A1AT (range, 10 to 80%). The majority of "positive" cases show extensive staining (Fig. 13–22).[656, 730]
- Keratin 34βE12: Less than 5% of HCCs stain with keratin 34βE12.[650, 651] We and others have found positive cells to be few and staining intensity to be weak.[1]
- EMA: Approximately 33% of well-differentiated and moderately differentiated HCCs, and 75% of poorly differentiated HCCs, stain

with EMA.[390, 444, 718, 723, 733] Staining in well-differentiated HCCs is usually focal (personal experience).

- BerEP4: Approximately 25 to 33% of HCCs stain with BerEP4 (personal experience). Staining is related to HCC grade; no well-differentiated, 33% of moderately differentiated, and 50% of poorly differentiated HCCs are positive.[332]
- Alpha inhibin: It has been reported that alpha inhibin can stain a significant number of HCCs. However, it has become clear that unless adequately blocked with biotin, alpha inhibin can produce a high rate of false-positive staining in hepatocytes (see earlier section on Biotin Blocking of Liver Tissue Specimens).[635] With the use of appropriate immunohistochemical staining techniques, HCCs do not or only extremely rarely (4%) stain with inhibin.[635, 734]
- Endothelial antibodies (CD34, CD31, factor

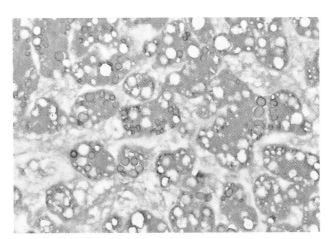

Figure 13–22. Almost all the neoplastic cells stain positively for alpha-1-antitrypsin in a hepatocellular carcinoma. (Intermediate-power magnification)

---

*References 8, 332, 643, 651, 653, 656, 715, 718, 726, 730, 732.

VIII, *Ulex*): Although hepatocytes (benign or malignant) do not stain with the endothelial antibodies, these antibodies can be used as ancillary antibodies to distinguish HCC from other carcinomas and from hepatocellular adenoma (see earlier section on Hepatocellular Adenomas), nodular hyperplasia (see earlier section on Focal Nodular Hyperplasia), or a regenerative cirrhotic nodule.[673, 674, 735–737]

HCC cords, trabecula, and acini are invested with an encircling endothelial cell layer, even in the absence of well-defined sinusoids (Fig. 13–23).[737] The endothelial cells that line the sinusoids or that surround nodules in the absence of well-defined sinusoids of HCCs stain with vascular antibodies, thus providing a useful discriminant ancillary immunohistochemical marker, because the sinusoidal endothelial lining around benign hepatic lesions either does not stain or only focally stains with these antibodies (see earlier).[674, 676, 677] This finding is thought to result from a transformation from normal endothelium-lined sinusoids to capillary structures, with its associated change in antigen expression.[677, 738] We have found this encirclement pattern of CD34+ endothelial cells around malignant hepatocytes to be a useful adjuvant staining pattern that establishes an HCC diagnosis, especially in cytologic specimens. CD34 shows the strongest reaction in HCC and stains the fewest endothelial cells in cirrhotic sinusoids.[676, 735]

Caution is advised in the use of these antibodies. One must restrict the examination to the presence or absence of an endothelial cell layer intimally wrapping around the malignant cells. The sinusoids adjacent to metastatic carcinoma nodules also undergo capillarization with expression of CD34 of their endothelial cells; however, individual nests and groups of metastatic carcinoma are not invested with an encircling endothelial cell layer.[675]

- HCV: Studies that have examined HCV staining patterns in HCV-associated HCCs have noted a random distribution of cytoplasmic staining of malignant hepatocytes and no correlation between staining response and the HCC grade.[693]

HEPATOCELLULAR CARCINOMA VARIANTS

Spindle Cell (Sarcomatoid) Hepatocellular Carcinoma

Spindle cell HCCs are occasionally observed in association with typical high-grade hepatocellular carcinoma.[653, 731, 739, 740] There can be an admixture with other types of sarcoma. Approximately 25% of spindle cell HCCs stain with AFP, a finding similar to the percentage of AFP+ high-grade typical HCCs. Also like typical (epithelioid) HCCs, the majority of spindle cell HCCs stain with keratin CAM5.2. Unlike typical HCCs, which do not stain with vimentin, the majority of spindle cell HCCs do. Coexpression with keratin CAM5.2 and vimentin in the same spindle cells occurs in approximately 50% of cases. A small minority of spindle cell HCCs have stained with S-100 protein, HHF-35, SMAs, and desmin.

Fibrolamellar Heptatocellular Carcinoma

Fibrolamellar HCCs stain with the characteristic HCC-specific antibodies, including keratin CAM5.2 (CK8 and CK18), and focally with CK19.[741, 742] Unlike most typical HCCs, these neoplasms diffusely and strongly stain with CK7.[742] Surprisingly, fibrolamellar HCCs, despite their relatively good prognosis, have a immunohistochemically demonstrable matrix antigen profile that is similar to that of clinically aggressive HCCs.[743, 744]

Fibrolamellar HCCs almost always stain with A1AT, in contrast to the 50% positivity rate in typical HCCs.[745–751]

HepPar 1 stains all fibrolamellar HCCs.[655]

The AFP staining response is positive in approximately 20% of fibrolamellar HCCs, a lower percentage than is reported for typical HCCs.[741, 745, 746, 748–751] In cases with admixed typical HCC and fibrolamellar HCC, there is a lack of AFP staining in the fibrolamellar regions, but staining does occur in the regions of typical HCC.[752, 753]

Occasional large eosinophilic globules (pale bodies) can be seen within the cytoplasm of fibrolamellar HCCs. These bodies do not stain with A1AT or AFP.[754]

Neuroendocrine differentiation has occasionally been described in fibrolamellar HCCs, with support from electron microscopic findings in some cases.[637, 755, 756]

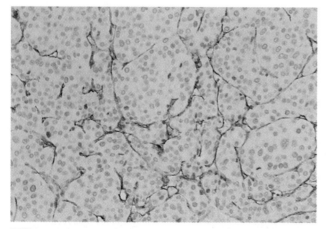

Figure 13–23. Positive CD34 staining of the encircling endothelial layer in a biopsy specimen of hepatocellular carcinoma. (Low-power magnification)

Small Cell Hepatocellular Carcinoma

A rare neoplasm, small cell HCC shares histologic features with high-grade neuroendocrine carcinoma (small cell carcinoma).[757] Immunohistochemical evaluation shows that small cell HCC stains diffusely with keratin AE1/AE3, keratin CAM5.2 (diffuse cytoplasmic staining with no perinuclear dots), and AFP. Neuroendocrine-related antibodies are negative.

Other Subtypes

Yolk sac carcinoma admixed with HCC has been described.[758] This case is interesting because it highlights the immunohistochemical overlap and differences between the two carcinomas. Both are AFP+. However, the yolk sac carcinoma showed positive CEA, placenta-like alkaline phosphatase (PLAP), and EMA, whereas the HCC cells did not stain with these antibodies. This case serves to characterize antibodies that distinguish the two AFP+ carcinomas.

Clear cell HCC, which can histologically mimic primary clear cell HCC as well as metastatic clear cell carcinomas from the kidney, thyroid, and gynecologic tract, has the same immunophenotype as typical HCC.[717]

Metaplastic HCCs with sarcomatous differentiation, including osteosarcoma and chondrosarcoma, are rare (carcinosarcomas). The immunophenotypes of the sarcomatous components that have identifiable cell lineage differentiation are identical to those of primary sarcomas of the same type occurring in the soft tissue.[759]

CHOLANGIOCARCINOMAS

The staining pattern of CCs with most antibodies is similar to that of extrahepatic pancreaticobiliary adenocarcinomas.[85] Given the bile duct differentiation in both lesions, this finding is not surprising. However, there are slight immunophenotypic differences between the two neoplasms. CK17 and CK20 are expressed more often in pancreaticobiliary adenocarcinomas than in CCs, according to the majority of authors (see later section on Pancreas), and a higher percentage of CCs than of extrahepatic pancreaticobiliary adenocarcinomas stain with CK7. This observation may reflect a difference in cell origin or differentiation of the malignant cells between the two neoplasms.[407]

One author has recommended that adenocarcinomas that arise from bile ducts or periductal glands be designated cholangiocarcinoma and those that arise from bile ductules formed by metaplastic hepatocytes be termed cholangiocellular adenocarcinoma.[685] Staining of CCs that arise in noncirrhotic livers has the same staining patterns as those that arise in cirrhotic livers, except the noncirrhotic CCs stain with A1AT but the cirrhotic CCs usually do not.[760] Some patients in the former group may have A1AT deficiency (see later discussion).

CC cells contain predominantly low and some high molecular weight cytokeratins, including CK7, CK8, CK18, and CK19.[644, 645, 650, 713, 725, 729] Accordingly, staining responses to AE1/AE3, CAM5.2, and 35βH11 are usually strongly positive. The staining response of CCs to cytokeratin 34βE12, a high molecular weight antibody that identifies CK5, CK10, CK11, and CK14, is usually negative or weakly positive unless the CC displays squamous differentiation.[9]

KEY DIAGNOSTIC POINTS (Table 13–27)

- Keratin 34βE12: Approximately 25% of CCs are positive with keratin 34βE12. "Positive" cases usually consist of rare, individual cells that stain weakly. Squamous differentiation, especially when modest amounts of keratin are present, is positive, showing moderate to strong staining intensity.[9]
- CK7: Approximately 98% of CCs stain with CK7 (range, 80 to 100%) (Fig. 13–24).[8, 85, 407, 679, 716, 761] In one study, 100% of 20 CCs had more than 50% positive CC cells.[716] Although this issue has not been extensively studied, one study noted a difference in CK7 positivity based on tumor location.[724] All of the central and large duct CCs stained with CK7, compared with only 50% of the peripheral CCs.
- CK20: Only about 20% of CCs stain with CK20 (range, 5 to 50%).[7, 8, 312, 326, 407, 761]
- CK7/CK20 coordinate staining patterns: Although few cases have been studied, 75% of CCs have a CK7+/CK20− pattern.[407]
- CK17: Fifty percent of CCs stain with CK17. "Positive" cases show a spectrum of staining, from scattered, individual cells to diffuse positivity.[327] These results differ from those in extrahepatic pancreaticobiliary adenocarcinomas, which show positivity in almost 90% of cases.[327]
- CK19: Approximately 98% of CCs stain with CK19 (range, 85 to 100%).* CK19 staining of CCs can be patchy. In one study, 15% of tumors had no staining, 25% showed focal staining, and 60% of CCs had staining in more than 50% of the neoplastic cells.[716]
- Monoclonal CEA: Approximately 75% of CCs stain with monoclonal CEA (range, 70 to 90%). The majority of studies report that almost all CCs uniformly stain in a diffuse cytoplasmic distribution.[8, 444, 651, 661, 662, 762, 763] Occasional reports have reported a smaller percentage of CCs staining with monoclonal CEA (approximately 60%); the variety in values may be a reflection of differences in CEA

---

*References 8, 85, 312, 407, 651, 679, 718, 724, 726, 729, 761.

Table 13-27. Antibody Staining of Cholangiocarcinoma

Antibody	Immunostaining	Comments and References*
Keratin AE1/AE3	+	Strong and diffuse cytoplasmic staining of all cases[444]
Keratin 35βH11	+	Strong and diffuse cytoplasmic staining of all cases[651]
Keratin CAM5.2	+	All cholangiocarcinomas (CCs) show strong and diffuse cytoplasmic staining[332, 656, 725, 726, 760, 761]
CK7	+	See text
CK20	R	See text
CK7+/CK20−	+	See text
CK7+/CK20+	R	
CK7−/CK20+	R	
CK7−/CK20−	R	
CK17	+/−	See text
CK19	+	See text
EMA	+	All CCs diffuse strong staining[444, 733, 761]
CA 19-9	+	See text
CEA		
Monoclonal	+	See text
Polyclonal	+	See text
CD 15 (LeuM1)	+	Approximately 80% of CCs respond positively (range, 75 to 100%)[332, 730]
BerEP4	+	Approximately 90% of CCs show diffuse, strong staining[332]
CA125	+/−	Approximately 60% of CCs show diffuse, strong staining[330]
Keratin 34βE12	R	See text
AFP	R	See text
HepPar 1	R	See text
A1AT	R	See text
Factor XIII	R	Positive staining in less than 10% of CCs[651, 730]
S-100	R	Rare "positive" tumors, usually as single cells[377]
B72.3	+	See text
Vimentin	R	See text
Synaptophysin	N	Ref 726
GCDFP-15	N	Ref 849

*Superscript numbers indicate chapter references.
+, almost always positive; N, negative; R, rare, +/−, more positive cases than negative.

clone or preprimary antibody procedures, including heat antigen retrieval versus enzyme digestion.[332, 726, 730]

- Polyclonal CEA: Polyclonal CEA stains a larger percentage of CCs compared with HCCs. Approximately 95% of CCs stain diffusely and strongly with polyclonal CEA (range, 85 to 100%).[332, 444, 656, 718, 726, 729, 732, 760]
- CA 19-9: Approximately 90% of CCs stain with

CA 19-9 (range, 50 to 100%). Staining of the majority of neoplastic cells has a moderate to strong intensity.[8, 329, 331, 651, 661, 662, 718, 760, 762, 763]

- B72.3: Approximately 50% of CCs are positive with B72.3 (range, 25 to 80%).[332, 730]
- AFP: The majority of CCs do not stain with AFP. Some studies note that approximately 10% of CCs do respond positively. The response in these cases consists of rare, indi-

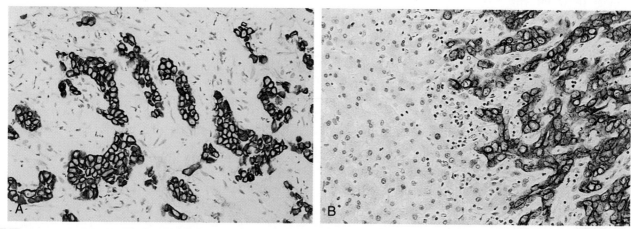

Figure 13-24. A, Cholangiocarcinoma demonstrating positive staining for CK7. (Low-power magnification) *B,* Poorly differentiated cholangiocarcinoma demonstrating intense positive staining of the malignant cells for CK7, whereas the nearby liver shows negative staining. (Intermediate-power magnification)

vidual tumor cells that stain with weak intensity.* Occasional studies note AFP positivity in 20 to 30% of CCs; however, there is no mention in these studies whether biotin blocks were employed prior to the application of the primary antibody.[8, 643, 656]

- HepPar 1: Staining with HepPar 1 occurs in 6 to 12% of CCs.[312, 655, 726] There is usually weak to moderate staining of rare, individual, mucin-secreting columnar cells in a coarse, diffuse cytoplasmic pattern.[312, 655, 726] The strong staining seen in HCCs has not been reported for CCs.
- A1AT: Approximately 10% of sporadic type CCs stain with A1AT (range, 0 to 33%).[656, 730, 760] In contrast, all the CCs that arise in association with A1AT deficiency show extensive staining.[679]
- Vimentin: Overall, approximately 40% of CCs stain with vimentin.[356] Importantly, definitions of tumor classification affect reported percentages. In our experience, vimentin staining of CCs is almost never seen in well-differentiated, moderately differentiated, and poorly differentiated CCs in which glandular differentiation can be observed. Neoplastic CC spindle cells almost always stain with vimentin (see later section on Spindle Cell [Sarcomatoid] CCs). In the clinical situation in which one is evaluating a carcinoma of unknown primary, a glandular or trabecular carcinoma that strongly stains with vimentin is almost never a CC (personal experience).

Spindle Cell (Sarcomatoid) Cholangiocarcinomas

Spindle cell (sarcomatoid) CCs usually have a histologic pattern that is admixed with poorly differentiated, typical CC. Spindled CC cells are usually CEA and AFP negative.[764, 765] Vimentin-positive rhabdoid cells can be admixed with spindle cells. Spindle cell foci can also stain focally with one of the keratins, including AE1/AE3, CAM5.2, and 35βH11, and are EMA+.[764, 766] As in any spindled carcinoma, spindle CC cells can focally express actin and, rarely, desmin (personal experience). S-100 protein and AFP are negative.[764–766]

Immunohistochemical distinction between pure spindled CC and pure spindled HCC is unreliable. Fortunately, the spindle cell pattern in both carcinomas is usually associated with high-grade typical (epithelioid architecture) HCC or CC. Tissue blocks chosen for immunohistochemistry should be from the epithelioid architecture regions rather than the spindled areas. See the later sections, Poorly Differentiated and Undifferentiated Carcinomas and Mixed Hepatocellular Carcinoma–Cholangiocarcinoma, for additional comments.

---

*References 332, 651, 718, 726, 730, 732, 760.

Mixed, Adenosquamous, and Clear Cell Cholangiocarcinomas

Mixed, adenosquamous, and clear cell variants of CC have been described that stain with antigens characteristic for each of their cellular constituents, including involucrin staining of the squamous regions.[717, 761, 767–770] Unlike typical CCs, some clear cell CCs have occasionally been noted to be negative with CEA.[767]

BILIARY CYSTADENOMAS AND CYSTADENOCARCINOMAS

Intrahepatic biliary cystadenomas and cystadenocarcinomas are similar in cytokeratin profile to their pancreaticobiliary counterparts. The phenotype of associated invasive adenocarcinomas in the pancreatobiliary counterparts is identical to that of pancreaticobiliary adenocarcinomas, although cytokeratin subset staining studies have not been performed, to our knowledge.

The epithelial cells stain diffusely and strongly with keratin AE1/AE3, CA 19-9, and CEA.[771–775] Admixed, single cells that stain with both chromogranin and synaptophysin are present in 50% of cases.[776] Some neoplasms have ovarian-like stroma that surrounds the epithelium-lined cysts. These stromal cells can stain with vimentin, SMA, and desmin but do not stain with cytokeratin, EMA, CEA, chromogranin, or synaptophysin.[771, 772] Estrogen and progesterone receptors have occasionally been demonstrated within the surrounding mesenchymal stromal cells of cystadenomas.[777, 778] Smooth muscle cells that display positivity to desmin, MSA, and SMA have also been reported to surround the biliary epithelium.[773] These smooth muscle cells were admixed with bland spindle cells that were unlike ovarian stromal cells.

MIXED HEPATOCELLULAR CARCINOMA– CHOLANGIOCARCINOMA

Mixed HCC-CCs are uncommon. Criteria for categorizing a hepatic carcinoma as mixed HCC-CC has differed among authors, making it difficult to summarize the immunohistochemical results. We restrict the immunohistochemical definition of mixed HCC-CCs to neoplasms with regions that have the global immunohistochemical profile characteristic of both HCC and CC. The definition of mixed HCC-CC carcinoma also depends to a great extent on a tumor's grade. There are well-differentiated, mixed neoplasms in which HCC and CC can be clearly distinguished on the basis of standard histologic features.[779] Less well-differentiated neoplasms have regions in which the tubular pattern of CC is contiguous to acinar, trabecular, or solid pattern HCC with zones of transitional-appearing cells.[779] Unlike some authors,[779] we do not regard as a mixed HCC-CC any primary hepatic carcinoma that is composed of undifferentiated cells such that it is impossible to classify histologically as CC or HCC. We label these neoplasms "undifferentiated carcinomas" (see later).

In those cases with well-defined regions of HCC and CC (collision type carcinomas), including the neoplasms with or without transition regions, the immunohistochemical phenotype of each morphologically classifiable region is identical to the phenotype of the corresponding pure neoplasm.[312, 724, 730, 779–781]

Tubules and transition regions in carcinomas in which the tubular pattern of CC is contiguous to HCC with a trabecular or solid pattern stain with CK7 and CK19 in most cases,[724, 779] indicating a bile duct differentiation, according to some authors.[779] However (and even though not directly related to immunohistochemistry), the cells forming the CK7+ and CK19+ tubular structures in HCC-CCs contain albumin mRNA, which is a feature of hepatocyte differentiation.[724] In contrast to findings in intrahepatic bile ducts and cholangiocarcinomas, CK20 has also been identified in approximately 50% of these tubular-transition regions.[312] AFP staining has been positive in tubular and transition regions in 0 to 50% of cases.[779, 782]

The authors of one study, with whom we agree, concluded that cells with mixed hepatocyte and biliary differentiation can be found in carcinomas that histologically are pure HCC, pure CC, or mixed HCC-CC.[649] Given the evidence of hepatic stem cells that can show differentiation toward hepatocytes, biliary cells, or both, a malignant counterpart can also be expected (see the earlier general comments about HCCs of the usual type). We do not label as mixed HCC-CC any carcinoma that has the characteristic histologic features of HCC or CC but is immunohistochemically shown to have cells that express a biliary or hepatic type immunophenotype.

POORLY DIFFERENTIATED AND UNDIFFERENTIATED CARCINOMAS

Poorly differentiated primary hepatic carcinoma has been classified as mixed HCC-CC by some authors.[779] Spindled cell regions can be admixed.[783] In the context that cytokeratin subset expression reflects, to a large extent, the degree of differentiation within carcinoma cells, expression of a small number of cytokeratin subtypes in poorly differentiated primary hepatic carcinoma cells does not necessarily imply true biliary differentiation. We believe that it is imprudent to diagnose this type of carcinoma definitively as HCC, CC, or mixed HCC-CC on the basis of immunohistochemistry. Electron microscopy may be beneficial in these instances as an additional ancillary test. Another alternative is to make the diagnosis "primary hepatic, poorly differentiated carcinoma."

These neoplasms usually are positive with CK7 and CK19 but do not stain with CEA, CA 19-9, AFP, or HepPar 1.[779] Vimentin is frequently positive, even within epithelioid carcinoma cells, a finding that is unusual in either HCC or CC (personal experience).

Primary hepatic undifferentiated "carcinoma" with rhabdoid cytologic features is rare. Such a tumor can arise in a child or, in our experience, can be seen as a component of a high-grade HCC. In children, the neoplastic cells stain diffusely and strongly with vimentin and cytokeratin CAM5.2. Staining with EMA and CD99 (MIC2) is patchy and variable.[784]

Primary hepatic undifferentiated carcinoma, or lymphoepithelioma-like carcinoma, has rarely been described in the liver.[785] The carcinoma cells stain with cytokeratin AE1/AE3 and EMA and do not stain with CEA, CD30 (BerH2), or S-100 protein.[785]

PRIMARY HEPATIC NEUROENDOCRINE NEOPLASMS

Most neuroendocrine carcinomas in the liver are metastatic. Rare primary hepatic neuroendocrine carcinomas of all grades have occasionally been reported, ranging from low-grade carcinoid to high-grade, small cell carcinoma.[786, 787] Their immunophenotype is identical to that of GI and pancreatic neuroendocrine carcinomas (Fig. 13–25).[788–799] AFP has been negative in the few characterized cases.[265] We have stained two primary hepatic high-grade neuroendocrine carcinomas (small cell carcinomas) with CK20, and both were negative.

Calcitonin positivity has occasionally been described in primary hepatic, pancreatic, and duodenal neuroendocrine carcinomas.[800] In the context of evaluating a potentially metastatic neuroendocrine carcinoma in the liver, calcitonin positivity does not always establish a diagnosis of metastatic thyroid medullary carcinoma.

Approximately 95% of pulmonary small cell carcinomas and 75% of pulmonary large cell neuroendocrine carcinomas are TTF-1+.[552] In our experience, TTF-1 did not stain two high-grade gallbladder-hepatic small cell carcinomas.

Although not strictly a neuroendocrine carcinoma, primary hepatic desmoplastic small round cell tumor has rarely been described.[801] This neoplasm should be considered in the immunohistochemical differential diagnosis of intermediate- and high-grade neuroendocrine (and rhabdoid) carcinomas, especially if the patient is young.

Rare adenocarcinoids of the liver, with an immunophenotype identical to that of such tumors occurring in the appendix, have been described, including within the goblet cell component (see earlier discussion in the GI section).[802]

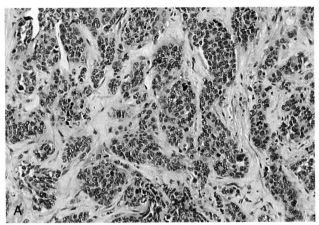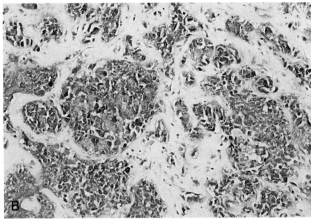

Figure 13–25. *A,* Metastatic, poorly differentiated malignancy in the liver showing histologic features of a large cell neuroendocrine carcinoma. (Intermediate-power magnification) *B,* Neuroendocrine differentiation was confirmed with a panel of immunoperoxidase stains, including positive staining of the cells for synaptophysin. A lung primary was found. (Intermediate-power magnification)

Differential Diagnostic Panels
Hepatocellular Carcinoma Versus Cholangiocarcinoma (Table 13–28)

Opinions differ regarding what antibody battery should be used to distinguish HCC and CC. A major reason for the differing opinions is that a large study using many antibodies and cases has not been performed. Another contributing reason is the grouping together of metastatic pancreaticobiliary adenocarcinomas and primary CCs in some studies. Some studies have suggested that although the staining patterns in primary hepatic CCs and metastatic pancreaticobiliary adenocarcinomas are identical for many antibodies, they may differ in regard to other antibodies, such as CK7, CK17, and CK20. This issue has not been extensively studied.

A third reason is that there are various definitions of poorly differentiated HCC, mixed HCC-CC, and poorly differentiated CC. As discussed previously, some authors choose to classify any primary hepatic carcinoma as a mixed HCC-CC if it displays biliary type cytokeratin or monoclonal CEA staining, whereas others, including us, consider the finding of such staining both permissible and not unexpected in HCCs, especially those that are poorly differentiated. Finally, as a primary hepatic carcinoma becomes less well-differentiated, the ability to distinguish between HCC and CC is increasingly difficult because of coexpression or lack of expression of antigens that are thought to represent hepatocyte or biliary differentiation. We diagnose these cases as primary hepatic undifferentiated carcinoma (see earlier section on Poorly Differentiated and Undifferentiated Carcinomas). We present the following diagnostic antibody panel with the intention that the reader keep our views on these issues in mind.

Antibodies: CK7, CK19, CEA (monoclonal and polyclonal), CA 19-9, HepPar 1, AFP, A1AT, B72.3

The stains that positively identify CCs are CK7, CK19, monoclonal CEA, CA 19-9, and B72.3. HCCs in general show no or weak patchy staining with CK7, CK19, and monoclonal CEA, whereas the overwhelming majority of CCs show diffuse strong cytoplasmic staining with these antibodies.[8, 444, 651, 718, 730] Few HCCs stain with CA 19-9 or B72.3, and those that are "positive" display patchy to weak cytoplasmic staining.[8] In contrast, at least 50% of CCs show diffuse strong staining with either antibody.[329, 332, 651, 718, 730] Because of this overlap, only diffuse strong staining is supportive of a diagnosis of CC; weak or no staining is diagnostically noncontributory.

The stains that positively identify HCC include polyclonal CEA, HepPar 1, AFP, and A1AT. Polyclonal CEA stains some to almost all HCCs in a canalicular pattern, compared with the diffuse cy-

Table 13–28. Hepatocellular Carcinoma (HCC) Versus Cholangiocarcinoma (CC)

Antibody	Result HCC	CC
AE1/AE3	R–N (useful if negative)	+
CK7	R	+
CK17	N	R–N (useful if positive)
CK19	R	+
CEA		
Monoclonal	R	+
Polyclonal, canalicular pattern	+/−	N
CA 19-9	N	+
B72.3	R	+
HepPar 1	+	R
AFP	+/− (useful if positive)	R
A1AT	+/− (useful if positive)	R

+, almost always positive; N, negative; R, rare; R–N, rare to negative; +/−, more positive cases than negative.

toplasmic staining pattern seen in almost all CCs. A minority of HCCs produce a diffuse cytoplasmic staining pattern with polyclonal CEA. Therefore, diffuse cytoplasmic staining of a neoplasm with polyclonal CEA does not contribute to a diagnosis, whereas a canalicular pattern points to HCC.[444, 651]

HepPar 1 stains almost all HCCs but only about 10% of CCs.[312, 655, 726] In our experience, HepPar 1 staining of CCs is usually on the single cell or small cell group level, compared with diffuse or regional type, patchy staining in HCCs.

Although AFP staining is not sensitive and is seen in approximately 50% of HCCs, it is extremely specific. Staining of typical CCs with use of biotin blocking prior to application of the primary antibody, as described earlier, has not been reported.

A1AT stains approximately 80% of HCCs but less than 10% of sporadic CCs. Caution regarding this antibody is advised if the A1AT deficiency status of the patient is unknown, because all CCs that arise in association with A1AT are diffuse and strongly A1AT+.

The utility of keratin CAM5.2 and factor XIII as components of a differential antibody panel is unclear, so we do not recommend their use at this time. One group of authors noted that most HCCs stain with keratin CAM5.2 in a membranous pattern but that most non-HCC adenocarcinomas do not.[726] We have observed that the distinction between cytoplasmic and membrane staining is not always clear. Some authors have suggested that factor XIII is a useful antibody for discriminating between HCC and CC.[730] However, other authors have reported significantly disparate staining results in HCCs (see earlier).

Hepatocellular Carcinoma Versus Adenocarcinomas Other Than Cholangiocarcinoma

Antibodies: CK7, CK19, CK20, HepPar 1, additional adenocarcinoma-specific antibodies

In general, HCCs do not stain with CK7, CK19, or CK20 but do stain with HepPar 1. Therefore, significant staining of a neoplasm with any of these cytokeratin antibodies and lack of staining with HepPar 1 constitute supportive evidence that the neoplasm is not an HCC. Additional, adenocarcinoma-specific antibodies are useful in the further characterization of the site of origin (see Chapter 7).

Hepatocellular Versus Neuroendocrine Carcinoma (Carcinoid–Small Cell Undifferentiated Carcinoma)

Antibodies: chromogranin, synaptophysin, CD57, CEA (monoclonal), HepPar 1, AFP, keratin CAM5.2, TTF

Primary hepatic or metastatic neuroendocrine carcinomas (carcinoids–small cell neuroendocrine carcinomas) and HCCs can be histologically simi-

lar, especially the small acinar pattern of HCC.[794] Neuroendocrine carcinomas usually stain with chromogranin, synaptophysin, PGP, or CD57 (Leu7) and do not stain with HepPar 1 or AFP.[15–30, 33, 503, 507, 509, 510, 516, 517, 655, 730, 803]

Metastatic pulmonary and foregut neuroendocrine carcinomas, including some primary hepatic neoplasms, stain with monoclonal CEA and TTF, features that also are not seen in HCCs (personal experience).[552] Staining of neuroendocrine carcinomas frequently occurs in a perinuclear dot distribution with cytokeratin CAM5.2.[517, 518] HCCs are usually positive with cytokeratin CAM5.2, in a diffusely cytoplasmic or membranous pattern rather than the perinuclear dot pattern seen in neuroendocrine carcinoma.

In contrast, HCCs usually stain with HepPar 1 and occasionally with AFP and do not stain or show only focal weak staining with synaptophysin, chromogranin, and CD57.[719]

CD56 (NCAM, Leu19) staining is not useful in distinguishing between the two neoplasms, because HCCs can respond positively to this antibody.

Hepatocellular Versus Renal Cell Carcinoma

Antibodies: HepPar 1, AFP

The immunophenotypes of HCC and RCC are similar. To date, no antibody positively stains only RCCs. HepPar 1 stains the majority of HCCs and (to date) does not stain RCCs. Caution is advised with this antibody in regard to RCCs that contain numerous cytoplasmic lysosomes or vesicles, which can nonspecifically stain with chromogens and produce false-positive results. Examination of "negative" control slides is mandatory in this situation.

HCCs usually stain with AFP (see earlier), in contrast to RCCs, in which AFP+ tumors constitute isolated case reports.[804]

Hepatocellular Versus Adrenal Cortical Carcinoma (Table 13–29)

Antibodies: HepPar 1, inhibin, melan-A (A103), keratin CAM5.2

HCCs stain with keratin CAM5.2 and HepPar 1 and do not stain with inhibin or melan-A.[734] Con-

Table 13–29. Hepatocellular Carcinoma (HCC) Versus Adrenal Cortical Carcinoma

Antibody	Result	
	HCC	*Adrenal Carcinoma*
HepPar 1	+	N
Keratin CAM5.2	+	R
Inhibin	N	+
Melan-A (A103)	N	+

+, almost always positive; N, negative; R, rare.

Table 13–30. Hepatocellular Carcinoma (HCC) Versus Ovarian Granulosa Cell Tumor

Antibody	Result	
	HCC	*Granulosa Cell Tumor*
HepPar 1	+	N
Keratin CAM5.2	+	R
Inhibin	N	+
Vimentin	N	+

+, almost always positive; N, negative; R, rare.

versely, approximately 50% and 75% of adrenal carcinomas stain with inhibin and melan-A, respectively, and do not stain with HepPar 1.[734] The latter neoplasms also show either no or extremely focal staining with keratin CAM5.2.[390]

Hepatocellular Carcinoma Versus Ovarian Granulosa Cell Tumor (Table 13–30)

Antibodies: inhibin, vimentin, HepPar 1, keratin CAM5.2

Ovarian granulosa cell tumors rarely metastasize. When they disseminate in the abdominal cavity, however, they frequently produce histologic challenges, especially if the primary ovarian neoplasm occurred many years prior to the metastases or was unknown. HCC and ovarian granulosa cell neoplasms can be histologically similar, and immunohistochemistry is frequently useful in distinguishing between them.[805] HCCs stain with HepPar 1 and cytokeratin CAM5.2 and do not stain with inhibin or vimentin; granulosa cell tumors display the opposite staining pattern. It is important to ensure a sufficient amount of biotin blockage in liver tissue, because false-positive staining with antibodies such as inhibin has been noted (see earlier discussion).

Cholangiocarcinoma Versus Colorectal Adenocarcinoma (Table 13–31)

Antibodies: CK7, CK20

CC and colorectal adenocarcinoma show opposite staining patterns with CK7 and CK20. Intrahepatic CC usually stains with CK7 and rarely with CK20.[8] Conversely, colorectal adenocarcinoma

Table 13–31. Cholangiocarcinoma (CC) Versus Colorectal Adenocarcinoma

Antibody	Result	
	CC	*Colorectal Adenocarcinoma*
CK7+/CK20−	+	N
CK7−/CK20+	R	+

+, almost always positive; N, negative; R, rare.

usually stains with CK20 and rarely with CK7. Approximately 75% of CCs expresses a CK7+/CK20− coordinate staining pattern, but no colorectal adenocarcinomas do so. Approximately 75% of colorectal adenocarcinomas express a CK7−/CK20+ staining pattern, compared with less than 10% of CCs. There is considerable overlap in the other staining patterns between the two neoplasms.[6, 370, 380, 407, 411]

Cholangiocarcinoma Versus Breast Carcinoma (Table 13–32)

Antibodies: ER, GCDFP-15, S-100 protein, CK17

Breast carcinomas can stain with ER, GCDFP-15, or S-100 protein. If these antibodies are positive, they are supportive of the diagnosis of a breast primary tumor. However, some breast carcinomas do not stain with these antibodies, so the lack of staining in a carcinoma is diagnostically noncontributory. Similarly, the CK17 response can be positive in CCs, a useful feature because breast carcinomas respond negatively. However, many CCs do not stain with CK17, making a negative response to this antibody also noncontributory.

Cholangiocarcinoma Versus Gastric Carcinoma

There is no reliable differential immunohistochemical profile that will separate CC from gastric carcinoma.[407]

Cholangiocarcinoma Versus Metastatic Pancreaticobiliary or Gallbladder Carcinoma

Although there are slight differences in the immunohistochemical phenotypes of CC and metastatic pancreaticobiliary or gallbladder carcinoma, an immunohistochemical distinction between them cannot be made.

Mesenchymal Lesions

ANGIOMYOLIPOMA

Angiomyolipoma (AML) can occasionally develop in the liver.[806–808] There is little need for

Table 13–32. Cholangiocarcinoma (CC) Versus Breast Ductal and Breast Lobular Carcinoma

Antibody	Result		
	CC	*Lobular*	*Ductal*
ER	N	+/−	+/−
GCDFP-15	N	+/−	+/−
S-100 protein	N	−/+	−/+
CK17	+/− (useful if positive)	N	N

N, negative; +/−, more positive cases than negative; −/+ more negative cases than positive.

immunohistochemical evaluation when the lesion is composed of an admixture of thick-walled vessels, adipose tissue, and spindled smooth muscle cells. However, immunohistochemical evaluation is especially helpful in dealing with an atypical AML, especially one composed predominantly of smooth muscle cells. Smooth muscle cells of AMLs can be spindled or epithelioid; the latter feature brings carcinoma, especially HCC, into the differential diagnosis. The "smooth muscle" cells of AMLs can display minimal smooth muscle differentiation and, therefore, may stain only focally with desmin or the actins.[510] These cells are cytokeratin-negative and vimentin-positive, distinguishing AML from HCC. They also characteristically stain in a patchy distribution with HMB-45 and MART-1 (melan-A).[510, 806, 809]

The difficult task with hepatic AML is to remember that AML can occur in the liver. Once the possibility of hepatic AML is raised, establishing or ruling out the diagnosis through the use of immunohistochemistry is straightforward.

EPITHELIOID HEMANGIOENDOTHELIOMA

Epithelioid hemangioendothelioma (EHE) is an intermediate-grade malignant vascular neoplasm. The neoplastic cells range in shape from epithelioid to dendritic.[810–812] The neoplastic cells, regardless of shape, stain with endothelium-related antibodies, including CD31, CD34, factor VIII, and *Ulex* 1.[811–828] Although some authors have found the staining prevalences of neoplastic vascular cells to be similar for the different vascular antibodies,[822] others have found that factor VIII monoclonal antibody stains a greater proportion of tumors than CD34 and CD31 (90%, 74%, and 33%, respectively).[812] We have found that staining with all of these antibodies can be patchy and variable within the same neoplasm; therefore, a panel of these antibodies is strongly recommended. *Ulex* is less useful because it stains hepatocytes in addition to the neoplastic cells, a finding that can produce problems in the distinction of neoplastic cells.[816]

EHE cells stain with factor XIIIa.[822] Benign dendritic cells likewise stain with factor XIIIa, and many of them are found admixed with the malignant EHE cells.[811] The admixed benign dendritic cells also stain with S-100 protein, MAC387, and CD68, which do not stain the neoplastic vascular cells.[811] CD1a stains neither EHE cells nor admixed benign dendritic cells.[811] Interestingly, primary hepatic EHEs have an immunohistochemically detected basement membrane component profile that closely resembles that of the normal liver, whereas the profile of pulmonary EHEs is similar to that of lung basement membranes.[815] These findings suggest that EHEs arise from local endothelial cell proliferation, and may represent multicentricity, rather than metastases, when multiple neoplasms are found.[815]

Approximately 15 to 50% of EHE cells stain with keratin AE1/AE3,[812] and approximately 30% are keratin CAM5.2+.[812, 813, 822] EHE cells also can focally and occasionally stain with S-100 protein and SMA.[812] EMA does not stain EHE cells.[812, 825]

The histologic distinction among EHE, HCC, and CC can be difficult because of the histologic and immunohistochemical phenotypic similarities. We believe that an appropriate antibody battery to distinguish EHE and HCC or CC consists of vimentin, CD31, CD34, factor VIII, and EMA.[813, 823] Vimentin and the endothelial antibodies stain EHE but not HCC or CC, whereas the latter two neoplasms do stain with EMA. Cytokeratin antibodies are not useful, because all three neoplasms may be positive.

ADDITIONAL MESENCHYMAL NEOPLASMS

Solitary fibrous tumor can rarely occur in the liver. Identical in immunophenotype to those neoplasms that arise in association with the pleura, solitary fibrous tumors usually stain with CD34 but do not stain with S-100 protein, NSE, desmin, smooth muscle actin, EMA, or cytokeratin CAM5.2.[829–833]

Follicular dendritic cell tumor can rarely involve the liver, as either a primary or metastatic process.[834–837] Follicular dendritic neoplasms usually stain with CD21 and several other antibodies, the responses to which are negative in inflammatory myofibroblastic neoplasms.[834]

Inflammatory myofibroblastic tumors (inflammatory pseudotumor) can occasionally arise in the liver.[535, 838] The spindle cells in these neoplasms are cytokeratin- and EMA-negative and show actin HHF-35 positivity. In our experience, they also can show focal positivity for CD34, SMA, and S-100 protein.

Infantile hemangioendothelioma is composed of immature endothelial cells and admixed hepatic parenchyma. The endothelial cells stain with vimentin, factor VIII, and CD31, suggesting that these cells differ from the endothelial cells of the normal adult liver, which rarely stain with the latter two antibodies.[839]

References

1. Gown AM. Immunohistochemical determination of primary sites of carcinomas. J Histotechnol 1999;22:209–215.
2. Gown AM. Uses of antibody panels in the analysis of metastatic carcinomas of unknown origin primary. Acta Histochem Cytochem 1999;32:153–159.
3. Moll R. Cytokeratins as markers of differentiation in the diagnosis of epithelial tumors. Subcell Biochem 1998;31:205–262.
4. Weber K, Osborn M, Moll R, et al. Tissue polypeptide antigen (TPA) is related to the non-epidermal keratins 8, 18 and 19 typical of simple and non-squamous epithelia: Re-evaluation of a human tumor marker. EMBO J 1984;3:2707–2714.
5. Woodcock-Mitchell J, Eichner R, Nelson WG, Sun TT. Im-

munolocalization of keratin polypeptides in human epidermis using monoclonal antibodies. J Cell Biol 1982;95:580–588.

6. Wang NP, Zee S, Zarbo RJ, et al. Coordinate expression of cytokeratins 7 and 20 defines unique subsets of carcinomas. Appl Immunohistochem 1995;3:99–107.

7. Alexander J, Krishnamurthy S, Kovacs D, Dayal Y. Cytokeratin profile of extrahepatic pancreaticobiliary epithelia and their carcinomas. Appl Immunohistochem 1997;5:216–222.

8. Maeda T, Kajiyama K, Adachi E, et al. The expression of cytokeratins 7, 19, and 20 in primary and metastatic carcinomas of the liver. Mod Pathol 1996;9:901–909.

9. Maeda T, Takenaka K, Taguchi K, et al. Adenosquamous carcinoma of the liver: Clinicopathologic characteristics and cytokeratin profile. Cancer 1997;80:364–371.

10. Watt SM, Sala-Newby G, Hoang T, et al. CD66 identifies a neutrophil-specific epitope within the hematopoietic system that is expressed by members of the carcinoembryonic antigen family of adhesion molecules. Blood 1991;78:63–74.

11. Grunert F, Daniel S, Nagel G, et al. CD66b, CD66c and carcinoembryonic antigen (CEA) are independently regulated markers in sera of tumor patients. Int J Cancer 1995;63:349–355.

12. Tsutsumi Y, Nagura H, Watanabe K. Immunohistochemical observations of carcinoembryonic antigen (CEA) and CEA-related substances in normal and neoplastic pancreas: Pitfalls and caveats in CEA immunohistochemistry. Am J Clin Pathol 1984;82:535–542.

13. Larsson A, Ghosh R, Hammarstrom S. Relative positions of some epitopes on carcinoembryonic antigen. Cancer Immunol Immunother 1989;30:92–96.

14. Lewin KJ, Ulich T, Yang K, Layfield L. The endocrine cells of the gastrointestinal tract. Tumors. Part II. Pathol Annu 1986;21(Part 2):181–215.

15. Capella C, Riva C, Rindi G, et al. Histopathology, hormone products, and clinico-pathologic profile of endocrine tumors of the upper small intestine: A study of 44 cases. Endocr Pathol 1991;2:92–110.

16. Thomas RM, Baybick JH, Elsayed AM, Sobin LH. Gastric carcinoids: An immunohistochemical and clinicopathologic study of 104 patients. Cancer 1994;73:2053–2058.

17. Gilligan CJ, Lawton GP, Tang LH, et al. Gastric carcinoid tumors: The biology and therapy of an enigmatic and controversial lesion. Am J Gastroenterol 1995;90:338–352.

18. Azzoni C, Doglioni C, Viale G, et al. Involvement of BCL-2 oncoprotein in the development of enterochromaffin-like cell gastric carcinoids. Am J Surg Pathol 1996;20:433–441.

19. Bordi C, Yu JY, Baggi MT, et al. Gastric carcinoids and their precursor lesions: A histologic and immunohistochemical study of 23 cases. Cancer 1991;67:663–672.

20. Burke AP, Federspiel BH, Sobin LH, et al. Carcinoids of the duodenum: A histologic and immunohistochemical study of 65 tumors. Am J Surg Pathol 1989;13:828–837.

21. Facer P, Bishop AE, Lloyd RV, et al. Chromogranin: A newly recognized marker for endocrine cells of the human gastrointestinal tract. Gastroenterology 1985;89:1366–1373.

22. Al-Khafaji B, Noffsinger AE, Miller MA, et al. Immunohistologic analysis of gastrointestinal and pulmonary carcinoid tumors. Hum Pathol 1998;29:992–999.

23. Hayashi H, Nakagawa M, Kitagawa S, et al. Immunohistochemical analysis of gastrointestinal carcinoids. Gastroenterol Jpn 1993;28:483–490.

24. Wiedenmann B, Waldherr R, Buhr H, et al. Identification of gastroenteropancreatic neuroendocrine cells in normal and neoplastic human tissue with antibodies against synaptophysin, chromogranin A, secretogranin I (chromogranin B), and secretogranin II. Gastroenterology 1988;95:1364–1374.

25. Le Gall F, Vallet VS, Thomas D, et al. Immunohistochemical study of secretogranin II in 62 neuroendocrine tumors of the digestive tract and of the pancreas in comparison with other granins. Pathol Res Pract 1997;193:179–185.

26. Wiedenmann B, Kuhn C, Schwechheimer K, et al. Synaptophysin identified in metastases of neuroendocrine tumors by immunocytochemistry and immunoblotting. Am J Clin Pathol 1987;88:560–569.

27. Gould VE, Wiedenmann B, Lee I, et al. Synaptophysin expression in neuroendocrine neoplasms as determined by immunocytochemistry. Am J Pathol 1987;126:243–257.

28. Mertz H, Vyberg M, Paulsen SM, Teglbjaerg PS. Immunohistochemical detection of neuroendocrine markers in tumors of the lungs and gastrointestinal tract. Appl Immunohistochem 1998;6:175–180.

29. Makhlouf HR, Burke AP, Sobin LH. Carcinoid tumors of the ampulla of Vater: A comparison with duodenal carcinoid tumors. Cancer 1999;85:1241–1249.

30. Capella C, Heitz PU, Hofler H, et al. Revised classification of neuroendocrine tumors of the lung, pancreas and gut. Virchows Arch 1995;425:547–560.

31. Cetin Y. Chromogranin A immunoreactivity and Grimelius' argyrophilia: A correlative study in mammalian endocrine cells. Anat Embryol (Berl) 1992;185:207–215.

32. Shipley WR, Hammer RD, Lennington WJ, Macon WR. Paraffin immunohistochemical detection of CD56, a useful marker for neural cell adhesion molecule (NCAM), in normal and neoplastic fixed tissues. Appl Immunohistochem 1997;5:87–93.

33. Kaufmann OK, George T, Dietel M. Utility of 123C3 monoclonal antibody against CD56 (NCAM) for the diagnosis of small cell carcinomas on paraffin sections. Hum Pathol 1997;28:1373–1378.

34. Moyana TN. Gastrointestinal endocrine cells and carcinoids: Histogenetic and pathogenetic considerations. Pathol Annu 1995;30(Part 1):227–246.

35. Raju GC. Occurrence and expression of cytokeratins in carcinoid tumors of the gastrointestinal tract and their probable precursor cells. Ann Acad Med Singapore 1989;18:298–301.

36. Hofler H, Denk H. Immunocytochemical demonstration of cytokeratin in gastrointestinal carcinoids and their probable precursor cells. Virchows Arch 1984;403:235–240.

37. Zhang PJ, Harris KR, Alobeid B, Brooks JJ. Immunoexpression of villin in neuroendocrine tumors and its diagnostic implications. Arch Pathol Lab Med 1999;123:812–816.

38. Gupta NM, Goenka MK, Atri A, Vaiphei K. Carcinoid tumour of the esophagus: A rare esophageal cancer. Eur J Surg 1996;162:841–844.

39. Brown RSJ, Peppercorn MA, Farraye FA, et al. Carcinoid tumor of the esophagus. J Clin Gastroenterol 1994;19:338–339.

40. Einspanier GR, Caleel RT, Milford AF. Carcinoid tumors of the esophagus: Report of a case. J Am Osteopath Assoc 1987;87:500–503.

41. Vaideeswar P, Sivaraman A, Deshpande JR. Primary malignant carcinoid of the esophagus. Indian J Gastroenterol 1994;13:67–68.

42. Muller J, Kirchner T, Muller-Hermelink HK. Gastric endocrine cell hyperplasia and carcinoid tumors in atrophic gastritis type A. Am J Surg Pathol 1987;11:909–917.

43. Berendt RC, Jewell LD, Shnitka TK, et al. Multicentric gastric carcinoids complicating pernicious anemia: Origin from the metaplastic endocrine cell population. Arch Pathol Lab Med 1989;113:399–403.

44. Fahrenkamp AG, Wibbeke C, Winde G, et al. Immunohistochemical distribution of chromogranins A and B and secretogranin II in neuroendocrine tumors of the gastrointestinal tract. Virchows Arch 1995;426:361–367.

45. Rindi G. Clinicopathologic aspects of gastric neuroendocrine tumors. Am J Surg Pathol 1995;19(Suppl 1):S20–S29.

46. Smith AM, Watson SA, Caplin M, et al. Gastric carcinoid expresses the gastrin autocrine pathway. Br J Surg 1998;85:1285–1289.

47. Wilander E. Diagnostic pathology of gastrointestinal and pancreatic neuroendocrine tumours. Acta Oncol 1989;28:363–369.

48. Solcia E, Capella C, Fiocca R, et al. Disorders of the endocrine system. In: Ming S-C, Goldman H, eds. Pathology of the Gastrointestinal Tract. Baltimore, Williams & Wilkins, 1998:295–322.

49. Lewin KJ, Riddell RH, Weinstein WM. Gastrointestinal Pathology and Its Clinical Implications. New York, Igaku-Shoin, 1992.

50. Solcia E, Bordi C, Creutzfeldt W, et al. Histopathological classification of nonantral gastric endocrine growths in man. Digestion 1988;41:185–200.

51. Dayal Y. Hyperplastic proliferations of the ECL cells. Yale J Biol Med 1992;65:805–825.

52. D'Adda T, Annibale B, Delle FG, Bordi C. Oxyntic endocrine cells of hypergastrinemic patients: Differential response to antrectomy or octreotide. Gut 1996;38:668–674.

53. Solcia E, Capella C, Fiocca R, et al. Disorders of the endocrine system. In: Ming S-C, Goldman H, eds. Pathology of the Gastrointestinal Tract. Baltimore, Williams & Wilkins, 1998:295–322.

54. Hirschowitz BI, Griffith J, Pellegrin D, Cummings OW. Rapid regression of enterochromaffin-like cell gastric carcinoids in pernicious anemia after antrectomy. Gastroenterology 1992;102:1409–1418.

55. Ordonez NG, Mackay B, El-Naggar A, et al. Clear cell carcinoid tumour of the stomach. Histopathology 1993;22:190–193.

56. Werbel GB, Nelson SP, Robinson PG, et al. A foregut carcinoid tumor causing Zollinger-Ellison syndrome. Arch Surg 1989;124:381–384.

57. Luk IS, Bhuta S, Lewin KJ. Clear cell carcinoid tumor of stomach: A variant mimicking gastric xanthelasma. Arch Pathol Lab Med 1997;121:1100–1103.

58. Klappenbach RS, Kurman RJ, Sinclair CF, James LP. Composite carcinoma-carcinoid tumors of the gastrointestinal tract: A morphologic, histochemical, and immunocytochemical study. Am J Clin Pathol 1985;84:137–143.

59. Sundler F, Hakanson R. Gastric endocrine cell typing at the light microscopic level. In: Hakason R, Sundler F, eds. The Stomach as an Endocrine Organ. Amsterdam, Elsevier Science Publishers, 1991:9–26.

60. Borch K, Renvall H, Kullman E, Wilander E. Gastric carcinoid associated with the syndrome of hypergastrinemic atrophic gastritis. Am J Surg Pathol 1987;11:435–444.

61. Kimura N, Sasano N, Namiki TS, Nakazato Y. Coexpression of cytokeratin, neurofilament, and vimentin in carcinoid tumors. Virchows Arch 1989;415:69–77.

62. Krishnamurthy S, Sarkar S, Palkar VM, et al. Gastric carcinoids—a clinicopathologic study. Indian J Gastroenterol 1998;17:90–92.

63. Moyana TN, Shukoor S. Gastrointestinal endocrine cell hyperplasia in celiac disease: A selective proliferative process of serotonergic cells. Mod Pathol 1991;4:419–423.

64. Pietroletti R, Bishop AE, Carlei F, et al. Gut endocrine cell population in coeliac disease estimated by immunocytochemistry using a monoclonal antibody to chromogranin. Gut 1986;27:838–843.

65. De Schryver-Kecskemeti K, Clouse RE, Kraus FT. Surgical pathology of gastric and duodenal neuroendocrine tumors masquerading clinically as common polyps. Semin Diagn Pathol 1984;1:5–12.

66. Lundqvist M, Eriksson B, Oberg K, Wilander E. Histogenesis of a duodenal carcinoid. Pathol Res Pract 1989;184:217–222.

67. Stamm B, Hedinger CE, Saremaslani P. Duodenal and ampullary carcinoid tumors: A report of 12 cases with pathological characteristics, polypeptide content and relation to the MEN I syndrome and von Recklinghausen's disease (neurofibromatosis). Virchows Arch 1986;408:475–489.

68. Watanabe W, Kurumada T, Shirai T, Tsutsumi Y. Aberrant insulinoma of the duodenal bulb. Pathol Int 1995;45:895–900.

69. Dayal Y, Tallberg KA, Nunnemacher G, et al. Duodenal carcinoids in patients with and without neurofibromatosis. Am J Surg Pathol 1986;10:348–357.

70. Taccagni GL, Carlucci M, Sironi M, et al. Duodenal somatostatinoma with psammoma bodies: An immunohistochemical and ultrastructural study. Am J Gastroenterol 1986;81:33–37.

71. Griffiths DFR, Jasani B, Newman GR, et al. Glandular duodenal carcinoid: A somatostatin rich tumor with neuroendocrine associations. J Clin Pathol 1984;37:163–169.

72. Burke AP, Sobin LH, Shekitka KM, et al. Somatostatin-producing duodenal carcinoids in patients with von Recklinghausen's neurofibromatosis: A predilection for black patients. Cancer 1990;65:1591–1595.

73. Ranaldi R, Bearzi I, Cinti S, Suraci V. Ampullary somatostatinoma: An immunohistochemical and ultrastructural study. Pathol Res Pract 1988;183:8–16.

74. Dayal Y, Doos WG, O'Brien MJ, et al. Psammomatous somatostatinomas of the duodenum. Am J Surg Pathol 1983;7:653–665.

75. Nagai E, Matsunaga H, Chijiiwa K, et al. Duodenal epithelial neoplasms complicating von Recklinghausen's disease: An immunohistochemical analysis in two patients. Int J Surg Pathol 1996;3:229–240.

76. Pai SA, Krishnamurthy S, Soman CS. Psammomatous carcinoid tumor of the duodenum. Indian J Gastroenterol 1994;13:26–27.

77. Burke AP, Thomas RM, Elsayed AM, Sobin LH. Carcinoids of the jejunum and ileum: An immunohistochemical and clinicopathologic study of 167 cases. Cancer 1997;79:1086–1093.

78. Wilander E, Lundqvist M, Oberg K. Gastrointestinal carcinoid tumours: Histogenetic, histochemical, immunohistochemical, clinical and therapeutic aspects. Prog Histochem Cytochem 1989;19:1–88.

79. Cai YC, Barnard G, Hiestand L, et al. Florid angiogenesis in mucosa surrounding an ileal carcinoid tumor expressing transforming growth factor-alpha. Am J Surg Pathol 1997;21:1373–1377.

80. Moyana TN, Zhang D, Xiang J. Single jejunoileal and right colonic carcinoids as midgut tumors: A study collating immunophenotypes and histogenesis. Ann Clin Lab Sci 1995;25:504–512.

81. Allibone RO, Hoffman J, Gosney JR, Helliwell TR. Granulation tissue polyposis associated with carcinoid tumours of the small intestine. Histopathology 1993;22:475–480.

82. Nash SV, Said JW. Gastroenteropancreatic neuroendocrine tumors: A histochemical and immunohistochemical study of epithelial (keratin proteins, carcinoembryonic antigen) and neuroendocrine (neuron-specific enolase, bombesin and chromogranin) markers in foregut, midgut, and hindgut tumors. Am J Clin Pathol 1986;86:415–422.

83. Venizelos ID, Shousha S. Carcinoid tumour of Meckel's diverticulum associated with cecal adenocarcinoma. Histopathology 1990;16:395–396.

84. Wilander E, Scheibenpflug L. Cytokeratin expression in small intestinal and appendiceal carcinoids: A basis for classification. Acta Oncol 1993;32:131–134.

85. Fischer HP, Altmannsberger M, Weber K, Osborn M. Keratin polypeptides in malignant epithelial liver tumors: Differential diagnostic and histogenetic aspects. Am J Pathol 1987;127:530–537.

86. Lundqvist M, Wilander E. A study of the histopathogenesis of carcinoid tumors of the small intestine and appendix. Cancer 1987;60:201–206.

87. Moyana TN, Satkunam NA. A comparative immunohistochemical study of jejunoileal and appendiceal carcinoids: Implications for histogenesis and pathogenesis. Cancer 1992;70:1081–1082.

88. Goddard MJ, Longsdale RN. The histogenesis of appendiceal carcinoid tumors. Histopathology 1992;20:345–349.

89. Berardi RS. Carcinoid tumors of the colon (exclusive of the rectum). Dis Colon Rectum 1972;15:383–391.

90. Rosenberg JM, Welch JP. Carcinoid tumors of the colon. Am J Surg 1985;149:775–779.

91. Azzoni C, Bonato M, D'Adda T, et al. Well-differentiated endocrine tumors of the middle ear and of the hindgut have immunohistochemical and ultrastructural features in common. Virchows Arch 1995;426:411–418.

92. Federspiel BH, Burke AP, Sobin LH, Shekitka KM. Rectal and colonic carcinoids: A clinicopathologic study of 84 cases. Cancer 1990;65:135–140.

93. Axumi N, Traweek ST, Battifora H. Prostatic acid phos-

phatase in carcinoid tumors: Immunohistochemical and immunoblot studies. Am J Surg Pathol 1991;15:785–790.

94. Matsui K, Iwase T, Kitagawa M. Small, polypoid-appearing carcinoid tumors of the rectum: Clinicopathologic study of 16 cases and effectiveness of endoscopic treatment. Am J Gastroenterol 1993;88:1949–1953.

95. Moyana TN, Satkunam NA. Crypt cell proliferative micronests in rectal carcinoids: An immunohistochemical study. Am J Surg Pathol 1993;17:350–356.

96. Le Marc'hadour F, Bost F, Peoc'h M, et al. Carcinoid tumour complicating inflammatory bowel disease: A study of two cases with review of the literature. Pathol Res Pract 1994;190:1185–1192.

97. Goris GA, Moscovic EA. Unlikely origin of trabecular hindgut carcinoids from crypt cell proliferative micronests. Am J Surg Pathol 1994;18:426–427.

98. Staren ED, Gould VE, Warren WH, et al. Neuroendocrine carcinomas of the colon and rectum: A clinicopathologic evaluation. Surgery 1988;104:1080–1089.

99. Saclarides TJ, Szeluga D, Staren ED. Neuroendocrine cancers of the colon and rectum: Results of a ten-year experience. Dis Colon Rectum 1994;37:635–642.

100. Lindberg GM, Molberg KH, Vuitch MF, Albores-Saavedra J. Atypical carcinoid of the esophagus: A case report and review of the literature. Cancer 1997;79:1476–1481.

101. Matsui T, Kataoka M, Sugita Y, et al. A case of small cell carcinoma of the stomach. Hepatogastroenterology 1997;44:156–160.

102. Chejfec G, Kovarick P, Graham G, et al. Neuroendocrine carcinoma of the stomach with extensive somatostatin immunoreactivity. Ultrastruct Pathol 1992;16:537–545.

103. Morikawa Y, Tohya K, Matsuura N, et al. Small cell carcinoma of the stomach: An immunohistochemical and electron microscopic study. Histol Histopathol 1992;7:629–634.

104. Haratake J, Horie A, Inoshita S. Gastric small cell carcinoma with squamous and neuroendocrine differentiation. Pathology 1992;24:116–120.

105. Matsui K, Kitagawa M, Miwa A, et al. Small cell carcinoma of the stomach: A clinicopathologic study of 17 cases. Am J Gastroenterol 1991;86:1167–1175.

106. Springall DR, Ibrahim NB, Rode J, et al. Endocrine differentiation of extra-pulmonary small cell carcinoma demonstrated by immunohistochemistry using antibodies to PGP 9.5, neuron-specific enolase and the C-flanking peptide of human pro-bombesin. J Pathol 1986;150:151–162.

107. Eichhorn JH, Young RH, Scully RE. Nonpulmonary small cell carcinomas of extragenital origin metastatic to the ovary. Cancer 1993;71:177–186.

108. Sarker AB, Hoshida Y, Akagi S, et al. An immunohistochemical and ultrastructural study of case of small-cell neuroendocrine carcinoma in the ampullary region of the duodenum. Acta Pathol Jpn 1992;42:529–535.

109. Zamboni G, Franzin G, Bonetti F, et al. Small-cell neuroendocrine carcinoma of the ampullary region: A clinicopathologic, immunohistochemical, and ultrastructural study of three cases. Am J Surg Pathol 1990;14:703–713.

110. Kaizaki Y, Fujii T, Kawai T, et al. Gastric neuroendocrine carcinoma associated with chronic atrophic gastritis type A. J Gastroenterol 1997;32:643–649.

111. Sarsfield P, Anthony PP. Small cell undifferentiated ('neuroendocrine') carcinoma of the colon. Histopathology 1990;16:357–363.

112. Fujiwara Y, Nakagawa K, Tanaka T, et al. Small cell carcinoma of the esophagus combined with superficial esophageal cancer. Hepatogastroenterology 1996;43:1360–1369.

113. O'Byrne KJ, Cherukuri AK, Khan MI, et al. Extrapulmonary small cell gastric carcinoma: A case report and review of the literature. Acta Oncol 1997;36:78–80.

114. Craig SR, Carey FA, Walker WS, Cameron EW. Primary small-cell cancer of the esophagus. J Thorac Cardiovasc Surg 1995;109:284–288.

115. Lechago J. Gastrointestinal neuroendocrine cell proliferations. Hum Pathol 1994;25:1114–1122.

116. Burke AP, Shekitka KM, Sobin LH. Small cell carcinomas of the large intestine. Am J Clin Pathol 1991;95:315–321.

117. Gaffey MJ, Mills SE, Lack EE. Neuroendocrine carcinoma of the colon and rectum: A clinicopathologic, ultrastructural, and immunohistochemical study of 24 cases. Am J Surg Pathol 1990;14:1010–1023.

118. Matsui K, Jin XM, Kitagawa M, Miwa A. Clinicopathologic features of neuroendocrine carcinomas of the stomach: Appraisal of small cell and large cell variants. Arch Pathol Lab Med 1998;122:1010–1017.

119. Tennvall J, Johansson L, Albertsson M. Small cell carcinoma of the esophagus: A clinical and immunohistopathological review. Eur J Cancer Clin Oncol 1990;6:109–115.

120. Hoda SA, Hajdu SI: Small cell carcinoma of the esophagus: Cytology and immunohistochemistry in four cases. Acta Cytol 1992;36:113–120.

121. Slavin J, Pitson G, Dowling JP. Neuroendocrine carcinoma arising in Barrett's esophagus. Int J Surg Pathol 1994;2:43–46.

122. Takubo K, Nakamura K-I, Sawabe M, et al. Primary undifferentiated small cell carcinoma of the esophagus. Hum Pathol 1999;30:216–221.

123. Rindi G, Azzoni C, La Rosa S, et al. ECL cell tumor and poorly differentiated endocrine carcinoma of the stomach: Prognostic evaluation by pathological analysis. Gastroenterology 1999;116:532–542.

124. Takaku H, Naoi Y, Santoh N, et al. Primary advanced gastric small cell carcinoma—a case report and review of the literature. Am J Gastroenterol 1999;94:1402–1404.

125. Kimura H, Konishi K, Maeda K, et al. Highly aggressive behavior and poor prognosis of small-cell carcinoma in the alimentary tract: Flow-cytometric analysis and immunohistochemical staining for the p53 protein and proliferating cell nuclear antigen. Dig Surg 1999;16:152–157.

126. Ulich TR, Kollin M, Lewin KJ. Composite gastric carcinoma: Report of a tumor of the carcinoma-carcinoid spectrum. Arch Pathol Lab Med 1988;112:91–93.

127. Chan JKC, Suster S, Wenig BM, et al. Cytokeratin 20 immunoreactivity distinguishes Merkel cell (primary cutaneous neuroendocrine) carcinomas and salivary gland small cell carcinomas from small cell carcinomas of various sites. Am J Surg Pathol 1997;21:226–234.

128. Wick MR, Weatherby RP, Weiland LH. Small cell neuroendocrine carcinoma of the colon and rectum: Clinical, histologic, and ultrastructural study and immunohistochemical comparison with cloacogenic carcinoma. Hum Pathol 1987;18:9–21.

129. Nagaoka S, Toyoshima H, Bandoh T, et al. Composite carcinoid-adenocarcinoma tumor of the stomach: Report of a case. Surg Today 1996;26:184–188.

130. Anderson NH, Somerville JE, Johnston CF, et al. Appendiceal goblet cell carcinoids: A clinicopathological and immunohistochemical study. Histopathology 1991;18:61–65.

131. Carr NJ, Remotti H, Sobin LH. Dual carcinoid/epithelial neoplasia of the appendix. Histopathology 1995;27:557–562.

132. Corsi A, Bosman C. Adenocarcinoma and atypical carcinoid: Morphological study of a gastric collision-type tumour in the carcinoma-carcinoid spectrum. Ital J Gastroenterol 1995;27:303–308.

133. Chejfec G, Capella C, Solcia E, et al. Amphicrine cells, dysplasias, and neoplasias. Cancer 1985;56:2683–2690.

134. Watson KJ, Shulkes A, Smallwood RA, et al. Watery diarrhea-hypokalemia-achlorhydria syndrome and carcinoma of the esophagus. Gastroenterology 1985;88:798–803.

135. Lyda MH, Fenoglio-Preiser C. Adenoma-carcinoid tumors of the colon. Arch Pathol Lab Med 1998;122:262–265.

136. Moyana TN, Qizilbash AH, Murphy F. Composite glandular-carcinoid tumors of the colon and rectum: Report of two cases. Am J Surg Pathol 1988;12:607–611.

137. Ambe K, Mori M, Enjoji M. Early gastric carcinoma with multiple endocrine cell micronests. Am J Surg Pathol 1987;11:310–315.

138. Caruso RA, Pilato FP, D'Adda T, et al. Composite carcinoid-adenocarcinoma of the stomach associated with multiple gastric carcinoids and nonantral gastric atrophy. Cancer 1989;64:1534–1539.

139. Yang GCH, Rotterdam H. Mixed (composite) glandular-endocrine cell carcinoma of the stomach: Report of a case and review of the literature. Am J Surg Pathol 1991;15:592–598.

140. Caruso RA, Heyman MF, Rigoli L, Inferrera C. Composite early carcinoma (ordinary adenocarcinoma, carcinoid, microglandular-goblet cell carcinoid, neuroendocrine mucinous carcinoma) of the stomach. Histopathology 1998;32:569–571.

141. Ikeda E, Tsutsumi Y, Yoshida H, Yanagi K. Goblet cell carcinoid of the vermiform appendix with ovarian metastasis mimicking mucinous cystadenocarcinoma. Acta Pathol Jpn 1991;41:455–460.

142. Bak M, Asschenfeldt P. Adenocarcinoid of the vermiform appendix: A clinicopathologic study of 20 cases. Dis Colon Rectum 1988;31:605–612.

143. Miller RT, Sarikaya H, Jenison EL. Adenocarcinoid tumor of appendix presenting as unilateral Krukenberg tumor. J Surg Oncol 1988;37:65–71.

144. Watson PH, Alguacil-Garcia A. Mixed crypt cell carcinoma: A clinicopathological study of the so-called 'goblet cell carcinoid'. Virchows Arch 1987;412:175–182.

145. Burke AP, Sobin LH, Federspiel BH, et al. Goblet cell carcinoids and related tumors of the vermiform appendix. Am J Clin Pathol 1990;94:27–35.

146. Burke AP, Sobin LH, Federspiel BH, Shekitka KM. Appendiceal carcinoids: Correlation of histology and immunohistochemistry. Mod Pathol 1989;2:630–636.

147. Battifora H. Quality assurance issues in immunohistochemistry. J Histotechnol 1999;22:169–175.

148. Shi S-R, Cote RJ, Taylor CR. Standardization and further development of antigen retrieval immunohistochemistry: Strategies and future goals. J Histotechnol 1999;22:177–192.

149. Mills SE, Allen MS Jr, Cohen AR. Small-cell undifferentiated carcinoma of the colon: A clinicopathological study of five cases and their association with colonic adenomas. Am J Surg Pathol 1983;7:643–651.

150. Fuller CE, Williams GT. Gastrointestinal manifestations of type 1 neurofibromatosis (von Recklinghausen's disease). Histopathology 1991;19:1–11.

151. Newman PL, Wadden C, Fletcher CD. Gastrointestinal stromal tumors: Correlation of immunophenotype with clinicopathological features. J Pathol 1991;164:107–117.

152. Antonioli DA. Gastrointestinal autonomic nerve tumors: Expanding the spectrum of gastrointestinal stromal tumors. Arch Pathol Lab Med 1989;113:831–833.

153. Chan GS, Shek TW. Test and teach No. 89: Gastrointestinal autonomic nerve tumor (GANT). Pathology 1998;30:156,207–208.

154. Herrera GA, Cerezo L, Jones JE, et al. Gastrointestinal autonomic nerve tumors: 'Plexosarcomas.' Arch Pathol Lab Med 1989;113:846–853.

155. Shanks JH, Harris M, Banerjee SS, Eyden BP. Gastrointestinal autonomic nerve tumors: A report of nine cases. Histopathology 1996;29:111–121.

156. Miettinen M, Virolainen M, Maarit SR. Gastrointestinal stromal tumors—value of CD34 antigen in their identification and separation from true leiomyomas and schwannomas. Am J Surg Pathol 1995;19:207–216.

157. Fernandez-Trigo V, Sugarbaker PH. Sarcomas involving the abdominal and pelvic cavity. Tumori 1993;79:77–91.

158. Isimbaldi G, Santangelo M, Cenacchi G, et al. Gastrointestinal autonomic nerve tumor (plexosarcoma): Report of a case with fine needle aspiration biopsy and histologic, immunocytochemical and ultrastructural study. Acta Cytol 1998;42:1189–1194.

159. Suster S, Fisher C, Moran CA. Expression of bcl-2 oncoprotein in benign and malignant spindle cell tumors of soft tissue, skin, serosal surfaces, and gastrointestinal tract. Am J Surg Pathol 1998;22:863–872.

160. Minni F, Casadei R, Santini D, et al. Gastrointestinal autonomic nerve tumor of the jejunum: Case report and review of the literature. Ital J Gastroenterol Hepatol 1997;29:558–563.

161. Garcia R, Montes DM, Garcia BF. Jejunal stromal tumor with skeinoid fibers or myenteric plexoma: A case report. Pathol Int 1997;47:794–800.

162. Pinedo MF, Martinez-Gonzalez MA, Ballestin CC, Vargas CJ. Gastrointestinal autonomic nerve tumors: A case report with ultrastructural and immunohistochemical studies. Histopathology 1992;20:323–329.

163. Donner LR. Gastrointestinal autonomic nerve tumor: A common type of gastrointestinal stromal neoplasm. Ultrastruct Pathol 1997;21:419–424.

164. MacLeod CB, Tsokos M. Gastrointestinal autonomic nerve tumor. Ultrastruct Pathol 1991;15:49–55.

165. Calderale SM, Marchioni L, Malizia A, et al. Malignant stromal tumor consistent with fibrosarcoma arising from Meckel's diverticulum: Clinicopathological study of an incidentally discovered tumor and review of the literature. Tumori 1997;83:703–708.

166. Tworek JA, Appelman HD, Singleton TP, Greenson JK. Stromal tumors of the jejunum and ileum. Mod Pathol 1997;10:200–209.

167. Ojanguren I, Ariza A, Navas-Palacios JJ. Gastrointestinal autonomic nerve tumor: Further observations regarding an ultrastructural and immunohistochemical analysis of six cases. Hum Pathol 1996;27:1311–1318.

168. Suster S. Gastrointestinal stromal tumors. Semin Diagn Pathol 1996;13:297–313.

169. Lam KY, Law SY, Chu KM, Ma LT. Gastrointestinal autonomic nerve tumor of the esophagus: A clinicopathologic, immunohistochemical, ultrastructural study of a case and review of the literature. Cancer 1996;78:1651–1659.

170. Ishida T, Wada I, Horiuchi H, et al. Multiple small intestinal stromal tumors with skeinoid fibers in association with neurofibromatosis 1 (von Recklinghausen's disease). Pathol Int 1996;46:689–695.

171. Segal A, Carello S, Caterina P, et al. Gastrointestinal autonomic nerve tumors: A clinicopathological, immunohistochemical and ultrastructural study of 10 cases. Pathology 1994;26:439–447.

172. Mentzel T, Katenkamp D. Gastrointestinal stromal tumour with skeinoid fibres and bidirectional immunohistochemical differentiation. Histopathology 1996;29:175–177.

173. Sakaguchi N, Sano K, Ito M, et al. A case of von Recklinghausen's disease with bilateral pheochromocytoma: Malignant peripheral nerve sheath tumors of the adrenal and gastrointestinal autonomic nerve tumors. Am J Surg Pathol 1996;20:889–897.

174. Suster S, Fletcher CD. Gastrointestinal stromal tumors with prominent signet-ring cell features. Mod Pathol 1996;9:609–613.

175. Vrettou E, Karkavelas G, Christoforidou B, et al. Immunohistochemical phenotyping and PCNA detection in gastrointestinal stromal tumors. Anticancer Res 1995;15:943–949.

176. Dhimes P, Lopez-Carreira M, Ortega-Serrano MP, et al. Gastrointestinal autonomic nerve tumors and their separation from other gastrointestinal stromal tumors: An ultrastructural and immunohistochemical study of seven cases. Virchows Arch 1995;426:27–35.

177. Kodet R, Snajdauf J, Smelhaus V. Gastrointestinal autonomic nerve tumor: A case report with electron microscopic and immunohistochemical analysis and review of the literature. Pediatr Pathol 1994;14:1005–1016.

178. Min KW. Gastrointestinal autonomic nerve tumors and skeinoid fibers: Clinicopathological, immunohistochemical, and ultrastructural investigations. Am J Surg Pathol 1994;16:145–155.

179. Ma CK, De Peralta MN, Amin MB, et al. Small intestinal stromal tumors: A clinicopathologic study of 20 cases with immunohistochemical assessment of cell differentiation and the prognostic role of proliferation antigens. Am J Clin Pathol 1997;108:641–651.

180. Lauwers GY, Erlandson RA, Casper ES, et al. Gastrointestinal autonomic nerve tumors: A clinicopathological, immunohistochemical, and ultrastructural study of 12 cases. Am J Surg Pathol 1993;17:887–897.

181. Franquemont DW, Frierson HF Jr: Muscle differentiation and clinicopathologic features of gastrointestinal stromal tumors. Am J Surg Pathol 1992;16:947−954.

182. Flinner RL, Hammond EH. Gastrointestinal stromal tumor of the duodenum: A case report. Ultrastruct Pathol 1991; 15:503−507.

183. Papla B, Urbanczyk K, Urban A, et al. Selected immunohistochemical markers in stromal neoplasms of the gastrointestinal tract. Folia Histochem Cytobiol 1991;29:31−36.

184. Tauchi K, Tsutsumi Y, Yoshimura S, Watanabe K. Immunohistochemical and immunoblotting detection of cytokeratin in smooth muscle tumors. Acta Pathol Jpn 1990;40: 574−580.

185. Brown DC, Theaker JM, Banks PM, et al. Cytokeratin expression in smooth muscle and smooth muscle tumours. Histopathology 1987;11:477−486.

186. Walsh NM, Bodurtha A. Auerbach's myenteric plexus: A possible site of origin for gastrointestinal stromal tumors in von Recklinghausen's neurofibromatosis. Arch Pathol Lab Med 1990;114:522−525.

187. Pike AM, Lloyd RV, Appelman HD. Cell markers in gastrointestinal stromal tumors. Hum Pathol 1988;19:830−834.

188. Miettinen M. Gastrointestinal stromal tumors: An immunohistochemical study of cellular differentiation. Am J Clin Pathol 1988;89:601−610.

189. Saul SH, Rast ML, Brooks JJ. The immunohistochemistry of gastrointestinal stromal tumors: Evidence supporting an origin from smooth muscle. Am J Surg Pathol 1987;11: 464−473.

190. Erlandson RA, Klimstra DS, Woodruff JM. Subclassification of gastrointestinal stromal tumors based on evaluation by electron microscopy and immunohistochemistry. Ultrastruct Pathol 1996;20:373−393.

191. Denk H, Krepler R, Artlieb U, et al. Proteins of intermediate filaments: An immunohistochemical and biochemical approach to the classification of soft tissue tumors. Am J Pathol 1983;110:193−208.

192. Rudolph P, Gloeckner K, Parwaresch R, et al. Immunophenotype, proliferation, DNA ploidy, and biological behavior of gastrointestinal stromal tumors: A multivariate clinicopathologic study. Hum Pathol 1998;29:791−800.

193. Donner LR, de Lanerolle P, Costa J. Immunoreactivity of paraffin-embedded normal tissues and mesenchymal tumors for smooth muscle myosin. Am J Clin Pathol 1983; 80:677−681.

194. Ueyama T, Guo K-J, Hashimoto H, et al. A clinicopathologic and immunohistochemical study of gastrointestinal stromal tumors. Cancer 1992;69:947−955.

195. Ma CK, Amin MB, Kintanar E, et al. Immunohistologic characterization of gastrointestinal stromal tumors: A study of 82 cases compared with 11 cases of leiomyomas. Mod Pathol 1993;6:139−144.

196. Hurlimann J, Gardiol D. Gastrointestinal stromal tumors: An immunohistochemical study of 165 cases. Histopathology 1991;19:311−320.

197. Hjermstad BM, Sobin LH, Helwig EB. Stromal tumors of the gastrointestinal tract: Myogenic or neurogenic? Am J Surg Pathol 1987;11:383−386.

198. Suster S, Sorace D, Moran CA. Gastrointestinal stromal tumors with prominent myxoid matrix: Clinicopathologic, immunohistochemical, and ultrastructural study of nine cases of a distinctive morphologic variant of myogenic stromal tumor. Am J Surg Pathol 1995;19:59−70.

199. Lee JSY, Nascimento AG, Farnell MB, et al. Epithelioid gastric stromal tumors (leiomyoblastomas): A study of 55 cases. Surgery 1995;118:653−661.

200. Mikhael AI, Bacchi CE, Zarbo RJ, et al. CD34 expression in stromal tumors of the gastrointestinal tract. Appl Immunohistochem 1994;2:89−93.

201. Monihan JM, Carr NJ, Sobin LH. CD34 immunoexpression in stromal tumors of the gastrointestinal tract and in mesenteric fibromatosis. Histopathology 1994;25:469−473.

202. Goldblum JR, Appelman HD. Stromal tumors of the duodenum: A histologic and immunohistochemical study of 20 cases. Am J Surg Pathol 1995;19:71−80.

203. Fukuda T, Ohnishi Y, Watanabe H, et al. Dedifferentiated leiomyosarcoma of the intestinal tract: Histological, ultrastructural, and immunohistochemical examinations. Virchows Arch 1992;420:313−320.

204. van de Rijn M, Hendrickson MR, Rouse RV. CD34 expression by gastrointestinal tract stromal tumors. Hum Pathol 1994;25:766−771.

205. Yao T, Aoyagi K, Hizawa K, et al. Gastric epithelioid stromal tumor (leiomyoma) with granular changes. Int J Surg Pathol 1996;4:37−42.

206. Shek TW, Luk IS, Loong F, et al. Inflammatory cell-rich gastrointestinal autonomic nerve tumor: An expansion of its histologic spectrum. Am J Surg Pathol 1996;20: 325−331.

207. Kerr JZ, Hicks MJ, Nuchtern JG, et al. Gastrointestinal autonomic nerve tumors in the pediatric population: Report of four cases and a review of the literature. Cancer 1999; 85:220−230.

208. Ferrer MD, Lloreta J. Signet ring epithelioid stromal tumor of the small intestine. Ultrastruct Pathol 1999;23:45−50.

209. Sicar K, Hewlett BR, Huizinga JD, et al. Interstitial cells of Cajal as precursors of gastrointestinal stromal tumors. Am J Surg Pathol 1999;23:377−389.

210. Tworek JA, Goldblum JR, Weiss SW, et al. Stromal tumors of the anorectum: A clinicopathologic study of 22 cases. Am J Surg Pathol 1999;23:946−954.

211. Tworek JA, Goldblum JR, Weiss SW, et al. Stromal tumors of the anorectum. Am J Surg Pathol 1999;23:946−954.

212. Miettinen M, Monihan JM, Sarlomo-Rikala M, et al. Gastrointestinal stromal tumors/smooth muscle tumors (GISTs) primary in the omentum and mesentery: Clinicopathologic and immunohistochemical study of 26 cases. Am J Surg Pathol 1999;23:1109−1118.

213. Diamiani S, Pasquinelli G, Eusebi V. GANT-like gastrointestinal pacemaker cell tumors with oncocytic features. Virchows Arch 1999;435:143−150.

214. Tornoczky T, Kalman E, Hegedus G, et al. High mitotic activity associated with poor prognosis in gastrointestinal autonomic nerve tumor. Histopathology 1999;35:121−128.

215. Miettinen M, Sarlomo-Rikala M, Lasota J. Gastrointestinal stromal tumors: Recent advances in understanding of their biology. Hum Pathol 1999;30:1213−1220.

216. Thompson EM, Evans DJ. The significance of PGP 9.5 in tumours—an immunohistochemical study of gastrointestinal stromal tumours. Histopathology 1990;17:175−177.

217. Miettinen M, Sarlomo-Rikala M, Kovatich AJ. Cell-type and tumor-type-related patterns of BCL-2 reactivity in mesenchymal cells and soft tissue tumors. Virchows Arch 1998;433:255−260.

218. Sarlomo-Rikala M, Kovatich AJ, Barusevicius BS, Miettinen M. CD 117: A sensitive marker for gastrointestinal stromal tumors that is more specific than CD 34. Mod Pathol 1998;11:728−734.

219. Hasegawa T, Yang P, Kagawa N, et al. CD34 expression by inflammatory fibroid polyps of the stomach. Mod Pathol 1997;10:451−456.

220. d'Amore ES, Manivel JC, Pettinato G, et al. Intestinal ganglioneuromatosis: Mucosal and transmural types: A clinicopathologic and immunohistochemical study of six cases. Hum Pathol 1991;22:276−286.

221. Beer TW. Solitary ganglioneuroma of the rectum: Report of two cases. J Clin Pathol 1992;45:353−355.

222. Dellinger GW, Lynch CA, Mihas AA. Colonic ganglioneuroma presenting as filiform polyposis. J Clin Gastroenterol 1996;22:66−70.

223. Sarlomo-Rikala M, Miettinen M. Gastric schwannoma—a clinicopathological analysis of six cases. Histopathology 1995;27:355−360.

224. Melvin WS, Wilkinson MG. Gastric schwannoma: Clinical and pathologic considerations. Am Surg 1993;59:293−296.

225. Arai T, Sugimura H, Suzuki M, et al. Benign schwannoma of the esophagus: Report of two cases with immunohistochemical and ultrastructural studies. Pathol Int 1994;44: 460−465.

226. Prevot S, Bienvenu L, Vaillant JC, De Saint Maur PP. Be-

nign schwannoma of the digestive tract: A clinicopathologic and immunohistochemical study of five cases, including a case of esophageal tumor. Am J Surg Pathol 1999;23: 431–436.

227. Schmid C, Beham A, Steindorfer P, et al. Non-functional malignant paraganglioma of the stomach. Virchows Arch 1990;417:261–266.

228. Linnoila RI, Lack EE, Steinberg SM, Keiser HR. Decreased expression of neuropeptides in malignant paragangliomas: An immunohistochemical study. Hum Pathol 1988;19: 41–50.

229. Schmid KW, Dockhorn-Dworniczak B, Ahrenkamp AG, et al. Chromogranin A, secretogranin II, and vasoactive intestinal peptide in pheochromocytomas and ganglioneuromas. Histopathology 1993;22:527–533.

230. Moran CA, Suster S, Fishback N, Koss MN. Mediastinal paraganglioma: A clinicopathologic and immunohistochemical study of 16 cases. Cancer 1993;72:2358–2364.

231. Googe PB, Ferry JA, Bhan AK, et al. A comparison of paraganglioma, carcinoid tumor, and small-cell carcinoma of the larynx. Arch Pathol Lab Med 1988;112:809–815.

232. Ulbright TM, Cummings OW. Retroperitoneal paraganglion: Distinction from metastatic germ cell tumor. J Urol Pathol 1995;3:269–278.

233. Laguette J, Matias-Guiu X, Rosai J. Thyroid paraganglioma: A clinicopathologic and immunohistochemical study of three cases. Am J Surg Pathol 1997;21:748–753.

234. Grignon DJ, Ro JY, Mackay B, et al. Paraganglioma of the urinary bladder: Immunohistochemical, ultrastructural, and DNA flow cytometric studies. Hum Pathol 1991;22: 1162–1169.

235. Burke AP, Helwig EB. Gangliocytic paraganglioma. Am J Clin Pathol 1989;92:1–9.

236. Barbareschi M, Frigo B, Aldovini D, et al. Duodenal gangliocytic paraganglioma: Report of a case and review of the literature. Virchows Arch 1989;416:81–89.

237. Inai K, Kobuke T, Yonehara S, Kuoka S. Duodenal gangliocytic paraganglioma with lymph node metastasis in a 17-year old boy. Cancer 1989;63:2540–2545.

238. Collina G, Maiorana A, Trentini GP. Duodenal gangliocytic paraganglioma: Case report with immunohistochemical study on the expression of keratin polypeptides. Histopathology 1991;19:476–478.

239. Hamid QA, Bishop AE, Rode J, et al. Duodenal gangliocytic paragangliomas: A study of 10 cases with immunohistochemical neuroendocrine markers. Hum Pathol 1986;17: 1151–1157.

240. Perrone T, Sibley RK, Rosai J. Duodenal gangliocytic paraganglioma: An immunohistochemical and ultrastructural study and hypothesis concerning its origin. Am J Surg Pathol 1985;9:31–41.

241. Scheithauer BW, Nora FE, Lechago J, et al. Duodenal gangliocytic paraganglioma: Clinicopathologic and immunocytochemical study of 11 cases. Am J Clin Pathol 1986;86: 559–565.

242. Evans JD, Wilson PG, Barber PC, Neoptolemos JP. Duodenal gangliocytic paraganglioma presenting as an ampullary tumor. Int J Pancreatol 1996;20:131–134.

243. Goldblum JR, Rice TW, Richter JE. Histopathologic features in esophagomyotomy specimens from patients with achalasia. Gastroenterology 1996;111:648–654.

244. Goldblum JR, Whyte RI, Orringer MB, Appelman HD. Achalasia: A morphologic study of 42 resected specimens. Am J Surg Pathol 1994;18:327–337.

245. Ormsby AH, Goldblum JR, Rice TW, et al. Cytokeratin subsets can reliably distinguish Barrett's esophagus from intestinal metaplasia of the stomach. Hum Pathol 1999;30: 288–294.

246. MacLennan AJ, Orringer MB, Beer DG. Identification of intestinal-type Barrett's metaplasia by using the intestine-specific protein villin and esophageal brush cytology. Mol Carcinog 1999;24:137–143.

247. Regalado SP, Nambu Y, Iannettoni MD, et al. Abundant expression of the intestinal protein villin in Barrett's metaplasia and esophageal adenocarcinomas. Mol Carcinog 1998;22:182–189.

248. Ouatu-Lascar R, Fitzgerald RC, Triadafilopoulos G. Differentiation and proliferation in Barrett's esophagus and the effects of acid suppression. Gastroenterology 1999;117: 327–335.

249. Kumble S, Omary MB, Fajardo LF, Triadafilopoulos G. Multifocal heterogeneity in villin and Ep-CAM expression in Barrett's esophagus. Int J Cancer 1996;66:48–54.

250. Fitzgerald RC, Omary MB, Triadafilopoulos G. Dynamic effects of acid on Barrett's esophagus: An ex vivo proliferation and differentiation model. J Clin Invest 1996;98: 2120–2128.

251. Ireland AP, Clark GW, DeMeester TR. Barrett's esophagus: The significance of p53 in clinical practice. Ann Surg 1997;225:17–30.

252. Symmans PJ, Linehan JM, Brito MJ, Filipe MI: p53 expression in Barrett's esophagus, dysplasia, and adenocarcinoma using antibody DO-7. J Pathol 1994;173:221–226.

253. Flejou JF, Paraf F, Potet F, et al. p53 protein expression in Barrett's adenocarcinoma: A frequent event with no prognostic significance. Histopathology 1994;24:487–489.

254. Flejou JF, Potet F, Muzeau F, et al. Overexpression of p53 protein in Barrett's syndrome with malignant transformation. J Clin Pathol 1993;46:330–333.

255. Rice TW, Goldblum JR, Falk GW, et al. p53 immunoreactivity in Barrett's metaplasia, dysplasia, and carcinoma. J Thorac Cardiovasc Surg 1994;108:1132–1137.

256. Krishnadath KK, Tilanus HW, van Blankenstein M, et al. Accumulation of p53 protein in normal, dysplastic, and neoplastic Barrett's oesophagus. J Pathol 1995;175: 175–180.

257. Younes M, Lebovitz RM, Lechago LV, Lechago J. p53 protein accumulation in Barrett's metaplasia, dysplasia, and carcinoma: A follow-up study. Gastroenterology 1993;105: 1637–1642.

258. Cawley HM, Meltzer SJ, De Benedetti VM, et al. Anti-p53 antibodies in patients with Barrett's esophagus or esophageal carcinoma can predate cancer diagnosis. Gastroenterology 1998;115:19–27.

259. Levine DS. Barrett's esophagus and p53. Lancet 1994;344: 212–213.

260. Kim R, Clarke MR, Melhem MF, et al. Expression of p53, PCNA, and C-erbB-2 in Barrett's metaplasia and adenocarcinoma. Dig Dis Sci 1997;42:2453–2462.

261. Fanberg-Smith JC, Meiss-Kindblom JM, Fante R, Kindblom L-G. Malignant granular cell tumor of soft tissue: Diagnostic criteria and clinicopathologic correlation. Am J Surg Pathol 1998;22:779–794.

262. Goldblum JR, Rice TW, Zuccaro G, Richter JE. Granular cell tumors of the esophagus: A clinical and pathologic study of 13 cases. Ann Thorac Surg 1996;62:860–865.

263. Mazur MT, Shultz JJ, Myers JL. Granular cell tumor: Immunohistochemical analysis of 21 benign tumors and one malignant tumor. Arch Pathol Lab Med 1990;114:692–696.

264. Junquera LM, de Vicente JC, Vega JA, et al. Granular-cell tumours: An immunohistochemical study. Br J Oral Maxillofac Surg 1997;35:180–184.

265. Ordonez NG, Mackay B. Granular cell tumor: A review of the pathology and histogenesis. Ultrastruct Pathol 1999;23: 207–222.

266. Steffelaar JW, Nap M, von Haelst UJ. Malignant granular cell tumor: Report of a case with special reference to carcinoembryonic antigen. Am J Surg Pathol 1982;6:665–672.

267. Ohmori T, Arita N, Uraga N, et al. Malignant granular cell tumor of the esophagus: A case report with light and electron microscopic, histochemical, and immunohistochemical study. Acta Pathol Jpn 1987;37:775–783.

268. Tateyama H, Eimoto T, Tada T, et al. Immunoreactivity of a new CD5 antibody with normal epithelium and malignant tumors including thymic carcinoma. Am J Clin Pathol 1999;111:235–240.

269. Kornstein MJ, Rosai J. CD5 labeling of thymic carcinomas and other nonlymphoid neoplasms. Am J Clin Pathol 1998;109:722–726.

270. Ordonez NG. Value of calretinin immunostaining in differ-

entiating epithelial mesothelioma from lung adenocarcinoma. Mod Pathol 1998;11:929–933.

271. Lam KY, Loke SL, Shen XC, Ma LT. Cytokeratin expression in non-neoplastic oesophageal epithelium and squamous cell carcinoma of the oesophagus. Virchows Arch 1995;426:345–349.

272. Takahashi H, Shikata N, Senzaki H, et al. Immunohistochemical staining patterns of keratins in normal esophageal epithelium and carcinoma of the esophagus. Histopathology 1995;26:45–50.

273. Shah KD, Tabibzadeh SS, Gerber MA. Comparison of cytokeratin expression in primary and metastatic carcinomas: Diagnostic application in surgical pathology. Am J Clin Pathol 1987;87:708–715.

274. Suo Z, Holm R, Nesland JM. Squamous cell carcinomas: An immunohistochemical study of cytokeratins and involucrin in primary and metastatic tumors. Histopathology 1993;23:45–54.

275. Moll R, Lowe A, Laufer J, Franke WW. Cytokeratin 20 in human carcinomas: A new histodiagnostic marker detected by monoclonal antibodies. Am J Pathol 1992;140: 427–447.

276. Ramaekers FC, van Niekerk CC, Poels L, et al. Use of monoclonal antibodies to keratin 7 in the differential diagnosis of adenocarcinomas. Am J Pathol 1990;136:641–655.

277. Clover J, Oates J, Edwards C. Anti-cytokeratin 5/6: A positive marker for epithelioid mesothelioma. Histopathology 1997;31:140–143.

278. Ordonez NG. Value of cytokeratin 5/6 immunostaining in distinguishing epithelial mesothelioma of the pleura from lung adenocarcinoma. Am J Surg Pathol 1998;22:1215–1221.

279. Tezuka Y, Yonezawa S, Maruyama I, et al. Expression of thrombomodulin in esophageal squamous cell carcinoma and its relationship to lymph node metastasis. Cancer Res 1995;55:4196–4200.

280. Lager DJ, Callaghan EJ, Worth SF, et al. Cellular localization of thrombomodulin in human epithelium and squamous malignancies. Am J Pathol 1995;146:933–943.

281. Chu P, Stagias J, West AB, Traube M. Diffuse pagetoid squamous cell carcinoma in situ of the esophagus: A case report. Cancer 1997;79:1865–1870.

282. Tsang WY, Chan JKC, Lee KC, et al. Basaloid-squamous carcinoma of the upper aerodigestive tract and so-called adenoid cystic carcinoma of the esophagus: The same tumor type? Histopathology 1991;19:35–46.

283. Barnes L, Ferlito A, Altavilla G, et al. Basaloid squamous cell carcinoma of the head and neck: Clinicopathological features and differential diagnosis. Ann Otol Rhinol Laryngol 1996;105:75–82.

284. Abe K, Sasano H, Itakura Y, et al. Basaloid-squamous carcinoma of the esophagus: A clinicopathologic, DNA ploidy, and immunohistochemical study of 7 cases. Am J Surg Pathol 1996;20:453–461.

285. Ishikawa Y, Asuwa N, Ishii T, et al. A case of basaloid-squamous carcinoma of the esophagus: Immunohistochemical and ultrastructural studies. Pathol Int 1994;44:466–474.

286. Sarbia M, Verreet P, Bittinger F, et al. Basaloid squamous cell carcinoma of the esophagus: Diagnosis and prognosis. Cancer 1997;79:1871–1878.

287. Koide N, Koike S, Adachi W, et al. Immunohistochemical expression of bcl-2 protein in squamous cell carcinoma and basaloid carcinoma of the esophagus. Surg Today 1997;27:685–691.

288. Takubo K, Mafune K, Tanaka Y, et al. Basaloid-squamous carcinoma of the esophagus with marked deposition of basement membrane substance. Acta Pathol Jpn 1991;41: 59–64.

289. Mafune K, Takubo K, Tanaka Y, Fujita K. Sclerosing mucoepidermoid carcinoma of the esophagus with intraepithelial carcinoma or dysplastic epithelium. J Surg Oncol 1995;58:184–190.

290. Sheahan K, O'Brien MJ, Burke B, et al. Differential reactivities of carcinoembryonic antigen (CEA) and CEA-related monoclonal and polyclonal antibodies in common epithelial malignancies. Am J Clin Pathol 1990;94:157–164.

291. Sauter ER, Keller SM, Erner S, Goldberg M. HER-2/neu: A differentiation marker in adenocarcinoma of the esophagus. Cancer Lett 1993;75:41–44.

292. Deamant FD, Pombo MT, Battifora H. Estrogen receptor immunohistochemistry as a predictor of site of origin in metastatic breast cancer. Appl Immunohistochem 1993;1: 188–192.

293. Sarbia M, Borchard F, Hengels KJ. Histogenetical investigations on adenocarcinomas of the esophagogastric junction: An immunohistochemical study. Pathol Res Pract 1993;189:530–535.

294. Morisaki Y, Yoshizumi Y, Hiroyasu S, et al. Adenoid cystic carcinoma of the esophagus: Report of a case and review of the Japanese literature. Surg Today 1996;26:1006–1009.

295. Cerar A, Jutersek A, Vidmar S. Adenoid cystic carcinoma of the esophagus: A clinicopathologic study of three cases. Cancer 1991;67:2159–2164.

296. Blaauwgeers JL, Allema JH, Bosma A, Brummelkamp WH. Early adenoid cystic carcinoma of the upper esophagus. Eur J Surg Oncol 1990;16:77–81.

297. Terada N, Yamamoto R, Ishiguro S, et al. Squamous cell carcinoma of the esophagus with cartilaginous metaplasia at metastatic lesions. Acta Pathol Jpn 1990;40:435–441.

298. Orsatti G, Corvalan AH, Sakurai H, Choi HS. Polypoid adenosquamous carcinoma of the esophagus with prominent spindle cells: Report of a case with immunohistochemical and ultrastructural studies. Arch Pathol Lab Med 1993;117:544–547.

299. Ooi A, Kawahara E, Okada Y, et al. Carcinosarcoma of the esophagus: An immunohistochemical and electron microscopic study. Acta Pathol Jpn 1986;36:151–159.

300. Linder J, Stein RB, Roggli VL, et al. Polypoid tumor of the esophagus. Hum Pathol 1987;18:692–700.

301. Guarino M, Reale D, Micoli G, Forloni B. Carcinosarcoma of the esophagus with rhabdomyoblastic differentiation. Histopathology 1993;22:493–498.

302. Rosty C, Prevot S, Tiret E, et al. Adenocarcinosarcoma in Barrett's esophagus: Report of a case. Int J Surg Pathol 1996;4:43–48.

303. Iezzoni JC, Mills SE. Sarcomatoid carcinomas (carcinosarcomas) of the gastrointestinal tract: A review. Semin Diag Pathol 1993;10:176–187.

304. Symmans WF, Grimes MM. Malignant melanoma of the esophagus: Histologic variants and immunohistochemical findings in four cases. Surg Pathol 1991;4:222–234.

305. de Mik JI, Kooijman CD, Hoekstra JBL, Tytgat GNJ. Primary malignant melanoma of the esophagus. Histopathology 1992;20:77–79.

306. Fetsch PA, Marincola FM, Filie A, et al. Melanoma-associated antigen recognized by T cells (MART-1). Cancer Cytopathol 1999;87:37–42.

307. Mizobuchi S, Tachimori Y, Kato H, et al. Metastatic esophageal tumors from distant primary lesions: Report of three esophagectomies and study of 1835 autopsy cases. Jpn J Clin Oncol 1997;27:410–414.

308. Kadakia SC, Parker A, Canales L. Metastatic tumors to the upper gastrointestinal tract: Endoscopic experience. Am J Gastroenterol 1992;87:1418–1423.

309. Fujii K, Nakanishi Y, Ochiai A, et al. Solitary esophageal metastasis of breast cancer with 15 years' latency: A case report and review of the literature. Pathol Int 1997;47: 614–617.

310. Herrera JL. Case report: Esophageal metastasis from breast carcinoma presenting as achalasia. Am J Med Sci 1992; 303:321–323.

311. Arakawa M, Kage M, Matsumoto S, et al. Frequency and significance of tumor thrombi in esophageal varices in hepatocellular carcinoma associated with cirrhosis. Hepatology 1986;6:419–422.

312. Leong AS, Sormunen RT, Tsui WM, Liew CT. Hep Par 1 and selected antibodies in the immunohistological distinction of hepatocellular carcinoma from cholangiocarcinoma,

combined tumors and metastatic carcinoma. Histopathology 1998;33:318–324.

313. Lee M, Munoz J, Duke EE. Metastatic papillary carcinoma of the thyroid to the esophagus. J Clin Gastroenterol 1995; 20:333–334.

314. Osborn M, Mazzoleni G, Santini D, et al. Villin, intestinal brush border hydrolases and keratin polypeptides in intestinal metaplasia and gastric cancer; an immunohistologic study emphasizing the different degrees of intestinal and gastric differentiation in signet ring cell carcinomas. Virchows Arch A Pathol Anat Histopathol 1988;413:303–312.

315. Waldum HL, Aase S, Kvetnoi I, et al. Neuroendocrine differentiation in human gastric carcinoma. Cancer 1998;83: 435–444.

316. Blumenfeld W, Chandhoke DK, Sagerman P, Turi GK. Neuroendocrine differentiation in gastric adenocarcinomas: An immunohistochemical study. Arch Pathol Lab Med 1996;120:478–481.

317. Park JG, Choe GY, Helman LJ, et al. Chromogranin-A expression in gastric and colon cancer tissues. Int J Cancer 1992;51:189–194.

318. Ooi A, Hayashi H, Katsuda S, Nakanishi I. Gastric carcinoma cells with endocrine differentiation show no evidence of proliferation. [see comments] Hum Pathol 1992; 23:736–741.

319. Berner A, Nesland JM. Endocrine profile in gastric carcinomas: An immunohistochemical study. Histol Histopathol 1991;6:317–323.

320. Waldum HL, Haugen OA, Isaksen C, et al. Enterochromaffin-like tumour cells in the diffuse but not the intestinal type of gastric carcinomas. Scand J Gastroenterol Suppl 1991;180:165–169.

321. Ikeda Y, Mori M, Haraguchi Y, et al. The incidence of chromogranin A defined endocrine cells decreases with tumour progression in gastric adenocarcinoma. Surg Oncol 1995;4:255–260.

322. Wauters CC, Smedts F, Gerrits LG, et al. Keratins 7 and 20 as diagnostic markers of carcinomas metastatic to the ovary. Hum Pathol 1995;26:852–855.

323. Tot T. Adenocarcinomas metastatic to the liver: The value of cytokeratins 20 and 7 in the search for unknown primary tumors. Cancer 1999;85:171–177.

324. Baars JH, De Ruijter JLM, Smedts F, et al. The applicability of a keratin 7 monoclonal antibody in routinely Papanicolaou-stained cytologic specimens for the differential diagnosis of carcinoma. Am J Clin Pathol 1994;101: 257–261.

325. Kaufmann OK, Deidesheimer T, Muehlenberg M, et al. Immunohistochemical differentiation of metastatic breast carcinomas from metastatic adenocarcinomas of other common primary sites. Histopathology 1996;29:233–240.

326. Miettinen M. Keratin 20: Immunohistochemical marker for gastrointestinal, urothelial, and Merkel cell carcinomas. Mod Pathol 1995;8:384–388.

327. Miettinen M, Nobel MP, Tuma BT, Kovatich AJ. Keratin 17: Immunohistochemical mapping of its distribution in human epithelial tumors and its potential applications. Appl Immunohistochem 1997;5:152–159.

328. McHugh M, Miettinen M. KP1 (CD68): Its limited specificity for histiocytic tumors. Appl Immunohistochem 1994;2: 186–190.

329. Loy TS, Sharp SC, Andershock CJ, Craig SB. Distribution of CA 19-9 in adenocarcinomas and transitional cell carcinomas: An immunohistochemical study of 527 cases. Am J Clin Pathol 1993;99:726–728.

330. Loy TS, Quesenberry JT, Sharp SC. Distribution of CA 125 in adenocarcinomas: An immunohistochemical study of 481 cases. Am J Clin Pathol 1992;98:175–179.

331. Gatalica D, Miettinen M. Distribution of carcinoma antigens CA 19-9 and CA 15-3: Immunohistochemical study of 400 tumors. Appl Immunohistochem 1994;2:205–211.

332. Ma CK, Zarbo RJ, Frierson HF Jr, Lee M. Comparative immunohistochemical study of primary and metastatic carcinomas of the liver. Am J Clin Pathol 1993;99: 551–557.

333. Fowler LJ, Maygarden SJ, Novotny DB. Human alveolar macrophage-56 and carcinoembryonic antigen monoclonal antibodies in the differential diagnosis between primary ovarian and metastatic gastrointestinal carcinomas. Hum Pathol 1994;25:666–670.

334. Chaubert P, Bouzourene H, Saraga E. Estrogen and progesterone receptors and pS2 and ERD5 antigens in gastric carcinomas from the European population. Mod Pathol 1996;9:189–193.

335. Kojima O, Takahashi T, Kawakami S, et al. Localization of estrogen receptors in gastric cancer using immunohistochemical staining of monoclonal antibody. Cancer 1991;67: 2401–2406.

336. Harrison JD, Jones JA, Ellis IO, Morris DL. Estrogen receptor D5 antibody is an independent negative prognostic factor in gastric cancer. Br J Surg 1991;78:334–336.

337. Theodoropoulos GE, Lazaris AC, Panoussopoulos D, et al. Significance of estrogen receptors and cathepsin D tissue detection in gastric adenocarcinoma. J Surg Oncol 1995;58: 176–183.

338. Cameron BL, Butler JA, Rutgers J, et al. Immunohistochemical determination of the estrogen receptor content of gastrointestinal adenocarcinomas. Am Surg 1992;58: 758–760.

339. Harrison JD, Morris DL, Ellis IO, et al. The effect of tamoxifen and estrogen receptor status on survival in gastric carcinoma. Cancer 1989;64:1007–1010.

340. Yokozaki H, Takekura N, Takanashi A, et al. Estrogen receptors in gastric adenocarcinoma: A retrospective immunohistochemical analysis. Virchows Arch 1988;413: 297–302.

341. Uehara Y, Takahashi T, Kojima O, et al. Peroxidase-antiperoxidase staining for estrogen and progesterone in scirrhous type of gastric cancer: Possible existence of the estrogen receptor. Jpn J Surg 1986;16:245–249.

342. Sica V, Nola E, Contieri E, et al. Estradiol and progesterone receptors in malignant gastrointestinal tumors. Cancer Res 1984;44:4670–4674.

343. Tokunaga A, Kojima N, Andoh T, et al. Hormone receptors in gastric cancer. Eur J Cancer Clin Oncol 1983;19: 687–689.

344. Tokunaga A, Nishi K, Matsukura N, et al. Estrogen and progesterone receptors in gastric cancer. Cancer 1986;57: 1376–1379.

345. Singh S, Poulsom R, Wright NA, et al. Differential expression of estrogen receptor and estrogen inducible genes in gastric mucosa and cancer. Gut 1997;40:516–520.

346. Johansson J, Thulin L, Ferno M, Andren-Sandberg A. Estrogen receptors in gastric cancer. Acta Oncol 1991;30: 870–872.

347. Linsalata M, Messa C, Russo F, et al. Estrogen receptors and polyamine levels in human gastric carcinoma. Scand J Gastroenterol 1994;29:67–70.

348. Wu CW, Tsay SH, Chang TJ, et al. Clinicopathologic comparisons between estrogen receptor-positive and -negative gastric cancers. J Surg Oncol 1992;51:231–235.

349. Matsui M, Kojima O, Uehara Y, Takahashi T. Characterization of estrogen receptor in human gastric cancer. Cancer 1991;68:305–308.

350. Wu CW, Chi CW, Chang TJ, et al. Sex hormone receptors in gastric cancer. Cancer 1990;65:1396–1400.

351. Mazoujian G, Pinkus GS, Davis S, Haagensen DE Jr. Immunohistochemistry of a gross cystic disease fluid protein (GCDFP-15) of the breast: A marker of apocrine epithelium and breast carcinomas with apocrine features. Am J Pathol 1983;110:105–112.

352. Wick MR, Lillemoe TJ, Copland GT, et al. Gross cystic disease fluid protein-15 as a marker for breast cancer: Immunohistochemical analysis of 690 human neoplasms and comparison with alpha-lactalbumin. Hum Pathol 1989;20: 281–287.

353. Raju U, Ma CK, Shaw A. Signet ring variant of lobular carcinoma of the breast: A clinicopathologic and immunohistochemical study. Mod Pathol 1993;6:516–520.

354. Koelma IA, Nap M, Rodenburg CJ, Fleuren GJ. The value

of tumor marker CA 125 in surgical pathology. Histopathology 1987;11:287–294.

355. Ueyama T, Nagai E, Yao T, Tsuneyoshi M. Vimentin-positive gastric carcinomas with rhabdoid features: A clinicopathologic and immunohistochemical study. [see comments] Am J Surg Pathol 1993;17:813–819.

356. Azumi N, Battifora H. The distribution of vimentin and keratin in epithelial and nonepithelial neoplasms. Am J Clin Pathol 1987;88:286–296.

357. Hyodo T, Kawamoto R. Double cancer of the stomach, one AFP-producing tumor. J Gastroenterol 1996;31:851–854.

358. Caruso RA, Tuccari G. A proposal of additional immunohistochemical markers for hepatoid carcinomas of the foregut. Pathology 1996;28:288.

359. Zamecnik M, Patrikova J, Gomolcak P. Yolk sac carcinoma of the stomach with gastrin positivity. Hum Pathol 1993; 24:927–928.

360. Puglisi F, Damante G, Pizzolitto S, et al. Combined yolk sac tumor and adenocarcinoma in a gastric stump. Cancer 1999;85:1910–1916.

361. Matsunou H, Konishi F, Jalal RE, et al. Alpha-fetoprotein producing gastric carcinoma with enteroblastic differentiation. Cancer 1994;73:534–540.

362. Roberts CC, Colby TV, Batts KP. Carcinoma of the stomach with hepatocyte differentiation (hepatoid adenocarcinoma). Mayo Clin Proc 1997;72:1154–1160.

363. Webb A, Scott-Mackie P, Cunningham D, et al. The prognostic value of serum and immunohistochemical tumour markers in advanced gastric cancer. Eur J Cancer 1996; 32A:63–68.

364. Jan YJ, Chen JT, Ho WL, et al. Primary coexistent adenocarcinoma and choriocarcinoma of the stomach: A case report and review of the literature. J Clin Gastroenterol 1997;25:550–554.

365. Herrera GA, Turbat-Herrera EA, Lott RL. S-100 protein expression by primary and metastatic adenocarcinomas. Am J Clin Pathol 1988;89:168–176.

366. Shimizu M, Matsumoto T, Hirokawa M, et al. Gastric metastasis from breast cancer: A pitfall in gastric biopsy specimens. Pathol Int 1998;48:240–241.

367. Briest S, Horn LC, Haupt R, et al. Metastasizing signet ring cell carcinoma of the stomach-mimicking bilateral inflammatory breast cancer. Gynecol Oncol 1999;74:491–494.

368. Battifora H. Metastatic breast carcinoma to the stomach simulating linitis plastica. Appl Immunohistochem 1994;2: 225–228.

369. Yim H, Jin YM, Shim C, Park HB. Gastric metastasis of mammary signet ring cell carcinoma—a differential diagnosis with primary gastric signet ring cell carcinoma. J Korean Med Sci 1997;12:256–261.

370. Perry A, Parisi JE, Kurtin PJ. Metastatic adenocarcinoma to the brain: An immunohistochemical approach. Hum Pathol 1997;28:938–943.

371. Brown RW, Campagna LB, Dunn JK, Cagle PT. Immunohistochemical identification of tumor markers in metastatic adenocarcinoma: A diagnostic adjunct in the determination of primary site. Am J Clin Pathol 1997;107: 12–19.

372. Ollayos CW, Riordan GP, Rushin JM. Estrogen receptor detection in paraffin sections of adenocarcinoma of the colon, pancreas, and lung. Arch Pathol Lab Med 1994;118: 630–632.

373. Cohen C, Guarner J, DeRose PB. Mammary Paget's disease and associated carcinoma: An immunohistochemical study. Arch Pathol Lab Med 1993;117:291–294.

374. Raab S, Berg LC, Swanson PE, Wick MR. Adenocarcinoma in the lung in patients with breast cancer: A prospective analysis of the discriminatory value of immunohistochemistry. Am J Clin Pathol 1993;100:27–35.

375. Wallace ML, Longacre TA, Smoller BR. Estrogen and progesterone receptors and anti-gross cystic disease fluid protein 15 (BRST-2) fail to distinguish metastatic breast carcinoma from eccrine neoplasms. Mod Pathol 1995;8: 897–901.

376. Bacchi CE, Gown AM. Distribution and pattern of expres-

377. Drier JK, Swanson PE, Cherwitz DL, Wick MR. S100 protein immunoreactivity in poorly differentiated carcinomas: Immunohistochemical comparison with malignant melanoma. Arch Pathol Lab Med 1987;111:447–452.

378. Savera AT, Torres FX, Lindin MD, et al. Primary versus metastatic pulmonary adenocarcinoma: An immunohistochemical study using villin and cytokeratins 7 and 20. Appl Immunohistochem 1996;4:86–94.

379. Harlamert HA, Mira J, Bejarano PA, et al. Thyroid transcription factor-1 and cytokeratins 7 and 20 in pulmonary and breast carcinoma. Acta Cytol 1998;42:1382–1388.

380. Loy TS, Calaluce RD. Utility of cytokeratin immunostaining in separating pulmonary adenocarcinomas from colonic adenocarcinomas. Am J Clin Pathol 1994;102: 764–767.

381. Moch H, Oberholzer M, Dalquen P, et al. Diagnostic tools for differentiating between pleural mesothelioma and lung adenocarcinoma in paraffin embedded tissue. Part I: Immunohistochemical findings. Virchows Arch 1993;423: 19–27.

382. Bejarano PA, Baughman RP, Biddinger PW, et al. Surfactant proteins and thyroid transcription factor-1 in pulmonary and breast carcinomas. Mod Pathol 1996;9:445–452.

383. Bohinski RJ, Bejarano PA, Balko G, et al. Determination of lung as the primary site of cerebral metastatic adenocarcinomas using monoclonal antibody to thyroid transcription factor-1. J Neurooncol 1998;40:227–231.

384. Di Loreto C, Puglisi F, Di Lauro V, et al. TTF-1 protein expression in pleural malignant mesotheliomas and adenocarcinomas of the lung. Cancer Lett 1998;124:73–78.

385. Di Loreto C, Di Lauro V, Puglisi F, et al. Immunocytochemical expression of tissue specific transcription factor-1 in lung carcinoma. J Clin Pathol 1997;50:30–32.

386. Holzinger A, Dingle S, Bejarano PA, et al. Monoclonal antibody to thyroid transcription factor-1: Production, characterization, and usefulness in tumor diagnosis. Hybridoma 1996;15:49–53.

387. Ro JY, El-Naggar A, Ayala AG, et al. Signet-ring-cell carcinoma of the prostate: Electron-microscopic and immunohistochemical studies of eight cases. Am J Surg Pathol 1988;12:453–460.

388. Ordonez NG. Role of immunohistochemistry in distinguishing epithelial peritoneal mesotheliomas from peritoneal and ovarian serous carcinomas. Am J Surg Pathol 1998;22:1203–1214.

389. Lin M, Hanai J, Wada A, et al. S-100 protein in ovarian tumors: A comparative immunohistochemical study of 135 cases. Acta Pathol Jpn 1991;41:233–239.

390. Gaffey MJ, Traweek ST, Mills SE, et al. Cytokeratin expression in adrenocortical neoplasia: An immunohistochemical and biochemical study with implications for the differential diagnosis of adrenocortical, hepatocellular, and renal cell carcinoma. Hum Pathol 1992;23:144–153.

391. Chivite A, Matias-Guiu X, et al. Inhibin A expression in adrenal neoplasms: A new immunohistochemical marker for adrenocortical tumors. Appl Immunohistochem 1998;6: 42–49.

392. McCluggage WC, Maxwell P. Adenocarcinomas of various sites may exhibit immunoreactivity with anti-inhibin antibodies. Histopathology 1999;35:216–220.

393. Utsunomiya T, Yao T, Masuda K, Tsuneyoshi M. Vimentin-positive adenocarcinomas of the stomach: Co-expression of vimentin and cytokeratin. Histopathology 1996;29: 507–516.

394. Lasota J, Hyjek E, Koo CH, et al. Cytokeratin-positive large-cell lymphomas of B-cell lineage: A study of five phenotypically unusual cases verified by polymerase chain reaction. Am J Surg Pathol 1996;20:346–354.

395. de Mascarel A, Merlio JP, Coindre JM, et al. Gastric large cell lymphoma expressing cytokeratin but no leukocyte common antigen: A diagnostic dilemma. Am J Clin Pathol 1989;91:478–481.

396. Swanson PE, Strickler JG. Gastric large cell lymphoma expressing cytokeratin but no leukocyte common antigen: An editorial dilemma. Am J Clin Pathol 1989;92:707–709.

397. Leong FJ, Leong AS. Malignant rhabdoid tumor in adults—heterogenous tumors with a unique morphological phenotype. Pathol Res Pract 1996;192:796–807.

398. Pinto JA, Gonzalez AJ, Gonzalez L, Stevenson N. Well differentiated gastric adenocarcinoma with rhabdoid areas: A case report with immunohistochemical analysis. Pathol Res Pract 1997;193:801–805.

399. Al Nafussi A, O'Donnell M. Poorly differentiated adenocarcinoma with extensive rhabdoid differentiation: Clinicopathological features of two cases arising in the gastrointestinal tract. Pathol Int 1999;49:160–163.

400. Cruz JJ, Paz JI, Cordero M, et al. Carcinosarcoma of the stomach with endocrine differentiation: A case report. Tumori 1991;77:355–357.

401. Fukuda T, Kamishima T, Ohnishi Y, Suzuki T. Sarcomatoid carcinoma of the small intestine: Histologic, immunohistochemical and ultrastructural features of three cases and its differential diagnosis. Pathol Int 1996;46:682–688.

402. Yamauchi H, Nitta A, Kakizaki K, et al. Different distribution of CA19-9 in carcinomas arising in the papilla of Vater: An immunohistochemical study. Tohoku J Exp Med 1993;170:235–244.

403. Abu-Alfa AK, Kuan S-F, West AB, Reyes-Mugica M. Cathepsin D in intestinal ganglion cells: A potential aid to diagnosis in suspected Hirschsprung's disease. Am J Surg Pathol 1997;21:201–205.

404. Mackenzie JM, Dixon MF. An immunohistochemical study of the enteric neural plexi in Hirschsprung's disease. Histopathology 1987;11:1055–1066.

405. Tan J, Sidhu G, Greco MA, et al. Villin, cytokeratin 7, and cytokeratin 20 expression in pulmonary adenocarcinoma with ultrastructural evidence of microvilli with rootlets. Hum Pathol 1998;29:390–396.

406. Berezowski K, Stastny JF, Kornstein MJ. Cytokeratins 7 and 20 and carcinoembryonic antigen in ovarian and colonic carcinoma. Mod Pathol 1996;9:426–429.

407. Sasaki A, Kawano K, Aramaki M, et al. Immunohistochemical expression of cytokeratins in intrahepatic cholangiocarcinoma and metastatic adenocarcinoma of the liver. J Surg Oncol 1999;70:103–108.

408. Fujisaki J, Shimoda T. Expression of cytokeratin subtypes in colorectal mucosa, adenoma, and carcinoma. Gastroenterol Jpn 1993;28:647–656.

409. Lagendijk JH, Mullink H, Van Diest PJ, et al. Tracing the origin of adenocarcinomas with unknown primary using immunohistochemistry: Differential diagnosis between colonic and ovarian carcinomas as primary sites. Hum Pathol 1998;29:491–497.

410. O'Hara BJ, Paetau A, Miettinen M. Keratin subsets and monoclonal antibody HMBE-1 in chordoma: Immunohistochemical differential diagnosis between tumors simulating chordoma. Hum Pathol 1998;29:119–126.

411. Loy TS, Calaluce RD, Keeney GL. Cytokeratin immunostaining in differentiating primary ovarian carcinoma from metastatic colonic adenocarcinoma. Mod Pathol 1996;9:1040–1044.

412. Millward C, Weidner N. CD30 (Ber-H2) expression in nonhematopoietic tumors. Appl Immunohistochem 1998;6:164–168.

413. Singh S, Poulsom R, Hanby AM, et al. Expression of estrogen receptor and estrogen-inducible genes pS2 and ERD5 in large bowel mucosa and cancer. J Pathol 1998;184:153–160.

414. Dawson PM, Shousha S, Blair SD, et al. Estrogen receptors in colorectal carcinoma. J Clin Pathol 1990;43:149–151.

415. Takeda H, Yamakawa M, Takahashi T, et al. An immunohistochemical study with an estrogen receptor-related protein (ER-D5) in human colorectal cancer. Cancer 1992;69:907–912.

416. Marugo M, Molinari F, Fazzuoli L, et al. Estradiol and progesterone receptors in normal and pathologic colonic mucosa in humans. J Endocrinol Invest 1985;8:117–119.

417. McClendon JE, Appleby D, Claudon DB, et al. Colonic neoplasms: Tissue estrogen receptor and carcinoembryonic antigen. Arch Surg 1977;112:240–241.

418. Di Leo A, Messa C, Russo F, et al. Prognostic value of cytosolic estrogen receptors in human colorectal carcinoma and surrounding mucosa: Preliminary results. Dig Dis Sci 1994;39:2038–2042.

419. Hendrickse CW, Jones CE, Donovan IA, et al. Oestrogen and progesterone receptors in colorectal cancer and human colonic cancer cell lines. Br J Surg 1993;80:636–640.

420. Meggouh F, Lointier P, Pezet D, Saez S. Status of sex steroid hormone receptors in large bowel cancer. Cancer 1991;67:1964–1970.

421. Sciascia C, Olivero G, Comandone A, et al. Estrogen receptors in colorectal adenocarcinomas and in other large bowel diseases. Int J Biol Markers 1990;5:38–42.

422. Francavilla A, Di Leo A, Polimeno L, et al. Nuclear and cytosolic estrogen receptors in human colon carcinoma and in surrounding noncancerous colonic tissue. Gastroenterology 1987;93:1301–1306.

423. Galandiuk S, Miseljic S, Yang A-R, et al. Expression of hormone receptors, cathepsin D, and HER-2/*neu* oncoprotein in normal colon and colonic disease. Arch Surg 1993;128:637–642.

424. Singh S, Sheppard MC, Langman MJ. Sex differences in the incidence of colorectal cancer: An exploration of estrogen and progesterone receptors. Gut 1993;34:611–615.

425. Brentani MM, Liberato MH, Macedo TM, et al. Steroid receptors in Brazilian patients with large bowel cancer. Braz J Med Biol Res 1993;26:277–284.

426. Taguchi T, Kijima H, Mitomi T, Osamura RY. Immunohistochemical study of colorectal adenocarcinomas and adenomas with antibodies against carcinoembryonic antigen (CEA), CA19-9, keratin, alpha-tubulin and secretory component (SC). Gastroenterol Jpn 1991;26:294–302.

427. Coffin CM, Swanson PE, Wick MR, Dehner LP. An immunohistochemical comparison of chordoma with renal cell carcinoma, colorectal adenocarcinoma, and myxopapillary ependymoma: A potential diagnostic dilemma in the diminutive biopsy. Mod Pathol 1993;6:531–538.

428. Ghoneim AHA, Brisson ML, Fuks A, et al. Monoclonal anti-CEA antibodies in the discrimination between primary pulmonary adenocarcinoma and colon carcinoma metastatic to the lung. Mod Pathol 1990;3:613–618.

429. Lash RH, Hart WR. Intestinal adenocarcinomas metastatic to the ovaries: A clinicopathologic evaluation of 22 cases. Am J Surg Pathol 1987;11:114–121.

430. Ordonez NG. Value of thrombomodulin immunostaining in the diagnosis of transitional cell carcinoma: A comparative study with carcinoembryonic antigen. Histopathology 1997;31:517–524.

431. Ascoli V, Scalzo CC, Taccogna S, Nardi F. The diagnostic value of thrombomodulin immunolocalization in serous effusions. Arch Pathol Lab Med 1995;119:1136–1140.

432. Hancock C, Allen BC, Herrera GA. HMB-45 detection in adenocarcinomas. Arch Pathol Lab Med 1991;115:886–890.

433. Bacchi CE, Bonetti F, Pea M, et al. HMB-45: A review. Appl Immunohistochem 1996;4:73–85.

434. Lapertosa G, Baracchini P, Delucchi F. Prevalence and prognostic significance of endocrine cells in colorectal adenocarcinomas. Pathologica 1994;86:170–173.

435. Syversen U, Halvorsen T, Marvik R, Waldum HL. Neuroendocrine differentiation in colorectal carcinomas. Eur J Gastroenterol Hepatol 1995;7:667–674.

436. Jansson D, Gould VE, Gooch GT, et al. Immunohistochemical analysis of colon carcinomas applying exocrine and neuroendocrine markers. APMIS 1988;96:1129–1139.

437. Mori M, Mimori K, Kamakura T, et al. Chromogranin positive cells in colorectal carcinoma and transitional mucosa. J Clin Pathol 1995;48:754–758.

438. Nicholson AG, McCormick CJ, Shimosato Y, et al. The value of PE-10, a monoclonal antibody against pulmonary surfactant, in distinguishing primary and metastatic lung tumors. Histopathology 1995;27:57–60.

439. Riopel MA, Klimstra DS, Godellas CV, et al. Intrabiliary growth of metastatic colonic adenocarcinoma: A pattern of intrahepatic spread easily confused with primary neoplasia of the biliary tract. Am J Surg Pathol 1997;21:1030–1036.

440. Young RH, Hart WR. Metastatic intestinal carcinomas simulating primary ovarian clear cell carcinoma and secretory endometrioid carcinoma: A clinicopathologic and immunohistochemical study of five cases. Am J Surg Pathol 1998;22:805–815.

441. Lagendijk JH, Mullink H, Van Diest PJ, et al. Immunohistochemical differentiation between primary adenocarcinomas of the ovary and ovarian metastases of colonic and breast origin: Comparison between a statistical and an intuitive approach. J Clin Pathol 1999;52:283–290.

442. Cagle PT, Brown RW, Lebovitz RM. p53 immunostaining in the differentiation of reactive processes from malignancy in pleural biopsy specimens. Hum Pathol 1994;25:443–448.

443. Delgado R, Vuitch F, Albores-Saavedra J. Salivary duct carcinoma. Cancer 1993;72:1503–1512.

444. Christensen WN, Boitnott JK, Kuhajda FP. Immunoperoxidase staining as a diagnostic aid for hepatocellular carcinoma. Mod Pathol 1989;2:8–12.

445. Han AC, Hovenden S, Rosenblum NG, Salazar H. Adenocarcinoma arising in extragonadal endometriosis: an immunohistochemical study. Cancer 1998;83:1163–1169.

446. DeCostanzo DC, Elias JM, Chumas JC. Necrosis in 84 ovarian carcinomas: A morphologic study of primary versus metastatic colonic carcinoma with a selective immunohistochemical analysis of cytokeratin subtypes and carcinoembryonic antigen. Int J Gynecol Pathol 1997;16:245–249.

447. Helle M, Krohn K. Immunohistochemical reactivity of monoclonal antibodies to human milk fat globule with breast carcinoma and with other normal and neoplastic tissues. Acta Pathol Microbiol Immunol Scand 1986;94:43–51.

448. Alpert LC, Truong LD, Bossart MI, Spjut HJ. Microcystic adenoma (serous cystadenoma) of the pancreas: A study of 14 cases with immunohistochemical and electron-microscopic correlation. Am J Surg Pathol 1988;12:251–263.

449. Bollinger DJ, Wick MR, Dehner LP, et al. Peritoneal malignant mesothelioma versus serous papillary adenocarcinoma: A histochemical and immunohistochemical comparison. Am J Surg Pathol 1989;13:659–670.

450. Gitsch G, Tabery U, Feigl W, Breitenecker G. The differential diagnosis of primary peritoneal papillary tumors. Arch Gynecol Obstet 1992;251:139–144.

451. Ueda G, Sawada M, Ogawa H, et al. Immunohistochemical study of cytokeratin 7 for the differential diagnosis of adenocarcinomas in the ovary. Gynecol Oncol 1993;51:219–223.

452. Guerrieri C, Franlund B, Fristedt S, et al. Mucinous tumors of the vermiform appendix and ovary, and pseudomyxoma peritonei: Histogenetic implications of cytokeratin 7 expression. Hum Pathol 1997;28:1039–1045.

453. Grignon DJ, Ro JY, Ayala AG, et al. Primary adenocarcinoma of the urinary bladder: A clinicopathologic analysis of 72 cases. Cancer 1991;67:2165–2172.

454. Renshaw AA, Corless CL. Papillary renal cell carcinoma: Histology and immunohistochemistry. Am J Surg Pathol 1995;19:842–849.

455. Akhtar M, Tulbah A, Kardar AH, Ali MA. Sarcomatoid renal cell carcinoma: The chromophobe connection. Am J Surg Pathol 1997;21:1188–1195.

456. Bonsib SM, Bromley C, Lager DJ. Renal oncocytoma: Diagnostic utility of cytokeratin containing globular filamentous bodies. Mod Pathol 1991;4:16–23.

457. Torbenson M, Dhir R, Nangia A, et al. Prostatic carcinoma with signet ring cells: A clinicopathologic and immunohistochemical analysis of 12 cases, with review of the literature. Mod Pathol 1998;11:552–559.

458. Papsidero LD, Croghan GA, Asirwatham J, et al. Immunohistochemical demonstration of prostate-specific antigen in metastases with the use of monoclonal antibody F5. Am J Pathol 1985;121:451–454.

459. Gaffney EF, O'Sullivan SN, O'Brian A. A major solid undifferentiated carcinoma pattern correlates with tumor progression in locally advanced prostatic carcinoma. Histopathology 1992;21:249–255.

460. Jones H, Anthony PP. Metastatic prostatic carcinoma presenting as left-sided cervical lymphadenopathy: A series of 11 cases. Histopathology 1992;21:149–154.

461. Weaver MG, Abdul-Karim FW, Srigley J, et al. Paneth cell-like metaplasia of the prostate gland: A histological, immunohistochemical, and electron microscopic study. Am J Surg Pathol 1992;16:62–68.

462. Nakayama H, Kimura A, Okumichi T, et al. Metaplastic shadow cells in rectal adenocarcinoma: Report of a case with immunohistochemical study. Jpn J Clin Oncol 1997;27:427–432.

463. Gibbs NM. Undifferentiated carcinoma of the large intestine. Histopathology 1977;1:77–84.

464. Kamel OW, Rouse RV, Warnke RA. Heterogeneity of epithelial marker expression in routinely processed poorly differentiated carcinomas. Arch Pathol Lab Med 1991;115:566–570.

465. Robey-Cafferty SS, Silva EG, Cleary KR. Anaplastic and sarcomatoid carcinoma of the small intestine: A clinicopathologic study. Hum Pathol 1988;20:858–863.

466. Staren ED, Gould VE, Jansson DS, et al. Neuroendocrine differentiation in "poorly differentiated" colon carcinomas. Am Surg 1990;56:412–419.

467. Jewell LD, Barr JR, McCaughey WTE, et al. Clear-cell epithelial neoplasms of the large intestine. Arch Pathol Lab Med 1988;112:197–199.

468. Reyes CV, Siddiqui MT. Anaplastic carcinoma of the colon: Clinicopathologic study of eight cases of a poorly recognized lesion. Ann Diagn Pathol 1997;1:19–25.

469. Bak M, Teglbjaerg PS. Pleomorphic (giant cell) carcinoma of the intestine: An immunohistochemical and electron microscopic study. Cancer 1989;64:2557–2564.

470. Weidner N, Zekan P. Carcinosarcoma of the colon: Report of a unique case with light and immunohistochemical studies. Cancer 1986;58:1126–1130.

471. Jones EA, Flejou JF, Molas G, Potet F. Pleomorphic carcinoma of the small bowel: The limitations of immunohistochemical specificity. Pathol Res Pract 1991;187:235–240.

472. Isimbaldi G, Sironi M, Assi A. Sarcomatoid carcinoma of the colon: Report of the second case with immunohistochemical study. Pathol Res Pract 1996;192:483–487.

473. Serio G, Aguzzi A. Spindle and giant cell carcinoma of the colon. Histopathology 1997;30:383–385.

474. Barnhill M, Hess E, Guccion JG, et al. Tripartite differentiation in a carcinoma of the duodenum. Cancer 1994;73:266–272.

475. Yang AH, Chen WYK, Chiang H. Malignant rhabdoid tumor of colon. Histopathology 1994;24:89–91.

476. Chetty R, Bhathal PS. Cecal adenocarcinoma with rhabdoid phenotype: An immunohistochemical and ultrastructural analysis. Virchows Arch 1993;422:179–182.

477. Ronnett BM, Shmookler BM, Diener-West M, et al. Immunohistochemical evidence supporting the appendiceal origin of pseudomyxoma peritonei in women. Int J Gynecol Pathol 1997;16:1–9.

478. Ronnett BM, Kurman RJ, Shmookler BM, et al. The morphologic spectrum of ovarian metastases of appendiceal adenocarcinomas: A clinicopathologic and immunohistochemical analysis of tumors often misinterpreted as primary ovarian tumors or metastatic tumors from other gastrointestinal sites. Am J Surg Pathol 1997;21:1144–1155.

479. Guerrieri C, Franlund B, Boeryd B. Expression of cytokeratin 7 in simultaneous mucinous tumors of the ovary and appendix. Mod Pathol 1995;8:573–576.

480. Kamoshida S, Tsutsumi Y. Extraprostatic localization of prostatic acid phosphatase and prostate-specific antigen: Distribution in cloacogenic glandular epithelium and sex-dependent expression in human anal gland. Hum Pathol 1990;21:1108–1111.

481. Iyer PV, Leong AS. Poorly differentiated squamous cell carcinomas of the skin can express vimentin. J Cutan Pathol 1992;19:34–39.

482. Levy R, Czernobilsky B, Geiger B. Cytokeratin polypeptide expression in a cloacogenic carcinoma and in the normal anal canal epithelium. Virchows Arch 1991;418:447–455.

483. Ordonez NG, Awalt H, Mackay B. Mammary and extramammary Paget's disease: An immunocytochemical and ultrastructural study. Cancer 1987;59:1173–1183.

484. Battles OE, Page DL, Johnson JE. Cytokeratins, CEA, and mucin histochemistry in the diagnosis and characterization of extramammary Paget's disease. Am J Clin Pathol 1997;108:6–12.

485. Helm KF, Goellner JR, Peters MS. Immunohistochemical stains in extramammary Paget's disease. Am J Dermatopathol 1992;14:402–407.

486. Smith KJ, Tuur S, Corvette D, et al. Cytokeratin 7 staining in mammary and extramammary Paget's disease. Mod Pathol 1997;10:1069–1074.

487. Nowak MA, Guerriere-Kovach P, Pathan A, et al. Perianal Paget's disease: Distinguishing primary and secondary lesions using immunohistochemical studies including gross cystic disease fluid protein-15 and cytokeratin 20 expression. Arch Pathol Lab Med 1998;122:1077–1081.

488. Goldblum JR, Hart WR. Perianal Paget's disease: A histologic and immunohistochemical study of 11 cases with and without associated rectal adenocarcinoma. Am J Surg Pathol 1998;22:170–179.

489. Lundquist K, Kohler S, Rouse RV. Intraepidermal cytokeratin 7 expression is not restricted to Paget cells but is also seen in Toker cells and Merkel cells. Am J Surg Pathol 1999;23:212–219.

490. Miller LR, McCunniff AJ, Randall ME. An immunohistochemical study of perianal Paget's disease: Possible origins and clinical implications. Cancer 1992;69:2166–2171.

491. Watson PH. Clear-cell carcinoma of the anal canal: A variant of anal transitional zone carcinoma. Hum Pathol 1990;21:350–352.

492. Kalogeropoulos NK, Antonakopoulos GN, Agapitos MB, Papacharalampous NX: Spindle cell carcinoma (pseudosarcoma) of the anus: A light, electron microscopic and immunocytochemical study of a case. Histopathology 1985;9:987–994.

493. Roncaroli F, Montironi R, Feliciotti F, et al. Sarcomatoid carcinoma of the anorectal junction with neuroendocrine and rhabdomyoblastic features. Am J Surg Pathol 1995;19:217–223.

494. Bouwens L. Cytokeratins and cell differentiation in the pancreas. J Pathol 1998;184:234–239.

495. Ectors N, Maillet B, Aerts R, et al. Non-alcoholic duct destructive chronic pancreatitis. Gut 1997;41:263–268.

496. Nishihara K, Nagai E, Tsuneyoshi M, Nagashima M. Small-cell carcinoma combined with adenocarcinoma of the gallbladder: A case report with immunohistochemical and flow cytometric studies. Arch Pathol Lab Med 1994;118:177–181.

497. Azzoni C, D'Adda T, Tamburrano G, et al. Functioning human insulinomas: An immunohistochemical analysis of intracellular insulin processing. Virchows Arch 1998;433:495–504.

498. Oikawa I, Hirata K, Katsuramaki T, et al. Neuroendocrine carcinoma of the extrahepatic biliary tract with positive immunostaining for gastrin-releasing peptide: Report of a case. Surg Today 1998;28:1192–1195.

499. Stokes MB, Kumar A, Symmans WF, et al. Pancreatic endocrine tumor with signet ring cell features: A case report with novel ultrastructural observations. Ultrastruct Pathol 1998;22:147–152.

500. Miettinen M, Lehto VP, Dahl D, Virtanen I: Varying expression of cytokeratin and neurofilaments in neuroendocrine tumors of human gastrointestinal tract. Lab Invest 1985;52:429–436.

501. Maurer CA, Glaser C, Reubi JC, Buchler MW. Carcinoid of the pancreas. Digestion 1997;58:410–414.

502. Ordonez NG, Cleary KR, Mackay B. Small cell undifferentiated carcinoma of the pancreas. Ultrastruct Pathol 1997;21:467–474.

503. Lam KY, Lo CY. Pancreatic endocrine tumour: A 22-year clinico-pathological experience with morphological, im-

504. munohistochemical observation and a review of the literature. Eur J Surg Oncol 1997;23:36–42.

504. Bordi C. Endocrine tumors of the pancreas: The pathologist's approach. Acta Biomed Ateneo Parmense 1993;64:195–204.

505. O'Connor TP, Wade TP, Sunwoo YC, et al. Small cell undifferentiated carcinoma of the pancreas: Report of a patient with tumor marker studies. Cancer 1992;70:1514–1519.

506. Yamaguchi K, Enjoji M. Endocrine neoplasms of the pancreas: A clinicopathologic study of 24 cases and immunohistochemical remarks. Surg Today 1992;22:305–312.

507. Davtyan H, Nieberg R, Reber HA. Pancreatic cystic endocrine neoplasms. Pancreas 1990;5:230–233.

508. Aletsee-Ufrecht MC, Langley OK, Gratzl M. NCAM expression in endocrine cells. Acta Histochem Suppl 1990;38:45–50.

509. Le Bodic M-F, Heyman MF, Lecomte M, et al. Immunohistochemical study of 100 pancreatic tumors in 28 patients with multiple endocrine neoplasia, type I. Am J Surg Pathol 1996;20:1378–1384.

510. Rindi G, Paolotti D, LaRosa S, Solcia E. The tumours of the endocrine pancreas. Eur J Histochem 1998;42(Spec No):63–66.

511. Lee CS, Machet D, Rode J. Small cell carcinoma of the ampulla of Vater. Cancer 1992;70:1502–1504.

512. Moller CJ, Christgau S, Williamson MR, et al. Differential expression of neural cell adhesion molecule and cadherins in pancreatic islets, glucagonomas, and insulinomas. Mol Endocrinol 1992;6:1332–1342.

513. Kotoulas C, Panayiotides J, Antiochos C, et al. Huge nonfunctioning pancreatic cystic neuroendocrine tumour: A case report. Eur J Surg Oncol 1998;24:74–76.

514. Aronsky D, Z'graggen K, Stauffer E, et al. Primary neuroendocrine tumors of the cystic duct. Digestion 1999;60:493–496.

515. Mount SL, Weaver DL, Taatjes DJ, et al. Von Hippel-Lindau disease presenting as pancreatic neuroendocrine tumour. Virchows Arch 1995;426:523–528.

516. Chejfec G, Falkmer S, Grimelius L, et al. Synaptophysin: A new marker for pancreatic neuroendocrine tumors. Am J Surg Pathol 1987;11:241–247.

517. Shah IA, Schlageter MO, Netto D. Immunoreactivity of neurofilament proteins in neuroendocrine neoplasms. Mod Pathol 1991;4:215–219.

518. Hoorens A, Prenzel K, Lemoine NR, Kloppel G. Undifferentiated carcinoma of the pancreas: Analysis of intermediate filament profile and Ki-ras mutations provides evidence of a ductal origin. J Pathol 1998;185:53–60.

519. Kimura N, Nakazato Y, Nagura H, Sasano N. Expression of intermediate filaments in neuroendocrine tumors. Arch Pathol Lab Med 1990;114:506–510.

520. Sessa F, Bonato M, Frigerio B, et al. Ductal cancers of the pancreas frequently express markers of gastrointestinal epithelial cells. Gastroenterology 1990;98:1655–1665.

521. Morikawa T, Kobayashi S, Yamadori I, et al. Three cases of extrapulmonary small cell carcinoma occurring in the prostate, stomach, and pancreas. Indian J Cancer 1994;31:268–273.

522. Kitajima T, Tomioka T, Tajima Y, et al. Small non-functioning endocrine tumor of pancreas: Comparison with solid cystic tumor. J Gastroenterol 1998;33:129–133.

523. Okada Y, Mori H, Tsutsumi A. Duct-acinar-islet cell tumor of the pancreas. Pathol Int 1995;45:669–676.

524. Kashiwabara K, Nakajima T, Shinkai H, et al. A case of malignant duct-islet cell tumor of the pancreas: Immunohistochemical and cytofluorometric study. Acta Pathol Jpn 1991;41:636–641.

525. Nonomura A, Mizukami Y, Matsubara F, et al. Duct-islet cell tumor of the pancreas: A case report with immunohistochemical and electron microscopic findings. Acta Pathol Jpn 1989;39:328–335.

526. Graham AR, Payne CM, Nagle RB, Angel E. The role of immunohistochemistry, electron microscopy, and ultrastructural cytochemistry in the diagnosis of mixed carcinoma-neuroendocrine neoplasms. Pathol Res Pract 1987;182:23–33.

527. Nishihara K, Tsuneyoshi M, Niiyama H, Ichimiya H. Composite glandular-endocrine cell carcinoma of the extrahepatic bile duct: Immunohistochemical study. Pathology 1993;25:90–94.

528. Kamisawa T, Fukayama M, Tabata I, et al. Neuroendocrine differentiation in pancreatic duct carcinoma: Special emphasis on duct-endocrine cell carcinoma of the pancreas. Pathol Res Pract 1996;192:901–908.

529. Laine VJ, Ekfors TO, Gullichsen R, Nevalainen TJ. Immunohistochemical characterization of an amphicrine mucinous islet-cell carcinoma of the pancreas: Case report. APMIS 1992;100:335–340.

530. Permert J, Mogaki M, Andren-Sandberg A, et al. Pancreatic mixed ductal-islet tumors: Is this an entity? Int J Pancreatol 1992;11:23–29.

531. Shankar KR, Losty PD, Khine MM, et al. Pancreatic inflammatory tumour: A rare entity in childhood. J R Coll Surg Edinb 1998;43:422–423.

532. Brown SZ, Owen DA, O'Connell JX, Scudamore CH. Schwannoma of the pancreas: A report of two cases and a review of the literature. Mod Pathol 1998;11:1178–1182.

533. Zalatnai A, Kovacs M, Flautner L, et al. Pancreatic leiomyosarcoma: Case report with immunohistochemical and flow cytometric studies. Virchows Arch 1998;432:469–472.

534. Fukushima N, Suzuki M, Abe T, Fukayama M. A case of inflammatory pseudotumour of the common bile duct. Virchows Arch 1997;431:219–224.

535. Walsh SV, Evangelista F, Khettry U: Inflammatory myofibroblastic tumor of the pancreaticobiliary region: Morphologic and immunocytochemical study of three cases. Am J Surg Pathol 1998;22:412–418.

536. Kroft SH, Stryker SJ, Winter JN, et al. Inflammatory pseudotumor of the pancreas. Int J Pancreatol 1995;18:277–283.

537. Yamaguchi K, Enjoji M, Tsuneyoshi M. Pancreatoduodenal carcinoma: A clinicopathologic study of 304 patients and immunohistochemical observation for CEA and CA19-9. J Surg Oncol 1991;47:148–154.

538. Yamaguchi K, Enjoji M. Carcinoma of the pancreas: A clinicopathologic study of 96 cases with immunohistochemical observations. Jpn J Clin Oncol 1989;19:14–22.

539. Albores-Saavedra J, Delgado R, Henson DE. Well-differentiated adenocarcinoma, gastric foveolar type, of the extrahepatic bile ducts: A previously unrecognized and distinctive morphologic variant of bile duct carcinoma. Ann Diagn Pathol 1999;3:75–80.

540. Shen DH, Ng TY, Khoo US, et al. Pseudomyxoma peritonei—a heterogenous disease. Int J Gynaecol Obstet 1998;62:173–182.

541. Luttges J, Vogel I, Menke M, et al. Clear cell carcinoma of the pancreas: An adenocarcinoma with ductal phenotype. Histopathology 1998;32:444–448.

542. Lonardo F, Cubilla AL, Klimstra DS. Microadenocarcinoma of the pancreas—morphologic pattern or pathologic entity? A reevaluation of the original series. Am J Surg Pathol 1996;20:1385–1393.

543. Ohshio G, Ogawa K, Kudo H, et al. Immunohistochemical studies on the localization of cancer associated antigens DU-PAN-2 and CA19-9 in carcinomas of the digestive tract. J Gastroenterol Hepatol 1990;5:25–31.

544. Toshkov I, Mogaki M, Kazakoff K, Pour PM. The patterns of coexpression of tumor-associated antigens CA 19-9, TAG-72, and DU-PAN-2 in human pancreatic cancer. Int J Pancreatol 1994;15:97–103.

545. Heyderman E, Larkin SE, O'Donnell PJ, et al. Epithelial markers in pancreatic carcinoma: Immunoperoxidase localisation of DD9, CEA, EMA and CAM 5.2. J Clin Pathol 1990;43:448–452.

546. Zhu L, Kim K, Domenico DR, et al. Adenocarcinoma of duodenum and ampulla of Vater: Clinicopathology study and expression of p53, c-neu, TGF-alpha, CEA, and EMA. J Surg Oncol 1996;61:100–105.

547. Klimstra DS, Lonardo F. Microglandular carcinoma of the pancreas. [letter] Am J Clin Pathol 1997;107:711–713.

548. Furukawa T, Chiba R, Kobari M, et al. Varying grades of epithelial atypia in the pancreatic ducts of humans: Classi-
fication based on morphometry and multivariate analysis and correlated with positive reactions of carcinoembryonic antigen. [see comments] Arch Pathol Lab Med 1994;118:227–234.

549. Loy TS, Nashelsky MB. Reactivity of B72.3 with adenocarcinomas: An immunohistochemical study of 476 cases. Cancer 1993;72:2495–2498.

550. Doglioni C, Dei Tos AP, Laurino L, et al. Calretinin: A novel immunocytochemical marker for mesothelioma. Am J Surg Pathol 1996;20:1037–1046.

551. Scheithauer W, Chott A, Knoflach P. Alpha-fetoprotein-positive adenocarcinoma of the pancreas. Int J Pancreatol 1989;4:99–103.

552. Folpe AL, Gown AM, Lamps LW, et al. Thyroid transcription factor-1: Immunohistochemical evaluation in pulmonary neuroendocrine tumors. Mod Pathol 1999;12:5–8.

553. Khoor A, Whitsett JA, Stahlman MT, et al. Utility of surfactant protein B precursor and thyroid transcription factor 1 in differentiating adenocarcinoma of the lung from malignant mesothelioma. Hum Pathol 1999;30:695–700.

554. Sheibani K, Shin SS, Kezirian J, Weiss LM. Ber-EP4 antibody as a discriminant in the differential diagnosis of malignant mesothelioma versus adenocarcinoma. Am J Surg Pathol 1991;15:779–784.

555. Gaffey MJ, Mills SE, Swanson PE, et al. Immunoreactivity for Ber-EP4 in adenocarcinomas, adenomatoid tumors, and malignant mesotheliomas. Am J Surg Pathol 1992;16:593–599.

556. Ordonez NG. The immunohistochemical diagnosis of mesothelioma. Am J Surg Pathol 1989;13:276–291.

557. Ordonez NG. The value of antibodies 44-3A6, SM3, HMBE-1, and thrombomodulin in differentiating epithelial pleural mesothelioma from lung adenocarcinoma: A comparative study with other commonly used antibodies. Am J Surg Pathol 1997;21:1399–1408.

558. Grove A, Paulsen SM, Gregersen M. The value of immunohistochemistry of pleural biopsy specimens in the differential diagnosis between malignant mesothelioma and metastatic carcinoma. Pathol Res Pract 1994;190:1044–1055.

559. Skov BG, Lauritzen AF, Hirsch FR, et al. Differentiation of adenocarcinoma of the lung and malignant mesothelioma: Predictive value and reproducibility of immunoreactive antibodies. Histopathology 1994;25:431–437.

560. Crotty TB, Myers JL, Katzenstein AL, et al. Localized malignant mesothelioma: A clinicopathologic and flow cytometric study. Am J Surg Pathol 1994;18:357–363.

561. Riera JR, Astengo-Osuna C, Longmate JA, Battifora H. The immunohistochemical diagnostic panel for epithelial mesothelioma: A reevaluation after heat-induced epitope retrieval. Am J Surg Pathol 1997;21:1409–1419.

562. Goldblum J, Hart WR. Localized and diffuse mesotheliomas of the genital tract and peritoneum in women: A clinicopathologic study of nineteen true mesothelial neoplasms, other than adenomatoid tumors, multicystic mesotheliomas, and localized fibrous tumors. [see comments] Am J Surg Pathol 1995;19:1124–1137.

563. Sosolik RC, McGaughy VR, De Young BR. Anti-MOC-31: A potential addition to the pulmonary adenocarcinoma versus mesothelioma immunohistochemistry panel. Mod Pathol 1997;10:716–719.

564. Jones MA, Young RH, Scully RE. Malignant mesothelioma of the tunica vaginalis: A clinicopathologic analysis of 11 cases with review of the literature. Am J Surg Pathol 1995;19:815–825.

565. Nascimento AG, Keeney GL, Fletcher CD. Deciduoid peritoneal mesothelioma: An unusual phenotype affecting young females. Am J Surg Pathol 1994;18:439–445.

566. Wick MR, Mills SE, Dehner LP, et al. Serous papillary carcinomas arising from the peritoneum and ovaries: A clinicopathologic and immunohistochemical comparison. Int J Gynecol Pathol 1989;8:179–188.

567. Nishihara K, Nagai E, Izumi Y, et al. Adenosquamous carcinoma of the gallbladder: A clinicopathological, immunohistochemical and flow-cytometric study of twenty cases. Jpn J Cancer Res 1994;85:389–399.

568. Motojima K, Tomioka T, Kohara N, et al. Immunohisto-chemical characteristics of adenosquamous carcinoma of the pancreas. J Surg Oncol 1992;49:58–62.

569. Yamaguchi K, Enjoji M. Adenosquamous carcinoma of the pancreas: A clinicopathologic study. J Surg Oncol 1991;47:109–116.

570. Deckard-Janatpour K, Kragel S, Teplitz RL, et al. Tumors of the pancreas with osteoclast-like and pleomorphic giant cells: An immunohistochemical and ploidy study. Arch Pathol Lab Med 1998;122:266–272.

571. Molberg KH, Heffess C, Delgado R, Albores-Saavedra J. Undifferentiated carcinoma with osteoclast-like giant cells of the pancreas and periampullary region. Cancer 1998;82:1279–1287.

572. Motoo Y, Kawashima A, Watanabe H, et al. Undifferentiated (anaplastic) carcinoma of the pancreas showing sarcomatous change and neoplastic cyst formation. Int J Pancreatol 1997;21:243–248.

573. Watanabe M, Miura H, Inoue H, et al. Mixed osteoclastic/pleomorphic-type giant cell tumor of the pancreas with ductal adenocarcinoma: Histochemical and immunohistochemical study with review of the literature. Pancreas 1997;15:201–208.

574. Gupta RK, Alansari AG. Aspiration cytology and immunocytochemical study of an unusual carcinoma of the pancreas with pleomorphic giant cells. Cytopathology 1994;5:306–309.

575. Marinho A, Nogueira R, Schmitt F, Sobrinho-Simoes M. Pancreatic mucinous cystadenocarcinoma with a mural nodule of anaplastic carcinoma. Histopathology 1995;26:284–287.

576. Imai Y, Morishita S, Ikeda Y, et al. Immunohistochemical and molecular analysis of giant cell carcinoma of the pancreas: A report of three cases. Pancreas 1999;18:308–315.

577. Nishihara K, Katsumoto F, Kurokawa Y, et al. Anaplastic carcinoma showing rhabdoid features combined with mucinous cystadenocarcinoma of the pancreas. Arch Pathol Lab Med 1997;121:1104–1107.

578. Gatteschi B, Saccomanno S, Bartoli FG, et al. Mixed pleomorphic-osteoclast-like tumor of the pancreas: Light microscopical, immunohistochemical, and molecular biological studies. Int J Pancreatol 1995;18:169–175.

579. Higashi M, Takao S, Sato E. Sarcomatoid carcinoma of the pancreas: A case report with immunohistochemical study. Pathol Int 1999;49:453–456.

580. Sun AP, Ohtsuki Y, Liang SB, et al. Osteoclast-like giant cell tumor of the pancreas with metastases to gallbladder and lymph nodes: A case report. Pathol Res Pract 1998;194:587–594.

581. Kijima H, Takeshita T, Suzuki H, et al. Carcinosarcoma of the ampulla of Vater: A case report with immunohistochemical and ultrastructural studies. Am J Gastroenterol 1999;94:3055–3059.

582. Kamisawa T, Tabata I, Isawa T, et al. A case of pleomorphic carcinoma of the pancreas showing sequential histological change by immunohistochemical study. Int J Pancreatol 1995;18:67–70.

583. Nishihara K, Tsuneyoshi M. Undifferentiated spindle cell carcinoma of the gallbladder: A clinicopathologic, immunohistochemical, and flow cytometric study of 11 cases. Hum Pathol 1993;24:1298–1305.

584. Adsay NV, Adair CF, Heffess CS, Klimstra DS. Intraductal oncocytic papillary neoplasms of the pancreas. Am J Surg Pathol 1996;20:980–994.

585. Thompson LD, Becker RC, Przygodzki RM, et al. Mucinous cystic neoplasm (mucinous cystadenocarcinoma of low-grade malignant potential) of the pancreas: A clinicopathologic study of 130 cases. Am J Surg Pathol 1999;23:1–16.

586. Nishihara K, Fukuda T, Tsuneyoshi M, et al. Intraductal papillary neoplasm of the pancreas. Cancer 1993;72:689–696.

587. Stommer P, Gebhardt C, Schultheiss KH. Adenocarcinoma of the pancreas with a predominant intraductal component: A special variety of ductal adenocarcinoma. Pancreas 1990;5:114–118.

588. Paal E, Thompson LD, Przygodzki RM, et al. A clinico-pathologic and immunohistochemical study of 22 intraductal papillary mucinous neoplasms of the pancreas, with a review of the literature. Mod Pathol 1999;12:518–528.

589. Zamboni G, Scarpa A, Bogina G, et al. Mucinous cystic tumors of the pancreas: Clinicopathological features, prognosis, and relationship to other mucinous cystic tumors. Am J Surg Pathol 1999;23:410–422.

590. Weihing RR, Shintaku IP, Geller SA, Petrovic LM. Hepatobiliary and pancreatic mucinous cystadenocarcinomas with mesenchymal stroma: Analysis of estrogen receptors/progesterone receptors and expression of tumor-associated antigens. Mod Pathol 1997;10:372–379.

591. Nagai E, Ueki T, Chijiiwa K, et al. Intraductal papillary mucinous neoplasms of the pancreas associated with so-called "mucinous ductal ectasia": Histochemical and immunohistochemical analysis of 29 cases. Am J Surg Pathol 1995;19:576–589.

592. Ohta T, Nagakawa T, Fukushima W, et al. Immunohistochemical study of carcinoembryonic antigen in mucinous cystic neoplasm of the pancreas. Eur Surg Res 1992;24:37–44.

593. Kawamori T, Tanaka T, Kawase Y, et al. An alpha-fetoprotein producing pancreatic cystadenocarcinoma. Clin Invest 1994;72:377–380.

594. Terada T, Ohta T, Kitamura Y, et al. Endocrine cells in intraductal papillary-mucinous neoplasms of the pancreas: A histochemical and immunohistochemical study. Virchows Arch 1997;431:31–36.

595. Friedman HD. Nonmucinous, glycogen-poor cystadenocarcinoma of the pancreas. Arch Pathol Lab Med 1990;114:888–891.

596. Tanno S, Obara T, Shudo R, et al. Alpha-fetoprotein producing mucin-producing carcinoma of the pancreas: A case report with immunohistochemical study and lectin-affinity profile. Dig Dis Sci 1997;42:2513–2518.

597. Fukushima N, Mukai K. 'Ovarian-type' stroma of pancreatic mucinous cystic tumor expresses smooth muscle phenotype. [letter] Pathol Int 1997;47:806–808.

598. Westra WH, Sturm P, Drillenburg P, et al. K-*ras* oncogene mutations in osteoclast-like giant cell tumors of the pancreas and liver: Genetic evidence to support origin from the duct epithelium. Am J Surg Pathol 1998;22:1247–1254.

599. Bergman S, Medeiros LJ, Radr T, et al. Giant cell tumor of the pancreas arising in the ovarian-like stroma of a mucinous cystadenocarcinoma. Int J Pancreatol 1995;18:71–75.

600. Wenig BM, Albores-Saavedra J, Buetow PC, Heffess CS. Pancreatic mucinous cystic neoplasm with sarcomatous stroma: A report of three cases. Am J Surg Pathol 1997;21:70–80.

601. Goldberg RD, Michelassi F, Montag AG. Osteoclast-like giant cell tumor of the pancreas: Immunophenotypic similarity to giant cell tumor of bone. Hum Pathol 1991;22:618–622.

602. Oehler U, Jurs M, Kloppel G, Helpap B. Osteoclast-like giant cell tumour of the pancreas presenting as a pseudocyst-like lesion. Virchows Arch 1997;431:215–218.

603. Newbould MJ, Benbow EW, Sene A, et al. Adenocarcinoma of the pancreas with osteoclast-like giant cells: A case report with immunocytochemistry. Pancreas 1992;7:611–615.

604. Kuerer H, Shim H, Pertsemlidis D, Unger P. Functioning pancreatic acinar cell carcinoma: Immunohistochemical and ultrastructural analyses. Am J Clin Oncol 1997;20:101–107.

605. Klimstra DS, Heffess CS, Oertel JE, Rosai J. Acinar cell carcinoma of the pancreas: A clinicopathologic study of 28 cases. Am J Surg Pathol 1992;16:815–837.

606. Caruso RA, Inferrera A, Tuccari G, Barresi G. Acinar cell carcinoma of the pancreas: A histologic, immunocytochemical and ultrastructural study. Histol Histopathol 1994;9:53–58.

607. Morohoshi T, Kanda M, Horie A, et al. Immunocytochemical markers of uncommon pancreatic tumors. Cancer 1987;59:739–747.

608. di Sant'Agnese PA. Acinar cell carcinoma of the pancreas. Ultrastruct Pathol 1991;15:573–577.

609. Shinagawa T, Tadokoro M, Maeyama S, et al. Alpha feto-protein-producing acinar cell carcinoma of the pancreas showing multiple lines of differentiation. Virchows Arch 1995;426:419–423.

610. Nojima T, Kojima T, Kato H, et al. Alpha-fetoprotein-producing acinar cell carcinoma of the pancreas. Hum Pathol 1992;23:828–830.

611. Kawamoto S, Hiraoka T, Kanemitsu K, et al. Alpha-fetoprotein-producing pancreatic cancer—a case report and review of 28 cases. Hepatogastroenterology 1992;39:282–286.

612. Frank M, Bittinger A, Rothmund M, Arnold R. Immunohistochemical analysis and clinical course of high-malignant composite endocrine-acinar cell carcinoma: A case report. [letter] Pancreas 1998;17:210–212.

613. Klimstra DS, Rosai J, Heffess CS. Mixed acinar-endocrine carcinomas of the pancreas. Am J Surg Pathol 1994;18:765–778.

614. Wunsch LP, Flemming P, Werner U, et al. Diagnosis and treatment of papillary cystic tumor of the pancreas in children. Eur J Pediatr Surg 1997;7:45–47.

615. Mao C, Guvendi M, Domenico DR, et al. Papillary cystic and solid tumors of the pancreas: A pancreatic embryonic tumor? Studies of three cases and cumulative review of the world's literature. Surgery 1995;118:821–828.

616. Yamaguchi K, Miyagahara T, Tsuneyoshi M, et al: Papillary cystic tumor of the pancreas: An immunohistochemical and ultrastructural study of 14 patients. Jpn J Clin Oncol 1989;19:102–111.

617. Pettinato G, Manivel JC, Ravetto C, et al. Papillary cystic tumor of the pancreas: A clinicopathologic study of 20 cases with cytologic, immunohistochemical, ultrastructural, and flow cytometric observations and a review of the literature. Am J Clin Pathol 1992;98:478–488.

618. Remadi S, MacGee GW, Doussis-Anagnostopoulou I, et al. Papillary-cystic tumor of the pancreas. Diagn Cytopathol 1996;15:398–402.

619. von Herbay A, Sieg B, Otto HF. Solid-cystic tumour of the pancreas: An endocrine neoplasm? Virchows Arch 1990;416:535–538.

620. Ohiwa K, Igarashi M, Nagasue N, et al. Solid and cystic tumor (SCT) of the pancreas in an adult man. HPB Surg 1997;10:315–321.

621. Morales A, Ruiz Molina JM, Esteves HO, et al. Papillary-cystic neoplasm of the pancreas: A sex-steroid dependent tumor. Int J Pancreatol 1998;24:219–225.

622. Ueda N, Nagakawa T, et al. Clinicopathological studies on solid and cystic tumors of the pancreas. Gastroenterol Jpn 1991;26:497–502.

623. Berho M, Blaustein A, Willis I, et al. Microglandular carcinoma of the pancreas: Immunohistochemical and ultrastructural study of an unusual variant of pancreatic carcinoma that may closely resemble a neuroendocrine neoplasm. Am J Clin Pathol 1996;105:727–732.

624. Suda K, Nobukawa B, Mogaki M, Fujii K. Variants of ductal adenocarcinoma of pancreas. Pancreas 1999;19:318–320.

625. Ono T, Komatsu M, Hoshino T, et al. Alpha-fetoprotein, carcinoembryonic antigen, and carbohydrate antigen 19-9-producing gallbladder cancer. J Gastroenterol 1996;31:742–746.

626. Vardaman C, Albores-Saavedra J. Clear cell carcinomas of the gallbladder and extrahepatic bile ducts. Am J Surg Pathol 1995;19:91–99.

627. Yano T, Ishikura H, Wada T, et al. Hepatoid adenocarcinoma of the pancreas. Histopathology 1999;35:90–92.

628. Zamboni G, Pea M, Martignoni G, et al. Clear cell "sugar" tumor of the pancreas: A novel member of the family of lesions characterized by the presence of perivascular epithelioid cells. Am J Surg Pathol 1996;20:722–730.

629. Ritter JH, Mills SE, Gaffey MJ, et al. Clear cell tumors of the alimentary tract and abdominal cavity. Semin Diag Pathol 1997;14:213–219.

630. Shorten SD, Hart WR, Petras RE. Microcystic adenomas (serous cystadenomas) of pancreas: A clinicopathologic investigation of eight cases with immunohistochemical and

631. Perez-Ordonez B, Naseem A, Lieberman PH, Klimstra DS. Solid serous adenoma of the pancreas: The solid variant of serous cystadenoma? Am J Surg Pathol 1996;20:1401–1405.

632. Ishikawa T, Nakao A, Nomoto S, et al. Immunohistochemical and molecular biological studies of serous cystadenoma of the pancreas. Pancreas 1998;16:40–44.

633. Fujii H, Kubo S, Hirohashi K, et al. Serous cystadenoma of the pancreas with atypical cells: Case report. Int J Pancreatol 1998;23:165–169.

634. Gafa R, Grandi E, Cavazzini L. Lymphoepithelial cyst of the pancreas. J Clin Pathol 1997;50:794–795.

635. Iezzoni JC, Mills SE, Pelkey TJ, Stoler MH. Inhibin is not an immunohistochemical marker for hepatocellular carcinoma: An example of the potential pitfall in diagnostic immunohistochemistry caused by endogenous biotin. Am J Clin Pathol 1999;111:229–234.

636. Bratthauer GL. The avidin-biotin complex (ABC) method and other avidin-biotin binding methods. Methods Mol Biol 1999;115:203–214.

637. Wang JH, Dhillon AP, Sankey EA, et al. 'Neuroendocrine' differentiation in primary neoplasms of the liver. J Pathol 1991;163:61–67.

638. Miller RT, Kubier P. Blocking of endogenous avidin-binding activity in immunohistochemistry: The use of egg whites. Appl Immunohistochem 1997;5:63–66.

639. Rodriguez-Soto J, Warnke RA, Rouse RV. Endogenous avidin-binding activity in paraffin-embedded tissue revealed after microwave treatment. Appl Immunohistochem 1997;5:59–62.

640. Dodson A, Campbell F. Biotin inclusions: A potential pitfall in immunohistochemistry avoided. Histopathology 1999;34:178–179.

641. Nayler SJ, Goetsch S, Cooper K. Biotin inclusions: A potential pitfall in immunohistochemistry. Histopathology 1998;33:87.

642. Bussolati G, Gugliotta P, Volante M, et al. Retrieved endogenous biotin: A novel marker and a potential pitfall in diagnostic immunohistochemistry. [see comments] Histopathology 1997;31:400–407.

643. McCluggage WC, Maxwell P, Patterson A, Sloan JM. Immunohistochemical staining of hepatocellular carcinoma with monoclonal antibody against inhibin. Histopathology 1997;30:518–522.

644. Denk H, Krepler R, Lackinger E, et al. Biochemical and immunocytochemical analysis of the intermediate filament cytoskeleton in human hepatocellular carcinomas and in hepatic neoplastic nodules of mice. Lab Invest 1982;46:584–596.

645. Moll R, Franke WW, Schiller DL, et al. The catalog of human cytokeratins: Patterns of expression in normal epithelia, tumors and cultured cells. Cell 1982;31:11–24.

646. Desmet VJ, Van Eyken P, Sciot R. Cytokeratins for probing cell lineage relationships in developing liver. Hepatology 1990;12:1249–1251.

647. Stosiek P, Kasper M, Karsten U: Expression of cytokeratin 19 during human organogenesis. Liver 1990;10:59–63.

648. Van Eyken P, Sciot R, van Damme B, et al. Keratin immunohistochemistry in normal human liver: Cytokeratin pattern of hepatocytes, bile ducts and acinar gradient. Virchows Arch A Pathol Anat Histopathol 1987;412:63–72.

649. Van Eyken P, Sciot R, Desmet VJ. Immunocytochemistry of cytokeratins in primary human liver tumors. APMIS Suppl 1991;23:77–85.

650. Lai Y-S, Thung SN, Gerber MA, et al. Expression of cytokeratins in normal and diseased livers and in primary liver carcinomas. Arch Pathol Lab Med 1989;113:134–138.

651. Hurlimann J, Gardiol D. Immunohistochemistry in the differential diagnosis of liver carcinomas. Am J Surg Pathol 1991;15:280–288.

652. Shah KD, Gerber MA. Development of intrahepatic bile ducts in humans: Immunohistochemical study using monoclonal cytokeratin antibodies. Arch Pathol Lab Med 1989;113:1135–1138.

653. Kakizoe S, Kojiro M, Nakashima K. Hepatocellular carcinoma with sarcomatous change: Clinicopathologic and immunohistochemical studies of 14 autopsy cases. Cancer 1987;59:310–316.

654. Demetris AJ, Seaberg EC, Wennerberg AE, et al. Ductular reaction after submassive necrosis in humans: Special emphasis on analysis of ductular hepatocytes. Am J Pathol 1996;149:439–448.

655. Wennerberg AE, Nalesnik MA, Coleman WB. Hepatocyte paraffin 1: A monoclonal antibody that reacts with hepatocytes and can be used for differential diagnosis of hepatic tumors. Am J Pathol 1993;143:1050–1054.

656. Johnson DE, Powers CN, Rupp G, Frable WJ. Immunocytochemical staining of fine-needle aspiration biopsies of the liver as a diagnostic tool for hepatocellular carcinoma. Mod Pathol 1992;5:117–123.

657. Theise ND, Fiel IM, Hytiroglou P, et al. Macroregenerative nodules in cirrhosis are not associated with elevated serum or stainable tissue alpha-fetoprotein. Liver 1995;15:30–34.

658. Goldstein NS, Blue DE, Hankin RH, et al. Serum alpha-fetoprotein levels in patients with chronic hepatitis C: Relationships with serum alanine amino transferase values, histologic activity index, and hepatocyte mib-1 scores. Am J Clin Pathol 1999;111:811–816.

659. Rubio CA. The detection of bile ducts in liver biopsies by cytokeratin 7. In Vivo 1998;12:183–186.

660. Ruck P, Xiao JC, Kaiserling E. Small epithelial cells and the histogenesis of hepatoblastoma: Electron microscopic, immunoelectron microscopic, and immunohistochemical findings. Am J Pathol 1996;148:321–329.

661. Terada T, Nakanuma Y. Pathological observations of intrahepatic peribiliary glands in 1,000 consecutive autopsy livers. II: A possible source of cholangiocarcinoma. Hepatology 1990;12:92–97.

662. Nakajima T, Kondo Y. Well-differentiated cholangiocarcinoma: Diagnostic significance of morphologic and immunohistochemical parameters. Am J Surg Pathol 1989;13:569–573.

663. Gerber MA, Thung SN. Liver stem cells and development. Lab Invest 1993;68:253–254.

664. Haque S, Haruna Y, Saito K, et al. Identification of bipotential progenitor cells in human liver regeneration. Lab Invest 1996;75:699–705.

665. Sell S. Is there a liver stem cell? Cancer Res 1990;50:3811–3815.

666. Thorgeirsson SS. Hepatic stem cells. Am J Pathol 1993;142:1331–1333.

667. Hsia CC, Evarts RP, Nakatsukasa H, et al. Occurrence of oval-type cells in hepatitis B virus-associated human hepatocarcinogenesis. Hepatology 1992;16:1327–1333.

668. Ruck P, Xiao JC, Pietsch T, et al. Hepatic stem-like cells in hepatoblastoma: Expression of cytokeratin 7, albumin and oval cell associated antigens detected by OV-1 and OV-6. Histopathology 1997;31:324–329.

669. Halme L, Karkkainen P, Isoniemi H, et al. Carbohydrate 19-9 antigen as a marker of non-malignant hepatocytic ductular transformation in patients with acute liver failure: A comparison with alpha-fetoprotein and carcinoembryonic antigen. Scand J Gastroenterol 1999;34:426–431.

670. Van Eyken P, Sciot R, Desmet VJ. A cytokeratin immunohistochemical study of cholestatic liver disease: Evidence that hepatocytes can express 'bile duct-type' cytokeratins. Histopathology 1989;15:125–135.

671. Van Eyken P, Sciot R, Callea F, Desmet VJ. A cytokeratin-immunohistochemical study of focal nodular hyperplasia of the liver: Further evidence that ductular metaplasia of hepatocytes contributes to ductular "proliferation." Liver 1989;9:372–377.

672. Van Eyken P, Sciot R, Desmet VJ. A cytokeratin immunohistochemical study of alcoholic liver disease: Evidence that hepatocytes can express 'bile duct-type' cytokeratins. Histopathology 1988;13:605–617.

673. Gottschalk-Sabag S, Ron N, Glick T. Use of CD34 and factor VIII to diagnose hepatocellular carcinoma on fine needle aspirates. Acta Cytol 1998;42:691–696.

674. Ruck P, Xiao JC, Kaiserling E. QBend 10 (CD34) in the diagnosis of hepatocellular carcinoma. Histopathology 1996;29:593–594.

675. Terayama N, Terada T, Nakanuma Y. An immunohistochemical study of tumour vessels in metastatic liver cancers and the surrounding liver tissue. Histopathology 1996;29:37–43.

676. Ruck P, Xiao JC, Kaiserling E. Immunoreactivity of sinusoids in hepatocellular carcinoma: An immunohistochemical study using lectin UEA-1 and antibodies against endothelial markers, including CD34. Arch Pathol Lab Med 1995;119:173–178.

677. Haratake J, Scheuer PJ. An immunohistochemical and ultrastructural study of the sinusoids of hepatocellular carcinoma. Cancer 1990;65:1985–1993.

678. Selby DM, Stocker T. Focal peliosis hepatis: A sequela of asphyxial death. Pediatr Pathol 1995;15:589–596.

679. Zhou H, Fischer HP. Liver carcinoma in PiZ alpha-1-antitrypsin deficiency. Am J Surg Pathol 1998;22:742–748.

680. Lohr HF, Schlaak JF, Dienes HP, et al. Liver cirrhosis associated with heterozygous alpha-1-antitrypsin deficiency type Pi MS and autoimmune features. Digestion 1995;56:41–45.

681. Iezzoni JC, Gaffey MJ, Stacy EK, Normansell D. Hepatocyte globules in end-stage hepatic disease: Relationship to alpha1-antitrypsin phenotype. Am J Clin Pathol 1997;107:692–697.

682. Hazan R, Denk H, Franke WW, et al. Change of cytokeratin organization during development of Mallory bodies as revealed by a monoclonal antibody. Lab Invest 1986;54:543–553.

683. Denk H, Gschnait F, Wolff K. Hepatocellar hyalin (Mallory bodies) in long term griseofulvin-treated mice: A new experimental model for the study of hyalin formation. Lab Invest 1975;32:773–776.

684. Zatloukal K, Bock G, Rainer I, et al. High molecular weight components are main constituents of Mallory bodies isolated with a fluorescence activated cell sorter. Lab Invest 1991;64:200–206.

685. Herrmann G. Immunohistochemical study of HBV antigens in 338 liver cell carcinomas. Z Gastroenterol 1999;37:329–342.

686. Suzuki K, Uchida T, Shikata T. Histopathological analysis of chronic hepatitis B virus (HBV) infection in relation to HBV replication. Liver 1987;7:260–270.

687. Suzuki K, Uchida T, Horiuchi R, Shikata T. Localization of hepatitis B surface and core antigens in human hepatocellular carcinoma by immunoperoxidase methods: Replication of complete virions of carcinoma cells. Cancer 1985;56:321–327.

688. Comanescu V, Ardeleanu C, Zaharia B, et al. Histopathologic and immunohistochemic correlations in virus B chronic hepatitis. Rom J Morphol Embryol 1997;43:169–172.

689. Guido M, Thung SN. The value of identifying hepatitis C virus in liver pathology specimens. Hepatology 1996;23:376–379.

690. Brody RI, Eng S, Melamed J, et al. Immunohistochemical detection of hepatitis C antigen by monoclonal antibody TORDJI-22 compared with PCR viral detection. Am J Clin Pathol 1998;110:32–37.

691. Chamlian A, Benkoel L, Sahel J, et al: Immunohistochemical detection of hepatitis C virus related C100-3 and core antigens in formalin-fixed liver tissue. Cell Mol Biol (Noisy-le-grand) 1996;42:557–566.

692. Sansonno D, Iacobelli AR, Cornacchiulo V, et al. Immunohistochemical detection of hepatitis C virus-related proteins in liver tissue. Clin Exp Rheumatol 1995;13 Suppl 13:S29–S32.

693. Uchida T, Shikata T. Hepatitis C virus appears to replicate not only in hepatocytes but also in hepatocellular carcinoma cells as demonstrated by immunostaining. Pathol Int 1994;44:832–836.

694. Uchida T, Shikata T, Tanaka E, Kiyosawa K. Immunoperoxidase staining of hepatitis C virus in formalin-fixed, paraffin-embedded needle liver biopsies. Virchows Arch 1994;424:465–469.

695. Asanza CG, Garcia-Monzon C, Clemente G, et al. Immunohistochemical evidence of immunopathogenetic mechanisms in chronic hepatitis C recurrence after liver transplantation. Hepatology 1997;26:755–763.

696. Dries V, von Both I, Muller M, et al. Detection of hepatitis C virus in paraffin-embedded liver biopsies of patients negative for viral RNA in serum. Hepatology 1999;29:223–229.

697. Gerber MA. Pathobiology of hepatitis C. Verh Dtsch Ges Pathol 1995;79:162–170.

698. Xiping Z, Dongliang Y, Lianjie H. Immunohistochemical detection and significance of hepatitis C virus antigen. Chin Med J (Engl) 1996;109:486–488.

699. Ohsawa M, Tomita Y, Hashimoto M, et al. Hepatitis C viral genome in a subset of primary hepatic lymphomas. Mod Pathol 1998;11:471–478.

700. Tanimoto K, Akbar SM, Michitaka K, Onji M. Immunohistochemical localization of antigen presenting cells in liver from patients with primary biliary cirrhosis; highly restricted distribution of CD83-positive activated dendritic cells. Pathol Res Pract 1999;195:157–162.

701. Desmet VJ. What more can we ask from the pathologist? J Hepatol 1996;25:25–29.

702. Washington K, Gottfried MR. Expression of p53 in adenocarcinoma of the gallbladder and bile ducts. Liver 1996;16:99–104.

703. Kaserer K, Exner M, Mosberger I, et al. Characterization of the inflammatory infiltrate in autoimmune cholangitis: A morphological and immunhistochemical study. Virchows Arch 1998;432:217–222.

704. Ponsioen CY, Kuiper H, Ten Kate FJ, et al. Immunohistochemical analysis of inflammation in primary sclerosing cholangitis. Eur J Gastroenterol Hepatol 1999;11:769–774.

705. Scott FR, el Refaie A, More L, et al. Hepatocellular carcinoma arising in an adenoma: Value of QBend 10 immunostaining in diagnosis of liver cell carcinoma. Histopathology 1996;28:472–474.

706. Bhathal PS, Hughes NR, Goodman ZD. The so-called bile duct adenoma is a peribiliary gland hamartoma. Am J Surg Pathol 1996;20:858–864.

707. Allaire GS, Rabin L, Ishak KG, Sesterhenn IA. Bile duct adenoma: A study of 152 cases. Am J Surg Pathol 1988;12:708–715.

708. Haas JE, Muczynski KA, Krailo M, et al. Histopathology and prognosis in childhood hepatoblastoma and hepatocarcinoma. Cancer 1989;64:1082–1095.

709. Warfel KA, Hull MT. Hepatoblastomas: An ultrastructural and immunohistochemical study. Ultrastruct Pathol 1992;16:451–461.

710. Schmidt D, Harms D, Lang W. Primary malignant hepatic tumours in childhood. Virchows Arch A Pathol Anat Histopathol 1985;407:387–405.

711. Van Eyken P, Sciot R, Callea F, et al. The development of the intrahepatic bile ducts in man: A keratin-immunohistochemical study. Hepatology 1988;8:1586–1595.

712. Fasano M, Theise ND, Nalesnik MA, et al. Immunohistochemical evaluation of hepatoblastomas with use of the hepatocyte-specific marker, hepatocyte paraffin 1, and the polyclonal anti-carcinoembryonic antigen. Mod Pathol 1998;11:934–938.

713. Osborn M, van Lessen G, Weber K, et al. Differential diagnosis of gastrointestinal carcinomas by using monoclonal antibodies specific for individual keratin polypeptides. Lab Invest 1986;55:497–504.

714. Van Eyken P, Sciot R, Paterson A, et al. Cytokeratin expression in hepatocellular carcinoma: An immunohistochemical study. Hum Pathol 1988;19:562–568.

715. Wu PC, Fang JW, Lau VK, et al. Classification of hepatocellular carcinoma according to hepatocellular and biliary differentiation markers: Clinical and biological implications. Am J Pathol 1996;149:1167–1175.

716. Maeda T, Adachi E, Kajiyama K, et al. Combined hepatocellular and cholangiocarcinoma: Proposed criteria according to cytokeratin expression and analysis of clinicopathologic features. Hum Pathol 1995;26:956–964.

717. Adamek HE, Spiethoff A, Kaufmann V, et al. Primary clear cell carcinoma of noncirrhotic liver: Immunohistochemical discrimination of hepatocellular and cholangiocellular origin. Dig Dis Sci 1998;43:33–38.

718. Tsuji M, Kashihara T, Terada N, Mori H. An immunohistochemical study of hepatic atypical adenomatous hyperplasia, hepatocellular carcinoma, and cholangiocarcinoma with alpha-fetoprotein, carcinoembryonic antigen, CA19-9, epithelial membrane antigen, and cytokeratins 18 and 19. Pathol Int 1999;49:310–317.

719. Zhao M, Zimmermann A. Apoptosis in hepatocellular carcinomas with neuroendocrine differentiation. Histol Histopathol 1997;12:973–980.

720. Zhao M, Laissue JA, Zimmermann A. "Neuroendocrine" differentiation in hepatocellular carcinomas (HCCs): Immunohistochemical reactivity is related to distinct tumor cell types, but not to tumor grade. Histol Histopathol 1993;8:617–626.

721. Listrom MB, Dalton LW. Comparison of keratin monoclonal antibodies MAK-6, AE1:AE3, and CAM-5.2. Am J Clin Pathol 1987;88:297–301.

722. Rosendale BE, Dusenbery D. Cytology of hepatocellular carcinoma in serous fluids: A report of three cases. Diagn Cytopathol 1996;15:127–131.

723. Thomas P, Battifora H. Keratins versus epithelial membrane antigen in tumor diagnosis: an immunohistochemical comparison of five monoclonal antibodies. Hum Pathol 1987;18:728–734.

724. D'Errico A, Baccarini P, Fiorentino M, et al. Histogenesis of primary liver carcinomas: Strengths and weaknesses of cytokeratin profile and albumin mRNA detection. Hum Pathol 1996;27:599–604.

725. Johnson DE, Herndier BG, Medeiros LJ, et al. The diagnostic utility of the keratin profiles of hepatocellular carcinoma and cholangiocarcinoma. Am J Surg Pathol 1988;12:187–197.

726. Minervini MI, Demetris AJ, Lee RG, et al. Utilization of hepatocyte-specific antibody in the immunocytochemical evaluation of hepatocyte-specific antibody in the immunocytochemical evaluation of liver tumors. Mod Pathol 1997;10:686–692.

727. Schwartz MZ: Unusual peptide-secreting tumors in adolescents and children. Semin Pediatr Surg 1997;6:141–146.

728. Spagnolo DV, Whitaker D, Carrello S, et al. The use of monoclonal antibody 44-3A6 in cell blocks in the diagnosis of lung carcinoma, carcinomas metastatic to lung and pleura, and pleural malignant mesothelioma. Am J Clin Pathol 1991;95:322–329.

729. Balaton AJ, Nehama-Sibony M, Gotheil C, et al. Distinction between hepatocellular carcinoma, cholangiocarcinoma, and metastatic carcinoma based on immunohistochemical staining for carcinoembryonic antigen and for cytokeratin 19 on paraffin sections. J Pathol 1988;156:305–310.

730. Fucich LF, Cheles MK, Thung SN, et al. Primary vs metastatic hepatic carcinoma: An immunohistochemical study of 34 cases. Arch Pathol Lab Med 1994;118:927–930.

731. Maeda T, Adachi E, Kajiyama K, et al. Spindle cell hepatocellular carcinoma: A clinicopathologic and immunohistochemical analysis of 15 cases. Cancer 1996;77:51–57.

732. Brumm C, Schulze C, Charels K, et al. The significance of alpha-fetoprotein and other tumour markers in differential immunocytochemistry of primary liver tumours. Histopathology 1989;14:503–513.

733. Pinkus GS, Kurtin PJ. Epithelial membrane antigen-A diagnostic discriminant in surgical pathology: Immunohistochemical profile in epithelial, mesenchymal, and hematopoietic neoplasms using paraffin sections and monoclonal antibodies. Hum Pathol 1985;16:929–940.

734. Renshaw AA, Granter SR. A comparison of A103 and inhibin reactivity in adrenal cortical tumors: Distinction from hepatocellular carcinoma and renal tumors. Mod Pathol 1998;11:1160–1164.

735. Kimura H, Nakajima T, Kagawa K, et al. Angiogenesis in hepatocellular carcinoma as evaluated by CD34 immunohistochemistry. Liver 1998;18:14–19.

736. Cui S, Hano H, Sakata A, et al. Enhanced CD34 expression

of sinusoid-like vascular endothelial cells in hepatocellular carcinoma. Pathol Int 1996;46:751–756.

737. Pitman MB, Szyfelbein WM. Significance of endothelium in the fine-needle aspiration biopsy diagnosis of hepatocellular carcinoma. Diagn Cytopathol 1995;12:208–214.

738. Park YN, Yang CP, Fernandez GJ, et al. Neoangiogenesis and sinusoidal "capillarization" in dysplastic nodules of the liver. Am J Surg Pathol 1998;22:656–662.

739. Akasofu M, Kawahara E, Kaji K, Nakanishi I. Sarcomatoid hepatocellular-carcinoma showing rhabdomyoblastic differentiation in the adult cirrhotic liver. Virchows Arch 1999;434:511–515.

740. Fayyazi A, Nolte W, Oestmann JW, et al. Carcinosarcoma of the liver. Histopathology 1998;32:385–387.

741. Andreola S, Audisio RA, Lombardi L. A light microscopic and ultrastructural study of two cases of fibrolamellar hepatocellular carcinoma. Tumori 1986;72:609–616.

742. Van Eyken P, Sciot R, Brock P, et al. Abundant expression of cytokeratin 7 in fibrolamellar carcinoma of the liver. Histopathology 1990;17:101–107.

743. Scoazec JY, Flejou JF, D'Errico A, et al. Fibrolamellar carcinoma of the liver: Composition of the extracellular matrix and expression of cell-matrix and cell-cell adhesion molecules. Hepatology 1996;24:1128–1136.

744. Nerlich AG, Majewski S, Hunzelmann N, et al. Excessive collagen formation in fibrolamellar carcinoma of the liver: A morphological and biochemical study. Mod Pathol 1992;5:580–585.

745. McCloskey JJ, Germain-Lee EL, Perman JA, et al. Gynecomastia as a presenting sign of fibrolamellar carcinoma of the liver. Pediatrics 1988;82:379–382.

746. Vecchio FM. Fibrolamellar carcinoma of the liver: A distinct entity within the hepatocellular tumors: A review. Appl Pathol 1988;6:139–148.

747. Caballero T, Aneiros J, Lopez-Caballero J, et al. Fibrolamellar hepatocellular carcinoma: An immunohistochemical and ultrastructural study. Histopathology 1985;9:445–456.

748. Berman MA, Burnham JA, Sheahan DG. Fibrolamellar carcinoma of the liver: An immunohistochemical study of nineteen cases and a review of the literature. Hum Pathol 1988;19:784–794.

749. Singson RC, Fraiman M, Geller SA. Hepatocellular carcinoma with fibrolamellar pattern in a patient with autoimmune cholangitis. Mt Sinai J Med 1999;66:109–112.

750. Eckstein RP, Bambach CP, Stiel D, et al. Fibrolamellar carcinoma as a cause of bile duct obstruction. Pathology 1988;20:326–331.

751. Mierau GW, Orsini EN Jr: Diagnosis of human tumors. Case 1: Hepatocarcinoma, fibrolamellar type. Ultrastruct Pathol 1983;5:273–279.

752. Okano A, Hajiro K, Takakuwa H, Kobashi Y. Fibrolamellar carcinoma of the liver with a mixture of ordinary hepatocellular carcinoma: A case report. Am J Gastroenterol 1998;93:1144–1145.

753. Okada K, Kim YI, Nakashima K, et al. Fibrolamellar hepatocellular carcinoma coexistent with a hepatocellular carcinoma of common type: Report of a case. Surg Today 1993;23:626–631.

754. Saul SH, Titelbaum DS, Gansler TS, et al. The fibrolamellar variant of hepatocellular carcinoma: Its association with focal nodular hyperplasia. Cancer 1987;60:3049–3055.

755. Payne CM, Nagle RB, Paplanus SH, Graham AR. Fibrolamellar carcinoma of liver: A primary malignant oncocytic carcinoid? Ultrastruct Pathol 1986;10:539–552.

756. Lloreta J, Vadell C, Fabregat X, Serrano S. Fibrolamellar hepatic tumor with neurosecretory features and systemic deposition of AA amyloid. Ultrastruct Pathol 1994;18:287–292.

757. Zanconati F, Falconieri G, Lamovec J, Zidar A. Small cell carcinoma of the liver: A hitherto unreported variant of hepatocellular carcinoma. Histopathology 1996;29:449–453.

758. Morinaga S, Nishiya H, Inafuku T. Yolk sac tumor of the liver combined with hepatocellular carcinoma. Arch Pathol Lab Med 1996;120:687–690.

759. Leger-Ravet MB, Borgonovo G, Amato A, et al. Carcinosarcoma of the liver with mesenchymal differentiation: A case report. Hepatogastroenterology 1996;43:255–259.

760. Terada T, Kida T, Nakanuma Y, et al. Intrahepatic cholangiocarcinomas associated with nonbiliary cirrhosis: A clinicopathologic study. J Clin Gastroenterol 1994;18:335–342.

761. Tihan T, Blumgart LH, Klimstra DS. Clear cell papillary carcinoma of the liver: An unusual variant of peripheral cholangiocarcinoma. [see comments] Hum Pathol 1998;29:196–200.

762. Yamato T, Sasaki M, Hoso M, et al. Intrahepatic cholangiocarcinoma arising in congenital hepatic fibrosis: Report of an autopsy case. J Hepatol 1998;28:717–722.

763. Sasaki M, Nakanuma Y, Shimizu K, Izumi R. Pathological and immunohistochemical findings in a case of mucinous cholangiocarcinoma. Pathol Int 1995;45:781–786.

764. Nakajima T, Tajima Y, Sugano I, et al. Intrahepatic cholangiocarcinoma with sarcomatous change: Clinicopathologic and immunohistochemical evaluation of seven cases. Cancer 1993;72:1872–1877.

765. Imazu H, Ochiai M, Funabiki T. Intrahepatic sarcomatous cholangiocarcinoma. J Gastroenterol 1995;30:677–682.

766. Honda M, Enjoji M, Sakai H, et al. Case report: Intrahepatic cholangiocarcinoma with rhabdoid transformation. J Gastroenterol Hepatol 1996;11:771–774.

767. Falta EM, Rubin AD, Harris JA. Peripheral clear cell cholangiocarcinoma: A rare histologic variant. Am Surg 1999;65:592–595.

768. Isa T, Kusano T, Muto Y, et al. Clinicopathologic features of resected primary adenosquamous carcinomas of the liver. J Clin Gastroenterol 1997;25:623–627.

769. Yamamoto K, Takenaka K, Kajiyama K, et al. A primary adenosquamous carcinoma of the liver with an elevated level of serum squamous cell carcinoma related antigen. Hepatogastroenterology 1996;43:658–662.

770. Shimonishi T, Sugawara H, Miyazaki K, Nakanuma Y. Intrahepatic cholangiocarcinoma showing mixed differentiation: A case report. Histopathology 1998;33:488–490.

771. Siren J, Karkkainen P, Luukkonen P, et al. A case report of biliary cystadenoma and cystadenocarcinoma. Hepatogastroenterology 1998;45:83–89.

772. Devaney K, Goodman ZD, Ishak KG. Hepatobiliary cystadenoma and cystadenocarcinoma: A light microscopic and immunohistochemical study of 70 patients. Am J Surg Pathol 1994;18:1078–1091.

773. Yanase M, Ikeda H, Ogata I, et al. Primary smooth muscle tumor of the liver encasing hepatobiliary cystadenoma without mesenchymal stroma. Am J Surg Pathol 1999;23:854–859.

774. Horsmans Y, Laka A, van Beers BE, et al. Hepatobiliary cystadenocarcinoma without ovarian stroma and normal CA 19-9 levels: Unusually prolonged evolution. Dig Dis Sci 1997;42:1406–1408.

775. Skopelitou A, Hadjiyannakis M. Hepatobiliary cystadenoma with mesenchymal stroma (CMS) in association with unilateral mucinous cystadenoma of the ovary (MCO): Case report and review of the literature. Eur J Gynaecol Oncol 1996;17:234–240.

776. Terada T, Kitamura Y, Ohta T, Nakanuma Y. Endocrine cells in hepatobiliary cystadenomas and cystadenocarcinomas. Virchows Arch 1997;430:37–40.

777. Scott FR, More L, Dhillon AP. Hepatobiliary cystadenoma with mesenchymal stroma: Expression of oestrogen receptors in formalin-fixed tissue. Histopathology 1995;26:555–558.

778. Grayson W, Teare J, Myburgh JA, Paterson AC. Immunohistochemical demonstration of progesterone receptor in hepatobiliary cystadenoma with mesenchymal stroma. Histopathology 1996;29:461–463.

779. Taguchi J, Nakashima O, Tanaka M, et al. A clinicopathological study on combined hepatocellular and cholangiocarcinoma. J Gastroenterol Hepatol 1996;11:758–764.

780. Dusenbery D. Combined hepatocellular-cholangiocarcinoma: Cytologic findings in four cases. Acta Cytol 1997;41:903–909.

781. Goodman ZD, Ishak KG, Langloss JM, et al. Combined hepatocellular-cholangiocarcinoma: A histologic and immunohistochemical study. Cancer 1985;55:124–135.

782. Ng IO, Shek TW, Nicholls J, Ma LT. Combined hepatocellular-cholangiocarcinoma: A clinicopathological study. J Gastroenterol Hepatol 1998;13:34–40.

783. Papotti M, Sambataro D, Marchesa P, Negro F. A combined hepatocellular/cholangiocellular carcinoma with sarcomatoid features. Liver 1997;17:47–52.

784. Scheimberg I, Cullinane C, Kelsey A, Malone M. Primary hepatic malignant tumor with rhabdoid features: A histological, immunocytochemical, and electron microscopic study of four cases and a review of the literature. Am J Surg Pathol 1996;20:1394–1400.

785. Vortmeyer AO, Kingma DW, Fenton RG, et al. Hepatobiliary lymphoepithelioma-like carcinoma associated with Epstein-Barr virus. Am J Clin Pathol 1998;109:90–95.

786. Oh YH, Kang GH, Kim OJ. Primary hepatic carcinoid tumor with a paranuclear clear zone: A case report. J Korean Med Sci 1998;13:317–320.

787. Krishnamurthy SC, Dutta V, Pai SA, et al. Primary carcinoid tumor of the liver: Report of four resected cases including one with gastrin production. J Surg Oncol 1996;62:218–221.

788. Pilichowska M, Kimura N, Ouchi A, et al. Primary hepatic carcinoid and neuroendocrine carcinoma: Clinicopathological and immunohistochemical study of five cases. Pathol Int 1999;49:318–324.

789. O'Hara BJ, McCue PA, Miettinen M. Bile duct adenomas with endocrine component: Immunohistochemical study and comparison with conventional bile duct adenomas. Am J Surg Pathol 1992;16:21–25.

790. Shetlar DJ, Font RL, Ordonez NG, et al. A clinicopathologic study of three carcinoid tumors metastatic to the orbit: Immunohistochemical, ultrastructural, and DNA flow cytometric studies. Ophthalmology 1990;97:257–264.

791. Miura K, Shirasawa H. Primary carcinoid tumor of the liver. Am J Clin Pathol 1988;89:561–564.

792. Fukunaga M. Neuroendocrine carcinoma of the liver: An autopsy case. Pathol Int 1998;48:481–485.

793. Yamamoto J, Abe Y, Nishihara K, et al. Composite glandular-neuroendocrine carcinoma of the hilar bile duct: Report of a case. Surg Today 1998;28:758–762.

794. Piatti B, Caspani B, Giudici C, Ferrario D. Fine needle aspiration biopsy of hepatocellular carcinoma resembling neuroendocrine tumor: A case report. Acta Cytol 1997;41:583–586.

795. Nakasuka H, Okada S, Okusaka T, et al. Undifferentiated carcinoma of the liver with neuroendocrine features: a case report. Jpn J Clin Oncol 1998;28:401–404.

796. Ruckert RI, Ruckert JC, Dorffel Y, et al. Primary hepatic neuroendocrine tumor: Successful hepatectomy in two cases and review of the literature. Digestion 1999;60:110–116.

797. Andreola S, Lombardi L, Audisio RA, et al. A clinicopathologic study of primary hepatic carcinoid tumors. Cancer 1990;65:1211–1218.

798. Sioutos N, Virta S, Kessimian N. Primary hepatic carcinoid tumor: An electron microscopic and immunohistochemical study. Am J Clin Pathol 1991;95:172–175.

799. Aoki K, Sakamoto M, Mukai K, et al. Signet-ring cell carcinoid: A primary hepatic carcinoid tumor with cytoplasmic inclusions comprising of aggregates of keratin. Jpn J Clin Oncol 1992;22:54–59.

800. Sugimoto F, Sekiya T, Saito M, et al. Calcitonin-producing pancreatic somatostatinoma: Report of a case. Surg Today 1998;28:1279–1282.

801. Ordonez NG. Desmoplastic small round cell tumor. I: A histopathologic study of 39 cases with emphasis on unusual histological patterns. Am J Surg Pathol 1998;22:1303–1313.

802. Papadogiannakis N, Gad A, Sjostedt S, et al. Adenocarcinoid of the liver arising within an area of hamartoma with predominant bile duct component. J Clin Gastroenterol 1996;23:145–151.

803. Prosser JM, Dusenbery D. Histocytologic diagnosis of neuroendocrine tumors in the liver: A retrospective study of 23 cases. Diagn Cytopathol 1997;16:383–391.

804. Hong SM, Yu E, Ahn H, Kim OJ. Alpha-fetoprotein producing renal cell carcinoma: A case report. J Korean Med Sci 1998;13:321–324.

805. Ali SZ: Metastatic granulosa-cell tumor in the liver: Cytopathologic findings and staining with inhibin. Diagn Cytopathol 1998;19:293–297.

806. Terris B, Flejou JF, Picot R, et al. Hepatic angiomyolipoma: A report of four cases with immunohistochemical and DNA-flow cytometric studies. Arch Pathol Lab Med 1996;120:68–72.

807. Cha I, Cartwright D, Guis M, et al. Angiomyolipoma of the liver in fine-needle aspiration biopsies: Its distinction from hepatocellular carcinoma. Cancer 1999;87:25–30.

808. Nonomura A, Mizukami Y, Kadoya M. Angiomyolipoma of the liver: A collective review. J Gastroenterol 1994;29:95–105.

809. Nonomura A, Minato H, Kurumaya H. Angiomyolipoma predominantly composed of smooth muscle cells: Problems in histological diagnosis. Histopathology 1998;33:20–27.

810. Gambacorta M, Bonacina E. Epithelioid hemangioendothelioma: Report of a case diagnosed by fine-needle aspiration. [see comments] Diagn Cytopathol 1989;5:207–210.

811. Demetris AJ, Minervini MI, Raikow RB, Lee RG. Hepatic epithelioid hemangioendothelioma: Biologic questions based on pattern of recurrence in an allograft and tumor immunophenotype. Am J Surg Pathol 1997;21:263–270.

812. Meis-Kindblom JM, Kindblom LG. Angiosarcoma of soft tissue: A study of 80 cases. Am J Surg Pathol 1998;22:683–697.

813. Hayashi Y, Inagaki K, Hirota S, et al. Epithelioid hemangioendothelioma with marked liver deformity and secondary Budd-Chiari syndrome: Pathological and radiological correlation. Pathol Int 1999;49:547–552.

814. Bralet MP, Terris B, Vilgrain V, et al. Epithelioid hemangioendothelioma, multiple focal nodular hyperplasias, and cavernous hemangiomas of the liver. Arch Pathol Lab Med 1999;123:846–849.

815. Nerlich A, Berndt R, Schleicher E. Differential basement membrane composition in multiple epithelioid haemangioendotheliomas of liver and lung. Histopathology 1991;18:303–307.

816. Anthony PP, Ramani P. Endothelial markers in malignant vascular tumours of the liver: Superiority of QB-END/10 over von Willebrand factor and *Ulex europaeus* agglutinin 1. J Clin Pathol 1991;44:29–32.

817. Kelleher MB, Iwatsuki S, Sheahan DG. Epithelioid hemangioendothelioma of liver: Clinicopathological correlation of 10 cases treated by orthotopic liver transplantation. Am J Surg Pathol 1989;13:999–1008.

818. Ruebner BH, Eggleston JC. What is new in epithelioid hemangioendothelioma of the liver? Pathol Res Pract 1987;182:110–112.

819. Weiss SW, Ishak KG, Dail DH, et al. Epithelioid hemangioendothelioma and related lesions. Semin Diagn Pathol 1986;3:259–287.

820. Dean PJ, Haggitt RC, O'Hara CJ. Malignant epithelioid hemangioendothelioma of the liver in young women: Relationship to oral contraceptive use. Am J Surg Pathol 1985;9:695–704.

821. Rojter S, Villamil FG, Petrovic LM, et al. Malignant vascular tumors of the liver presenting as liver failure and portal hypertension. Liver Transpl Surg 1995;1:156–161.

822. Makhlouf HR, Ishak KG, Goodman ZD. Epithelioid hemangioendothelioma of the liver: A clinicopathologic study of 137 cases. Cancer 1999;85:562–582.

823. Soslow RA, Yin P, Steinberg CR, Yang GC. Cytopathologic features of hepatic epithelioid hemangioendothelioma. Diagn Cytopathol 1997;17:50–53.

824. Cho NH, Lee KG, Jeong MG. Cytologic evaluation of primary malignant vascular tumors of the liver: One case each of angiosarcoma and epithelioid hemangioendothelioma. Acta Cytol 1997;41:1468–1476.

825. Scoazec JY, Degott C, Reynes M, et al. Epithelioid heman-

gioendothelioma of the liver: An ultrastructural study. Hum Pathol 1989;20:673–681.

826. Dietze O, Davies SE, Williams R, Portmann B. Malignant epithelioid haemangioendothelioma of the liver: A clinico-pathological and histochemical study of 12 cases. Histopathology 1989;15:225–237.

827. Eckstein RP, Ravich RB. Epithelioid hemangioendothelioma of the liver: Report of two cases histologically mimicking veno-occlusive disease. Pathology 1986;18:459–462.

828. Ferrell L. Malignant liver tumors that mimic benign lesions: Analysis of five distinct lesions. Semin Diagn Pathol 1995;12:64–76.

829. Guglielmi A, Frameglia M, Iuzzolino P, et al. Solitary fibrous tumor of the liver with CD 34 positivity and hypoglycemia. J Hepatobiliary Pancreat Surg 1998;5:212–216.

830. Coffin CM, Humphrey PA, Dehner LP. Extrapulmonary inflammatory myofibroblastic tumor: A clinical and pathological survey. Semin Diagn Pathol 1998;15:85–101.

831. Levine TS, Rose DS. Solitary fibrous tumour of the liver. [letter; comment] Histopathology 1997;30:396–397.

832. Moran CA, Ishak KG, Goodman ZD. Solitary fibrous tumor of the liver: A clinicopathologic and immunohistochemical study of nine cases. Ann Diagn Pathol 1998;2:19–24.

833. Barnoud R, Arvieux C, Pasquier D, Letoublin C. Solitary fibrous tumor of the liver with CD 34 expression. Histopathology 1996;28:551–554.

834. Perez-Ordonez B, Rosai J. Follicular dendritic cell tumor: Review of the entity. Semin Diagn Pathol 1998;15:144–154.

835. Selves J, Meggetto F, Brousset P, et al. Inflammatory pseudotumor of the liver: Evidence for follicular dendritic reticulum cell proliferation associated with clonal Epstein-Barr virus. Am J Surg Pathol 1996;20:747–753.

836. Shek TW, Liu CL, Peh WC, et al. Intra-abdominal follicular dendritic cell tumour: A rare tumour in need of recognition. Histopathology 1998;33:465–470.

837. Shek TW, Ho FC, Ng IO, et al. Follicular dendritic cell tumor of the liver: Evidence for an Epstein-Barr virus-related clonal proliferation of follicular dendritic cells. Am J Surg Pathol 1996;20:313–324.

838. Nonomura A, Minato H, Shimizu K, et al. Hepatic hilar inflammatory pseudotumor mimicking cholangiocarcinoma with cholangitis and phlebitis—a variant of primary sclerosing cholangitis? Pathol Res Pract 1997;193:519–525.

839. Cerar A, Dolenc-Strazar ZD, Bartenjev D. Infantile hemangioendothelioma of the liver in a neonate: Immunohistochemical observations. Am J Surg Pathol 1996;20:871–876.

840. La Rosa S, Uccella S, Billo P, et al. Immunohistochemical localization of alpha- and beta-A-subunits of inhibin/activin in human normal endocrine cells and related tumors of the digestive system. Virchows Arch 1999;434:29–36.

841. Murata T, Nakashima Y, Takeuchi M, Sueishi K. The diagnostic use of low molecular weight keratin expression in sebaceous carcinoma. Pathol Res Pract 1993;189:888–893.

842. McKinley M, Listrom MB, Fenoglio-Preiser C. Cytokeratin 19: A potential marker of colonic differentiation. Surg Pathol 1990;3:107–113.

843. Yeh KH, Chen YC, Yeh SH, et al. Detection of circulating cancer cells by nested reverse transcription-polymerase chain reaction of cytokeratin-19 (K19)—possible clinical significance in advanced gastric cancer. Anticancer Res 1998;18:1283–1286.

844. Stevenson AJ, Chatten J, Bertoni F, Miettinen M. CD99 (p30/32^{MIC2}) neuroectodermal/Ewing's sarcoma antigen as an immunohistochemical marker: Review of more than 600 tumors and literature experience. Appl Immunohistochem 1994;2:231–240.

845. El-Habashi A, El-Morsi B, Freeman SM, et al. Tumor oncogenic expression in malignant effusions as a possible method to enhance cytologic diagnostic sensitivity: An immunocytochemical study of 87 cases. Am J Clin Pathol 1995;103:206–214.

846. Wick MR, Swanson PE, Manivel JC. Placental-like alkaline phosphatase reactivity in human tumors: An immunohistochemical study of 520 cases. Hum Pathol 1987;18:946–954.

847. Van Krieken JHJM. Prostate marker immunoreactivity in salivary gland neoplasms: A rare pitfall in immunohistochemistry. Am J Surg Pathol 1993;17:410–414.

848. Ordonez NG. Thrombomodulin expression in transitional cell carcinoma. Am J Clin Pathol 1998;110:385–390.

849. Akasofu M, Kawahara E, Kurumaya H, Nakanishi I. Immunohistochemical detection of breast specific antigens and cytokeratins in metastatic breast carcinoma in the liver. Acta Pathol Jpn 1993;43:736–744.

Immunohistochemistry of the Prostate and Bladder, Testis, and Renal Tumors

Prostate and Bladder

David G. Bostwick, M.D., Junqi Qian, M.D., and Dharamdas M. Ramnani, M.D.

PROSTATE

Markers of Prostatic Cells

PROSTATE-SPECIFIC ANTIGEN

Prostate-specific antigen (PSA) is a 34-kd, single-chain glycoprotein of 237 amino acids produced almost exclusively by prostatic epithelial cells.[1] PSA, a serine protease, is a member of the kallikrein gene family and has a high sequence homology with human glandular kallikrein 2. It exhibits chymotrypsin-like, trypsin-like, and esterase-like activity. In serum, PSA is present mainly in complex with alpha-1-antichymotrypsin. It is secreted in seminal plasma and is responsible for gel dissolution in freshly ejaculated semen by proteolysis of the major gel-forming proteins semenogelin I and II and fibronectin. A small amount of PSA in semen is complexed. The free, noncomplexed form of PSA constitutes a minor fraction of serum PSA, and derivatives of PSA such as free to total ratio of PSA may be superior to PSA alone.[2] Production of PSA appears to be under the control of circulating androgens acting through the androgen receptors.

Serum PSA may become elevated by conditions other than benign prostatic hyperplasia (BPH) and cancer, including prostatitis, prostatic intraepithelial neoplasia (PIN), acute urinary retention, renal failure, and sialadenitis. In the normal and hyperplastic prostate, PSA is uniformly present at the apical portion of the glandular epithelium of secretory cells (Fig. 14–1A). The intensity of the staining decreases in poorly differentiated adenocarcinoma (see Fig. 14–1B). PSA immunoreactivity has been described in extraprostatic tissues and tumors, but these sites are usually patchy and weak in immunoreactivity (Table 14–1). PSA is particularly sensitive and accurate in the detection of residual cancer, recurrence, and cancer progression after treatment, irrespective of the treatment modality. Earlier detection through screening for elevated levels of PSA, while controversial, has been proposed as a way to decrease prostate cancer mortality.[3] PSA accurately predicts cancer status and can detect recurrence several months before detection by any other method.[4] PSA is also a sensitive and specific immunohistochemical marker for tumors of prostatic origin.

Serum PSA concentration exceeding 0.2 ng/mL after radical prostatectomy is often considered as evidence of biochemical tumor recurrence. However, in 26 to 29% of radical prostatectomy specimens, the surgical margin contains benign prostatic glands with or without tumor. In 45% of whole mounted prostatectomies, only benign glands were present at the margins. In one third of these patients, postoperative serum PSA was measurable, and in half of these cases, the PSA concentration indicated recurrence. This apparent PSA elevation depends on the normal working ranges of the clinical laboratory providing the analysis and cannot be assumed as an absolute value.

PROSTATIC ACID PHOSPHATASE

The immunohistochemical localization and distribution of prostatic acid phosphatase (PAP) in normal, hyperplastic, and cancerous human prostate has been used as a prostate-specific marker for many years.[5-26] In the normal and hyperplastic prostate, PAP was uniformly present at the apical portion of the glandular epithelium of secretory cells. There was more intense and uniform staining of cancer cells and the glandular epithelium of well-differentiated adenocarcinoma, whereas less intense and more variable staining was seen in moderately and poorly differentiated adenocarcinoma (Fig. 14–2). Today, examination of PAP expression has been replaced by examination of other tissue markers, including PSA, other human glandular kallikreins, and prostate-specific membrane antigen (PSMA).

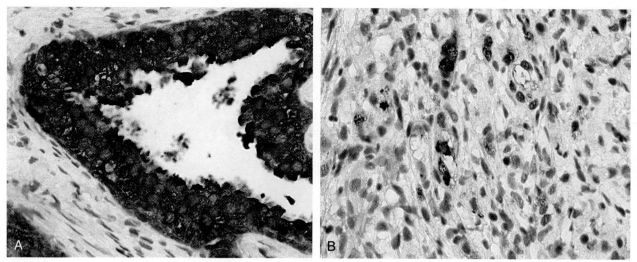

Figure 14–1. *A,* Normal prostate epithelium labeled with prostate-specific antibody (PSA). *B,* The intensity of PSA staining is decreased in poorly differentiated prostatic adenocarcinoma cells.

PROSTATE-SPECIFIC MEMBRANE ANTIGEN

PSMA is a membrane-bound antigen that is highly specific for benign and malignant prostatic epithelial cells.[27–36] It is present in the serum of normal men, according to studies with monoclonal antibody 7E11.C5, and an elevated concentration is associated with the presence of prostatic adenocarcinoma, clinical progression of carcinoma, and hormone-refractory carcinoma.[27, 33, 37] PSMA may be superior to PSA in predicting patient outcome for some patients (Table 14–2).[27–29, 31–33, 38]

PSMA has partial homology with the transferrin receptor, and its extracellular domain also possesses properties of the NAALADase enzyme activity.[39] The antibody that we used in this study, 7E11.C5, recognizes the first six N-terminal amino acids of the cytoplasmic domain. Another antibody to PSMA, 3F5.4G6, recognizes an eight amino acid region near the C-terminal portion of the extracellular domain.[40] The 7E11.C5 antibody has been successfully used with single photon emission computed tomography (SPECT) to detect soft tissue and bone metastatic prostate cancer, as well as cancer in the preoperative and postoperative prostate and prostate bed.[27–30, 35, 41, 42]

There is intense cytoplasmic epithelial immunoreactivity for PSMA in every prostate.[31, 36, 37] The number of immunoreactive cells increased from benign epithelium to high-grade PIN and prostatic adenocarcinoma. High-grade PIN displayed intermediate immunoreactivity, suggesting that this microscopic finding has some but not all of the phenotypic features of carcinoma, similar to studies of other secretory markers.[32] The most extensive and intense staining for PSMA was observed in high-grade carcinoma, with immunoreactivity in virtually every cell in Gleason primary patterns of 4 or 5. One study noted greater heterogeneity of stain-

Table 14–1. Prostate-Specific Antigen Immunoreactivity in Extraprostatic Tissues and Tumors

Extraprostatic tissues
  Urethra and periurethral glands (male and female)
  Bladder, including cystitis cystica and glandularis
  Anus, including anal glands (male)
  Urachal remnants
  Neutrophils
Extraprostatic tumors
  Urethral and periurethral gland adenocarcinoma (female)
  Villous adenoma and adenocarcinoma of the bladder
  Extramammary Paget's disease of the male external genitals
  Pleomorphic adenoma of the salivary glands (male)
  Carcinoma of the salivary glands (male)
  Breast carcinoma
  Mature teratoma

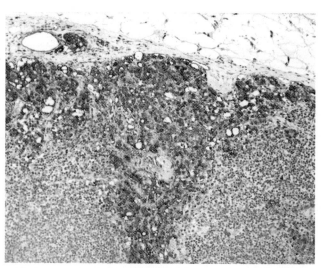

Figure 14–2. Immunoreactivity for PSA in prostate cancer lymph node metastasis.

Table 14–2. Comparative Immunoreactivity of Prostate-Specific Membrane Antigen and Prostate-Specific Antigen in the Benign and Neoplastic Prostate in 184 Radical Prostatectomies

	Percent Immunoreactive Cells Plus Standard Deviation (Range)
PSMA	
Benign	69.5 + 17.3 (20–90)
High-grade PIN	77.9 + 13.7 (30–100)
Cancer	80.2 + 13.7 (30–100)
PSA	
Benign	81.3 + 11.8 (20–90)
High-grade PIN	64.8 + 17.3 (10–90)
Cancer	74.2 + 16.2 (10–90)

PSMA, prostate-specific membrane antigen; PSA, prostate-specific antigen, PIN, prostatic intraepithelial neoplasia.

ing in high-grade cancer than in lower grade cancer,[31] in contrast with our findings.[32] PSMA expression is up-regulated in prostate cancer, and the ratio of the mRNA encoding PSMA is nearly 100-fold greater than its splice variant, PSMA′, in cancer.

Extraprostatic expression of PSMA is highly restricted and has been reported in the duodenal mucosa, a subset of proximal renal tubules, a subset of colonic crypt neuroendocrine cells, lactating breast, and salivary and submaxillary glands.[27, 31, 36] One report described immunoreactivity in capillary endothelial cells,[43, 44] but we were unable to confirm this finding in the prostate.[29, 32] Extraprostatic cancer is invariably negative for PSMA, including renal cell carcinoma (RCC), urothelial carcinoma, and colonic adenocarcinoma.[31]

PSMA immunoreactivity in cancer cells was not predictive of PSA biochemical failure or recurrence in a cohort of organ-confined margin-negative cancers treated by surgery[32]; these findings differ from serum studies in which elevated concentration of PSMA indicated surgical treatment failure.[27]

PSMA is clinically useful for diagnostic and therapeutic applications. PSMA is expressed in lymph node[31, 36] and bone marrow metastases[31] of prostate cancer (Fig. 14–3), underscoring its utility in identifying cancer of unknown primary site. Serum PSMA was of prognostic significance, especially in the presence of metastases, and correlated well with cancer stage in a screened population. It is also useful in reverse transcriptase-polyermase chain reaction (RT-PCR) assays that detect circulating PSMA-containing cells (presumptive tumor cells), providing positive results in 42%[45] and 75%[46] of patients with localized prostate cancer.[47, 48] Such PSMA-containing cells apparently spill into the circulation during radical prostatectomy,[49] but decline in number after androgen deprivation therapy.[31, 50] Antibody-radionuclide con-

jugates to PSMA have been used to localize metastastic prostate cancer successfully in animals and humans[28–30, 38, 41, 42, 51] and to treat human cancer in nude mice.[35]

HUMAN GLANDULAR KALLIKREIN 2

The human kallikrein family consists of three members; hK1, hK2, and hK3 (PSA). The mRNA for hK2 and PSA are located predominantly in prostatic epithelium and are regulated by androgens.[52–55] In addition, hK2 has 78% amino acid homology with PSA and is expressed predominantly in the prostate, suggesting that it may be a clinically useful marker for the diagnosis and monitoring of prostate cancer.[54, 55] The intensity and extent of hK2 expression was greater in cancer than in PIN, which, in turn, was greater than in benign epithelium. Gleason primary grades 4 and 5 cancers showed hK2 staining in almost every cell, whereas there was greater heterogeneity of staining in lower grades of cancer. In marked contrast to hK2, PSA and PAP immunoreactivity was most intense in benign epithelium and stained to a lesser extent in PIN and carcinoma.[56] The number of immunoreactive cells for hK2 and PSA was not predictive of cancer recurrence. Tissue expression of hK2 appears to be regulated independently of PSA and PAP.

KERATIN 34β-E12 (KERATIN 903, HIGH MOLECULAR WEIGHT KERATIN)

Monoclonal basal cell-specific anti–keratin 34β-E12 stains virtually all the normal basal cells of the prostate, with continuous intact circumferential staining in most instances (Fig. 14–4). There is no staining in the secretory and stromal cells.

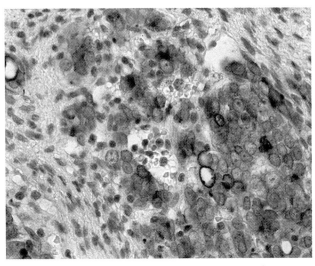

Figure 14–3. Positive prostate-specific membrane antigen (PSMA) staining in prostate cancer lymph node metastasis.

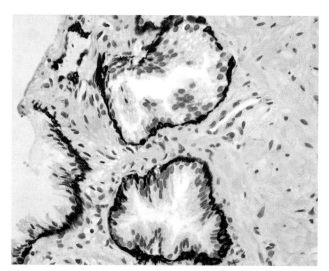

Figure 14–4. Immunostaining with 34βE12 reveals intact basal cell layer in normal prostatic acini.

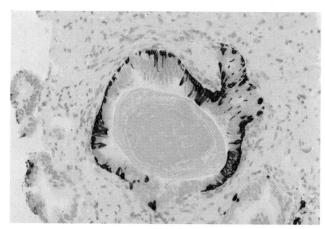

Figure 14–5. Basal cell layer labeled with 34βE12 is disrupted in high-grade prostatic intraepithelial neoplasia (PIN).

This marker is the most commonly used immunostain for prostatic basal cells,[57–59] and methods of use with paraffin-embedded sections have been optimized.[60] Keratin 34β-E12 is formalin-sensitive and requires pretreatment by enzymes or heat if formalin-based fixatives are used. After pepsin predigestion or microwaving, there is progressive loss of immunoreactivity of 1 week or longer of formalin fixation. Heat-induced epitope retrieval with a hot plate yielded consistent results with no decrease in immunoreactivity with as long as 1 month of formalin fixation.[60] The staining intensity was consistently stronger at all periods of formalin fixation when the hot plate method was used, compared with pepsin predigestion or microwaving. Weak immunoreactivity was rarely observed in cancer cells after hot plate treatment but was not seen with pepsin predigestion or microwave antigen retrieval. Our laboratory reported that steam-ethylenediaminetetraacetic acid (EDTA) in combination with protease significantly enhanced basal cell immunoreactivity compared with protease treatment alone in noncancerous prostatic epithelium.[61] Nonreactive benign acini were always the most peripheral acini in a lobule, a small cluster of outpouched acini furthest from a large duct, or the terminal end of a large duct.[62] More proximal acini had a discontinuous pattern of immunoreactivity. Electron microscopy showed occasional acini with luminal cells abutting the basement membrane, without the interposition of basal cell cytoplasm, and other acini with extremely attenuated basal cell cytoplasmic processes containing sparse bundles of intermediate filaments.

Increasing grades of PIN are associated with progressive disruption of the basal cell layer, according to studies using anti–keratin 34β-E12 (Fig. 14–5). Basal cell layer disruption is present in 56% of cases of high-grade PIN and is more frequent in acini adjacent to invasive carcinoma than in distant acini. The amount of disruption increases with increasing grades of PIN. Early invasive carcinoma occurs at sites of glandular outpouching and basal cell discontinuity in association with PIN (Fig. 14–6).[63] The cribriform pattern of PIN may be mistaken for cribriform adenocarcinoma, and the use of antikeratin staining is invaluable in making this distinction.[64]

Cancer cells consistently fail to react with this antibody, although admixed benign acini may be misinterpreted as cancerous staining (Fig. 14–7). Thus, immunohistochemical stains for anti–keratin 34β-E12 may show the presence or absence of basal cells in a small focus of atypical glands, helping to establish a benign or malignant diagnosis, respectively. We believe that this antibody can be used successfully if one judiciously interprets the results in combination with the light microscopic findings; relying solely on the *absence* of

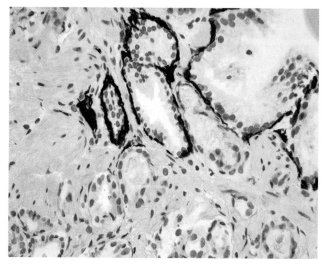

Figure 14–6. Early invasive carcinoma occurs at sites of glandular outpouching and basal cell discontinuity in association with PIN.

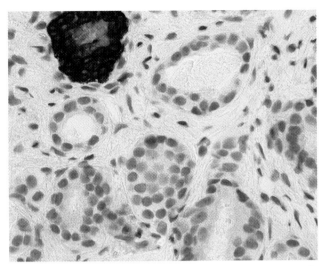

Figure 14–7. Immunostaining with 34βE12 reveals the absence of a basal cell layer in prostate cancer acini.

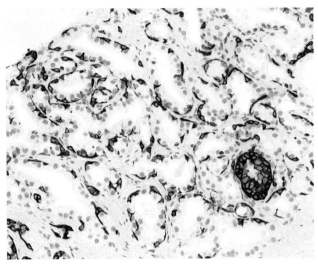

Figure 14–8. Atypical adenomatous hyperplasia labeled with antibody 34βE12, demonstrating the basal cells.

immunoreactivity (absence of basal cell staining) to render the diagnosis of cancer is without precedent in diagnostic immunohistochemistry and is discouraged.[65] Nonetheless, reports have noted that the rate of equivocal cases can be reduced considerably,[66] by 68%,[57] or from 5.1 to 1.0,[67] by addition of this immunohistochemical marker. Evaluation of prostate biopsy results after therapy such as radiation therapy may be one of the most useful roles for anti–keratin 34β-E12 (see further on).[68]

In addition to PIN and cancer, basal cell layer disruption or loss also occurs in inflamed acini, atypical adenomatous hyperplasia (Fig. 14–8), and postatrophic hyperplasia (Fig. 14–9), and may be misinterpreted as cancer if one relies exclusively on the immunohistochemical profile of a suspicious focus.[63, 65, 69] Furthermore, basal cells of Cowper's glands may not express keratin 34β-E12,[70] although this has been disputed.[71] Rare (0.2%) cases of adenocarcinoma have been reported that express keratin 34β-E12, including foci of metastatic high-grade adenocarcinoma; these cases did not appear phenotypically to be basal cell–adenoid cystic carcinoma.[72]

Basal cell hyperplasia is a histologic mimic of cancer, and the use of anti–keratin 34β-E12 is recommended in any equivocal case that includes this lesion in the differential diagnosis.[73–75]

CK5 and CK14 mRNA and protein are expressed in the basal cells of benign acini and PIN, and CK14 mRNA is present in low levels in the luminal cells in most of the foci of PIN; thus, if PIN is derived from basal cells, as currently believed, CK14 translation is depressed, and a low level of CK14 mRNA may persist.[76] CK8 mRNA and protein were constitutively expressed in all epithelia of normal and abnormal prostate tissues. CK19 mRNA and protein were expressed in both basal and luminal cells of benign acini. CK16 mRNA

was expressed in a pattern similar to that of CK19, but CK16 protein was not detected.[76]

We routinely generate unstained intervening sections of all prostate biopsy specimens for possible immunohistochemical staining, recognizing that small foci of concern are often lost when the tissue block is recut; one study reported loss of the suspicious focus in 31 of 52 cases.[77]

OTHER MARKERS OF BASAL CELLS

Numerous immunohistochemical markers have been identified in the prostate, and many of these are preferentially found in the basal cell layer of the epithelium (Table 14–3). These markers include proliferation markers, differentiation markers, and genetic markers. The preferential localization of many of these markers in basal cells but not in secretory cells suggests that they play a role in growth regulation.

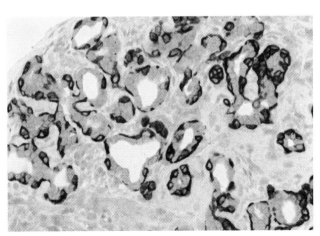

Figure 14–9. Prostatic postatrophic hyperplasia shows 34βE12 immunoreactivity in basal cells.

Table 14–3. Markers of Basal Cell Differentiation in the Prostate

Biomarker	Function	Findings
PCNA	Cell proliferation marker	Up to 70% of labeled cells are basal cells
MIB-1	Cell proliferation marker	Up to 77% of labeled cells are basal cells
Ki-67	Cell proliferation marker	Up to 81% of labeled cells are basal cells
Androgen receptors	Nuclear receptors that are necessary for prostatic epithelial growth	Strong immunoreactivity; also present in cancer cells
Prostate-specific antigen	Enzyme that liquifies the seminal coagulum	Present in rare basal cells; mainly in secretory luminal cells
CK8.12	CK13, CK16	Strong immunoreactivity
CK4.62	CK19	Moderate immunoreactivity
CK PKK1	CK7, CK8, CK17, CK18	Moderate immunoreactivity
CK312C8-1	CK14	Strong immunoreactivity
CK34β-E12	CK5, CK10, CK11	Strong immunoreactivity; most commonly used for diagnostic purposes
Epidermal growth factor receptor	Membrane-bound 170-kd glycoprotein that mediates the activity of EGF	Strong immunoreactivity; rare in cancer
CuZn-superoxide dismutase	Enzyme that catalyzes superoxide anion radicals	Strong immunoreactivity
Type IV collagenase	Enzyme involved in extracellular matrix degradation	Strong immunoreactivity; decreased in cancer
Type VII collagen	Part of the hemidesmosomal complex	Strong immunoreactivity; lost in cancer
Integrins alpha 1, 2, 4, 6, and v; Beta 1 and 4	Extracellular matrix adhesion molecules	Strong immunoreactivity; decreased in most with cancer, although alpha 6 and beta 1 are retained
Estrogen receptors	Hormone receptor	Moderate immunoreactivity
bcl-2	Oncoprotein that suppresses apoptosis	Strong immunoreactivity; also found in most cancers
c-*erb*-B2	Oncogene protein in the EGF family	Strong immunoreactivity; also found in most cancers
Glutathione S-transferase gene (GSTP1)	Enzyme that inactivates electrophilic carcinogens	Strong immunoreactivity; rare in cancer
C-CAM	Epithelial cell adhesion molecule	Strong immunoreactivity; absent in cancer
TGF-β	Growth factor that regulates cell proliferation and differentiation	Strong immunoreactivity; absent in cancer
Cathepsin B	Enzyme that degrades basement membranes; may be involved in tumor invasion and metastases	Present in many basal cells, and rarely in luminal secretory cells; also found in cancer cells
Progesterone receptors	Hormone receptor	Moderate immunoreactivity

Refer to text for selected references.
PCNA, proliferating cell nuclear antigen; CK; cytokeratin; E-CAM, epithelial-cell adhesion molecule; TGF-β, transforming growth factor-β.

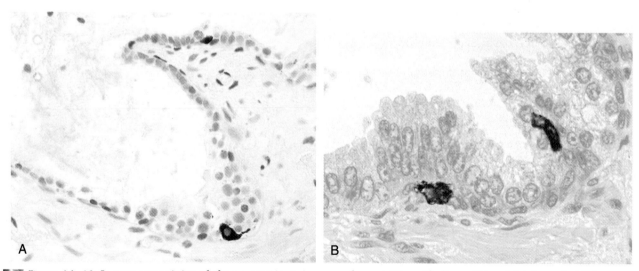

▨▧ *Figure 14-10.* Immunoreactivity of chromogranin A in normal prostatic epithelium *(A)* and high-grade PIN cells *(B)*.

Basal cells display immunoreactivity at least focally for CK5, CK10, CK11, CK13, CK14, CK16, and CK19; of these, only CK19 is also found in secretory cells.[63, 69, 78–86] Keratins found exclusively in the secretory cells include CK7, CK8, and CK18.

Basal cells usually do not display immunoreactivity for PSA, PAP, and S-100 protein, and only rare single cells stain with chromogranin and neuron-specific enolase (NSE). Conversely, the normal secretory luminal cells invariably stain with PSA and PAP. Prostatic basal cells do not usually display myoepithelial differentiation,[85, 87] in contrast to basal cells in the breast, salivary glands, pancreas, and other sites.

Neuroendocrine Markers

Neuroendocrine cells are part of the widely dispersed diffuse neuroendocrine regulatory system, also known as *endocrine-paracrine cells.* In the human prostate, subpopulations of neuroendocrine cells have been identified based on morphologic features and secretory products (Fig. 14–10A).[88–94] In LNCaP cell lines, the paracrine-endocrine phenotype can be induced by agents that increase intracellular dibutyryl $3',5'$-cyclic adenosine monophosphate (dbcAMP) levels (such as forskolin, isoproterenol, and epinephrine). Withdrawal of these differentiating agents resulted in reversal of the paracrine-endocrine differentiation in vitro.[95] Most neuroendocrine cells of the prostate contain serotonin,[96] chromogranin A,[97–99] and other neuroendocrine markers that are not consistently expressed. Neuroendocrine cells in the prostate are probably involved in regulation of growth, differentiation, and secretory functions (see Fig. 14–10B). The absence of chromogranin A–immunoreactive neuroendocrine cells in the rat, guinea pig, cat, and dog prostate challenge the validity of these animal models for physiologic studies of neuroendocrine cells in the human prostate.[100]

In humans, there are three patterns of neuroendocrine differentiation in prostatic carcinoma: as (1) infrequent small cell neuroendocrine carcinoma (Fig. 14–11); (2) rare carcinoid-like cancer; and (3) conventional prostatic cancer with focal neuroendocrine differentiation. Virtually all prostatic adenocarcinomas contain at least a small number of neuroendocrine cells, but special studies such as histochemistry and immunohistochemistry are usually necessary to identify these cells.[91–93, 98, 99, 101–105] Neuroendocrine differentiation typically consists of scattered cells that are inapparent by light microscopy but are revealed by immunoreactivity for one or more markers. Neuroendocrine cells in prostate cancer are malignant and lack androgen receptor expression.[91, 92, 98, 106, 107] About 10% of adenocarcinomas contain cells with large eosinophilic granules (formerly referred to as *adenocarcinoma with Paneth cell-like change),* usually consisting of only rare foci of scattered cells and small clusters that may be overlooked.[108, 109] Cells with large

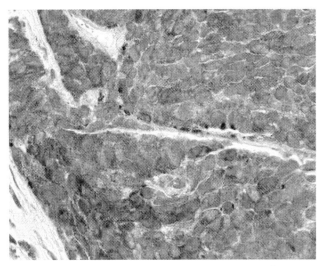

Figure 14–11. Immunoreactivity of synaptophysin in small cell prostate cancer cells.

eosinophilic granules in the normal epithelium and adenocarcinoma resemble Paneth cells of the intestine and other sites by light microscopy, but they differ from Paneth cells by their neuroendocrine differentiation (producing chromogranin, NSE, and serotonin) and their lack of lysozyme expression.[108] The number of neuroendocrine cells in benign prostatic epithelium and adenocarcinoma is substantially greater than the number of cells with large eosinophilic granules, indicating that most neuroendocrine cells are not apparent on hematoxylin and eosin–stained sections.

Most cases of neuroendocrine carcinoma have typical local signs and symptoms of prostatic adenocarcinoma, although paraneoplastic syndromes are frequent in these patients. Cushing's syndrome is most common, invariably in association with adrenocorticotropic hormone immunoreactivity in tumor cells[110–113]; other clinical conditions include malignant hypercalcemia,[114] syndrome of inappropriate antidiuretic hormone (SIADH) secretion, and myasthenic (Eaton-Lambert) syndrome. Small cell carcinoma is aggressive and rapidly fatal.[109, 115–117] Neuroendocrine carcinoma of the prostate varies histopathologically from carcinoid-like pattern (low-grade neuroendocrine carcinoma) to small cell undifferentiated (oat cell) carcinoma (high-grade neuroendocrine carcinoma).[118] These tumors are morphologically identical to their counterparts in the lung and other sites. Typical acinar adenocarcinoma is present, at least focally, in many cases, and transition patterns may be seen. In cases with solid grade 5 pattern suggestive of neuroendocrine carcinoma, immunohistochemical stains are recommended. Mixed patterns may be observed, including one case with small cell carcinoma, adenocarcinoma, typical carcinoid, and spindle cell carcinoma.[109] A wide variety of secretory products may be detected within the malignant cells, including serotonin, calcitonin, adrenocorticotropic hormone, human chorionic gonadotropin, thyroid-

stimulating hormone, bombesin, calcitonin gene-related peptide, and inhibin. The same cells may
express peptide hormones and PSA and PAP, but
pure small cell carcinoma does not usually display
immunoreactivity for PSA. Serotonin, chromogranin, and synaptophysin are the most useful
markers of neuroendocrine cells in formalin-fixed
sections of prostate.[99, 119-126] Ultrastructurally, small
cell carcinoma and carcinoid tumor of the prostate
contain a variable number of round regular membrane-bound neurosecretory granules.[119-125] Well-
defined cytoplasmic processes are usually present
that contain neurosecretory granules. The cells are
small, with dispersed chromatin and small, inconspicuous nucleoli.

Neuroendocrine cells have no apparent clinical
or prognostic significance in benign epithelium,
primary prostatic adenocarcinoma, and lymph
node metastases, according to most but not all reports (Table 14–4).* Aprikian and colleagues
found no correlation of neuroendocrine differentiation with pathologic stage or metastases.[137] We previously found no apparent relationship between
the number of immunoreactive neuroendocrine
cells in high-grade PIN and cancer and a variety of
clinical and pathologic factors, including stage.[126]
Allen and associates studied 120 patients and
found no significant association between neuroendocrine differentiation and patient prognosis.[138]
Conversely, Weinstein and colleagues studied 104
patients with clinically localized prostate cancer
and found that neuroendocrine differentiation was
associated with patient survival, although they restricted their study to cancers with Gleason scores
of 5 and 6, so their findings may be influenced by
selection bias.[136] Frierson and colleagues showed
that neuroendocrine differentiation predicted patient survival, but this was only true for the analysis with one variable model.[139] Krijnen and associates reported that neuroendocrine differentiation
was associated with early hormone therapy failure,
indicating that these cells are androgen-independent.[107] Their findings suggested that the presence
of large numbers of neuroendocrine cells in cancer
may indicate a poor prognosis, perhaps because of
insensitivity to hormonal growth regulation, but
this has been refuted by most studies (see Table
14–4). We reported that lymph node metastases
contain fewer chromogranin- and serotonin-immu-
noreactive cells than do benign prostatic epithelium and primary prostate cancer, suggesting that
decreased expression of neuroendocrine markers is
involved in cancer progression.[105] Neuroendocrine
expression was not clinically useful for predicting
outcome in patients with node-positive prostate
cancer treated by radical prostatectomy.

Prostatic Immune Response

The immune response in the prostate is primarily cell-mediated. Lymphocytes were more numer-

ous in the stroma, and T cells represent more than
90% of the total number of prostatic lymphocytes
present in both stromal and intraepithelial compartments. Stromal T cells are mainly helper-inducer, whereas intraepithelial T cells are mainly
cytotoxic-suppressor cells (inverted CD4/CD8
ratio), findings that concur with previous reports.[140-142] The inverted CD4/CD8 ratio in the intraepithelial compartment indicates that cytotoxic-
suppressor T cells may represent the first line of
defense against luminal foreign agents reaching the
prostate through the urethra by retrograde flow. Interestingly, there is no significant difference in the
number of lymphocytes (either T or B cells,
stromal or intraepithelial) according to patient age,
race, or anatomic zone (peripheral, central, or transition zones).[141] These findings indicate that the
regulation of lymphocyte function and distribution
is tightly controlled and that there is a relatively
constant level of immunosurveillance in the prostate from birth to at least the seventh decade of
life.

Proliferation Antigens

PROLIFERATING CELL NUCLEAR ANTIGEN

The proliferating cell nuclear antigen (PCNA) labeling index is lowest in benign normal prostatic
epithelium and organ-confined cancer, but increases
progressively from well-differentiated through
poorly differentiated cancer,[143] although there is
wide variance.[73, 135, 144-154] The correlation of PCNA
index with cancer stage is strong.[146, 155, 156] Hence,
high PCNA labeling indices may indicate progression of prostate cancer[157] and may be an independent prognostic indicator.[145] However, PCNA measures DNA repair in nondividing cells and thus
may not be not an optimal method for assessing
proliferation.

KI-67 AND MIB-I

In prostate cancer, a high proliferation index for
Ki-67 or MIB-1 appears to add little predictive information for patient outcome above the traditional
indicators of Gleason score, pathologic stage, and
DNA ploidy.[158] However, the Ki-67 labeling index
may discriminate between organ-confined and
metastatic cancer (Fig. 14–12).[146] Hence, elevation
in the proliferation indices of Ki-67–MIB-1 appears to reflect progression.[131, 159, 160] This is further
reflected in an association between expression of
Ki-67 and epidermal growth factor receptor,[161] mutant p53,[161-163] particular chromosomal aberrations,[164] and perineural invasion.[165] In combination, these findings suggest that Ki-67 expression
may be a weak predictor of recurrence, progression,[131, 159, 160] and survival.[162, 166-168]

OTHER KERATINS

In prostatic epithelium, three cell types are distinguished according to location, morphologic

---

*References 89–91, 97–99, 101, 102, 106, 108, 111, 116, 126–
137.

Text continued on page 419

Table 14–4. Predictive Value of Neuroendocrine Differentiation by Immunohistochemistry in Prostatic Adenocarcinoma: Collected Works

	No. Patients	Patient Population	Tissue Studied	Neuroendocrine Markers	Cancer Cases Stained (%)	Quantitation of Neuroendocrine Staining	Outcome Variables	Multivariate Analysis	Mean Length of Follow-Up	Comments
(Study Not Predictive of Outcome)										
Aprikian et al, 1993[137]	78	31 primary cancers, 16 metastases, 21 diethylstilbestrol-treated cancers, 10 hormone-refractory cancers	Radical prostatectomy and TURP specimens	Chromogranin A, NSE, serotonin, calcitonin, ACTH, somatostatin, gastrin-releasing peptide, TSH	77% of primary untreated cancer, 56% of metastatic lesions	No positive cells (−); occasionally identified NE cells (+), numerous cells (++), majority of cells (+++)	Recurrence or metastasis, hormone-independent, cancer progression	Yes, factors including cancer grade, stage, progression, hormone-independent	Not given	NE cells were not associated with cancer stage or metastasis
Cohen et al, 1994[642]	38	Clinical stage II, III cancers	Retropubic prostatectomy specimens	Chromogranin A, NSE	29% for chromogranin A; 24% for NSE	No positive cells identified (−); positive cells identified occasionally (+), 1–3 per acinar structure (++); >3 cells per acinar structure (+++)	PSA failure, recurrence or metastasis in tissue biopsy, positive bone scan or radiograph	Yes, cancer grade, stage, NE staining	4.2 yr (range, 4–6 yr)	Chromogranin A is not useful in predicting cancer progression
Bostwick et al, 1994[125]	26	1 stage pT1b, 10 stage pT2a + b, 13 stage pT2c, 1 stage pT3a, 1 stage T3c cancers; no clinical history of androgen-deprivation therapy or radiation therapy before surgery	Whole-mounted, totally-embedded, radical prostatectomy specimens	Chromogranin A, NSE, serotonin, HCG, calcitonin, ACTH, TSH, prolactin, glucagon	92%	Mean percent of positive high power field (×640)	Cancer grade, stage	Yes, stepwise regression, analysis including cancer grade, stage, volume, microvascular invasion	Not given	NE differentiation was down-regulated in prostate cancer, no correlation of NE differentiation with various clinical and pathologic factors
Noordzij et al, 1995[134]	90	22 stage pT2 cancers, 66 stage pT3 cancers, 2 pT4 cancers, 5 stage pN1 cancers, 2 stage PN.2 cancers	Radical prostatectomy specimens	Chromogranin A, chromogranin B	78%	No positive cell visible (−); a few positive cells, widely scattered (±); some positive cells, more regularly distributed or small clusters (++); numerous positive cells or large clusters (+++)	Histologically local cancer recurrence or metastasis, cancer-specific death	Yes, Cox's regression model, which included cancer grade, stage	7.2 yr (range, 0.1–16.9 yr)	NE differentiation was not associated with Gleason sum, pathologic stage, or cancer-specific death

Table continued on following page

Table 14–4. Predictive Value of Neuroendocrine Differentiation by Immunohistochemistry in Prostatic Adenocarcinoma: Collected Works *Continued*

Study	No. Patients	Patient Population	Tissue Studied	Neuroendocrine Markers	Cancer Cases Stained (%)	Quantitation of Neuroendocrine Staining	Outcome Variables	Multivariate Analysis	Mean Length of Follow-Up	Comments
Allen et al, 1995[138]	120	17 stage T0, 6 stage T1, 17 stage T2, 38 stage T3, 42 stage T4 cancers	Needle biopsy, TURP, radical prostatectomy specimens	Chromogranin A, NSE	31%	Positive (any stained cells), negative (no positive cell)	Systemic progression, cancer-specific survival	Yes, factors included grade, stage, survival	>5 yr (range not given)	NE cells; was not associated with cancer grade, stage, and patient survival
Speights et al, 1997[643]	33	23 high-grade, high-stage cancers; 10 stage T1a, low-grade cancers; all diagnosed by TURP; some received androgen deprivation therapy	TURP specimens	Chromogranin A, NSE, synaptophysin (also included MIB-1)	High-grade cancers: "nearly all"; low-grade: 50%	Counted 1000 cells of benign and cancer per marker	PSA failure (not defined), biopsy-proven recurrence; clinical failure or metastases (imaging)—14 of 23 high grade cancers progressed	Yes; Cox's regression models, which accounted for variable length of follow-up and Gleason scores	13.4 mo for high-grade cancers (range, 1–42 mo)	Greater number of NE cells and higher proliferative index (MIB-1 staining) in high-stage high-grade cancer than in low-grade cancer
McWilliam et al, 1997[102]	92	64 stage T1–2, 9 stage T3, 19 stage M1	TURP specimens	Chromogranin A, NSE	52%	Positive (>10% tumor cells); negative (<10% tumor cells)	Cancer-specific survival (33 patients died of cancer, cancer metastasis (5 cases)	Yes; factors including cancer grade, stage, vascular invasion, bone metastasis	9 yr (7–13 yr)	Positive correlation of NE differentiation with worsening tumor differentiation; no association with cancer stage and cancer-specific survival
Pruneri et al, 1998[98]	64	7 stage A, 13 stage B, 30 stage C, 14 stage D; 57 patients underwent preoperative hormonal therapy	Prostatectomy (5 cases), radical prostatectomy (28 cases), TURP (31 cases)	Chromogranin A, chromogranin B, secretogranin II	86%	Number of positive cells was counted in at least 50 cancer fields	Overall and disease-free survival	Yes; generalized savage analysis, which included stage	3.6 yr (range, 1.5–7.3 yr)	NE differentiation was associated with high Gleason score, but not with stage and patient survival
Casella et al, 1998[132]	105	T2 and higher; patients selected "according to availability of follow-up information"; wide variety of treatments	Needle biopsies	Chromogranin A	25% (limited biopsy samples)	Subjectively as "few" or "numerous"	Cancer-specific survival	3-group analysis of variance; Gleason score and Ki-67 index were predictive, but not NE	Not given	NE differentiation was more frequent and intense in hormone-resistant cancer
Tan et al, 999[90]	41	Clinical stages: A, 6 cases; B, 10 cases; C, 1 case; D, 24 cases	Prostatectomy, TURP specimens	Chromogranin A, NSE	53.6%	No staining (–); rare scattered individual positive cells (+); small clusters of stained cells (++); large, sometimes confluent foci of stained cells (+++)	Systemic progression, cancer-specific survival	Yes, parameters including cancer grade, stage, systemic progression	5 yr (range, not given)	NE differentiation was not associated with high Gleason score, stage and patient survival

416

No. Patients	Patient Population	Tissue Studied	Neuroendocrine Markers	Cancer Cases Stained (%)	Quantitation of Neuroendocrine Staining	Outcome Variables	Multivariate Analysis	Mean Length of Follow-Up	Comments
Bostwick et al, in press — 196	Node-positive prostate cancer treated primarily by radical prostatectomy	Single section of radical prostatectomy or lymph node metastasis	Chromogranin A, serotonin	98.5% for chromogranin A; 94.9% for serotonin	Subjective in 10% increments; intensity measured independently	Systemic progression, cancer-specific survival, and all-cause survival	Yes, Cox's proportional hazards models, which included cancer grade, ploidy, volume, progression, survival	6.8 yr (range, 0.3–11 yr)	No significant association between the level of chromogranin A with cancer specific or all-cause survival; level of serotonin expression was associated with cancer-specific survival, but not for all-cause survival
(Study Predictive of Outcome)									
Abrahamsson et al, 1989[99] — 25	TURP-detected cancer followed by androgen deprivation therapy (stages A1, A2, B1)	TURP or enucleation prostate specimens	Chromogranin A	92%	Subjectively as negative (0), isolated single cells (±); rather few squattered cells (+); moderate numbers of cells (++); numerous cells (+++)	Cancer grade in subsequent TURP specimens	No	5.5 yr (range, 1–11 yr)	Most of the 25 tumors underwent marked tumor progression, whereas the number of NE cells concomitantly increased
Cohen et al, 1990, 1992[644,645] — 90	TURP or needle biopsy–detected stages B (22 cases), C (20 cases), and D (48 cases)	TURP or needle biopsy specimens	Chromogranin A, NSE	52%	Negative (no NE cells present); positive (individual cells or groups of NE cells)	Cancer-specific survival	Yes; grade and NE staining were predictive of tumor progression	>4 yr (range 4–7 yr)	NE differentiation was a more important prognostic factor than Gleason score
Weinstein et al, 1996[136] — 104	Clinically localized prostate cancer (T1–2) treated by radical prostatectomy	Single section of radical prostatectomy	Chromogranin A	62%	Maximal number of NE cells at per ×100 field	PSA failure	Yes; Cox's proportional hazards models, which included Gleason grade, NE staining, and tumor progression	8 yr (range, 7–10 yr)	NE differentiation may be a prognostic marker for tumors with intermediate Gleason sum
Krijnen et al, 1993[107] — 72	TURP-detected cancer followed by androgen deprivation therapy; included 12 stage T1b, 3 stage T2, 36 stage T3, 21 stage T4 cancers	TURP specimens	Chromogranin A	55%	Number of positive cells and clusters per 1 mm² tumor area	Progression-free survival	Yes; Cox's proportional hazards models, grade and NE staining were predictive	3 yr (range, 0.1–7.9 yr)	Density of NE cells and Gleason score were independent prognostic factors for cancer progression

Table continued on following page

417

Table 14–4. Predictive Value of Neuroendocrine Differentiation by Immunohistochemistry in Prostatic Adenocarcinoma: Collected Works *Continued*

	No. Patients	Patient Population	Tissue Studied	Neuroendocrine Markers	Cancer Cases Stained (%)	Quantitation of Neuroendocrine Staining	Outcome Variables	Multivariate Analysis	Mean Length of Follow-Up	Comments
Theodorescu et al, 1997[646]	71	T1–2 cancer treated by radical prostatectomy without adjuvant treatment until recurrence	Single section of radical prostatectomy specimen	Chromogranin A (also included cathepsin D)	24%	Subjectively as negative (0), rare positive cancer cells (1), <1% (2), 1–10% (3), 11–25% (4), 26–50% (5), or >50% (6); number of cells counted not given; for analyses, only 2–6 were considered positive; semiquantitatively scored as weak, moderate, and strong staining	Cancer-specific survival—51% of patients had recurrence; 24% died of prostate cancer	Yes; Cox's proportional hazards models, which included Gleason grade, stage, % cancer in specimen	Median follow-up interval of 10.6 yr; 53% had more than 10 yr of follow-up	Chromogranin A significant in univariate analysis and multivariate analysis with one-variable model, but not two-variable model; cathepsin D was not predictive of survival in univariate or multivariate analysis
Borre et al, 2000[249]	221	Patients treated by watchful waiting	Diagnostic biopsy specimens	VEGF and NE markers	VEGF expression correlates with microvessel density and neuroendocrine differentiation		Cancer-specific survival—57% died of prostate cancer	Yes; models included VEGF expression and microvessel density	Median follow-up of 15 yr	NE differentiation significantly correlated with microvessel density, VEGF expression, and survival

NE, neuroendocrine; NSE, neuron-specific enolase; TURP, transurethral resection of the prostate; ACTH, adrenocorticotropic hormone; TSH, thyroid-stimulating hormone; PSA, prostate-specific antigen; HCG, human chorionic gonadotropin; VEGF, vascular endothelial growth factor.

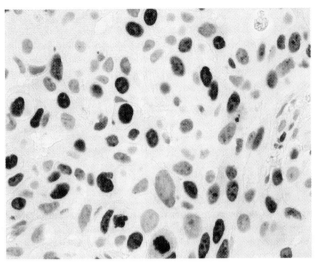

Figure 14–12. Immunoreactivity for MIB-1 in poorly differentiated prostate cancer cells.

characteristics, degree of differentiation, and cell-specific markers: (1) luminal secretory cells, (2) basal cells, and (3) endocrine-paracrine cells.[169, 170] The luminal and basal cells have characteristic patterns of cytokeratin (CK) expression.[171] The phenotypic plasticity of basal cells suggests that they contain a subset of stem cells that gives rise to all epithelial cells.[170, 172]

According to the stem cell model, there are at least three cell types, including stem cells, amplifying cells, and transit cells. Antikeratin immunoreactivity reveals at least three subpopulations of cells, one putatively representing amplifying cells.[169] The candidate stem cell population appears to be absent in prostatic carcinoma. Amplifying cells are defined in the stem cell model as precursors of transit (luminal) cells in the hierarchic pathway of prostatic epithelium differentiation, so the keratin expression profile led to the concept that this subpopulation might be the target of neoplastic transformation.[85, 173–177]

There is differential expression of CK polypeptides in normal, hyperplastic, and malignant prostatic epithelial cells.[177] Immunoblot analysis of prostate cancer cell lines PC3, DU145, and LNCaP showed expression of CK8 and CK18 but not CK5, CK7, and CK15, which were observed in benign prostatic tissue. Simultaneous labeling with CK18 and PSA detected metastatic prostate cancer cells in 50% of bone marrow aspirates.[178] Assays of fragments of CK8 and CK18 identify patients with high-grade and metastatic cancer.[179]

Extracellular Matrix Proteins

LAMININ

Laminin localization occurs in an intense and uniform manner in the basement membranes of acini, blood vessels, smooth muscle, and nerve fibers in normal prostate, BPH, and well-differentiated carcinoma. The basement membrane of poorly differentiated carcinoma does not contain laminin reactivity. However, in common with many other proteins, high-grade cancers exhibit laminin reactivity in the cytoplasm, on the surface, and in secretory material.[180–183]

INTEGRINS

Cell adhesion and migration are important features of tumor invasion and are mediated in part by integrins. The integrins are a large family of homologous linker proteins that interact with a variety of extracellular matrix components. These receptor proteins bind and respond to the extracellular matrix. They are composed of two noncovalently associated transmembrane glycoprotein subunits called alpha and beta, both of which contribute to the binding to matrix proteins. Integrin binding is dependent on divalent cations. Many extracellular matrix components, including laminin and fibronectin, recognize and bind multiple forms of integrin heterodimers. Reciprocal expression of E-cadherin and beta 1 integrin in higher grades of prostate cancer[184] has been demonstrated by parallel immunohistochemical analysis. Although integrins are significantly decreased in human prostate cancer, an exception is alpha 6 integrin (laminin receptor), which persists during prostate tumor progression.[185] Progression of prostate carcinoma may be influenced by the biochemical nature of the basal lamina surrounding the primary carcinoma cells.[186]

Normal basal cells form focal adhesions with hemidesmosomal-like structures and exhibit a polarized distribution of hemidesmosomal-associated proteins, including BP180, BP230, HD1, plectin, laminin gamma2, collagen VII, and the corresponding integrin-laminin receptors alpha 6 beta 1 and alpha 6 beta 4. The expression and distribution pattern of these proteins is retained in PIN. In contrast, carcinoma uniformly lacked hemidesmosomal structures, integrin alpha 6 beta 4, BP180, laminin gamma2, and collagen VII, but expressed BP230, plectin, HD1, and the integrin-laminin receptors alpha 3 beta 1 and alpha 6 beta 1. These results suggest that although a detectable basal lamina is present in carcinoma, its composition and cellular attachments are abnormal. Hemidesmosomal proteins and the alpha 3 beta 1 and alpha 6 beta 1 integrins are retained in PIN. The apparently anomalous production of alpha 6 beta 1 and laminin in cancer may contribute to the invasive phenotype.[186, 187]

Laminin 5 is an extracellular matrix protein integral to the formation of the hemidesmosomes that attach normal basal cells to the underlying basal lamina. These hemidesmosomal complexes are lost in prostatic carcinoma, probably causing reduced adhesion of malignant cells from anchoring structures and thus allowing them to invade and migrate through the adjacent tissues. Failure of hemidesmosome formation results in less stable epithelial-stromal junctions, which may allow malignant cells to invade and spread.[188] Prostate cancer also contains a cell surface receptor for entactin, a glycoprotein found in basement membranes in complex with laminin. The heterodimeric receptor was identified as the integrin alpha 3 beta 1.[189] Purified entactin promotes attachment and spreading of cells.

Differential expression of integrins may be clinically useful. The alpha 4 subunit of integrins is expressed only on nontumorigenic cells, whereas prostate cancer expresses alpha 2b beta 3 integrin.[190] Integrin beta 1C is expressed in benign prostate but is undetectable in cancer, consistent with its in vitro growth-inhibitory properties.[191, 192] Selective cleavage of the beta 4 integrin by matrilysin may explain its loss in cancer.[182, 193]

OSTEOPONTIN

Osteopontin is an acidic, reversibly phosphorylated, adhesive glycoprotein secreted by bone and by all glandular luminal epithelial cells, including prostate. In the latter, it is concentrated at the apical surfaces.[194–197] It is a Ca^{2+}-binding protein shown to promote cell attachment and spreading through its Gly-Arg-Gly-Asp-Ser binding domain.[198] Cell attachment to osteopontin is mediated, in part, through cell surface integrin[199] that is also a receptor for other adhesive agents, including vitronectin, fibrinogen, von Willebrand factor, thrombospondin, and fibronectin. Osteopontin expression is increased after neoplastic transformation. Studies have demonstrated a direct correlation between levels of osteopontin messenger RNA (mRNA) and metastatic potential in different cell types within the Dunning model of rat prostate cancer. In human tissues, immunohistochemistry has confirmed high levels of osteopontin protein expression in invasive prostate cancer cells.

COLLAGEN

Collagen is an important component of the extracellular matrix. More than 19 types have been identified and are encoded by 33 genes. Types I, II, III, V, and XI constitute the fibrillar collagens, whereas types IV, VI to X, and XII to XIX represent the structurally diverse, nonfibrillar members. In addition to their role in basement membrane–stroma interactions, the pronounced vascular association with collagen type XIX suggests involvement of this and related collagen types with angiogenesis and cancer.[200] Type IV collagen, a major component of basement membranes, is organized in a network responsible for mechanical resistance. It also plays a key role in epithelial cell adhesion to basement membranes. The distribution of collagen type IV alpha chains in benign prostate, PIN, and cancer basement membranes reveals specific loss of the alpha 5 (IV) and alpha 6 (IV) chains in cancer, whereas the classic alpha 1 (IV) and alpha 2 (IV) chains are consistently retained. Additionally, type VII collagen colocalize with alpha 5 (IV) collagen chains.[201]

OTHER EXTRACELLULAR MATRIX PROTEINS

Other components of the extracellular matrix that have been examined in prostatic tissue include fibronectin, which demonstrated higher levels in cancer patients[202]; perlecan, a multidomain heparan sulfate proteoglycan[203]; and proteoglycans, macromolecules that contain bound glycosaminoglycans. Tenascin is a hexameric glycoprotein component in the extracellular matrix of stromal tissue. High expression was found in embryonic development and during carcinogenesis in almost all organs and in prostate cancer.[204] Tenascin is distributed preferentially in the peripheral zone during postnatal development.[183, 205–207]

Cadherins

The cadherins are responsible for calcium-dependent cell-cell adhesion. The three main cadherins are E-cadherins (associated with many types of epithelial cells), N-cadherins (nerve and muscle cells), and P-cadherins (cells in the placenta and epidermis). All are found transiently in other tissues during development. In the absence of calcium, the cadherins undergo conformational changes and are rapidly degraded by proteolytic enzymes. E-cadherins are concentrated in the adhesion belts (zonula adherens) in mature epithelial cells where they connect to the actin cytoskeleton through intracellular catenins.

Dysfunction of the cadherin pathway is involved in cancer invasion and progression.[184, 208–223] E-cadherin expression inversely correlates with cancer grade, stage, metastasis, recurrence, and survival.[184, 213, 216, 220, 224–229] P-cadherin is not expressed in prostatic cancer, probably reflecting loss of the basal cell layer rather than a transcriptional down-regulation. Catenins, particularly alpha-catenin, also play an important role in the dysfunction of the cell adhesion complex. Epithelial cells of prostatic acini, ejaculatory ducts, and seminal vesicles expressed E-cadherin but not N-cadherin. P-cadherin expression was limited to the basal cells, and P-cadherin–immunoreactive cells were negative for PSA. Prostatic cancer was usually P-cadherin–negative, but some tumors had focal positive areas frequently located close to ejaculatory ducts that were negative for PSA. The mutually exclusive expression of P-cadherin and PSA suggests that these proteins are involved in differential mechanisms of cell regulation.[230]

Cluster Differentiation Proteins

Another family of transmembrane glycoproteins, the CD (cluster of differentiation) proteins, display extracellular matrix adhesion properties. One of these proteins, CD44, and its isoforms may be involved in malignant progression of prostate cancer.[228, 231, 232] Epithelial cell populations were separated by flow cytometry using antibodies to differentially expresssed CD44 (basal cells) and CD57 (secretory cells).[233] PSA expression by CD57+ cells was abolished after prostate tissue was dispersed by collagenase into single cells. Expression of PSA was restored when CD57+ cells were reconstituted with stromal cells. Both cell types expressed a novel prostate marker, CD38.[234] Complete loss of CD38 expression was found in BPH and cancer.

Matrix Proteases

Localized degradation of the extracellular matrix is required for tissue remodeling, cell migration through the basal lamina, and metastasis. This degradation is accomplished through the action of proteases. The proteolytic enzymes comprise two main classes, including the metalloproteinases such as collagenases and matrilysin, and serine proteases such as the kallikreins and urokinase-type plasminogen activator (u-PA). uPA converts plasminogen into plasmin and thus mediates pericellular proteolysis during cell migration and tissue remodeling. uPA is secreted as an enzymatically inactive proenzyme (pro-uPA) by cancer and stromal cells. Active uPA converts plasminogen to plasmin, which, in turn, degrades components of the cancer stroma such as fibrin, fibronectin, proteoglycans, and laminin; it may also activate procollagenase type IV that degrades collagen type IV, a major part of the basement membrane. Primary cancer and metastases contain an elevated concentration of uPA compared with that found in benign tissues.[235–239] Expression of type IV collagenase was minimal in benign tissue but was consistently strong in PIN and cancer of all Gleason grades.[240]

A proteolytic cascade may occur during initiation and invasion of cancer cells.[236] The actions of proteases such as matrix metalloproteinases (MMPs) are often confined to specific areas by secreted protease inhibitors such as the tissue inhibitors of matrix metalloproteinases (TIMPs). MMP activity was greater in cancer than in BPH. Pro-MMP-9, in its 92-kd form, was exclusively expressed by cancer, particularly those cancers with an aggressive and metastatic phenotype.[241, 242] Many isoforms of these proteases and their inhibitors are present in the prostate. Expression of TIMP-1, TIMP-2, MMP-2, and MMP-9 appear to be independent predictors of outcome for prostate cancer.

Matrilysin, another member of the MMP family, is involved in tissue remodeling. It is expressed in epithelial cells of BPH and cancer, in contrast with the majority of MMPs that are produced by the stroma.[243]

Growth Factors and Receptors

Progression of prostate cancer is accompanied by modification of expression of growth factors and their receptors. A characteristic of the transformation process is that the cancer cells exhibit multiple and concurrent modifications in the expression of growth factors, receptors, oncogenes, and tumor suppressor genes. Hence, many of the modifications that occur in cancer cells may be interdependent or caused by one or more common processes of transformation.

Androgen Receptor

Androgen receptor gene mutations are present in prostate cancer before hormonal therapy and in hormone-refractory cancer. The activation of mutant androgen receptor by estrogen and weak androgens may confer on cancer cells an ability to survive testicular androgen deprivation by allowing activation of the androgen receptor by adrenal androgens or exogenous estrogen. Such mutations might confer a growth advantage even without androgen deprivation, since prostate cancer has lower levels of 5α-reductase and dihydrotestosterone than does normal tissue.

Microvessel Density

Microvessel density is a promising prognostic factor in the management of patients with prostate cancer. Unlike cancer cell–based factors, microvessel density is a host stromal factor that has apparently limited heterogeneity within a cancer. Its predictive value for pathologic stage has been demonstrated in most but not all reports. Further, studies reveal that microvessel density may be predictive of cancer recurrence and perhaps survival in some patients. Inhibition of angiogenesis may be an effective chemopreventive approach, particularly for men at high risk of prostate cancer. Standards have been proposed for analysis of microvessel density in prostate cancer and other cancers.[244–246] Immunohistochemical studies using CD34 appear to be more accurate than those using CD31 in prostate cancer.[247]

There are two putative phases of angiogenesis in prostatic carcinogenesis. The presumptive *prevas-*

cular phase may last for years; during this time, epithelial cells undergo limited growth that may progress to high-grade PIN and small foci of invasive cancer. The presumptive *angiogenic phase* of growth occurs when new blood vessel development is enhanced within the cancer, augmenting growth and perhaps clinical aggressiveness. This angiogenic "switch" may be regulated in part by tissue factor and its ability to induce vascular endothelial growth factor (VEGF), an angiogenic molecule, and inhibit thrombospondin 2, an antiangiogenic molecule. Prostate cancer expresses high levels of tissue factor, and this expression correlates with microvessel density and serum PSA.[248] Further, VEGF expression correlates with microvessel density, cancer stage, and cancer-specific survival in patients treated by watchful waiting.[249]

Microvessel density is higher at the geographic center of prostate cancer than at the periphery (Fig. 14–13A), but the variance is modest (106/mm² versus 50/mm², respectively).[250–252] Studies of the area of maximal density, termed the *hot spot*, suggest that sampling variation may lead to differences in microvessel density between biopsy and matched radical prostatectomy specimens,[250, 251] but this has been refuted empirically.[253, 254] Optimized microvessel density, calculated from the computer-analyzed microvessel density after subtracting glandular lumen spaces, is probably more accurate than manual counts of overall number of blood vessels per unit area.[253] A novel method was described to visualize and analyze prostate microvessels in three dimensions from serially sectioned prostate specimens.[255] This method included routine tissue preparation, computer reconstruction of digitized serial histologic sections into three-dimensional volumes, and calculation of geometric characteristics and microvessel density. The total length of vessels in a given volume, referred to as *vessel length density*, discriminated between be-

nign prostatic tissue and cancer better than did microvessel density. Results indicated that microvessels associated with cancer have a more homogeneous distribution in location, size, and tortuosity than do those in benign tissue.

Data are limited regarding microvessel density in benign prostatic disease and nodular hyperplasia. In one study, microvessel density averaged 99/mm² in hyperplastic nodules,[256] similar to cancer (see Fig. 14–13B) and significantly greater than that in the normal transition zone (70/mm²).[257] Vascular density was also increased in small stromal nodules. Expansion of established hyperplastic nodules beyond 1 mm³ may include an "angiogenic switch" similar to that found in carcinoma,[258] resulting in increased microvessel density concomitant with proliferative growth. Comparison of cancer to the benign tissue within the same specimen may be flawed because those with cancer may have increased vessel density in the benign areas,[257] although most investigators reject this possibility.[253]

High-grade PIN, the most likely precursor of invasive cancer,[259] is virtually always accompanied by a proliferation of small capillaries in the stroma. Microvessel density is higher in high-grade PIN than in adjacent benign prostatic tissue,[250, 251] and the capillaries are shorter and more widely spaced, have more open lumina and undulated external contours, and are lined by a greater number of endothelial cells.[260] The degree of microvessel density in PIN is intermediate between benign epithelium and cancer, lending support to the concept of PIN as the precursor of prostate cancer.

Microvessel density analysis offers promise for predicting pathologic stage and patient outcome in prostate cancer. The microvessels associated with prostate cancer are shorter than those in benign or hyperplastic prostatic tissue, with more undulating vessel walls.[260, 261] The cumulative evidence suggests that there is an important role for microvessel

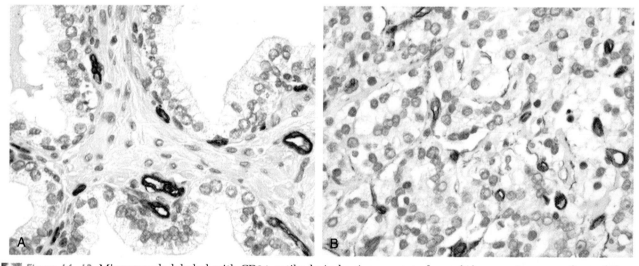

Figure 14–13. Microvessels labeled with CD34 antibody in benign prostate focus *(A)* versus in cancer focus *(B)*.

density analysis in the management of select patients with prostate cancer. Multiple studies have investigated the relationship of microvessel density and cancer stage (Table 14–5).[250, 253, 254, 256, 261–272] Most compared microvessel density in prostatectomy specimens with pathologic stage, probably because of the ease of evaluation and abundance of available tissue. Two assessed microvessel density in contemporary needle biopsies and correlated it with pathologic stage at prostatectomy.[273] Others compared microvessel density in transurethral resections from patients undergoing irradiation[265] or predominantly watchful waiting[264] with clinical stage; however, clinical stage is prone to serious staging error when compared with pathologic stage, so these findings should be interpreted with caution.[274] Many of the prostatectomy studies found a positive correlation of microvessel density with pathologic stage.[256, 271, 274] However, in one study, the important difference in microvessel density between stage pT2 and pT3 was observed only among low-grade cancer, whereas the reverse was true in another study. Silberman and colleagues found no correlation of microvessel density and stage,[270] but that study was limited to patients with Gleason scores 6 and 7; the authors then, surprisingly, combined this cohort with another that had different selection criteria. Barth and colleagues found no significant correlation of microvessel density and stage.[261] Biopsy results showed a positive correlation with matched prostatectomies regarding microvessel density in cancer, which was an independent predictor of extraprostatic extension.[253, 271] When optimized microvessel density was added to the Gleason score and serum PSA concentration, the predictive value of these measures for stage increased significantly. Microvascular invasion also correlated with stage, grade, and other parameters,[263] although other reports refute these findings. The bulk of evidence favors the relationship of microvessel density and cancer stage, although variance exists among methods and patient cohorts.[272]

There is generally good agreement that microvessel density is not an optimal predictor of prostate cancer recurrence (Table 14–6).* In studies in which patients were treated by surgery or external beam radiation therapy,[265] microvessel density[266, 269, 270] and microvascular invasion[282] predicted biochemical (PSA) failure. However, in patients treated with radiation therapy, microvessel density was not analyzed independently of grade.[265] When most patients were treated with palliative hormonal manipulation only, microvessel density did not predict progression independent of grade.[264] Microvessel density did not correlate with biochemical failure after controlling for stage (pT2) and grade (Gleason grade 6 and higher) in patients

treated by radical prostatectomy.[280] These authors found similar results for stage pT3 patients.[276] Other studies addressed the potential of microvessel density[264, 281] or microvascular invasion[283] to predict cancer-specific survival and found no independent predictive value (see Table 14–6). The predictive value on univariate analysis was negated by inclusion of grade[264, 283] or stage.[281]

Diagnosis of Prostatic Adenocarcinoma After Therapy

PROSTATE-SPECIFIC ANTIGEN, PROSTATIC ACID PHOSPHATASE, AND KERATIN 34βE12

Immunohistochemical studies for PSA, PAP, and basal cell–specific keratin 34βE12 are useful in identifying carcinoma after therapy. PSA and PAP are retained in tumor cells after therapy, and keratin 34βE12 assays remain negative, indicating an absent basal cell layer (Fig. 14–14).

NEUROENDOCRINE MARKERS

No differences were found in expression of neuroendocrine differentiation markers such as chromogranin, NSE, β-human chorionic gonadotropin (HCG), and serotonin after androgen deprivation therapy.[98, 284]

PROLIFERATING CELL NUCLEAR ANTIGEN

PCNA immunoreactivity declines after androgen deprivation therapy, indicating that androgens regulate cyclically expressed proteins involved in cell proliferation.[285, 286]

ANDROGEN AND ESTROGEN RECEPTORS

Androgen receptors are present within androgen-responsive and androgen-unresponsive cells in prostate cancer, suggesting that development of androgen independence is unlikely to be a consequence of loss of androgen receptor expression. These receptors are widely distributed immunohistochemically in secretory cells of the normal prostate, BPH, high-grade PIN,[287–293] and localized and metastatic prostatic carcinoma.[294–298] The percentage of cancer cells with androgen receptors is not predictive of time to progression after androgen deprivation therapy, although there is greater heterogeneity of immunoreactivity in cancers that respond poorly to therapy. Immunoreactivity is higher in specimens with amino acid substitutions in the receptor protein.

Estrogen receptors are present at low levels within nuclei of normal prostatic stromal cells, according to immunohistochemical studies, but increase significantly after combination androgen

---

*References 133, 246, 247, 249, 254, 264, 265, 270, 272, 275–281.

Table 14–5. Relation of Microvessel Density or Microvessel Invasion Analysis to Prostate Cancer Stage

Reference	Patient Population	No. of Patients	Antibody or Stain	Quantitation	Findings
Wakui et al, 1992[267]	Underwent TURP, prostatectomy, or autopsy, including 43 with and 58 without bone metastases	101	Vimentin	DIA	For stages pT2, pT3, MVD was lower in low-grade than in intermediate- or high-grade cancer; for stage pT4, there was no difference among grades
Bigler et al, 1993[257]	Underwent prostatectomy, with organ-confined or metastatic cancer	15	FVIII	DIA; expressed as ratio of capillary area to tumor area	Ratio increased twofold in high-grade, but not in low- or intermediate-grade cancer
Fregene et al, 1993[266]	Underwent prostatectomy, with or without LN metastases	34	FVIII	Stereology	MVD: no difference between stages T2 and T3, but increased in patients with LN metastases; control group included 34 benign biopsy specimens
Weidner et al, 1993[269]	Underwent prostatectomy, including 29 with and 45 without metastases or elevated postoperative PSA	74	FVIII	Stereology, "hot spots"	MVD higher (77) in patients with than without (39) metastases; by multivariate analysis, MVD was superior to Gleason score in prediction of metastases
Hall et al, 1994[265]	pT1–T2, diagnosed by TURP, treated with external beam radiation	25	FVIII	Stereology, hot spots	MVD higher in patients with EPE than in those without EPE; patients who progressed after radiotherapy had higher MVD than those who did not (97 versus 46 at 200×); results not analyzed independently of cancer grade
Brawer et al, 1994[250]	Underwent prostatectomy, with (9) and without (19) positive margins or LN (4) or bone (5) metastases	37	FVIII	DIA	MVD superior to Gleason score for predicting stage; MVD higher in patients with positive margins and LN or bone metastases than in those with negative margins
Vesalainen et al, 1994[264]	pT1–2, diagnosed by TURP; in most cases, watchful waiting and follow-up at 11 yr; 2 prostatectomy, 1 radiation therapy, 2 estrogen, and 23 orchiectomy	88	Type IV collagen	Hot spots; DIA for vascular surface density (mm^2 per mm^3 of tissue)	Vascular surface density did not differ among stages
Salomao et al, 1995[263]	Underwent prostatectomy; stages pT2 and pT3	210	Hematoxylin and eosin stain	N/A	MV invasion present in 53% and correlates with stage, grade, volume and margin status
Barth et al, 1996[261]	Underwent prostatectomy; stages pT2–4; grades low, intermediate, and high	41	FVIII	DIA for vascular surface density (mm^2 per mm^3 of tissue)	Microvessel number increased with stage and grade, but MVD decreased; normal tissue used as control (unspecified source)
Bostwick et al, 1996[253]	Quantitation based on biopsies of 115 pT2 and 71 pT3 patients who underwent prostatectomy	186	FVIII	DIA; optimized microvessel density subtracted glandular lumen space from tissue area	MVD independently predicted EPE
Silberman et al, 1997[270]	Underwent prostatectomy; grades 6 and 7 only; stages pT2 (31%), pT3 (69%)	109	CD31	Stereology, hot spots	MVD had no relation to stage, but did correlate with EPE
Rogatsch et al, 1997[271]	Underwent prostatectomy, biopsy compared with prostatectomy for pT2 and pT3	36	CD31	Stereology, hot spots	MVD correlated with stage; positive correlation between biopsy and prostatectomy
Rubin et al, 1999[272]	Underwent radical prostatectomy for clinically localized cancer	87	CD31; good interobserver agreement	Hot spots	MVD did not correlate with Gleason score, stage, surgical margin status, seminal vesicle invasion, or PSA failure

TURP, transurethral resection of prostate; FVIII, factor VIII–related antigen; hot spots, see text; DIA, computer-assisted digital image analysis; LN, lymph nodes; MV, microvascular; MVD, microvessel density; EPE, extraprostatic extension; grade represents Gleason grade.

Table 14-6. Relation of Microvessel Invasion Analysis to Prostate Cancer Recurrence, Progression, and Survival

Reference	Patient Population	No. of Patients	Antibody	Quantitation	Findings
Bahnson et al, 1989[283]	Underwent radical prostatectomy	55		Microvascular invasion	Patients with microvascular invasion had a fourfold greater probability of clinical cancer progression
Hall et al, 1994[265]	pT1–T2, diagnosed by TUR, treated with external beam radiation	25	FVIII	Stereology, hot spots	MVD higher in patients with EPE than in those without EPE; patients who progressed after radiation therapy had higher MVD than those who did not (97 versus 46 at 200×); results not analyzed independently of cancer grade
Vesalainen et al, 1994[264]	pT1–2; in most cases, watchful waiting and follow-up at 11 yr	88	Type IV collagen	Hot spots, DIA for vascular surface density (mm² per mm³ of tissue)	Vascular surface density not an independent predictor of clinical progression; dependent on grade
McNeal and Yemoto, 1996[282]	Patients with >0.5 cm³ cancer undergoing prostatectomy	357	CD34		MV invasion in 7% of cancers <4 cc and 24% of cancers >4 cc; MV invasion was an independent predictor of PSA failure (rise to >0.07 ng/mL), along with tumor grade and volume
Silberman et al, 1997[270]	Underwent prostatectomy; grades 5–7 only; stages pT2 (75%) and pT3 (25%)	87	CD31	Hot spots	MVD was an independent predictor of progression (43 in progressors and 29 in nonprogressors)
Gettman et al, 1998[280]	pT2 cancer patients treated by radical prostatectomy; only those with grade 6 or higher	148	FVIII	DIA; optimized microvessel density subtracted glandular lumen space from tissue area	MVD was not a significant univariate or multivariate predictor of clinical or biochemical recurrence, or both, in this select cohort
Gettman et al, 1999[276]	pT3 cancer patients treated by radical prostatectomy	211	FVIII	DIA; optimized microvessel density subtracted glandular lumen space from tissue area	MVD was not a significant multivariate predictor of clinical or biochemical recurrence in this select cohort.
de la Taille et al, 2000[247]	Underwent radical prostatectomy	102	CD31 versus CD34		MVD with CD34 was a multivariate predictor of biochemical failure
Bahnson et al, 1989[283]	Localized cancer, stages pT2–pT3	55	Hematoxylin and eosin stain	N/A	MV invasion present in 38%; conferred 4× risk of progression and death; but this variable is dependent on grade by multivariate analysis
Vesalainen et al, 1994[264]	pT1–2; in most cases, watchful waiting and follow-up at 11 yr	88	Type IV collagen	Hot spots; DIA for vascular surface density (mm² per mm³ of tissue)	MVD had no independent predictive value for survival; dependent on grade
Lissbrant et al, 1997[281]	Cancer detected by TURP; most patients followed by watchful waiting	98	FVIII	Hot spots	MVD predicted survival (56% died); independent predictive value negated by including the presence of metastases in the analysis
Borre et al, 2000[249]	Patients followed by watchful waiting; median follow-up of 15 yr	221	FVIII and VEGF	Semiquantitative scoring	MVD and VEGF expression correlated with each other, stage, and cancer-specific survival; however, VEGF was not predictive in multivariate analysis for survival in patients with localized cancer at diagnosis

TUR, transurethral resection; FVIII, factor VIII–related antigen; hot spots, see text; DIA, computer-assisted digital image analysis; LN, lymph nodes; MV, microvascular; MVD, microvessel density; EPE, extraprostatic extension; grade represents Gleason grade; VEGF, vascular endothelial growth factor.

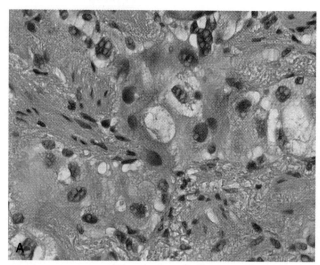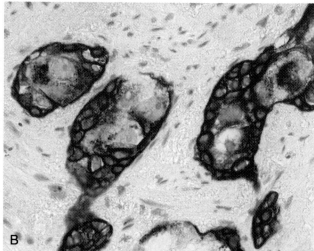

Figure 14–14. *A,* Benign prostate tissue with radiation changes. *B,* Immunostaining shows the basal cell staining.

deprivation therapy, particularly around prostatic acini.[299–307] Cancer cells are unreactive.

A-80 MUCIN GLYCOPROTEIN

Gould and colleagues demonstrated specific and intense immunoreactivity for high molecular weight mucin glycoprotein A-80 in neoplastic prostatic epithelium, with virtually every cell staining after androgen deprivation therapy.[308] Colloid pools and hemangiopericytoma-like areas were also immunoreactive, suggesting that some of these spaces represent remnants of ruptured malignant acini. The remarkable stability of this marker and its apparent specificity for dysplastic and malignant epithelial cells increase its value for routine use, but it is not yet commercially available.

MICROVESSEL DENSITY

The mean number of microvessels after androgen deprivation therapy for clinically localized prostatic adenocarcinoma is lower than in untreated cancer, according to immunohistochemical studies.[309]

Immunophenotype After Radiation Therapy

The biologic nature of cancer that persists at the primary site despite radiation administered with curative intent is not fully understood. Although locally persistent or recurrent cancer may be associated with an adverse outcome, the contemporary use of PSA monitoring, transrectal ultrasonographically guided prostatic biopsy, and early "salvage" intervention after therapy provides the opportunity to identify locally persistent cancer at an earlier and (potentially) more curable stage. The

prognostic significance of various biomarkers in prostate cancer has been studied previously, but little is known about the biologic characteristics associated with cancer that persists after radiation therapy.

PROSTATIC ACID PHOSPHATASE, PROSTATE-SPECIFIC ANTIGEN, AND KERATIN 34βE12

No definitive method exists for the assessment of tumor viability after irradiation. PAP expression usually persists,[310] suggesting that tumor cells capable of protein production probably retain the potential for cell division and consequent metastatic spread. PSA and keratin 34βE12 expression also persist after radiation therapy[310] and are often of value in distinguishing treated adenocarcinoma from some of its mimics. Most reports claim that if prostatic carcinoma is not histologically ablated by external beam radiation therapy after 12 months, it is probably biologically active.[311–314]

P53 AND PROLIFERATION MARKERS

A large proportion of cancers showed p53 nuclear accumulation after radiation therapy (Fig. 14–15), and overexpression of the p53 protein was associated with increased cellular proliferation of prostate cancer cells. p53 nuclear accumulation was also associated with adverse outcome after radiation therapy and may be increased in recurrent prostate cancer after irradiation.[315–327] p53 mutations are associated with decreased sensitivity to DNA damaging agents, and loss of p53 function may be associated with radiation resistance.[315–327]

Prendergast and coworkers studied 18 patients with locally recurrent prostate cancer after therapy and found that 72% had p53 nuclear immunoreactivity; among 5 patients with available pretreatment biopsy results, all had p53 immunoreactivity.[323] The immunohistochemical findings correlated with single strand conformational polymorphism and DNA sequencing analysis.[323] This observation suggested that p53 alterations may be present before therapy and may serve as a pretherapy marker for cancer recurrence. Retention of PCNA immunoreactivity in post-treatment prostatic biopsies correlated with local cancer recurrence.[318] Among postirradiation salvage prostatectomy patients, most (96%) had histologically evident prostate cancer that was proliferative, as demonstrated by MIB-1 immunostaining.[318, 326] The mean Ki-67 labeling index in recurrent prostate cancer was increased (mean, 7.0%) compared with those from prostatectomy series without prior radiation therapy at our institution (mean, 2.7%, unpublished data). Patients with higher cellular proliferative rates also had increased p53 protein overexpression, which suggested that these tumors were biologically active.

Our study design did not allow determination of whether the biologic characteristics of cancer changed over time (i.e, time-dependent cancer "clonal evolution") or whether cancer recurrence was an expression of an innately aggressive tumor (i.e., tumor "selection") prone to recurrence.[318] Indeed, the observation that p53 immunoreactivity was also present in the pretherapy specimens of patients with cancer recurrence after therapy as well as the association of abnormal p53 protein expression with adverse patient outcome may suggest that these patients had unfavorable cancer types before the inception of radiation therapy.

GLYCOPROTEIN A-80

The A-80 glycoprotein appears remarkably durable and is readily demonstrable in postradiation prostatic carcinoma despite profound architectural and cytologic changes.[328] In one study, all cases showed readily detectable and often intense staining in the cytoplasm of cancer cells and in intralu-

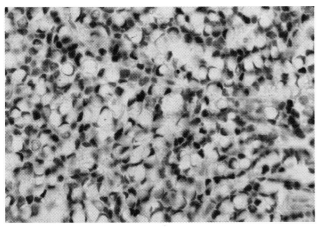

Figure 14–15. Imunoreactivity for p53 in poorly differentiated prostate cancer cells.

minal material of malignant acini. The extent and intensity of the reactions were independent of cancer size and grade. Strong reactions were seen in preserved and distorted acini, clear cell areas, single cancer cells, and colloid pools with few or no recognizable cancer cells. PIN was present in 53% of cases, of which 79% stained strongly for A-80; atrophic and hyperplastic acini generally did not stain, irrespective of the degree of cellular atypia.[328]

Immunohistochemical Studies in Benign Tumors of the Prostate

SCLEROSING ADENOSIS

Sclerosing adenosis was originally described two decades ago as adenomatoid or pseudoadenomatoid tumor and consists of a benign circumscribed proliferation of small acini set in a dense spindle cell stroma. In our study of overdiagnosis of prostate cancer in transurethral resection specimens, sclerosing adenosis accounted for 10% of cases.[329] Sclerosing adenosis is an incidental finding in transurethral resection specimens for benign prostatic hyperplasia and is present in less than 2% of specimens; rare cases are associated with elevated serum PSA concentrations. Sclerosing adenosis is usually solitary and microscopic but may be multifocal and extensive. The acini are predominantly well formed and small to medium-sized, but they may form minute cellular nests or clusters with abortive lumens. The cells lining the acini display a moderate amount of clear to eosinophilic cytoplasm, often with distinct cell margins. The basal cell layer may be focally prominent and hyperplastic, particularly in acini thickly rimmed by cellular stroma. In some foci, the acini merge with the exuberant stroma of fibroblasts and loose ground substance. There is usually no significant cytologic atypia of the epithelial cells or stromal cells, but in some cases there may be prominent cytologic atypia (DG Bostwick, unpublished observations). Sclerosing adenosis is distinguished from adenocarcinoma by the presence of distinctive fibroblastic stroma, which is rarely seen in carcinoma; benign cytologic features, with epithelial cells and stromal cells that lack prominent nucleomegaly; hyalinized periacinar stroma occasionally seen in sclerosing adenosis; an intact basal cell layer; frequent association with nodular hyperplasia; a unique immunophenotype of S-100 protein and actin reactivity (Fig. 14–16); and ultrastructural studies demonstrating myoepithelial differentiation.[330–334]

Immunohistochemical Studies in Variants of Prostatic Carcinoma

The biologic behavior of histologic variants of adenocarcinoma may differ from typical acinar adenocarcinoma, and proper clinical management de-

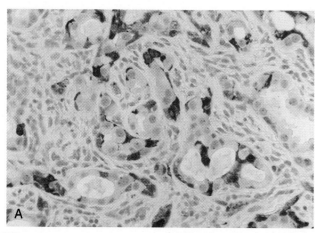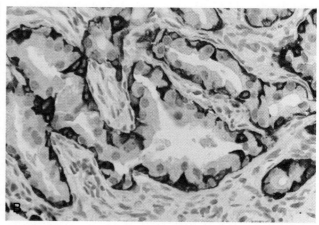

Figure 14–16. *A,* Sclerosing adenosis with intense S-100 protein immunoreactivity in the basal cells. *B,* Sclerosing adenosis with intense smooth muscle actin protein immunoreactivity in the basal cells.

pends on accurate diagnosis and separation from tumors arising in other sites. Unusual tumors arising in the prostate also raise questions of histogenesis. In this section, emphasis is placed on those variants of adenocarcinoma that display distinctive immunophenotypes; the reader is referred to specialized texts of urologic pathology for additional information regarding the clinical behavior and other pathologic features of these uncommon tumors.

DUCTAL CARCINOMA (ADENOCARCINOMA WITH ENDOMETRIOID FEATURES; PAPILLARY CARCINOMA; ENDOMETRIOID CARCINOMA)

Ductal carcinoma accounts for about 0.8% of prostatic adenocarcinomas. It typically arises as a polypoid or papillary mass within the prostatic urethra and large periurethral prostatic ducts. Most authors refer to this tumor as *adenocarcinoma with endometrioid features* or simply *ductal carcinoma.* The term *endometrial* should not be used in the prostate.

At the time of presentation, most patients have tumors confined to the prostate or urethra, with concurrent invasive acinar prostatic adenocarcinoma in at least 77% of cases. The prognosis of ductal carcinoma appears to be the same as typical acinar adenocarcinoma, although conflicting results have been found. Serum concentrations of PSA may be normal at the time of diagnosis except in patients with bone metastases.

Ductal carcinoma usually involves the large periurethral prostatic ducts and verumontanum, consisting of masses of complex papillae or acini lined by variably stratified columnar epithelium. Two architectural patterns have been observed: papillary and cribriform. These patterns coexist in about half of cases, and both have nuclear abnormalities and frequent mitotic figures. Ductal carcinoma invaria-

bly displays intense cytoplasmic immunoreactivity for PAP and PSA; focal carcinoembryonic antigen (CEA) immunoreactivity is occasionally present.[335–338]

The differential diagnosis of ductal carcinoma includes urothelial carcinoma of the prostate, large gland variant of Gleason pattern 3 adenocarcinoma, ectopic prostatic tissue, benign polyp, nephrogenic metaplasia, proliferative papillary urethritis, inverted papilloma, and accentuated mucosal folds. There is usually evidence of acinar differentiation in ductal carcinoma, allowing separation from urothelial carcinoma; in difficult cases or in those with small samples, immunohistochemical stains for PSA and PAP are useful (positive in ductal carcinoma and negative in urothelial carcinoma). The presence of urothelial abnormalities in the adjacent urethral mucosa is strong evidence of urothelial cancer, but is not definitive.

MUCINOUS CARCINOMA (COLLOID CARCINOMA)

Pure mucinous carcinoma of the prostate is rare, although typical acinar adenocarcinoma often produces mucin focally, particularly after high-dose estrogen therapy.[339–342] This tumor may not respond well to endocrine therapy or radiation therapy and is highly aggressive.

Focal mucinous differentiation is observed in at least one third of cases of prostatic carcinoma, but the diagnosis of mucinous carcinoma requires that at least 25% of the tumor consist of pools of extracellular mucin. Mucinous carcinoma consists of tumor cell nests and clusters floating in mucin, similar to mucinous carcinoma of the breast. Three patterns of mucinous carcinoma have been described: acinar carcinoma with luminal distention, cribriform carcinoma with luminal distention, and "colloid carcinoma" with cell nests embedded in mucinous lakes. Other histologic patterns of adenocarcinoma are usually present, including cribriform and comedocarcinoma patterns. Collagenous micronodules are an incidental finding in mucin-producing carcinoma and probably result from extracellular acid mucin.

Mucinous carcinoma stains with periodic acid–Schiff, alcian blue, and mucicarmine, similar to other prostatic mucin, but we rarely use these in practice. Most studies have found neutral mucin in benign acini and acidic mucin in malignant acini, although benign acini rarely produce small quantities of acidic mucin. Acidic mucin has also been described in atypical adenomatous hyperplasia, mucinous metaplasia, PIN, sclerosing adenosis, and basal cell hyperplasia. The cells of mucinous carcinoma contain PSA and PAP but usually do not produce CEA. The differential diagnosis includes mucinous carcinoma of the rectum, urinary bladder, or Cowper's glands. These distinctions are important because of significant differences in treatment and prognosis. Immunohistochemical stains for PSA and PAP are positive, at least focally, in mucinous carcinoma of the prostate and confirm prostatic origin.

SIGNET-RING CELL CARCINOMA

Signet-ring cell carcinoma of the prostate is rare.[341, 343–349] The clinical presentation is similar to typical acinar adenocarcinoma except that all are high stage. The prognosis is poor.

The diagnosis of signet-ring cell carcinoma requires that 25% or more of the tumor be composed of signet-ring cells, although some authors require 50%. Most often, it is a minor component of Gleason pattern 5 carcinoma. Tumor cells show distinctive nuclear displacement by clear cytoplasm. Signet-ring cells are present in 2.5% of cases of acinar adenocarcinoma, but rarely in sufficient numbers to be considered signet-ring cell carcinoma.[346] Histochemical and immunohistochemical results with mucin, lipid, PSA, PAP, and CEA stains are variable, and the signet-ring cell appearance may result from cytoplasmic lumens, mucin granules, and fat vacuoles.

The differential diagnosis of signet-ring cell carcinoma of the prostate includes similar tumors arising in other sites, particularly the gastrointestinal tract and stomach. Prostatic origin should be considered in metastatic signet-ring cell carcinoma of supraclavicular lymph nodes, which exhibits negative mucin staining; PSA and PAP immunostaining may be useful. Artifactual changes that mimic signet-ring cell carcinoma can occur in lymphoma, benign lymphocytes, and vacuolated smooth muscle cells, causing diagnostic difficulty. In these cases, PSA and PAP staining of the suspicious cells is negative, and CD45 (leukocyte common antigen) and smooth muscle actin immunoreactivity is observed within the inflammatory cells and smooth muscle cells, respectively.

SARCOMATOID CARCINOMA (CARCINOSARCOMA; METAPLASTIC CARCINOMA)

Sarcomatoid carcinoma is considered by many to be synonymous with carcinosarcoma.[111, 350–353] Authors who separate these tumors define sarcomatoid carcinoma as an epithelial tumor showing spindle cell (mesenchymal) differentiation and carcinosarcoma as adenocarcinoma intimately admixed with heterologous malignant soft tissue elements. Regardless of terminology, these tumors are rare.

Patients tend to be older men who present with symptoms of urinary outlet obstruction, similar to typical adenocarcinoma. Serum PSA concentration may be normal at the time of diagnosis. About half of patients have a prior history of typical acinar adenocarcinoma treated by radiation therapy or androgen deprivation therapy. Treatment is variable and has no apparent influence on the poor prognosis.

Pathologically, the distinction between sarcomatoid carcinoma and carcinosarcoma is often difficult and of no apparent clinical significance. However, metastases may consist of carcinoma or sarcoma, or both, so careful search of the primary tumor is useful to identify a component of carcinoma. Coexistent adenocarcinoma is almost always high grade (Gleason score 9 or 10). According to Dundore and colleagues, the most common soft tissue elements are osteosarcoma, with or without cartilaginous differentiation, and leiomyosarcoma.[350] The epithelial component displays cytoplasmic immunoreactivity for keratin, PSA, and PAP, similar to typical prostatic adenocarcinoma. The soft tissue component usually displays immunoreactivity for vimentin, with variable staining for desmin, actin, and S-100 protein. Ultrastructurally, tumor cells within the sarcomatoid areas occasionally display desmosomes and filaments that apparently represent CK.

The differential diagnosis includes sarcoma, and this distinction may be difficult and clinically unimportant, although immunohistochemical stains and electron microscopy are helpful. Keratin immunoreactivity has been identified in some cases of leiomyosarcoma, so this finding alone may not be sufficient to determine epithelial differentiation.

ADENOID CYSTIC CARCINOMA–BASAL CELL CARCINOMA

Adenoid cystic carcinoma–basal cell carcinoma consists of basal cell nests of varying size infiltrating the stroma (Fig. 14–17A). The malignant potential of adenoid cystic carcinoma–basal cell carcinoma is uncertain because of the small number of reported cases and limited follow-up, but some cases are malignant with extraprostatic extension and distant metastases. At present, adenoid basal cell tumor is probably best considered a tumor of low malignant potential.[74, 75, 354]

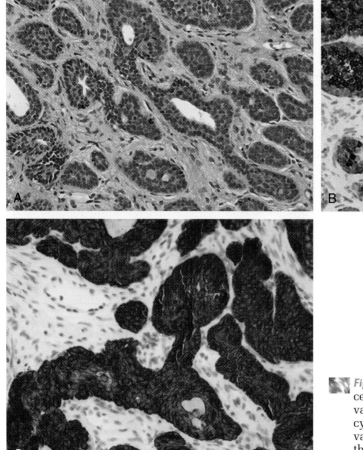

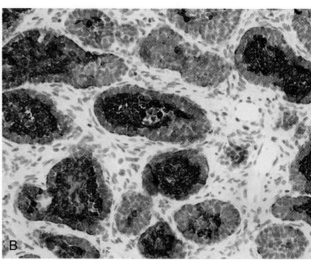

Figure 14–17. Adenoid cystic carcinoma–basal cell carcinoma consists of basal cell nests of varying size infiltrating the stroma *(A)*. Adenoid cystic carcinoma–basal cell carcinoma displays variable immunoreactivity with keratin 34βE12; there is luminal cell staining *(B)* as well as peripheral basal cell staining *(C)*.

There are two architectural patterns of adenoid cystic carcinoma–basal cell carcinoma: adenoid cystic and basaloid.[74, 75, 354] The adenoid cystic pattern consists of irregular clusters of crowded basal cells punctated by rounded fenestrations, many of which contain mucinous material resembling salivary gland adenoid cystic carcinoma. The basaloid pattern consists of variably sized rounded basaloid cell nests with prominent peripheral palisading. These patterns frequently coexist, although pure forms have been described.

Both patterns are histologically similar to basal cell hyperplasia and basal cell adenoma, but the tumor involves large areas of the prostate with little or no circumscription and often displays perineural invasion.[74, 75, 354] Adenoid cystic carcinoma–basal cell carcinoma displays variable immunoreactivity with keratin 34βE12; there may be luminal cell staining (see Fig. 14–17*B*) or peripheral basal cell staining (see Fig. 14–17*C*). Rare scattered cells show PSA and PAP immunoreactivity, but these may represent entrapped residual secretory luminal cells; other cells may show chromogranin staining. S-100 protein and NSE stains produce

negative results. The amorphous luminal material is negative with all stains.

Immunohistochemical Studies of Soft Tissue Tumors of the Prostate

Soft tissue tumors of the prostate have an immunophenotype similar to their counterparts arising in other parts of the body. Unusual tumors such as postoperative spindle cell nodule, inflammatory pseudotumor, and rhabdomyosarcoma are more often observed in the bladder and are described in that section further on. In this section, we emphasize soft tissue tumors of the prostate with a common or distinctive immunophenotype.

LEIOMYOSARCOMA

Leiomyosarcoma presents as a large bulky mass that replaces the prostate and periprostatic tissues. It is the most common sarcoma in adults and accounts for 26% of all prostatic sarcomas. Patients range in age from 40 to 71 years (mean, 59 years), with sporadic reports in younger patients.[350, 355, 356] Although the criteria for separating leiomyoma from low-grade leiomyosarcoma have not been precisely defined in the prostate, they are probably similar to those in other organs, including the degree of cellularity, cytologic anaplasia, number of mitotic figures, amount of necrosis, vascular invasion, and size.

Tumor cells usually display intense cytoplasmic immunoreactivity for smooth muscle–specific actin and vimentin and weak desmin immunoreactivity. Most are negative for CK (AE1/AE3) and S-100 protein, but exceptions have been described, particularly in those with epithelioid features in which keratin immunoreactivity may be seen.[355]

Local recurrence and distant metastasis are frequent, and the prognosis is poor. Mean survival after diagnosis was less than 3 years in one series (range, 0.2 to 6.5 years), and most patients died of tumor.[355] Rare long-term survivors have been reported. Radical surgery is the preferred treatment, although limited data are available.[355]

PHYLLODES TUMOR (CYSTOSARCOMA PHYLLODES)

Phyllodes tumor of the prostate is a rare lesion that should be considered a neoplasm rather than atypical hyperplasia because of the frequent early recurrences, infiltrative growth, and potential for extraprostatic spread in some cases.[357–364] Dedifferentiation with multiple recurrences in some cases is further evidence of the potentially aggressive nature of this tumor.[364] Although a benign clinical course has been emphasized in some reports,[365] the cumulative evidence in the literature indicates that some patients develop local recurrence.[364]

Patients with prostatic phyllodes tumor typically present with urinary obstruction, hematuria, and dysuria. There may be severe urinary obstruction, often occurring at a younger age than expected for typical prostatic hyperplasia. Most tumors range in size from 4 to 25 cm, with one report of a 58-cm tumor weighing 11.2 kg.[366] At the time of transurethral resection, the urologist may note an unusual spongy or cystic texture of the involved prostate.

Prostatic phyllodes tumor exhibits a spectrum of histologic features, similar to its counterpart in the breast. It may be subdivided into low-grade, intermediate-grade, and high-grade groups, but even low-grade tumors may recur.[364] High-grade prostatic phyllodes tumor has a high stromal to epithelial ratio, prominent stromal cellularity and overgrowth, marked cytologic atypia, and increased mitotic activity. A sarcomatous component may arise within a low-grade tumor over time, invariably after multiple recurrences over many years.[364] One reported case consisted of phyllodes tumor containing an incidental focus of well-differentiated adenocarcinoma.[366]

Immunohistochemical studies reveal intense cytoplasmic immunoreactivity in most stromal cells for vimentin and actin, in luminal epithelial cells for PSA, PAP, and keratin AE1/AE3, and in basal epithelial cells for high molecular weight keratin 34βE12; no staining was observed for desmin and S-100 protein (Table 14–7).

The histogenesis is uncertain but is not considered müllerian for the following reasons: (1) no müllerian remnants exist in the adult prostate and the müllerian epithelium in the prostatic utricle is replaced by the urogenital sinus early in life; (2) PSA and PAP are present in the epithelium of the adult utricle, indicating the endodermal (prostatelike) nature of this tissue; and (3) PSA is present in the epithelium of prostate phyllodes tumors.

Phyllodes tumor must be considered potentially aggressive, and an individualized approach to complete excision of the tumor is needed. Low-grade tumors may be treated conservatively, recognizing that recurrences may be higher grade and require complete excision.[364] Rarely, tumors with overtly malignant stroma give rise to lung, bone, and abdominal wall metastases of sarcoma. Lymph node metastases have not been observed.

The differential diagnosis of phyllodes tumor includes stromal hyperplasia with bizarre nuclei, giant multilocular prostatic cystadenoma, hyperplasia with cystic acini, and cysts such as müllerian duct cyst and congenital and acquired seminal vesicle cyst (Table 14–8). Phyllodes tumor may also arise in the seminal vesicle as a supraprostatic retrovesicular mass, but it is separated from its prostatic counterpart by the absence of PSA and PAP immunoreactivity in the epithelium. Stromal hyperplasia with bizarre nuclei is a cellular lesion with enlarged hyperchromatic degenerative-appearing nuclei occurring in the stroma adjacent to typical hyperplastic acini or within nodular hyperplasia. Giant multilocular cystadenoma of the prostate is a solitary tumor with cysts lined by prostatic epithelium surrounded by dense fibrous stroma. Cystic adenoma of the prostate has also been described, consisting of complex inward growth of papillary epithelial fronds with scant stroma. Nodular hyperplasia commonly contains small cystic acini within hyperplastic nodules, and small fibroadenoma-like foci may infrequently be misinterpreted as phyllodes tumor. Müllerian duct cyst (typically midline) and seminal vesicle cyst (typically lateral) are usually unilocular and lack the prostatic epithelial lining and stromal cellularity of phyllodes tumor. Primary sarcoma of the prostate, such as leiomyosarcoma, is also a diagnostic consideration, but this tumor consists of a monophasic, densely cellular proliferation of spindle cells that lacks the epithelial component of phyllodes tumor. Sarcomatoid carcinoma is a concern when an overtly malignant spindle cell component is present, but it is distinguished by the presence of a malignant epithelial component or evidence of

Table 14–7. Prostatic Phyllodes Tumor: Immunohistochemical Findings in Seven Cases*

Case No.*	Prostate-Specific Antigen	Prostatic Acid Phosphatase	Keratin AE1/AE3	Keratin 34βE12	S-100 Protein	Chromogranin	Serotonin	Estrogen Receptors	Progesterone Receptors	Androgen Receptors	Vimentin	Desmin	Actin
1	++	+++	++	+	–	–	–	–	–	++	++	–	+++
2†	++	+++	+++	+++	–	–	–	–	–	–	+++	+++	+++
3	+++	+++	++	+	–	–	–	–	–	–	+++	–	++
4	+++	+++	+	++	–	–	–	–	–	+++	+++	–	+
5	++	++	+++	+	–	–	–	–	–	–	+	–	+
6	+++	+++	++	+	–	–	–	–	–	–	+++	–	+
7	+++	+++	++	+++	–	–	–	NT	NT	NT	+++	–	+

* Tissue not available for staining in case No. 7.
† All but case No. 2 were run in a single batch for each antibody to avoid inter-run variation.
NT, Not tested.
Scale from – to +++ based on number of cells staining (+ = <25%; ++ = 25–50%; +++ = >50%).

Table 14–8. Phyllodes Tumor of the Prostate or Seminal Vesicles: Differential Diagnosis

Characteristic Features	Phyllodes Tumor	Stromal Hyperplasia with Atypia (Leiomyoma-like Pattern)*	Stromal Hyperplasia with Atypia (Infiltrative Pattern)*	Leiomyosarcoma†
Clinical features				
Mean patient age (range)		68 yr (57–80)	69 yr (59–80)	61 yr (41–78)
Presenting symptoms	Urinary obstructive symptoms, hematuria, or incidental finding	Urinary obstructive symptoms or incidental finding	Urinary obstructive symptoms or incidental finding	Urinary obstructive symptoms; perineal pain
Cystoscopic-macroscopic		Stromal nodule	Stromal nodule	Mass measuring 3 to 21 cm. in diameter (mean, 9 cm)
Serum PSA	Normal range	Normal range	Normal range	Normal range
Architecture	Biphasic pattern, including distorted cystically dilated or slit-like epithelial glands, often with leaf-like projections, together with condensed stroma	Solid circumscribed expansile stromal nodule with abundant smooth muscle and atypical stromal cells	Ill-defined hyperplastic stromal nodule with atypical cells diffusely and uniformly infiltrating around typical hyperplasia acini; hypocellular loose myxoid matrix with large ectatic vessels	Large bulky nodular tumor composed of spindle cells
Cytologic features	Benign epithelium; variable number of bizarre stromal cells with vacuolated nuclei and multinucleation; mitotic figures and necrosis indicate higher grade	Bizarre giant stromal cells with vacuolated nuclei and frequent multinucleation; no mitotic figures or necrosis	Bizarre giant stromal cells with vacuolated nuclei and frequent multinucleation; no mitotic figures or necrosis	Spindle or epithelioid tumor cells with variable pleomorphism, mitotic figures, and frequent necrosis
Immunohistochemistry				
Vimentin	Usually +++	+	+++	++
Desmin	Usually –; rare +++	+++	Usually +	Usually –; rare +
Actin	+	+++	+	Usually –; rare +
Estrogen receptors	–	–	–	NT
Progesterone receptors	Usually –; rare +	Usually ++	Usually +++	NT
Androgen receptors	Usually –; rare ++	+++	+++	NT
Keratin AE1/AE3	++ (epithelium)	–	–	Usually – (+ in 27% of cases)
Keratin 34βE12	++ (epithelium)	–	–	NT
PSA	+++	–	–	–
PAP	+++	–	–	–
S-100 protein	–	–	–	–
Follow-up	Frequent recurrences with late onset of stromal overgrowth, indicating significant malignant potential	Benign; very rare solitary recurrences	Benign; very rare solitary recurrences	Malignant; mean of 22 months to death (3–72 months)

* Data from Bostwick D, Qian J, Ramnani D, et al. Prostatic phyllodes tumor: Long-term follow-up study of 23 cases. Cancer, in press.
† Data from Cheville JC, Dundore PA, Nascimento AG, et al. Leiomyosarcoma of the prostate: Report of 23 cases. Cancer 1995; 76: 1422–1427.
PSA, prostate-specific antigen; PAP, prostatic acid phosphatase; NT, not tested.

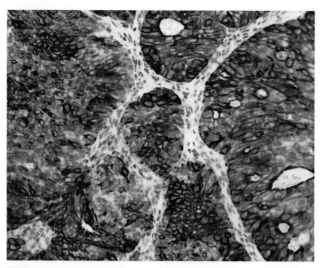

Figure 14–18. Immunoreactivity for cytokeratin 7 (CK7) in urothelial carcinoma cells.

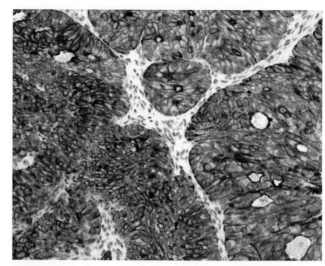

Figure 14–19. Immunoreactivity for CK20 in urothelial carcinoma cells.

epithelial differentiation within the neoplastic spindle cells.

BLADDER

Markers of Bladder Cells

CYTOKERATINS 7 AND 20

Cytokeratin 7 (CK7) is present in a wide variety of simple epithelia, including the lung, cervix, breast, bile ducts, collecting ducts of the kidney, urothelium, and mesothelium. However, it is largely absent in gastrointestinal epithelium, hepatocytes, proximal and distal tubules of the kidney, and squamous cell epithelia. The major utility of antibody to CK7 is in identifying nongastrointestinal adenocarcinoma. Conversely, CK20 is present in human intestinal epithelium, gastric foveolar cells, urothelial umbrella cells, and Merkel cells of the epidermis. This relatively limited tissue distribution of CK20 is useful in the differential diagnosis of carcinoma of unknown primary, especially in combination with CK7.

Most cases of urothelial carcinoma are strongly positive for both keratins (Figs. 14–18 and 14–19).[367–374] Conversely, hepatocellular carcinoma, prostatic adenocarcinoma, RCC, squamous cell car-

cinoma, and neuroendocrine carcinoma are usually negative for both CK7 and CK20. The immunophenotype CK7−/CK20+ is highly specific for colorectal adenocarcinomas, whereas CK7+/CK20− is found in the vast majority of carcinomas arising from other sites, including ovary, endometrium, breast, and lung, as well as malignant mesothelioma (Table 14–9).[375]

The discriminant value of CK7 and CK20 is further enhanced by use of other organ-specific markers. For example, Bassily and associates studied the expression of CK7, CK20, and PSA in 59 prostate adenocarcinoma specimens and 28 urothelial carcinoma specimens.[376] In the prostate adenocarcinoma specimens, 5 cases had CK7 positivity only, 5 had CK20 focal positivity only, 1 stained for both markers, and 48 were negative for both; PSA was positive in all but 1 poorly differentiated prostatic carcinoma. For urothelial tumors, CK7 was the sole positive marker in 6 cases, and CK20 was positive in 1 case; 17 cases were positive for both markers, and 4 were negative for both. All urothelial carcinomas were negative for PSA. They concluded that PSA was useful for differentiating prostatic from urothelial carcinoma, and CK7 and CK20 were helpful when both were positive, supporting the diagnosis of urothelial carcinoma. However, if only one marker was positive or both

Table 14–9. Utility of Cytokeratins 7 and 20 in the Differential Diagnosis of Urothelial Carcinoma

CK7+/CK20+	CK7−/CK20−	CK7+/CK20−	CK7−/CK20+
Urothelial carcinoma	Hepatocellular carcinoma	Breast cancer	Colorectal adenocarcinoma
Pancreatic carcinoma	Renal cell carcinoma	Lung non–small cell carcinoma	
Ovarian mucinous carcinoma	Prostatic adenocarcinoma	Primary seminal vesicle adenocarcinoma	
	Squamous cell carcinoma	Ovarian serous carcinoma	
	Neuroendocrine carcinoma	Mesothelioma (all forms)	
		Endometrial adenocarcinoma	

were negative, they had limited usefulness for distinguishing these carcinomas. Ormsby and coworkers evaluated the utility of cancer antigen 125 (CA 125), CK7, and CK20 for distinguishing primary seminal vesicle adenocarcinoma from other neoplasms.[377] They found a unique immunophenotype for seminal vesicle cancer that was CK7+, CK20−, CA 125+, and PSA− and PAP−. This combination, in conjunction with histomorphologic features, distinguished seminal vesicle cancer from other tumors, including prostatic adenocarcinoma (CA 125−, PSA+, PAP+), bladder urothelial carcinoma (CK20+, CA 125−), rectal adenocarcinoma (CA 125−, CK7−, CK20+), bladder adenocarcinoma (CA 125−), and adenocarcinoma arising in müllerian duct cyst (CA 125−). Urothelial carcinoma of the bladder and transitional cell carcinoma of the ovary are immunophenotypically distinct; the ovarian cancer rarely expresses CEA and never expresses CK20 or thrombospondin, in contrast with the bladder cancer.[378, 379] Cheng and associates reported that atypical nephrogenic metaplasia was positive for high molecular weight CK, CK7, and EMA, and was usually negative for CK20 and CEA.[380]

The expression of CK20 is restricted to superficial "umbrella" cells and occasional intermediate cells in the benign and reactive urothelium, even in the presence of severe inflammation. However, there is usually complete loss of this cellular restriction at least focally in dysplasia and carcinoma in situ, with positive expression in all layers of the urothelium seen in 31 of 36 cases in one study.[369] Thus, abnormal expression of CK20 is a useful adjunct to morphologic characteristics in the diagnosis of dysplasia and may be of greatest utility in distinguishing it from reactive states in which diagnostic difficulties are greatest. Abnormal expression of CK20 also predicted recurrence in patients with urothelial dysplasia, although this finding has not been independently confirmed.[368]

Experimental Markers in Urothelial Carcinoma

PROLIFERATION MARKERS

Ki-67 and MIB-1. Ki-67 and MIB-1 expression, measured as the number of immunoreactive cells in frozen tissue specimens, correlated with cancer grade and stage and was usually predictive of recurrence of urothelial carcinoma (Fig. 14–20).[381–399] MIB-1 expression is significantly associated with p53 expression.[400]

Proliferating Cell Nuclear Antigen (Cyclin). The PCNA labeling index in bladder cancer varies from 5 to 92% and was predictive of genetic instability,[401] cancer recurrence,[402–404] response to radiation therapy,[405] and survival.[389, 406–408] Conversely, some reports found that PCNA was not predictive of clinical outcome.[395, 409] Diploid urothelial cancer

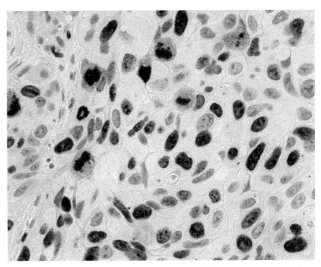

Figure 14–20. Immunoreactivity for MIB-1 in urothelial carcinoma cells.

with a PCNA labeling index less than 30% of cells did not recur, whereas aneuploid cancer with a PCNA index greater than 30% usually recurred.[410] PCNA expression correlated with nuclear morphometric findings in bladder cancer cells.[411]

Oncogenes, Tumor Suppressor Genes, and Mutator Genes. Several oncogenes and tumor suppressor genes appear to play a significant role in urothelial carcinogenesis (Table 14–10). The most likely factors include p53, retinoblastoma, Her-2/neu, and the ras family of genes.

p53 Gene. p53 is a 53-kd DNA-binding phosphoprotein that is coded for by a tumor suppressor gene located on the short arm of chromosome 17 (17p13.1). This transcription factor regulates cell growth and inhibits cells from entering the S phase. Mutations of p53 or functional inactivation with intact p53 genes are common in many human cancers, reflecting loss of normal growth regulation.[412] Mutations result in prolonged half-life and accumulation of the p53 protein to a level that makes it detectable immunohistochemically in cancer cell nuclei.[413] Overexpression of p53 protein is associated with a poor prognosis in a variety of cancers.[414, 415]

Most antibodies for p53 require antigen retrieval procedures when used with deparaffinized formalin-fixed sections. Staining results may vary because of differences in fixation, specimen pretreatment, and antibody binding sites.[416] Immunohistochemical methods rely on the accumulation of p53 protein in cells with p53 missense mutations. The cause of this is unknown, and studies indicate that immunoreactivity is not always indicative of p53 mutations. Wild-type p53 protein may accumulate in the setting of p53 activation, including hypoxia and DNA damage. In addition, not all p53 missense mutations result in protein accumulation, and they may cause false-negative immunohistochemical results. Finally, there may be a gradient

Table 14–10. Select Markers in Urothelial Cancer

Propietary commercial markers
  BTA
  NMP22
  Immunocyt
Proliferation markers
  Proliferating cell nuclear antigen (PCNA)
  Ki-67
  MIB-1
Oncogenes, tumor suppressor genes, and mutator genes
  p53
  Retinoblastoma gene (Rb)
  Her-2/neu
  ras
  bcl-2
Growth factors and receptors
  Epidermal growth factor receptor (EGFr)
  Acidic fibroblastic growth factor
  Basic fibrobast growth factor
Cell adhesion markers
  E-cadherin
  Integrins
  Cyclin D1
  CD44
  F and G actin
Telomerase
Angiogenic markers
  Microvessel density
  Vascular endothelial growth factor
Miscellaneous markers
  Autocrine motility factor
  Luminal epithelial antigen (LEA.135)
  Androgen receptor
  Urokinase-type plasminogen activator factor
  FHIT gene
  Cytokeratin (CK)20
  T138
  Hyaluronic acid

of p53 inactivation that varies according to the site and extent of the mutation. Nonetheless, there is a strong positive correlation of immunoreactivity and p53 mutations.[417] Benign urothelium rarely if ever displays staining, whereas expression in carcinoma is observed in 18 to 78% of cases.[418–422] Different cut-off points have been used for positive and negative staining, most commonly being 0% of cells,[423, 424] 10% of cells,[390, 422, 425, 426] and 20% of cells.[400, 414, 415, 419, 420, 427, 428] Intratumoral heterogeneity is reflected in the heterogeneous expression of staining. The cellular urine sediment may be used for genetic analysis of p53 mutations.[429]

In urothelial carcinoma, nuclear p53 protein immunoreactivity correlates with high grade (Fig. 14–21),[390, 430–434] high stage,[390, 431–433, 435, 436] vascular invasion,[431] cancer recurrence and progression,[414, 415, 425, 430] survival,[397, 414, 415, 420, 437–441] and p53 mutations, including 17p deletion and 17 polysomy.* Immunoreactivity may have independent prognostic significance,† but this has been re-

---

*References 390, 394, 400, 420, 427, 428, 434, 442–445.

†References 394, 400, 414, 415, 420, 424, 428, 437, 438, 445–450.

futed.[390, 418, 423, 432, 451–453] Stage T1 bladder carcinoma with more than 20% p53-immunoreactive cells had a higher progression rate than cancer with fewer stained cells (21% versus 3% progression per year, respectively).[438] Similarly, carcinoma in situ with more than 20% p53-immunoreactive cells had a higher progression rate than cases with fewer stained cells (86% versus 16% per year, respectively).[437] These results have been confirmed by other authors.[420, 425, 454, 455] Conversely, a recent study showed that cancer grade and stage were the only independent predictive factors for patient survival when p53 and bcl-2 were included in the analysis.[390] p53 status is not predictive of initial clinical response to bacillus Calmette-Guérin therapy in T1 cancer treated by transurethral resection, regardless of grade.[456, 457]

The predictive value of p53 may be increased when combined with other factors. p53 immunoreactivity and DNA aneuploidy are closely associated and, when found in combination, predict a very poor outcome for patients with invasive cancer[436]; conversely, another study found no correlation of p53 expression and DNA ploidy status.[452]

p53 alterations in urothelial carcinoma may result in increased sensitivity to chemotherapeutic agents that damage DNA, including doxorubicin and cisplatin.[458, 459] In patients with p53 mutations, adjuvant chemotherapy resulted in a threefold decreased risk of recurrence and a 2.6-fold increased chance of survival with median follow-up of about 9 years.[458, 459] Patients without p53 mutations derived no survival advantage with chemotherapy. These results suggest that patients at greatest risk of progression and death (those with p53 mutations) may also derive the maximal benefit from adjuvant chemotherapy and that p53 status may identify such patients.

Wild-type p53 leads to apoptotic cell death, whereas mutant p53 inhibits apoptotic death, simi-

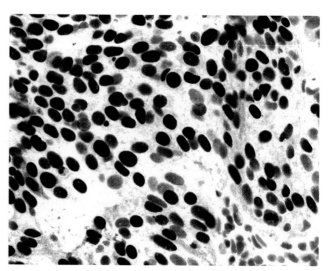

Figure 14–21. Immunoreactivity for p53 in urothelial carcinoma cells.

lar to bcl-2. Thus, it is interesting to note that bcl-2 is expressed more frequently in low-grade and low-stage urothelial cancer, whereas mutant p53 is more frequent in high-grade and high-stage cancer. One possible explanation is that mutant p53 prolongs survival of cells with established genetic defects, allowing them to become more unstable and clinically aggressive; conversely, the presence of bcl-2 may be an early event that prolongs survival of cells, allowing them to acquire initial genetic defects.[390]

p53 protein can be inactivated by viral proteins such as the E6 protein of human papillomavirus (HPV) 16. HPV is detected in occasional cases of papillary noninvasive and invasive cancer, and the presence of HPV correlates with higher stage and grade.[460–463] p53 mutations are rarely observed in patients with HPV-positive cancer, suggesting separate etiologic pathways.[464] Also, p53 can activate the proto-oncogene nuclear protein MDM2.[465, 466] This protein is increased in 67% of cases of noninvasive and early invasive bladder cancer but is present in only 27% of cases of muscle-invasive carcinoma. The p16 gene, present on chromosome 9, is abnormal in up to 60% of cases of squamous cell carcinoma associated with schistosomiasis but in only 18% of cases of urothelial carcinoma.[467–469] Moreover, anomalies of p16 and p53 are mutually exclusive, suggesting a complementary role in the pathogenesis of bladder cancer.[468, 470] Synchronous p53 and nm23 H-1 detection showed significant correlation with poor patient survival.[471]

p53 induces p53-dependent genes. A prototype of this class of genes, Cip-1 (WAF1), encodes a 21-kd protein that inhibits cyclin-dependent kinases responsible for initiation of the G1 phase of the cell cycle. Mutations in the p53 gene result in failure to stimulate Cip-1, with subsequent loss of inhibition of cyclin-dependent kinase complexes and initiation of G1.[435] The discovery of p53-dependent cyclin-dependent kinase inhibitors linked this gene to the basic enzyme mechanisms operative in cell cycle regulation. Mutations in p53 are usually missense substitutions that cluster in one particular region of the gene product between amino acids 130 and 290, involving residues 117 to 142, 171 to 181, 239 to 258, and 270 to 286. These regions are highly conserved among species and are probably necessary for normal p53 function. The regions encompassing codons 280 and 285 are a hot spot for p53 mutations.[472–474]

Loss of heterozygosity of the p53 locus occurs in many human cancers. Therefore, p53 most likely contributes to human carcinogenesis when its normal allele is deleted or inactivated. Transforming activity in the heterozygous state may be a result of formation of an oligomeric complex between mutant and wild-type p53. In cells transformed with mutant p53 gene, the altered protein complex remains in the cytoplasm.

Mutated p53 genes can cooperate with ras genes to transform primary cultured fibroblasts in the presence of endogenous wild-type p53 protein.[417] In some cancers, deletion of chromosome 17 loci occurs simultaneously with other chromosomal abnormalities, suggesting that p53 mutation is a late event in carcinogenesis. Cancer cell aneuploidy, reflecting chromosomal instability, may play a role in selection of cancer cells with p53 gene mutations. This process could lead to loss of the remaining wild-type allele and inactivation of growth control function of the normal p53 protein.[412]

About 65% of cases of carcinoma in situ contain p53 mutations,[466, 475] considerably greater than the 28 to 33% of cases of atypia and dysplasia.[421, 422] This high frequency of mutations is similar to that found in invasive urothelial carcinoma and may explain on a genetic basis the great propensity of carcinoma in situ to progress.[466] Moreover, germ line transmission of p53 mutations occurs in cancer-prone families, including those with Li-Fraumeni syndrome. p53 gene mutations were present in 11 of 18 invasive bladder cancers, and the most common mutation was single base-pair substitution. Missense mutations were present in 7 of 11 cases, and nonsense mutations were seen in 3 cases. Mutations of p53 are also detectable in urine sediment[476] and may be predictive of progression.[429, 477–483] In a study of 25 bladder cancers from 23 patients, the incidence of p53 mutations was significantly higher in muscle-invasive than in non–muscle-invasive cancer (58% versus 8%, respectively).[444] High-grade bladder cancer contained diverse p53 mutations in 36% of cases in one study.[417] These molecular studies confirm the immunohistochemical observations of p53 protein expression in bladder carcinoma. The identification of mutations of Cip-1 and MTS1 genes in urothelial carcinoma and other human cancers indicates that similar biologic effects can be the result of alterations of different genes in the p53 regulatory pathway.

Retinoblastoma Gene. The retinoblastoma (Rb) gene on chromosome 13p14 encodes a 105-kd protein that regulates transcription in all adult cells. The normal gene product suppresses expression of genes required for cell cycle progression. Cyclin and cyclin-dependent kinases inactivate the Rb gene product by phosphorylation. pRb can be inactivated by the protein corresponding to the open reading frames E6 of HPV 16 without mutation of the Rb gene.[460] Loss of function of the MTS-1 gene, which encodes the p16 protein, is an upstream regulator of Rb maintaining the Rb in its active or hypophosphorylated state. Absence of p16 correlates with functional inactivation of the Rb protein, perhaps accounting for the equal prognosis in patients with Rb absence or overexpression in some studies.[484]

pRb is expressed in all human tissues. Mutational inactivation of the Rb gene and reduction of pRb expression occurs in retinoblastoma and other cancers. The two main types of alteration of Rb in human cancer are deletion and mutation. Major deletions of large segments of the gene result in the absence of a properly functioning gene product.[485] Mutations, including nucleotide substitutions that alter gene function, create improperly located initiation signals, splicing sites, stop codons, amino acid substitutions, and other changes that destabilize transcription, producing a truncated gene product or otherwise modifying the mRNA. These changes cause absence of a functional Rb protein.[486, 487] Rb alterations in bladder cancer appear to be subtle point mutations rather than major deletions. The Rb gene is one of the major genetic factors responsible for the development and progression of high-grade muscle-invasive bladder cancer.[381, 425, 453, 484, 488–498] Loss of Rb function occurs in 30% of high-grade papillary and nonpapillary urothelial carcinomas. Loss of Rb correlates with loss of heterozygosity at the Rb gene locus, as well as high-grade and muscle invasion.

Altered expression of pRb is associated with decreased survival of patients with urothelial carcinoma.[425, 487] Benign urothelial mucosa and noninvasive urothelial carcinoma have pRb immunoreactivity in most cells.[499] Immunohistochemical detection of pRb appears to be a useful marker of cancer progression but is not routinely used.[430, 489, 500, 501]

Her-2/neu; p185 (c-*erb*-B2). Her-2/neu immunoreactivity in urothelial carcinoma is usually present on the cell membrane (Fig. 14–22),[502] although cytoplasmic reactivity has also been reported.[503] Stained cells are distributed diffusely, with no preference for superficial or basal cells. The frequency of Her-2/neu protein expression varies from 2 to 65% in the normal and inflamed urothelium and is present in 19% of cases of dysplasia and 64% of cases of carcinoma in situ.[504] Immunoreactivity increases with urothelial cancer stage, recurrence,[505] and survival,[506, 507] although some reports found no correlation of Her-2/neu staining and outcome.[508]

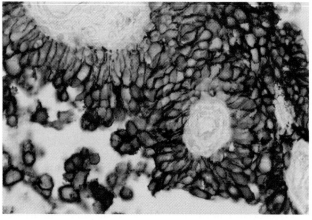

Figure 14–22. Immunoreactivity for Her-2/neu in urothelial carcinoma cells.

Purely superficial Her-2/neu positivity was present in both normal and dysplastic biopsy specimens. However, diffuse positivity and p53 overexpression were both associated with advanced dysplasia. Analysis by fluorescence in situ hybridization showed Her-2/neu gene amplification and p53 deletions in selected cases of carcinoma in situ, as well as a marked chromosome 17 copy number heterogeneity in all six cases of carcinoma in situ examined. These findings indicate a considerable genomic instability in bladder carcinoma in situ. They show that both erbB-2 and p53 are altered.[509]

bcl-2. bcl-2 immunoreactivity was observed in benign and dysplastic urothelium and in about half of cases of urothelial carcinoma, but was negative in carcinoma in situ.[390, 510] There was decreased expression with higher stage and higher grade cancer.[390, 394, 407, 446, 454, 511–526] bcl-2 expression offers promise as a marker of response to neoadjuvant chemotherapy in patients treated by radiation therapy for cancer.[382, 493, 527]

CELL ADHESION MARKERS

E-Cadherin. The normal human urothelium displays homogeneous immunohistochemical expression of E-cadherin, with membranous staining at cell borders.[528, 529] The luminal membrane of superficial cells was devoid of staining, as was the part of the cells in contact with the basement membrane. Abnormal staining is present in 21% of low-stage cancers and 76% of invasive cancers.[530] The strong correlation of E-cadherin expression with cancer stage indicates that it plays a role in invasion.[531] There is also a strong correlation between E-cadherin expression and survival; conversely, the presence of normal E-cadherin staining appears to indicate a good prognosis, even if the cancer is high stage.[214, 528, 529, 531–539] Serum concentration of E-cadherin correlated with cancer grade, number of cancers at presentation, and cancer recurrence, but not with immunoreactivity in tissue sections.[540]

Integrins. Normal urothelium does not express alpha 1, alpha 4, and alpha 5 subunits but shows cell membrane staining for alpha 2 and alpha 3 that is stronger in the basal cell layer than in luminal cells.[536, 541–543] There is progressive loss of alpha 2 beta 1 expression and, to a lesser extent, alpha 3 beta 1 in progression from Ta and T1 cancer to T2–3 cancer.[543] In normal urothelium, the alpha 6 beta 4 integrin colocalizes with type VII collagen at the junction of the basal cell and the lamina propria.[543] Minimal expression of this member of the integrin family in urothelial carcinoma was predictive of better survival than were those with strong staining or absence of staining in a series of 57 patients.[541] In 83% of noninvasive bladder cancers, integrin expression is present on the suprabasal and basal cells, whereas type VII collagen remains at the hemidesmosomal anchoring complex. This finding suggests that the anchoring complex in low-stage cancer is normal or only slightly altered, whereas in 83% of invasive cancers, loss of integrin or type VII collagen, or both, indicates abnormalities.[543]

Cyclin D1. Benign and dysplastic urothelium, including inverted papilloma, do not express cyclin D1.[544] Conflicting results have been obtained with immunohistochemical studies of cyclin D1 expression in urothelial carcinoma. One study identified nuclear cyclin D1 only in stage Ta and T1 papillary urothelial cancer but not in invasive cancer or nonpapillary cancer, and there was a marked decline with cancer grade.[544] There was an inverse correlation of cyclin D1 expression and PCNA and p53 expression, suggesting that cyclin D1 plays a role in negatively controlling cellular proliferation and allowing cancer differentiation. Conversely, other studies found no correlation of cyclin D1 expression with grade and stage, although cyclin D1–immunoreactive cancers recurred more rapidly than did unreactive cancer.[545, 546] Overexpression of cyclin D1 mRNA was found in 81% of non–muscle-invasive cancer and 38% of muscle-invasive cancer.[547, 548] For comparison, about 10 to 15% of bladder cancers have amplification of the 11q13 region.[547] The cumulative results indicate that genetic alterations in cyclin D1 are probably early events in urothelial carcinogenesis.[545, 549, 550]

CD44. The normal urothelium expresses CD44, but the greatest expression is present in early noninvasive papillary urothelial carcinoma, with progressive loss with invasion.[529, 551–561] CD44 protein isoforms and mRNA species are also detectable in exfoliated cancer cells in urine specimens.[551, 554] Soluble CD44 proteins are detectable in serum, with lower levels in men with bladder cancer than in matched healthy controls.[562] CD44v6 immunostaining discriminates small cell carcinoma of the bladder (negative) from poorly differentiated urothelial carcinoma (usually positive).

MICROVESSEL DENSITY

Increased microvessel density in urothelial carcinoma is predictive of lymph node metastases,[563] recurrence, and survival,[477, 564–569] and appears to be an independent prognostic factor.[564, 565]

VASCULAR ENDOTHELIAL GROWTH FACTOR

VEGF and, to a lesser extent, basic fibroblast growth factor, are the primary inducers of angiogenesis in bladder cancer cells.[570–574] VEGF mRNA and protein levels are higher in cancer than in benign urothelium,[573] and high VEGF predicts a poor prognosis.[575–578] An inhibitor of VEGF, thrombospondin-1, appears to play a key role in angiogenesis; its down-regulation is associated with the switch from an antiangiogenic to an angiogenic phenotype that occurs early in urothelial carcinoma.[570]

MISCELLANEOUS MARKERS

A variety of other markers have been evaluated in limited series. Autocrine motility factor (AMF-R, or gp78) was not expressed by benign urothelium, whereas its expression in urothelial carcinoma was an independent predictor of outcome in patients treated surgically.[579] Expression of the surface glycoprotein luminal epithelial antigen (LEA.135) in immunohistochemical assays showed progressive loss with high-grade and higher stage cancer.[580] Androgen receptor, a member of the steroid hormone nuclear receptor superfamily, is expressed in the majority of cases of urothelial carcinoma[581] but not in benign urothelium. Urokinase-type plasminogen activator is a serine protease whose expression was an independent predictor of survival in node-negative muscle-invasive bladder cancer but not in upper urinary tract carcinoma.[235, 582–585] The fragile histidine triad (FHIT) gene on chromosome 3p14.2 is aberrantly expressed in most primary urothelial cancers.[586] CK20 is expressed in neoplastic urothelial cells but apparently not in normal urothelium, and mRNA extraction from urine samples of patients with bladder cancer revealed a sensitivity of 91% and specificity of 67%.[587] Progression marker T138 detected a surface antigen that, together with cancer stage, was an independent predictor of metastases.[588] The glycosaminoglycan hyaluronic acid promotes cell migration and adhesion, and levels in the urine, when measured by enzyme-linked immunoabsorption assay, are elevated three- to fivefold in patients with urothelial carcinoma.[589–593]

Unusual Tumors and Tumor-like Conditions of the Bladder and Urothelium

VARIANTS OF UROTHELIAL CARCINOMA

There are a variety of unique variants of urothelial carcinoma, including those with mixed differentiation (Table 14–11). Recognition of some of these variants may be prognostically valuable. Two variants with a unique or unexpected immunophenotype are described in the following sections; the reader is referred to specialized texts of urologic pathology for details regarding the other variants.[594]

Small Cell Carcinoma (High-Grade Neuroendocrine Carcinoma). Urothelial carcinoma composed partially or completely of small cell undifferentiated carcinoma is rare, the likelihood increasing

Table 14–11. Variants of Urothelial Carcinoma

Nested
Micropapillary
Microcystic
Lymphoepithelioma-like
Lymphoma-like or plasmacytoma-like
Inverted papilloma–like
Urothelial carcinoma with syncytiotrophoblastic giant cells
Giant cell
Clear cell (glycogen-rich)
Sarcomatoid
Mixed differentiation
Carcinoma with tumor-associated stromal reaction

after therapy such as radiation therapy, similar to prostatic small cell carcinoma. The immunohistochemical findings are typical of small cell carcinoma at other sites, as is the aggressive clinical course (Table 14–12).[555, 595–598]

Immunoreactivity for CD44v6 was absent in 25 of 27 cases of small cell carcinoma, with two showing only weak staining of less than 10% of cells; in contrast, all cases of moderately or poorly differentiated urothelial carcinoma displayed moderately intense reactivity in 50 to 100% of cells. CD44v6 immunostaining discriminated cases of poorly differentiated urothelial carcinoma from small cell carcinoma and highlighted the presence of mixed small cell urothelial differentiation, when present.[555]

Small cell carcinoma of the bladder has a high number of genomic alterations (mean: 11.3 per tumor).[599] Deletions are most frequent at 10q (7 of 10 tumors deleted), 4q, 5q (5 of 10 each), and 13q (4 of 10). These regions may carry tumor suppressor genes with relevance for this particular tumor type. Gains of DNA sequences were most prevalent at 8q (5 of 10) 5p, 6p, and 20q (4 of 10 each). High-level amplifications were found at 1p22-32, 3q26.3, 8q24, and 12q14-21. These loci may pinpoint the localization of oncogenes with relevance for small cell bladder cancer. The analysis of one tumor having areas of both small cell and urothelial carcinoma strongly suggests that small cell carcinoma can develop from urothelial carcinoma through the acquisition of additional genetic alterations.[599]

Urothelial Carcinoma with Syncytiotrophoblastic Giant Cells. Giant cells are present in about 12% of cases of urothelial carcinoma, occasionally producing substantial amounts of immunoreactive β-HCG, indicative of syncytiotrophoblastic differentiation.[600] The number of HCG-immunoreactive cells is inversely associated with cancer grade.[601] Secretion of HCG into the serum may be associated with a poor response to radiation therapy.[602] The most important differential diagnostic consideration is choriocarcinoma; most but not all cases previously reported as primary choriocarcinoma of the bladder represent urothelial carcinoma with syncytiotrophoblastic cells.

Soft Tissue Tumors and Spindle Cell Lesions of the Bladder

Soft tissue tumors in the urinary bladder are immunohistochemically similar to their counterparts in other organs of the body. The most common adult sarcoma, leiomyosarcoma, may be mistaken for sarcomatoid (spindle cell) carcinoma, and routine immunohistochemical studies described elsewhere in this text are often useful in making this clinically important separation (Table 14–13).

Two unique mimics of malignancy, postoperative spindle cell tumor and inflammatory myofibroblastic tumor, have characteristic immunohistochemical profiles that can be exploited in distinguishing these from sarcoma and sarcomatoid carcinoma.

POSTOPERATIVE SPINDLE CELL NODULE

Postoperative spindle cell nodule (PSCN) is an uncommon lesion in the lower genitourinary tract that usually develops within about 3 months of a surgical procedure. It appears as a friable vegetant mass, consisting of intersecting fascicles of spindle cells that often display conspicuous numbers of mitotic figures, but none is atypical.[603–608] Reactive atypia may be present, but the cells do not exhibit marked cytologic abnormalities. PSCN shows a marked resemblance to leiomyosarcoma, but other sarcomas such as Kaposi's sarcoma should also be considered. PSCN is easily distinguished from intermediate or high-grade leiomyosarcoma because of the absence of cytologic abnormalities, but it is most difficult to separate from low-grade leiomyosarcoma. Both may involve the muscularis propria, and both may display myxoid change, although extensive and prominent myxoid change favors leiomyosarcoma.

Table 14–12. Immunohistochemistry of Small Cell Carcinoma of the Urinary Bladder

Antibody	% Cases Staining
Neuron-specific enolase (NSE)	90
Neurofilament	84
Human milk fat globulin	67
Epithelial membrane antigen (EMA)	63
Keratin AE1/AE3; CAM5.2	61
Carcinoembryonic antigen (CEA)	50
Synaptophysin	46
LeuM1	43
Chromogranin	41
Serotonin	38
Leu7	35
S-100 protein	34
Serotonin	31
Vasoactive intestinal peptide (VIP)	17
Vimentin	17
Adrenocorticotropic hormone (ACTH)	9

Table 14–13. Comparative Immunohistochemistry of Soft Tissue Tumors of the Urinary Bladder

	Postoperative Spindle Cell Nodule	Inflammatory Pseudotumor*	Spindle Cell Carcinoma	Leiomyosarcoma	Rhabdomyosarcoma
Keratin	+	− (rare aberrant expression)	+	−	−
EMA	−	−	+	−	−
Vimentin	+	+	+	+	+
Desmin	+	−	−	+	+
MSA	+	−	−	+	+

* Inflammatory myofibroblastic tumor.
   EMA, epithelial membrane antigen; MSA, muscle-specific actin.

The clinical history is of great diagnostic utility, as is the distinctive delicate network of small blood vessels in PSCN.

Immunocytochemistry is of value in the diagnosis of PSCN. This tumor-like proliferation displays CK immunoreactivity in 80% of cases, whereas this is less common in leiomyosarcoma of the bladder.

INFLAMMATORY PSEUDOTUMOR (PSEUDOSARCOMATOUS MYOFIBROBLASTIC TUMOR; INFLAMMATORY MYOFIBROBLASTIC TUMOR; PSEUDOSARCOMATOUS FIBROMYXOID TUMOR)

Inflammatory pseudotumor may occur at all ages, with a mean of about 30 years; there is a female predominance. It may be mistaken for rhabdomyosarcoma in children and leiomyosarcoma or sarcomatoid carcinoma in adults.[595, 609–615] Some cases occur after urinary tract infection, but most have no demonstrable cause. Inflammatory pseudotumor is composed of proliferating myofibroblasts, fibroblastic cells, and endothelial cells set in an acid-mucopolysaccharide–rich stroma that suggests active granulation tissue, similar to nodular fasciitis.[595] Tumor cells do not show anaplasia and nuclear hyperchromasia, effectively excluding intermediate- and high-grade sarcoma. Infiltration into the muscularis propria is frequent and should not be considered strong evidence of malignancy. Sarcomatoid carcinoma may have foci resembling inflammatory pseudotumor, and caution is warranted with small or limited samples. Variants include cases with a storiform pattern or those with hyalinization that produces a sclerosing pattern. The spindle cells are immunoreactive for vimentin (10 of 10 cases in one study) and muscle-specific actin (10 of 10 cases). A few cases exhibit immunoreactivity for smooth muscle–specific actin (3 of 8 cases), CK (2 of 10 cases), desmin (2 of 9 cases), and EMA (2 of 8 cases).[595] Aberrant expression of keratin is observed at least focally in some cases.[595, 615] DNA content analysis by flow cytometry yielded diploid histograms (6 of 6 cases).[595]

BENIGN SOFT TISSUE TUMORS

Paraganglioma (pheochromocytoma) is a rare but important tumor that probably arises from normal paraganglionic tissue within the bladder wall.[616–622] It appears at any age and is equally common in men and women. Rare cases are associated with neurofibromatosis,[623] intestinal carcinoid[619] and, curiously, long-term dialysis.[624] The diagnosis is usually confirmed by measurement of catecholamines and metabolites in urine and serum. Paraganglioma is intramural, with a predilection for the trigone, anterior wall, and dome. The overlying mucosa may be intact or ulcerated.

Microscopically, paraganglioma of the bladder is identical to that occurring elsewhere and is composed of cells arranged in discrete nests ("zellballen") separated by a prominent sinusoidal vascular network (Fig. 14–23). Pathologic predictors of behavior for these tumors are not well defined. Features associated with aggressive behavior in paraganglioma arising at other sites, including mitotic figures, necrosis, and vascular invasion, have not been studied in urinary bladder tumors. Immunohistochemically, the most useful features are the lack of immunoreactivity for CK, EMA, and CEA, and positive reaction with antibodies to neuroen-

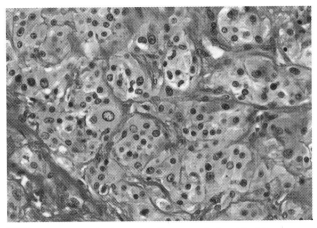

Figure 14–23. Paraganglioma of the bladder, composed of cells arranged in discrete nests ("zellballen") separated by a prominent sinusoidal vascular network.

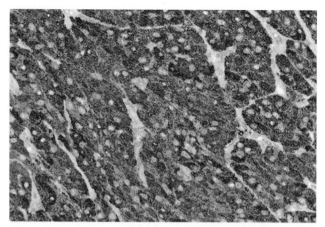

Figure 14–24. Paraganglioma of the bladder, immunoreactivity for chromogranin in tumor cells.

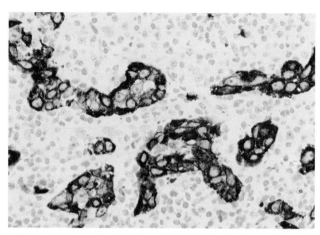

Figure 14–26. Immunoreactivity for AE1/AE3 in lymphoepithelioma-like urothelial carcinoma cells.

docrine markers, including NSE, chromogranin (Fig. 14–24), synaptophysin, serotonin, somatostatin, and others. Sustentacular cells stain positively for S-100 protein (Fig. 14–25).[616–622, 625–627]

SOLITARY FIBROUS TUMOR

Solitary fibrous tumor, previously referred to as *localized fibrous mesothelioma,* rarely arises within the bladder wall.[628–630] Immunohistochemical studies are useful in separating solitary fibrous tumor from other soft tissue tumors of the bladder; it is characteristically immunoreactive for CD34 and negative for keratin and S-100 protein. Rare cells may display actin and muscle-specific actin, but this finding is inconsistent.

GRANULAR CELL TUMOR

Granular cell tumor of the urinary bladder is rare, invariably arising in adults. This tumor is considered neurogenic (Schwann cell) in origin and is S-100 protein immunoreactive, similar to granular cell tumor elsewhere.[631–633]

Malignant Lymphoma of Bladder

Primary malignant lymphoma in the bladder is rare, with less than 100 reported cases, accounting for only 0.2% of extranodal lymphomas.[634–640] Most examples have been reported as single cases, and histologic classification has varied greatly, with only a small number having immunologic studies to phenotype the lymphoma.[636]

Microscopically, the tumor consists of a diffuse infiltrate of lymphoid cells surrounding and permeating normal structures rather than replacing them. Lymphoepithelial lesions are often frequent. The most common types of lymphoma are mucosa-associated lymphoid tissue type lymphoma (MALT), diffuse large cell lymphoma, and small lymphocytic lymphoma.[636] Rare cases of lymphoma arise synchronously in association with adenocarcinoma and urothelial carcinoma.

Immunohistochemically, almost all bladder lymphomas are of B-cell origin and display monoclonality. The most common type of primary lymphoma is low-grade lymphoma of MALT type.[636] Primary Hodgkin's disease and immunoblastic sarcoma are extremely rare.

The major differential diagnostic considerations are florid chronic cystitis, small cell carcinoma, lymphoepithelioma-like carcinoma (Fig. 14–26), and lymphoma-like carcinoma. Overall survival for bladder lymphoma is estimated to be 68 to 73% at 1 year and 27 to 64% at 5 years.[636]

References

1. Bostwick DG. Prostate-specific antigen: Current role in diagnostic pathology of prostate cancer. Am J Clin Pathol 1994;102(4 Suppl 1):S31–37.
2. Akdas A, Cevik I, Tarcan T, et al. The role of free prostate-specific antigen in the diagnosis of prostate cancer. Br J Urol 1997;79:920–923.
3. Ablin RJ. A retrospective and prospective overview of prostate-specific antigen. J Cancer Res Clin Oncol 1997;123:583–594.
4. Brawer MK, Benson MC, Bostwick DG, et al. Prostate-spe-

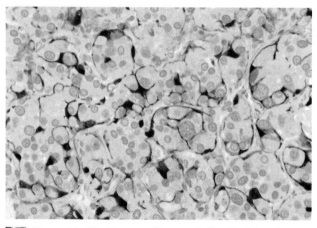

Figure 14–25. Paraganglioma of the bladder; immunoreactivity for S-100 in tumor cells.

cific antigen and other serum markers: Current concepts from the World Health Organization Second International Consultation on Prostate Cancer. Semin Urol Oncol 1999; 17:206–221.

5. Romas NA. Prostatic acid phosphatase: Current concepts. Semin Urol 1983;1:177–185.

6. Lippert MC, Bensimon H, Javadpour N. Immunoperoxidase staining of acid phosphatase in human prostatic tissue. J Urol 1982;128:1114–1116.

7. Ordonez NG, Ayala AG, von Eschenbach AC, et al. Immunoperoxidase localization of prostatic acid phosphatase in prostatic carcinoma with sarcomatoid changes. Urology 1982;19:210–214.

8. Nadji M, Morales AR. Immunohistochemistry of prostatic acid phosphatase. Ann NY Acad Sci 1982;390:133–141.

9. Jobsis AC, De Vries GP, Meijer AE, Ploem JS. The immunohistochemical detection of prostatic acid phosphatase: Its possibilities and limitations in tumour histochemistry. Histochem J 1981;13:961–973.

10. Ablin RJ. Immunohistological localization of prostatic acid phosphatase. Allergol Immunopathol (Madr) 1979;7:361–364.

11. Stein BS, Vangore S, Petersen RO. Immunoperoxidase localization of prostatic antigens: Comparison of primary and metastatic sites. Urology 1984;24:146–152.

12. Pollen JJ, Dreilinger A. Immunohistochemical identification of prostatic acid phosphatase and prostate specific antigen in female periurethral glands. Urology 1984;23:303–304.

13. Broghamer WL Jr, Richardson ME, Faurest S, Parker JE. Prostatic acid phosphatase immunoperoxidase staining of cytologically positive effusions associated with adenocarcinomas of the prostate and neoplasms of undetermined origin. Acta Cytol 1985;29:274–278.

14. Song GX, Lin CT, Wu JY, et al. Immunoelectron microscopic demonstration of prostatic acid phosphatase in human hyperplastic prostate. Prostate 1985;7:63–71.

15. Mori K, Wakasugi C. Immunocytochemical demonstration of prostatic acid phosphatase: Different secretion kinetics between normal, hyperplastic and neoplastic prostates. J Urol 1985;133:877–883.

16. Kumar PP, Good RR, Newland JR. Immunodiagnosis by prostatic acid phosphatase to differentiate primary male breast cancer from metastatic prostate cancer. J Natl Med Assoc 1986;78:782–784; 786.

17. Keillor JS, Aterman K. The response of poorly differentiated prostatic tumors to staining for prostate specific antigen and prostatic acid phosphatase: A comparative study. J Urol 1987;137:894–896.

18. van Dieijen-Visser MP, Delaere KP, Gijzen AH, Brombacher PJ. A comparative study on the diagnostic value of prostatic acid phosphatase (PAP) and prostatic specific antigen (PSA) in patients with carcinoma of the prostate gland. Clin Chim Acta 1988;174:131–140.

19. Ersev A, Ersev D, Turkeri L, et al. The relation of prostatic acid phosphatase and prostate specific antigen with tumour grade in prostatic adenocarcinoma: An immunohistochemical study. Prog Clin Biol Res 1990;357:129–134.

20. Sakai H, Shiraishi K, Minami Y, et al. Immunohistochemical prostatic acid phosphatase level as a prognostic factor of prostatic carcinoma. Prostate 1991;19:265–272.

21. Garde SV, Sheth AR, Porter AT, Pienta KJ. A comparative study on expression of prostatic inhibin peptide, prostate acid phosphatase and prostate specific antigen in androgen independent human and rat prostate carcinoma cell lines. Cancer Lett 1993;70:159–166.

22. Grob BM, Schellhammer PF, Brassil DN, Wright GL Jr. Changes in immunohistochemical staining of PSA, PAP, and TURP-27 following irradiation therapy for clinically localized prostate cancer. Urology 1994;44:525–529.

23. Sauvageot J, Epstein JI. Immunoreactivity for prostate-specific antigen and prostatic acid phosphatase in adenocarcinoma of the prostate: Relation to progression following radical prostatectomy. Prostate 1998;34:29–33.

24. Moul JW, Connelly RR, Perahia B, McLeod DG. The contemporary value of pretreatment prostatic acid phosphatase to predict pathological stage and recurrence in radical prostatectomy cases. J Urol 1998;159:935–940.

25. Sinha AA, Quast BJ, Wilson MJ, et al. Immunocytochemical localization of an immunoconjugate (antibody IgG against prostatic acid phosphatase conjugated to 5-fluoro-2′-deoxyuridine) in human prostate tumors. Anticancer Res 1998;18:1385–1392.

26. Epstein JI. PSA and PAP as immunohistochemical markers in prostate cancer. Urol Clin North Am 1993;20:757–770.

27. Murphy GP, Elgamal AA, Su SL, et al. Current evaluation of the tissue localization and diagnostic utility of prostate specific membrane antigen. Cancer 1998;83:2259–2269.

28. Gregorakis AK, Holmes EH, Murphy GP. Prostate-specific membrane antigen: Current and future utility. Semin Urol Oncol 1998;16:2–12.

29. Elgamal AA, Holmes EH, Su SL, et al. Prostate-specific membrane antigen (PSMA): Current benefits and future value. Semin Surg Oncol 2000;18:10–16.

30. Gong MC, Chang SS, Sadelain M, et al. Prostate-specific membrane antigen (PSMA)–specific monoclonal antibodies in the treatment of prostate and other cancers. [in process citation] Cancer Metastasis Rev 1999;18:483–490.

31. Silver DA, Pellicer I, Fair WR, et al. Prostate-specific membrane antigen expression in normal and malignant human tissues. Clin Cancer Res 1997;3:81–85.

32. Sweat SD, Pacelli A, Murphy GP, Bostwick DG. Prostate-specific membrane antigen expression is greatest in prostate adenocarcinoma and lymph node metastases. Urology 1998;52:637–640.

33. Troyer JK, Beckett ML, Wright GL Jr. Detection and characterization of the prostate-specific membrane antigen (PSMA) in tissue extracts and body fluids. Int J Cancer 1995;62:552–558.

34. Zhang S, Zhang HS, Cordon-Cardo C, et al. Selection of tumor antigens as targets for immune attack using immunohistochemistry: Protein antigens. Clin Cancer Res 1998; 4:2669–2676.

35. Axelrod HRR, D'Aleo CJ, Petrylack D, et al. Preclinical results and human immunohistochemical studies with 90Y-CYT-356. J Urol 1992;147:361A.

36. Wright GL Jr, Beckett ML, Schelhammer PF. Expression of prostate-specific membrane antigen in normal, benign, and malignant tissues. Urol Oncol 1995;1:18–28.

37. Lopes AD, David WL, Rosenstraus MJ, et al. Immunohistochemical and pharmakokinetic characterization of the site-specific immunoconjugate CYT-356 derived from anti-prostate monoclonal antibody 7E11-C5. Cancer Res 1990; 50:6423–6429.

38. Murphy G, Tjoa B, Ragde H, et al. Phase I clinical trial: T-cell therapy for prostate cancer using autologous dendritic cells pulsed with HLA-A0201-specific peptides from prostate-specific membrane antigen. Prostate 1996;29:371–380.

39. Carter RE, Feldman AR, Coyle JT. Prostate-specific membrane antigen is a hydrolase with substrate and pharmacologic characteristics of a neuropeptidase. Proc Natl Acad Sci U S A 1996;3:749–753.

40. Murphy GP, Tino WT, Holmes EH. Measurement of prostate-specific membrane antigen in the serum with a new antibody. Prostate 1996;28:266–271.

41. Salgaller ML, Lodge PA, McLean JG, et al. Report of immune monitoring of prostate cancer patients undergoing T-cell therapy using dendritic cells pulsed with HLA-A2-specific peptides from prostate-specific membrane antigen (PSMA). Prostate 1998;35:144–151.

42. Zhang S, Zhang HS, Reuter VE, et al. Expression of potential target antigens for immunotherapy on primary and metastatic prostate cancers. Clin Cancer Res 1998;4:295–302.

43. Chang SS, O'Keefe DS, Bacich DJ, et al. Prostate-specific membrane antigen is produced in tumor-associated neovasculature. Clin Cancer Res 1999;5:2674–2681.

44. Liu H, Moy P, Kim S, et al. Monoclonal antibodies to the extracellular domain of prostate-specific membrane antigen also react with tumor vascular endothelium. Cancer Res 1997;57:3629–3634.

45. Loric S, Dumas F, Eschwege P, et al. Enhanced detection of hematogenous circulating prostatic cells in patients with prostatic adenocarcinoma by using nested reverse transcription polymerase chain reaction assay base on prostate-specific membrane antigen. Clin Chem 1995;41:1698–1704.

46. Israeli R, Miller W, Su S, et al. Sensitive nested reverse transcription polymerase chain reaction detection of circulating prostatic tumor cells: Comparison of prostate-specific membrane antigen and prostate-specific antigen-based assays. Cancer Res 1994;54:6306–6310.

47. Israeli R, Miller W, Su S, et al. Sensitive detection of prostatic hematogenous tumor cell dissemination using prostate specific membrane-derived primers in the polymerase chain reaction. J Urol 1995;153:573–577.

48. Cama C, Olsson CA, Raffo A, et al. Molecular staging of prostate cancer. II: A comparison of the application of an enhanced reverse transcriptase polymerase chain reaction assay for prostate specific antigen versus prostate specific membrane antigen. J Urol 1995;153:1373–1378.

49. Eschwege P, Dumas F, Blanchet P, et al. Haematogenous dissemination of prostatic epithelial cells during radical prostatectomy. Lancet 1995;346:1528–1530.

50. Su S, Heston W, Perroti M, et al. Evaluating neoadjuvant therapy effectiveness on systemic disease: Use of a prostate-specific membrane reverse transcription polymerase chain reaction. Urology 1997;49(Suppl 3A):95–101.

51. Troyer JK, Beckett ML, Wright GL Jr. Location of prostate-specific membrane antigen in the LNCaP prostate carcinoma cell line. Prostate 1997;30:232–242.

52. Partin AW, Catalona WJ, Finlay JA, et al. Use of human glandular kallikrein 2 for the detection of prostate cancer: Preliminary analysis. Urology 1999;54:839–845.

53. Tremblay RR, Deperthes D, Tetu B, Dube JY. Immunohistochemical study suggesting a complementary role of kallikreins hK2 and hK3 (prostate-specific antigen) in the functional analysis of human prostate tumors. Am J Pathol 1997;150:455–459.

54. Darson MF, Pacelli A, Roche P, et al. Human glandular kallikrein 2 (hK2) expression in prostatic intraepithelial neoplasia and adenocarcinoma: A novel prostate cancer marker. Urology 1997;49:857–862.

55. Darson MF, Pacelli A, Roche P, et al. Human glandular kallikrein 2 expression in prostate adenocarcinoma and lymph node metastases. Urology 1999;53:939–944.

56. Chang SS, Reuter VE, Heston WD, et al. Short term neoadjuvant androgen deprivation therapy does not affect prostate specific membrane antigen expression in prostate tissues. Cancer 2000;88:407–415.

57. Novis DA, Zarbo RJ, Valenstein PA. Diagnostic uncertainty expressed in prostate needle biopsies: A College of American Pathologists Q-probes Study of 15,753 prostate needle biopsies in 332 institutions. Arch Pathol Lab Med 1999;123:687–692.

58. Wojno KJ, Epstein JI. The utility of basal cell-specific anticytokeratin antibody (34 beta E12) in the diagnosis of prostate cancer: A review of 228 cases. Am J Surg Pathol 1995;19:251–260.

59. Kahane H, Sharp JW, Shuman GB, et al. Utilization of high molecular weight cytokeratin on prostate needle biopsies in an independent laboratory. Urology 1995;45:981–986.

60. Varma M, Linden MD, Amin MB. Effect of formalin fixation and epitope retrieval techniques on antibody 34betaE12 immunostaining of prostatic tissues. [see comments] Mod Pathol 1999;12:472–478.

61. Iczkowski KA, Cheng L, Crawford BG, Bostwick DG. Steam heat with an EDTA buffer and protease digestion optimizes immunohistochemical expression of basal cell-specific antikeratin 34betaE12 to discriminate cancer in prostatic epithelium. Mod Pathol 1999;12:1–4.

62. Goldstein NS, Underhill J, Roszka J, Neill JS. Cytokeratin 34-beta-E12 immunoreactivity in benign prostatic acini: Quantitation, pattern assessment, and electron microscopic study. Am J Clin Pathol 1999;112:69–74.

63. Bostwick DG, Brawer MK. Prostatic intra-epithelial neoplasia and early invasion in prostate cancer. Cancer 1987;59:788–794.

64. Amin MB, Schultz DS, Zarbo RJ. Analysis of cribriform morphology in prostatic neoplasia using antibody to high-molecular-weight cytokeratins. Arch Pathol Lab Med 1994;118:260–264.

65. Ramnani DM, Bostwick DG. Basal cell-specific anti-keratin antibody 34betaE12: Optimizing its use in distinguishing benign prostate and cancer. [editorial; comment] Mod Pathol 1999;12:443–444.

66. Shin M, Fujita MQ, Yasunaga Y, et al. Utility of immunohistochemical detection of high molecular weight cytokeratin for differential diagnosis of proliferative conditions of the prostate. Int J Urol 1998;5:237–242.

67. Freibauer C. Diagnosis of prostate carcinoma on biopsy specimens improved by basal-cell-specific anti-cytokeratin antibody (34-beta-E12). Wien Klin Wochenschr 1998;110:608–611.

68. Brawer MK, Nagle RB, Pitts W, et al. Keratin immunoreactivity as an aid to the diagnosis of persistent adenocarcinoma in irradiated human prostates. Cancer 1989;63:454–460.

69. Hedrick L, Epstein JI. Use of keratin 903 as an adjunct in the diagnosis of prostate carcinoma. Am J Surg Pathol 1989;13:389–396.

70. Saboorian MH, Huffman H, Ashfaq R, et al. Distinguishing Cowper's glands from neoplastic and pseudoneoplastic lesions of prostate: Immunohistochemical and ultrastructural studies. Am J Surg Pathol 1997;21:1069–1074.

71. Cina SJ, Silberman MA, Kahane H, Epstein JI. Diagnosis of Cowper's glands on prostate needle biopsy. Am J Surg Pathol 1997;21:550–555.

72. Yang XJ, Lecksell K, Gaudin P, Epstein JI. Rare expression of high-molecular-weight cytokeratin in adenocarcinoma of the prostate gland: A study of 100 cases of metastatic and locally advanced prostate cancer. Am J Surg Pathol 1999;23:147–152.

73. Bonkhoff H, Stein U, Remberger K. The proliferative function of basal cells in the normal and hyperplastic human prostate. Prostate 1994;24:114–118.

74. Epstein JI, Armas OA. Atypical basal cell hyperplasia of the prostate. Am J Surg Pathol 1992;16:1205–1214.

75. Devaraj LT, Bostwick DG. Atypical basal cell hyperplasia of the prostate: Immunophenotypic profile and proposed classification of basal cell proliferations. Am J Surg Pathol 1993;17:645–659.

76. Yang Y, Hao J, Liu X, et al. Differential expression of cytokeratin mRNA and protein in normal prostate, prostatic intraepithelial neoplasia, and invasive carcinoma. Am J Pathol 1997;150:693–704.

77. Green R, Epstein JI. Use of intervening unstained slides for immunohistochemical stains for high molecular weight cytokeratin on prostate needle biopsies. Am J Surg Pathol 1999;23:567–570.

78. Kitajima K, Tokes ZA. Immunohistochemical localization of keratin in human prostate. Prostate 1986;9:183–190.

79. Purnell DM, Heatfield BM, Anthony RL, Trump BF. Immunohistochemistry of the cytoskeleton of human prostatic epithelium: Evidence for disturbed organization in neoplasia. Am J Pathol 1987;126:384–395.

80. Dhom G, Seitz G, Wernert N. Histology and immunohistochemistry studies in prostate cancer. Am J Clin Oncol 1988;11(Suppl 2):S37–S42.

81. Wernert N, Luchtrath H, Seeliger H, et al. Papillary carcinoma of the prostate, location, morphology, and immunohistochemistry: The histogenesis and entity of so-called endometrioid carcinoma. Prostate 1987;10:123–131.

82. Guinan P, Shaw M, Targonski P, et al. Evaluation of cytokeratin markers to differentiate between benign and malignant prostatic tissue. J Surg Oncol 1989;42:175–180.

83. Nagle RB, Ahmann FR, McDaniel KM, et al. Cytokeratin characterization of human prostatic carcinoma and its derived cell lines. Cancer Res 1987;47:281–286.

84. O'Malley FP, Grignon DJ, Shum DT. Usefulness of immunoperoxidase staining with high-molecular-weight cytokeratin in the differential diagnosis of small-acinar lesions of the prostate gland. Virchows Arch A Pathol Anat Histopathol 1990;417:191–196.

85. Srigley JR, Dardick I, Hartwick RW, Klotz L. Basal epithelial cells of human prostate gland are not myoepithelial cells: A comparative immunohistochemical and ultrastructural study with the human salivary gland. Am J Pathol 1990;136:957–966.

86. Shah IA, Schlageter MO, Stinnett P, Lechago J. Cytokeratin immunohistochemistry as a diagnostic tool for distinguishing malignant from benign epithelial lesions of the prostate. [see comments] Mod Pathol 1991;4:220–224.

87. Howat AJ, Mills PM, Lyons TJ, Stephenson TJ. Absence of S-100 protein in prostatic glands. Histopathology 1988;13:468–470.

88. Xue Y, van der Laak J, Smedts F, et al. Neuroendocrine cells during human prostate development: Does neuroendocrine cell density remain constant during fetal as well as postnatal life? Prostate 2000;42:116–123.

89. Mucci NR, Akdas G, Manely S, Rubin MA. Neuroendocrine expression in metastatic prostate cancer: Evaluation of high throughput tissue microarrays to detect heterogeneous protein expression. Hum Pathol 2000;31:406–414.

90. Tan MO, Karaoglan U, Celik B, et al. Prostate cancer and neuroendocrine differentiation. Int Urol Nephrol 1999;31:75–82.

91. Helpap B, Kollermann J, Oehler U. Neuroendocrine differentiation in prostatic carcinomas: Histogenesis, biology, clinical relevance, and future therapeutical perspectives. Urol Int 1999;62:133–138.

92. Bonkhoff H, Stein U, Remberger K. Endocrine-paracrine cell types in the prostate and prostatic adenocarcinoma are postmitotic cells. [see comments] Hum Pathol 1995;26:167–170.

93. Bonkhoff H, Stein U, Welter C, Remberger K. Differential expression of the pS2 protein in the human prostate and prostate cancer: Association with premalignant changes and neuroendocrine differentiation. Hum Pathol 1995;26:824–828.

94. Schmid KW, Helpap B, Totsch M, et al. Immunohistochemical localization of chromogranins A and B and secretogranin II in normal, hyperplastic and neoplastic prostate. Histopathology 1994;24:233–239.

95. Djakiew D, Delsite R, Pflug B, et al. Regulation of growth by a nerve growth factor-like protein which modulates paracrine interactions between a neoplastic epithelial cell line and stromal cells of the human prostate. Cancer Res 1991;51(12):3304–3310.

96. di Sant'Agnese PA, de Mesy KL, Jensen CJ et al. Human prostatic endocrine-paracrine (APUD) cells: Distributional analysis with a comparison of serotonin and neuron-specific enolase immunoreactivity and silver stains. Arch Pathol Lab Med 1985;109:607–612.

97. Wu JT, Wu TL, Chang CP, et al. Different patterns of serum chromogranin A in patients with prostate cancer with and without undergoing hormonal therapy. J Clin Lab Anal 1999;13:308–311.

98. Pruneri G, Galli S, Rossi RS, et al. Chromogranin A and B and secretogranin II in prostatic adenocarcinomas: Neuroendocrine expression in patients untreated and treated with androgen deprivation therapy. Prostate 1998;34:113–120.

99. Abrahamsson PA, Falkmer S, Falt K, Grimelius L. The course of neuroendocrine differentiation in prostatic carcinomas: An immunohistochemical study testing chromogranin A as an "endocrine marker." Pathol Res Pract 1989;185:373–380.

100. Angelsen A, Mecsei R, Sandvik AK, Waldum HL. Neuroendocrine cells in the prostate of the rat, guinea pig, cat, and dog. Prostate 1997;33:18–25.

101. Falkmer S, Askensten U, Grimelius L, Abrahamsson PA. Cytochemical markers and DNA content of neuroendocrine cells in carcinoma of the prostate gland during tumour progression. Acta Histochem Suppl 1990;38:127–132.

102. McWilliam LJ, Manson C, George NJ. Neuroendocrine differentiation and prognosis in prostatic adenocarcinoma. Br J Urol 1997;80:287–290.

103. Xue Y, Verhofstad A, Lange W, et al. Prostatic neuroendocrine cells have a unique keratin expression pattern and do not express Bcl-2: Cell kinetic features of neuroendocrine cells in the human prostate. Am J Pathol 1997;151:1759–1765.

104. Guy L, Begin LR, Al-Othman K, et al. Neuroendocrine cells of the verumontanum: A comparative immunohistochemical study. Br J Urol 1998;82:738–743.

105. Bostwick D, Qian J, Pacelli A, et al. Neuroendocrine expression in node-positive prostate cancer: Correlation with systemic progression and patient survival. J Urol, in press.

106. Chen X, Okada H, Gotoh A, et al. Neuroendocrine cells in the prostatic carcinomas after neoadjuvant hormonal therapy. Kobe J Med Sci 1997;43:71–81.

107. Krijnen JL, Janssen PJ, Ruizeveld de Winter JA, et al. Do neuroendocrine cells in human prostate cancer express androgen receptor? Histochemistry 1993;100:393–398.

108. Adlakha H, Bostwick DG. Paneth cell–like change in prostatic adenocarcinoma represents neuroendocrine differentiation: Report of 30 cases. [see comments] Hum Pathol 1994;25:135–139.

109. Weaver MG, Abdul-Karim FW, Srigley JR. Paneth cell–like change and small cell carcinoma of the prostate: Two divergent forms of prostatic neuroendocrine differentiation. Am J Surg Pathol 1992;16:1013–1016.

110. Fjellestad-Paulsen A, Abrahamsson PA, Bjartell A, et al. Carcinoma of the prostate with Cushing's syndrome: A case report with histochemical and chemical demonstration of immunoreactive corticotropin-releasing hormone in plasma and tumoral tissue. Acta Endocrinol (Copenh) 1988;119:506–516.

111. Frkovic-Grazio S, Kraljic I, Trnski D, Tarle M. Immunohistochemical staining and serotest markers during development of a sarcomatoid and small cell prostate tumor. Anticancer Res 1994;14:2151–2156.

112. Hagood PG, Johnson FE, Bedrossian CW, Silverberg AB. Small cell carcinoma of the prostate. Cancer 1991;67:1046–1050.

113. Watanabe K, Hoshi N, Hiraki H, et al. Neoplastic endocrine cells in prostatic carcinoma: A case report with immunocytochemical and electron microscopic findings. Fukushima J Med Sci 1995;41:51–60.

114. Iwamura M, Wu G, Abrahamsson PA, et al. Parathyroid hormone–related protein is expressed by prostatic neuroendocrine cells. Urology 1994;43:667–674.

115. Helpap B, Kollermann J. Undifferentiated carcinoma of the prostate with small cell features: Immunohistochemical subtyping and reflections on histogenesis. Virchows Arch 1999;434:385–391.

116. Oesterling JE, Hauzeur CG, Farrow GM. Small cell anaplastic carcinoma of the prostate: A clinical, pathological and immunohistological study of 27 patients. J Urol 1992;147(3 Pt 2):804–807.

117. Schron DS, Gipson T, Mendelsohn G. The histogenesis of small cell carcinoma of the prostate: An immunohistochemical study. Cancer 1984;53:2478–2480.

118. Ro JY, Tetu B, Ayala AG, Ordonez NG. Small cell carcinoma of the prostate. II: Immunohistochemical and electron microscopic studies of 18 cases. Cancer 1987;59:977–982.

119. di Sant'Agnese PA. Neuroendocrine differentiation in prostatic adenocarcinoma does not represent true Paneth cell differentiation. [editorial; comment] Hum Pathol 1994;25:115–116.

120. di Sant'Agnese PA. Neuroendocrine differentiation in human prostatic carcinoma. Hum Pathol 1992;23:287–296.

121. di Sant'Agnese PA. Neuroendocrine differentiation in car-

cinoma of the prostate: Diagnostic, prognostic, and therapeutic implications. Cancer 1992;70(1 Suppl):254–268.

122. di Sant'Agnese PA, Cockett AT. Neuroendocrine differentiation in prostatic malignancy. Cancer 1996;8:357–361.

123. di Sant'Agnese PA, Cockett AT. The prostatic endocrine-paracrine (neuroendocrine) regulatory system and neuroendocrine differentiation in prostatic carcinoma: A review and future directions in basic research. [see comments] J Urol 1994;152(5 Pt 2):1927–1931.

124. di Sant'Agnese PA. Neuroendocrine differentiation in prostatic carcinoma: An update. Prostate Suppl 1998;8:74–79.

125. di Sant'Agnese PA. Neuroendocrine cells of the prostate and neuroendocrine differentiation in prostatic carcinoma: A review of morphologic aspects. Urology 1998;51(5A Suppl):121–124.

126. Bostwick DG, Dousa MK, Crawford BG, Wollan PC. Neuroendocrine differentiation in prostatic intraepithelial neoplasia and adenocarcinoma. Am J Surg Pathol 1994;18:1240–1246.

127. Abrahamsson PA, Cockett AT, di Sant'Agnese PA. Prognostic significance of neuroendocrine differentiation in clinically localized prostatic carcinoma. Prostate Suppl 1998;8:37–42.

128. Angelsen A, Syversen U, Stridsberg M, et al. Use of neuroendocrine serum markers in the follow-up of patients with cancer of the prostate. Prostate 1997;31:110–117.

129. Angelsen A, Syversen U, Haugen OA, et al. Neuroendocrine differentiation in carcinomas of the prostate: Do neuroendocrine serum markers reflect immunohistochemical findings? Prostate 1997;30:1–6.

130. Berner A, Waere H, Nesland JM, et al. DNA ploidy, serum prostate specific antigen, histological grade and immunohistochemistry as predictive parameters of lymph node metastases in T1-T3/M0 prostatic adenocarcinoma. Br J Urol 1995;75:26–32.

131. Bubendorf L, Sauter G, Moch H, et al. Ki67 labelling index: An independent predictor of progression in prostate cancer treated by radical prostatectomy. J Pathol 1996;178:437–441.

132. Casella R, Bubendorf L, Sauter G, et al. Focal neuroendocrine differentiation lacks prognostic significance in prostate core needle biopsies. J Urol 1998;160:406–410.

133. Krupski T, Petroni GR, Frierson HF Jr, Theodorescu JU. Microvessel density, p53, retinoblastoma, and chromogranin A immunohistochemistry as predictors of disease-specific survival following radical prostatectomy for carcinoma of the prostate. Urology 2000;55:743–749.

134. Noordzij MA, van der Kwast TH, van Steenbrugge GJ, et al. The prognostic influence of neuroendocrine cells in prostate cancer: Results of a long-term follow-up study with patients treated by radical prostatectomy. Int J Cancer 1995;62:252–258.

135. Van de Voorde WM, Elgamal AA, Van Poppel HP, et al. Morphologic and immunohistochemical changes in prostate cancer after preoperative hormonal therapy: A comparative study of radical prostatectomies. Cancer 1994;74:3164–3175.

136. Weinstein MH, Partin AW, Veltri RW, Epstein JI. Neuroendocrine differentiation in prostate cancer: Enhanced prediction of progression after radical prostatectomy. Hum Pathol 1996;27:683–687.

137. Aprikian AG, Cordon-Cardo C, Fair WR, Reuter VE. Characterization of neuroendocrine differentiation in human benign prostate and prostatic adenocarcinoma. Cancer 1993;71:3952–3965.

138. Allen FJ, Van Velden DJ, Heyns CF. Are neuroendocrine cells of practical value as an independent prognostic parameter in prostate cancer? Br J Urol 1995;75:751–754.

139. Frierson HF Jr, Theodorescu D, Mills SE, Hanigan MH. Gamma-glutamyl transpeptidase in normal and neoplastic prostate glands. Mod Pathol 1997;10:1–6.

140. el-Demiry MI, Hargreave TB, Busuttil A, et al. Lymphocyte sub-populations in the male genital tract. Br J Urol 1985;57:769–774.

141. Bostwick D, Corica F, de la Roza G, et al. Intraepithelial and stromal lymphocytes in the normal human prostate. Prostate, in press.

142. Theyer G, Kramer G, Assmann I, et al. Phenotypic characterization of infiltrating leukocytes in benign prostatic hyperplasia. Lab Invest 1992;66:96–107.

143. Nemoto R, Kawamura H, Miyakawa I, et al. Immunohistochemical detection of proliferating cell nuclear antigen (PCNA)/cyclin in human prostate adenocarcinoma. J Urol 1993;149:165–169.

144. Chan PK, Frakes R, Tan EM, et al. Indirect immunofluorescence studies of proliferating cell nuclear antigen in nucleoli of human tumor and normal tissues. Cancer Res 1983;43:3770–3777.

145. Botticelli AR, Casali AM, Botticelli L, Zaffe D. Immunohistochemical detection of cell-cycle associated markers on paraffin embedded and formalin fixed needle biopsies of prostate cancer: Correlation of p120 protein expression with AgNOR, PCNA/cyclin, Ki-67/MIB1 proliferation-scores and Gleason gradings. Eur J Histochem 1998;42:41–48.

146. Cher ML, Chew K, Rosenau W, Carroll PR. Cellular proliferation in prostatic adenocarcinoma as assessed by bromodeoxyuridine uptake and Ki-67 and PCNA expression. Prostate 1995;26:87–93.

147. Helpap B. Cell kinetic studies on prostatic intraepithelial neoplasia (PIN) and atypical adenomatous hyperplasia (AAH) of the prostate. Pathol Res Pract 1995;191:904–907.

148. Hepburn PJ, Glynne-Jones E, Goddard L, et al. Cell proliferation in prostatic carcinoma: Comparative analysis of Ki-67, MIB-1 and PCNA. Histochem J 1995;27:196–203.

149. Igawa M, Urakami S, Shiina H, et al. Immunohistochemical evaluation of proliferating cell nuclear antigen, prostate-specific antigen and alpha 1-antichymotrypsin in human prostate cancer. Br J Urol 1996;77:107–112.

150. Ljung G, Egevad L, Norberg M, et al. Assessment of proliferation indicators in residual prostatic adenocarcinoma cells after radical external beam radiotherapy. Prostate 1996;29:303–310.

151. Montironi R, Galluzzi CM, Diamanti L, et al. Proliferating cell nuclear antigen (PCNA) in prostatic invasive adenocarcinoma: Is the proliferation state in the marginal zone of the tumour higher than in the central part? Anticancer Res 1993;13:129–132.

152. Naito S, Sakamoto N, Kotoh S, et al. Proliferating cell nuclear antigen in needle biopsy specimens of prostatic carcinoma. Eur Urol 1994;26:164–169.

153. Sakr WA, Sarkar FH, Sreepathi P, et al. Measurement of cellular proliferation in human prostate by AgNOR, PCNA, and SPF. Prostate 1993;22:147–154.

154. Visakorpi T. Proliferative activity determined by DNA flow cytometry and proliferating cell nuclear antigen (PCNA) immunohistochemistry as a prognostic factor in prostatic carcinoma. J Pathol 1992;168:7–13.

155. Limas C, Frizelle SP. Proliferative activity in benign and neoplastic prostatic epithelium. J Pathol 1994;174:201–208.

156. Carroll PR, Waldman FM, Rosenau W, et al. Cell proliferation in prostatic adenocarcinoma: In vitro measurement by 5-bromodeoxyuridine incorporation and proliferating cell nuclear antigen expression. J Urol 1993;149:403–407.

157. Idikio HA. Expression of proliferating cell nuclear antigen in node-negative human prostate cancer. Anticancer Res 1996;16:2607–2611.

158. Coetzee LJ, Layfield LJ, Hars V, Paulson DF. Proliferative index determination in prostatic carcinoma tissue: Is there any additional prognostic value greater than that of Gleason score, ploidy and pathological stage? [see comments] J Urol 1997;157:214–218.

159. Bubendorf L, Tapia C, Gasser TC, et al. Ki67 labeling index in core needle biopsies independently predicts tumor-specific survival in prostate cancer. Hum Pathol 1998;29:949–954.

160. Sadi MV, Barrack ER. Determination of growth fraction in advanced prostate cancer by Ki-67 immunostaining and its

relationship to the time to tumor progression after hormonal therapy. Cancer 1991;67:3065–3071.

161. Glynne-Jones E, Goddard L, Harper ME. Comparative analysis of mRNA and protein expression for epidermal growth factor receptor and ligands relative to the proliferative index in human prostate tissue. Hum Pathol 1996;27:688–694.

162. Moul JW. Angiogenesis, p53, bcl-2 and Ki-67 in the progression of prostate cancer after radical prostatectomy. Eur Urol 1999;35:399–407.

163. Thompson SJ, Mellon K, Charlton RG, et al. P53 and Ki-67 immunoreactivity in human prostate cancer and benign hyperplasia. Br J Urol 1992;69:609–613.

164. Henke RP, Kruger E, Ayhan N, et al. Numerical chromosomal aberrations in prostate cancer: Correlation with morphology and cell kinetics. Virchows Arch A Pathol Anat Histopathol 1993;422:61–66.

165. Aaltomaa S, Lipponen P, Vesalainen S, et al. Value of Ki-67 immunolabelling as a prognostic factor in prostate cancer. Eur Urol 1997;32:410–415.

166. Moul JW, Bettencourt MC, Sesterhenn IA, et al. Protein expression of p53, bcl-2, and KI-67 (MIB-1) as prognostic biomarkers in patients with surgically treated, clinically localized prostate cancer. Surgery 1996;120:159–166; discussion 166–167.

167. Bettencourt MC, Bauer JJ, Sesterhenn IA, et al. Ki-67 expression is a prognostic marker of prostate cancer recurrence after radical prostatectomy. [see comments] J Urol 1996;156:1064–1068.

168. Mashal RD, Lester S, Corless C, et al. Expression of cell cycle–regulated proteins in prostate cancer. Cancer Res 1996;56:4159–4163.

169. Verhagen AP, Aalders TW, Ramaekers FC, et al. Differential expression of keratins in the basal and luminal compartments of rat prostatic epithelium during degeneration and regeneration. Prostate 1988;13:25–38.

170. Bonkhoff H, Stein U, Remberger K. Multidirectional differentiation in the normal, hyperplastic, and neoplastic human prostate: Simultaneous demonstration of cell-specific epithelial markers. Hum Pathol 1994;25:42–46.

171. Soeffing WJ, Timms BG. Localization of androgen receptor and cell-specific cytokeratins in basal cells of rat ventral prostate. J Androl 1995;16:197–208.

172. Foster CS, Ke Y. Stem cells in prostatic epithelia. Int J Exp Pathol 1997;78:311–329.

173. Foster BA, Gingrich JR, Kwon ED et al. Characterization of prostatic epithelial cell lines derived from transgenic adenocarcinoma of the mouse prostate (TRAMP) model. Cancer Res 1997;57:3325–3330.

174. Robinson EJ, Neal DE, Collins AT. Basal cells are progenitors of luminal cells in primary cultures of differentiating human prostatic epithelium. Prostate 1998;37:149–160.

175. Wang X, Hsieh JT. Androgen repression of cytokeratin gene expression during rat prostate differentiation: Evidence for an epithelial stem cell-associated marker. Chin Med Sci J 1994;9:237–241.

176. Verhagen AP, Ramaekers FC, Aalders TW, et al. Colocalization of basal and luminal cell-type cytokeratins in human prostate cancer. Cancer Res 1992;52:6182–6187.

177. Sherwood ER, Theyer G, Steiner G, et al. Differential expression of specific cytokeratin polypeptides in the basal and luminal epithelia of the human prostate. Prostate 1991;18:303–314.

178. Oberneder R, Riesenberg R, Kriegmair M, et al. Immunocytochemical detection and phenotypic characterization of micrometastatic tumour cells in bone marrow of patients with prostate cancer. Urol Res 1994;22:3–8.

179. Silen A, Wiklund B, Norlen BJ, Nilsson S. Evaluation of a new tumor marker for cytokeratin 8 and 18 fragments in healthy individuals and prostate cancer patients. Prostate 1994;24:326–332.

180. Fuchs ME, Brawer MK, Rennels MA, Nagle RB. The relationship of basement membrane to histologic grade of human prostatic carcinoma. Mod Pathol 1989;2:105–111.

181. Sinha AA, Gleason DF, Wilson MJ, et al. Immunohisto chemical localization of laminin in the basement membranes of normal, hyperplastic, and neoplastic human prostate. Prostate 1989;15:299–313.

182. Nagle RB, Knox JD, Wolf C, et al. Adhesion molecules, extracellular matrix, and proteases in prostate carcinoma. J Cell Biochem Suppl 1994;19:232–237.

183. Xue Y, Li J, Latijnhouwers MA, et al. Expression of periglandular tenascin-C and basement membrane laminin in normal prostate, benign prostatic hyperplasia and prostate carcinoma. Br J Urol 1998;81:844–851.

184. Murant SJ, Handley J, Stower M, et al. Co-ordinated changes in expression of cell adhesion molecules in prostate cancer. Eur J Cancer 1997;33:263–271.

185. Rabinovitz I, Nagle RB, Cress AE. Integrin alpha 6 expression in human prostate carcinoma cells is associated with a migratory and invasive phenotype in vitro and in vivo. Clin Exp Metastasis 1995;13:481–491.

186. Nagle RB, Hao J, Knox JD, et al. Expression of hemidesmosomal and extracellular matrix proteins by normal and malignant human prostate tissue. Am J Pathol 1995;146:1498–1507.

187. Knox JD, Mack CF, Powell WC, et al. Prostate tumor cell invasion: A comparison of orthotopic and ectopic models. Invasion Metastasis 1993;13:325–331.

188. Hao J, Yang Y, McDaniel KM, et al. Differential expression of laminin 5 (alpha 3 beta 3 gamma 2) by human malignant and normal prostate. Am J Pathol 1996;149:1341–1349.

189. Dedhar S, Saulnier R, Nagle R, Overall CM. Specific alterations in the expression of alpha 3 beta 1 and alpha 6 beta 4 integrins in highly invasive and metastatic variants of human prostate carcinoma cells selected by in vitro invasion through reconstituted basement membrane. Clin Exp Metastasis 1993;11:391–400.

190. Trikha M, Raso E, Cai Y, et al. Role of alphaII(b)beta3 integrin in prostate cancer metastasis. Prostate 1998;35:185–192.

191. Fornaro M, Manzotti M, Tallini G, et al. Beta1C integrin in epithelial cells correlates with a nonproliferative phenotype: Forced expression of beta1C inhibits prostate epithelial cell proliferation. Am J Pathol 1998;153:1079–1087.

192. Fornaro M, Tallini G, Bofetiado CJ, et al. Down-regulation of beta 1C integrin, an inhibitor of cell proliferation, in prostate carcinoma. Am J Pathol 1996;149:765–773.

193. von Bredow DC, Nagle RB, Bowden GT, Cress AE. Cleavage of beta 4 integrin by matrilysin. Exp Cell Res 1997;236:341–345.

194. Tozawa K, Yamada Y, Kawai N, et al. Osteopontin expression in prostate cancer and benign prostatic hyperplasia. Urol Int 1999;62:155–158.

195. Thalmann GN, Sikes RA, Devoll RE, et al. Osteopontin: Possible role in prostate cancer progression. Clin Cancer Res 1999;5:2271–2277.

196. Devoll RE, Pinero GJ, Appelbaum ER, et al. Improved immunohistochemical staining of osteopontin (OPN) in paraffin-embedded archival bone specimens following antigen retrieval: Anti-human OPN antibody recognizes multiple molecular forms. Calcif Tissue Int 1997;60:380–386.

197. Brown LF, Papadopoulos-Sergiou A, Berse B, et al. Osteopontin expression and distribution in human carcinomas. Am J Pathol 1994;45:610–623.

198. Oldberg A, Antonsson P, Hedbom E, Heinegard D. Structure and function of extracellular matrix proteoglycans. Biochem Soc Trans 1990;18:789–792.

199. Ross FP, Chappel J, Alvarez JI, et al. Interactions between the bone matrix proteins osteopontin and bone sialoprotein and the osteoclast integrin alpha v beta 3 potentiate bone resorption. J Biol Chem 1993;268:9901–9907.

200. Myers JC, Li D, Bageris A, et al. Biochemical and immunohistochemical characterization of human type XIX defines a novel class of basement membrane zone collagens. Am J Pathol 1997;151:1729–1740.

201. Dehan P, Waltregny D, Beschin A, et al. Loss of type IV collagen alpha 5 and alpha 6 chains in human invasive prostate carcinomas. Am J Pathol 1997;151:1097–1104.

202. Suer S, Sonmez H, Karaaslan I, et al. Tissue sialic acid and fibronectin levels in human prostatic cancer. Cancer Lett 1996;99:135–137.
203. Murdoch AD, Liu B, Schwarting R, et al. Widespread expression of perlecan proteoglycan in basement membranes and extracellular matrices of human tissues as detected by a novel monoclonal antibody against domain III and by in situ hybridization. J Histochem Cytochem 1994;42:239–249.
204. Schenk S, Muser J, Vollmer G, Chiquet-Ehrismann R. Tenascin-C in serum: A questionable tumor marker. Int J Cancer 1995;61:443–449.
205. Shiraishi T, Kato H, Komada S, et al. Tenascin expression and postnatal development of the human prostate. Int J Dev Biol 1994;38:391–395.
206. Ibrahim SN, Lightner VA, Ventimiglia JB, et al. Tenascin expression in prostatic hyperplasia, intraepithelial neoplasia, and carcinoma. Hum Pathol 1993;24:982–989.
207. Xue Y, Smedts F, Latijnhouwers MA, et al. Tenascin-C expression in prostatic intraepithelial neoplasia (PIN): A marker of progression? Anticancer Res 1998;18:2679–2684.
208. Bryden AA, Freemont AJ, Clarke NW, George NJ. Paradoxical expression of E-cadherin in prostatic bone metastases. BJU Int 1999;84:1032–1034.
209. Aaltomaa S, Lipponen P, Ala-Opas M, et al. Alpha-catenin expression has prognostic value in local and locally advanced prostate cancer. Br J Cancer 1999;80:477–482.
210. Brewster SF, Oxley JD, Trivella M, et al. Preoperative p53, bcl-2, CD44 and E-cadherin immunohistochemistry as predictors of biochemical relapse after radical prostatectomy. J Urol 1999;161:1238–1243.
211. Bussemakers MJ, van Moorselaar RJ, Giroldi LA, et al. Decreased expression of E-cadherin in the progression of rat prostatic cancer. Cancer Res 1992;52:2916–2922.
212. Cheng L, Nagabhushan M, Pretlow TP, et al. Expression of E-cadherin in primary and metastatic prostate cancer. Am J Pathol 1996;148:1375–1380.
213. De Marzo AM, Knudsen B, Chan-Tack K, Epstein JI. E-cadherin expression as a marker of tumor aggressiveness in routinely processed radical prostatectomy specimens. Urology 1999;53:707–713.
214. Giroldi LA, Bringuier PP, Schalken JA. Defective E-cadherin function in urological cancers: Clinical implications and molecular mechanisms. Invasion Metastasis 1994;14:71–81.
215. Jarrard DF, Paul R, van Bokhoven A, et al. P-Cadherin is a basal cell-specific epithelial marker that is not expressed in prostate cancer. Clin Cancer Res 1997;3:2121–2128.
216. Kuczyk M, Serth J, Machtens S, et al. Expression of E-cadherin in primary prostate cancer: Correlation with clinical features. Br J Urol 1998;81:406–412.
217. Morita N, Uemura H, Tsumatani K, et al. E-cadherin and alpha-, beta- and gamma-catenin expression in prostate cancers: Correlation with tumour invasion. Br J Cancer 1999;79:1879–1883.
218. Pan Y, Matsuyama H, Wang N, et al. Chromosome 16q24 deletion and decreased E-cadherin expression: Possible association with metastatic potential in prostate cancer. Prostate 1998;36:31–38.
219. Rembrink K, Otto T, Goepel M, et al. E-cadherin: Expression of the epithelial cell-cell-adhesion molecule in prostatic carcinoma and normal prostate. Invest Urol 1994;5:24–27.
220. Ross JS, Figge HL, Bui HX, et al. E-cadherin expression in prostatic carcinoma biopsies: Correlation with tumor grade, DNA content, pathologic stage, and clinical outcome. Mod Pathol 1994;7:835–841.
221. Ruijter E, van de Kaa C, Aalders T, et al. Heterogeneous expression of E-cadherin and p53 in prostate cancer: Clinical implications. BIOMED-II Markers for Prostate Cancer Study Group. Mod Pathol 1998;11:276–281.
222. Umbas R, Schalken JA, Aalders TW, et al. Expression of the cellular adhesion molecule E-cadherin is reduced or absent in high-grade prostate cancer. Cancer Res 1992;52:5104–5109.

223. Umbas R, Isaacs WB, Bringuier PP, et al. Relation between aberrant alpha-catenin expression and loss of E-cadherin function in prostate cancer. Int J Cancer 1997;74:374–377.
224. Schalken J. Molecular diagnostics and therapy of prostate cancer: New avenues. Eur Urol 1998;34(Suppl 3):3–6.
225. Rennie PS, Nelson CC. Epigenetic mechanisms for progression of prostate cancer. Cancer Metastasis Rev 1998;17:401–409.
226. Richmond PJ, Karayiannakis AJ, Nagafuchi A, et al. Aberrant E-cadherin and alpha-catenin expression in prostate cancer: Correlation with patient survival. Cancer Res 1997;57:3189–3193.
227. Otto T, Rembrink K, Goepel M, et al. E-cadherin: A marker for differentiation and invasiveness in prostatic carcinoma. Urol Res 1993;21:359–362.
228. Cohen MB, Griebling TL, Ahaghotu CA, et al. Cellular adhesion molecules in urologic malignancies. Am J Clin Pathol 1997;107:56–63.
229. Schalken JA. New perspectives in the treatment of prostate cancer. Eur Urol 1997;31(Suppl 2):20–23.
230. Soler AP, Harner GD, Knudsen KA, et al. Expression of P-cadherin identifies prostate-specific antigen-negative cells in epithelial tissues of male sexual accessory organs and in prostatic carcinomas: Implications for prostate cancer biology. Am J Pathol 1997;151:471–478.
231. Bourrguignon LY, Iida N, Welsh CF, et al. Involvement of CD44 and its variant isoforms in membrane-cytoskeleton interaction, cell adhesion and tumor metastasis. J Neurooncol 1995;26:201–208.
232. Terpe HJ, Stark H, Prehm P, Gunthert U. CD44 variant isoforms are preferentially expressed in basal epithelial of non-malignant human fetal and adult tissues. Histochemistry 1994;101:79–89.
233. Liu AY, True LD, LaTray L, et al. Cell-cell interaction in prostate gene regulation and cytodifferentiation. Proc Natl Acad Sci U S A 1997;94:10705–10710.
234. Kramer G, Steiner G, Fodinger D, et al. High expression of a CD38-like molecule in normal prostatic epithelium and its differential loss in benign and malignant disease. J Urol 1995;154:1636–1641.
235. Schmitt M, Janicke F, Moniwa N, et al. Tumor-associated urokinase-type plasminogen activator: Biological and clinical significance. Biol Chem Hoppe Seyler 1992;373:611–622.
236. Frenette G, Tremblay RR, Lazure C, Dube JY. Prostatic kallikrein hK2, but not prostate-specific antigen (hK3), activates single-chain urokinase-type plasminogen activator. Int J Cancer 1997;71:897–899.
237. Reese JH, McNeal JE, Redwine EA, et al. Tissue type plasminogen activator as a marker for functional zones, within the human prostate gland. Prostate 1988;12:47–53.
238. Lyon PB, See WA, Xu Y, Cohen MB. Diversity and modulation of plasminogen activator activity in human prostate carcinoma cell lines. Prostate 1995;27:179–186.
239. Van Veldhuizen PJ, Sadasivan R, Cherian R, Wyatt A. Urokinase-type plasminogen activator expression in human prostate carcinomas. Am J Med Sci 1996;312:8–11.
240. Stearns ME, Wang M. Type IV collagenase (M(r) 72,000) expression in human prostate: Benign and malignant tissue. Cancer Res 1993;53:878–883.
241. Hamdy FC, Fadlon EJ, Cottam D, et al. Matrix metalloproteinase 9 expression in primary human prostatic adenocarcinoma and benign prostatic hyperplasia. Br J Cancer 1994;69:177–182.
242. Still K, Robson CN, Autzen P, et al. Localization and quantification of mRNA for matrix metalloproteinase-2 (MMP-2) and tissue inhibitor of matrix metalloproteinase-2 (TIMP-2) in human benign and malignant prostatic tissue. Prostate 2000;42:18–25.
243. Wilson CL, Matrisian LM. Matrilysin: An epithelial matrix metalloproteinase with potentially novel functions. Int J Biochem Cell Biol 1996;28:123–136.
244. Siegal JA, Yu E, Brawer MK. Topography of neovascularity in human prostate carcinoma. Cancer 1995;75:2545–2551.
245. Weidner N. Intratumoral vascularity as a prognostic factor

in cancers of the urogenital tract. Eur J Cancer 1996;32A: 2506–2512.

246. Bostwick DG, Grignon DJ, Hammond ME, et al., Prognostic factors in prostate cancer: College of American Pathologists Consensus Statement 1999. Arch Pathol Lab Med 2000;124:995–1000.

247. de la Taille A, Katz AE, Bagiella E, et al. Microvessel density as a predictor of PSA recurrence after radical prostatectomy: A comparison of CD34 and CD31. Am J Clin Pathol 2000;113:555–562.

248. Abdulkadir SA, Carvalhal GF, Kaleem Z, et al. Tissue factor expression and angiogenesis in human prostate carcinoma. [see comments] Hum Pathol 2000;31:443–447.

249. Borre M, Nerstrom B, Overgaard J. Association between immunohistochemical expression of vascular endothelial growth factor (VEGF), VEGF-expressing neuroendocrine-differentiated tumor cells, and outcome in prostate cancer patients subjected to watchful waiting. Clin Cancer Res 2000;6:1882–1890.

250. Brawer MK, Deering RE, Brown M, et al. Predictors of pathologic stage in prostatic carcinoma. The role of neovascularity. Cancer 1994;73:678–687.

251. Brawer MK. Quantitative microvessel density: A staging and prognostic marker for human prostatic carcinoma. Cancer 1996;78:345–349.

252. Eberhard A, Kahlert S, Goede V, et al. Heterogeneity of angiogenesis and blood vessel maturation in human tumors: Implications for antiangiogenic tumor therapies. Cancer Res 2000;60:1388–1393.

253. Bostwick DG, Wheeler TM, Blute M, et al. Optimized microvessel density analysis improves prediction of cancer stage from prostate needle biopsies. Urology 1996;48:47–57.

254. Yorukoglu K, Sagol O, Ozkara E, et al. Comparison of microvascularization in diagnostic needle biopsies and radical prostatectomies in prostate carcinoma. Eur Urol 1999;35:109–112.

255. Kay PA, Robb RA, Bostwick DG. Prostate cancer microvessels: A novel method for three-dimensional reconstruction and analysis. Prostate 1998;37:270–277.

256. Deering RE, Bigler SA, Brown M, Brawer MK. Microvascularity in benign prostatic hyperplasia. Prostate 1995;26: 111–115.

257. Bigler SA, Deering RE, Brawer MK. Comparison of microscopic vascularity in benign and malignant prostate tissue. Hum Pathol 1993;24:220–226.

258. Folkman J, Watson K, Ingber D, Hanahan D. Induction of angiogenesis during the transition from hyperplasia to neoplasia. Nature 1989;339:58–61.

259. Bostwick DG. Progression of prostatic intraepithelial neoplasia to early invasive adenocarcinoma. Eur Urol 1996;30: 145–152.

260. Montironi R, Diamanti L, Thompson D, et al. Analysis of the capillary architecture in the precursors of prostate cancer: Recent findings and new concepts. Eur Urol 1996;30: 191–200.

261. Barth PJ, Weingartner K, Kohler HH, Bittinger A. Assessment of the vascularization in prostatic carcinoma: A morphometric investigation. Hum Pathol 1996;27:1306–1310.

262. Volavsek M, Masera A, Ovcak Z. Tumor neoangiogenesis in rebiopsied patients with prostatic carcinoma. Acta Med Croatica 1999;53:73–78.

263. Salomao DR, Graham SD, Bostwick DG. Microvascular invasion in prostate cancer correlates with pathologic stage. Arch Pathol Lab Med 1995;119:1050–1054.

264. Vesalainen S, Lipponen P, Talja M, et al. Tumor vascularity and basement membrane structure as prognostic factors in T1-2M0 prostatic adenocarcinoma. Anticancer Res 1994; 14:709–714.

265. Hall MC, Troncoso P, Pollack A, et al. Significance of tumor angiogenesis in clinically localized prostate carcinoma treated with external beam radiotherapy. Urology 1994;44:869–875.

266. Fregene TA, Khanuja PS, Noto AC, et al. Tumor-associated

267. Wakui S, Furusato M, Itoh T, et al., Tumour angiogenesis in prostatic carcinoma with and without bone marrow metastasis: A morphometric study. J Pathol 1992;168:257–262.

268. Furusato M, Wakui S, Sasaki H, et al. Tumour angiogenesis in latent prostatic carcinoma. Br J Cancer 1994;70: 1244–1246.

269. Weidner N, Carroll PR, Flax J, et al. Tumor angiogenesis correlates with metastasis in invasive prostate carcinoma. Am J Pathol 1993;143:401–409.

270. Silberman MA, Partin AW, Veltri RW, Epstein JI. Tumor angiogenesis correlates with progression after radical prostatectomy but not with pathologic stage in Gleason sum 5 to 7 adenocarcinoma of the prostate. Cancer 1997;79:772–779.

271. Rogatsch H, Hittmair A, Reissigl A, et al. Microvessel density in core biopsies of prostatic adenocarcinoma: A stage predictor? J Pathol 1997;182:205–210.

272. Rubin MA, Buyyounouski M, Bagiella E, et al. Microvessel density in prostate cancer: Lack of correlation with tumor grade, pathologic stage, and clinical outcome. Urology 1999;53:542–547.

273. Offersen BV, Borre M, Overgaard J. Immunohistochemical determination of tumor angiogenesis measured by the maximal microvessel density in human prostate cancer. Apmis 1998;106:463–469.

274. Bostwick DG, Myers RP, Oesterling JE. Staging of prostate cancer. Semin Surg Oncol 1994;10:60–72.

275. Strohmeyer D, Rossing C, Strauss F, et al. Tumor angiogenesis is associated with progression after radical prostatectomy in pT2/pT3 prostate cancer. Prostate 2000;42:26–33.

276. Gettman MT, Pacelli A, Slezak J, et al. Role of microvessel density in predicting recurrence in pathologic stage T3 prostatic adenocarcinoma. Urology 1999;54:479–485.

277. Cetinkaya M, Gunce S, Ulusoy E, et al. Relationship between prostate specific antigen density, microvessel density and prostatic volume in benign prostatic hyperplasia and advanced prostatic carcinoma. Int Urol Nephrol 1998; 30:581–585.

278. Borre M, Offersen BV, Nerstrom B, Overgaard J. Microvessel density predicts survival in prostate cancer patients subjected to watchful waiting. Br J Cancer 1998;78:940–944.

279. Bettencourt MC, Bauer JJ, Sesterhenn IA, et al. CD34 immunohistochemical assessment of angiogenesis as a prognostic marker for prostate cancer recurrence after radical prostatectomy. J Urol 1998;160:459–465.

280. Gettman MT, Bergstralh EJ, Blute M, et al. Prediction of patient outcome in pathologic stage T2 adenocarcinoma of the prostate: Lack of significance for microvessel density analysis. Urology 1998;51:79–85.

281. Lissbrant IF, Stattin P, Damber JE, Bergh A. Vascular density is a predictor of cancer-specific survival in prostatic carcinoma. Prostate 1997;33:38–45.

282. McNeal JE, Yemoto CE. Significance of demonstrable vascular space invasion for the progression of prostatic adenocarcinoma. Am J Surg Pathol 1996;20:1351–1360.

283. Bahnson RR, Dresner SM, Gooding W, Becich MJ. Incidence and prognostic significance of lymphatic and vascular invasion in radical prostatectomy specimens. Prostate 1989;15:149–155.

284. Berruti A, Dogliotti L, Mosca A, et al. Circulating neuroendocrine markers in patients with prostate carcinoma. Cancer 2000;88:2590–2597.

285. Bostwick DG, Aquilina JW. Prostatic intraepithelial neoplasia (PIN) and other prostatic lesions as risk factors and surrogate endpoints for cancer chemoprevention trials. J Cell Biochem Suppl 1996;25:156–164.

286. Polito M, Muzzonigro G, Minardi D, Montironi R. Effects of neoadjuvant androgen deprivation therapy on prostatic cancer. Eur Urol 1996;30(Suppl 1):26–31; discussion 38–39.

287. van der Kwast TH, Labrie F, Tetu B. Persistence of high-

grade prostatic intra-epithelial neoplasia under combined androgen blockade therapy. Hum Pathol 1999;30:1503–1507.

288. Tsuji M, Kanda K, Murakami Y, et al. Biologic markers in prostatic intraepithelial neoplasia: Immunohistochemical and cytogenetic analyses. J Med Invest 1999;46:35–41.

289. Harper ME, Glynne-Jones E, Goddard L, et al. Expression of androgen receptor and growth factors in premalignant lesions of the prostate. J Pathol 1998;186:169–177.

290. Magi-Galluzzi C, Xu X, Hlatky L, et al. Heterogeneity of androgen receptor content in advanced prostate cancer. Mod Pathol 1997;10:839–845.

291. Lyne JC, Melhem MF, Finley GG, et al. Tissue expression of neu differentiation factor/heregulin and its receptor complex in prostate cancer and its biologic effects on prostate cancer cells in vitro. Cancer J Sci Am 1997;3:21–30.

292. Leav I, McNeal JE, Kwan PW, et al. Androgen receptor expression in prostatic dysplasia (prostatic intraepithelial neoplasia) in the human prostate: An immunohistochemical and in situ hybridization study. Prostate 1996;29:137–145.

293. van der Kwast TH, Tetu B. Androgen receptors in untreated and treated prostatic intraepithelial neoplasia. Eur Urol 1996;30:265–268.

294. Takeda H, Akakura K, Masai M, et al. Androgen receptor content of prostate carcinoma cells estimated by immunohistochemistry is related to prognosis of patients with stage D2 prostate carcinoma. Cancer 1996;77:934–940.

295. Hobisch A, Culig Z, Radmayr C, et al. Androgen receptor status of lymph node metastases from prostate cancer. Prostate 1996;28:129–135.

296. Hobisch A, Culig Z, Radmayr C, et al. Distant metastases from prostatic carcinoma express androgen receptor protein. Cancer Res 1995;55:3068–3072.

297. Loda M, Fogt F, French FS, et al. Androgen receptor immunohistochemistry on paraffin-embedded tissue. Mod Pathol 1994;7:388–391.

298. Sadi MV, Barrack ER. Androgen receptors and growth fraction in metastatic prostate cancer as predictors of time to tumour progression after hormonal therapy. Cancer Surv 1991;11:195–215.

299. Hiramatsu M, Maehara I, Orikasa S, Sasano H. Immunolocalization of oestrogen and progesterone receptors in prostatic hyperplasia and carcinoma. Histopathology 1996;28:163–168.

300. Ehara H, Koji T, Deguchi T, et al. Expression of estrogen receptor in diseased human prostate assessed by non-radioactive in situ hybridization and immunohistochemistry. Prostate 1995;27:304–313.

301. Bodker A, Balslev E, Juul BR, et al. Estrogen receptors in the human male bladder, prostatic urethra, and prostate: An immunohistochemical and biochemical study. Scand J Urol Nephrol 1995;29:161–165.

302. Kirschenbaum A, Ren M, Erenburg I, et al. Estrogen receptor messenger RNA expression in human benign prostatic hyperplasia: Detection, localization, and modulation with a long-acting gonadotropin-releasing hormone agonist. J Androl 1994;15:528–533.

303. Konishi N, Nakaoka S, Hiasa Y, et al. Immunohistochemical evaluation of estrogen receptor status in benign prostatic hypertrophy and in prostate carcinoma and the relationship to efficacy of endocrine therapy. Oncology 1993;50:259–263.

304. Brolin J, Skoog L, Ekman P. Immunohistochemistry and biochemistry in detection of androgen, progesterone, and estrogen receptors in benign and malignant human prostatic tissue. Prostate 1992;20:281–295.

305. Schulze H, Claus S. Histological localization of estrogen receptors in normal and diseased human prostates by immunocytochemistry. Prostate 1990;16:331–343.

306. Mobbs BG, Liu Y. Immunohistochemical localization of progesterone receptor in benign and malignant human prostate. Prostate 1990;16:245–251.

307. Seitz G, Wernert N. Immunohistochemical estrogen recep-

tor demonstration in the prostate and prostate cancer. Pathol Res Pract 1987;182:792–796.

308. Gould VE, Doljanskaia V, Gooch GT, Bostwick DG. Stability of the glycoprotein A-80 in prostatic carcinoma subsequent to androgen deprivation therapy. Am J Surg Pathol 1997;21:319–326.

309. Matsushima H, Goto T, Hosaka Y, et al. Correlation between proliferation, apoptosis, and angiogenesis in prostate carcinoma and their relation to androgen ablation. Cancer 1999;85:1822–1827.

310. Ljung G, Norberg M, Holmberg L, et al. Characterization of residual tumor cells following radical radiation therapy for prostatic adenocarcinoma; immunohistochemical expression of prostate-specific antigen, prostatic acid phosphatase, and cytokeratin 8. Prostate 1997;31:91–97.

311. Bostwick DG, Egbert BM, Fajardo LF. Radiation injury of the normal and neoplastic prostate. Am J Surg Pathol 1982;6:541–551.

312. Cheng L, Sebo TJ, Slezak J, et al. Predictors of survival for prostate carcinoma patients treated with salvage radical prostatectomy after radiation therapy. Cancer 1998;83:2164–2171.

313. Cheng L, Cheville JC, Pisansky TM, et al. Prevalence and distribution of prostatic intraepithelial neoplasia in salvage radical prostatectomy specimens after radiation therapy. Am J Surg Pathol 1999;23:803–808.

314. Cheng L, Cheville JC, Bostwick DG. Diagnosis of prostate cancer in needle biopsies after radiation therapy. Am J Surg Pathol 1999;23:1173–1183.

315. Larson TR, Bostwick DG, Corica A. Temperature-correlated histopathologic changes following microwave thermoablation of obstructive tissue in patients with benign prostatic hyperplasia. Urology 1996;47:463–469.

316. Scherr DS, Vaughan ED Jr, Wei J, et al. BCL-2 and p53 expression in clinically localized prostate cancer predicts response to external beam radiotherapy [published erratum appears in J Urol 1999;162:503]. J Urol 1999;162:12–16; discussion 16–17.

317. Rakozy C, Grignon DJ, Li Y, et al. p53 gene alterations in prostate cancer after radiation failure and their association with clinical outcome: A molecular and immunohistochemical analysis. Pathol Res Pract 1999;195:129–135.

318. Cheng L, Sebo TJ, Cheville JC, et al. p53 protein overexpression is associated with increased cell proliferation in patients with locally recurrent prostate carcinoma after radiation therapy. Cancer 1999;85:1293–1299.

319. Rakozy C, Grignon DJ, Sarkar FH, et al. Expression of bcl-2, p53, and p21 in benign and malignant prostatic tissue before and after radiation therapy. Mod Pathol 1998;11:892–899.

320. Kyprianou N, Rock S. Radiation-induced apoptosis of human prostate cancer cells is independent of mutant p53 overexpression. Anticancer Res 1998;18:897–905.

321. Huang A, Gandour-Edwards R, Rosenthal SA, et al. p53 and bcl-2 immunohistochemical alterations in prostate cancer treated with radiation therapy. Urology 1998;51:346–351.

322. Grignon DJ, Caplan R, Sarkar FH, et al. p53 status and prognosis of locally advanced prostatic adenocarcinoma: A study based on RTOG 8610. J Natl Cancer Inst 1997;89:158–165.

323. Prendergast NJ, Atkins MR, Schatte EC, et al. p53 immunohistochemical and genetic alterations are associated at high incidence with post-irradiated locally persistent prostate carcinoma. J Urol 1996;155:1685–1692.

324. Stattin P, Damber JE, Modig H, Bergh A. Pretreatment p53 immunoreactivity does not infer radioresistance in prostate cancer patients. Int J Radiat Oncol Biol Phys 1996;35:885–889.

325. Ljung G, Egevad L, Norberg M, et al. Expression of p21 and mutant p53 gene products in residual prostatic tumor cells after radical radiotherapy. Prostate 1997;32:99–105.

326. Grossfeld GD, Olumi AF, Connolly JA, et al. Locally recurrent prostate tumors following either radiation therapy or radical prostatectomy have changes in Ki-67 labeling in-

dex, p53 and bcl-2 immunoreactivity. J Urol 1998;159: 1437–1443.

327. Kim HE, Han SJ, Kasza T, et al. Platelet-derived growth factor (PDGF)–signaling mediates radiation-induced apoptosis in human prostate cancer cells with loss of p53 function. Int J Radiat Oncol Biol Phys 1997;39:731–736.

328. Magi-Galluzzi C, Nagy S, Bostwick DG, et al. Demonstrability of the glycoprotein A-80 in postradiation prostatic carcinoma. Hum Pathol 1999;30:1474–1478.

329. Bostwick DG, Chang L. Overdiagnosis of prostatic adenocarcinoma. Semin Urol Oncol 1999;17:199–205.

330. Collina G, Botticelli AR, Martinelli AM, et al. Sclerosing adenosis of the prostate: Report of three cases with electronmicroscopy and immunohistochemical study. Histopathology 1992;20:505–510.

331. Grignon DJ, Ro JY, Srigley JR, et al. Sclerosing adenosis of the prostate gland: A lesion showing myoepithelial differentiation. Am J Surg Pathol 1992;16:383–391.

332. Jones EC, Clement PB, Young RH. Sclerosing adenosis of the prostate gland: A clinicopathological and immunohistochemical study of 11 cases. Am J Surg Pathol 1991;15: 1171–1180.

333. Sakamoto N, Tsuneyoshi M, Enjoji M. Sclerosing adenosis of the prostate: Histopathologic and immunohistochemical analysis. Am J Surg Pathol 1991;15:660–667.

334. Young RH, Clement PB. Sclerosing adenosis of the prostate. Arch Pathol Lab Med 1987;111:363–366.

335. Oxley JD, Abbott CD, Gillatt DA, MacIver AG. Ductal carcinomas of the prostate: A clinicopathological and immunohistochemical study. Br J Urol 1998;81:109–115.

336. Grizzle WE, Myers RB, Arnold MM, Srivastava S. Evaluation of biomarkers in breast and prostate cancer. J Cell Biochem Suppl 1994;19:259–266.

337. Millar EK, Sharma NK, Lessells AM. Ductal (endometrioid) adenocarcinoma of the prostate: A clinicopathological study of 16 cases. Histopathology 1996;29:11–19.

338. Bock BJ, Bostwick DG. Does prostatic ductal adenocarcinoma exist? Am J Surg Pathol 1999;23:781–785.

339. Van de Voorde W, Van Poppel H, Haustermans K, et al. Mucin-secreting adenocarcinoma of the prostate with neuroendocrine differentiation and Paneth-like cells. Am J Surg Pathol 1994;18:200–207.

340. McNeal JE, Alroy J, Villers A, et al. Mucinous differentiation in prostatic adenocarcinoma. Hum Pathol 1991;22: 979–988.

341. Uchijima Y, Ito H, Takahashi M, Yamashina M. Prostate mucinous adenocarcinoma with signet ring cell. Urology 1990;36:267–268.

342. Ro JY, Grignon DJ, Ayala AG, et al. Mucinous adenocarcinoma of the prostate: Histochemical and immunohistochemical studies. Hum Pathol 1990;21:593–600.

343. Dodson MK, Cliby WA, Pettavel PP, et al. Female urethral adenocarcinoma: Evidence for more than one tissue of origin? Gynecol Oncol 1995;59:352–357.

344. Skodras G, Wang J, Kragel PJ. Primary prostatic signet-ring cell carcinoma. Urology 1993;42:338–342.

345. Segawa T, Kakehi Y. Primary signet ring cell adenocarcinoma of the prostate: A case report and literature review. Hinyokika Kiyo 1993;39:565–568.

346. Guerin D, Hasan N, Keen CE. Signet ring cell differentiation in adenocarcinoma of the prostate: A study of five cases. Histopathology 1993;22:367–371.

347. Ben-Izhak O, Lichtig C. Signet-ring cell carcinoma of the prostate mimicking primary gastric carcinoma. J Clin Pathol 1992;45:452–454.

348. Ro JY, el-Naggar A, Ayala AG, et al. Signet-ring-cell carcinoma of the prostate: Electron-microscopic and immunohistochemical studies of eight cases. Am J Surg Pathol 1988;12:453–460.

349. Torbenson M, Dhir R, Nangia A, et al. Prostatic carcinoma with signet ring cells: A clinicopathologic and immunohistochemical analysis of 12 cases, with review of the literature. Mod Pathol 1998;11:552–559.

350. Dundore PA, Cheville JC, Nascimento AG, et al. Carcino-sarcoma of the prostate: Report of 21 cases. Cancer 1995; 76:1035–1042.

351. Lindboe CF, Mjones J. Carcinosarcoma of prostate: Immunohistochemical and ultrastructural observations. Urology 1992;40:376–380.

352. Delahunt B, Eble JN, Nacey JN, Grebe SK. Sarcomatoid carcinoma of the prostate: Progression from adenocarcinoma is associated with p53 over-expression. Anticancer Res 1999;19:4279–4283.

353. Ro JY, el-Naggar AK, Amin MB, et al. Pseudosarcomatous fibromyxoid tumor of the urinary bladder and prostate: Immunohistochemical, ultrastructural, and DNA flow cytometric analyses of nine cases. Hum Pathol 1993;24:1203–1210.

354. Grignon DJ, Ro JY, Ordonez NG, et al. Basal cell hyperplasia, adenoid basal cell tumor, and adenoid cystic carcinoma of the prostate gland: An immunohistochemical study. Hum Pathol 1988;19:1425–1433.

355. Cheville JC, Dundore PA, Nascimento AG, et al. Leiomyosarcoma of the prostate: Report of 23 cases. Cancer 1995; 76:1422–1427.

356. Nazeer T, Barada JH, Fisher HA, Ross JS. Prostatic carcinosarcoma: Case report and review of literature. J Urol 1991; 146:1370–1373.

357. Kim HS, Lee JH, Nam JH, et al. Malignant phyllodes tumor of the prostate. Pathol Int 1999;49:1105–1108.

358. Umekita Y, Yoshida H. Immunohistochemical study of hormone receptor and hormone-regulated protein expression in phyllodes tumour: Comparison with fibroadenoma. Virchows Arch 1998;433:311–314.

359. Cacic M, Petrovic D, Tentor D, et al. Cystosarcoma phyllodes of the prostate. Scand J Urol Nephrol 1996;30:501–502.

360. Lopez-Beltran A, Gaeta JF, Huben R, Croghan GA. Malignant phyllodes tumor of prostate. Urology 1990;35:164–167.

361. Ito H, Ito M, Mitsuhata N, Tahara E. Phyllodes tumor of the prostate: A case report. Jpn J Clin Oncol 1989;19:299–304.

362. Manivel C, Shenoy BV, Wick MR, Dehner LP. Cystosarcoma phyllodes of the prostate: A pathologic and immunohistochemical study. Arch Pathol Lab Med 1986;110: 534–538.

363. Yokota T, Yamashita Y, Okuzono Y, et al. Malignant cystosarcoma phyllodes of prostate. Acta Pathol Jpn 1984;34: 663–668.

364. Bostwick D, Qian J, Ramnani D, et al. Prostatic phyllodes tumor. Long term follow-up study of 23 cases. Cancer, in press.

365. Reese JH, Lombard CM, Krone K, Stamey TA. Phyllodes type of atypical prostatic hyperplasia: A report of 3 new cases. J Urol 1987;138:623–626.

366. Kerley SW, Pierce P, Thomas J. Giant cystosarcoma phyllodes of the prostate associated with adenocarcinoma. Arch Pathol Lab Med 1992;116:195–197.

367. Wang N, Bacchi C, Gown A. Coordinate expression of cytokeratins 7 and 20 define unique subsets of carcinomas. Appl Immunohistochem 1995;3:88–107.

368. Harnden P, Mahmood N, Southgate J. Expression of cytokeratin 20 redefines urothelial papillomas of the bladder. Lancet 1999;353:974–977.

369. Harnden P, Eardley I, Joyce AD, Southgate J. Cytokeratin 20 as an objective marker of urothelial dysplasia. Br J Urol 1996;78:870–875.

370. Harnden P, Allam A, Joyce AD, et al. Cytokeratin 20 expression by non-invasive transitional cell carcinomas: Potential for distinguishing recurrent from non-recurrent disease. Histopathology 1995;27:169–174.

371. Baars JH, De Ruijter JL, Smedts F, et al. The applicability of a keratin 7 monoclonal antibody in routinely Papanicolaou-stained cytologic specimens for the differential diagnosis of carcinomas. [see comments] Am J Clin Pathol 1994;101:257–261.

372. Mortimer G, Jones DN, Assaf H, al-Ahmadi T. Patterns of

cytokeratin expression by neoplastic and non-neoplastic epithelium. Ir J Med Sci 1993;162:77–81.

373. Vojtesek B, Staskova Z, Nenutil R, et al. A panel of monoclonal antibodies to keratin no. 7: Characterization and value in tumor diagnosis. Neoplasma 1990;37:333–342.

374. Reedy EA, Heatfield BM, Trump BF, Resau JH. Correlation of cytokeratin patterns with histopathology during neoplastic progression in the rat urinary bladder. Pathobiology 1990;58:15–27.

375. Gown A. Immunohistochemical detection of primary sites of carcinomas. J Histotechnol 1999;22:209–215.

376. Bassily NH, Vallorosi CJ, Akdas G, et al. Coordinate expression of cytokeratins 7 and 20 in prostate adenocarcinoma and bladder urothelial carcinoma. Am J Clin Pathol 2000;113:383–388.

377. Ormsby AH, Haskell R, Jones D, Goldblum JR. Primary seminal vesicle carcinoma: An immunohistochemical analysis of four cases. Mod Pathol 2000;13:46–51.

378. Ordonez NG. Transitional cell carcinomas of the ovary and bladder are immunophenotypically different. Histopathology 2000;36:433–438.

379. Soslow RA, Rouse RV, Hendrickson MR, et al. Transitional cell neoplasms of the ovary and urinary bladder: A comparative immunohistochemical analysis. Int J Gynecol Pathol 1996;15:257–265.

380. Cheng L, Cheville JC, Sebo TJ, et al. Atypical nephrogenic metaplasia of the urinary tract: A precursor lesion? Cancer 2000;88:853–861.

381. Korkolopoulou P, Christodoulou P, Konstantinidou AE, et al. Cell cycle regulators in bladder cancer: A multivariate survival study with emphasis on p27Kip1. Hum Pathol 2000;31:751–760.

382. Rodel C, Grabenbauer GG, Rodel F, et al. Apoptosis, p53, bcl-2, and Ki-67 in invasive bladder carcinoma: Possible predictors for response to radiochemotherapy and successful bladder preservation. Int J Radiat Oncol Biol Phys 2000;46:1213–1221.

383. Zlotta AR, Schulman CC. Biological markers in superficial bladder tumors and their prognostic significance. Urol Clin North Am 2000;27:179–189.

384. Pfister C, Lacombe L, Vezina MC, et al. Prognostic value of the proliferative index determined by Ki-67 immunostaining in superficial bladder tumors. Hum Pathol 1999;30:1350–1355.

385. Zlotta AR, Noel JC, Fayt I, et al. Correlation and prognostic significance of p53, p21WAF1/CIP1 and Ki-67 expression in patients with superficial bladder tumors treated with bacillus Calmette-Guerin intravesical therapy. [see comments] J Urol 1999;161:792–798.

386. Osen I, Fossa SD, Majak B, et al. Prognostic factors in muscle-invasive bladder cancer treated with radiotherapy: An immunohistochemical study. Br J Urol 1998;81:862–869.

387. Lianes P, Charytonowicz E, Cordon-Cardo C, et al. Biomarker study of primary nonmetastatic versus metastatic invasive bladder cancer: National Cancer Institute Bladder Tumor Marker Network. Clin Cancer Res 1998;4:1267–1271.

388. Pfister C, Buzelin F, Casse C, et al. Comparative analysis of MiB1 and p53 expression in human bladder tumors and their correlation with cancer progression. Eur Urol 1998;33(3):278–284.

389. Korkolopoulou P, Christodoulou P, Kapralos P, et al. The role of p53, MDM2 and c-erb B-2 oncoproteins, epidermal growth factor receptor and proliferation markers in the prognosis of urinary bladder cancer. Pathol Res Pract 1997;193:767–775.

390. Nakopoulou L, Vourlakou C, Zervas A, et al. The prevalence of bcl-2, p53, and Ki-67 immunoreactivity in transitional cell bladder carcinomas and their clinicopathologic correlates. Hum Pathol 1998;29:146–154.

391. Leonardi E, Cristofori A, Reich A, Dalla Palma P. Bivariate analysis DNA/cytokeratin 7 and flow cytometric measurement of MIB-1 in superficial transitional carcinoma of the bladder (TCC): Methodological aspects and prognostic implications. Eur J Histochem 1997;41(Suppl 2):133–134.

392. Siu LL, Banerjee D, Khurana RJ, et al. The prognostic role of p53, metallothionein, P-glycoprotein, and MIB-1 in muscle-invasive urothelial transitional cell carcinoma. Clin Cancer Res 1998;4:559–565.

393. Lee E, Park I, Lee C. Prognostic markers of intravesical bacillus Calmette-Guerin therapy for multiple, high-grade, stage T1 bladder cancers. Int J Urol 1997;4:552–556.

394. Vollmer RT, Humphrey PA, Swanson PE, et al. Invasion of the bladder by transitional cell carcinoma: Its relation to histologic grade and expression of p53, MIB-1, c-erb B-2, epidermal growth factor receptor, and bcl-2. Cancer 1998;82:715–723.

395. Vorreuther R, Hake R, Borchmann P, et al. Expression of immunohistochemical markers (PCNA, Ki-67, 486p and p53) on paraffin sections and their relation to the recurrence rate of superficial bladder tumors. Urol Int 1997;59:88–94.

396. Popov Z, Hoznek A, Colombel M, et al. The prognostic value of p53 nuclear overexpression and MIB-1 as a proliferative marker in transitional cell carcinoma of the bladder. Cancer 1997;80:1472–1481.

397. Tsuji M, Kojima K, Murakami Y, et al. Prognostic value of Ki-67 antigen and p53 protein in urinary bladder cancer: Immunohistochemical analysis of radical cystectomy specimens. Br J Urol 1997;79:367–372.

398. Hake R, Vorreuther R, Borchmann P, et al. Monoclonal antibodies (MIB 1, PC 10, 486p and p53) as prognostic factors for recurrent urothelial carcinoma of the urinary bladder. Verh Dtsch Ges Pathol 1993;77:236–240.

399. Pich A, Chiusa L, Comino A, Navone R. Cell proliferation indices, morphometry and DNA flow cytometry provide objective criteria for distinguishing low and high grade bladder carcinomas. Virchows Arch 1994;424:143–148.

400. Liukkonen T, Rajala P, Raitanen M, et al. Prognostic value of MIB-1 score, p53, EGFr, mitotic index and papillary status in primary superficial (stage pTa/T1) bladder cancer: A prospective comparative study: The Finnbladder Group. Eur Urol 1999;36:393–400.

401. Shiina H, Igawa M, Yagi H, et al. Relationship of genetic instability with immunoreactivities for p53 protein and proliferating cell nuclear antigen in transitional cell carcinoma of the bladder. Eur Urol 1996;30:80–88.

402. Blasco-Olaetxea E, Belloso L, Garcia-Tamayo J. Superficial bladder cancer: Study of the proliferative nuclear fraction as a prognostic factor. Eur J Cancer 1996;32A:444–446.

403. Chen G, Lin MS, Li RC. Expression and prognostic value of proliferating cell nuclear antigen in transitional cell carcinoma of the urinary bladder. Urol Res 1997;25:25–30.

404. Iizumi T, Iiyama T, Tanaka W, et al. Immunohistochemical studies of proliferating cell nuclear antigen and cathepsin D in transitional cell carcinoma of the urinary bladder. Urol Int 1997;59:81–87.

405. Ogura K, Habuchi T, Yamada H, et al. Immunohistochemical analysis of p53 and proliferating cell nuclear antigen (PCNA) in bladder cancer: Positive immunostaining and radiosensitivity. Int J Urol 1995;2:302–308.

406. Shiina H, Igawa M, Nagami H, et al. Immunohistochemical analysis of proliferating cell nuclear antigen, p53 protein and nm23 protein, and nuclear DNA content in transitional cell carcinoma of the bladder. Cancer 1996;78:1762–1774.

407. Plastiras D, Moutzouris G, Barbatis C, et al. Can p53 nuclear over-expression, Bcl-2 accumulation and PCNA status be of prognostic significance in high-risk superficial and invasive bladder tumours? Eur J Surg Oncol 1999;25:61–65.

408. Lipponen PK, Eskelinen MJ. Cell proliferation of transitional cell bladder tumours determined by PCNA/cyclin immunostaining and its prognostic value. Br J Cancer 1992;66:171–176.

409. Skopelitou A, Hadjiyannakis M, Dimopoulos D, et al. p53 and c-jun expression in urinary bladder transitional cell carcinoma: Correlation with proliferating cell nuclear antigen (PCNA) histological grade and clinical stage. Eur Urol 1997;31:464–471.

410. Pantazopoulos D, Ioakim-Liossi A, Karakitsos P, et al. DNA content and proliferation activity in superficial transitional cell carcinoma of the bladder. Anticancer Res 1997;17:781–786.

411. Ogura K, Fukuzawa S, Habuchi T, et al. Correlation of nuclear morphometry and immunostaining for p53 and proliferating cell nuclear antigen in transitional cell carcinoma of the bladder. Int J Urol 1997;4:561–566.

412. Dalbagni G, Cordon-Cardo C, Reuter V, Fair WR. Tumor suppressor gene alterations in bladder carcinoma: Translational correlates to clinical practice. Surg Oncol Clin North Am 1995;4:231–240.

413. Underwood MA, Reeves J, Smith G, et al. Overexpression of p53 protein and its significance for recurrent progressive bladder tumours. Br J Urol 1996;77:659–666.

414. Cordon-Cardo C, Sheinfeld J, Dalbagni G. Genetic studies and molecular markers of bladder cancer. Semin Surg Oncol 1997;13:319–327.

415. Cordon-Cardo C, Reuter VE. Alterations of tumor suppressor genes in bladder cancer. Semin Diagn Pathol 1997;14:123–132.

416. McShane LM, Aamodt R, Cordon-Cardo C, et al. Reproducibility of p53 immunohistochemistry in bladder tumors: National Cancer Institute, Bladder Tumor Marker Network. Clin Cancer Res 2000;6:1854–1864.

417. Cordon-Cardo C, Dalbagni G, Saez GT, et al. p53 mutations in human bladder cancer: Genotypic versus phenotypic patterns. Int J Cancer 1994;56:347–353.

418. Burkhard FC, Markwalder R, Thalmann GN, Studer UE. Immunohistochemical determination of p53 overexpression: An easy and readily available method to identify progression in superficial bladder cancer? Urol Res 1997;25(Suppl 1):S31–S35.

419. Caliskan M, Turkeri LN, Mansuroglu B, et al. Nuclear accumulation of mutant p53 protein: A possible predictor of failure of intravesical therapy in bladder cancer. Br J Urol 1997;79:373–377.

420. Esrig D, Elmajian D, Groshen S, et al. Accumulation of nuclear p53 and tumor progression in bladder cancer. [see comments] N Engl J Med 1994;331:1259–1264.

421. Sinik Z, Alkibay T, Ataoglu O, et al. Nuclear p53 overexpression in bladder, prostate, and renal carcinomas. Int J Urol 1997;4:546–551.

422. Sinik Z, Alkibay T, Ataoglu O, et al. Correlation of nuclear p53 over-expression with clinical and histopathological features of transitional cell bladder cancer. Int Urol Nephrol 1997;29:25–31.

423. Vatne V, Maartmann-Moe H, Hoestmark J. The prognostic value of p53 in superficially infiltrating transitional cell carcinoma. Scand J Urol Nephrol 1995;29:491–495.

424. Casetta G, Gontero P, Russo R, et al. p53 expression compared with other prognostic factors in OMS grade-I stage-Ta transitional cell carcinoma of the bladder. Eur Urol 1997;32:229–236.

425. Grossman HB, Liebert M, Antelo M, et al. p53 and RB expression predict progression in T1 bladder cancer. Clin Cancer Res 1998;4:829–834.

426. Gardiner RA, Walsh MD, Allen V, et al. Immunohistological expression of p53 in primary pT1 transitional cell bladder cancer in relation to tumour progression. Br J Urol 1994;73:526–532.

427. Liukkonen TJ, Lipponen PK, Helle M, Jauhiainen KE. Immunoreactivity of bcl-2, p53 and EGFr is associated with tumor stage, grade and cell proliferation in superficial bladder cancer: Finnbladder III Group. Urol Res 1997;25:1–7.

428. Raitanen MP, Tammela TL, Kallioinen M, Isola J. p53 accumulation, deoxyribonucleic acid ploidy and progression of bladder cancer. J Urol 1997;157:1250–1253.

429. Friedrich MG, Erbersdobler A, Schwaibold H, et al. Detection of loss of heterozygosity in the p53 tumor-suppressor gene with PCR in the urine of patients with bladder cancer. J Urol 2000;163:1039–1042.

430. Lipponen PK, Liukkonen TJ. Reduced expression of retinoblastoma (Rb) gene protein is related to cell proliferation and prognosis in transitional-cell bladder cancer. J Cancer Res Clin Oncol 1995;121:44–50.

431. Dalbagni G, Presti JC Jr, Reuter VE, et al. Molecular genetic alterations of chromosome 17 and p53 nuclear overexpression in human bladder cancer. Diagn Mol Pathol 1993;2:4–13.

432. Inagaki T, Ebisuno S, Uekado Y, et al. PCNA and p53 in urinary bladder cancer: Correlation with histological findings and prognosis. Int J Urol 1997;4:172–177.

433. Miyamoto H, Kubota Y, Shuin T, et al. Analyses of p53 gene mutations in primary human bladder cancer. Oncol Res 1993;5:245–249.

434. Oyasu R, Nan L, Szumel RC, et al. p53 gene mutations in human urothelial carcinomas: Analysis by immunohistochemistry and single-strand conformation polymorphism. Mod Pathol 1995;8:170–176.

435. Miyamoto H, Shuin T, Ikeda I, et al. Loss of heterozygosity at the p53, RB, DCC and APC tumor suppressor gene loci in human bladder cancer. J Urol 1996;155:1444–1447.

436. Nakopoulou L, Constantinides C, Papandropoulos J, et al. Evaluation of overexpression of p53 tumor suppressor protein in superficial and invasive transitional cell bladder cancer: Comparison with DNA ploidy. Urology 1995;46:334–340.

437. Sarkis AS, Dalbagni G, Cordon-Cardo C, et al. Association of p53 nuclear overexpression and tumor progression in carcinoma in situ of the bladder. J Urol 1994;152(2 Pt 1):388–392.

438. Sarkis AS, Dalbagni G, Cordon-Cardo C, et al. Nuclear overexpression of p53 protein in transitional cell bladder carcinoma: A marker for disease progression. J Natl Cancer Inst 1993;85:53–59.

439. Llopis J, Alcaraz A, Ribal MJ, et al. p53 expression predicts progression and poor survival in T1 bladder tumours. Eur Urol 2000;37:644–653.

440. Gao JP, Uchida T, Wang C, et al. Relationship between p53 gene mutation and protein expression: Clinical significance in transitional cell carcinoma of the bladder. Int J Oncol 2000;16:469–475.

441. Uchida T, Wada C, Ishida H, et al. p53 mutations and prognosis in bladder tumors. J Urol 1995;153:1097–1104.

442. Mayr B, Reifinger M, Alton K, Schaffner G. Novel p53 tumour suppressor mutations in cases of spindle cell sarcoma, pleomorphic sarcoma and fibrosarcoma in cats. Vet Res Commun 1998;22:249–255.

443. Okamoto M, Hattori K, Fujimoto K, et al. Antisense RNA-mediated reduction of p53 induces malignant phenotype in nontumorigenic rat urothelial cells. Carcinogenesis 1998;19:73–79.

444. Fujimoto K, Yamada Y, Okajima E, et al. Frequent association of p53 gene mutation in invasive bladder cancer. Cancer Res 1992;52:1393–1398.

445. Spruck CH 3rd, Ohneseit PF, Gonzalez-Zulueta M, Esrig D, et al. Two molecular pathways to transitional cell carcinoma of the bladder. Cancer Res 1994;54:784–788.

446. Tzai TS, Chow NH, Lin JS, et al. The expression of p53 and bcl-2 in superficial bladder transitional cell carcinoma and its role in the outcome of postoperative intravesical chemotherapy. Anticancer Res 1998;18:4717–4721.

447. Aprikian AG, Sarkis AS, Reuter VE, et al. Biological markers of prognosis in transitional cell carcinoma of the bladder: Current concepts. Semin Urol 1993;11:137–144.

448. Cordon-Cardo C, Dalbagni G, Sarkis AS, Reuter VE. Genetic alterations associated with bladder cancer. Important Adv Oncol 1994;pp 71–83.

449. Sarkis AS, Bajorin DF, Reuter VE, et al. Prognostic value of p53 nuclear overexpression in patients with invasive bladder cancer treated with neoadjuvant MVAC. J Clin Oncol 1995;13:1384–1390.

450. Esrig D, Spruck CH 3d, Nichols PW, et al. p53 nuclear protein accumulation correlates with mutations in the p53 gene, tumor grade, and stage in bladder cancer. Am J Pathol 1993;143:1389–1397.

451. Lipponen PK. Over-expression of p53 nuclear oncoprotein

in transitional-cell bladder cancer and its prognostic value. Int J Cancer 1993;53:365–370.

452. al-Abadi H, Nagel R, Neuhaus P. Immunohistochemical detection of p53 protein in transitional cell carcinoma of the bladder in correlation to DNA ploidy and pathohistological stage and grade. Cancer Detect Prev 1998;22:43–50.

453. Niehans GA, Kratzke RA, Froberg MK, et al. G1 checkpoint protein and p53 abnormalities occur in most invasive transitional cell carcinomas of the urinary bladder. Br J Cancer 1999;80:1175–1184.

454. Glick SH, Howell LP, White RW. Relationship of p53 and bcl-2 to prognosis in muscle-invasive transitional cell carcinoma of the bladder. J Urol 1996;155:1754–1757.

455. Watanabe R, Tomita Y, Nishiyama T, et al. Correlation of p53 protein expression in human urothelial transitional cell cancers with malignant potential and patient survival. Int J Urol 1994;1:43–48.

456. Lebret T, Becette V, Barbagelatta M, et al. Correlation between p53 over expression and response to bacillus Calmette-Guerin therapy in a high risk select population of patients with T1G3 bladder cancer. J Urol 1998;59:788–791.

457. Pages F, Flam TA, Vieillefond A, et al. p53 status does not predict initial clinical response to bacillus Calmette-Guerin intravesical therapy in T1 bladder tumors. J Urol 1998;159:1079–1084.

458. Cote RJ, Esrig D, Groshen S, et al. p53 and treatment of bladder cancer. [letter; comment] Nature 1997;385:123–125.

459. Grossfeld GD, Mouchizadeh J, Stein JP, et al. Thrombospondin-1 expression in bladder cancer: Association with p53 alterations, tumor angiogenesis, and tumor progression. J Natl Cancer Inst 1997;89:219–227.

460. Lopez-Beltran A, Escudero AL. Human papillomavirus and bladder cancer. Biomed Pharmacother 1997;51:252–257.

461. Lopez-Beltran A, Escudero AL, Carrasco-Aznar JC, Vicioso-Recio L. Human papillomavirus infection and transitional cell carcinoma of the bladder: Immunohistochemistry and in situ hybridization. Pathol Res Pract 1996;192:154–159.

462. Lopez-Beltran A, Escudero AL, Vicioso-Recio L, et al. Human papillomavirus DNA as a factor determining the survival of bladder cancer patients. Br J Cancer 1996;73:124–127.

463. Lopez-Beltran A, Munoz E. Transitional cell carcinoma of the bladder: Low incidence of human papillomavirus DNA detected by the polymerase chain reaction and in situ hybridization. Histopathology 1995;26:565–569.

464. Simoneau M, LaRue H, Fradet Y. Low frequency of human papillomavirus infection in initial papillary bladder tumors. Urol Res 1999;27:180–184.

465. Lianes P, Orlow I, Zhang ZF, et al. Altered patterns of MDM2 and TP53 expression in human bladder cancer. [see comments] J Natl Cancer Inst 1994;86:1325–1330.

466. Schmitz-Drager BJ, Kushima M, Goebell P, et al. p53 and MDM2 in the development and progression of bladder cancer. Eur Urol 1997;32:487–493.

467. Warren W, Biggs PJ, el-Baz M, et al. Mutations in the p53 gene in schistosomal bladder cancer: A study of 92 tumours from Egyptian patients and a comparison between mutational spectra from schistosomal and non-schistosomal urothelial tumours. Carcinogenesis 1995;16:1181–1189.

468. Orlow I, Lacombe L, Hannon GJ, et al. Deletion of the p16 and p15 genes in human bladder tumors. [see comments] J Natl Cancer Inst 1995;87:1524–1529.

469. Gonzalez-Zulueta M, Bender CM, Yang AS, et al. Methylation of the 5' CpG island of the p16/CDKN2 tumor suppressor gene in normal and transformed human tissues correlates with gene silencing. Cancer Res 1995;55:4531–4535.

470. Orlow I, LaRue H, Osman I, et al. Deletions of the INK4A gene in superficial bladder tumors: Association with recurrence. Am J Pathol 1999;155:105–113.

471. Nakopoulou LL, Constandinides CA, Tzonou A, et al. Immunohistochemical evaluation of nm23-H1 gene product

in transitional cell carcinoma of the bladder. Histopathology 1996;28:429–435.

472. Xu X, Stower MJ, Reid IN, et al. A hot spot for p53 mutation in transitional cell carcinoma of the bladder: Clues to the etiology of bladder cancer. Cancer Epidemiol Biomarkers Prev 1997;6:611–616.

473. Ahrendt SA, Decker PA, Doffek K, et al. Microsatellite instability at selected tetranucleotide repeats is associated with p53 mutations in non-small cell lung cancer. Cancer Res 2000;60:2488–2491.

474. Xu X, Stower MJ, Reid IN, et al. Molecular screening of multifocal transitional cell carcinoma of the bladder using p53 mutations as biomarkers. Clin Cancer Res 1996;2:1795–1800.

475. Spruck CH 3rd, Gonzalez-Zulueta M, Shibata A, et al. p16 gene in uncultured tumours. [letter; see comments] Nature 1994; 370:183–184.

476. Sidransky D, Von Eschenbach A, Tsai YC, et al. Identification of p53 gene mutations in bladder cancers and urine samples. Science 1991;252:706–709.

477. Krupski T, Moskaluk C, Boyd JC, Theodorescu D. A prospective pilot evaluation of urinary and immunohistochemical markers as predictors of clinical stage of urothelial carcinoma of the bladder. BJU Int 2000;85:1027–1032.

478. Brown FM. Urine cytology: Is it still the gold standard for screening? Urol Clin North Am 2000;27:25–37.

479. Righi E, Rossi G, Ferrari G, et al. Does p53 immunostaining improve diagnostic accuracy in urine cytology? Diagn Cytopathol 1997;17:436–439.

480. Sugano K, Tsutsumi M, Nakashima Y, et al. Diagnosis of bladder cancer by analysis of the allelic loss of the p53 gene in urine samples using blunt-end single-strand conformation polymorphism. Int J Cancer 1997;74:403–406.

481. Mao L. Genetic alterations as clonal markers for bladder cancer detection in urine. J Cell Biochem Suppl 1996;25:191–196.

482. Walther PJ. "Wildcatting" for breakthroughs in urothelial cancer detection and management—a frustrating business [editorial; comment] J Urol 1995;154:1348–1350.

483. Hruban RH, van der Riet P, Erozan YS, Sidransky D. Brief report: Molecular biology and the early detection of carcinoma of the bladder—the case of Hubert H. Humphrey. [see comments] N Engl J Med 1994;330:1276–1278.

484. Benedict WF, Lerner SP, Zhou J, et al. Level of retinoblastoma protein expression correlates with p16 (MTS-1/INK4A/CDKN2) status in bladder cancer. Oncogene 1999;18:1197–1203.

485. Ishikawa J, Xu HJ, Hu SX, et al. Inactivation of the retinoblastoma gene in human bladder and renal cell carcinomas. Cancer Res 1991;51:5736–5743.

486. Miyamoto H, Shuin T, Torigoe S, et al. Retinoblastoma gene mutations in primary human bladder cancer. Br J Cancer 1995;71:831–835.

487. Kubota Y, Miyamoto H, Noguchi S, et al. The loss of retinoblastoma gene in association with c-myc and transforming growth factor-beta 1 gene expression in human bladder cancer. [see comments] J Urol 1995;154(2 Pt 1):371–374.

488. Diaz-Cano SJ, Blanes A, Rubio J, et al. Molecular evolution and intratumor heterogeneity by topographic compartments in muscle-invasive transitional cell carcinoma of the urinary bladder. Lab Invest 2000;80:279–289.

489. Cordon-Cardo C. Molecular alterations in bladder cancer. Cancer Surv 1998;32:115–131.

490. de Vere White RW, Stapp E. Predicting prognosis in patients with superficial bladder cancer. Oncology (Huntingt) 1998;12:1717–1723; discussion 1724–1726.

491. Ow K, Delprado W, Fisher R, et al. Relationship between expression of the KAI1 metastasis suppressor and other markers of advanced bladder cancer. J Pathol 2000;191:39–47.

492. Wada T, Louhelainen J, Hemminki K, et al. Bladder cancer: allelic deletions at and around the retinoblastoma tumor suppressor gene in relation to stage and grade. Clin Cancer Res 2000;6:610–615.

493. Pollack A, Wu CS, Czerniak B, et al. Abnormal bcl-2 and pRb expression are independent correlates of radiation response in muscle-invasive bladder cancer. Clin Cancer Res 1997;3:1823–1829.

494. Adshead JM, Kessling AM, Ogden CW. Genetic initiation, progression and prognostic markers in transitional cell carcinoma of the bladder: A summary of the structural and transcriptional changes, and the role of developmental genes. Br J Urol 1998;82:503–512.

495. Orntoft TF, Wolf H. Molecular alterations in bladder cancer. [editorial] Urol Res 1998;26:223–233.

496. Jahnson S, Karlsson MG. Predictive value of p53 and pRb immunostaining in locally advanced bladder cancer treated with cystectomy. J Urol 1998;160:1291–1296.

497. Pollack A, Czerniak B, Zagars GK, et al. Retinoblastoma protein expression and radiation response in muscle-invasive bladder cancer. Int J Radiat Oncol Biol Phys 1997;39:687–695.

498. Cordon-Cardo C, Zhang ZF, Dalbagni G, et al. Cooperative effects of p53 and pRB alterations in primary superficial bladder tumors. Cancer Res 1997;57:1217–1221.

499. Goodrich DW, Chen Y, Scully P, Lee WH. Expression of the retinoblastoma gene product in bladder carcinoma cells associates with a low frequency of tumor formation. Cancer Res 1992;52:1968–1973.

500. Wright C, Thomas D, Mellon K, et al. Expression of retinoblastoma gene product and p53 protein in bladder carcinoma: Correlation with Ki67 index. Br J Urol 1995;75:173–179.

501. Geradts J, Hu SX, Lincoln CE, et al. Aberrant RB gene expression in routinely processed, archival tumor tissues determined by three different anti-RB antibodies. Int J Cancer 1994;58:161–167.

502. Gorgoulis VG, Barbatis C, Poulias I, Karameris AM. Molecular and immunohistochemical evaluation of epidermal growth factor receptor and c-erb-B-2 gene product in transitional cell carcinomas of the urinary bladder: A study in Greek patients. Mod Pathol 1995;8:758–764.

503. Tetu B, Allard P, Fradet Y, et al. Prognostic significance of nuclear DNA content and S-phase fraction by flow cytometry in primary papillary superficial bladder cancer. Hum Pathol 1996;27:922–926.

504. Underwood M, Bartlett J, Reeves J, et al. C-erbB-2 gene amplification: A molecular marker in recurrent bladder tumors? Cancer Res 1995;55:2422–2430.

505. Mellon JK, Lunec J, Wright C, et al. C-erbB-2 in bladder cancer: Molecular biology, correlation with epidermal growth factor receptors and prognostic value. [see comments] J Urol 1996;155:321–326.

506. Lonn U, Lonn S, Friberg S, et al. Prognostic value of amplification of c-erb-B2 in bladder carcinoma. Clin Cancer Res 1995;1:1189–1194.

507. Miyamoto H, Kubota Y, Noguchi S, et al. C-ERBB-2 gene amplification as a prognostic marker in human bladder cancer. Urology 2000;55:679–683.

508. Moch H, Sauter G, Mihatsch MJ, et al. p53 but not erbB-2 expression is associated with rapid tumor proliferation in urinary bladder cancer. Hum Pathol 1994;25:1346–1351.

509. Wagner U, Sauter G, Moch H, et al. Patterns of p53, erbB-2, and EGF-r expression in premalignant lesions of the urinary bladder. Hum Pathol 1995;26:970–978.

510. Li B, Kanamaru H, Noriki S, et al. Reciprocal expression of bcl-2 and p53 oncoproteins in urothelial dysplasia and carcinoma of the urinary bladder. Urol Res 1998;26:235–241.

511. Kelly JD, Williamson KE, Irvine AE, et al. Apoptosis and its clinical significance for bladder cancer therapy. BJU Int 1999;83:1–10.

512. Miyake H, Hara I, Yamanaka K, et al. Overexpression of Bcl-2 enhances metastatic potential of human bladder cancer cells. Br J Cancer 1999;79:1651–1656.

513. Kong G, Shin KY, Oh YH, et al. Bcl-2 and p53 expressions in invasive bladder cancers. Acta Oncol 1998;37:715–720.

514. Wu TT, Chen JH, Lee YH, Huang JK. The role of bcl-2, p53, and ki-67 index in predicting tumor recurrence for

515. Gazzaniga P, Gradilone A, Vercillo R, et al. Bcl-2/bax mRNA expression ratio as prognostic factor in low-grade urinary bladder cancer. Int J Cancer 1996;69:100–104.

516. Keegan PE, Lunec J, Neal DE. p53 and p53-regulated genes in bladder cancer. [see comments] Br J Urol 1998;82:710–720.

517. Atug F, Turkeri L, Ozyurek M, Akdas A. Bcl-2 and p53 overexpression as associated risk factors in transitional cell carcinoma of the bladder. Int Urol Nephrol 1998;30:455–461.

518. Ye D, Li H, Qian S, et al. bcl-2/bax expression and p53 gene status in human bladder cancer: Relationship to early recurrence with intravesical chemotherapy after resection. J Urol 1998;160(6 Pt 1):2025–2028; discussion 2029.

519. Okamura T, Akita H, Kawai N, et al. Immunohistochemical evaluation of p53, proliferating cell nuclear antigen (PCNA) and bcl-2 expression during bacillus Calmette-Guerin (BCG) intravesical instillation therapy for superficial bladder cancers. Urol Res 1998;26:161–164.

520. Eissa S, Seada LS. Quantitation of bcl-2 protein in bladder cancer tissue by enzyme immunoassay: Comparison with Western blot and immunohistochemistry. Clin Chem 1998;44:1423–1429.

521. Bilim VN, Tomita Y, Kawasaki T, et al. Variable Bcl-2 phenotype in benign and malignant lesions of urothelium. [see comments] Cancer Lett 1998;128:87–92.

522. Gazzaniga P, Gradilone A, Silvestri I, et al. Variable levels of bcl-2, bcl-x and bax mRNA in bladder cancer progression. Oncol Rep 1998;5:901–904.

523. Kirsh EJ, Baunoch DA, Stadler WM. Expression of bcl-2 and bcl-X in bladder cancer. J Urol 1998;159:1348–1353.

524. Shiina H, Igawa M, Urakami S, et al. Immunohistochemical analysis of bcl-2 expression in transitional cell carcinoma of the bladder. J Clin Pathol 1996;49:395–399.

525. Lipponen PK, Aaltomaa S, Eskelinen M. Expression of the apoptosis suppressing bcl-2 protein in transitional cell bladder tumours. Histopathology 1996;28:135–140.

526. King ED, Matteson J, Jacobs SC, Kyprianou N. Incidence of apoptosis, cell proliferation and bcl-2 expression in transitional cell carcinoma of the bladder: Association with tumor progression. [see comments] J Urol 1996;155:316–320.

527. Cooke PW, James ND, Ganesan R, et al. Bcl-2 expression identifies patients with advanced bladder cancer treated by radiotherapy who benefit from neoadjuvant chemotherapy. BJU Int 2000;85:829–835.

528. Ross JS, del Rosario AD, Figge HL, et al. E-cadherin expression in papillary transitional cell carcinoma of the urinary bladder. Hum Pathol 1995;26:940–944.

529. Ross JS, del Rosario AD, Bui HX, et al. Expression of the CD44 cell adhesion molecule in urinary bladder transitional cell carcinoma. Mod Pathol 1996;9:854–860.

530. Lipponen PK, Eskelinen MJ. Reduced expression of E-cadherin is related to invasive disease and frequent recurrence in bladder cancer. J Cancer Res Clin Oncol 1995;121:303–308.

531. Wakatsuki S, Watanabe R, Saito K, et al. Loss of human E-cadherin (ECD) correlated with invasiveness of transitional cell cancer in the renal pelvis, ureter and urinary bladder. Cancer Lett 1996;103:11–17.

532. Popov Z, Gil-Diez de Medina S, Lefrere-Belda MA, et al. Low E-cadherin expression in bladder cancer at the transcriptional and protein level provides prognostic information. Br J Cancer 2000;83:209–214.

533. Garcia del Muro X, Torregrosa A, Munoz J, et al. Prognostic value of the expression of E-cadherin and beta-catenin in bladder cancer. Eur J Cancer 2000;36:357–362.

534. Syrigos KN, Karayiannakis A, Syrigou EI, et al. Abnormal expression of p120 correlates with poor survival in patients with bladder cancer. Eur J Cancer 1998;34:2037–2040.

535. Mialhe A, Louis J, Montlevier S, et al. Expression of E-cadherin and alpha-, beta- and gamma-catenins in human

bladder carcinomas: Are they good prognostic factors? Invasion Metastasis 1997;17:124–137.

536. Mialhe A, Louis J, Pasquier D, et al. Expression of three cell adhesion molecules in bladder carcinomas: Correlation with pathological features [published erratum appears in Anal Cell Pathol 1997;14(2):1225–1227]. Anal Cell Pathol 1997;13:125–136.

537. Shimazui T, Schalken JA, Giroldi LA, et al. Prognostic value of cadherin-associated molecules (alpha-, beta-, and gamma-catenins and p120cas) in bladder tumors. Cancer Res 1996;56:4154–4158.

538. Fujisawa M, Miyazaki J, Takechi Y, et al. The significance of E-cadherin in transitional-cell carcinoma of the human urinary bladder. World J Urol 1996;14(Suppl 1):S12–S15.

539. Ross JS, Cheung C, Sheehan C, et al. E-cadherin cell-adhesion molecule expression as a diagnostic adjunct in urothelial cytology. Diagn Cytopathol 1996;14:310–315.

540. Griffiths TR, Brotherick I, Bishop RI, et al. Cell adhesion molecules in bladder cancer: Soluble serum E-cadherin correlates with predictors of recurrence. Br J Cancer 1996; 74:579–584.

541. Grossman HB, Lee C, Bromberg J, Liebert M. Expression of the alpha6beta4 integrin provides prognostic information in bladder cancer. Oncol Rep 2000;7:13–16.

542. Wilson CB, Leopard J, Cheresh DA, Nakamura RM. Extracellular matrix and integrin composition of the normal bladder wall. World J Urol 1996;14(Suppl 1):S30–S37.

543. Liebert M, Washington R, Wedemeyer G, et al. Loss of co-localization of alpha 6 beta 4 integrin and collagen VII in bladder cancer. Am J Pathol 1994;144:787–795.

544. Lee CC, Yamamoto S, Morimura K, et al. Significance of cyclin D1 overexpression in transitional cell carcinomas of the urinary bladder and its correlation with histopathologic features. Cancer 1997;79:780–789.

545. Shin KY, Kong G, Kim WS, et al. Overexpression of cyclin D1 correlates with early recurrence in superficial bladder cancers. Br J Cancer 1997;75:1788–1792.

546. Wagner U, Suess K, Luginbuhl T, et al. Cyclin D1 overexpression lacks prognostic significance in superficial urinary bladder cancer. J Pathol 1999;188:44–50.

547. Bringuier PP, Tamimi Y, Schuuring E, Schalken J. Expression of cyclin D1 and EMS1 in bladder tumours; relationship with chromosome 11q13 amplification. Oncogene 1996;12:1747–1753.

548. Suwa Y, Takano Y, Iki M, et al. Cyclin D1 protein overexpression is related to tumor differentiation, but not to tumor progression or proliferative activity, in transitional cell carcinoma of the bladder. J Urol 1998;160(3 Pt 1):897–900.

549. Takaba K, Saeki K, Suzuki K, et al. Significant overexpression of metallothionein and cyclin D1 and apoptosis in the early process of rat urinary bladder carcinogenesis induced by treatment with N-butyl-N-(4-hydroxybutyl)-nitrosamine or sodium L-ascorbate. Carcinogenesis 2000; 21:691–700.

550. Rabbani F, Cordon-Cardo C. Mutation of cell cycle regulators and their impact on superficial bladder cancer. Urol Clin North Am 2000;27:83–102.

551. Woodman AC, Goodison S, Drake M, et al. Noninvasive diagnosis of bladder carcinoma by enzyme-linked immunosorbent assay detection of CD44 isoforms in exfoliated urothelia. Clin Cancer Res 2000;6:2381–2392.

552. Miyake H, Hara I, Arakawa S, Kamidono S. Utility of competitive reverse transcription-polymerase chain reaction analysis of specific CD44 variant RNA for detecting upper urinary tract transitional-cell carcinoma. Mol Urol 1999;3: 365–370.

553. Lipponen P, Aaltoma S, Kosma VM, et al. Expression of CD44 standard and variant-v6 proteins in transitional cell bladder tumours and their relation to prognosis during a long-term follow-up. J Pathol 1998;186:157–164.

554. Miyake H, Hara I, Gohji K, et al. Urinary cytology and competitive reverse transcriptase-polymerase chain reaction analysis of a specific CD44 variant to detect and monitor bladder cancer. [see comments] J Urol 1998;160(6 Pt 1):2004–2008.

555. Iczkowski KA, Shanks JH, Bostwick DG. Loss of CD44 variant 6 expression differentiates small cell carcinoma of urinary bladder from urothelial (transitional cell) carcinoma. Histopathology 1998;32:322–327.

556. Muller M, Heicappell R, Habermann F, et al. Expression of CD44V2 in transitional cell carcinoma of the urinary bladder and in urine. Urol Res 1997;25:187–192.

557. Naot D, Sionov RV, Ish-Shalom D. CD44: Structure, function, and association with the malignant process. Adv Cancer Res 1997;71:241–319.

558. Sugino T, Gorham H, Yoshida K, et al. Progressive loss of CD44 gene expression in invasive bladder cancer. Am J Pathol 1996;149:873–882.

559. Takada S, Namiki M, Matsumiya K, et al. Expression of CD44 splice variants in human transitional cell carcinoma. Eur Urol 1996;29:370–373.

560. Kan M, Furukawa A, Aki M, et al. Expression of CD44 splice variants in bladder cancer. Int J Urol 1995;2:295–301.

561. Matsumura Y, Sugiyama M, Matsumura S, et al. Unusual retention of introns in CD44 gene transcripts in bladder cancer provides new diagnostic and clinical oncological opportunities. J Pathol 1995;177:11–20.

562. Lein M, Jung K, Weiss S, et al. Soluble CD44 variants in the serum of patients with urological malignancies. Oncology 1997;54:226–230.

563. Jaeger TM, Weidner N, Chew K, et al. Tumor angiogenesis correlates with lymph node metastases in invasive bladder cancer. J Urol 1995;154:69–71.

564. Dickinson AJ, Fox SB, Persad RA, et al. Quantification of angiogenesis as an independent predictor of prognosis in invasive bladder carcinomas. Br J Urol 1994;74:762–766.

565. Bochner BH, Cote RJ, Weidner N, et al. Angiogenesis in bladder cancer: Relationship between microvessel density and tumor prognosis. J Natl Cancer Inst 1995;87:1603–1612.

566. Hawke CK, Delahunt B, Davidson PJ. Microvessel density as a prognostic marker for transitional cell carcinoma of the bladder. Br J Urol 1998;81:585–590.

567. Dinney CP, Babkowski RC, Antelo M, et al. Relationship among cystectomy, microvessel density and prognosis in stage T1 transitional cell carcinoma of the bladder. J Urol 1998;160:1285–1290.

568. Ozer E, Mungan MU, Tuna B, et al. Prognostic significance of angiogenesis and immunoreactivity of cathepsin D and type IV collagen in high-grade stage T1 primary bladder cancer. Urology 1999;54:50–55.

569. Chaudhary R, Bromley M, Clarke NW, et al. Prognostic relevance of micro-vessel density in cancer of the urinary bladder. Anticancer Res 1999;19:3479–3484.

570. Campbell SC, Volpert OV, Ivanovich M, Bouck NP. Molecular mediators of angiogenesis in bladder cancer. Cancer Res 1998;58:1298–1304.

571. Crew JP. Vascular endothelial growth factor: An important angiogenic mediator in bladder cancer. Eur Urol 1999;35: 2–8.

572. Sato K, Sasaki R, Ogura Y, et al. Expression of vascular endothelial growth factor gene and its receptor (flt-1) gene in urinary bladder cancer. Tohoku J Exp Med 1998;185: 173–184.

573. Brown LF, Berse B, Jackman RW, et al. Increased expression of vascular permeability factor (vascular endothelial growth factor) and its receptors in kidney and bladder carcinomas. Am J Pathol 1993;143:1255–1262.

574. Chow NH, Liu HS, Chan SH, et al. Expression of vascular endothelial growth factor in primary superficial bladder cancer. Anticancer Res 1999;19:4593–4597.

575. Jones A, Crew J. Vascular endothelial growth factor and its correlation with superficial bladder cancer recurrence rates and stage progression. Urol Clin North Am 2000;27:191–197.

576. Crew JP, O'Brien T, Bicknell R, et al. Urinary vascular endothelial growth factor and its correlation with bladder cancer recurrence rates. [see comments] J Urol 1999;161: 799–804.

577. Droller MJ. Vascular endothelial growth factor is a predictor of relapse and stage progression in superficial bladder cancer. J Urol 1998;160:1932.

578. Crew JP, O'Brien T, Bradburn M, et al. Vascular endothelial growth factor is a predictor of relapse and stage progression in superficial bladder cancer. Cancer Res 1997;57: 5281–5285.
579. Otto T, Bex A, Schmidt U, et al. Improved prognosis assessment for patients with bladder carcinoma. Am J Pathol 1997;150:1919–1923.
580. Jones HL, Delahunt B, Bethwaite PB, Thornton A. Luminal epithelial antigen (LEA.135) expression correlates with tumor progression for transitional carcinoma of the bladder. Anticancer Res 1997;17:685–687.
581. Zhuang YH, Blauer M, Tammela T, Tuohimaa P. Immunodetection of androgen receptor in human urinary bladder cancer. Histopathology 1997;30:556–562.
582. Hasui Y, Osada Y. Urokinase-type plasminogen activator and its receptor in bladder cancer. [editorial; see comments] J Natl Cancer Inst 1997;89:678–679.
583. Hasui Y, Marutsuka K, Asada Y, Osada Y. Prognostic value of urokinase-type plasminogen activator in patients with superficial bladder cancer. Urology 1996;47:34–37.
584. Hasui Y, Marutsuka K, Nishi S, et al. The content of urokinase-type plasminogen activator and tumor recurrence in superficial bladder cancer. J Urol 1994;151:16–19; discussion 19–20.
585. Hasui Y, Suzumiya J, Marutsuka K, et al. Comparative study of plasminogen activators in cancers and normal mucosae of human urinary bladder. Cancer Res 1989;49: 1067–1070.
586. Baffa R, Gomella LG, Vecchione A, et al. Loss of FHIT expression in transitional cell carcinoma of the urinary bladder. Am J Pathol 2000;156:419–424.
587. Klein A, Zemer R, Buchumensky V, et al. Expression of cytokeratin 20 in urinary cytology of patients with bladder carcinoma. [see comments] Cancer 1998;82:349–354.
588. Ravery V, Colombel M, Popov Z, et al. Prognostic value of epidermal growth factor-receptor, T138 and T43 expression in bladder cancer. Br J Cancer 1995;71:196–200.
589. Lokeshwar VB, Obek C, Pham HT, et al. Urinary hyaluronic acid and hyaluronidase: Markers for bladder cancer detection and evaluation of grade. J Urol 2000;163:348–356.
590. Lokeshwar VB, Block NL. HA-HAase urine test: A sensitive and specific method for detecting bladder cancer and evaluating its grade. Urol Clin North Am 2000;27:53–61.
591. Lokeshwar VB, Soloway MS, Block NL. Secretion of bladder tumor-derived hyaluronidase activity by invasive bladder tumor cells. Cancer Lett 1998;131:21–27.
592. Pham HT, Block NL, Lokeshwar VB. Tumor-derived hyaluronidase: A diagnostic urine marker for high-grade bladder cancer (published erratum appears in Cancer Res 1997; 57:1622). Cancer Res 1997;57:778–783.
593. Lokeshwar VB, Obek C, Soloway MS, Block NL. Tumor-associated hyaluronic acid: A new sensitive and specific urine marker for bladder cancer (published erratum appears in Cancer Res 1998;58:3191). Cancer Res 1997;57: 773–777.
594. Bostwick D, Lopez-Beltran A. Bladder Biopsy Interpretation. Glen Allen, VA: United Pathologists Press, 1999.
595. Jones EC, Clement PB, Young RH. Inflammatory pseudotumor of the urinary bladder: A clinicopathological, immunohistochemical, ultrastructural, and flow cytometric study of 13 cases. [see comments] Am J Surg Pathol 1993; 17:264–274.
596. Yamaguchi T, Imamura Y, Shimamoto T, et al. Small cell carcinoma of the bladder: Two cases diagnosed by urinary cytology. Acta Cytol 2000;44:403–409.
597. Eusebi V, Damiani S, Pasquinelli G, et al. Small cell neuroendocrine carcinoma with skeletal muscle differentiation: Report of three cases. Am J Surg Pathol 2000;24:223–230.
598. Ali SZ, Reuter VE, Zakowski MF. Small cell neuroendocrine carcinoma of the urinary bladder: A clinicopathologic study with emphasis on cytologic features. Cancer 1997;79:356–361.
599. Terracciano L, Richter J, Tornillo L, et al. Chromosomal imbalances in small cell carcinomas of the urinary bladder. J Pathol 1999;189:230–235.
600. Grammatico D, Grignon DJ, Eberwein P, et al. Transitional cell carcinoma of the renal pelvis with choriocarcinomatous differentiation: Immunohistochemical and immunoelectron microscopic assessment of human chorionic gonadotropin production by transitional cell carcinoma of the urinary bladder. Cancer 1993;71:1835–1841.
601. Yamase HT, Wurzel RS, Nieh PT, Gondos B. Immunohistochemical demonstration of human chorionic gonadotropin in tumors of the urinary bladder. Ann Clin Lab Sci 1985;15:414–417.
602. Martin JE, Jenkins BJ, Zuk RJ, et al. Human chorionic gonadotrophin expression and histological findings as predictors of response to radiotherapy in carcinoma of the bladder. Virchows Arch A Pathol Anat Histopathol 1989; 414:273–277.
603. Biyani CS, Sharma N, Nicol A, Heal MR. Postoperative spindle cell nodule of the bladder: A diagnostic problem. Urol Int 1996;56:119–121.
604. Allen PW, Allen LJ. Perce the permissive pathologist: A cautionary tale of one who misdiagnosed a pseudosarcoma, killed the patient and was found out. Aust NZ J Surg 1994;64:273–274.
605. Lo JW, Fung CH, Yonan T, DiMauro J. Postoperative spindle-cell nodule of urinary bladder with unusual intracytoplasmic inclusions. Diagn Cytopathol 1992;8:171–176.
606. Young RH. Spindle cell lesions of the urinary bladder. Histol Histopathol 1990;5:505–512.
607. Vekemans K, Vanneste A, Van Oyen P, et al. Postoperative spindle cell nodule of bladder. Urology 1990;35:342–344.
608. Huang WL, Ro JY, Grignon DJ, et al. Postoperative spindle cell nodule of the prostate and bladder. J Urol 1990;143: 824–826.
609. Lopez-Beltran A, Lopez-Ruiz J, Vicioso L. Inflammatory pseudotumor of the urinary bladder: A clinicopathological analysis of two cases. Urol Int 1995;55:173–176.
610. Wanibuchi H, Iwata H, Washida H, et al. A case report of inflammatory pseudotumor of the urinary bladder. Osaka City Med J 1995;41:31–39.
611. Foschini MP, Scarpellini F, Rinaldi P, et al. Inflammatory pseudotumor of the urinary bladder: Study of 4 cases and review of the literature. Pathologica 1995;87:653–658.
612. Jones EC, Young RH. Myxoid and sclerosing sarcomatoid transitional cell carcinoma of the urinary bladder: A clinicopathologic and immunohistochemical study of 25 cases. Mod Pathol 1997;10:908–916.
613. Horn LC, Reuter S, Biesold M. Inflammatory pseudotumor of the ureter and the urinary bladder. Pathol Res Pract 1997;193:607–612.
614. Coffin CM, Humphrey PA, Dehner LP. Extrapulmonary inflammatory myofibroblastic tumor: A clinical and pathological survey. Semin Diagn Pathol 1998;15:85–101.
615. Sonobe H, Okada Y, Sudo S, et al. Inflammatory pseudotumor of the urinary bladder with aberrant expression of cytokeratin: Report of a case with cytologic, immunocytochemical and cytogenetic findings. Acta Cytol 1999;43: 257–262.
616. Moyana TN, Kontozoglou T. Urinary bladder paragangliomas: An immunohistochemical study. Arch Pathol Lab Med 1988;112):70–72.
617. Salo JO, Miettinen M, Makinen J, Lehtonen T. Pheochromocytoma of the urinary bladder: Report of 2 cases with ultrastructural and immunohistochemical analyses. Eur Urol 1989;16:237–239.
618. Grignon DJ, Ro JY, Mackay B, et al. Paraganglioma of the urinary bladder: Immunohistochemical, ultrastructural, and DNA flow cytometric studies. Hum Pathol 1991;22: 1162–1169.
619. Lam KY, Chan AC. Paraganglioma of the urinary bladder: An immunohistochemical study and report of an unusual association with intestinal carcinoid. Aust NZ J Surg 1993; 63:740–745.
620. Shono T, Sakai H, Minami Y, et al. Paraganglioma of the urinary bladder: A case report and review of the Japanese literature. Urol Int 1999;62:102–105.
621. Kato H, Suzuki M, Mukai M, Aizawa S. Clinicopathological study of pheochromocytoma of the urinary bladder: Immunohistochemical, flow cytometric and ultrastructural

findings with review of the literature. Pathol Int 1999;49:
1093–1099.

622. Cheng L, Leibovich BC, Cheville JC, et al. Paraganglioma of the urinary bladder: Can biologic potential be predicted? Cancer 2000;88:844–852.

623. Burton EM, Schellhammer PF, Weaver DL, Woolfitt RA. Paraganglioma of urinary bladder in patient with neurofibromatosis. Urology 1986;27:550–552.

624. Misawa T, Shibasaki T, Toshima R, et al. A case of pheochromocytoma of the urinary bladder in a long-term hemodialysis patient. Nephron 1993;64:443–446.

625. Nesi G, Vezzosi V, Amorosi A, et al. Paraganglioma of the urinary bladder. Urol Int 1996;56:250–253.

626. Honma K. Paraganglia of the urinary bladder: An autopsy study. Zentralbl Pathol 1994;139:465–469.

627. Hacker GW, Bishop AE, Terenghi G, et al. Multiple peptide production and presence of general neuroendocrine markers detected in 12 cases of human phaeochromocytoma and in mammalian adrenal glands. Virchows Arch A Pathol Anat Histopathol 1988;412:399–411.

628. Mentzel T, Bainbridge TC, Katenkamp D. Solitary fibrous tumour: Clinicopathological, immunohistochemical, and ultrastructural analysis of 12 cases arising in soft tissues, nasal cavity and nasopharynx, urinary bladder and prostate. Virchows Arch 1997;430:445–453.

629. Bainbridge TC, Singh RR, Mentzel T, Katenkamp D. Solitary fibrous tumor of urinary bladder: Report of two cases. Hum Pathol 1997;28:1204–1206.

630. Westra WH, Grenko RT, Epstein J. Solitary fibrous tumor of the lower urogenital tract: A report of five cases involving the seminal vesicles, urinary bladder, and prostate. Hum Pathol 2000;31:63–68.

631. Park SH, Kim TJ, Chi JG. Congenital granular cell tumor with systemic involvement: Immunohistochemical and ultrastructural study. Arch Pathol Lab Med 1991;115:934–938.

632. Kontani K, Okaneya T, Takezaki T. Recurrent granular cell tumour of the bladder in a patient with von Recklinghausen's disease. BJU Int 1999;84:871–872.

633. Fletcher MS, Aker M, Hill JT, et al. Granular cell myoblastoma of the bladder. Br J Urol 1985;57:109–110.

634. Ando K, Matsuno Y, Kanai Y, et al. Primary low-grade lymphoma of mucosa-associated lymphoid tissue of the urinary bladder: A case report with special reference to the use of ancillary diagnostic studies. Jpn J Clin Oncol 1999;29:636–639.

635. Yuille FA, Angus B, Roberts JT, Vadanan BS. Low grade MALT lymphoma of the urinary bladder. Clin Oncol 1998; 10:265–266.

636. Kempton CL, Kurtin PJ, Inwards DJ, et al. Malignant lymphoma of the bladder: Evidence from 36 cases that low-grade lymphoma of the MALT-type is the most common primary bladder lymphoma. Am J Surg Pathol 1997;21: 1324–1333.

637. Fernandez Acenero MJ, Martin Rodilla C, Lopez Garcia-Asenjo J, et al. Primary malignant lymphoma of the bladder: Report of three cases. Pathol Res Pract 1996;192:160–163; discussion 164–165.

638. Ohsawa M, Aozasa K, Horiuchi K, Kanamaru A. Malignant lymphoma of bladder: Report of three cases and review of the literature. Cancer 1993;72:1969–1974.

639. Pawade J, Banerjee SS, Harris M, et al. Lymphomas of mucosa-associated lymphoid tissue arising in the urinary bladder. Histopathology 1993;23:147–151.

640. Siegel RJ, Napoli VM. Malignant lymphoma of the urinary bladder: A case with signet-ring cells simulating urachal adenocarcinoma. Arch Pathol Lab Med 1991;115:635–637.

641. Alanen KA, Kuopio T, Collan YU, et al. Immunohistochemical labelling for prostate-specific antigen in breast carcinomas. Breast Cancer Res Treat 1999;56:169–176.

642. Cohen MK, Arber DA, Coffield KS, et al. Neuroendocrine differentiation in prostatic adenocarcinoma and its relationship to tumor progression. Cancer 1994;74:1899–1903.

643. Speights VO Jr, Cohen MK, Riggs MW, et al. Neuroendocrine stains and proliferative indices of prostatic adenocarcinomas in transurethral resection samples. Br J Urol 1997; 80:281–286.

644. Cohen RJ, Glezerson G, Haffejee Z. Prostate-specific antigen and prostate-specific acid phosphatase in neuroendocrine cells of prostate cancer. Arch Pathol Lab Med 1992; 116:65–66.

645. Cohen RJ, Glezerson G, Haffejee Z, Afrika D. Prostatic carcinoma: Histological and immunohistological factors affecting prognosis. Br J Urol 1990;66:405–410.

646. Theodorescu D, Broder SR, Boyd JC, et al. Cathepsin D and chromogranin A as predictors of long term disease specific survival after radical prostatectomy for localized carcinoma of the prostate. Cancer 1997;80:2109–2119.

Immunohistochemistry of the Testis

Dharamdas M. Ramnani, M.D., Junqi Qian, M.D., and David G. Bostwick, M.D.

TESTIS, ADNEXAL STRUCTURES, AND EXTERNAL GENITALS

Testicular neoplasms are extremely uncommon, composing about 1% of malignant neoplasms in males; however, they are most common in men between the ages of 15 and 44 years.[1] The current incidence of testicular cancer in white males in the United States is 6 cases per 100,000 population.[2] The vast majority of testicular neoplasms are germ cell tumors. Tremendous advances have been made since the 1980s in our understanding of the pathogenesis of testicular cancer. Intratubular germ cell neoplasia is now considered to be the precursor of most germ cell tumors.[3–7] Advances in immunohistochemistry, cytogenetics, DNA ploidy, and other molecular testing methods have supplemented routine light microscopy, which remains the mainstay in the diagnosis of testicular cancer. The classification of sex cord–stromal tumors, which compose approximately 4% of testicular neoplasms, has undergone considerable evolution, with description of several new morphologic variants of the more established entities.

The following discussion first deals with the immunohistochemical markers that have a special role in testicular pathology followed by immunohistochemical profiles of the tumors of the testis, adnexal structures, and external genitals. Other immunohistochemical markers, such as keratins and mesenchymal markers that may be useful in the diagnosis of tumors arising in these locations, have been discussed elsewhere in this book.

Markers

PLACENTAL-LIKE ALKALINE PHOSPHATASE

Human alkaline phosphatase activity results from three genetically distinct isoenzymes produced in tissues such as liver, bone, intestine, and placenta. The proteins of these three isoenzymes are encoded by multilocus genes derived from a common ancestral gene.[8] The placental fraction of alkaline phosphatase is a membrane-bound enzyme of 120 kd, normally synthesized by placental syncytiotrophoblastic cells and released into maternal circulation after the 12th week of pregnancy.[9] However, it is also produced by many neoplasms and is a useful tumor marker.[10] Physiologically, this enzyme is involved in cellular transport, proliferation, and differentiation, as well as regulation of metabolism and gene transcription.[11]

Placental-like alkaline phosphatase (PLAP) is not unique to germ cell tumors and has been detected by biochemical and immunohistochemical methods in the serum and tissues of patients with a variety of tumors, including gastrointestinal, gynecologic, hematologic, lung, breast, and urologic tumors.[12, 13] In fact, tumor-associated PLAP was first demonstrated in the serum of a patient with small cell carcinoma of the lung and was named Regan's isoenzyme after the patient.[14] Among germ cell tumors, PLAP immunoreactivity was reported in 98% of seminomas, 98% of intratubular germ cell neoplasia, 97% of embryonal carcinomas, and 85% of yolk sac tumors in a study.[12] The germ cell elements in the majority of gonadoblastomas are also positive for PLAP. The immunoreactivity for PLAP in other germ cell tumors such as choriocarcinoma and teratoma is variable and may be seen in about half of the cases. The presence of PLAP has also been reported in ovarian germ cell tumors.[15] Normal testis contains only trace amounts of PLAP, which cannot be demonstrated immunohistochemically in the majority of cases. In the absence of intratubular germ cell neoplasia, dysgenetic gonads, cryptorchid testis, or testicular biopsies from infertile men rarely show immunoreactivity for PLAP.[12]

The staining reaction product for PLAP is localized mainly to the cell membrane and occasionally in the cytoplasm. The distribution and intensity of staining for PLAP varies between different tumors as well as between different areas of the same tumor. This is due to the underlying heterogeneity both of the quantity of the enzyme in tumor cells and of the enzyme itself from an immunohistochemical point of view.[13]

ALPHA FETOPROTEIN

Alpha fetoprotein, which resembles albumin in many physicochemical properties, is a major fetal serum protein normally produced by fetal yolk sac, fetal and regenerating adult liver, and the fetal gastrointestinal epithelium. AFP is elevated in up to 75% of patients with nonseminomatous germ cell tumors and can be demonstrated in the tumor tissue immunohistochemically.[16] AFP is never produced by pure classic seminoma.[17] Testicular tumors with elevation of serum AFP should be treated as nonseminomatous germ cell tumors even if AFP cannot be demonstrated in the tumor tissue immunohistochemically.[18] AFP is also the most useful marker for the diagnosis and management of hepatocellular carcinoma.

KEY DIAGNOSTIC POINTS

* Elevated in up to 75% of nonseminomatous germ cell tumors
* Never produced by pure classic seminoma

HUMAN CHORIONIC GONADOTROPIN

Human chorionic gonadotropin (HCG), the first pregnancy-specific protein to be described, is a 37-kd glycoprotein composed of an alpha and a beta subunit. The alpha subunit is identical to its counterpart in several other hormones, including thyroid-stimulating hormone, luteinizing hormone, and follicle-stimulating hormone. It is the beta subunit that imparts target organ specificity. β-HCG is synthesized by syncytiotrophoblastic cells in both benign and malignant chorionic tissue and is excreted in urine. It first appears in maternal serum 8 days after ovulation, reaches its peak level in the eighth week of pregnancy, followed by a rapid decline and maintenance of low levels for the remainder of pregnancy.[19]

As a marker of viable trophoblastic tissue, serum assays of β-HCG have played an important role in the diagnosis, staging, therapeutic monitoring, and follow-up of patients with gestational trophoblastic disease and testicular tumors.[17, 20] Serum β-HCG is elevated in the majority of cases of choriocarcinoma and in up to 10% of patients with seminoma. When assayed in conjunction with AFP, as many as 50 to 90% of men with nonseminomatous germ cell tumors have elevated levels of β-HCG.[21] β-HCG has been localized to syncytiotrophoblastic giant cells in seminomas, embryonal carcinomas, yolk sac tumors and to syncytiotrophoblastic cells in choriocarcinoma.

KEY DIAGNOSTIC POINTS

* Elevated in 50 to 90% of men with nonseminomatous germ cell tumors
* Localized to syncytiotrophoblastic giant cells in seminomas, embryonal carcinomas, yolk sac tumors, and choriocarcinoma

HUMAN PLACENTAL LACTOGEN

Human placental lactogen (HPL), also known previously as *human chorionic somatomammotropin,* is a 22-kd protein with partial homology to growth hormone.[22] HPL is first detectable in the maternal serum in the 5th week of gestation and reaches a plateau by the 34th week. HPL has been demonstrated by immunohistochemistry in the syncytiotrophoblastic cells of choriocarcinoma. A rare variant of trophoblastic tumor has been reported in the testis with resemblance to uterine placental site trophoblastic tumor.[115] It consisted purely of intermediate trophoblasts, which were diffusely positive for HPL and focally positive for β-HCG.

KEY DIAGNOSTIC POINTS

- Positive in the syncytiotrophoblastic cells of choriocarcinoma
- Diffusely positive in a variant of trophoblastic tumor consisting of intermediate trophoblast

INHIBIN

Inhibin is a 32-kd dimeric glycoprotein composed of an alpha and a beta subunit.[23] It is produced mainly by ovarian granulosa cells and testicular Sertoli cells with an additional small contribution from Leydig cells.[24] It inhibits the release of follicle-stimulating hormone from the pituitary, inhibiting folliculogenesis.[25] Inhibin has proved to be a sensitive immunohistochemical marker of ovarian sex cord–stromal tumors in general and of granulosa cell tumors in particular.[26–30]

Inhibin has now been shown to be expressed within sex cord–stromal tumors arising in the testis as well.[31–33] In one study, immunoreactivity for inhibin was demonstrated in 15 of 16 Leydig cell tumors, 4 of 6 testicular sex cord–stromal tumors with varying degrees of Sertoli or granulosa cell differentiation, and 2 of 3 sex cord–stromal tumors of unclassified type.[32] The majority of positive cases had diffuse, strong cytoplasmic staining. In all cases, non-neoplastic Leydig and Sertoli cells also stained with antiinhibin antibodies, although the staining is less intense than in neoplastic Sertoli and Leydig cells. Immunostaining for inhibin was not found in cases of seminoma, melanoma, lymphoma, malignant teratoma of undifferentiated type, or metastatic carcinoma used as controls in this study.[32]

In another study, inhibin A was found in 10 of 11 Sertoli cell tumors, all Sertoli cell adenomas, and all the benign and malignant Leydig cell tumors. In this study, six seminomas, one embryonal carcinoma, and three mixed germ cell tumors were not reactive for inhibin.[31] Syncytiotrophoblastic cells stain positively with antiinhibin antibodies.[34, 35] This may create a diagnostic dilemma in seminomas containing syncytiotrophoblastic cells because of the presence of areas of focal positivity for inhibin. Inhibin is now also considered to be a useful immunohistochemical marker for intermediate trophoblastic and syncytiotrophoblastic cells in hydatidiform mole, placental site trophoblastic tumor, and choriocarcinoma.[35–37]

KEY DIAGNOSTIC POINTS

- Positive in sex cord–stromal tumors arising in the testis
- Positive in intermediate trophoblastic and syncytiotrophoblastic cells
- Largely negative in seminoma, melanoma, lymphoma, malignant teratoma of undifferentiated type, or metastatic carcinoma

Testicular Tumors

GERM CELL TUMORS

Intratubular Germ Cell Neoplasia

Intratubular germ cell neoplasia, unclassified type (IGCNU) is the precursor of most types of germ cell tumors, except spermatocytic seminoma and pediatric germ cell tumors (Fig. 14–27). Its role in the pathogenesis of invasive germ cell tumors was first recognized by elegant observations made by Skakkebaek and colleagues.[3–7] IGCNU can be found in testicular biopsy specimens in cryptorchidism, oligospermic infertility, dysgenetic testes, and in the contralateral testis of patients with germ cell tumor. Invasive germ cell tumor develops within 5 years in approximately 50% of patients with IGCNU on testicular biopsy results.[38] IGCNU is less commonly found in prepubertal testes removed for germ cell tumors. In the absence of an invasive component, IGCNU is asymptomatic and is a microscopic finding in the testicular biopsies of men in the high-risk groups mentioned.

The seminiferous tubules involved by IGCNU rarely show spermatogenesis and often have de-

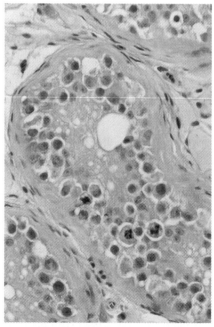

Figure 14–27. Intratubular germ cell neoplasia, unclassified type (IGCNU).

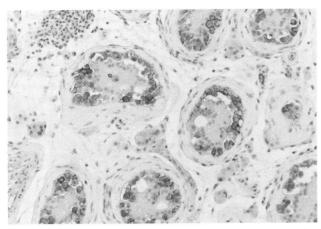

▼ *Figure 14–28.* Intratubular germ cell neoplasia; the tumor cells show membrane staining for placental-like alkaline phosphatase (PLAP).

creased tubular diameter with thickening of peritubular basement membrane. The tumor cells are basally located and have enlarged hyperchromatic nuclei with one or more nucleoli, clear cytoplasm containing periodic acid–Schiff–positive material (glycogen), and distinct cytoplasmic borders.[39] PLAP is a sensitive and specific marker for IGCNU. The tumor cells show membrane staining with this marker in between 85% and 98% of cases (Fig. 14–28), whereas the normal germ cells and Sertoli cells are usually negative.[40–43] Rarely, tumors metastasizing to the testis may invade seminiferous tubules and mimic IGCNU. PLAP is helpful in distinguishing them from IGCNU. Immunohistochemical stains for AFP, β-HCG, CEA, and HPL are usually negative in IGCNU.[44–46] Ferritin was found to be positive in 83% of cases of IGCNU by Jacobsen and coworkers.[47] They also found immunoreactivity for ferritin in IGCNU adjacent to invasive seminoma or nonseminomatous germ cell tumors in 94% of 189 orchiectomy specimens.[48] However, others have been unable to replicate these results.[49] Neuron-specific enolase (NSE), a marker of neuroendocrine differentiation, has also been reported with high frequency in IGCNU and invasive germ cell tumors.[50] Overexpression of the protein product of tumor suppressor gene p53 seen by immunohistochemistry has been detected in IGCNU adjacent to mature teratoma.[51, 52] Numerous other antigens have been identified in IGCNU by immunohistochemical methods, including TRA-1-60, c-kit proto-oncogene protein product (Kit), insulin-like growth factor I, M2A, 43-9F, glutathione-S-transferase π, and glycolipid globotriaosylceramide.[53–60] These markers are present to varying degrees in invasive germ cell tumors and have not found their way yet into the diagnostic armamentarium of surgical pathology.

Classic Seminoma

Seminoma is the most common germ cell tumor, composing 27 to 56% of all germ cell tumors.[61, 62]

The mean age at diagnosis is about 40 years, and most patients present with a testicular mass. Serum β-HCG is elevated in between 5% and 40% of cases of localized pure seminoma and in 13 to 61% of patients with metastatic disease.[63] Serum AFP is normal. Grossly, it is a soft pink-tan, diffuse or multinodular mass, which may contain small foci of necrosis and hemorrhage. The tumor cells have abundant clear cytoplasm, distinct cytoplasmic membranes, round vesicular nuclei, and prominent nucleoli. The fibrous septa separating tumor cell clusters contain lymphoplasmacytic infiltrate.

Immunohistochemical stains are useful in distinguishing seminoma from its benign and malignant mimics. PLAP is a sensitive marker for seminoma, with a cytoplasmic membrane staining pattern in 90 to 100% of cases.[64–66] PLAP is not specific for seminoma and stains other germ cell tumors and carcinomas.[65] Immunohistochemical staining for PLAP is especially helpful in distinguishing seminoma with exuberant granulomatous response (PLAP+) from idiopathic granulomatous orchitis (PLAP−). Tubular seminoma, a histologic variant of seminoma mimicking Sertoli cell tumor, is PLAP+, whereas Sertoli cell tumor is PLAP−, as are other sex cord–stromal tumors.

A significant minority of seminomas are associated with elevation of serum β-HCG levels. Such cases usually reveal clusters of syncytiotrophoblastic giant cells that are immunoreactive for β-HCG.[66–69] In some seminomas, β-HCG+ cells are not recognizable as syncytiotrophoblastic, and they perhaps represent intermediate trophoblasts. AFP, a marker for yolk sac tumor, is not expressed in seminoma. CD30 is negative in the majority of seminomas and is usually positive in embryonal carcinoma.[70–72] It has been suggested that CD30 expression seen in the rare cases of seminoma might reflect their incipient transformation to embryonal carcinomas.[71] Seminoma lacks immunoreactivity for inhibin, a sensitive and specific marker for testicular sex cord–stromal tumors.[73]

Up to 40% of seminomas may exhibit expression of cytokeratin, although the percentage of positivity reported in the literature ranges from 0 to 73%.[66, 74–77] Staining is usually weak and is seen in isolated cells or in small clusters. Rare cases may be diffusely positive for cytokeratin. The intermingled syncytiotrophoblastic cells may show strong immunoreactivity for cytokeratin (CK) AE1/AE3. CK8 and CK18 have been demonstrated in seminomas.[78, 87] CK19, a marker diffusely present in embryonal carcinomas, is generally absent.[79, 80] Rare cases of seminoma also show CK4 and CK17.[81] Epithelial membrane antigen is not expressed.[66] Vimentin, desmin, neurofilament protein, NSE, ferritin, lactate dehydrogenase (LDH), Leu7, and alpha-1-antitrypsin are also expressed to varying degrees in seminoma, but they are not diagnostically useful.[48, 66, 74, 81, 82]

The published reports on p53 immunohistochemistry in seminomas range from negative to overexpression in 90% of cases.[83] Primary mediastinal seminomas appear to be different from testicular seminomas in their K-ras and p53 immunohistochemical profiles (less frequently positive).[83] Significant differences have been observed between testicular and mediastinal seminomas in the expression of other markers by immunohistochemistry. Mediastinal seminomas showed strong dot-like positivity for CAM5.2 in 80% of cases, as compared with only 20% positivity in testicular seminomas.[84]

In summary, seminoma shows cytoplasmic membrane immunoreactivity for PLAP and is generally negative or only weakly positive for EMA, cytokeratins, β-HCG, AFP, CD30, and inhibin. No differences, with the exception of high proliferating cell nuclear antigen (PCNA) expression, have been noted between typical seminoma and seminoma with a high mitotic index (formerly referred to as *anaplastic seminoma).*[85]

PLAP is a sensitive marker for seminoma, with a cytoplasmic membrane staining pattern in 90 to 100% of cases.

Immunohistochemical staining for PLAP is especially helpful in distinguishing seminoma with exuberant granulomatous response (PLAP+) from idiopathic granulomatous orchitis (PLAP−). Tubular seminoma, a histologic variant of seminoma mimicking Sertoli cell tumor, is PLAP+, whereas Sertoli cell tumor is PLAP−, as are other sex cord–stromal tumors.

Spermatocytic Seminoma

Spermatocytic seminoma is an uncommon testicular neoplasm that behaves in an indolent fashion. It composes about 5% of testicular seminomas.[86] The histogenesis, clinical presentation, morphologic features, and the biologic behavior of spermatocytic seminoma bear no resemblance to classic seminoma. It usually arises in older men, with the mean age at diagnosis of 54 years (range 25 to 87 years) and has not been reported in prepubertal children or adolescents.[88] It does not arise in cryptorchid testes, extratesticular sites, or in association with other germ cell tumors. The biologic behavior is benign except in rare cases that undergo sarcomatous transformation.[89] Microscopically, it contains three cell types: abundant intermediate-sized cells and scant numbers of small lymphocyte-like cells and larger cells.

Spermatocytic seminoma does not show immunoreactivity for any specific marker, and the diagnosis is based largely on routine light microscopy; however, immunohistochemical stains are valuable in diagnostically challenging cases in which unusual morphologic patterns produce resemblance to other germ cell tumors. Lymphocytic infiltrate in some cases of spermatocytic seminoma may produce resemblance to classic seminoma. Microcystic

areas reminiscent of yolk sac tumor are seen in some cases. An anaplastic variant of spermatocytic seminoma resembling embryonal carcinoma with a solid growth pattern has also been described.[90] Spermatocytic seminoma is negative for antibodies directed against AFP, β-HCG, CD30, CEA, HPL, NSE, S-100 protein, leukocyte common antigen, desmin, vimentin, and actin. Cytoplasmic and membrane positivity for PLAP may be seen in scattered cells in rare cases.[91] EPA and AE1/AE3 are negative, whereas low molecular weight cytokeratins (CAM5.2, CK18) may show inclusion-like positivity in about 40% of cases, reminiscent of the pattern seen in Merkel cell carcinoma.[92] p53 overexpression by immunohistochemistry was documented in two of four cases of anaplastic variant of spermatocytic seminoma in a study.[90] Positivity for c-kit proto-oncogene protein product has been found in 40% of cases of spermatocytic seminoma. All cases of classic seminoma were positive for c-kit in that study.[93]

Embryonal Carcinoma

Pure embryonal carcinoma composes less than 5% of testicular germ cell tumors and is seen more often as a component of mixed germ cell tumors (about 45% of cases).[61, 62] It is a tumor of young males with a mean age at diagnosis of 30 years. Most patients present with a testicular mass; rare cases show distant metastases at initial presentation. Microscopically, embryonal carcinoma is composed of polygonal cells with abundant cytoplasm and indistinct cytoplasmic borders, enlarged vesicular nuclei, prominent nucleoli, and brisk mitotic activity. The cells are arranged in sheets, glands, papillary, or tubular structures. Primitive mesenchyme may be associated with the tumor cells and is not a reflection of immature teratoma.

The majority of embryonal carcinomas are immunoreactive for CKs AE1/AE3 and CAM5.2 as well as CK8, CK18, and CK19. Some cases also show immunoreactivity for CK4 and CK17.[64–66, 94, 95] EMA, CEA, and vimentin are generally negative. Immunoreactivity for PLAP has been reported in 86 to 97% of embryonal carcinomas.[64, 66] The staining for PLAP in embryonal carcinomas is both cytoplasmic and membranous and tends to be more intense and focal than in seminomas.

More than 80% of embryonal carcinomas are positive for CD30 (Ki-1, BerH2).[70–72] CD30 immunoreactivity is rarely seen in other germ cell tumors and is useful in separating somatic carcinoma from embryonal carcinoma at metastatic sites. Immunoreactivity for PLAP, pancytokeratin, and CD30 and negativity for EMA favors embryonal carcinoma over somatic carcinoma when dealing with a poorly differentiated neoplasm in an extratesticular location.

Immunoreactivity for AFP and β-hCG may be seen in scattered tumor cells in 33% and 21% of cases, respectively.[66] A variety of reasonable hypotheses have been suggested to explain staining for AFP in embryonal carcinoma: true staining in rare tumor cells, staining of intermixed yolk sac tumor elements, and early transformation to yolk sac tumor.[96]

Many other immunohistochemical markers have been demonstrated in embryonal carcinoma but are not useful in daily practice. Ferritin, monoclonal antibody 43-9F, LDH-1, p53, alpha-1-antitrypsin, Leu7, vimentin, and HPL may be seen in embryonal carcinoma.[66, 82, 97–99]

KEY DIAGNOSTIC POINTS OF EMBRYONAL CARCINOMA

* PLAP+ (86 to 97% of cases; sensitive, not specific)
* Pancytokeratin-positive
* CD30+
* EMA−

Yolk Sac Tumor

Yolk sac tumor is the most common testicular neoplasm of children, accounting for almost 80% of all prepubertal germ cell tumors.[100] In adults, pure yolk sac tumor composes approximately 1.5% of testicular germ cell tumors but is present as a component in about 40% of mixed germ cell tumors.[101, 102] There is a strong correlation between the presence of yolk sac elements in pure or mixed forms (as a component of mixed germ cell tumor) and the elevation of serum AFP.[103, 104] Grossly, they are pink-tan, homogeneous lobulated tumors with a glistening, mucoid surface that frequently shows microcystic areas. Foci of necrosis or hemorrhage are frequent. A variety of histologic patterns have been described that create resemblance to other germ cell tumors or extratesticular malignancies. The microcystic (reticular) pattern is the most common.

Immunoreactivity for AFP in yolk sac tumors is reported in between 55% and 100% of cases in various studies.[44, 66, 105] The staining is usually cytoplasmic and may be weak and focal in many cases. The hepatoid variant may show intense staining for AFP. Cytoplasmic and extracellular eosinophilic hyaline globules, a characteristic histologic feature of yolk sac tumor, show variable immunoreactivity for AFP, alpha-1-antitrypsin, albumin, and transferrin.[61, 106] CK is intensely positive in most cases.[66, 75] EMA is negative and this can be helpful in distinguishing yolk sac tumor from somatic carcinoma in extratesticular sites.[66] PLAP is positive in more than half the cases.[42, 66, 107] The spindle cell component shows staining with vimentin.[75] The enteric glands may be positive for CEA in a small number of cases.[108, 109] Alpha-1-antitrypsin immunoreactivity is reported in about

50% of cases.[44, 66] Laminin, NSE, Leu7, p53, and CD34 are some additional markers that are expressed in a variable proportion of cases.[66, 97, 108, 110] CD30 is not expressed, unlike in embryonal carcinoma.[70, 72]

KEY DIAGNOSTIC POINTS OF YOLK SAC TUMOR

* PLAP+ (>50% of cases)
* AFP+ (55 to 100% of cases)
* Cytokeratin-positive (most of cases)
* Alpha-1-antitrypsin−positive (>50% of cases)
* CD30−
* EMA−

Choriocarcinoma

Pure choriocarcinoma represents only about 0.3% of testicular germ cell tumors but may be seen as a component in almost 8% of mixed germ cell tumors.[111] It is a highly aggressive tumor, and patients often present initially with distant metastases. Marked elevations of serum β-HCG associated with this tumor may cause gynecomastia in about 10% of patients. Grossly, it is a hemorrhagic and necrotic mass. Microscopically, most cases have a typical biphasic appearance consisting of syncytiotrophoblast intimately associated with and capping the cytotrophoblast (Fig. 14−29).

The correct diagnosis in many cases may be hampered by the presence of extensive necrosis. Small foci of viable tumor may be found at the periphery of the necrotic area. Immunostaining for β-HCG will often identify syncytiotrophoblastic cells in the necrotic foci. Syncytiotrophoblastic cells are strongly immunoreactive for β-HCG in all cases (Fig. 14−30); cytotrophoblast is negative or weakly positive.[44, 66, 112] HPL and pregnancy-specific β-1-glycoprotein (SP-1) are also expressed in syncytiotrophoblastic and intermediate cytotropho-

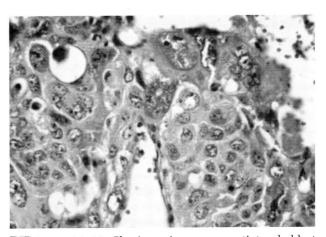

Figure 14–29. Choriocarcinoma, syncytiotrophoblast intimately associated with capping cytotrophoblast.

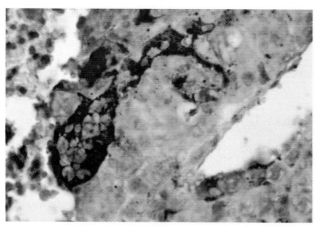

◥ Figure 14–30. Choriocarcinoma, syncytiotrophoblast is strongly immunoreactive for β-human chorionic gonadotropin (β-HCG).

blastic cells.[112] Cytokeratin is strongly expressed in both cytotrophoblastic and syncytiotrophoblastic cells.[66, 113] Immunoreactivity for EMA is seen in syncytiotrophoblastic cells in a significant percentage of cases, unlike seminoma, embryonal carcinoma, and yolk sac tumor.[66] About half the cases show immunoreactivity for PLAP.[66] CEA is expressed in both cytotrophoblastic and syncytiotrophoblastic cells.[114] Inhibin, a marker of sex cord–stromal tumors, is strongly positive in syncytiotrophoblastic cells.

Rare cases of choriocarcinoma consisting predominantly of cytotrophoblast, with only scant syncytiotrophoblastic elements, have been designated monophasic choriocarcinoma.[115] They may be confused with seminoma or a solid variant of yolk sac tumor. Immunostains can be helpful in arriving at the correct diagnosis. In one case report of so-called monophasic choriocarcinoma, both the cytotrophoblast and the rare syncytiotrophoblast were diffusely positive for β-HCG. HPL was found by immunostaining only in the syncytiotrophoblastic cells. Another rare variant of a trophoblastic tumor has been reported in the testis with resemblance to uterine placental site trophoblastic tumor.[115] It consisted purely of intermediate trophoblastic cells that were diffusely positive for HPL and focally for β-HCG.

Teratoma

Teratoma is the second most common germ cell tumor in the pediatric population, composing 14 to 20% of cases.[116–118] Pure teratoma is uncommon in adults but is seen as a component in 50% of mixed germ cell tumors.[101, 119] Its biologic behavior in children is benign; adults may develop metastases that contain nonteratomatous germ cell tumor.[120–122] Gross and microscopic features are varied, depending on the tissue present.

Immunohistochemistry is of limited diagnostic

use in these tumors. The immunohistochemical profile is a reflection of the tissue components produced by the tumor. Cells with hepatic differentiation and glandular structures with respiratory or intestinal-type epithelium may stain with antibodies directed against AFP.[44, 61] AFP immunoreactivity has been reported in 19 to 36% of teratomas.[61, 108] Alpha-1-antitrypsin, CEA, ferritin, and PLAP have been reported in the glandular component in a variable number of cases.[108] Actin, vimentin, and desmin are often found in the surrounding stroma. In teratomas with sarcomatous change, these markers can be useful in subtyping the sarcoma. Intratubular germ cell neoplasia is absent in prepubertal testis removed for teratoma. Atypical germ cells that are present adjacent to prepubertal mature teratoma lack immunoreactivity for PLAP and may represent a precursor other than IGCNU.[123]

Mixed Germ Cell Tumor

Mixed germ cell tumors contain more than one type of germ cell tumor and compose between 30% and 60% of all germ cell tumors.[62, 101, 124, 125] The most frequent pattern is embryonal carcinoma with one or more components of seminoma, teratoma, yolk sac tumor, or choriocarcinoma. Virtually all possible combinations have been reported to date. By convention, seminoma with syncytiotrophoblastic giant cells only is not considerd a mixed germ cell tumor. The clinical features of mixed germ cell tumors are similar to nonseminomatous germ cell tumors. AFP and β-HCG levels are often elevated and reflect the constituent components.

The diagnosis of mixed germ cell tumor is usually straightforward and rarely requires the use of immunohistochemical stains. In some cases, immunostaining for AFP may be helpful to confirm the presence of microscopic foci of yolk sac tumor that are often overlooked on routine light microscopy.

Sex Cord–Stromal Tumors

Sex cord–stromal tumors account for approximately 5% of all testicular tumors.[31] In prepubertal males, they account for a slightly higher proportion of testicular tumors. The well-differentiated tumors in this category resemble non-neoplastic Leydig cells, Sertoli cells, or the stromal cells. The sex cord–stromal tumors can display a wide spectrum of histologic patterns, often creating confusion with germ cell neoplasms or other tumors arising in this location. Immunohistochemical stains can be invaluable in separating difficult cases from these mimics.

Leydig Cell Tumor

Leydig cell tumor is the most common type of sex cord–stromal tumor, accounting for up to 3%

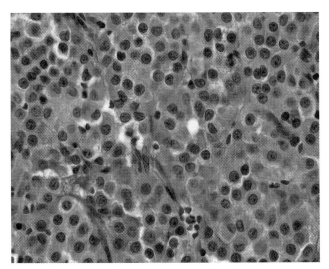

Figure 14–31. Leydig cell tumor shows large polygonal cells with abundant eosinophilic cytoplasm and indistinct cytoplasmic borders.

of testicular neoplasms.[39, 126] Although they occur both in children and adults, more than 55% of cases occur in men older than 30 years.[39] Children often have small, unpalpable tumors and present with isosexual precocity due to elaboration of androgens. Adults present with testicular mass, gynecomastia, decreased libido or potency, and occasionally with infertility. Usually, the tumors are well circumscribed and yellow or tan-white, frequently with areas of necrosis and hemorrhage. They are composed of large polygonal cells with abundant eosinophilic cytoplasm and indistinct cytoplasmic borders (Fig. 14–31). The nuclei are round and vesicular with small punctate nucleoli. Crystalloids of Reinke are found in approximately 30% of cases, and lipochrome pigment is seen in about 20% of cases.

Leydig cell tumor generally has characteristic histologic features, but it may be confused with a wide variety of benign and malignant lesions arising in the testis, including Leydig cell hyperplasia in cryptorchidism, testicular "tumor" arising in adrenogenital syndrome, malakoplakia, malignant lymphoma, plasmacytoma, seminoma, and metastatic carcinoma. Immunohistochemical stain for inhibin has proved to be of immense value in separating Leydig cell tumor from its many mimics.[29–33] In one study, immunoreactivity for inhibin was found in all the benign and malignant Leydig cell tumors tested.[31] Ten cases of testicular germ cell tumors used as controls were not reactive for inhibin. Another study demonstrated inhibin immunoreactivity in 15 of 16 Leydig cell tumors.[32] The staining is usually strong, diffuse, and cytoplasmic in positive cases (Fig. 14–32). Non-neoplastic Sertoli and Leydig cells are also positive for inhibin, although the intensity of staining is lower than in tumor cells. None of the cases (total 18 cases) of seminoma, malignant melanoma, testicular lymphoma, malignant teratoma of undifferentiated type, and testicular metastatic carcinoma was positive for inhibin.[32] Seminomas with syncytiotrophoblastic giant cells may show focal positivity for inhibin because the latter component stains with anti-inhibin antibodies.[34, 35]

Leydig cell tumors lack PLAP immunoreactivity, allowing their distinction from seminoma in difficult cases. Immunoreactivity for a number of antibodies has been found in Leydig cell tumors, including CAM5.2, vimentin, S-100 protein, desmin, and EMA.[32] These results are similar to those shown in ovarian lipid cell tumors, including Leydig cell tumors.[127] Immunoreactivity for cytokeratin, when present, is usually weak and focal. An immunohistochemical profile consisting of positivity for inhibin and vimentin, lack of reactivity for EMA, and variable cytokeratin immunoreactivity support the diagnosis of Leydig cell tumor over metastatic carcinoma. S-100 protein is sometimes present in Leydig cell tumors and is therefore unhelpful in its distinction from malignant melanoma, a rare differential diagnostic consideration. Leydig cell tumor is negative for HMB-45.

A rare variant of Leydig cell tumor with microcystic areas mimicking yolk sac tumor has been described.[128] By immunohistochemistry, all four cases in this study were diffusely positive for vimentin; two of three were positive for inhibin, and one was focally positive for CAM5.2. All cases were negative for PLAP and AFP. The MIB-1 labeling index, a measure of the proliferative activity, has been found to correlate with the metastatic behavior of Leydig cell tumors.[129]

A subset of normal Leydig cells are now considered to be part of a dispersed neuroendocrine system and are immunoreactive for synaptophysin and chromogranin.[130] Immunoreactivity for S-100 has also been demonstrated in non-neoplastic and

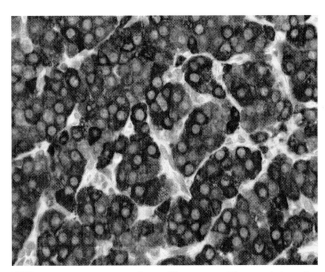

Figure 14–32. Leydig cell tumor. The staining for inhibin is usually strong, diffuse, and cytoplasmic in tumor cells.

neoplastic Leydig cells, as discussed earlier. In one study, chromogranin was present in 24 of 26 benign Leydig cell tumors but only 3 of 7 malignant Leydig cell tumors.[31] The staining in malignant cells was focal and less intense. Synaptophysin was demonstrated in 23 of 33 Leydig cell tumors.

KEY DIAGNOSTIC POINTS OF LEYDIG CELL TUMORS

* Positivity for inhibin and vimentin
* Lack of reactivity for EMA
* Variable cytokeratin immunoreactivity

Sertoli Cell Tumor

Sertoli cell tumors compose less than 1% of testicular tumors.[131] They can be subdivided into three types: Sertoli cell tumor, not otherwise specified (NOS), sclerosing variant, and large cell calcifying Sertoli cell tumor. Sertoli cell tumor, not otherwise specified, is the most common type and it usually presents with a testicular mass. The mean age at presentation in the largest series of Sertoli cell tumors published to date was 46 years.[131] Only 2 of 60 patients were less than 20 years. Sclerosing Sertoli cell tumor, an exceedingly rare variant, is characterized by cords, sheets, and solid tubules of Sertoli cells in dense sclerotic stroma.[132] Large cell calcifying Sertoli cell tumor may occur sporadically or may be seen in the setting of hereditary endocrine anomalies such as Carney's and Peutz-Jeghers syndromes or androgen insensitivity syndrome.

Inhibin A is a sensitive marker of Sertoli cell differentiation.[31, 32] In one study, 10 of 11 (91%) Sertoli cell tumors and all of Sertoli cell adenomas in patients with cryptorchidism demonstrated immunoreactivity for inhibin.[31] Non-neoplastic Sertoli cells in these cases showed greater intensity of staining than did tumor cells. A case of Sertoli cell tumor with a heterologous sarcomatous component has been reported.[133] Sertoli cell differentiation in this rare biphasic malignant testicular tumor was demonstrated by strong diffuse inhibin and vimentin immunoreactivity in the epithelial component. Cytokeratin AE1/AE3 and CAM5.2 were focally positive; EMA, monoclonal and polyclonal CEA, S-100 protein, CA19-9, and PLAP were negative in the epithelial component.

Sertoli cell tumors, including the large cell calcifying variant, stain positively with antibodies to vimentin, cytokeratin, S-100, synaptophysin, chromogranin, and NSE.[134–137] Cytokeratin immunoreactivity in Sertoli cell tumors is usually stronger than that seen in Leydig cell tumors. Immunoreactivity for PLAP is not seen in Sertoli cell tumors. Tubular seminoma, which often mimics Sertoli cell tumor architecturally, can be separated from Sertoli cell tumor by PLAP immunoreactivity and lack of staining for inhibin and cytokeratin.

KEY DIAGNOSTIC POINTS OF SERTOLI CELL TUMORS

* Inhibin A is a sensitive marker
* Positive for cytokeratin
* Negative for PLAP
* Positive for vimentin
* Positive for S-100, synaptophysin, chromogranin, and NSE

Granulosa Cell Tumor, Juvenile Type

Juvenile granulosa cell tumor is an uncommon testicular tumor, most frequently seen in newborns and infants younger than age 2.[138–140] Histologically, these rare tumors contain irregular cysts lined by granulosa cells arranged in single or multiple layers. Call-Exner bodies and nuclear grooves are not seen, unlike in the adult type. The tumor cells show dual epithelial-mesenchymal differentiation and stain with low molecular weight cytokeratins (CK8, CK18, and CK19) as well as smooth muscle actin, desmin, and vimentin.[139, 140]

Granulosa Cell Tumor, Adult Type

The adult variant of granulosa cell tumor is also extremely rare and usually presents with a testicular mass, sometimes accompanied by gynecomastia.[141, 142] Microscopically, their features are identical to those seen in the ovaries, characterized by sheets of neoplastic cells with longitudinal nuclear grooves. The data on immunohistochemical profile of this tumor are scant. They are positive for vimentin and inhibin but lack immunoreactivity for CKs and EMA.[28, 32, 142, 143] S-100 protein and smooth muscle actin have also been demonstrated in rare cases.[32, 144] The immunohistochemical profile of sex cord–stromal tumors, unclassified type, is similar to that of granulosa cell tumor, with reactivity for smooth muscle actin and S-100 protein.[144]

Fibroma-Thecoma

Tumors in the fibroma-thecoma group can arise rarely from the stroma in the testis.[145, 146] They are indistinguishable from their counterparts arising in the ovary. Immunohistochemical stains are rarely required for their diagnosis in routine practice. They show strong immunoreactivity for vimentin and focal positivity for actin and desmin.[146] Immunostains for keratin, S-100 protein, and CD34 were negative in this study. Rare examples of sex cord–stromal tumors of the testis have a predominant spindle cell component. The immunohistochemical profile of these tumors is similar to that of granulosa cell tumors, consisting of positivity for S-100 protein and smooth muscle actin.[144] An immunohistochemical study of ovarian tumors showed the presence of inhibin immunoreactivity in 10 of 11 thecomas and 3 of 11 fibromas.[147]

Mixed Sex Cord–Stromal and Germ Cell Tumors

Gonadoblastoma. Gonadoblastoma is a unique testicular neoplasm that contains nests of germ cells and cells resembling Sertoli cells or granulosa cells.[148–150] It arises in dysgenetic gonads and is associated with an increased risk of the development of germ cell tumors. One immunohistochemical study showed the presence of all the markers of intratubular germ cell neoplasia (ITGCN), including PLAP, antibodies M2A, 43-9F, and TRA-1-60.[148] However, the germ cell populations are usually heterogeneous, resulting in variable staining within the tumor. Sertoli-like cells in these tumors react with antibodies to CK and vimentin. The hyaline material surrounding the cell clusters stains with laminin.[149] One study demonstrated positivity for Wilms' tumor gene (WT1), müllerian-inhibiting substance, inhibin, and p53 in two of two cases.[150] Inhibin was noted in the sex cord component and not in the germ cells, müllerian-inhibiting substance was present in both components, WT1 was found only in the sex cord region, and p53 was noted in the germ cells.

KEY DIAGNOSTIC POINTS OF GONADOBLASTOMA

- Gonadoblastoma cells are positive for all the markers of ITGCN; however, the germ cell populations are usually heterogeneous

Hematopoietic Tumors, Metastases, and Other Rare Testicular Tumors

Müllerian Papillary Serous Tumors. A number of ovarian-type epithelial tumors have been reported in the testis, including serous papillary cystic tumor of low malignant potential, serous papillary carcinoma, mucinous cystadenoma, Brenner's tumor, endometrioid adenocarcinoma, mucinous cystadenocarcinoma, and clear cell adenocarcinoma.[151–155] The serous papillary cystic tumors of low malignant potential are the most common in this group and they are morphologically indistinguishable from their ovarian counterpart. LeuM1, CA 125, estrogen receptors, progesterone receptors, CK7, and weak CK20 immunoreactivity was reported in one case.[151] CEA was negative. In the same study, all of the nine ovarian papillary serous tumors expressed CK7, CA 125, and estrogen receptors. Eight of the nine tumors expressed progesterone receptors. Five of the nine were positive for LeuM1 and two of the nine expressed weak CK20. Another study of paratesticular papillary serous carcinoma reported immunoreactivity for cytokeratin AE1/AE3, S-100 protein, EMA, Ber-EP4, LeuM1, B72.3, CEA, and PLAP.[152]

Primary Carcinoid Tumor. Primary testicular carcinoid tumor is a rare indolent tumor with metastatic potential.[156, 157] The histologic and im-

munohistochemical features are identical to those seen in lung, gastrointestinal tract, and other locations. Immunoreactivity for chromogranin, serotonin, NSE, CK, gastrin, substance P, and vasoactive intestinal peptide have been demonstrated in these tumors.[156] About 25% of testicular carcinoids occur in association with teratoma.[156, 158] Carcinoid syndrome has not been reported in testicular carcinoids.

KEY DIAGNOSTIC POINTS

- Immunoreactivity for chromogranin, serotonin, NSE, CK, gastrin, substance P, and vasoactive intestinal peptide has been demonstrated in primary carcinoid tumor of testis

Lymphoma. Testicular lymphoma accounts for about 5% of all testicular tumors, including more than half the cases of testicular neoplasms in older men.[159, 160] Lymphoma should be considered in the differential diagnosis of testicular tumors in older men, along with spermatocytic seminoma and metastases. The majority of cases in testes are B-cell lymphomas but T-cell lymphomas and T/NK cell lymphoma have also been reported.[161–163] The distinction of testicular lymphoma from classic seminoma, spermatocytic seminoma, and embryonal carcinoma is usually straightforward in most cases. Lymphomas have a predominant interstitial pattern of growth. In rare cases, the tumor cells invade seminiferous tubules and may display an intratubular pattern of growth. Conversely, some cases of seminomas may show a predominant intertubular pattern of growth at their periphery. In difficult cases, immunohistochemical staining for leukocyte common antigen and B- and T-cell markers is helpful in separating lymphomas from primary germ cell tumors. Lymphomas are negative for PLAP and CK.

The distinction of anaplastic large cell lymphoma from embryonal carcinoma may be especially difficult. Anaplastic large cell lymphoma may show an intratubular pattern of growth with necrosis, mimicking embryonal carcinoma.[160] Immunoreactivity for CD45, CD3, CD45RO, and CD43, and lack of positivity for B-cell markers, PLAP, and CK is helpful in arriving at the correct diagnosis.

KEY DIAGNOSTIC POINTS

- Lymphomas: leukocyte common antigen–positive, positive for B- or T-cell markers, PLAP− and CK−
- Anaplastic large cell lymphoma: CD45+, CD3+, CD45RO+, CD43+; negative for B-cell markers; PLAP−, CK−

Plasmacytoma. The incidence of testicular plasmacytoma appears to be 1 in 1000 testicular tumors.[164] Most testicular plasmacytomas represent either metastatic spread from another site or a manifestation of systemic plasma cell dyscrasia.[165] Because of its rarity, most cases have initially been considered to be seminoma, spermatocytic seminoma, or lymphoma. Immunohistochemically, most plasmacytomas express monotypic cytoplasmic immunoglobulins (usually IgG or IgA type) and usually lack B-cell markers such as CD20. Many cases do not express CD45.[166] UCHL-1 (CD45RO) is commonly seen in plasmacytoma. Expression of EMA may raise the question of an epithelial tumor, but CK is usually negative. PLAP immunoreactivity has not been reported in testicular plasmacytomas.

Leukemia. Secondary testicular involvement in acute leukemia is common. About 5% of boys with acute lymphoblastic leukemia develop testicular disease either at initial presentation or during the disease course or as the first site of relapse.[167] At autopsy, 64% of patients with acute leukemia and 22% of those with chronic leukemia show infiltrates in the testis.[168] Granulocytic sarcoma has also been reported in the testis and causes significant diagnostic difficulties, because it is often not entertained in the differential diagnosis.[169-171] Most cases are initially misdiagnosed as malignant lymphoma or plasmacytoma. In some cases, the presence of eosinophilic granules in eosinophilic myelocytes suggests the correct diagnosis. Granulocytic sarcomas are positive for stains for chloroacetate esterase and immunohistochemical stains for lysozyme, myeloperoxidase, and leukocyte common antigen. B- and T-cell markers and CKs are usually negative.[169]

Metastases. Testes may rarely be involved by metastases.[172-174] The correct diagnosis may initially be missed when the testicular mass is the first manifestation of disease. The most common primary tumors originate from the prostate and lung.[172] Six percent of orchiectomy specimens in men with prostate cancer harbor metastatic deposits.[175] Other primary tumors and sites include melanoma, colon, kidney, stomach, pancreas, bladder, ureter, bile duct, salivary glands, and thyroid. Neuroblastoma, carcinoid tumor, retinoblastoma, and mesothelioma have also metastasized to the testes. The tumor morphologic features depend on the primary site and may mimic primary germ cell tumor. Older age at presentation, bilaterality and multifocality, relevant clinical history (if available), interstitial growth pattern, and the presence of lymphovascular invasion support metastases over primary germ cell tumor. In difficult cases, a basic immunohistochemical panel consisting of CK, EMA, PLAP, PSA, leukocyte common antigen, and HMB-45 should be helpful. Additional markers, such as inhibin, CD30, and B- and T-cell antigens may be indicated based on the results of initial studies. A rare case of prostatic adenocarcinoma metastasizing to epididymis and mimicking adenomatoid tumor has been reported.[176] The correct

diagnosis was established by immunostaining for PAP and PSA.

Tumors of Adnexal Structures and External Genitals

ADENOMATOID TUMOR

Adenomatoid tumor is the most common benign tumor of the adnexal structures of the testis and represents 60% of the cases.[39] In a typical case, it consists of round, oval, or slit-like tubules lined by cuboidal or flattened cells. However, this mesothelial neoplasm is capable of displaying a wide variety of histologic patterns that may mimic sex cord–stromal tumors, signet-ring cell adenocarcinoma, malignant mesothelioma, and yolk sac tumor. Adenomatoid tumor reacts uniformly with antibodies to CK, EMA, and vimentin.[177, 178] CEA, Ber-EP4, B72.3, LeuM1, factor VIII–related antigen, and CD34 have been reported to be negative. Lack of immunoreactivity for vascular markers allows its distinction from histiocytoid hemangioma, a rare mimic arising in this location.[39, 179] Histiocytoid hemangioma reacts with antibodies to vimentin, factor VIII–related antigen, and *Ulex europaeus* I lectin but not CK or EMA. The distinction of adenomatoid tumor from malignant mesothelioma can be accomplished in most cases on the basis of gross and microscopic appearance. Large bulky tumor with poorly circumscribed margins and biphasic appearance on light microscopy is more likely to be malignant mesothelioma. The presence of cytologic atypia and a prominent papillary component also support mesothelioma. Some cases of adenomatoid tumor display a solid growth pattern with prominent eosinophilic cytoplasm and lack vacuoles, creating a resemblance to sex cord–stromal tumors. The features supporting the latter include abundant lipofuscin pigment, foamy cytoplasm, Reinke's crystalloids, strong immunoreactivity for inhibin, and negativity or weak positivity for CK. The immunoreactivity of adenomatoid tumors for antibodies against inhibin is unknown.

KEY DIAGNOSTIC POINTS

- Uniformly positive for CK, EMA, and vimentin
- Negative for CEA, Ber-EP4, B72.3, LeuM1, factor VIII–related antigen, and CD34
- Negative for vascular markers

EXTRAMAMMARY PAGET'S DISEASE

Extramammary Paget's disease may arise from intradermal apocrine cells and can be regarded as intraepidermal adenocarcinoma with potential for dermal invasion.[39] Many cases also arise secondary to pagetoid spread from underlying urogenital or colorectal malignancies.[180–182] Histologically, it consists of large vacuolated cells with pale eosinophilic cytoplasm in the basal portion of the epidermis. The main differential diagnostic considerations include melanoma and squamous cell carcinoma in situ. The tumor cells show immunoreactivity for CK, EMA, and CEA; S-100 protein and HMB-45 are absent.[182] The vacuolated cytoplasm also stains with mucicarmine and alcian blue.

MESOTHELIOMA

Malignant mesothelioma of tunica vaginalis is an extremely rare tumor that usually presents with hydrocele or a paratesticular mass.[183–185] The mean age at presentation is 53.5 years. The histologic features are similar to those encountered in the pleural and peritoneal cavities. In one study, eight of eight tumors were positive for CK, and four of five were positive for EMA and vimentin.[183] All tumors tested were negative for CEA, B72.3, LeuM1, and Ber-EP4. Calretinin, a calcium-binding protein, has been recognized as a specific marker of mesothelial differentiation and has been reported to be positive in 87.5 to 92% of cases tested in various studies.[186–188] The staining pattern is cytoplasmic and nuclear with or without intense membranous staining resulting in a characteristic "fried egg" appearance.[186] It also stains reactive mesothelial cells and other benign mesothelial proliferations. There are no significant differences between the immunohistochemical profiles of adenomatoid tumor and malignant mesothelioma.[184] The distinction is based largely on gross and light microscopic features. Thrombomodulin, CK5/CK6, and CD44H have also been found useful in distinguishing mesothelioma from metastatic adenocarcinoma, especially when involving pleura.[187]

DESMOPLASTIC SMALL ROUND CELL TUMOR

Desmoplastic small round cell tumor (DSRCT) typically occurs in the abdomen but may also present in the paratesticular region.[189, 190] It usually presents as a scrotal mass at a young age (mean 28 years) involving the paratesticular soft tissue, the tunica, or epididymis. The tumor is composed of nests and islands of small uniform cells divided into multiple nodules by desmoplastic stroma. They show immunohistochemical evidence of multilineage differentiation, including epithelial, mesenchymal, and neuronal features. The tumor cells are positive for CK, vimentin, desmin, and NSE, and negative for HBA-71. Three other tumors enter into the differential diagnosis of DSRCT: embryonal rhabdomyosarcoma, malignant lymphoma, and retinal anlage tumor; all are composed of "small round blue cells." Embryonal rhabdomyosarcoma has myxoid stroma and occurs at a much younger age. Rhabdomyoblasts with densely eosinophilic abundant cytoplasm and cross-striations, when present, are helpful in diagnosing rhabdomyosarcoma. Malignant lymphomas lack the nests and clusters formed by the tumor cells in DSRCT. They also lack the sclerotic stroma and the immunohistochemical profile of DSRCT. In challenging cases, reverse transcriptase–polymerase chain reaction analysis of paraffin sections for demonstration of EWS/WT1 chimeric mRNA is conclusive for DSRCT.[190]

RETINAL ANLAGE TUMOR

Retinal anlage tumor is a rare neoplasm that is known by a variety of names, including *melanotic neuroectodermal tumor* and *melanotic hemartoma*.[191–193] The typical patient is less than 1 year old and presents with involvement of maxilla or mandible. Rare cases involving epididymis have been reported.[193] There is one case report of melanotic neuroectodermal tumor arising as a major component of an immature testicular teratoma.[194] Histologically, it is composed of two cell populations: large columnar or cuboidal epithelial-like cells with vesicular nuclei and prominent nucleoli and a population of small neuroblast-like cells with scant cytoplasm and hyperchromatic nuclei. This tumor shows polyphenotypic differentiation with expression of epithelial and neural markers, melanin production, occasional glial markers, and rhabdomyoblastic markers.[192] Both cell populations are positive for NSE, synaptophysin, and HMB-45.[192] S-100 protein has been observed in the large cells. Immunoreactivity for EMA, glial fibrillary acidic protein, desmin, and Leu7 has been observed in a variable number of cases. The majority of large cells express CK and vimentin. The biologic behavior of this tumor is generally benign. Retinal anlage tumor may occasionally resemble DSRCT, a tumor with a more ominous prognosis. The distinction between the two is based on the presence of two cell types and melanin in the former. In difficult cases, especially when melanin pigment and the two cell populations are inconspicuous and the stroma is sclerotic, the presence of HMB-45 and S-100 immunoreactivity supports retinal anlage tumor.

Benign, Locally Aggressive, and Malignant Soft Tissue Tumors of the Testis

Virtually the entire spectrum of mesenchymal tumors has been observed mainly in the paratesticular soft tissues.[39] In rare cases, testicular parenchyma itself may be involved. Benign or locally aggressive soft tissue tumors reported in this region include leiomyoma, lipoma, lipoblastoma, rhabdomyoma, fibromas (excluding those of sex cord–stromal origin), capillary hemangioma, cavernous hemangioma, histiocytoid hemangioma, angiomyofibroblastoma, and aggressive angiomyxoma.[39, 195–197] The most common sarcoma arising in this region in adults is liposarcoma[198]; in children it is rhabdomyosarcoma.[199, 200] Leiomyosarcoma, malignant fibrous histiocytoma, rhabdoid tumor, and fibromatosis have also been reported. The histologic and immunohistochemical features of these soft tissue tumors are discussed elsewhere in this book.

References

1. Brown LM, Pottern LM, Hoover RN, et al. Testicular cancer in the United States: Trends in incidence and mortality. Int J Epidemiol 1986;15:164–170.
2. Muir C, Waterhouse J, Mack T, et al. Cancer incidence in five continents, vol 5. Lyon, France: International Agency for Research on Cancer, 1987.
3. Skakkebaek NE. Possible carcinoma-in-situ of the undescended testis. Lancet 1972;2:516–517.
4. Skakkebaek NE. Carcinoma-in-situ of the testis: Frequency and relationship to invasive germ cell tumors in infertile men. Histopathology 1978;2:157–170.
5. Berthelsen JG, Skakkebaek NE. Value of testicular biopsy in diagnosing carcinoma in situ of testis. Scand J Urol Nephrol 1981;15:165–168.
6. Muller J, Skakkebaek NE. Abnormal germ cells in maldescended testes: A study of cell density, nuclear size and deoxyribonucleic acid content in testicular biopsies from 50 boys. J Urol 1984;131:730–733.
7. Skakkebaek NE, Berthelsen JG, Giwercman A, Müller J. Carcinoma-in-situ of the testis: Possible origin from gonocytes and precursor of all types of germ cell tumours except spermatocytoma. Int J Androl 1987;10:19–28.
8. Fishman WH. Oncotrophoblast gene expression: Placental alkaline phosphatase. Adv Cancer Res 1987;48:1.
9. Fishman WH, Bardawil WA, Habib HG, et al. The placental isoenzyme of alkaline phosphatase in sera of normal pregnancy. Am J Clin Pathol 1972;57:65.
10. Fishman WH, Inglis NI, Stolbach LL, Krant MJ. A serum alkaline phosphatase isoenzyme of human neoplastic cell origin. Cancer Res 1968;28:150–154.
11. Benham F, Cotell DC, Franks LM, Wilson PD. Alkaline phosphatase activity in human bladder tumor cell lines. J Histochem Cytochem 1977;25:266–274.
12. Manivel JC, Jessurun J, Wick MR, Dehner LP. Placental alkaline phosphatase immunoreactivity in testicular germ-cell neoplasms. Am J Surg Pathol 1987;11:21–29.
13. Koshida K, Wahren B. Placental-like alkaline phosphatase in seminoma. Urol Res 1990;18:87–92.
14. Fishman WH, Inglis NR, Stolbach LL, Krant MJ. A serum alkaline phosphatase isoenzyme of human neoplastic cell origin. Cancer Res 1968;28:150.
15. Aguirre P, Scully RE, Dayal Y, DeLellis RA. Placenta-like alkaline phosphatase in germ cell tumors of the ovary and testis. [abstract] Lab Invest 1986;54:2A.
16. Javadpour N. The role of biologic tumor markers in testicular cancer. Cancer 1980;45:1755–1761.
17. Bosl GJ, Chaganti RSK. The use of tumor markers in germ cell malignancies. In: Tumor markers in adult solid malignancies. Hematol Oncol Clin North Am 1994;8:573–587.
18. Grossman BH. Tumor markers in urology. Semin Urol 1985;3:10–17.
19. Wilson RB, Albert A, Randall M. Quantitative studies on the production, destruction and elimination of chorionic gonadotrophin in normal pregnancy. Am J Obstet Gynecol 1949;58:960–967.
20. Horne CHW, Rankin R, Bremner RD. Pregnancy-specific proteins as markers for gestational trophoblastic disease. Int J Gynecol Pathol 1984;3:27–39.
21. Hussa RO. Human chorionic gonadotropin, a clinical marker: Review of its biosynthesis. Ligand Rev 1981;3:1.
22. Sherwood LM, Handwerger S, McLauren WD, Pang EC. Comparison of the structure and function of HPL and human GH. In: Pecile A, Muller EE, eds. Second International Symposium on Growth Hormone. Amsterdam: Excerpta Medica, 1971:8–9.
23. McCluggage WG, Shanks JH, Whiteside C, et al. Immunohistochemical study of testicular sex cord-stromal tumors, including staining with anti-inhibin antibody. Am J Surg Pathol 1998;22:615–619.
24. Roberts V, Meunier H, Sanchenko PE, Vale W. Differential production and regulation of inhibin subunits in rat testicular cell types. Endocrinology 1989;125:2350–2359.
25. McLachlan RI, Robertson DM, Burger HG, de Kretser DM. Circulating immunoreactive inhibin levels during the normal menstrual cycle. J Clin Endocrinol Metab 1987;65:954–961.
26. Arora DS, Cooke IE, Ganesan TS, et al. Immunohistochemical expression of inhibin/activin subunits in epithelial and granulosa cell tumors of the ovary. J Pathol 1997;181:413–418.
27. Flemming P, Wellmann A, Maschek H, Lang H, et al. Monoclonal antibodies against inhibin represent key markers of adult granulosa tumors of the ovary even in their metastases. Am J Surg Pathol 1995;19:927–933.
28. McCluggage WG, Maxwell P, Sloan JM. Immunohistochemical staining of ovarian granulosa cell tumors with monoclonal antibody against inhibin. Hum Pathol 1997;28:1034–1038.
29. Rishi M, Howard L, Bratthauer GL, Tavassoli F. Use of monoclonal antibody against inhibin as a marker for sex cord-stromal tumors of the ovary. Am J Surg Pathol 1997;21:583–589.
30. Stewart CJR, Jeffers MD, Kennedy A. Diagnostic value of inhibin immunoreactivity in ovarian gonadal stromal tumors and their histological mimics. Histopathology 1997;31:67–74.
31. Iczkowski KA, Bostwick DG, Roche PC, Cheville JC. Inhibin A is a sensitive and specific marker for testicular sex cord-stromal tumors. Mod Pathol 1998;11:774–779.
32. McCluggage WG, Shanks JH, Whiteside C, et al. Immunohistochemical study of testicular sex cord-stromal tumors, including staining with anti-inhibin antibody. Am J Surg Pathol 1998;22:615–619.
33. Amin MB, Young RH, Scully RE. Immunohistochemical profile of Sertoli and Leydig cell tumors of the testis. [abstract] Mod Pathol 1998;11:78A.
34. McCluggage WB, Ashe P, McBride H, et al. Localization of the cellular expression of inhibin in trophoblastic tissue. Histopathology 1998;32:252–256.
35. Pelkey TJ, Frierson HF Jr, Mills SE, Stoler MH. Detection of the alpha-subunit of inhibin in trophoblastic neoplasia. Hum Pathol 1999;30:26–31.
36. Minami S, Yamoto M, Nakano R. Immunohistochemical localization of inhibin/activin subunits in human placenta. Obstet Gynecol 1992;80:410–414.
37. Minami S, Yamoto M, Nakano R. Immunohistochemical localization of inhibin/activin subunits in hydatidiform mole and invasive mole. Obstet Gynecol 1993;82:414–418.
38. Skakkebaek NE, Berthelsen JG, Muller J. Carcinoma-in-situ of the undescended testis. Urol Clin North Am 1982;9:377.
39. Ulbright TM, Amin MB, Young RH. Tumors of the testis, adnexa, spermatic cord, and scrotum. Washington, D.C.: Armed Forces Institute of Pathology Fascicle 25, 1999:41–58.
40. Beckstead JH. Alkaline phosphatase histochemistry in human germ cell neoplasms. Am J Surg Pathol 1983;7:341–349.
41. Jacobsen GK, Norgaard-Pedersen B. Placental alkaline phosphatase in testicular germ cell tumors and carcinoma-in-situ of the testis: An immunohistochemical study. Acta Pathol Microbiol Immunol Scand (A) 1984;92:323–329.

42. Manivel JC, Jessurun J, Wick MR, Dehner LP. Placental alkaline phosphatase immunoreactivity in testicular germ cell tumors. Am J Surg Pathol 1987;11:21–29.

43. Burke AP, Mostofi FK. Intratubular malignant germ cells in testicular biopsies: Clinical course and identification by staining for placental alkaline phosphatase. Mod Pathol 1988;1:475–479.

44. Jacobsen GK, Jacobsen M. Alpha-fetoprotein (AFP) and human chorionic gonadotropin (HCG) in testicular germ cell tumors: A prospective immunohistochemical study. Acta Pathol Microbiol Scand 1983;91:165–176.

45. Jacobsen GK, Jacobsen M, Claussen PP, et al. Immunohistochemical demonstration of tumor-associated antigens in carcinoma-in-situ of the testis. Int J Androl 1981;4(Suppl):203.

46. Sigg C, Hedinger C. Atypical germ cells of the testis: Comparative, ultrastructural and histochemical investigations. Virchows Arch 1984;402:439.

47. Jacobsen GK, Jacobsen M, Praetorius C. Ferritin as a possible marker protein of carcinoma-in-situ of the testis. Lancet 1980;2:533–534.

48. Jacobsen GK, Jacobsen M. Ferritin in testicular germ cell tumors: An immunohistochemical study. Acta Pathol Microbiol Immunol Scand (A) 1983;91:177–181.

49. Coffin CM, Ewing S, Dehner LP. Frequency of the intratubular germ cell neoplasia with invasive testicular germ cell tumors: Histologic and immunocytochemical features. Arch Pathol Lab Med 1985;109:555–559.

50. Kang JL, Meyts E, Skakkebaek NE. Immunoreactive neuron-specific enolase is expressed in testicular carcinoma-in-situ. J Pathol 1996;178:161–165.

51. Kuczyk MA, Serth J, Bokemeyer C, et al. Overexpression of the p53 oncoprotein in carcinoma-in-situ of the testis. Pathol Res Pract 1994;190:993–998.

52. Kuczyk MA, Serth J, Bokemeyer C, et al. Alterations in the p53 tumor suppressor gene in carcinoma-in-situ of the testis. Cancer 1996;78:1958–1966.

53. Giwercman A, Andrews PW, Jorgensen N, et al. Immunohistochemical expression of embryonal marker TRA-1-60 in carcinoma-in-situ and germ cell tumors of the testis. Cancer 1993;72:1308–1314.

54. Giwercman A, Lindenberg S, Kimber SJ, et al. Monoclonal antibody 43-9-F as a sensitive immunohistochemical marker of carcinoma-in-situ of human testis. Cancer 1990;65:1135–1142.

55. Rajpert-De Meyts E, Kvist M, Skakkebaek NE. Heterogeneity of expression of immunohistochemical tumor markers in testicular carcinoma-in-situ: Pathogenetic relevance. Virchows Arch 1996;428:133–139.

56. Drescher B, Lauke H, Hartmann M, et al. Immunohistochemical pattern of insulin-like growth factor (IGF) I, IGF II and IGF-binding proteins 1 to 6 in carcinoma-in-situ of the testis. Mol Pathol 1997;50:298–303.

57. Giwercman A, Cantell L, Marks A. Placental-like alkaline phosphatase as a marker of carcinoma-in-situ of the testis: Comparison with monoclonal antibodies M2A and 43-9F. APMIS 1991;99:586–594.

58. Jorgensen N, Giwercman A, Muller J, Skakkebaek NE. Immunohistochemical markers of carcinoma-in-situ of the testis are also expressed in normal infantile germ cells. Histopathology 1993;22:373–378.

59. Klys HS, Whillis D, Howard G, Harrison DJ. Glutathione-S-transferase expression in the human testis and testicular germ cell neoplasia. Br J Cancer 1992;66:589–593.

60. Kang JL, Rajpert-De Meyts E, Wiels J, Skakkebaek NE. Expression of the glycolipid globotriaosylceramide (Gb3) in testicular carcinoma-in-situ. Virchows Arch 1995;426:369–374.

61. Mostofi FK, Sesterhenn IA. Pathology of germ cell tumors of testes. Prog Clin Biol Res 1985;203:1–34.

62. Mostofi FK, Spaander P, Grigor K, et al. Consensus on pathological classifications of testicular tumors. Prog Clin Biol Res 1990;357:267.

63. Rustin GJS, Vogelzand NJ, Sleijfer DT, et al. Consensus statement on circulating tumor markers and staging patients with germ cell tumors. Prog Clin Biol Res 1990;357:277.

64. Manivel JC, Jesserun J, Wick MR, Dehner LP. Placental alkaline phosphatase immunoreactivity in testicular germ cell neoplasms. Am J Surg Pathol 1987;11:21–29.

65. Wick MR, Swanson PE, Manivel JC. Placental alkaline-like phosphatase reactivity in human tumors. Hum Pathol 1987;18:946–954.

66. Niehans GA, Manival JC, Copland GT, et al. Immunohistochemistry of germ cell and trophoblastic neoplasms. Cancer 1988;62:1113–1123.

67. Bosman FT, Giard RW, Kruseman AC, et al. Human chorionic gonadotropin and alpha-fetoprotein in testicular germ cell tumors: A retrospective immunohistochemical study. Histopathology 1980;4:673–684.

68. Jacobsen GK, Jacobsen M. Alpha-fetoprotein (AFP) and human chorionic gonadotropin in testicular germ cell tumors: A prospective immunohistochemical study. Acta Pathol Microbiol Scand (A) 1983;91:165–176.

69. von Hochstetter AR, Sigg C, Saremaslani P, et al. The significance of giant cells in human testicular seminomas: A clinicopathological study. Virchows Arch A Pathol Anat Histopathol 1985;407:309–322.

70. Ferreiro JA. Ber-H2 expression in testicular germ cell tumors. Hum Pathol 1994;25:522–524.

71. Hittmair A, Rogatsch H, Hobisch A, et al. CD30 expression in seminoma. Hum Pathol 1996;27:1166–1171.

72. Pallesen G, Hamilton-Dutoit SJ. Ki-1 (CD30) antigen is regularly expressed in tumor cells of embryonal carcinoma. Am J Pathol 1988;133:446–450.

73. Iczkowski KA, Bostwick DG, Roche PC, et al. Inhibin A is a sensitive and specific marker for testicular sex cord-stromal tumors. Mod Pathol 1998;11:774.

74. Eglen DE, Ulbright TM. The differential diagnosis of cytokeratin, alpha-fetoprotein, and alpha-1-antitrypsin immunoperoxidase reactions. Am J Surg Pathol 1987;88:328.

75. Miettinen M, Virtanen I, Talerman A. Intermediate filament proteins in human testis and testicular germ cell tumors. Am J Surg Pathol 1985;120:402.

76. Rao S, Iczkowski KA, Cheville JC. Cytokeratin expression in seminoma and embryonal carcinoma of the testis. [abstract] Mod Pathol 1998;11:92A.

77. Cheville JC, Rao S, Iczkowski KA, et al. Cytokeratin expression in seminoma of the human testis. Am J Clin Pathol 2000;113:583–588.

78. Moll F, Franke WW, Schiller DR, et al. The catalog of human cytokeratins: Patterns of expression in normal epithelia, tumors, and cultured cells. Cell 1982;31:11–14.

79. Denk H, Moll R, Weybora W, et al. Intermediate filaments and desmosomal plaque proteins in testicular seminomas and non-seminomatous germ cell tumors as revealed by immunohistochemistry. Virchows Arch A Pathol Anat Histopathol 1987;410:295–307.

80. Bartkova J, Rejthar A, Bartek J, Kovarik J. Differentiation patterns in testicular germ cell tumors as revealed by a panel of monoclonal antibodies. Tumor Biol 1987;49:196–202.

81. Fogel M, Lifschitz-Mercer B, Moll R, et al. Heterogeneity of intermediate filament expression in human testicular seminomas. Differentiation 1990;45:242–249.

82. Murakami SS, Said JW. Immunohistochemical localization of lactate dehydrogenase isoenzyme 1 in the germ cell tumors of the testis. Am J Clin Pathol 1984;81:293–296.

83. Przygodzki RM, Moran CA, Suster S, et al. Primary mediastinal and testicular seminomas: A comparison of K-ras-2 gene sequence and p53 immunoperoxidase analysis of 26 cases. Hum Pathol 1996;27:975–979.

84. Suster S, Moran CA, Dominguez-Malagon H, Quevedo-Blanco P. Germ cell tumors of the mediastinum and testis: A comparative immunohistochemical study of 120 cases. Hum Pathol 1998;29:737–742.

85. Suzuki T, Sasano H, Aoki H, et al. Immunohistochemical comparison between anaplastic seminoma and typical seminoma. Acta Pathol Jpn 1993;43:751–757.

86. Talerman A. Spermatocytic seminoma: A clinicopathologic study of 22 cases. Cancer 1980;45:2169–2176.
87. Ramaekers F, Feitz W, Moesker O, et al. Antibodies to cytokeratin and vimentin in testicular tumor diagnosis. Virchows Arch A Pathol Anat Histopathol 1985;408:127–142.
88. Eble JN. Spermatocytic seminoma. Hum Pathol 1994;25:1035–1042.
89. Burke AP, Mostofi FK. Spermatocytic seminoma, a clinicopathologic study of 79 cases. J Urol Pathol 1993;1:21–32.
90. Albores-Saavedra J, Huffman H, Alvarado-Cabrero I, et al. Anaplastic variant of spermatocytic seminoma. Hum Pathol 1996;27:650–655.
91. Dekker I, Rozeboom T, Delemarre J, et al. Placental-like alkaline phosphatase and DNA flow cytometry in spermatocytic seminoma. Cancer 1992;69:993–996.
92. Cummings OW, Ulbright TM, Eble JN, et al. Spermatocytic seminoma: An immunohistochemical study. Hum Pathol 1994;25:54–59.
93. Kraggerud SM, Berner A, Bryne M, et al. Spermatocytic seminoma as compared to classical seminoma: An immunohistochemical and DNA flow cytometric study. APMIS 1999;107:297–302.
94. Battifora H, Sheibani K, Tubbs RR, et al. Antikeratin antibodies in tumor diagnosis: Distinction between seminoma and embryonal carcinoma. Cancer 1984;54:843–848.
95. Lifschitz-Mercer B, Fogel M, Moll R, et al. Intermediate filament protein profiles of human testicular non-seminomatous germ cell tumors: Correlation of cytokeratin synthesis to cell differentiation. Differentiation 1991;48:191–198.
96. Stiller D, Bahn H, Pressler H. Immunohistochemical demonstration of alpha-fetoprotein in testicular germ cell tumors. Acta Histochem Suppl 1986;33:225–231.
97. Bartkova J, Bartek J, Lukas J, et al. p53 protein alterations in human testicular cancer including preinvasive intratubular germ cell neoplasia. Int J Cancer 1991;49:196–202.
98. Visfeldt J, Giwercman A, Skakkebaek NE. Monoclonal antibody 43-9F: An immunohistochemical marker of embryonal carcinoma of the testis. APMIS 1992;100:63–70.
99. Ulbright TM, Orazi A, de Riese W, et al. The correlation of p53 protein expression with proliferative activity and occult metastases in clinical stage I non-seminomatous germ cell tumors of the testis. Mod Pathol 1994;7:64–68.
100. Brown NJ. Yolk-sac tumour ("orchioblastoma") and other testicular tumours of childhood. In: Pugh RC, ed. Pathology of the testis. Oxford: Blackwell Scientific, 1976:356–370.
101. von Hochstetter AR, Hedinger CE. The differential diagnosis of testicular germ cell tumors in theory and in practice: A critical analysis of two major systems of classification and review of 389 cases. Virchows Arch A Pathol Anat Histopathol 1982;396:247.
102. Talerman A. Endodermal sinus (yolk sac) tumor elements in testicular germ cell tumors in adults: Comparison of prospective and retrospective studies. Cancer 1980;46:1213.
103. Talerman A, Haije WG, Baggerman L. Histological patterns in germ cell tumors associated with raised serum alpha fetoprotein (AFP). Scand J Immunol Suppl 1978;8:97.
104. Talerman A, Haije WG, Baggerman L. Serum alpha fetoprotein (AFP) in patients with germ cell tumors of the gonads and extragonadal sites: Correlation between endodermal sinus (yolk sac) tumor and raised serum AFP. Cancer 1980;46:380.
105. Mostofi FK, Sesterhenn IA, Davis CJ Jr. Immunopathology of germ cell tumors of the testis. Semin Diagn Pathol 1987;4:320–341.
106. Wold LE, Kramer SA, Farrow GM. Testicular yolk sac and embryonal carcinomas in pediatric patients: Comparative immunohistochemical and clinicopathologic study. Am J Clin Pathol 1984;81:427.
107. Burke AP, Mostofi FK. Placental alkaline phosphatase immunohistochemistry of intratubular malignant germ cells and associated testicular germ cell tumors. Hum Pathol 1988;19:663–670.
108. Jacobsen GK, Jacobsen M, Clausen PP. Distribution of tumor-associated antigens in the various histologic components of germ cell tumors of the testis. Am J Surg Pathol 1981;5:257–266.
109. Ulbright TM, Roth LM, Brodhecker CA. Yolk sac differentiation in germ cell tumors: A morphologic study of 50 cases with emphasis on hepatic, enteric and parietal yolk sac features. Am J Surg Pathol 1986;10:151–164.
110. Visfeldt J, Jorgensen N, Muller J, et al. Testicular germ cell tumors of childhood in Denmark 1943–1989: Incidence and evaluation of histology using immunohistochemical techniques. J Pathol 1994;174:39–47.
111. Ulbright TM, Amin MB, Young RH. Tumors of the testis, adnexa, spermatic cord, and scrotum: Atlas of Tumor Pathology, 3rd Series, Fascicle 25. Washington, D.C.: Armed Forces Institute of Pathology, 1999.
112. Manivel JC, Niehans G, Wick MR, Dehner LP. Intermediate trophoblast in germ cell neoplasms. Am J Surg Pathol 1987;11:693–701.
113. Clark RK, Damjanov I. Intermediate filaments of human trophoblast and choriocarcinoma cell lines. Virchows Arch A Pathol Anat Histopathol 1985;407:203–208.
114. Lind HM, Haghighi P. Carcinoembryonic antigen staining in choriocarcinoma. Am J Clin Pathol 1986;86:538–540.
115. Ulbright TM, Young RH, Scully RE. Trophoblastic tumors of the testis other than classic choriocarcinoma: "Monophasic" choriocarcinoma and placental site trophoblastic tumor: A report of two cases. Am J Surg Pathol 1997;21:282–288.
116. Brosman SA. Testicular tumors in prepubertal children. Urology 1979;13:581–588.
117. Grady RW, Ross JH, Kay R. Epidemiological features of testicular teratomas in prepubertal population. J Urol 1997;158:1191–1192.
118. Kay R. Prepubertal testicular tumor registry. J Urol 1993;150:671–674.
119. Barsky SH. Germ cell tumors of the testis. In: Javadpour N, Barsky SH, eds. Surgical Pathology of Urologic Diseases. Baltimore: Williams & Wilkins, 1987:224–246.
120. Leibovitch I, Foster RS, Ulbright TM, Donohue JP. Adult primary pure teratoma of the testis: The Indiana experience. Cancer 1995;75:2244–2250.
121. Simmonds PD, Lee AH, Theaker JM, et al. Primary pure teratoma of the testis. J Urol 1996;155:939–942.
122. Stevens MJ, Normal AR, Fisher C, et al. Prognosis of testicular teratoma differentiated. Br J Urol 1994;73:701–706.
123. Jorgensen N, Muller J, Giwercman A, et al. DNA content and expression of tumour markers in germ cells adjacent to germ cell tumours in childhood: Probably a different origin for infantile and adolescent germ cell tumors. J Pathol 1995;176:269–278.
124. Mostofi FK. Testicular tumors: Epidemiologic, etiologic and pathologic features. Cancer 1973;32:1186.
125. Mostofi FK, Sesterhenn IA, Davis DJ. Developments in histopathology of testicular germ cell tumors. Semin Urol 1988;6:171.
126. Kim I, Young RH, Scully RE. Leydig cell tumors of the testis: A clinicopathologic study of 40 cases and review of the literature. Am J Surg Pathol 1985;9:177.
127. Seidman JD, Abbondanzo SL, Bratthauer GL. Lipid cell (steroid cell) tumor of the ovary: Immunophenotype with analysis of potential pitfall due to endogenous biotin-like activity. Int J Gynecol Pathol 1995;14:331–338.
128. Billings SD, Roth LM, Ulbright TM. Microcystic Leydig cell tumors mimicking yolk sac tumor: A report of four cases. Am J Surg Pathol 1999;23:546–551.
129. Cheville JC, Sebo TJ, Lager DG, et al. Leydig cell tumor of the testis: A clinicopathologic, DNA content, and MIB-1 comparison of nonmetastasizing and metastasizing tumors. Am J Surg Pathol 1998;22:1361–1367.
130. Middendorff R, Davidoff MS, Mayer H, Holstein AF. Neuroendocrine characteristics of human Leydig cell tumors. Andrologia 1995;27:351–355.

131. Young RH, Koelliker DD, Scully RE. Sertoli cell tumors of the testis, not otherwise specified: A clinicopathologic analysis of 60 cases. Am J Surg Pathol 1998;22:709–721.

132. Zukerberg LR, Young RH, Scully RE. Sclerosing Sertoli cell tumor of the testis: A report of 10 cases. Am J Surg Pathol 1991;15:829–834.

133. Gilcrease MZ, Delgado R, Albores-Saavedra J. Testicular Sertoli cell tumor with a heterologus sarcomatous component: Immunohistochemical assessment of Sertoli cell differentiation. Arch Pathol Lab Med 1998;122:907–911.

134. Cano-Valdez AM, Chanona-Vilchis J, Dominguez-Malagon H. Large cell calcifying Sertoli cell tumor of the testis: A clinicopathological, immunohistochemical, and ultrastructural study of two cases. Ultrastruct Pathol 1999;23:259–265.

135. Plata C, Algaba F, Andujar M, et al. Large cell calcifying sertoli cell tumor of the testis. Histopathology 1995;26:255–259.

136. Kratzer SS, Ulbright TM, Talerman A, et al. Large cell calcifying Sertoli cell tumor of the testis: Contrasting features of six malignant and six benign tumors and a review of the literature. Am J Surg Pathol 1997;21:1271–1280.

137. Bufo P, Pennella A, Serio G, et al. Malignant large cell calcifying Sertoli cell tumor of the testis: Report of a case in an elderly man and review of the literature. Pathologica 1999;91:107–114.

138. Lawrence WD, Young RH, Scully RE: Juvenile granulosa cell tumor of the infantile testis: A report of 14 cases. Am J Surg Pathol 1985;9:87.

139. Groisman GM, Dische MR, Fine EM, Unger PD. Juvenile granulosa cell tumor of the testis: A comparative immunohistochemical study with normal infantile gonads. Pediatr Pathol 1993;13:389–400.

140. Perez-Atayde AR, Joste N, Mulhern H. Juvenile granulosa cell tumor of the infantile testis: Evidence of a dual epithelial–smooth muscle differentiation. Am J Surg Pathol 1996;20:72–79.

141. Talerman A. Pure granulosa cell tumor of the testis: Report of a case and review of the literature. Appl Pathol 1985;3:117.

142. Jiminez-Quintero LP, Ro JY, Zavala-Pompa A, et al. Granulosa cell tumor of the adult testis: A clinicopathologic study of seven cases and a review of the literature. Hum Pathol 1993;24:1120–1125.

143. Morgan DR, Brame KG. Granulosa cell tumor of the testis displaying immunoreactivity for inhibin. BJU Int 1999;83:731–732.

144. Renshaw AA, Gordon M, Corless CL. Immunohistochemistry of unclassified sex cord-stromal tumors of the testis with a predominance of spindle cells. Mod Pathol 1997;10:693–700.

145. Nistal M, Martinez-Garcia C, Paniagua R. Testicular fibroma. J Urol 1992;147:1617–1619.

146. Jones MA, Young RH, Scully RE. Benign fibromatous tumors of the testis and paratesticular region: A report of 9 cases with a proposed classification of fibromatous tumors and tumor-like lesions. Am J Surg Pathol 1997;21:296–305.

147. Kommoss F, Oliva E, Bhan AK, et al. Inhibin expression in ovarian tumors and tumor-like lesions: An immunohistochemical study. Mod Pathol 1998;11:656–664.

148. Jorgensen N, Muller J, Jaubert F, Clausen OP, et al. Heterogeneity of gonadoblastoma germ cells: Similarities with immature germ cells, spermatogonia and testicular carcinoma in situ cells. Histopathology 1997;30:177–186.

149. Roth LM, Eglen DE. Gonadoblastoma: Immunohistochemical and ultrastructural observations. Int J Gynecol Pathol 1989;8:72–81.

150. Hussong J, Crussi FG, Chou PM. Gonadoblastoma: Immunohistochemical localization of müllerian-inhibiting substance, inhibin, WT-1, and p53. Mod Pathol 1997;10:1101–1105.

151. Carano KS, Soslow RA. Immunophenotypic analysis of ovarian and testicular müllerian papillary serous tumors. Mod Pathol 1997;10:414–420.

152. Jones MA, Young RH, Srigley JR, Scully RE. Paratesticular serous papillary carcinoma: A report of six cases. Am J Surg Pathol 1995;19:1359–1365.

153. Caccamo D, Social M, Truchet C. Malignant Brenner tumor of the testis and epididymis. Arch Pathol Lab Med 1991;115:524–527.

154. Elbadawi A, Batchvarov MM, Linke CA. Intratesticular papillary mucinous cystadenocarcinoma. Urology 1970;26:853–865.

155. Young RH, Scully RE. Testicular and paratesticular tumors and tumor-like lesions of ovarian common epithelium and mullerian types: A report of 4 cases and review of the literature. Am J Clin Pathol 1986;86:146–152.

156. Zavala-Pompa A, Ro JY, el-Naggar A, et al. Primary carcinoid tumor of testis: Immunohistochemical, ultrastructural, and DNA flow cytometric study of three cases with a review of the literature. Cancer 1993;72:1726–1732.

157. Kim HJ, Cho MY, Park YN, Kie JH. Primary carcinoid tumor of the testis: Immunohistochemical, ultrastructural and DNA flow cytometric study of two cases. J Korean Med Sci 1999;14:57–62.

158. Miliauskas JR. Carcinoid tumor occurring in a mature testicular teratoma. Pathology 1991;23:72–74.

159. Ferry JA, Harris NL, Young RH, et al. Malignant lymphoma of the testis, epididymis, and spermatic cord: A clinicopathological study of 69 cases with immunophenotypic analysis. Am J Surg Pathol 1994;18:376–390.

160. Ferry JA, Ulbright TM, Young RH. Anaplastic large cell lymphoma of the testis: A lesion that may be confused with embryonal carcinoma. J Urol Pathol 1996;5:139–147.

161. Akhtar M, Al-Dayel F, Siegrist K, Ezzat A. Neutrophil-rich Ki-1-positive anaplastic large cell lymphoma presenting as a testicular mass. Mod Pathol 1996;9:812–815.

162. Hsueh C, Gonzalez-Crussi F, Murphy SB. Testicular angiocentric lymphoma of post-thymic T-cell type in a child with T-cell acute lymphoblastic leukemia in remission. Cancer 1993;72:1801–1805.

163. Guler G, Altinok G, Uner AH, Sungur A. CD56+ lymphoma presenting as a testicular tumor. Leuk Lymphoma 1999;36:207–211.

164. Levin HS, Mostofi FK. Symptomatic plasmacytoma of the testis. Cancer 1970;25:1193–1203.

165. Chica G, Johnson DE, Ayala AG. Plasmacytoma of testis presenting as primary testicular tumor. Urology 1978;11:90–92.

166. Ferry JA, Young RH, Scully RE. Testicular and epididymal plasmacytoma: A report of 7 cases, including three that were the initial manifestation of plasma cell myeloma. Am J Surg Pathol 1997;21:590–598.

167. Gutjahr P, Humpl T. Testicular lymphoblastic leukemia/lymphoma. World J Urol 1995;13:230–232.

168. Givler RL. Testicular involvement in leukemia and lymphoma. Cancer 1969;23:1290–1295.

169. Ferry JA, Srigley JR, Young RH. Granulocytic sarcoma of the testis: A report of two cases of a neoplasm prone to misinterpretation. Mod Pathol 1997;10:320–325.

170. Economopoulos T, Alexopoulos C, Anagnostou D, et al. Primary granulocytic sarcoma of the testis. Leukemia 1994;8:199–200.

171. Neiman RS, Barcos M, Berard C, et al. Granulocytic sarcoma: A clinicopathologic study of 61 biopsied cases. Cancer 1981;48:1426–1437.

172. Pater SR, Richardson RL, Kvols L. Metastatic cancer to the testes: A report of 20 cases and review of the literature. J Urol 1989;142:1003–1005.

173. Haupt HM, Mann RB, Trump DL, Abeloff MD. Metastatic carcinoma involving the testis: Clinical and pathologic distinction from primary testicular neoplasms. Cancer 1984;54:709–714.

174. Meacham RB, Mata JA, Espada R, et al. Testicular metastasis as the first manifestation of colon carcinoma. J Urol 1988;140:621–622.

175. Johansson JE, Lannes P. Metastases to the spermatic cord, epididymis and testicles from carcinoma of the prostate—five cases. Scand J Urol Nephrol 1983;17:249–251.

176. Rizk CC, Scholes J, Chen SK, et al. Epididymal metastasis from prostatic adenocarcinoma mimicking adenomatoid tumor. Urology 1990;36:526–530.
177. Detassis C, Pusiol T, Piscioli F, Luciani F. Adenomatoid tumor of the epididymis: Immunohistochemical study of 8 cases. Urol Int 1986;41:232–234.
178. Delahunt B, Eble JN, King D, et al. Immunohistochemical evidence for mesothelial origin of paratesticular adenomatoid tumor. Histopathology 2000;36:109–115.
179. Banks ER, Mills SE. Histiocytoid (epithelioid) hemangioma of the testis: The so-called vascular variant of "adenomatoid tumor." Am J Surg Pathol 1990;14:584–589.
180. Hoch WH. Adenocarcinoma of the scrotum (extramammary Paget's disease): Case report and review of the literature. J Urol 1984;132:137–139.
181. Koh KB, Nazarina AR. Paget's disease of the scrotum: Report of a case with underlying carcinoma of the prostate. Br J Dermatol 1995;133:306–307.
182. Ordonez NG, Awalt H, Mackay B. Mammary and extramammary Paget's disease: An immunocytochemical and ultrastructural study. Cancer 1987;59:1173–1183.
183. Jones MA, Young RH, Scully RE. Malignant mesothelioma of the tunica vaginalis: A clinicopathologic analysis of 11 cases with review of the literature. Am J Surg Pathol 1995;19:815–825.
184. Moch H, Ohnacker H, Epper R, et al. A new case of malignant mesothelioma of the tunica vaginalis testis: Immunohistochemistry in comparison with an adenomatoid tumor of the testis. Pathol Res Pract 1994;190:400–404.
185. Kamiya M, Eimoto T. Malignant mesothelioma of the tunica vaginalis. Pathol Res Pract 1990;186:680–684.
186. Chhieng DC, Yee H, Schaefer D, et al. Calretinin staining pattern aids in the differentiation of mesothelioma from adenocarcinoma in serous effusions. Cancer 2000;90:194–200.
187. Cury PM, Butcher DN, Fisher C, et al. Value of the mesothelium-associated antibodies thrombomodulin, cytokeratin 5/6, calretinin, and CD44H in distinguishing epithelioid pleural mesothelioma from adenocarcinoma metastatic to the pleura. Mod Pathol 2000;13:107–112.
188. Doglioni C, Dei Tos AP, Laurino L, et al. Calretinin: A novel immunocytochemical marker for mesothelioma. Am J Surg Pathol 1996;20:1037–1046.
189. Cummings OW, Ulbright TM, Young RH, et al. Desmoplastic small round cell tumors of the paratesticular region: A report of six cases. Am J Surg Pathol 1997;21:219–225.
190. Kawano N, Inayama Y, Nagashima Y, et al. Desmoplastic small round-cell tumor of the paratesticular region: Report of an adult case with demonstration of EWS and WT1 gene fusion using paraffin-embedded tissue. Mod Pathol 1999;12:729–734.
191. Johnson RE, Scheithauer BW, Dahlin DC. Melanotic neuroectodermal tumor of infancy: A review of seven cases. Cancer 1983;52:661–666.
192. Pettinato G, Manivel JC, d'Amore ES, et al. Melanotic neuroectodermal tumor of infancy: A reexamination of histogenetic problem based on immunohistochemical, ultrastructural, and flow cytometric study of 10 cases. Am J Surg Pathol 1991;15:233–245.
193. Jurincic-Winkler C, Metz KA, Klippel KF. Melanotic neuroectodermal tumor of infancy (MNTI) in the epididymis: A case report with immunohistological studies and special consideration of malignant features. Zentrabl Pathol 1994;140:181–185.
194. Anagnostaki L, Krag JG, Horn T, et al. Melanotic neuroectodermal as a predominant component of an immature testicular teratoma: Case report with immunohistochemical investigations. APMIS 1992;100:809–816.
195. Ulbright TM. Neoplasms of the testis. In: Bostwick DG, Eble JN, eds. Urologic Surgical Pathology. St. Louis: CV Mosby, 1997.
196. Lioe TF, Biggart JD. Tumors of the spermatic cord and paratesticular tissue: A clinicopathological study. Br J Urol 1993;71:600–606.
197. Srigley JR, Hartwick RW. Tumors and cysts of the paratesticular region. Pathol Annu 1990;25:51–108.
198. Schwartz SL, Swierzewski SJ III, Sondak VK, Grossman HB. Liposarcoma of the spermatic cord: Report of 6 cases and review of the literature. J Urol 1995;153:154–157.
199. Leuschner I, Newton WA Jr, Schmidt D, et al. Spindle cell variants of embryonal rhabdomyosarcoma in the paratesticular region: A report of the Intergroup Rhabdomyosarcoma Study. Am J Surg Pathol 1993;17:221–230.
200. Loughlin KR, Retik AB, Weinstein JT, et al. Genitourinary rhabdomyosarcoma in children. Cancer 1989;63:1600–1606.

Immunohistochemistry of Kidney Tumors

Junqi Qian, M.D., Dharamdas M. Ramnani, M.D., and David G. Bostwick, M.D.

There is a wide variety of benign and malignant neoplasms in the kidney, many of which pose a diagnostic challenge to the pathologist. The most common tumors in the kidney are RCC in adults and nephroblastoma (Wilms' tumor) in children.

RENAL CELL TUMORS IN ADULTS

Renal Cell Carcinoma

Renal cell carcinoma (RCC) is the third most common genitourinary neoplasm. In the United States, it is estimated that 31,200 new cases of kidney cancer will be diagnosed in the year 2000, resulting in approximately 11,900 deaths. There is a two- to threefold male predominance of this disease; no obvious racial predilection has been noted. The peak age is in the fifth and sixth decades of life, and it is rare under the age of 35 years.[1] Table 14–14 summarizes the classification of renal epithelial tumors.[2–4]

Table 14–14. Classification of Renal Epithelial Tumors

World Health Organization (1981)	World Health Organization (1998)
Renal cell adenoma (RCA)	
RCA, metanephric type	Metanephric adenoma
RCA, papillary type (chromophil)	Tubule papillary adenoma
RCA, oncocytic type	Oncocytic adenoma
Renal cell carcinoma (RCC)	
RCC, clear cell type	Clear cell carcinoma
RCC, papillary type (chromophil)	Papillary carcinoma
RCC, chromophobe type	Chromophobe carcinoma
RCC, collecting duct type	Collecting duct carcinoma
RCC, neuroendocrine type	Granular cell carcinoma
RCC, unclassified	Spindle cell carcinoma
	Cyst-associated RCC

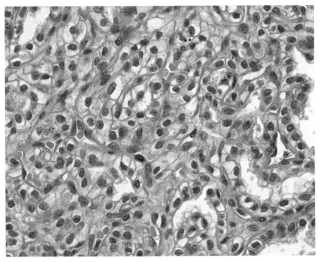

Figure 14-33. Clear cell renal cell carcinoma (RCC); the cytoplasm of the clear cell type appears clear and empty.

high molecular weight keratin (34βE12, CK19),[18-20] CEA,[21] S-100 protein,[7, 22] HMB-45,[21] and inhibin.[23, 24]

The positive rate of these markers varies in different studies. For example, Medeiros and associates found 48 of 55 RCCs expressed keratins. CAM5.2 stained 46 tumors (84%) and AE1 stained 37 neoplasms (67%). AE1 reacted with two CAM5.2− tumors. EMA was expressed by 35 carcinomas (64%), including 3 of the CAM5.2− neoplasms. Vimentin was expressed by 26 tumors (47%), and S-100 was expressed by one.[25, 26]

When there is difficulty diagnosing metastatic RCC, urothelial cell carcinoma, or other tumors, the immunohistochemical findings can assist in the differential diagnosis. Urothelial cell carcinoma was positive for all the cytokeratins and CEA and was negative for vimentin. Paragangliomas were positive for chromogranin and showed scattered positivity for the S-100 protein in the sustentacular

CONVENTIONAL (CLEAR CELL) RENAL CELL CARCINOMA

The most common type of renal cell carcinoma is clear cell renal cell carcinoma (RCC).[2-4] Clear cell RCCs are characterized by multinodular and multicolored tumor mass, with a predominantly yellow cut surface and additional gray and white foci. Under the light microscope, the cytoplasm of the clear cell type appears clear and empty (Fig. 14-33).[2-4] Clear cell RCCs have partial or complete loss of chromosome 3 or a gene mutation on the short arm of chromosome 3, resulting in the loss of one or more tumor suppressor genes. The VHL gene is located at 3p25-26, which is often deleted in clear cell RCC.[5, 6]

The majority of renal neoplasms can be distinguished on the basis of histologic examination alone; however, there are morphologic similarities between clear cell RCC and chromophobe cell carcinoma, as well as between the granular-eosinophilic variants of these tumors and renal oncocytoma.[2-4] Only a limited number of histochemical markers are available to aid in the differential diagnosis of these neoplasms. Table 14-15 summarizes the immunohistochemical findings in clear cell RCC.[7-18]

MARKERS FOR RENAL CELL CARCINOMA

Cytokeratin, Epithelial Membrane Antigen, and Vimentin

Using a panel of antibodies including CK, EMA, and vimentin has been reported useful for the differential diagnosis of RCC.[7-18] Clear cell RCC is usually positive for low molecular weight keratin (CAM5.2), CK18, AE1/AE3, EMA (Fig. 14-34), and vimentin (Fig. 14-35), but negative for CK7, CK20,

---

Table 14-15. Clear Cell Renal Cell Carcinoma: Immunohistochemical Profile

Histochemical Markers for Clear Cell RCC

Low molecular weight cytokeratin−positive
Epithelial membrane antigen (EMA)−positive
Vimentin-positive
Carbonic anhydrase (G250)−positive
CD10+
RCC antibody−positive
Placental alkaline phosphatase (PLAP)−positive
Periodic acid−Schiff (PAS)/glycogen−positive
High molecular weight cytokeratin−negative
Carcinoembryonic antigen (CEA)−negative
S-100 protein−negative
Band 3 protein−negative
Inhibin-negative
Mucin-negative
Oil red O (lipid)−positive
Hale's colloidal iron stain−negative

Histochemical Markers of Differential Diagnosis

Adrenocortical carcinoma
  Inhibin-positive
  Epithelial membrane antigen (EMA)−negative
  Cytokeratin (CK)-negative
Urothelial carcinoma of the renal pelvis
  Carcinoembryonic antigen (CEA)−positive
  High molecular weight cytokeratin−positive
  CK7+
  CK20+
  Vimentin-negative
Papillary renal cell carcinoma
  Carbonic anhydrase (G250)−negative
Chromophobe carcinoma
  Hale's colloidal iron stain (acid mucopolysaccharides)−positive
  High molecular weight cytokeratin−positive or negative
  CK7+
  Vimentin-negative
  Lipid and glycogen (periodic acid−Schiff)−negative
Oncocytoma
  Band 3 protein−positive
Melanoma
  S-100+, HMB-45+, CK− EMA−

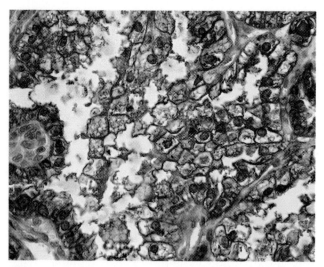

Figure 14–34. Immunoreactivity of epithelial membrane antigen (EMA) in clear cell RCC cells.

cells. Metastatic melanomas were positive for S-100 protein and HMB-45.[7, 21, 24, 27, 28]

ANTIBODIES OF RENAL CELL CARCINOMA AND CD10

The antibody of RCC binds to a 200-kd glycoprotein expressed in renal proximal tubule epithelial cells. Yoshida and coworkers[29] reported that this antibody was positive in 93% of primary and 84% of metastatic RCC, but the paper was published without information of tumor subtypes. CD10 (acute lymphocyte leukemia antigen, CALLA) is expressed on the brush border of renal tubular epithelial cells. Avery and colleagues used antibodies to RCC and CD10 in the differential diagnosis of common renal tumor.[8] They observed that 85% of clear cell carcinomas (53 of 62) had detectable surface membrane staining for RCC, and 94% (58 of 62) were positive for CD10. Papillary carcinomas were likewise strongly positive for RCC and CD10 in nearly all cases (13 of 14 each). In contrast, all 19 chromophobe cell carcinomas examined were completely negative for surface membrane staining with both these markers. Oncocytomas were also negative for RCC (0 of 9), but CD10 was detectable in some cases (3 of 9). These results suggest that the presence of surface membrane staining for RCC and CD10 may be used to confirm a diagnosis of suspected clear cell or papillary renal carcinoma. Chromophobe cell carcinomas should be negative for both markers. The absence of RCC staining may also be helpful in the diagnosis of renal oncocytoma. Furthermore, CK7 can be used to distinguish oncocytoma (CK7−) from chromophobe cell carcinoma (CK7+).[8–10, 29–36] Applying a panel of antibodies including vimentin, EMA, CEA, RCC, CD10, and CK7 is helpful for the differential diagnosis of renal cell neoplasms.

OTHER DIAGNOSTIC MARKERS IN CLEAR CELL RENAL CELL CARCINOMA

The utility of cadherin in RCC is controversial. Taki and colleagues reported that E-cadherin was negative in clear cell RCC but positive in chromophobe RCC and oncocytoma.[37] However, Fischer and coworkers reported the expression of E-cadherin is associated with RCC progression.[38]

G250 is an antibody that recognizes carbonic anhydrase IX (CA IX).[39, 40] Carbonic anhydrase is normally suppressed in normal renal epithelium by the pVHL gene. In clear cell RCC, loss of VHL function led to the expression of CA IX antigen and reactivity with antibody G250.[39, 40] The CA IX antigen is expressed by clear cell RCC but not by normal kidney cells and papillary RCC. However, G250 is not a RCC-specific antibody; it also stains normal gastric mucosa and biliary ductules.[39, 40]

Anti–alpha inhibin, an antibody directed against a peptide hormone, has been reported to be a useful diagnostic aid in distinguishing between adrenocortical carcinoma (inhibin-positive) and clear cell RCC (inhibin-negative).[41] The FHIT gene on human chromosome 3p14.2 is deleted in a variety of malignant tumors, including clear cell RCCs, resulting in a loss of expression of FHIT protein.[42–44] Other markers such as CD44 and IL-6 were also reported to be positive in clear cell RCC.[15, 16, 38, 45, 46]

PAPILLARY RENAL CELL CARCINOMA

Papillary RCC is an uncommon subtype of RCC that has distinctive gross, histologic, and cytogenetic features.[47–49] The gross features include a ball-shaped outline and dotted pattern.[2–4, 50] On light microscopy, the basic chromophilic cell type exhibits a less basophilic-stained cytoplasm and overlapping, centrally located, small nuclei (Fig. 14–36). Cytogenetic features include a gain of chromosomes 16, 12, and the long arm of chromo-

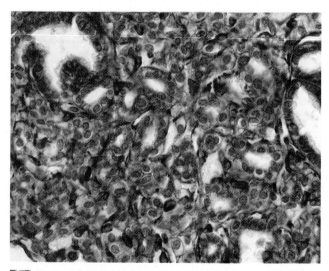

Figure 14–35. Immunoreactivity of vimentin in clear cell RCC cells.

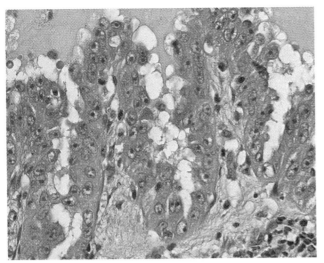

Figure 14–36. Papillary RCC exhibiting a less basophilic-stained cytoplasm and overlapping, centrally located, small nuclei.

Table 14–16. **Papillary Renal Cell Carcinoma: Immunohistochemical Profile**

Immunohistochemistry

Cytokeratin (CK) AE1/AE3+
Vimentin-positive
Mucin-positive
Glycogen-positive
Low molecular weight (CK7)–positive
High molecular weight CK–negative
Ulex europaeus lectin–negative
Carbonic anhydrase (G250)–negative

Differential Diagnosis

Collecting duct carcinoma
    Mucin-positive, high molecular weight CK–positive
Metanephric adenoma
    Closely packed tubules lined by cells with uniform nuclei
        and scant cytoplasm; lacks extensive papillae with fibrovas-
        cular cores

some 3 q; trisomy 10; and mutation of the *met* oncogene.[5, 6]

Only limited immunohistochemistry data have been reported on this type of tumor. Table 14–16 summarizes the immunohistochemical findings in papillary RCC.[42, 47, 48, 51, 52] Renshaw and coworkers studied 36 papillary RCCs using a variety of antibodies to keratin and CEA. They found 100% (36 of 36 cases) of the papillary tumors were positive for AE1/AE3 (Fig. 14–37), and 92% (33 of 36 cases) were positive for callus keratins (Fig. 14–38); only 3% (one of 36 cases) stained for 34βE12, and 11% (4 of 36 cases) stained weakly for CEA.[48, 52]

CHROMOPHOBE RENAL CELL CARCINOMA

Chromophobe RCC is a newly established category of RCC composed histologically of characteristic "chromophobe" tumor cells, characterized by a large polygonal shape with a transparent or slightly reticulated cytoplasm and prominent cell membranes (Fig. 14–39).[2–4] Another diagnostic feature is the lack of cytoplasmic coloring with routine dyes, but a diffuse cytoplasmic staining reaction with Hale's iron stain).[2–4] Cytogenetic features include a massive loss of chromosomes (i.e., 1, 2, 6, 10, 13, 17, and 21). These data were confirmed by fluorescence in situ hybridization and comparative genomic hybridization analyses.[5, 6]

Although ultrastructural and immunohistochemical studies showed that these tumor cells present several features similar to those found in the intercalated cells of the collecting duct, immunohistochemical studies using antibody panels on a large number of cases are limited (Table 14–17).[27, 34, 51, 53–56] Taki and associates performed an immunohistochemical study of 21 cases of chromophobe RCC, along with cases of clear RCC and

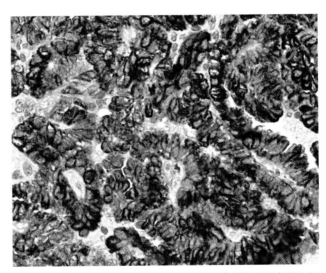

Figure 14–37. Immunoreactivity of CK AE1/AE3 in papillary RCC cells.

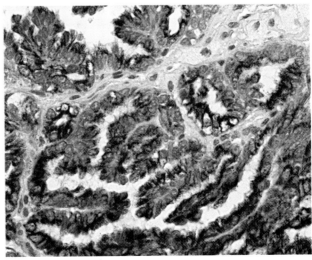

Figure 14–38. Immunoreactivity of CK CAM5.2 in papillary RCC cells.

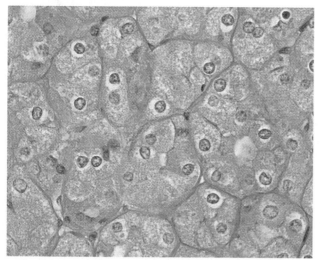

Figure 14–39. Chromophobe RCC exhibiting large polygonal cells with a transparent or slightly reticulated cytoplasm and prominent cell membranes.

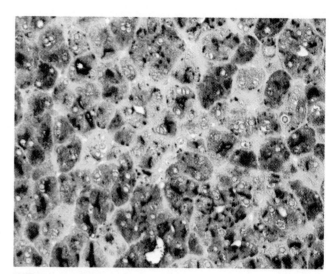

Figure 14–40. Immunoreactivity of EMA in chromophobe RCC cells.

renal oncocytoma.[37] They found that chromophobe RCC was positive for EMA (Fig. 14–40) but negative for vimentin. CKs did not show constant immunoreactivity in the three types of renal tumors. Furthermore, all the chromophobe RCCs and renal oncocytomas were positive for E-cadherin but not for N-cadherin, whereas all the clear RCCs were negative for E-cadherin, but 58% were positive for N-cadherin. Immunoreaction for E-cadherin, vimentin, and Hale's iron stain can be useful for distinguishing chromophobe RCC from clear cell RCC.[37] Leroy and colleagues reported that immunostaining with CK7 is useful for the differential diagnosis of renal oncocytomas (CK7−) and chromophobe RCCs (CK7+) (Fig. 14–41) when results from Hale's colloidal iron staining are uncertain.[33]

COLLECTING DUCT CARCINOMA

Collecting duct carcinoma (CDC) of the kidney is a rare but distinctive renal cancer. It may arise from the medullary collecting ducts.[2–4] The tumor mass is typically centered on the medulla of the kidney and extends into the cortex. The histologic appearance has been described as tubulopapillary, tubular, solid, and sarcomatoid (Fig. 14–42). Prominent stromal desmoplasia, angiolymphatic invasion, and neutrophil infiltrate are usually present. Intracytoplasmic mucin may be present.[2–4] The cytogenetic features include a loss of chromosome 8p and chromosome 13. Monosomy 1, 6, 14, 15, and 22 were also observed in this type of tumor.[5, 6]

Table 14–17. Chromophobe Renal Cell Carcinoma: Immunohistochemical Profile

Immunohistochemistry

Hale's colloidal iron stain−positive
Low molecular weight cytokeratin (CK)−negative
High molecular weight cytokeratin−positive or negative
Cytokeratin AE1/AE3−positive
E-cadherin−positive
Epithelial membrane antigen (EMA)−positive
Lipid and glycogen (periodic acid−Schiff)−negative
CK7+
Vimentin-negative
CD10−
RCC antibody−negative
Carbonic anhydrase C−negative or positive
N-cadherin−negative
Band 3 protein−negative
Alcian blue−positive

Differential Diagnosis

Oncocytoma
    CK7−, Hale's colloidal iron stain−negative, band 3 protein-positive
Clear cell renal cell carcinoma
    Vimentin-positive, Hale's colloidal iron stain−negative, RCC antibody−positive, CD10+

RCC, renal cell carcinoma.

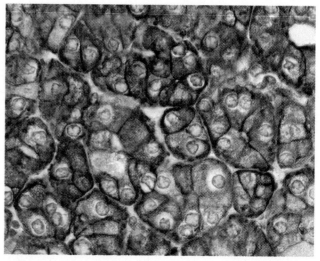

Figure 14–41. Immunoreactivity of CK7 in chromophobe RCC cells.

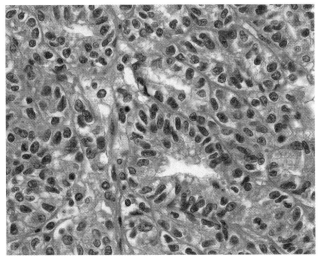

▶¶ *Figure 14–42.* Collecting duct carcinoma (CDC), tubular pattern.

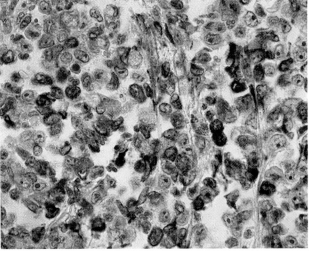

▶¶ *Figure 14–44.* Immunoreactivity for vimentin in CDC cells.

The typical immunohistochemical profile is positive staining with antibodies for pankeratin (AE1/AE3), low (CAM5.2) and high molecular weight keratin (CK19 and 34βE12) (Fig. 14–43), EMA, vimentin (Fig. 14–44) and with the lectin *Ulex europaeus* agglutinin (UEAI). The staining for CEA is not consistent in CDC (Table 14–18). Immunohistochemical as well as mucinocarminic and periodic acid–Schiff staining studies are necessary for the diagnosis of CDC. The prognosis of CDC is poor; most patients have developed metastases or died[49, 50, 57, 58] within 2 years of presentation.

Benign Epithelial Neoplasms

PAPILLARY ADENOMA

The tumor most frequently considered as being adenoma is small and is located in the superficial cortex. It is composed of small cells with little cytoplasm and a papillary or tubular architecture.[2–4] Cytogenetically, papillary renal cell adenomas show trisomy 7 or 17 or tetrasomy 17. There are a limited number of studies on immunohistochemistry of this tumor.[5, 6]

RENAL ONCOCYTOMA

Renal oncocytoma is a neoplasm of the renal cortex. The most macroscopic feature of oncocytoma is its mahogany brown color, which contrasts with the bright yellow color of clear cell RCC.[8, 36, 59] Light microscopically, this basic cell type is characterized by isomorphic tumor cells with a coarsely granulated eosinophilic cytoplasm (Fig. 14–45). Round, vesicular, centrally located

▶¶ *Figure 14–43.* Immunoreactivity for high molecular weight CK (34βE12) in CDC cells.

Table 14–18. Collecting Duct Carcinoma: Immunohistochemical Profile

Immunohistochemistry

Mucin-positive
Epithelial membrane antigen (EMA)–positive
Low molecular weight cytokeratin (CK)–positive
High molecular weight CK–positive
CK13–
Vimentin-positive
Peanut lectin–positive
UEAI+
CEA focal–positive
LeuM1–

Differential Diagnosis

Papillary renal cell carcinoma
  Ulex europaeus lectin–negative
  High molecular weight CK–negative
Clear cell renal cell carcinoma
  Ulex europaeus lectin–negative
  High molecular weight CK–negative
Urothelial carcinoma of the renal pelvis
  Vimentin-negative, CK13+, CK19+

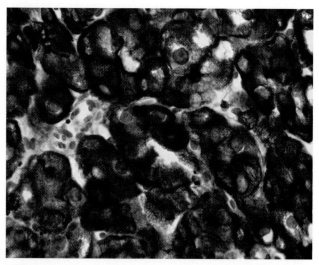

Figure 14–45. Renal oncocytoma exhibiting isomorphic tumor cells with a coarsely granulated eosinophilic cytoplasm.

nuclei usually can be found. Focally, they become polymorphic as a result of polyploidization. An increase of binucleated cells with overlapping nuclei is of differential diagnostic importance.[2–4] The cytogenetic features include a heterogeneous group of tumors with consistent loss of chromosomes Y and 1, telomeric associations, and a few cases with reciprocal translocation t(5;11)(q35;q13).[5, 6]

Immunohistochemically, oncocytomas are positive for CK AE1/AE3 (Fig. 14–46) and low molecular weight CK.[8, 10, 18, 33, 35–37, 56, 60] It is negative for CK7, which can be used to differentiate oncocytoma from chromophobe RCC.[33] Band 3 protein was reported positive in oncocytoma but not in other types of renal epithelial tumors. When the interpretation of Hale's colloidal iron stain is uncertain, CK7 and band 3 protein can be used for

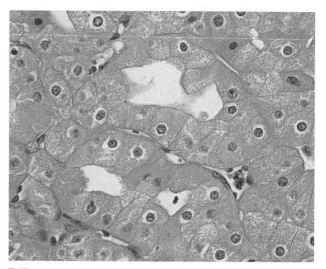

Figure 14–46. Immunoreactivity for keratin (AE1) in oncocytoma cells.

the differential diagnosis.[61] Oncocytomas were also negative for RCC antibody, but CD10 was detectable in some cases.[8]

METANEPHRIC ADENOMA

Metanephric adenoma of the kidney is a newly recognized entity of renal adenoma.[62–74] Metanephric adenoma has a diploid DNA pattern.[75, 76] Studies done in the late 1990s revealed *met* oncogene mutation in this type of tumor.[5, 6]

The immunohistochemical features of the tumor have not yet been well elucidated (Table 14–19).[69, 73, 74] Several studies have suggested that renal metanephric adenoma is composed of immature renal epithelial cells. For example, Nonomura and colleagues reported that the cytoplasm of the majority of the tumor cells was positive for S-100 and occasionally for alpha-1-antitrypsin and vimentin.[77, 78] The predominant cell membrane staining for CK, lysozyme, and Leu7 was also observed in tumor cells. Only tumor cells arranged in papillary or large tubular patterns were positive for EMA. Tumor cells were negative for LeuM1 and HMB-45. Tsuji and associates reported that metanephric adenoma cells were positive for vimentin, CK, and Leu7.[79]

OTHER BENIGN RENAL TUMORS AND TUMOR-LIKE CONDITIONS

Table 14–20 summarizes the immunohistochemical findings in benign renal tumors and tumor-like conditions.[64] For example, cystic hamartoma of the pelvis shows immunoreactivity for CK, EMA, and smooth muscle actin.[80] Juxtaglomerular cell tumor is usually positive for rennin.[81–87] Angiomyoli-

---

Table 14–19. Renal Oncocytoma: Immunohistochemical Profile

Immunohistochemistry

Vimentin-negative
Cytokeratin (CK) AE1/AE3+
Carbonic anhydrase-positive
CK7−
RCC antibody−negative
Periodic acid−Schiff (PAS)-negative
Low molecular weight CK−positive
Band 3 anion exchange protein−positive
Hale's colloidal iron stain−negative
CD10 −/+

Differential Diagnosis

Chromophobe RCC:
   Hale's colloidal iron stain−positive, CK7+, band 3 protein−negative
Clear cell RCC:
   Vimentin-positive, band 3 protein−negative, CD10+, RCC antibody−positive

RCC, renal cell carcinoma.

Table 14–20. Metanephric Adenoma: Immunohistochemical Profile

Immunohistochemistry

Cytokeratin (CK)–positive
Leu7+
Epithelial membrane antigen (EMA)–positive or negative
Smooth muscle actin–positive or negative
Glycogen (PAS)–negative
HMB-45–
Chromogranin-negative
Vimentin-positive
S-100 protein–positive or negative
Carcinoembryonic antigen (CEA)–negative
Desmin-negative
Oil red O–negative
Neuron-specific enolase–negative
Neurofilament-negative

Differential Diagnosis

Adult Wilms' tumor
    Vimentin-positive, NSE+, CK+
Renal adenoma
    Epithelial membrane antigen (EMA)–positive
Papillary renal cell carcinoma
    CK7+
Carcinoid
    Neuroendocrine markers are positive

NSE, neuron-specific enolase.

poma shows immunoreactivity for HMB-45 in smooth muscle.[88–92]

RENAL CELL TUMORS IN CHILDREN

Wilms' Tumor (Nephroblastoma)

Wilms' tumor composes more than 80% of renal tumors of childhood. It is usually large, more than 5 cm in diameter.[2–4] The cut surface is typically solid, soft, and gray or pink, resembling brain tissue. Microscopically, Wilms' tumor is typically composed of a variable mixture of blastema, epithelium, and stroma. Blastema is commonly arranged in three patterns: serpentine, nodular, and diffuse. The epithelial component usually consists of small tubules or cysts lined by primitive columnar or cuboidal cells. Various types of soft tissue can be observed in the stroma of Wilms' tumor.[2–4]

The immunohistologic findings in the blastemal tissue component of Wilms' tumor include both characteristics of embryonic tissue and signs of early epithelial differentiation, suggesting blastemal cells are capable of differentiating into tubular epithelial cells and stromal cells.[93–98] Undifferentiated blastemal cells contain exclusively vimentin intermediate filaments, better differentiated blastemal cells contain vimentin and cytokeratin, and stromal cells contain exclusively vimentin. NSE is also positive in blastema (Table 14–21).[93, 96, 98–100] In addition, the histologically apparent transition

between blastema and tubules was reflected in a concurrently occurring and gradual increase in the number of expressed epithelial antigens.[96, 98, 101] The differential diagnosis of Wilms' tumor from other malignancies is summarized in Table 14–22.[98, 101–104]

Clear Cell Sarcoma of Kidney (Bone-Metastasizing Renal Tumor of Childhood)

Clear cell sarcoma is a highly malignant neoplasm. Mean age at diagnosis is 36 months with a range of 2 months to 14 years. The male to female ratio is 2:1. Typical gross features include large size, a mucoid texture, foci of necrosis, and prominent cyst formation. Nine major histologic patterns have been identified (classic, myxoid, sclerosing, cellular, epithelioid, palisading, spindle, storiform,

Table 14–21. Benign Renal Tumors and Tumor-Like Conditions

Tumor or Tumor-like Lesion	Immunohistochemical Profile
Multilocular cyst	Cytokeratin (CK)–positive EMA+
Mesoblastic nephroma	Vimentin-positive Desmin-positive or -negative Muscle-specific actin–positive or negative CK– Desmin-negative
Oncocytoma	CKAE1/AE3+ Low molecular weight keratin–positive Carbonic anhydrase–positive Band 3 anion exchange protein–positive Vimentin-positive
Angiomyolipoma	HMB-45+ (in smooth muscle) Muscle-specific antigen–positive Desmin-positive Vimentin-positive CK– S-100 protein–positive
Metanephric adenoma	Cytokeratin-positive Vimentin-positive Smooth muscle actin–positive or negative CEA–, S-100 protein–negative, NSE–, chromogranin-negative, neurofilament-negative, EMA–
Cystic hamartoma of pelvis	CK+ EMA+ Smooth muscle actin–positive
Juxtaglomerular cell tumor	Rennin-positive Smooth muscle actin–positive Muscle-specific actin–positive Vimentin-positive CK–, NSE–, desmin-negative, S-100 protein-negative

EMA, epithelial membrane antigen; CEA, carcinoembryonic antigen; NSE, neuron-specific enolase.

Table 14–22. Characteristic Immunophenotype and Differential Diagnosis of Wilms' Tumor, Clear Cell Sarcoma, and Rhabdoid Tumor

Tumor	Immunohistochemical Marker	Differential Diagnosis
Wilms' tumor (blastema)	Vimentin-positive NSE+ CK+	*Neuroblastoma:* Vimentin-negative, neurofilament-positive, synaptophysin-positive, NSE+ *Ewing's sarcoma:* MIC2 (HBA71)+ *Rhabdomyosarcoma:* Desmin-positive *Lymphoma:* LCA+
Clear cell sarcoma	CK− Vimentin-positive or -negative Alpha-1-antichymotrypsin-positive EMA− MSA− Desmin-negative	*Wilms' tumor:* Vimentin-positive, NSE+, CK+ *Rhabdoid tumor:* CK+/−, vimentin-positive, EMA+
Rhabdoid tumor	CK+/− Vimentin-positive EMA+ S-100 protein−positive or negative Actin-negative Desmin-positive or -negative Myoglobin-negative	*Wilms' tumor:* Vimentin-positive, NSE+, CK+ *Clear cell sarcoma:* CK−, vimentin-positive or -negative, EMA−

and anaplastic); virtually all tumors contain multiple patterns that blend with one another. In studies, only vimentin was consistently immunoreactive immunohistochemically. Consistently negative results with other antibodies helped exclude other tumors in the differential diagnosis. Clear cell sarcomas were CK−, including epithelioid tumors that mimicked Wilms' tumor, and MIC2-negative, including cellular tumors that mimicked primitive neuroectodermal tumor (see Table 14–22).[7, 105–107] Alpha-1-antichymotrypsin was reported to be positive in this tumor.[108, 109]

Rhabdoid Tumor of the Kidney

Rhabdoid tumor is the most malignant renal neoplasm of childhood; usually it metastasizes widely and causes death within 12 months of diagnosis.[2–4] Macroscopically, these tumors are yellow-gray or light tan with indistinct borders and fragment easily. Histologically, rhabdoid tumor is diffuse and monotonous, consisting of medium or large polygonal cells with abundant eosinophilic cytoplasm and round nuclei with thick nuclear membranes and large nucleoli.[2–4] Immunohistochemical studies showed vimentin positivity in this type of tumor.[110] Low molecular weight keratin (CAM5.2), EMA, NSE, S-100 protein, and desmin are positive in some cases of rhabdoid tumors.[111–115] The differential diagnosis is summarized in Table 14–22.[111–115]

Mesoblastic Nephroma

Although composing less than 3% of primary renal tumors in children, mesoblastic nephroma is the most common type of renal tumor in the first 3

months of life.[2–4] The tumor is unencapsulated, and the cut surface resembles that of a leiomyoma. The classic histologic appearance is a moderately cellular proliferation of thick interlacing bundles of spindle cells with elongated nuclei that usually infiltrate renal and perirenal tissues. Another pattern has been called *cellular mesoblastic nephroma.*[2–4] Immunohistochemically, this type of tumor is positive for vimentin (see Table 14–21).[116–119]

The malignancies of soft tissue, lymphoma, and metastatic tumors in kidney are not discussed in this chapter. They share the immunohistochemical phenotypes with the same type of tumors in other organs, and are discussed in other chapters.

References

1. Greenlee RT, Murray T, Bolden S, Wingo PA. Cancer statistics, 2000. CA Cancer J Clin 2000;50:7–33.
2. Bostwick DG, Murphy GP. Diagnosis and prognosis of renal cell carcinoma: Highlights from an international consensus workshop. Semin Urol Oncol 1998;16:46–52.
3. Bostwick DG, Eble JN. Diagnosis and classification of renal cell carcinoma. Urol Clin North Am 1999;26:627–635.
4. Storkel S, Eble JN, Adlakha K, et al. Classification of renal cell carcinoma: Workgroup No. 1: Union Internationale Contre le Cancer (UICC) and the American Joint Committee on Cancer (AJCC). Cancer 1997;80:987–989.
5. Storkel S. Epithelial tumors of the kidney: Pathological subtyping and cytogenetic correlation. Urologe A 1999;38:425–432.
6. van den Berg E, Dijkhuizen T, Oosterhuis JW, et al. Cytogenetic classification of renal cell cancer. Cancer Genet Cytogenet 1997;95:103–107.
7. Amin MB, de Peralta-Venturina MN, Ro JY, et al. Clear cell sarcoma of kidney in an adolescent and in young adults: A report of four cases with ultrastructural, immunohistochemical, and DNA flow cytometric analysis. Am J Surg Pathol 1999;23:1455–1463.
8. Avery AK, Beckstead J, Renshaw AA, Corless CL. Use of antibodies to RCC and CD10 in the differential diagnosis of renal neoplasms. Am J Surg Pathol 2000;24:203–210.

9. Beham A, Ratschek M, Zatloukal K, et al. Immunohistochemical analysis of 42 renal cell carcinomas and one oncocytoma with mono- and polyclonal antibodies against vimentin and cytokeratin. Verh Dtsch Ges Pathol 1989;73: 392–395.

10. Bonsib SM, Bromley C, Lager DJ. Renal oncocytoma: Diagnostic utility of cytokeratin-containing globular filamentous bodies. Mod Pathol 1991;4:16–23.

11. Bonsib SM, Bray C. Cytokeratin-containing globular filamentous bodies in renal oncocytoma. Ultrastruct Pathol 1991;15:521–529.

12. Chu P, Arber DA. Paraffin-section detection of CD10 in 505 nonhematopoietic neoplasms: Frequent expression in renal cell carcinoma and endometrial stromal sarcoma. Am J Clin Pathol 2000;113:374–382.

13. Coffin CM, Swanson PE, Wick MR, Dehner LP. An immunohistochemical comparison of chordoma with renal cell carcinoma, colorectal adenocarcinoma, and myxopapillary ependymoma: A potential diagnostic dilemma in the diminutive biopsy. Mod Pathol 1993;6:531–538.

14. Gerharz CD, Moll R, Storkel S, et al. Ultrastructural appearance and cytoskeletal architecture of the clear, chromophilic, and chromophobe types of human renal cell carcinoma in vitro. Am J Pathol 1993;142:851–859.

15. Gilcrease MZ, Guzman-Paz M, Niehans G, et al. Correlation of CD44S expression in renal clear cell carcinomas with subsequent tumor progression or recurrence. [see comments] Cancer 1999;86:2320–2326.

16. Heider KH, Ratschek M, Zatloukal K, Adolf GR. Expression of CD44 isoforms in human renal cell carcinoma. Virchows Arch 1996;428:267–273.

17. Jin TX, Kakehi Y, Moroi S, Yoshida O. E-cadherin expression and histopathological features in renal cell carcinomas. Hinyokika Kiyo 1995;41:653–657.

18. Markovic-Lipkovski J, Brasanac D, Todorovic V, et al. Immunomorphological characteristics of renal cell carcinoma. Histol Histopathol 1995;10:651–659.

19. Waldherr R, Schwechheimer K. Co-expression of cytokeratin and vimentin intermediate-sized filaments in renal cell carcinomas: Comparative study of the intermediate-sized filament distribution in renal cell carcinomas and normal human kidney. Virchows Arch A Pathol Anat Histopathol 1985;408:15–27.

20. Martin de las Mulas J, Espinosa de los Monteros A, Carrasco L, et al. Immunohistochemical distribution pattern of intermediate filament proteins in 50 feline neoplasms. Vet Pathol 1995;32:692–701.

21. Sim SJ, Ro JY, Ordonez NG, et al. Metastatic renal cell carcinoma to the bladder: A clinicopathologic and immunohistochemical study. Mod Pathol 1999;12:351–355.

22. Banner BF, Burnham JA, Bahnson RR, et al. Immunophenotypic markers in renal cell carcinoma. Mod Pathol 1990; 3:129–134.

23. Gaffey MJ, Mills SE, Askin FB, et al. Clear cell tumor of the lung: A clinicopathologic, immunohistochemical, and ultrastructural study of eight cases. [see comments] Am J Surg Pathol 1990;14:248–259.

24. Amo-Takyi BK, Handt S, Gunawan B, et al. A cytogenetic approach to the differential diagnosis of metastatic clear cell renal carcinoma. Histopathology 1998;32:436–443.

25. Medeiros LJ, Gelb AB, Weiss LM. Low-grade renal cell carcinoma: A clinicopathologic study of 53 cases. Am J Surg Pathol 1987;11:633–642.

26. Medeiros LJ, Michie SA, Johnson DE, et al. An immunoperoxidase study of renal cell carcinomas: Correlation with nuclear grade, cell type, and histologic pattern. Hum Pathol 1988;19:980–987.

27. Akhtar M, Kardar H, Linjawi T, et al. Chromophobe cell carcinoma of the kidney: A clinicopathologic study of 21 cases. Am J Surg Pathol 1995;19:1245–1256.

28. Kletscher BA, Qian J, Bostwick DG, et al. Prospective analysis of the incidence of ipsilateral adrenal metastasis in localized renal cell carcinoma. J Urol 1996;155:1844–1846.

29. Yoshida K, Moriguchi H, Sumi S, et al. Alterations of asparagine-linked sugar chains of N-acetyl beta-D-hexosaminidase during human renal oncogenesis: A preliminary study using serial lectin affinity chromatography. J Chromatogr B Biomed Sci Appl 1999;723:75–80.

30. Yoshida K, Hosoya Y, Sumi S, et al. Studies of the expression of epidermal growth factor receptor in human renal cell carcinoma: A comparison of immunohistochemical method versus ligand binding assay. Oncology 1997;54: 220–225.

31. Yoshida SO, Imam A. Monoclonal antibody to a proximal nephrogenic renal antigen: Immunohistochemical analysis of formalin-fixed, paraffin-embedded human renal cell carcinomas. Cancer Res 1989;49:1802–1809.

32. Yoshida K, Sumi S, Honda M, et al. Serial lectin affinity chromatography demonstrates altered asparagine-linked sugar chain structures of gamma-glutamyltransferase in human renal cell carcinoma. J Chromatogr B Biomed Appl 1995;672:45–51.

33. Leroy X, Moukassa D, Copin MC, et al. Utility of cytokeratin 7 for distinguishing chromophobe renal cell carcinoma from renal oncocytoma. Eur Urol 2000;37:484–487.

34. Cochand-Priollet B, Molinie V, Bougaran J, et al. Renal chromophobe cell carcinoma and oncocytoma: A comparative morphologic, histochemical, and immunohistochemical study of 124 cases. Arch Pathol Lab Med 1997;121: 1081–1086.

35. Beham A, Ratschek M, Zatloukal K, et al. Distribution of cytokeratins, vimentin and desmoplakins in normal renal tissue, renal cell carcinomas and oncocytoma as revealed by immunofluorescence microscopy. Virchows Arch A Pathol Anat Histopathol 1992;421:209–215.

36. Cohen C, McCue PA, Derose PB. Histogenesis of renal cell carcinoma and renal oncocytoma: An immunohistochemical study. Cancer 1988;62:1946–1951.

37. Taki A, Nakatani Y, Misugi K, et al. Chromophobe renal cell carcinoma: An immunohistochemical study of 21 Japanese cases. Mod Pathol 1999;12:310–317.

38. Fischer C, Georg C, Kraus S, et al. CD44s, E-cadherin and PCNA as markers for progression in renal cell carcinoma. Anticancer Res 1999;19:1513–1517.

39. Oosterwijk E, Bander NH, Divgi CR, et al. Antibody localization in human renal cell carcinoma: A phase I study of monoclonal antibody G250. J Clin Oncol 1993;11:738–750.

40. Uemura H, Nakagawa Y, Yoshida K, et al. MN/CA IX/G250 as a potential target for immunotherapy of renal cell carcinomas. Br J Cancer 1999;81:741–746.

41. Renshaw AA, Granter SR. A comparison of A103 and inhibin reactivity in adrenal cortical tumors: Distinction from hepatocellular carcinoma and renal tumors. Mod Pathol 1998;11:1160–1164.

42. Eyzaguirre EJ, Miettinen M, Norris BA, Gatalica Z. Different immunohistochemical patterns of FHIT protein expression in renal neoplasms. Mod Pathol 1999;12:979–983.

43. Hadaczek P, Siprashvili Z, Markiewski M, et al. Absence or reduction of Fhit expression in most clear cell renal carcinomas. Cancer Res 1998;58:2946–2951.

44. Hadaczek P, Kovatich A, Gronwald J, et al. Loss or reduction of Fhit expression in renal neoplasias: Correlation with histogenic class. Hum Pathol 1999;30:1276–1283.

45. Fujita J, Takenawa J, Kaneko Y, et al. Anti-interleukin-6 (IL-6) therapy of IL-6-producing renal cell carcinoma. Hinyokika Kiyo 1992;38:1333–1336.

46. Li N, Tsuji M, Kanda K, et al. Analysis of CD44 isoform v10 expression and its prognostic value in renal cell carcinoma. BJU Int 2000;85:514–518.

47. Amin MB, Corless CL, Renshaw AA, et al. Papillary (chromophil) renal cell carcinoma: Histomorphologic characteristics and evaluation of conventional pathologic prognostic parameters in 62 cases. [see comments] Am J Surg Pathol 1997;21:621–635.

48. Renshaw AA, Corless CL. Papillary renal cell carcinoma: Histology and immunohistochemistry. Am J Surg Pathol 1995;19:842–849.

49. Delahunt B, Eble JN. Papillary renal cell carcinoma: A clinicopathologic and immunohistochemical study of 105 tumors. Mod Pathol 1997;10:537–544.

50. Srigley JR, Eble JN. Collecting duct carcinoma of kidney. Semin Diagn Pathol 1998;15:54–67.

51. Mai KT, Burns BF. Chromophobe cell carcinoma and renal cell neoplasms with mucin-like changes. Acta Histochem 2000;102:103–113.

52. Renshaw AA, Zhang H, Corless CL, et al. Solid variants of papillary (chromophil) renal cell carcinoma: Clinicopathologic and genetic features. Am J Surg Pathol 1997;21:1203–1209.

53. Wechsel HW, Petri E, Feil G, et al. Renal cell carcinoma: Immunohistological investigation of expression of the integrin alpha v beta 3. Anticancer Res 1999;19:1529–1532.

54. Morell-Quadreny L, Gregori-Romero M, Llombart-Bosch A. Chromophobe renal cell carcinoma: Pathologic, ultrastructural, immunohistochemical, cytofluorometric and cytogenetic findings. Pathol Res Pract 1996;192:1275–1281; discussion 1282.

55. Weiss LM, Gaffey MJ, Warhol MJ, et al. Immunocytochemical characterization of a monoclonal antibody directed against mitochondria reactive in paraffin-embedded sections. Mod Pathol 1991;4:596–601.

56. Storkel S, Steart PV, Drenckhahn D, Thoenes W. The human chromophobe cell renal carcinoma: Its probable relation to intercalated cells of the collecting duct. Virchows Arch B Cell Pathol Mol Pathol 1989;56:237–245.

57. MacLennan GT, Farrow GM, Bostwick DG. Low-grade collecting duct carcinoma of the kidney: Report of 13 cases of low-grade mucinous tubulocystic renal carcinoma of possible collecting duct origin. Urology 1997;50:679–684.

58. Tickoo SK, Amin MB, Linden MD, Zarbo RJ. The MIB-1 tumor proliferation index in adult renal epithelial tumors with granular cytoplasm: Biologic implications and differential diagnostic potential. Mod Pathol 1998;11:1115–1121.

59. Eble JN, Hull MT. Morphologic features of renal oncocytoma: A light and electron microscopic study. Hum Pathol 1984;15:1054–1061.

60. van den Berg E, van der Hout AH, Oosterhuis JW, et al. Cytogenetic analysis of epithelial renal-cell tumors: Relationship with a new histopathological classification. Int J Cancer 1993;55:223–227.

61. Bonsib SM, Bromley C. Immunocytochemical analysis of band 3 protein in renal cell carcinoma, nephroblastoma, and oncocytoma. Arch Pathol Lab Med 1994;118:702–704.

62. Keshani de Silva V, Tobias V, Kainer G, Beckwith B. Metanephric adenoma with embryonal hyperplasia of Bowman's capsular epithelium: Previously unreported association. Pediatr Dev Pathol 2000;3:472–478.

63. Renshaw AA, Freyer DR, Hammers YA. Metastatic metanephric adenoma in a child. Am J Surg Pathol 2000;24:570–574.

64. Tamboli P, Ro JY, Amin MB, et al. Benign tumors and tumor-like lesions of the adult kidney. Part II: Benign mesenchymal and mixed neoplasms, and tumor-like lesions. Adv Anat Pathol 2000;7:47–66.

65. Birgisson H, Einarsson GV, Steinarsdottir M, Jonasson JG. Metanephric adenoma. Scand J Urol Nephrol 1999;33:340–343.

66. Monge Mirallas JM, Asensio Lahoz A, Martinez Bretones F, Acinas Garcia O. Metanephric adenoma of the kidney and chronic myeloproliferative syndrome: An unusual association. Actas Urol Esp 1999;23:359–362.

67. Patankar T, Punekar S, Madiwale C, et al. Metanephric adenoma in a solitary kidney. Br J Radiol 1999;72:80–81.

68. Imamoto T, Furuya Y, Ueda T, Ito H. Metanephric adenoma of the kidney. Int J Urol 1999;6:200–202.

69. Martin L, Justrabo E, Michel F, et al. Metanephric adenoma of the kidney; A clinicopathologic, immunohistochemical and electron microscopic study of two cases. Ann Pathol 1998;18:120–124.

70. Grignon DJ, Eble JN. Papillary and metanephric adenomas of the kidney. Semin Diagn Pathol 1998;15:41–53.

71. Granter SR, Fletcher JA, Renshaw AA. Cytologic and cytogenetic analysis of metanephric adenoma of the kidney: A report of two cases. Am J Clin Pathol 1997;108:544–549.

72. Renshaw AA, Maurici D, Fletcher JA. Cytologic and fluorescence in situ hybridization (FISH) examination of metanephric adenoma. Diagn Cytopathol 1997;16:107–111.

73. Ban S, Yoshii S, Tsuruta A, et al. Metanephric adenoma of the kidney: Ultrastructural, immunohistochemical and lectin histochemical studies. Pathol Int 1996;46:661–666.

74. Gatalica Z, Grujic S, Kovatich A, Petersen RO. Metanephric adenoma: Histology, immunophenotype, cytogenetics, ultrastructure. Mod Pathol 1996;9:329–333.

75. Brown JA, Anderl KL, Borell TJ, et al. Simultaneous chromosome 7 and 17 gain and sex chromosome loss provide evidence that renal metanephric adenoma is related to papillary renal cell carcinoma. J Urol 1997;158:370–374.

76. Brown JA, Sebo TJ, Segura JW. Metaphase analysis of metanephric adenoma reveals chromosome Y loss with chromosome 7 and 17 gain. Urology 1996;48:473–475.

77. Nonomura A, Mizukami Y, Hasegawa T, Ohkawa M. Metanephric adenoma of the kidney: An electron microscopic and immunohistochemical study with quantitative DNA measurement by image analysis. Ultrastruct Pathol 1995;19:481–488.

78. Nonomura A, Mizukami Y, Hasegawa T, et al. Metanephric adenoma of the kidney. Pathol Int 1995;45:160–164.

79. Tsuji M, Murakami Y, Kanayama H, et al. A case of renal metanephric adenoma: Histologic, immunohistochemical and cytogenetic analyses. Int J Urol 1999;6:203–207.

80. Mensch LS, Trainer TD, Plante MK. Cystic hamartoma of the renal pelvis: A rare pathologic entity. Mod Pathol 1999;12:417–421.

81. Kuroda N, Moriki T, Komatsu F, et al. Adult-onset giant juxtaglomerular cell tumor of the kidney. Pathol Int 2000;50:249–254.

82. Hashimoto Y, Nakazawa H, Okuda H, et al. A juxtaglomerular cell tumor: Analysis of immunohistochemistry, electron microscopy and in situ hybridization. Nippon Hinyokika Gakkai Zasshi 1998;89:907–910.

83. Hayami S, Sasagawa I, Suzuki H, et al. Juxtaglomerular cell tumor without hypertension. Scand J Urol Nephrol 1998;32:231–233.

84. Caregaro L, Menon F, Gatta A, et al. Juxtaglomerular cell tumor of the kidney. Clin Exp Hypertens 1994;16:41–53.

85. Kodet R, Taylor M, Vachalova H, Pycha K. Juxtaglomerular cell tumor: An immunohistochemical, electron-microscopic, and in situ hybridization study. Am J Surg Pathol 1994;18:837–842.

86. Lopez GAJA, Blanco Gonzalez J, Ortega Medina L, Sanz Esponera J. Juxtaglomerular cell tumor of the kidney: Morphological, immunohistochemical and ultrastructural studies of a new case. Pathol Res Pract 1991;187:354–359; discussion 360–361.

87. Lindop GB, Stewart JA, Downie TT. The immunocytochemical demonstration of renin in a juxtaglomerular cell tumour by light and electron microscopy. Histopathology 1983;7:421–431.

88. L'Hostis H, Deminiere C, Ferriere JM, Coindre JM. Renal angiomyolipoma: A clinicopathologic, immunohistochemical, and follow-up study of 46 cases. Am J Surg Pathol 1999;23:1011–1020.

89. Watanabe K, Suzuki T. Mucocutaneous angiomyolipoma: A report of 2 cases arising in the nasal cavity. Arch Pathol Lab Med 1999;123:789–792.

90. Jungbluth AA, Busam KJ, Gerald WL, et al. A103: An anti-melan-A monoclonal antibody for the detection of malignant melanoma in paraffin-embedded tissues. [see comments] Am J Surg Pathol 1998;22:595–602.

91. Gupta RK, Nowitz M, Wakefield SJ. Fine-needle aspiration cytology of renal angiomyolipoma: Report of a case with immunocytochemical and electron microscopic findings. Diagn Cytopathol 1998;18:297–300.

92. Gyure KA, Prayson RA. Subependymal giant cell astrocytoma: A clinicopathologic study with HMB45 and MIB-1 immunohistochemical analysis. Mod Pathol 1997;10:313–317.

93. Nagao T, Sugano I, Ishida Y, et al. Cystic partially differentiated nephroblastoma in an adult: An immunohistochemical, lectin histochemical and ultrastructural study. Histopathology 1999;35:65–73.

94. Froberg K, Brown RE, Gaylord H, Manivel C. Intra-abdominal desmoplastic small round cell tumor: Immunohisto-

chemical evidence for up-regulation of autocrine and para-crine growth factors. Ann Clin Lab Sci 1999;29:78–85.

95. Eble JN, Bonsib SM. Extensively cystic renal neoplasms: Cystic nephroma, cystic partially differentiated nephroblastoma, multilocular cystic renal cell carcinoma, and cystic hamartoma of renal pelvis. Semin Diagn Pathol 1998; 15:2–20.

96. Folpe AL, Patterson K, Gown AM. Antibodies to desmin identify the blastemal component of nephroblastoma. Mod Pathol 1997;10:895–900.

97. Ellison DA, Silverman JF, Strausbauch PH, et al. Role of immunocytochemistry, electron microscopy, and DNA analysis in fine-needle aspiration biopsy diagnosis of Wilms' tumor. Diagn Cytopathol 1996;14:101–107.

98. Leuschner I, Harms D, Schmidt D. Renal cell carcinoma in children: Histology, immunohistochemistry, and follow-up of 10 cases. Med Pediatr Oncol 1991;19:33–41.

99. Juszkiewicz P. Immunohistochemical evaluation of the percentage of proliferating neoplastic cells of Wilms' tumor in children by means of the MIB-1 monoclonal antibody. Ann Acad Med Stetin 1997;43:113–127.

100. Tarnowski BI, Hazen-Martin DJ, Garvin AJ, et al. Characterization of a monoclonal antibody recognizing the blastemal element of Wilms' tumors and fetal kidneys. Pediatr Pathol 1994;14:849–862.

101. Domagala W, Chosia M, Bedner E, et al. Immunocytochemistry in fine needle aspirates of small cell-, round-, blue-cell malignant tumors of childhood (neuroblastoma, nephroblastoma, lymphoma, Ewing's sarcoma, rhabdomyosarcoma). Patol Pol 1991;42:79–82.

102. Ohshio G, Ogawa K, Kudo H, et al. Immunohistochemical distribution of CA19-9 in normal and tumor tissues of the kidney. Urol Int 1990;45:1–3.

103. Schmidt D, Harms D, Pilon VA. Small-cell pediatric tumors: Histology, immunohistochemistry, and electron microscopy. Clin Lab Med 1987;7:63–89.

104. Takagi M, Takakuwa T, Ushigome S, et al. Sarcomatous variants of Wilms' tumor: Immunohistochemical and ultrastructural comparison with classical Wilms' tumor. Cancer 1987;59:963–971.

105. Choi YJ, Jung WH, Jung SH, Park C. Clear cell sarcoma of the kidney—immunohistochemical study and flow cytometric DNA analysis of 7 cases. Yonsei Med J 1994;35: 336–343.

106. Oda H, Shiga J, Machinami R. Clear cell sarcoma of kidney: Two cases in adults. Cancer 1993;71:2286–2291.

107. Ogawa K, Nakashima Y, Yamabe H, Hamashima Y. Clear cell sarcoma of the kidney: An immunohistochemical study. Acta Pathol Jpn 1986;36:681–689.

108. Altmannsberger M, Osborn M, Schafer H, et al. Distinction of nephroblastomas from other childhood tumors using antibodies to intermediate filaments. Virchows Arch B Cell Pathol Mol Pathol 1984;45:113–124.

109. Fleming S, Gibson AA. Proteinase inhibitors in the kidney and its tumours. Histopathology 1986;10:1303–1313.

110. Weeks DA, Beckwith JB, Mierau GW, Luckey DW. Rhabdoid tumor of kidney: A report of 111 cases from the National Wilms' Tumor Study Pathology Center. Am J Surg Pathol 1989;13:439–458.

111. Hirose M, Yamada T, Toyosaka A, et al. Rhabdoid tumor of the kidney: A report of two cases with respective tumor markers and a specific chromosomal abnormality, del(11p13). Med Pediatr Oncol 1996;27:174–178.

112. Kaiserling E, Ruck P, Handgretinger R, et al. Immunohistochemical and cytogenetic findings in malignant rhabdoid tumor. Gen Diagn Pathol 1996;141:327–337.

113. Liu Y, Li P, Liu S. Malignant rhabdoid tumor of kidney: A clinicopathologic and immunohistochemical study of 15 patients). Chung Hua Ping Li Hsueh Tsa Chih 1995;24:72–74.

114. Ueyama T, Nagai E, Yao T, Tsuneyoshi M. Vimentin-positive gastric carcinomas with rhabdoid features: A clinicopathologic and immunohistochemical study. [see comments] Am J Surg Pathol 1993;17:813–819.

115. Fischer HP, Thomsen H, Altmannsberger M, Bertram U. Malignant rhabdoid tumour of the kidney expressing neurofilament proteins: Immunohistochemical findings and histogenetic aspects. Pathol Res Pract 1989;184:541–547.

116. Bisceglia M, Carosi I, Vairo M, et al. Congenital mesoblastic nephroma: Report of a case with review of the most significant literature. Pathol Res Pract 2000;196:199–204.

117. Siracusano S, Bosincu L, Onida A, et al. Congenital mesoblastic nephroma (CMN) with an unusual immunohistochemical feature. Arch Esp Urol 1999;52:299–303.

118. Nadasdy T, Roth J, Johnson DL, et al. Congenital mesoblastic nephroma: An immunohistochemical and lectin study. Hum Pathol 1993;24:413–419.

119. Boccon-Gibod L, Ben Lagha N. Atypical congenital mesoblastic nephroma (atypical Bolande's tumor). Arch Anat Cytol Pathol 1992;40:333–336.

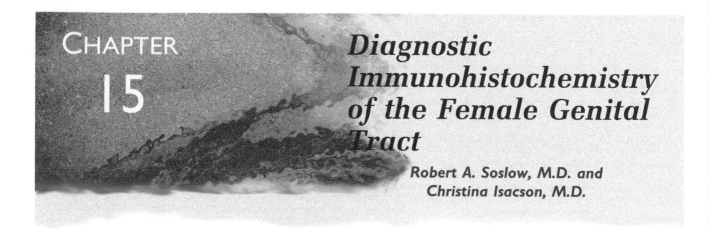

CHAPTER

15

Diagnostic Immunohistochemistry of the Female Genital Tract

Robert A. Soslow, M.D. and
Christina Isacson, M.D.

This chapter represents our approach to the use of immunohistochemistry in the setting of diagnostic gynecologic pathology. The 1990s ushered in the application of antibody panels commonly used in nongynecologic neoplasms for diagnosing complex gynecologic lesions. The use of cytokeratin 7 (CK7) and CK20 in the differential diagnosis of primary versus metastatic carcinoma is one notable example. Other important advances of this type include proliferation markers in vulvar and cervical squamous intraepithelial lesions, p53 in endometrial carcinoma, calretinin and CK5 and CK6 in mesothelioma, and epithelial membrane antigen and melan-A in sex-cord stromal tumors. Inhibin is an example of an antibody developed for use in gynecologic lesions predominantly.

This chapter is divided into four sections: vulva, vagina, and cervix; uterus; gestational trophoblastic disease; and ovary, fallopian tube, and peritoneum. The first part of each section includes a description of the properties and applications of the relevant antibodies. Please refer to the table of commonly used antibodies that are discussed in the text (Table 15–1). In the second section, we discuss the use of antibody panels in the context of the differential diagnosis of problematic gynecologic lesions.

Although the focus of this chapter is diagnostic immunohistochemistry, we wish to emphasize that the proper use of antibodies and the interpretation of results is dependent on careful morphologic assessment and clinicopathologic correlation.

VULVA, VAGINA, AND CERVIX

General Considerations

Commonly used cytokeratins for evaluating lesions of the stratified squamous epithelium of the vulva, vagina, and cervix include AE1/AE3 (pancytokeratin), CAM5.2 (low molecular weight cytokeratin), and CK7 and CK20. The stratified squamous epithelium of all sites normally expresses

AE1/AE3,[1, 2] whereas low molecular weight keratin is negative.[1, 2] With preneoplastic (vulvar intraepithelial neoplasia [VIN], vaginal intraepithelial neoplasm [VAIN], cervical intraepithelial neoplasia [CIN]) and neoplastic (carcinoma) transformation, there is the appearance of low molecular weight keratin expression[3–6]; however, this has not been found to be specific for dysplasia and is not diagnostically useful.[7, 8] CK7 and CK20 are not normally expressed in squamous epithelium. In the endocervix, the glandular cells express CK7 but not CK20, which is similar to the expression seen in the upper genital tract (endometrium, fallopian tubes, and ovaries).[1] Evaluation of CK7 and CK20 expression has emerged as a useful combination for both the differential diagnosis of Paget's disease of the vulva and identifying tumors of nongynecologic origin involving the lower genital tract, such as direct extension from colonic or urologic tumors.

Cell Proliferation Markers

Markers of cell proliferation, such as proliferating cell nuclear antigen (PCNA) and Ki-67 antigen, have been used by pathologists to obtain objective data with which to categorize tumors and other diseases. The Ki-67 antigen is a nuclear nonhistone protein that is present in all stages of the cell cycle except G0. MIB-1 is a monoclonal antibody raised against a recombinant part of the Ki-67 antigen.[9] Both MIB-1 and polyclonal anti–Ki-67 antibody (DAKO, Carpenteria, CA) recognize the Ki-67 antigen in fixed material. Ki-67 antibodies are preferred over PCNA antibodies because Ki-67 antigen is rapidly degraded as the cell leaves the cell cycle, whereas PCNA may continue to be expressed.[10]

When using MIB-1 immunohistochemical analysis, the percentage and distribution of cells that express Ki-67 antigen, rather than merely their presence or absence, is evaluated. MIB-1 expression in normal skin and squamous mucosa is lim-

Table 15–1. Antibodies Used in Diagnostic Gynecologic Pathology

Antibody	Clone	Vendor	Dilution	Retrieval	Control	Pattern
AE1/AE3	AE1,AE3	B-M	1:8000	T 10 min	Colon	Cytoplasmic
AFP	C3	BioGenex	1:300	NT	Fetal liver	Cytoplasmic
B72.3	B72.3	BioGenex	1:100	MW 10 min	Lung carcinoma	Membrane
BerEP4	BerEP4	DAKO	1:200	T 10 min	Breast	Membrane
BRST-2	GCDFP-15	Signet	1:50	NT	Breast carcinoma	Cytoplasmic
CD15	MMA	Becton-Dickinson	1:150	PC	Hodgkin disease	Membrane
CD30	BerH2	DAKO	1:25	MW 15 min	Hodgkin disease	Cytoplasmic
CD44	A308	NeoMarkers	1:100	MW 10 min	Tonsil	Membrane
CD44v6	VFF7	Bender Med	1:20	MW 10 min	Colon	Membrane
CD99	O13	Signet	1:200	PC	Thymus	Membrane
CEA (mono)	B01-94-11M	BioGenex	1:1000	NT	Colon	Cytoplasmic/membrane
CK7	OV-TL 12/30	DAKO	1:100	MW 10 min	Breast	Cytoplasmic
CK20	KS 20.8	DAKO	1:1000	MW 20 min	Colon	Cytoplasmic
Caldesmon	h-CD	DAKO	1:100	WB 40 min	Smooth muscle	Cytoplasmic
Calretinin	Polyclonal	BioGenex	1:100	MW 20 min	Mesothelioma	Cytoplasmic/nuclear
Chromo	LK2H10	BioGenex	1:400	NT	Pancreas	Cytoplasmic
Desmin	D33	DAKO	1:300	MW 10 min	Colon	Cytoplasmic
EMA	E29	DAKO	1:200	PC	Tonsil	Cytoplasmic/membrane
ER	1D5	DAKO	1:25	PC	Breast	Nuclear
HCG	Polyclonal	DAKO	1:1000	NT	Placenta	Cytoplasmic
HMB-45	HMB-45	Enzo	1:50	NT	Melanoma	Cytoplasmic
hPL	Polyclonal	BioGenex	1:200	NT	Placenta	Cytoplasmic
Inhibin	R1	Serotec	1:20	PC	Ovary	Cytoplasmic
Melan-A	A103	DAKO	1:400	MW 20 min	Melanoma	Cytoplasmic
MIB-1	7B11	Zymed	1:50	PC	Breast cancer	Nuclear
p53	1801	BioGenex	1:150	PC	Ovarian cancer	Nuclear
PLAP	Polyclonal	DAKO	1:500	NT	Placenta	Cytoplasmic
PR	PR88	BioGenex	1:50	PC	Breast cancer	Nuclear
S-100	Polyclonal	DAKO	1:4000	NT	Skin	Cytoplasmic/nuclear
SMA	1A4	DAKO	1:400	NT	Colon cancer	Cytoplasmic
Synaptophysin	Sy 38	DAKO	1:100	NT	Brain	Cytoplasmic
Vimentin	V9	DAKO	1:100	MW 10 min	Colon cancer	Cytoplasmic

NT, no treatment; WB, water bath; MW, microwave (followed by time in minutes); PC, pressure cooker; AFP, alpha fetoprotein; CEA, carcinoembryonic antigen; CK, cytokeratin; EMA, epithelial membrane antigen; T, trypsin; hPL, human placental lactogen; PLAP, placental alkaline phosphatase; PR, progesterone receptor; SMA, smooth muscle actin.

ited to the parabasal cells. In intraepithelial neoplasia, MIB-1+ cells progressively increase in quantity and height within the epithelium with increasing lesion grade.[11, 12] However, Ki-67 expression has also been identified in benign and reactive conditions in which there is loss of normal squamous maturation.[13] The utility of cell proliferation markers as a diagnostic aid may provide an objective method with which to diagnose lesions or provide quality assurance in specific circumstances. Expression of Ki-67 antigen is not a positive or negative finding. As Ki-67 expression does not lend itself well to image analysis because of the stratified architectural pattern, a labeling index (i.e., the percentage of cells stained per full epithelial thickness in which between 300 and 500 cells must be counted) can be performed, but is tedious and time-consuming. Ki-67 may be most useful when mitotic figures are not readily apparent or when features of the lesion examined are equivocal. MIB-1 expression is readily detectable with routine antigen enhancement (microwave) and is easily interpretable, as the nuclear staining is crisp and clear. In addition, there is always a positive control on the slide, either within the epithelium or within lymphocytes. There is only rare, occasional staining of normal endocervical cells.[14]

Monoclonal carcinoembryonic antigen (CEA) antibodies are useful in the characterization of glandular lesions of the lower genital tract such as in Paget's disease and endocervical adenocarcinoma. CEA stains the cytoplasm or the luminal border of glandular cells, or both. Normal endocervical glandular epithelium does not stain with CEA.[15]

Mesenchymal markers that are useful in the lower genital tract include vimentin, desmin, and smooth muscle–specific actin (SMSA). Mesenchymal neoplasms are less common in the lower genital tract than are epithelial lesions. The differentiation of vulvar-specific spindle cell lesions such as angiomyofibroblastoma and aggressive angiomyxoma is based on histologic characteristics such as the circumscription of the border and cytologic atypia. Markers of smooth muscle differentiation (vimentin, actin, and desmin) are expressed in these tumors as well as in other smooth muscle neoplasms.[16] S-100 protein is useful when considering myxoid melanoma, liposarcoma, or neural tumors. Myogenin and MyoD1 are useful in identifying skeletal muscle differentiation, for example, in malignant rhabdoid tumors of the vulva or in embryonal rhabdomyosarcoma of the vagina.

The neuroendocrine markers chromogranin, synaptophysin, and serotonin are useful in the diagnosis of neuroendocrine tumors of the cervix, including carcinoid tumor, large cell neuroendocrine carcinoma, and small cell carcinoma.[17] Isolated neuroendocrine cells can also be identified in adenoma malignum,[18] cervical adenocarcinomas, squamous carcinomas,[19] and endometrial adenocarcinomas.[20]

BRST-2, or gross cystic disease fluid protein (GCDFP), is often expressed in breast carcinomas and has also been found to be useful in identifying Paget cells in the vulva.[21, 22] Markers of melanocytic differentiation include S-100 and HMB-45. The latter is highly specific for the detection of melanoma cells, but it lacks sensitivity, and some nodular melanomas can be negative. S-100 is a more sensitive marker but less specific, as it can also stain non-melanocytic tumors.

Differential Diagnosis

PRIMARY PAGET'S DISEASE VERSUS SECONDARY PAGET'S DISEASE VERSUS SUPERFICIAL SPREADING MELANOMA VERSUS PAGETOID VULVAR INTRAEPITHELIAL NEOPLASIA (Table 15–2 and Fig. 15–1)

Immunohistochemistry can assist in the differentiation of extramammary Paget's disease from superficial spreading melanoma and pagetoid VIN and also can suggest the presence of underlying pelvic malignancy with spread to the epidermis (secondary Paget's disease). A valuable immunohistochemical panel in the differential diagnosis of extramammary Paget's disease includes keratins (AE1/AE3, CK7/CK20), CEA, GCDFP, and S-100.

The most useful antibody in the differential diagnosis of pagetoid vulvar lesions is CK7. It uniformly and diffusely stains the cytoplasm of Paget cells and does not stain the stratified squamous epithelial cells.[23, 24] CK7 can be used to identify Paget cells at surgical margins and also to highlight areas of early stromal invasion. However, CK7 can also mark intraepithelial Merkel cells that can mimic the cells of Paget's disease.[25] Therefore, identification of CK7+ cells within the skin and mucosa of the vulva is a sensitive marker for

Paget's disease, but it is not absolutely specific. CK20 should also be included in the diagnostic antibody panel, especially when secondary involvement of the epithelium by an underlying malignancy is considered. Positivity for CK20 is seen in association with rectal adenocarcinoma or transitional cell carcinoma as well as in a minority of cases of primary extramammary Paget's disease.[21-23]

Antibodies less useful in the setting of suspected Paget's disease include pan-cytokeratins, CEA, and GCDFP, or BRST-2. For example, antibodies against cytokeratins AE1/AE3 mark both squamous epithelial cells and Paget cells, which limits their utility in this setting. Monoclonal CEA expression is positive in most cases of Paget's disease, but its expression can be weak.[23] GCDFP is a useful marker, although it is not as sensitive for Paget's disease as is CK7. Like CK7, though, GCDFP is more commonly expressed in primary vulvar Paget's disease when compared with cases associated with an internal malignancy.[23, 26] Underlying malignancy should be ruled out in cases with CK20 expression or lack of GCDFP reactivity. The finding of CK20+/GCDFP− Paget cells suggests the presence of an underlying carcinoma in the lower gastrointestinal or urinary tract.[22]

Virtually all nondesmoplastic melanomas are S-100+. As S-100 reactivity can occasionally be seen in Paget cells, HMB-45 should be used as a confirmatory antibody for melanoma if there is a positive reaction with any of the other antibodies in the panel.[26] Another lesion with pagetoid characteristics is cutaneous T-cell lymphoma. This should be considered if the cytokeratins are negative.[26]

CONDYLOMA ACUMINATUM VERSUS SQUAMOUS PAPILLOMA OR FIBROEPITHELIAL POLYP (Fig. 15–2)

Cell proliferation markers may be a diagnostic aid in the detection of human papillomavirus (HPV)-associated lesions, as immunohistochemical methods were developed for HPV, but have a low sensitivity.[27] The differential diagnosis of common exophytic vulvar lesions includes condyloma acu-

Table 15–2. Pagetoid Lesions of the Vulva
Suggested antibody panel: AE1/AE3, CK7, CK20, mCEA, GCDFP and S-100

	AE1/AE3	CK7	CK20	CEA	GCDFP	S-100
Paget's disease	+/−	+	−/+	+/−	+/−	R
Secondary Paget's disease	+	+	+/−	+	N	N
Pagetoid vulvar intraepithelial neoplasia	+	N	N	N	N	N
Superficial spreading melanoma	R	N	N	N	N	+

+, almost always strong, diffuse reactivity; +/−, variable, mostly positive reactivity; −/+, variable, mostly negative reactivity; R, rare cells may be positive; N, almost always negative.

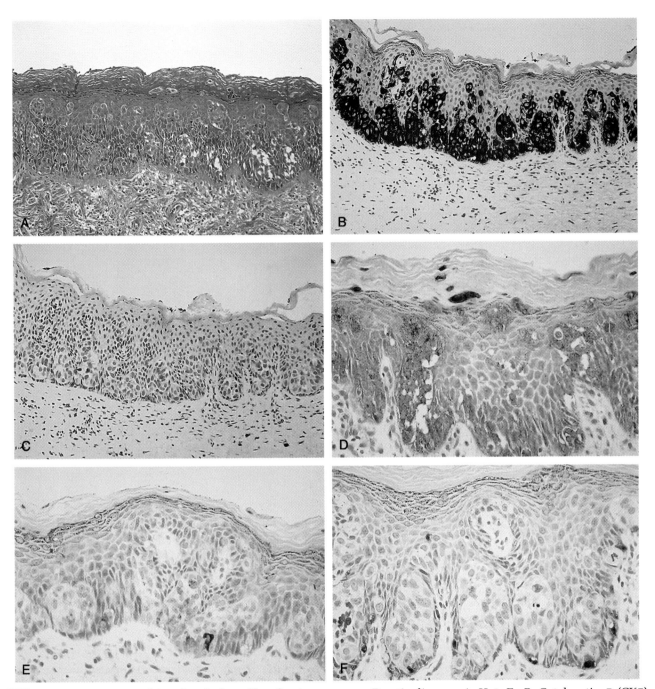

Figure 15–1. Immunohistochemical profile of extramammary Paget's disease. *A*, H & E. *B*, Cytokeratin 7 (CK7) shows intense positive staining that clearly highlights the lesional cells. *C*, CK20 shows negative staining. *D*, Carcinoembryonic antigen (CEA) shows moderate, granular cytoplasmic staining. *E*, Gross cystic disease fluid protein (GCDFP) shows weak, focal staining. *F*, S-100 shows staining of dendritic cells, not the lesional cells.

minatum, fibroepithelial polyp, and squamous papilloma. Although koilocytosis is considered to be a pathognomonic feature of HPV-associated lesions, this finding often is not present in vulvar condylomata, and the diagnosis is based on nonspecific features such as papillomatosis, acanthosis, parakeratosis, and dyskeratosis. MIB-1 and Ki-67 expression in normal vulvar skin and mucosa is limited to the parabasal cells, whereas in VIN and condylomata, MIB-1 positivity extends to the up-

per two thirds of the epithelial thickness.[12, 28] In a study evaluating the differential diagnosis of these lesions, all condyloma acuminatum cases demonstrated MIB-1+ cells in the upper two thirds of the epithelium and in the same region as HPV DNA detected by in situ hybridization.[29] In contrast, MIB-1+ cells were not seen above the parabasal cell layer in any of the 10 cases of squamous papilloma nor in 12 of 14 cases of fibroepithelial polyps. In equivocal cases of condylomata, MIB-1

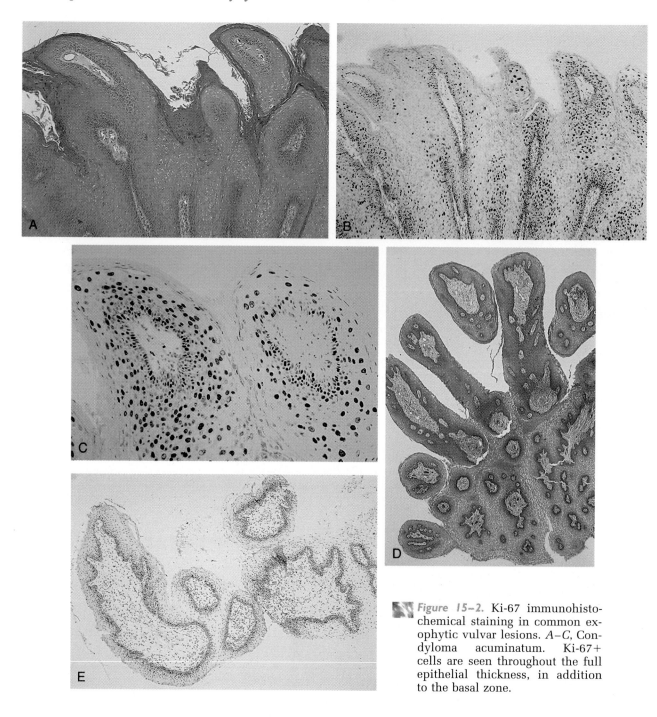

Figure 15-2. Ki-67 immunohisto-chemical staining in common exophytic vulvar lesions. *A–C*, Condyloma acuminatum. Ki-67+ cells are seen throughout the full epithelial thickness, in addition to the basal zone.

staining was useful in identifying both overdiagnoses (HPV DNA− cases) and, occasionally, underdiagnoses (HPV DNA+ cases).

SQUAMOUS AND GLANDULAR INTRAEPITHELIAL LESIONS (Fig. 15–3)

Studies have also examined the expression of the cell proliferation marker Ki-67 (MIB-1), in cervical neoplasia.[11, 14, 30–33] All have demonstrated that high-grade squamous intraepithelial lesions (HSILs) have uniform and diffuse nuclear expression of Ki-67 throughout all cell layers of the le-

sion. In low-grade squamous intraepithelial lesions (LSILs), the percentage of positive cells is not as high in the superficial layers. The proliferative appearance of HPV-associated lesions is most likely due to the increased cell division from the mitogenic effects of HPV protein expression, specifically HPV early proteins E6 and E7.

Although histologic features are still the most valuable tool for the diagnosis of intraepithelial lesions, there may be a role for using Ki-67 expression in equivocal cases. In normal cervical mucosa, there is uniform linear staining of nuclei in the parabasal region. Notably, the basal cells in normal mucosa fail to stain. In regions of squamous meta-

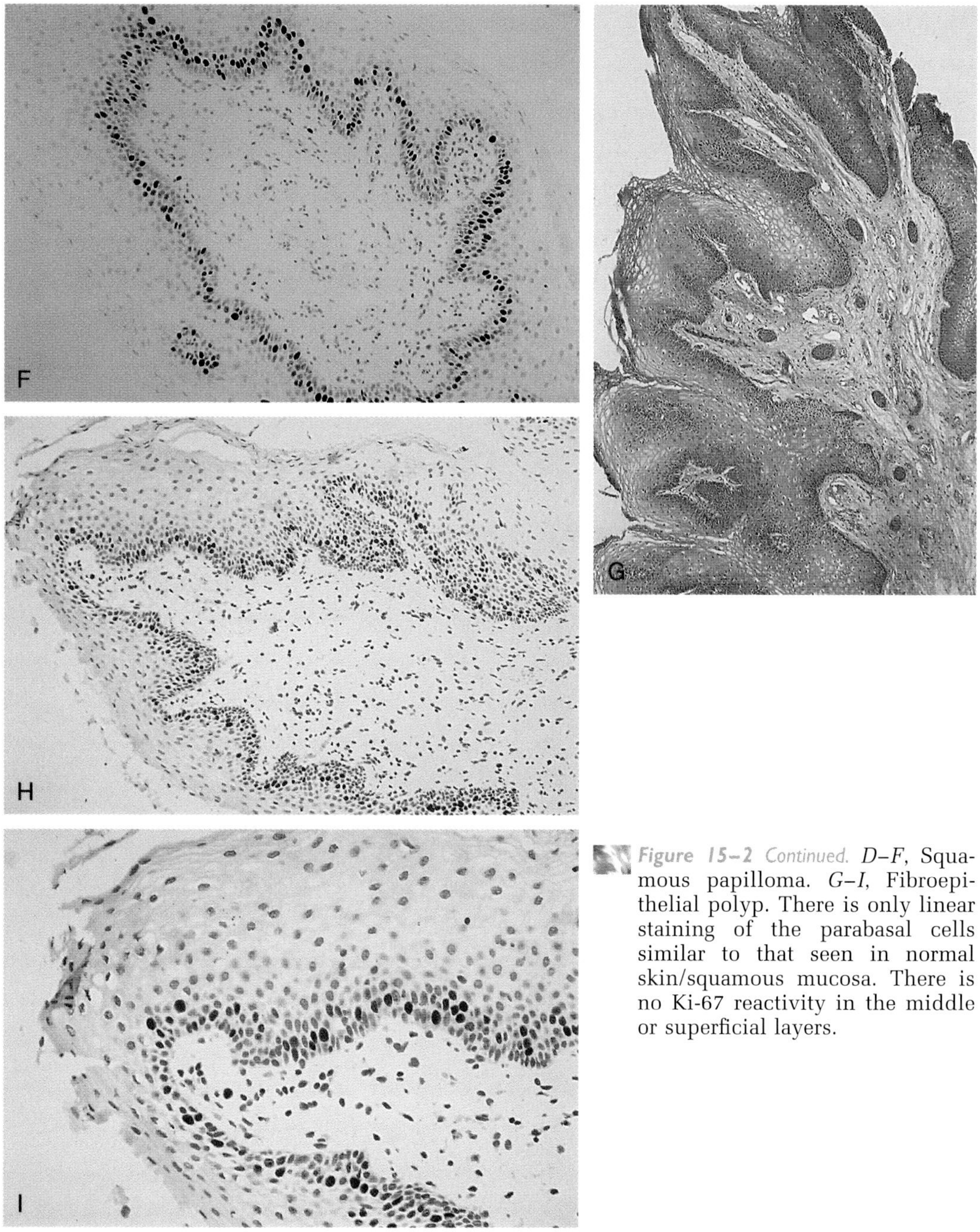

Figure 15-2 *Continued.* *D–F*, Squamous papilloma. *G–I*, Fibroepithelial polyp. There is only linear staining of the parabasal cells similar to that seen in normal skin/squamous mucosa. There is no Ki-67 reactivity in the middle or superficial layers.

plasia, there is parabasal as well as focal involvement of the basal cells, but there is no significant difference in Ki-67 antigen immunostaining between normal squamous mucosa and regions of squamous metaplasia,[11, 30] including regions with inflammation.[32] In SILs, the staining is markedly increased in the parabasal and basal layers, and Ki-67+ cells are also distributed in the intermediate (LSILs) or all layers of the epithelium (HSILs).

Atrophy can be a mimicker for HSILs because of its lack of maturation. Typically, the bland nuclear features and lack of mitotic activity resolve this problem, but absence of Ki-67 expression could be used for confirmation.[31, 33] Atypical immature

metaplasia (AIM) may also mimic HSILs. In one study, the Ki-67 index of AIM was increased when compared with normal, but the range overlapped those of normal cervix, LSILs, and HSILs, suggesting that AIM represents a heterogeneous group of lesions.[13] Overall, in lesions that lack squamous maturation but show proliferative activity, the distinction can be difficult.

MIB-1 reactivity can also be useful in distinguishing glandular neoplastic lesions such as adenocarcinoma in situ (AIS) and adenocarcinoma from endocervicitis, microglandular hyperplasia, and tuboendometrioid metaplasia.[34, 35] Neoplastic glands demonstrate an increase in the percentage

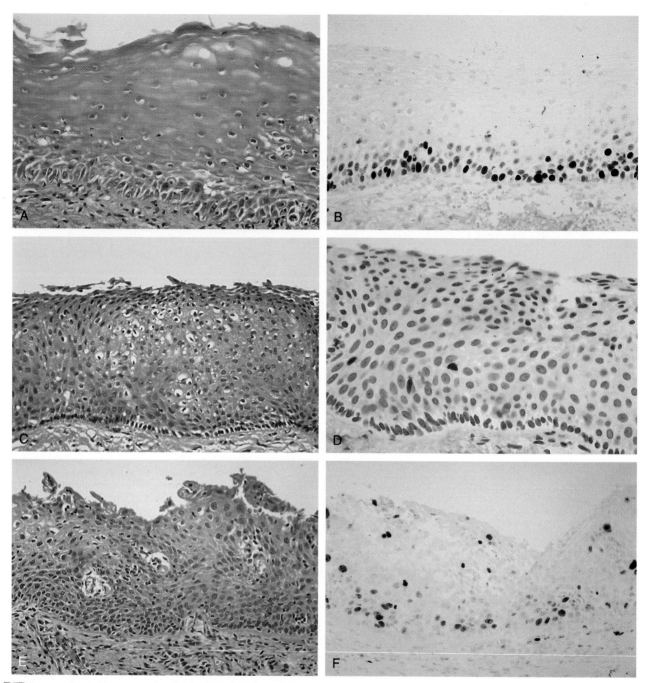

Figure 15–3. Ki-67 immunohistochemical staining in normal cervix *(A and B)*, postmenopausal atrophy *(C and D)*, and squamous metaplasia with inflammation *(E and F)*.

and distribution of positively staining cells similar to that seen with HSILs and squamous carcinoma. Caution is advised, however, because the use of MIB-1 in this setting has not been as widely tested as in squamous intraepithelial lesions.

Immunohistochemistry may also be performed on cervical smears and thin-layer specimens.[36, 37] The application of Ki-67 antigen antibodies for the identification of squamous intraepithelial lesions on cervical smears was examined in one study. They found that air-dried smears stained with avidin-biotin peroxidase and blocked with 0.3% H_2O_2

and phosphate-buffered saline gave the best results for identification of Ki-67 expression in SILs.[36]

ADENOMA MALIGNUM AND WELL-DIFFERENTIATED ADENOCARCINOMA VERSUS BENIGN GLANDULAR LESIONS
(Table 15–3)

At times it can be difficult to distinguish between benign and malignant glandular lesions of the cervix, especially if the tumors are well differ-

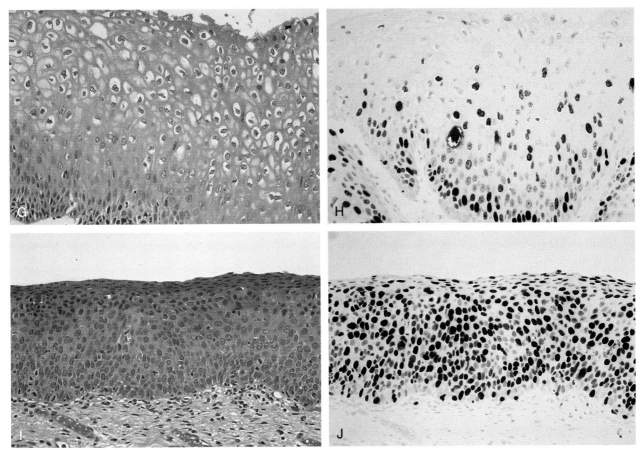

Figure 15-3 Continued. Ki-67 immunohistochemical staining in low-grade squamous intraepithelial lesions (LSILs) *(G* and *H)* and high-grade squamous intraepithelial lesions (HSILs) *(I* and *J).* Ki-67–reactive cells are confined to the parabasal region in the normal cervix, and they are less conspicuous in atrophy. The Ki-67 pattern in reactive lesions and LSILs shows a passing resemblance, especially because both contain superficial immunoreactive cells, but the proliferative zone in LSILs is significantly wider. The superficial immunoreactive cells in reactive lesions are mostly, if not entirely, activated intraepithelial lymphocytes. HSILs demonstrate the widest proliferative zone with extensively immunoreactive superficial cells.

entiated, as is the case with adenoma malignum. It has been proposed that CEA, Ki-67, and p53 immunostaining can be contributory to narrowing the differential diagnosis. Numerous studies have suggested a role for CEA in this setting, as it is expressed in the cytoplasm of most cervical adenocarcinomas, whereas it is absent in normal cervix.[18, 38–40] However, CEA positivity in adenoma malignum can be focal or diffuse, and it may be absent in small biopsy or curettage specimens in which only a small portion of the tumor is represented.[18] CEA, in combination with Ki-67 and p53, has been found to be useful in the differential diagnosis of these lesions.[40] A high proliferative index or CEA positivity, or both, was limited to cases of adenocarcinoma, adenoma malignum, and AIS as compared with normal endocervix and benign glandular mimickers such as tunnel clusters and microglandular hyperplasia. In addition, p53 overexpression (defined as 10% of the glandular nuclei staining) was seen only in neoplastic glandular lesions, with the exception of florid microglandular hyperplasia.

Table 15-3. Cervical Lesions

Differential Diagnosis	Suggested Antibody Panel
Squamous metaplasia versus LSILs	Ki-67
Squamous atrophy versus HSILs	Ki-67
Normal, benign glandular lesions versus preneoplastic, neoplastic lesions	p53, Ki-67, CEA
Endocervical adenocarcinoma versus endometrial adenocarcinoma	CK, vimentin, CEA
Small cell neuroendocrine carcinoma versus poorly differentiated squamous cell carcinoma versus lymphoma	CK, chromogranin, synaptophysin, LCA

LSILs, low-grade squamous intraepithelial lesions; HSILs, high-grade intraepithelial lesions; CEA, carcinoembryonic antigen; CK, cytokeratin; LCA, leukocyte common antigen.

ENDOCERVICAL ADENOCARCINOMA VERSUS ENDOMETRIAL ADENOCARCINOMA (see Table 15–3)

The distinction of adenocarcinoma of endocervical versus endometrial origin can usually be made on histologic grounds by identifying their respective precursor lesions (AIS and complex atypical hyperplasia) or by the predominance of tumor in either the endocervical or endometrial component of the specimen. CEA is more commonly expressed in endocervical adenocarcinomas (up to 100%) than in endometrial adenocarcinomas (up to 50%); however, the great degree of overlap precludes its clinical utility on an individual case basis.[15, 41, 42] Vimentin staining may be a more useful immunohistochemical aid, as coexpression of low molecular weight cytokeratin and vimentin is seen in the majority of endometrial adenocarcinomas, but not in endocervical adenocarcinomas.[43]

LARGE CELL NEUROENDOCRINE CARCINOMA VERSUS SMALL CELL CARCINOMA VERSUS SQUAMOUS CARCINOMA VERSUS LYMPHOMA

(see Table 15–3)

Confirmation of neuroendocrine differentiation is required for the diagnosis of large cell neuroendocrine carcinoma in order to distinguish it from other poorly differentiated carcinomas.[17] These tumors show expression of either chromogranin or synaptophysin.[44] Immunohistochemical stains are not required for the diagnosis of small cell carcinoma, however, especially if the lesion in question demonstrates *all* the characteristic morphologic features of small cell carcinoma; up to 60% of cervical small cell carcinomas do not show reactivity for either chromogranin or synaptophysin.[17] However, expression of neuroendocrine markers in a tumor with *most* of the histologic features of small cell carcinoma favors a neuroendocrine origin. Cytokeratin expression alone without neuroendocrine marker reactivity in such borderline lesions favors small cell squamous cell carcinoma over small cell neuroendocrine carcinoma.[45] In addition to chromogranin and synaptophysin, small cell carcinomas have been reported to express adrenocorticotropic hormone (ACTH), somatostatin, and serotonin.[46] Because the differential diagnosis of small cell neoplasms of the cervix also includes lymphomas, an appropriate immunohistochemical panel should include leukocyte common antigen.

UTERUS

General Considerations

To confirm an epithelial origin in tumors of most organ systems, expression of cytokeratins (AE1/AE3 and CAM5.2) is usually sufficient. However, in the uterus, cytokeratin expression is not limited to epithelial cells. Both endometrial stromal and smooth muscle cells have been shown to have focal cytokeratin expression, although it is much weaker than in epithelial cells.[47–49] This finding is particularly highlighted in the sarcomatous portion of malignant mixed müllerian tumors (MMMTs), which also can coexpress cytokeratins in addition to mesenchymal markers. Other epithelial markers include epithelial membrane antigen (EMA) and CK7. Vimentin, an intermediate filament, is expressed in normal proliferative endometrial epithelial cells and also in the majority of endometrial carcinomas.[15, 43] The coexpression of vimentin and low molecular weight cytokeratin can aid in the differential diagnosis of an endocervical versus an endometrial adenocarcinoma, as discussed in the previous section. There are no known immunohistochemical stains that reliably distinguish between complex atypical hyperplasia and well-differentiated endometrioid adenocarcinoma.

Overexpression of the p53 tumor suppressor protein is seen in the majority (>80%) of uterine serous carcinomas and their putative precursor lesion, endometrial intraepithelial carcinoma (EIC).[50–52] The pattern of staining is dramatic— >75% of the tumor cells stain with strong intensity, and there is an abrupt cut-off with the adjacent uninvolved atrophic endometrium. Complex atypical hyperplasia and grade 1 endometrioid adenocarcinomas rarely demonstrate p53 immunoreactivity, and if present, the pattern is weak and focal.[53–56] There is increasing expression of p53 in endometrioid adenocarcinomas with increasing grade and some grade 3 endometrioid adenocarcinomas will stain intensely.[53–55, 57]

Estrogen and progesterone receptor expression is seen in normal uterine elements, benign tumors and malignant processes, but these stains are not commonly used for diagnostic purposes. Of note, ER/PR expression is moderate in endometrioid carcinomas as compared to negative or only occasional weak staining in clear cell carcinomas and uterine serous carcinomas.[53, 58] However, ER/PR expression is just as weak in poorly differentiated endometrioid carcinomas as compared to serous and clear cell.[59–61]

The muscle actins (MSA and SMSA) and desmin are useful in identifying smooth muscle cells. Normal endometrial stromal cells express vimentin and muscle actins, but lack expression of cytokeratins and epithelial membrane antigen.[48] Some authors have found desmin expression in normal endometrial stromal cells and endometrial stromal neoplasms, but others have found desmin to be a reliable indicator for differentiating smooth muscle from endometrial stromal cells.[49, 62, 63] Sex-cord-like elements in uterine mesenchymal tumors show immunohistochemical evidence of sex-cord differentiation with inhibin, a peptide hormone normally expressed by ovarian granulosa cells.[64] Smooth muscle cells can express keratins, but despite their high rate of keratin positivity, uterine smooth muscle tumors, even those with epithelioid features, will still show frequent reactivity for muscle markers making their identification less difficult.[65] Endometrial stromal tumors have been reported to express keratins as well, but there is usually not expression of epithelial membrane antigen.[47–49, 62] Antidesmin antibodies can be used to highlight rhabdoid differentiation in malignant mixed müllerian tumors. However, in the absence of heterologous elements, distinction of MMMT from poorly differentiated carcinoma is not immunohistochemically possible as their immunophenotypes overlap.[66]

Differential Diagnosis

ENDOMETRIAL INTRAEPITHELIAL CARCINOMA VERSUS METAPLASIA
(Fig. 15–4)

The p53 tumor suppressor gene is frequently altered in uterine serous carcinoma and its putative precursor lesion, EIC. The alteration in p53 often results in its overexpression in an intense, diffuse pattern. This feature may be used to distinguish

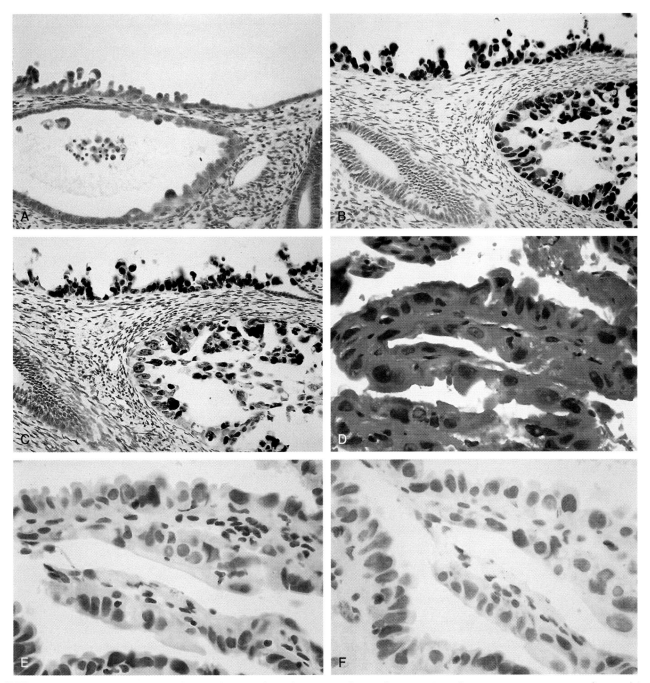

Figure 15–4. p53 and Ki-67 in endometrial surface metaplastic-degenerative change versus serous surface carcinoma endometrial intraepithelial carcinoma (EIC). EIC *(A–C)* contrasts with metaplastic-degenerative change *(D–F)* by virtue of uniform and intense nuclear expression for p53 *(B and E)* and Ki-67 *(C and F)* in EIC.

surface uterine serous carcinoma or EIC from its benign mimics.[50, 52] Endometrial surface lesions with severe cytologic atypia may be found in either curettage or hysterectomy specimens. In the absence of myometrial invasion, the differential diagnosis includes EIC and surface serous carcinoma and endometrial metaplastic surface changes, including eosinophilic, tubal change, or degenerative processes. The combination of Ki-67 and p53 antibodies can aid the differential diagnosis, as the addition of Ki-67 antigen helps highlight the atypical proliferative cells in these endometrial lesions.

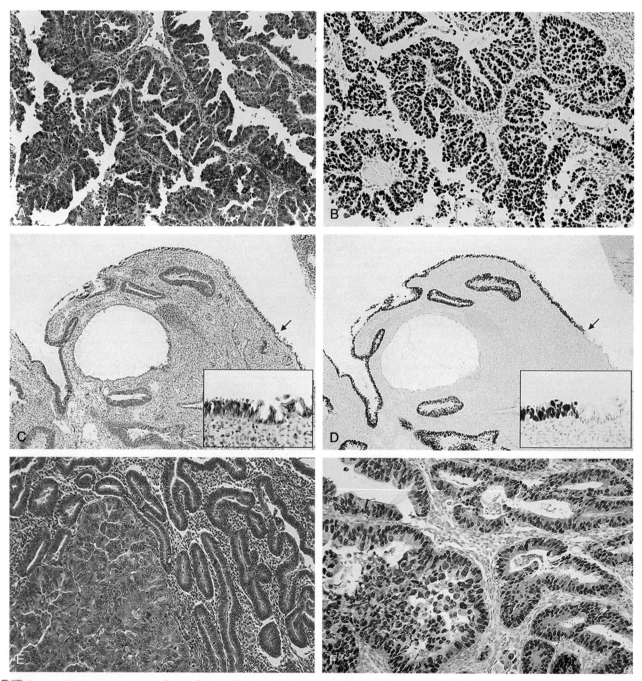

Figure 15–5. p53 immunohistochemical staining in uterine serous carcinoma (USC) versus uterine endometrioid carcinoma (UEC). USC shows diffuse and intense nuclear immunoreactivity for p53 *(A and B),* as does the USC precursor EIC *(C and D).* Not infrequently, USC can demonstrate a glandular architectural pattern *(E).* Diffuse and intense p53 immunoreactivity in glandular USC *(F)* can provide support for this entity when simple hyperplasia with atypia and endometrioid adenocarcinoma are considerations.

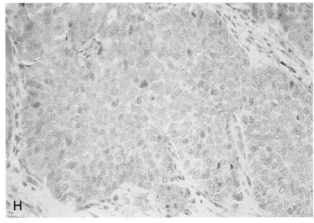

Figure 15–5 *Continued.* Although low-grade endometrioid adenocarcinomas rarely overexpress p53, high-grade examples *(G)* can show significant p53 overexpression *(H)*. p53 expression in International Federation of Gynecology and Obstetrics (FIGO) grade 3 endometrioid adenocarcinoma is usually less diffuse and less intense when compared with USC. (*A–D* from Tashiro H, Isacson C, Levine R, et al. p53 gene mutations are common in uterine serous carcinomas and occur early in their pathogenesis. Am J Pathol 1997;150:177–185.)

UTERINE SEROUS CARCINOMA VERSUS UTERINE ENDOMETRIOID CARCINOMA

(Figs. 15–5 and 15–6)

The two major histologic types of endometrial carcinoma, endometrioid and serous, exhibit unique biologic behaviors and arise in different clinical settings. Immunohistochemistry has been used to highlight their divergent pathways and may be useful diagnostically. The distinction of uterine serous carcinoma (USC) from uterine endometrioid carcinoma (UEC) is important because of the aggressive behavior of USCs that results in a disproportionate number of endometrial cancer-related deaths.[67, 68] When USCs are separated from UECs, strong p53 immunoreactivity is seen in greater than 80% of cases. In contrast, p53 immunohistochemical studies have demonstrated positive immunostaining in only approximately 20% of endometrioid carcinomas.[54] Expression of p53 in UECs is negative to weak in grade 1 to grade 2 tumors, and it is not seen in complex atypical hyperplasia, the putative precursor to UEC. These results are confirmed by molecular analyses that have demonstrated p53 gene mutations in the majority (90%) of serous carcinomas,[51] whereas in contrast, p53 mutations occur in only 10 to 20% of endometrioid carcinomas and usually are found in those of higher grade.[54] Misclassification of USC as an endometrioid carcinoma can occur when a glandular architectural pattern predominates. A combination of p53, Ki-67, and estrogen receptor/progesterone receptor (ER/PR) may help identify these two tumor types. Certainly, mixed cases can occur.

CD44v6, E-cadherin, and beta-catenin expression also correlates with histologic subtype, but their use in routine clinical practice is limited because negative results are common in both endometrioid and serous carcinomas.[69, 70] CD44 is a cell membrane glycoprotein that is associated with cell adhesion, lymphocyte activation, and homing functions; expression of the v6 isoform (splice variant) has been reported to vary with aggressive clinical disease and metastasis. Serous carcinomas do not express CD44v6 or nuclear beta-catenin, but significant numbers of endometrioid carcinomas do. These differences in cell adhesion molecule expression may account for differences in patterns of tumor dissemination.

ENDOMETRIAL STROMAL TUMORS VERSUS SMOOTH MUSCLE TUMORS (Fig. 15–7)

A common dilemma in mesenchymal tumors of the uterus is the distinction of endometrial stromal origin from that of smooth muscle origin. Cellular leiomyomas can be easily confused with endometrial stromal nodules,[49] and the immunohistochemical profiles of endometrial stromal sarcomas and leiomyomas and leiomyosarcomas can overlap.[47, 48] Smooth muscle actin (SMA) and SMSA can be expressed in both stromal and smooth muscle cells, but a lack of desmin expression is usually, but not always, sufficient to support endometrial stromal differentiation. h-caldesmon, an actin and tropomyosin binding protein, has also been reported to be helpful in the identification of smooth muscle tumors in the uterine corpus.[71, 72] Two studies have found that h-caldesmon, which is significantly more specific for smooth muscle differentiation when compared with desmin, distinguishes uterine smooth muscle neoplasms from endometrial stromal neoplasms, which uniformly lack h-caldesmon reactivity. The utility of h-caldesmon in the evaluation of mixed endometrial stromal and smooth muscle tumors[62] has not yet been studied.

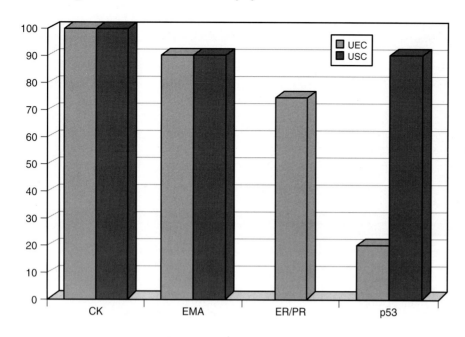

Figure 15–6. Comparative immunohistochemical profiles of uterine endometrioid carcinoma (UEC) and uterine serous carcinoma (USC).

LEIOMYOMA VERSUS LEIOMYOSARCOMA

One of the most difficult differential diagnoses in gynecologic pathology concerns the distinction of leiomyomas from leiomyosarcomas. Classic morphologic criteria are useful, but the relative deficiencies of this approach are well known. Unfortunately, the contributions of immunohistochemistry to the differentiation of leiomyoma from leiomyosarcoma are limited. Investigators have studied the expression of ER/PR, p53, BCL-2 and MIB-1 in

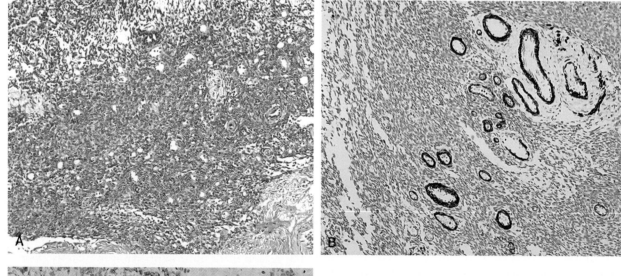

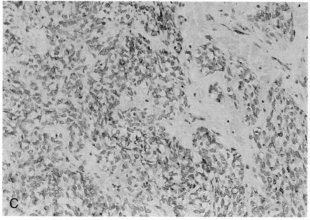

Figure 15–7. Endometrial stromal tumor versus cellular leiomyoma. Cellular mesenchymal proliferations, endometrial stromal tumors (nodules and sarcomas), and cellular leiomyomas can show significant morphologic similarity. Although desmin reactivity can frequently distinguish among these entities, the newly described h-caldesmon antibody appears to be much more specific for smooth muscle differentiation. *A* shows an endometrial stromal sarcoma that is not immunoreactive for h-caldesmon *(B). C* shows a striking and unexpected degree of desmin expression in an endometrial stromal sarcoma.

uterine smooth muscle tumors.[73-75] Leiomyosarcomas express more p53 and MIB-1 than leiomyomas, but less BCL-2 and ER/PR. h-caldesmon expression is also much less strong and diffuse in leiomyosarcomas than in leiomyomas.[72] We do not find this immunohistochemical panel to be clinically useful because the results indicate a broad gradient of expression in leiomyomas, atypical smooth muscle tumors, and leiomyosarcomas, instead of sharp cutoff points that facilitate quantitation. MIB-1 expression, however, is useful in confirming the impression of mitotic activity, especially in poorly preserved specimens in which the distinction of mitotic figures from apoptotic bodies is not straightforward.

GESTATIONAL TROPHOBLASTIC DISEASE

General Considerations

Trophoblasts, including cytotrophoblasts, intermediate trophoblasts, and syncytiotrophoblasts, stain strongly and diffusely with cytokeratins (AE1/AE3).[76] Additional markers can help distinguish the different types of trophoblast. Syncytiotrophoblasts will stain strongly with human chorionic gonadotropin (hCG) in early gestation and show a progressive decrease in intensity towards term.[77] Human placental lactogen (hPL) stains intermediate trophoblasts in the implantation site strongly throughout gestation. hPL also stains syncytiotrophoblasts, but is weaker in intensity in early gestation, with increasing expression toward term.[77] Placental lactogen alkaline phosphatase (PLAP) also stains intermediate cells[78] and syncytiotrophoblast cells in a manner similar to that of hPL, but it is more often positive in the chorionic-type intermediate trophoblast with clear cytoplasm as opposed to the intermediate trophoblast with eosinophilic cytoplasm, which is often more positive for hPL.[77, 79] A new marker for intermediate trophoblastic cells has been identified. Mel-CAM (also known as CD146) is a membrane glycoprotein of the immunoglobulin gene superfamily involved in cell-to-cell interaction.[80] Antibodies to this protein have been shown to stain intermediate trophoblast cells specifically and to demonstrate an increase in intensity from the base to the tip of the trophoblastic column.[80] Mel-CAM expression is not seen in either syncytiotrophoblasts or cytotrophoblasts. Mel-CAM can be used in a manner similar to that of hPL for help in identifying intermediate trophoblasts. There are two Mel-CAM antibodies: MN-4 mouse monoclonal and Mel-CAM rabbit polyclonal antibodies. Neither antibody is commercially available yet.

One pitfall in the evaluation of gestational endometrium is optical clearing of endometrial nuclei. These nuclei are clear and can mimic a herpes simplex virus (HSV) nuclear inclusion.[81] However, these nuclei have been found to contain biotin and may result in a positive immunohistochemical reaction if an avidin-biotin-peroxidase complex is used.[82] Evaluation of the negative control will solve this problem, as it will be positive as well.

Differential Diagnosis

Trophoblastic lesions include hydatidiform mole (partial, complete, and invasive), choriocarcinoma, placental site trophoblastic tumor, epithelioid trophoblastic tumor, exaggerated placental site, and placental site nodule. Immunohistochemistry is rarely used for the diagnosis of hydatidiform moles. Ki-67 immunostaining has been demonstrated to aid in the differential diagnosis of trophoblastic lesions. Caution is advised, however, because Ki-67 can mark normally proliferating lymphocytes that infiltrate the lesion in question. In light of this finding, Shih and Kurman have advocated double staining with a trophoblast marker, such as Mel-CAM, in addition to Ki-67 for the differential diagnosis of exaggerated placental site, placental site trophoblastic tumor, and choriocarcinoma.[83] Table 15–4 presents the immunophenotype of trophoblast lesions and potential mimickers.

PLACENTAL SITE NODULE VERSUS SQUAMOUS INTRAEPITHELIAL LESIONS AND SQUAMOUS CELL CARCINOMA
(see Table 15–4)

Placental site nodules are composed of intermediate trophoblast cells within a nodular, hyalinized stroma. In curettage specimens, these lesions can be confused with either squamous intraepithelial lesions or invasive, keratinizing squamous carcinoma. Immunostaining with PLAP has been reported to be useful by some investigators, as PLAP highlights the placental site nodule.[78, 84] An immunohistochemical panel with PLAP, cytokeratin, Ki-67, and hPL or Mel-CAM is suggested. The Ki-67 index of HSILs and carcinomas is greater than 60%,[11] whereas the Ki-67 index in a placental site nodule is not more than 15%.[85]

PLACENTAL SITE TROPHOBLASTIC TUMOR VERSUS PLACENTAL SITE NODULE
(see Table 15–4)

Both placental site trophoblastic tumor cells and normal intermediate cells in a placental site nodule stain with cytokeratin, hPL, and Mel-CAM. Studies have shown that double staining with both Ki-67 and Mel-CAM can aid in distinguishing these two lesions.[80] The Ki-67 index (percentage of positively staining cells) is close to zero in placental site nodules, whereas placental site trophoblastic tumors have an index of 14% ± 7%. Exaggerated implantation sites also have a low Ki-67 index.

Table 15–4. Trophoblastic Lesions and Mimickers
Suggested antibody panel: Ki-67, hPL or Mel-CAM, or both, and PLAP

	Exaggerated Placental Site	Placental Site Nodule	Placental Site Trophoblastic Tumor	Squamous Intraepithelial Lesion/Carcinoma
CK	+	+	+	+
Ki-67	N	−/+	+/−	+
hPL	+	R	+/−	N
Mel-CAM	+	R	+	N
PLAP	+	+	NA	N

+, almost always strong, diffuse reactivity; +/− variable, mostly positive reactivity; −/+, variable, mostly negative reactivity; R, rare cells may be positive; N, almost always negative; NA, data not available.
hPL, human placental lactogen; PLAP, placental lactogen alkaline phosphatase.

EXAGGERATED PLACENTAL SITE VERSUS IMPLANTATION SITE ASSOCIATED WITH A MOLAR PREGNANCY

Although immunohistochemistry has a limited role in the distinction of hydropic placental tissue from hydatidiform moles, evaluation of the implantation site with Ki-67 may be useful. The implantation site of a hydatidiform mole is mitotically active and has an increased Ki-67 labeling index of 5% ± 4% in contrast to a labeling index of 0 in the exaggerated implantation site of a nonmolar gestation.[80]

TROPHOBLAST CELLS VERSUS DECIDUA

(see Table 15–4)

Immunohistochemical staining with hPL or Mel-CAM can be useful in identifying intermediate trophoblast cells in decidua when determining an intrauterine pregnancy in a curettage specimen.[80, 86] In addition, pan-cytokeratins highlight the distinction of trophoblast cells from decidualized stromal cells with degenerative changes.[76]

CHORIOCARCINOMA VERSUS POORLY DIFFERENTIATED NEOPLASM VERSUS PLACENTAL SITE TROPHOBLASTIC TUMOR

Choriocarcinoma is a biphasic tumor consisting of syncytiotrophoblast cells and mononuclear cells that can be either intermediate trophoblasts or cytotrophoblasts. At times, its appearance can mimic a poorly differentiated carcinoma, especially if multinucleated giant cells are present. A placental site trophoblastic tumor may also enter the differential diagnosis. Immunohistochemical staining with a panel of cytokeratin, hPL or Mel-CAM, and hCG is recommended. One pitfall in immunohistochemical staining with hCG alone is that hCG expression has been reported in other tumors that could involve the uterus, such as cervical squamous carcinoma[87] and transitional cell carcinoma of the bladder.[88] In addition, evaluation of the Ki-67 index is helpful as placental site trophoblastic tumors have a low index of 14% ± 7%, whereas choriocarcinoma and carcinomas frequently have an index greater than 60%.[11, 80]

OVARY, FALLOPIAN TUBE, AND FEMALE PELVIC PERITONEUM

General Considerations

Immunohistochemical study of ovarian, fallopian tube, and female pelvic peritoneal neoplasms is a valuable adjunct to thorough histologic examination; using current immunohistochemical panels, the practicing pathologist can use immunohistochemistry to distinguish between primary and metastatic ovarian neoplasms and to separate surface epithelial from sex cord stromal and germ cell tumors. Since neoplasms of the ovary, fallopian tube, and female pelvic peritoneum show considerable histologic and immunohistochemical overlap, this discussion is limited to ovarian tumors in general, unless otherwise specified.

Epithelial Markers

Non-neoplastic fallopian tube epithelium and mesothelium (ovarian surface epithelium and pelvic peritoneum) express cytokeratins. Evaluation for pan-cytokeratins (AE1/AE3) in the context of ovarian tumors is useful only in specific instances: the identification of epithelial differentiation in an apparently undifferentiated neoplasm, the distinction of dysgerminoma from nondysgerminomatous germ cell tumors,[89–93] and when support for mesothelial differentiation is required to distinguish an adenomatoid tumor from lymphangioma or lipoleiomyoma. Nondysgerminomatous germ cell tumors characteristically express cytokeratins diffusely and strongly, whereas dysgerminoma either does not express pan-cytokeratins or shows only focal and weak expression.[89–93]

EMA expression is useful in the distinction of epithelial proliferations from sex cord stromal tumors that mimic true epithelial neoplasms.[94–100] Although EMA can be expressed in both primary surface epithelial ovarian tumors and metastatic carcinomas, it is only rarely expressed in sex cord stromal tumors.[94–100] In this respect, EMA is far more specific for epithelial differentiation than are pan-cytokeratins, because cytokeratins can be expressed by many varied ovarian tumors, including primary surface epithelial tumors, metastatic carcinomas, granulosa cell tumors,[94–102] Sertoli-Leydig cell tumors,[97, 98, 101] and nondysgerminomatous germ cell tumors.

Although most adenocarcinomas do not demonstrate specific immunophenotypes, use of CK7 and CK20 permits separation into groups used to narrow the differential diagnosis of primary ovarian tumors and metastatic lesions involving the ovary.[103–112]

Adenocarcinomas of the lung[107, 112–115] and breast[103, 107, 112–114, 116] as well as nonmucinous müllerian tumors[103–112] and mesotheliomas demonstrate the CK7+/CK20− immunophenotype.[112] Non-neoplastic fallopian tube epithelium and mesothelium (ovarian surface epithelium and pelvic peritoneum) also express this phenotype. Rare pulmonary adenocarcinomas, however, can express both CK7 and CK20.[117] Strong and diffuse cytoplasmic monoclonal CEA (mCEA) reactivity can permit distinction of pulmonary adenocarcinoma from other possibilities in this category.[118, 119] Breast, ovarian, and endometrial carcinomas also frequently express ER or PR, or both. In addition, at least 40% to 50% of breast carcinomas express BRST-2 (GCDFP).[118, 120, 121]

Transitional cell carcinoma,[107, 108, 112, 122] pancreatic-biliary adenocarcinoma,[112, 123] and many gastric,[110, 112, 123] appendiceal,[124, 125] and ovarian mucinous proliferations[103–107, 109–112, 124, 125] characteristically express the CK7+/CK20+ immunophenotype. These tumors often express mCEA and CA 19-9 as well.[104] Evaluation for expression of ERs and PRs can be contributory for the purposes of distinguishing among these tumors.[104]

Colorectal adenocarcinoma is characteristically CK7−/CK20+.* Hepatocellular and small cell pulmonary carcinomas as well as some renal cell carcinomas are CK7−/CK20−.[112]

LeuM1, which recognizes the CD15 antigen, is an antibody that is reactive in neutrophils, histiocytes, immunoblasts,[128] classic Reed-Sternberg cells,[129–133] anaplastic large cell lymphoma,[134–136] and various adenocarcinomas.[137–144] The latter attribute is shared with BerEP4, B72.3, and mCEA. LeuM1,[137–144] BerEP4,[137, 145, 146] B72.3,[137–139, 141–144, 147] and mCEA[138, 145, 148–150] are markers that can be used to support epithelial differentiation when distinction from mesothelioma is sought. A preponderance of adenocarcinomas expresses these markers, but expression in both pleural and peritoneal mesotheliomas is unusual.[137–144] BerEP4 and B72.3 are more sensitive for female genital surface epithelial differentiation than are LeuM1 and CEA. The relevance of evaluation for the expression of CA 125 (OC125) in the context of diagnostic immunohistochemistry is limited because female genital surface epithelial proliferations, metastatic carcinomas from extragenital sites, and mesothelial proliferations can all express CA 125.[151–155]

---

*References 103, 104, 107, 109, 110, 112, 123, 126, and 127.

Mesothelial Markers

The calcium-binding protein calretinin is useful in the identification of mesothelial differentiation.[156] Diffuse nuclear expression of calretinin[156–159] and cytoplasmic expression of CK5 and CK6[137, 160] are indicative of mesothelial differentiation in the appropriate context. CK5 and CK6 expression is also commonly encountered in squamous cell carcinomas,[161, 162] but only rarely in adenocarcinomas.[137, 160] Although some adenocarcinomas have been reported to express calretinin,[156–159] mesothelial cells are much more likely to express the antigen diffusely and in a nuclear distribution. Therefore, using a panel that combines the affinity of LeuM1, B72.3, and BerEP4 for epithelial differentiation and calretinin and CK5 and CK6 for mesothelial differentiation can enable the pathologist to distinguish one entity from the other confidently.

Neuroendocrine and Neural-Associated Markers

The demonstration of chromogranin, synaptophysin, CD57, and glial fibrillary acidic protein (GFAP) expression can be useful in the identification of carcinoids[163–166]; neuroendocrine carcinomas, including small cell carcinoma of pulmonary type[163, 167, 168]; and the rare primary neuroectodermal tumors of the ovary, including ependymoma.[169–171]

Germ Cell–Associated Markers

Evaluation with antibodies against these antigens can be useful in support of a germ cell tumor. Ovarian neoplasms that express alpha fetoprotein (AFP) include yolk sac tumors[172–176] and tumors showing hepatoid differentiation, including hepatoid yolk sac tumor,[100, 173, 174, 177] the rare ovarian hepatoid carcinoma,[173, 177, 178] and metastatic hepatocellular carcinoma.[179–181] Among germ cell tumors, AFP expression is almost entirely confined to yolk sac tumors,[172–176] although focal expression can be seen in the rare embryonal carcinoma. Also, expression in clear cell carcinomas without hepatoid features has been reported.[182] Therefore, AFP expression in ovarian surface epithelial tumors is generally considered to be definitive support for a yolk sac tumor given the appropriate morphologic context. This is particularly important in the distinction of true endometrioid proliferations from the endometrioid yolk sac tumor.[174, 177] Among germ cell tumors, hCG expression is essentially limited to syncytiotrophoblasts and a subpopulation of extravillous (intermediate) trophoblasts.[77, 183] Primary ovarian tumors that contain syncytiotrophoblasts, including choriocarcinoma by definition, and other germ cell tumors, including dysgerminoma and embryonal carcinoma, express hCG on occasion.[77, 184] Numerous poorly differentiated carcinomas that neither represent germ cell tumors nor contain syncytiotrophoblasts have also been reported to express hCG.[185–195] hCG expression has also been documented in functioning ovarian stroma surrounding primary and secondary ovarian epithelial tumors.[196]

PLAP is generally considered a useful marker for dysgerminoma[93, 104] and neoplasms that contain related cells, such as gonadoblastoma, but expression in numerous other tumors has also been reported.[197–200] Absence of PLAP expression is unusual in dysgerminoma, but expression of PLAP generally is not helpful; nondysgerminomatous germ cell tumors and several carcinomas have been reported to express PLAP.[197–200]

Sex Cord Stromal Markers

The demonstration of inhibin[97, 201–207] and CD99 expression (MIC2 antigen)[101, 201] is useful to support sex cord stromal differentiation in the proper context. Inhibins are peptide hormones that participate in the regulation of the pituitary-gonadal feedback system. The MIC2 antigen is the product of a pseudoautosomal gene[208] that is expressed on the cell surface and thought to be involved in cell-to-cell interactions; it is best known for its expression in immature lymphoid cells, including lymphoblastic lymphoma, and in the Ewing's sarcoma/primitive neuroectodermal tumor (ES/PNET) group of neoplasms. A significant diagnostic pitfall can be avoided if attention is paid to the morphology of cells that express the antigen in question. Luteinized stromal cells that accompany carcinomas can express inhibin,[196, 202, 204, 209] which can lead to the erroneous interpretation that a carcinoma expresses inhibin. In general, inhibin expression in carcinomas is encountered uncommonly, and when it is, the pattern is only exceptionally strong and diffuse.[201, 202, 204, 209]

Aside from its use in support of sex cord stromal differentiation, CD99 can be used in the evaluation of primitive small round cell tumors, including lymphoblastic lymphoma[210] and ES/PNET,[169, 211–213] each of which can involve the ovary. Therefore, expression of CD99 alone is not pathognomonic of any one entity. Close morphologic evaluation and the use of a panel of diagnostic antibodies are recommended.

Lymphoid Markers

Malignant lymphomas can affect the ovary both primarily and secondarily. Although there are certain types of lymphomas that occur more frequently in the ovary than elsewhere, especially Burkitt's lymphoma, the antibodies used and the diagnostic algorithms are similar to those used for lymphomas in other sites. CD45 (leukocyte common antigen) is a useful first-line antibody that recognizes most, but not all, hematolymphoid proliferations. Evaluation with antibodies against T- and B-cell–associated antigens can also be contributory.

CD30 (Ki-1) is probably best known for its expression in hematolymphoid proliferations, particularly but not exclusively Hodgkin's disease and anaplastic large cell lymphoma. Fortunately, this marker is also useful in the distinction of embryonal carcinoma from other carcinomas and other germ cell tumors.[214–216] Although CD30 can be expressed in small foci of dysgerminoma,[214] it is almost never expressed in nongerminomatous carcinomas and germ cell tumors other than embryonal carcinoma. These data are based on testicular germ cell tumors; embryonal carcinomas of the ovary are rare, and CD30 expression in this setting has not been studied.

Melanocyte-Associated Markers

Malignant melanoma always features prominently in a discussion of apparently poorly differentiated metastatic neoplasms, and the ovary is no exception. In fact, metastatic melanoma is a known mimic of several primary and metastatic ovarian neoplasms, including juvenile granulosa cell tumor[102, 217–219] and small cell carcinoma of hypercalcemic type.[220–226] The S-100 protein can be identified in numerous neoplasms, including both carcinomas and melanomas in addition to many others, and in dendritic cells that frequently accompany neoplasms; therefore, confirmation of melanocytic differentiation can be accomplished with antibodies against HMB-45 and melan-A (A103).[227, 228] These latter two markers are significantly more specific for melanoma than is S-100, but they are not entirely specific and are only partially sensitive. HMB-45 is expressed in the tuberous sclerosis–associated proliferations, including lymphangioleiomyomatosis and angiomyolipoma.[229–232] Melan-A's relative lack of specificity in relation to melanocytes, however, is useful in ovarian lesions because it is expressed in luteinized cells, Leydig cells, and ectopic adrenal tissue.[227, 228]

Muscle-Associated Markers

Muscle-associated markers have a limited role in the work-up of ovarian proliferations; evaluation for desmin, for example, is indicated only for the recognition of the rare primary or metastatic ovarian mesenchymal proliferations, such as small, round desmoplastic tumor[233–236] and rhabdomyosarcoma.[225, 237, 238] Desmin can also be used in the identification of muscle differentiation (usually skeletal muscle) in primary and metastatic ovarian tumors that show heterologous differentiation,

Table 15–5. Surface Epithelial Proliferations Versus Mesothelioma
Suggested antibody panel: CD15 (LeuM1), BerEP4 or B72.3, or both, CK5/CK6 or calretinin, or both

Antibody	Surface Epithelial (Adenocarcinoma)	Mesothelial
CD15	+/−	N
BerEP4	+	N
B72.3	+	N
CK5/CK6	N	+
Calretinin	R	+

+, almost always strong, diffuse reactivity; +/−, variable, mostly positive reactivity; R, rare cells may be positive; N, almost always negative.

such as carcinosarcoma (MMMTs), heterologous Sertoli-Leydig cell tumors,[239–245] and teratomas. Antibodies that are more specific for skeletal muscle differentiation are available, including MyoD1[246, 247] and myogenin,[248] but this group of

markers has limited applications in the female genital tract.

Differential Diagnosis

SURFACE EPITHELIAL LESIONS VERSUS MESOTHELIOMA (Table 15–5 and Figs. 15–8 and 15–9)

Primary ovarian surface epithelial proliferations can demonstrate serous, intestinal mucinous, müllerian mucinous, endometrioid, clear cell, transitional and, rarely, squamous differentiation. Serous proliferations that can be confused with metastases include atypically proliferating tumors (low malignant potential or borderline tumors) and carcinomas, which by definition show significant stromal invasion. Using strict morphologic criteria for serous differentiation, however, should make confusion with a metastasis a rare event. However, since

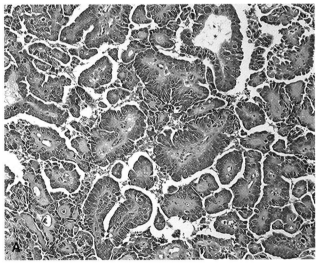

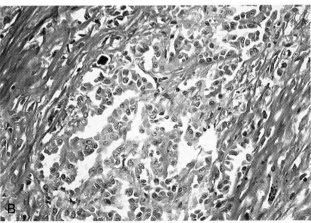

Figure 15–8. Serous carcinoma versus mesothelioma. Serous carcinoma *(A)* and mesothelioma *(B)* can show a remarkable degree of histologic similarity. Both examples exhibit papillary and micropapillary architecture.

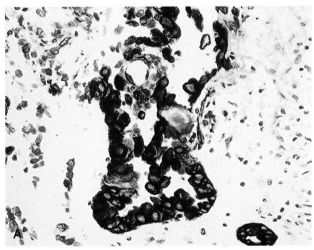

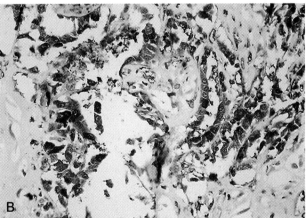

Figure 15–9. Serous carcinoma versus mesothelioma. Although both serous carcinoma and mesothelioma express pan-cytokeratins, CK7 *(A),* and epithelial membrane antigen (EMA), only serous carcinoma expresses LeuM1, BerEP4, and B72.3 (not shown). Epithelial mesotheliomas are characterized by strong nuclear and cytoplasmic expression of calretinin *(B).*

Table 15–6. Surface Epithelial Versus Metastatic Carcinoma
Suggested antibody panel: CK7, CK20, mCEA, ER, PR

Antibody	Surface Epithelial, Nonmucinous	Surface Epithelial, Mucinous	Lower Gastrointestinal Tract*	Upper Gastrointestinal Tract†	Breast	Lung
CK7	+	+	R	+	+	+
CK20	N	+/−	+	+	N	−/+
mCEA	−/+	+/−	+	+	R	+
ER	+/−	+/−	N	N	+/−	N
PR	+/−	+/−	N	N	+/−	−/+

Algorithm

CK7−	CK20+			Lower gastrointestinal tract
CK7+	CK20+	ER/PR+		Surface epithelial, mucinous
		ER/PR−		Upper gastrointestinal tract
	CK20−		mCEA+	Lung
			mCEA−	Surface epithelial, nonmucinous

*Colon.
†Stomach and pancreatobiliary.
+, almost always strong, diffuse reactivity; +/− variable, mostly positive reactivity; −/+, variable, mostly negative reactivity; R, rare cells may be positive; N, almost always negative.
mCEA, monoclonal carcinoembryonic antigen; ER, estrogen receptor; PR, progesterone receptor.

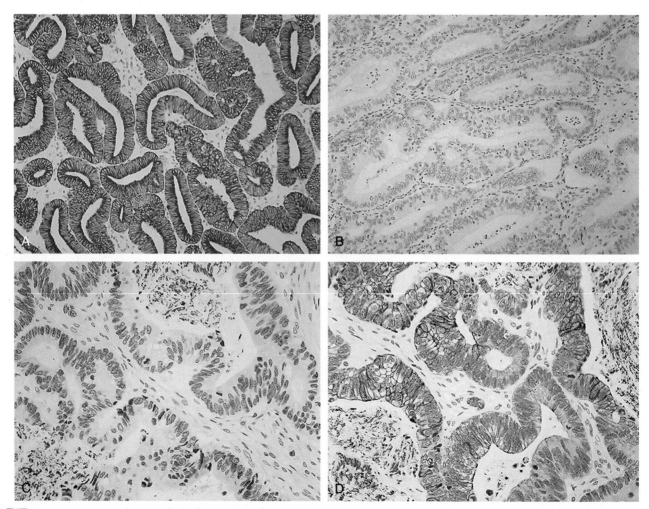

Figure 15–10. Surface epithelial tumor versus metastasis. Antibodies against CK7 and CK20 enable the pathologist to distinguish between surface epithelial proliferations and metastases, especially when support for a lower gastrointestinal tract primary is sought. Surface epithelial proliferations, including endometrioid adenocarcinomas, express CK7 *(A)*, but not CK20 *(B)*. In contrast, most colonic adenocarcinomas express CK20 *(D)*, but not CK7 *(C)*.

Table 15–7. Surface Epithelial Versus Sex Cord Stromal Lesions
Suggested antibody panel: EMA, inhibin or melan A, or both, or CD99 (MIC2), or both

Antibody	Surface Epithelial	Thecoma/Fibrothecoma	Adult and Juvenile Granulosa Cell Tumor	Sertoli-Leydig Cell Tumor	Female Adnexal/Ovarian Tumor of Probable Wolffian Origin
EMA	+	R	N	N	N
Inhibin	R	+	+	+/−	+
Melan-A	−	NA	+/−	+	NA

+, almost always strong, diffuse reactivity; +/−, variable, mostly positive reactivity; −/+, variable, mostly negative reactivity; R, rare cells may be positive; N, almost always negative; NA, data not available.

serous tumors arise not only within intraovarian surface epithelial inclusions but also on the ovarian surface and on peritoneal surfaces, they may raise clinical suspicion for mesothelioma. Serous carcinomas involving the ovarian and mesothelial surfaces can also overlap with mesotheliomas histologically,[138, 143, 145, 146] so evaluation with an antibody panel against CD15 (LeuM1),[137–144] BerEP4,[137, 145, 146] or B72.3, or a combination,[137–139, 141–144, 147] along with calretinin[156–159] and CK5/CK6[137, 160] can be contributory.

SURFACE EPITHELIAL VERSUS METASTASIS
(Table 15–6 and Fig. 15–10)

The differentiation of a primary surface epithelial tumor of the female genital tract from an extragenital primary is seldom straightforward, especially when the surgeon or the pathologist, or both, do not know the patient's clinical history. Morphologic clues are useful, although there are many instances in which the histopathologic appearance is misleading; immunohistochemistry can be particularly valuable in these cases. Unfortunately, in contrast to the situation regarding distant metastases, neither the histopathologic findings nor immunohistochemical data reliably distinguish between primary ovarian surface epithelial proliferations and metastases from other genital sites.

In contrast to serous proliferations, both mucinous and endometrioid tumors are commonly confused with metastases. Since intestinal mucinous tumors[124, 125, 249–254] and endometrioid tumors[255] affect both ovaries, any bilateral proliferation that is thought to be intestinal mucinous or endometrioid, or both, should be evaluated for the possibility of

metastasis. This rule of thumb applies not only to obviously invasive tumors (carcinomas) but also to apparently noninvasive tumors (atypically proliferating, borderline, low malignant potential tumors); this is particularly true of metastatic mucinous neoplasms from the appendix, colon, pancreas, and gallbladder, which on occasion can show remarkable morphologic overlap with atypically proliferating mucinous and endometrioid tumors.* Evaluation of tumors suspicious for metastases from these sites should include antibodies against CK7 and CK20.† Clear cell carcinomas may be confused with metastases from the gastrointestinal tract as well.[105] In this case, also, evaluation with antibodies against CK7 and CK20 can be helpful. Immunohistochemical distinction of metastatic clear cell carcinoma of the kidney from a primary ovarian clear cell carcinoma can be difficult, although renal clear cell carcinomas may not express either CK7 or CK20.[112] Finally, when transitional cell tumors do not contain a benign Brenner component, distinction from a metastatic urothelial tumor is important; this can also be accomplished with antibodies against CK7 and CK20.[108]

SURFACE EPITHELIAL LESIONS VERSUS SEX CORD STROMAL AND GERM CELL TUMORS (Tables 15–7 and 15–8 and Figs. 15–11 to 15–14)

Once a metastasis is excluded, one must consider the possibility that a primary ovarian neo-

---

*References 105, 124, 125, 249–251, 253, 254, 256, and 257.
†References 1, 103, 104, 109, 111–113, 124, and 257.

Table 15–8. Surface Epithelial Versus Germ Cell Tumors
Suggested antibody panel: pan-cytokeratin (CK), AFP, hCG, CD30

Antibody	Surface Epithelial	Dysgerminoma	Yolk	Embryonal Carcinoma	Choriocarcinoma
CK	+	R	+	+	+
AFP	N	N	+	−/+	NA
hCG	−/+	R	R	R	+
CD30	−	R	R	+	N

+, almost always strong, diffuse reactivity; +/−, variable, mostly positive reactivity; −/+, variable, mostly negative reactivity; R, rare cells may be positive; N, almost always negative; NA, data not available.
CK, cytokeratin; AFP, alpha fetoprotein; hCG, human chorionic gonadotropin.

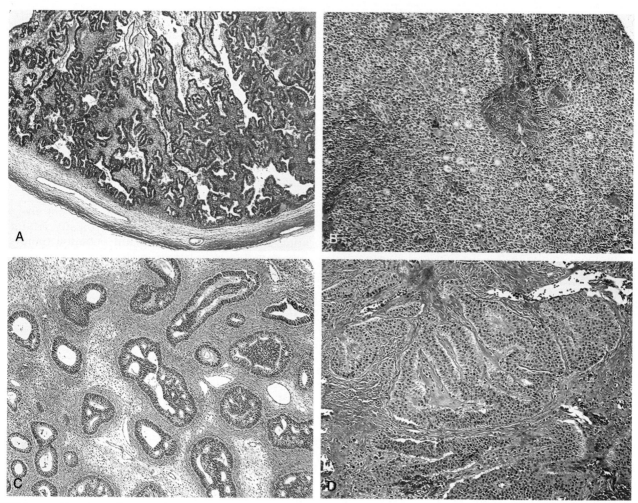

Figure 15–11. Surface epithelial versus sex cord stromal versus germ cell tumors. Illustrated here are mimics of primary and metastatic ovarian carcinomas and atypically proliferating tumors, including atypically proliferating endometrioid tumor *(A)*, adult granulosa cell tumor *(B)*, endometrioid yolk sac tumor *(C)*, carcinoid tumor *(D)*, and Leydig cell tumor (see Figure 15–13). Each of these tumors can be composed of tubules, islands, and trabeculae set in a fibromatous stroma. *(A courtesy of Danielle Lu; C courtesy of Ruoqing Huang.)*

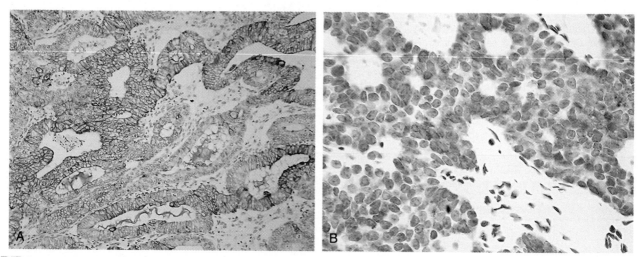

Figure 15–12. Surface epithelial versus sex cord stromal versus germ cell tumors. Evaluation with antibodies against EMA, inhibin, alpha fetoprotein (AFP), and chromogranin can assist in making the correct diagnosis. With only rare exceptions, EMA is expressed only in carcinomas and atypically proliferating tumors *(A)*. Inhibin reactivity is characteristic of sex cord stromal tumors, such as granulosa cell tumor *(B)*, whereas AFP expression

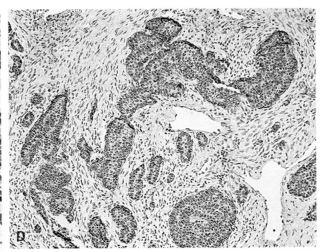

Figure 15–12 *Continued.* supports a diagnosis of yolk sac tumor *(C)*, even when there is histologic similarity to endometrioid proliferations. Chromogranin reactivity permits a diagnosis of carcinoid tumor in the appropriate context *(D)*.

plasm represents a sex cord stromal tumor or a germ cell tumor. This is particularly important when the patient's age falls outside the characteristic range for surface epithelial tumors. As an exam-

ple, the finding of tubules surrounded by fibrous stroma raises the differential diagnosis of an atypically proliferating endometrioid tumor (borderline or low malignant potential tumor,[255] Brenner tu-

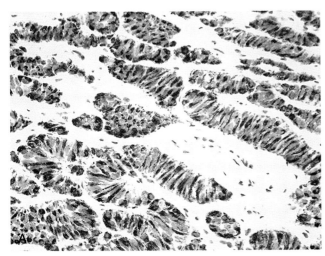

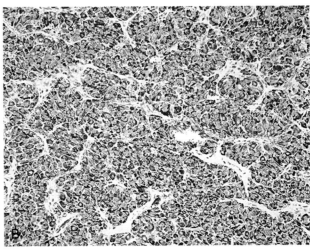

Figure 15–13. Surface epithelial versus sex cord stromal tumor. Examples in both groups can express pan-cytokeratin, as illustrated in this Leydig cell tumor *(A)*. However, sex cord stromal tumors do not generally express EMA. Sex cord stromal tumors, including Leydig cell tumors, commonly express inhibin *(B)* and melan-A *(C)*. Melan-A expression is usually strongest in the Leydig cell component, but it can also be seen in Sertoli cells and granulosa cells.

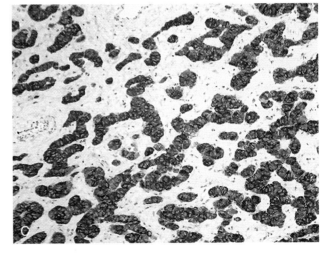

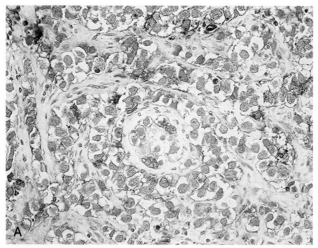

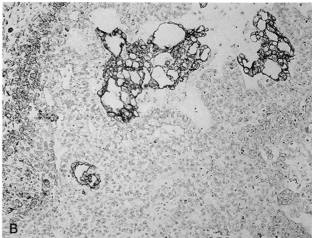

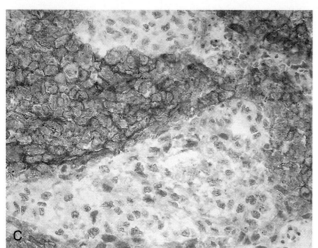

Figure 15–14. Germ cell tumors. Evaluation with antibodies against pan-cytokeratins, AFP, human chorionic gonadotropin (hCG), and CD30 permits distinction among germ cell tumors. Although placenta-like alkaline phosphatase (PLAP) expression is characteristic of dysgerminoma *(A),* it is by no means specific. In contrast, strong cytokeratin expression distinguishes nondysgerminomatous elements from dysgerminoma, which usually does not show strong pan-cytokeratin expression *(B).* Note the focal pan-cytokeratin expression in the yolk sac component of this mixed dysgerminomatous and nondysgerminomatous germ cell tumor *(B).* CD30 is usually strong and diffuse in embryonal carcinoma, whereas generally it is not expressed in other germ cell tumors *(C).* Note the use of anti-CD30 for the distinction of embryonal carcinoma from dysgerminoma in this mixed germ cell tumor. AFP expression is characteristic of yolk sac tumors (see Figure 15–12C).

mors, carcinoid,[163–166] the endometrioid variant of yolk sac tumor tumors,[172–176] Sertoli-Leydig cell tumors,[239–245] and even tumors of probable wolffian origin.[258–261] Other difficult differential diagnoses include clear cell carcinoma versus dysgerminoma, yolk sac tumor, juvenile granulosa cell tumor,[102, 217, 218] steroid cell tumors,[262–264] and fallopian tube–adnexal and ovarian tumors;[258–261] primary

Table 15–9. Small Blue Cell Tumors
Suggested antibody panel: pan-cytokeratins, EMA, CD45, S-100, inhibin, chromogranin, desmin, CD99

Antibody	Carcinoma	Malignant Lymphoma	Melanoma	Adult and Juvenile Granulosa Cell Tumor	Small Cell Carcinoma (Pulmonary Type)	Small Cell Carcinoma (Hypercalcemic Type)	Desmoplastic Small Round Cell Tumor
CK	+	N	N	+/−	+	+/−	+
EMA	+	−/+*	N	N	+	+/−	+
CD45	N	+*	N	N	N	N	N
S-100	−/+	N	+	−/+	R	N	R
Inhibin	R	N	N	+	NA	N	pN
Chromogranin	−/+	N	N	N	+/−	+/−†	−/+
Desmin	N	N	N	−/+	N	N	+/−
CD99	N	−/+*	N	+/−	−/+	−/+	−/+

*Certain subtypes possess different immunophenotypes.
†These cases might represent small cell neuroendocrine carcinomas (SCCPs) that were misclassified as SCCCs.
+, almost always strong, diffuse reactivity; +/−, variable, mostly positive reactivity; −/+, variable, mostly negative reactivity; R, rare cells may be positive; N, almost always negative; NA, data not available; pN, probably negative (only very rare cases studied).
CK, cytokeratin; EMA, epithelial membrane antigen.

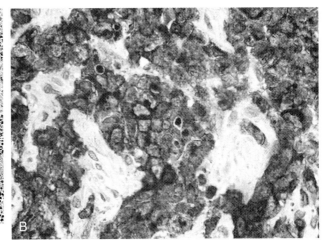

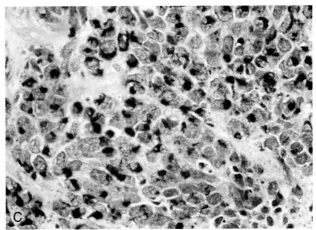

▨ *Figure 15–15.* Small blue cell tumors. Desmoplastic small round cell tumor (DSRCT) is rare, but it is prototypical of a small blue cell tumor that can involve the ovary. Despite the striking clinical differences between DSRCT and primary surface epithelial carcinoma, there can be significant histologic overlap *(A). A* demonstrates its characteristic nested pattern of growth and prominent desmoplastic stroma. Both carcinoma and DSRCT express pancytokertatins and EMA *(B);* DSRCT, however, is well known for its coexpression of mesenchymal markers, including desmin *(C). C* illustrates the paranuclear dot-like pattern of reactivity for desmin in DSRCT. *(A–C* courtesy of Anjali Saqi, M.D.)

ovarian carcinoma versus mucinous and heterologous Sertoli-Leydig cell tumors,[239–245] and selected germ cell tumors; and serous tumors versus the retiform variant of Sertoli-Leydig cell tumor.[239–245] Using a panel of antibodies against EMA, chromogranin, synaptophysin, AFP, inhibin and A103 can help significantly in making the correct diagnosis. Antibodies also useful in the diagnosis of ovarian germ cell tumors include PLAP, hCG, AFP and CD30.

SMALL ROUND CELL TUMORS
(Table 15–9 and Fig. 15–15)

The differential diagnosis of small round cell tumors is extensive, but can be narrowed with attention to clinical data. For the purposes of this discussion, one could consider the following entities in the differential diagnosis: undifferentiated carcinoma (both primary and metastatic), lymphoma, melanoma, granulosa cell tumor, small cell carcinoma of pulmonary (neuroendocrine) type,[163, 165, 168] small cell carcinoma of hypercalcemic type,[97, 220–226, 265] desmoplastic small round cell tumor,[233–236] ES/PNET,[169, 211–213] and primary and

metastatic round cell sarcomas, including embryonal and alveolar rhabdomyosarcomas.[219, 225, 237, 238] Antibodies useful in the differential diagnosis include pan-cytokeratins, EMA, CD45 and related markers, S-100 and related markers, inhibin, CD99, chromogranin, synaptophysin and related markers, and desmin.

ACKNOWLEDGMENTS

We appreciate the contributions of Drs. Demaretta Rush and Erika Resetkova to the discussion of uterine mesenchymal tumors. Drs. Ronald DeLellis and Dennis Frisman deserve thanks for their helpful comments and provision of background materials.

References

1. Moll R, Levy R, Czernobilsky B, et al. Cytokeratins of normal epithelia and some neoplasms of the female genital tract. Lab Invest 1983;49:599–610.
2. Puts JJ, Moesker O, Aldeweireldt J, et al. Application of antibodies to intermediate filament proteins in simple and

complex tumors of the female genital tract. Int J Gynecol Pathol 1987;6:257–274.

3. Bobrow LG, Makin CA, Law S, et al. Expression of low molecular weight cytokeratin proteins in cervical neoplasia. J Pathol 1986;148:135–140.

4. Raju GC. Expression of the cytokeratin marker CAM5.2 in cervical neoplasia. Histopathology 1988;12:437–443.

5. Esquius J, Brisigotti M, Matias-Guiu X, et al. Keratin expression in normal vulva, non-neoplastic epithelial disorders, vulvar intraepithelial neoplasia, and invasive squamous cell carcinoma. Int J Gynecol Pathol 1991;10:341–355.

6. Smedts F, Ramaekers F, Leube RE, et al. Expression of keratins 1, 6, 15, 16, and 20 in normal cervical epithelium, squamous metaplasia, cervical intraepithelial neoplasia, and cervical carcinoma. Am J Pathol 1993;142:403–412.

7. Malecha MJ, Miettinen M. Patterns of keratin subsets in normal and abnormal uterine cervical tissues: An immunohistochemical study. Int J Gynecol Pathol 1992;11:24–29.

8. Gernow A, Nielsen B, Holund B, et al. Immunohistochemical study of possible changes in keratin expression during neoplastic transformation of the uterine mucosa. Virchows Arch A Pathol Anat Histopathol 1990;416:287–293.

9. Cattoretti G, Becker MH, Key G, et al. Monoclonal antibodies against recombinant parts of the Ki-67 antigen (MIB 1 and MIB 3) detect proliferating cells in microwave-processed formalin-fixed paraffin sections. J Pathol 1992;168:357–363.

10. Bravo R, Macdonald-Bravo H. Changes in the nuclear distribution of cyclin (PCNA) but not its synthesis depend on DNA replication. EMBO J 1985;4:655–661.

11. Isacson C, Kessis TD, Hedrick L, et al. Both cell proliferation and apoptosis increase with lesion grade in cervical neoplasia but do not correlate with human papillomavirus type. Cancer Res 1996;56:669–674.

12. van Hoeven KH, Kovatich AJ. Immunohistochemical staining for proliferating cell nuclear antigen, BCL2, and Ki-67 in vulvar tissues. Int J Gynecol Pathol 1996;15:10–16.

13. Geng L, Connolly DC, Isacson C, et al. Atypical immature metaplasia (AIM) of the cervix: Is it related to high-grade squamous intraepithelial lesion (HSIL)? [see comments] Hum Pathol 1999;30:345–351.

14. Resnick M, Lester S, Tate JE, et al. Viral and histopathologic correlates of MN and MIB-1 expression in cervical intraepithelial neoplasia. [see comments] Hum Pathol 1996;27:234–239.

15. Dabbs DJ, Geisinger KR, Norris HT. Intermediate filaments in endometrial and endocervical carcinomas: The diagnostic utility of vimentin patterns. Am J Surg Pathol 1986;10:568–576.

16. Ockner DM, Sayadi H, Swanson PE, et al. Genital angiomyofibroblastoma: Comparison with aggressive angiomyxoma and other myxoid neoplasms of skin and soft tissue. [see comments] Am J Clin Pathol 1997;107:36–44.

17. Albores-Saavedra J, Gersell D, Gilks CB, et al. Terminology of endocrine tumors of the uterine cervix: Results of a workshop sponsored by the College of American Pathologists and the National Cancer Institute. Arch Pathol Lab Med 1997;121:34–39.

18. Gilks CB, Young RH, Aguirre P, et al. Adenoma malignum (minimal deviation adenocarcinoma) of the uterine cervix: A clinicopathological and immunohistochemical analysis of 26 cases. Am J Surg Pathol 1989;13:717–729.

19. Savargaonkar PR, Hale RJ, Mutton A, et al. Neuroendocrine differentiation in cervical carcinoma. J Clin Pathol 1996;49:139–141.

20. Aguirre P, Scully RE, Wolfe HJ, et al. Endometrial carcinoma with argyrophil cells: A histochemical and immunohistochemical analysis. Hum Pathol 1984;15:210–217.

21. Goldblum JR, Hart WR. Vulvar Paget's disease: A clinicopathologic and immunohistochemical study of 19 cases. Am J Surg Pathol 1997;21:1178–1187.

22. Goldblum JR, Hart WR. Perianal Paget's disease: A histologic and immunohistochemical study of 11 cases with and without associated rectal adenocarcinoma. Am J Surg Pathol 1998;22:170–179.

23. Battles OE, Page DL, Johnson JE. Cytokeratins, CEA, and mucin histochemistry in the diagnosis and characterization of extramammary Paget's disease. Am J Clin Pathol 1997;108:6–12.

24. Smith KJ, Tuur S, Corvette D, et al. Cytokeratin 7 staining in mammary and extramammary Paget's disease. Mod Pathol 1997;10:1069–1074.

25. Lundquist K, Kohler S, Rouse RV. Intraepidermal cytokeratin 7 expression is not restricted to Paget cells but is also seen in Toker cells and Merkel cells. Am J Surg Pathol 1999;23:212–219.

26. Kohler S, Rouse RV, Smoller BR. The differential diagnosis of pagetoid cells in the epidermis. Mod Pathol 1998;11:79–92.

27. Kadish AS, Burk RD, Kress Y, et al. Human papillomaviruses of different types in precancerous lesions of the uterine cervix: histologic, immunocytochemical and ultrastructural studies. Hum Pathol 1986;17:384–392.

28. Scurry J, Beshay V, Cohen C, et al. Ki67 expression in lichen sclerosus of vulva in patients with and without associated squamous cell carcinoma. Histopathology 1998;32:399–404.

29. Pirog EC, Chen YT, Isacson C. Mib-1 immunostaining is a beneficial addition for the accurate diagnosis of vulvar condyloma acuminatum. Mod Pathol 1999;12:122A.

30. al-Saleh W, Delvenne P, Greimers R, et al. Assessment of Ki-67 antigen immunostaining in squamous intraepithelial lesions of the uterine cervix: Correlation with the histologic grade and human papillomavirus type. Am J Clin Pathol 1995;104:154–160.

31. McCluggage WG, Buhidma M, Tang L, et al. Monoclonal antibody MIB1 in the assessment of cervical squamous intraepithelial lesions. Int J Gynecol Pathol 1996;15:131–136.

32. Mittal K, Palazzo J. Cervical condylomas show higher proliferation than do inflamed or metaplastic cervical squamous epithelium. Mod Pathol 1998;11:780–783.

33. Mittal K, Mesia A, Demopoulos RI. MIB-1 expression is useful in distinguishing dysplasia from atrophy in elderly women. Int J Gynecol Pathol 1999;18:122–124.

34. McCluggage WG, Maxwell P, McBride HA, et al. Monoclonal antibodies Ki-67 and MIB1 in the distinction of tuboendometrial metaplasia from endocervical adenocarcinoma and adenocarcinoma in situ in formalin-fixed material. Int J Gynecol Pathol 1995;14:209–216.

35. van Hoeven KH, Ramondetta L, Kovatich AJ, et al. Quantitative image analysis of MIB-1 reactivity in inflammatory, hyperplastic, and neoplastic endocervical lesions. Int J Gynecol Pathol 1997;16:15–21.

36. van Hoeven KH, Kovatich AJ, Oliver RE, et al. Protocol for immunocytochemical detection of SIL in cervical smears using MIB-1 antibody to Ki-67 [corrected] [published erratum appears in Mod Pathol 1996;9:790]. Mod Pathol 1996;9:407–412.

37. Dabbs DJ, Abendroth CS, Grenko RT, et al. Immunocytochemistry on the Thinprep processor. Diagn Cytopathol 1997;17:388–392.

38. Speers WC, Picaso LG, Silverberg SG. Immunohistochemical localization of carcinoembryonic antigen in microglandular hyperplasia and adenocarcinoma of the endocervix. Am J Clin Pathol 1983;79:105–107.

39. Michael H, Grawe L, Kraus FT. Minimal deviation endocervical adenocarcinoma: Clinical and histologic features, immunohistochemical staining for carcinoembryonic antigen, and differentiation from confusing benign lesions. Int J Gynecol Pathol 1984;3:261–276.

40. Cina SJ, Richardson MS, Austin RM, et al. Immunohistochemical staining for Ki-67 antigen, carcinoembryonic antigen, and p53 in the differential diagnosis of glandular lesions of the cervix. Mod Pathol 1997;10:176–180.

41. Kudo R, Sasano H, Koizumi M, et al. Immunohistochemical comparison of new monoclonal antibody 1C5 and carcinoembryonic antigen in the differential diagnosis of ade-

nocarcinoma of the uterine cervix. Int J Gynecol Pathol 1990;9:325–336.

42. Maes G, Fleuren GJ, Bara J, et al. The distribution of mucins, carcinoembryonic antigen, and mucus-associated antigens in endocervical and endometrial adenocarcinomas. Int J Gynecol Pathol 1988;7:112–122.

43. Dabbs DJ, Sturtz K, Zaino RJ. The immunohistochemical discrimination of endometrioid adenocarcinomas. Hum Pathol 1996;27:172–177.

44. Gilks CB, Young RH, Gersell DJ, et al. Large cell neuroendocrine [corrected] carcinoma of the uterine cervix: A clinicopathologic study of 12 cases. [published erratum appears in Am J Surg Pathol 1997;21:1260] Am J Surg Pathol 1997;21:905–914.

45. Ambros RA, Park JS, Shah KV, et al. Evaluation of histologic, morphometric, and immunohistochemical criteria in the differential diagnosis of small cell carcinomas of the cervix with particular reference to human papillomavirus types 16 and 18. [published erratum appears in Mod Pathol 1992;5:40] Mod Pathol 1991;4:586–593.

46. Gersell DJ, Mazoujian G, Mutch DG, et al. Small-cell undifferentiated carcinoma of the cervix: A clinicopathologic, ultrastructural, and immunocytochemical study of 15 cases. Am J Surg Pathol 1988;12:684–698.

47. Farhood AI, Abrams J. Immunohistochemistry of endometrial stromal sarcoma. Hum Pathol 1991;22:224–230.

48. Franquemont DW, Frierson HF Jr, Mills SE. An immunohistochemical study of normal endometrial stroma and endometrial stromal neoplasms: Evidence for smooth muscle differentiation. Am J Surg Pathol 1991;15:861–870.

49. Oliva E, Young RH, Clement PB, et al. Cellular benign mesenchymal tumors of the uterus: A comparative morphologic and immunohistochemical analysis of 33 highly cellular leiomyomas and six endometrial stromal nodules, two frequently confused tumors. Am J Surg Pathol 1995; 19:757–768.

50. Sherman ME, Bur ME, Kurman RJ. p53 in endometrial cancer and its putative precursors: Evidence for diverse pathways of tumorigenesis. Hum Pathol 1995;26:1268–1274.

51. Tashiro H, Isacson C, Levine R, et al. p53 gene mutations are common in uterine serous carcinoma and occur early in their pathogenesis. Am J Pathol 1997;150:177–185.

52. Zheng W, Khurana R, Farahmand S, et al. p53 immunostaining as a significant adjunct diagnostic method for uterine surface carcinoma: Precursor of uterine papillary serous carcinoma. Am J Surg Pathol 1998;22:1463–1473.

53. Lax SF, Pizer ES, Ronnett BM, et al. Comparison of estrogen and progesterone receptor, Ki-67, and p53 immunoreactivity in uterine endometrioid carcinoma and endometrioid carcinoma with squamous, mucinous, secretory, and ciliated cell differentiation. Hum Pathol 1998;29:924–931.

54. Lax SF, Kendall B, Tashiro H, et al. The frequency of p53, K-ras mutations, and microsatellite instability differs in uterine endometrioid and serous carcinoma: Evidence of distinct molecular genetic pathways. Cancer 2000;88:814–824.

55. Kohler MF, Nishii H, Humphrey PA, et al. Mutation of the p53 tumor-suppressor gene is not a feature of endometrial hyperplasias. Am J Obstet Gynecol 1993;169:690–694.

56. Yu CC, Wilkinson N, Brito MJ, et al. Patterns of immunohistochemical staining for proliferating cell nuclear antigen and p53 in benign and neoplastic human endometrium. Histopathology 1993;23:367–371.

57. Soslow RA, Shen PU, Chung MH, et al. Distinctive p53 and mdm2 immunohistochemical expression profiles suggest different pathogenetic pathways in poorly differentiated endometrial carcinoma. Int J Gynecol Pathol 1998;17:129–134.

58. Lax SF, Pizer ES, Ronnett BM, et al. Clear cell carcinoma of the endometrium is characterized by a distinctive profile of p53, Ki-67, estrogen, and progesterone receptor expression. Hum Pathol 1998;29:551–558.

59. Soslow RA, Shen PUF, Chung MH, et al. Cyclin D1 expression in high grade uterine carcinomas—association

with estrogen receptor expression in endometrioid but not serous carcinoma. unpublished observations 2000.

60. Chambers JT, Carcangiu ML, Voynick IM, et al. Immunohistochemical evaluation of estrogen and progesterone receptor content in 183 patients with endometrial carcinoma. Part II: Correlation between biochemical and immunohistochemical methods and survival. Am J Clin Pathol 1990;94:255–260.

61. Carcangiu ML, Chambers JT, Voynick IM, et al. Immunohistochemical evaluation of estrogen and progesterone receptor content in 183 patients with endometrial carcinoma. Part I: Clinical and histologic correlations. Am J Clin Pathol 1990;94:247–254.

62. Oliva E, Clement PB, Young RH, Scully RE. Mixed endometrial stromal and smooth muscle tumors of the uterus: A clinicopathologic study of 15 cases. Am J Surg Pathol 1998;22:997–1005.

63. Oliva E, Young RH, Clement PB, et al. Myxoid and fibrous endometrial stromal tumors of the uterus: A report of 10 cases. Int J Gynecol Pathol 1999;18:310–319.

64. Baker RJ, Hildebrandt RH, Rouse RV, et al. Inhibin and CD99 (MIC2) expression in uterine stromal neoplasms with sex-cord–like elements. Hum Pathol 1999;30:671–679.

65. Rizeq MN, van de Rijn M, Hendrickson MR, Rouse RV. A comparative immunohistochemical study of uterine smooth muscle neoplasms with emphasis on the epithelioid variant. Hum Pathol 1994;25:671–677.

66. Meis JM, Lawrence WD. The immunohistochemical profile of malignant mixed mullerian tumor: Overlap with endometrial adenocarcinoma. [see comments] Am J Clin Pathol 1990;94:1–7.

67. Carcangiu ML, Chambers JT. Uterine papillary serous carcinoma: A study on 108 cases with emphasis on the prognostic significance of associated endometrioid carcinoma, absence of invasion, and concomitant ovarian carcinoma. Gynecol Oncol 1992;47:298–305.

68. Sherman ME, Bitterman P, Rosenshein NB, et al. Uterine serous carcinoma: A morphologically diverse neoplasm with unifying clinicopathologic features. Am J Surg Pathol 1992;16:600–610.

69. Soslow RA, Shen PU, Isacson C, et al. The CD44v6-negative phenotype in high-grade uterine carcinomas correlates with serous histologic subtype. [published erratum appears in Mod Pathol 1998;11:375] Mod Pathol 1998;11:194–199.

70. Schlosshauer PW, Hedrick Ellenson L, Soslow RA. Expression of beta-catenin and e-cadherin in high grade endometrial cancers is associated with histological subtype. Mod Pathol 2000;13:131A.

71. Nucci MR, O'Connell JT, Cviko A, et al. h-Caldesmon expression distinguishes endometrial stromal neoplasms from smooth muscle tumors. Mod Pathol 2000;13:129A.

72. Rush DS, Baergen RN, Soslow RA. h-Caldesmon, a novel smooth muscle–specific antibody, distinguishes between cellular leiomyomas and endometrial stromal sarcomas. Mod Pathol 2000;13:131A.

73. Zhai YL, Kobayashi Y, Mori A, et al. Expression of steroid receptors, Ki-67, and p53, in uterine leiomyosarcomas. Int J Gynecol Pathol 1999;18:20–28.

74. Nordal RR, Kristensen GB, Stenwig AE, et al. Immunotochemical analysis of p53 protein in uterine sarcomas. Gynecol Oncol 1997;70:45–48.

75. Blom R, Guerrieri C, Stal O, et al. Leiomyosarcoma of the uterus: A clinicopathologic, DNA flow cytometric, p53, and mdm-2 analysis of 49 cases. Gynecol Oncol 1998;68:54–61.

76. Daya D, Sabet L. The use of cytokeratin as a sensitive and reliable marker for trophoblastic tissue. Am J Clin Pathol 1991;95:137–141.

77. Kurman RJ, Young RH, Norris HJ, et al. Immunocytochemical localization of placental lactogen and chorionic gonadotropin in the normal placenta and trophoblastic tumors, with emphasis on intermediate trophoblast and the placental site trophoblastic tumor. Int J Gynecol Pathol 1984;3:101–121.

78. Huettner PC, Gersell DJ. Placental site nodule: A clinico-pathologic study of 38 cases. Int J Gynecol Pathol 1994;13:191–198.

79. Yeh IT, O'Connor DM, Kurman RJ. Vacuolated cytotropho-blast: A subpopulation of trophoblast in the chorion laeve. Placenta 1989;10:429–438.

80. Shih IM, Kurman RJ. Expression of melanoma cell adhe-sion molecule in intermediate trophoblast. Lab Invest 1996;75:377–388.

81. Mazur MT, Hendrickson MR, Kempson RL. Optically clear nuclei: An alteration of endometrial epithelium in the presence of trophoblast. Am J Surg Pathol 1983;7:415–423.

82. Yokoyama S, Kashima K, Inoue S, et al. Biotin-containing intranuclear inclusions in endometrial glands during ges-tation and puerperium. [see comments] Am J Clin Pathol 1993;99:13–17.

83. Shih IM, Kurman RJ. Ki-67 labeling index in the differen-tial diagnosis of exaggerated placental site, placental site trophoblastic tumor, and choriocarcinoma: A double im-munohistochemical staining technique using Ki-67 and Mel-CAM antibodies. Hum Pathol 1998;29:27–33.

84. Shitabata PK, Rutgers JL. The placental site nodule: An immunohistochemical study. Hum Pathol 1994;25:1295–1301.

85. Shih IM, Seidman JD, Kurman RJ. Placental site nodule and characterization of distinctive types of intermediate trophoblast. Hum Pathol 1999;30:687–694.

86. Angel E, Davis JR, Nagle RB. Immunohistochemical dem-onstration of placental hormones in the diagnosis of uter-ine versus ectopic pregnancy. Am J Clin Pathol 1985;84:705–709.

87. Hameed A, Miller DS, Muller CY, et al. Frequent expres-sion of beta-human chorionic gonadotropin (beta-hCG) in squamous cell carcinoma of the cervix. Int J Gynecol Pathol 1999;18:381–386.

88. Bacchi CE, Coelho KI, Goldberg J. Expression of beta-hu-man chorionic gonadotropin (beta-hCG) in non-trophoblas-tic elements of transitional cell carcinoma of the bladder: Possible relationship with prognosis. Rev Paul Med 1993;111:412–416.

89. Battifora H, Sheibani K, Tubbs RR, et al. Antikeratin anti-bodies in tumor diagnosis: Distinction between seminoma and embryonal carcinoma. Cancer 1984;54:843–848.

90. Ramaekers F, Feitz W, Moesker O, et al. Antibodies to cytokeratin and vimentin in testicular tumour diagnosis. Virchows Arch A Pathol Anat Histopathol 1985;408:127–142.

91. Miettinen M, Virtanen I, Talerman A. Intermediate fila-ment proteins in human testis and testicular germ-cell tu-mors. Am J Pathol 1985;120:402–410.

92. Eglen DE, Ulbright TM. The differential diagnosis of yolk sac tumor and seminoma: Usefulness of cytokeratin, alpha-fetoprotein, and alpha-1-antitrypsin immunoperoxidase re-actions. Am J Clin Pathol 1987;88:328–332.

93. Lifschitz-Mercer B, Walt H, Kushnir I, et al. Differentiation potential of ovarian dysgerminoma: An immunohistochem-ical study of 15 cases. Hum Pathol 1995;26:62–66.

94. Aguirre P, Thor AD, Scully RE. Ovarian endometrioid car-cinomas resembling sex cord-stromal tumors: An immu-nohistochemical study. Int J Gynecol Pathol 1989;8:364–373.

95. Costa MJ, Morris RJ, Wilson R, et al. Utility of immunohis-tochemistry in distinguishing ovarian Sertoli-stromal cell tumors from carcinosarcomas. Hum Pathol 1992;23:787–797.

96. McCluggage WG, Date A, Bharucha H, et al. Endometrial stromal sarcoma with sex cord-like areas and focal rhab-doid differentiation. [see comments] Histopathology 1996;29:369–374.

97. Riopel MA, Perlman EJ, Seidman JD, et al. Inhibin and epithelial membrane antigen immunohistochemistry assist in the diagnosis of sex cord-stromal tumors and provide clues to the histogenesis of hypercalcemic small cell carci-nomas. Int J Gynecol Pathol 1998;17:46–53.

98. Guerrieri C, Franlund B, Malmstrom H, et al. Ovarian en-dometrioid carcinomas simulating sex cord-stromal tu-mors: A study using inhibin and cytokeratin 7. Int J Gyne-col Pathol 1998;17:266–271.

99. Ordi J, Schammel DP, Rasekh L, et al. Sertoliform endo-metrioid carcinomas of the ovary: A clinicopathologic and immunohistochemical study of 13 cases. Mod Pathol 1999;12:933–940.

100. Devouassoux-Shisheboran M, Schammel DP, Tavassoli FA. Ovarian hepatoid yolk sac tumours: Morphological, immu-nohistochemical and ultrastructural features. Histopathol-ogy 1999;34:462–469.

101. Gordon MD, Corless C, Renshaw AA, et al. CD99, keratin, and vimentin staining of sex cord-stromal tumors, normal ovary, and testis. Mod Pathol 1998;11:769–773.

102. Biscotti CV, Hart WR. Juvenile granulosa cell tumors of the ovary. Arch Pathol Lab Med 1989;113:40–46.

103. Lagendijk JH, Mullink H, van Diest PJ, et al. Immunohisto-chemical differentiation between primary adenocarcino-mas of the ovary and ovarian metastases of colonic and breast origin: Comparison between a statistical and an in-tuitive approach. J Clin Pathol 1999;52:283–290.

104. Lagendijk JH, Mullink H, van Diest PJ, et al. Tracing the origin of adenocarcinomas with unknown primary using immunohistochemistry: Differential diagnosis between co-lonic and ovarian carcinomas as primary sites. Hum Pathol 1998;29:491–497.

105. Young RH, Hart WR. Metastatic intestinal carcinomas sim-ulating primary ovarian clear cell carcinoma and secretory endometrioid carcinoma: A clinicopathologic and immu-nohistochemical study of five cases. Am J Surg Pathol 1998;22:805–815.

106. DeCostanzo DC, Elias JM, Chumas JC. Necrosis in 84 ovar-ian carcinomas: A morphologic study of primary versus metastatic colonic carcinoma with a selective immunohis-tochemical analysis of cytokeratin subtypes and carcino-embryonic antigen. Int J Gynecol Pathol 1997;16:245–249.

107. Sack MJ, Roberts SA. Cytokeratins 20 and 7 in the differ-ential diagnosis of metastatic carcinoma in cytologic speci-mens. Diagn Cytopathol 1997;16:132–136.

108. Soslow RA, Rouse RV, Hendrickson MR, et al. Transitional cell neoplasms of the ovary and urinary bladder: A com-parative immunohistochemical analysis. Int J Gynecol Pathol 1996;15:257–265.

109. Berezowski K, Stastny JF, Kornstein MJ. Cytokeratins 7 and 20 and carcinoembryonic antigen in ovarian and co-lonic carcinoma. Mod Pathol 1996;9:426–429.

110. Wauters CC, Smedts F, Gerrits LG, et al. Keratins 7 and 20 as diagnostic markers of carcinomas metastatic to the ovary. Hum Pathol 1995;26:852–855.

111. Moll R, Lowe A, Laufer J, et al. Cytokeratin 20 in human carcinomas: A new histodiagnostic marker detected by monoclonal antibodies. Am J Pathol 1992;140:427–447.

112. Wang N, Zee S, Zarbo R, et al. Coordinate expression of cytokeratins 7 and 20 defines unique subsets of carcino-mas. Appl Immunohistochem 1995;3:99–107.

113. Blumenfeld W, Turi GK, Harrison G, et al. Utility of cyto-keratin 7 and 20 subset analysis as an aid in the identifica-tion of primary site of origin of malignancy in cytologic specimens. Diagn Cytopathol 1999;20:63–66.

114. Harlamert HA, Mira J, Bejarano PA, et al. Thyroid tran-scription factor-1 and cytokeratins 7 and 20 in pulmonary and breast carcinoma. Acta Cytol 1998;42:1382–1388.

115. Loy TS, Calaluce RD. Utility of cytokeratin immunostain-ing in separating pulmonary adenocarcinomas from co-lonic adenocarcinomas. Am J Clin Pathol 1994;102:764–767.

116. Tot T. Patterns of distribution of cytokeratins 20 and 7 in special types of invasive breast carcinoma: A study of 123 cases. Ann Diagn Pathol 1999;3:350–356.

117. Ritter JH, Boucher LD, Wick MR. Peripheral pulmonary adenocarcinomas with bronchioloalveolar features: Immu-nophenotypes correlate with histologic patterns. Mod Pathol 1998;11:566–572.

118. Raab SS, Berg LC, Swanson PE, et al. Adenocarcinoma in the lung in patients with breast cancer: A prospective analysis of the discriminatory value of immunohistology. [see comments] Am J Clin Pathol 1993;100:27–35.

119. Brown RW, Campagna LB, Dunn JK, et al. Immunohisto-

chemical identification of tumor markers in metastatic adenocarcinoma: A diagnostic adjunct in the determination of primary site. Am J Clin Pathol 1997;107:12–19.

120. Wick MR, Lillemoe TJ, Copland GT, et al. Gross cystic disease fluid protein-15 as a marker for breast cancer: Immunohistochemical analysis of 690 human neoplasms and comparison with alpha-lactalbumin. Hum Pathol 1989;20: 281–287.

121. Monteagudo C, Merino MJ, LaPorte N, et al. Value of gross cystic disease fluid protein-15 in distinguishing metastatic breast carcinomas among poorly differentiated neoplasms involving the ovary. Hum Pathol 1991;22:368–372.

122. Han AC, Duszak R Jr. Coexpression of cytokeratins 7 and 20 confirms urothelial carcinoma presenting as an intrarenal tumor. Cancer 1999;86:2327–2330.

123. Tot T. Adenocarcinomas metastatic to the liver: The value of cytokeratins 20 and 7 in the search for unknown primary tumors. Cancer 1999;85:171–177.

124. Ronnett BM, Kurman RJ, Shmookler BM, et al. The morphologic spectrum of ovarian metastases of appendiceal adenocarcinomas: A clinicopathologic and immunohistochemical analysis of tumors often misinterpreted as primary ovarian tumors or metastatic tumors from other gastrointestinal sites. Am J Surg Pathol 1997;21:1144–1155.

125. Ronnett BM, Shmookler BM, Sugarbaker PH, et al. Pseudomyxoma peritonei: New concepts in diagnosis, origin, nomenclature, and relationship to mucinous borderline (low malignant potential) tumors of the ovary. Anat Pathol 1997;2:197–226.

126. Tan J, Sidhu G, Greco MA, et al. Villin, cytokeratin 7, and cytokeratin 20 expression in pulmonary adenocarcinoma with ultrastructural evidence of microvilli with rootlets. Hum Pathol 1998;29:390–396.

127. Torenbeek R, Lagendijk JH, van Diest PJ, et al. Value of a panel of antibodies to identify the primary origin of adenocarcinomas presenting as bladder carcinoma. Histopathology 1998;32:20–27.

128. Valente AM, Taatjes DJ, Mount SL. Comparison of the pattern of expression of Leu-M1 antigen in adenocarcinomas, neutrophils and Hodgkin's disease by immunoelectron microscopy. Histochem Cell Biol 1995;103:181–186.

129. Hsu SM, Jaffe ES. Leu M1 and peanut agglutinin stain the neoplastic cells of Hodgkin's disease. Am J Clin Pathol 1984;82:29–32.

130. Hsu SM, Yang K, Jaffe ES. Phenotypic expression of Hodgkin's and Reed-Sternberg cells in Hodgkin's disease. Am J Pathol 1985;118:209–217.

131. Pinkus GS, Thomas P, Said JW. Leu-M1—a marker for Reed-Sternberg cells in Hodgkin's disease: An immunoperoxidase study of paraffin-embedded tissues. Am J Pathol 1985;119:244–252.

132. Frierson HF Jr, Innes DJ Jr. Sensitivity of anti–Leu-M1 as a marker in Hodgkin's disease. Arch Pathol Lab Med 1985; 109:1024–1028.

133. Norton AJ, Isaacson PG. Granulocyte and HLA-D region specific monoclonal antibodies in the diagnosis of Hodgkin's disease. J Clin Pathol 1985;38:1241–1246.

134. Rosso R, Paulli M, Magrini U, et al. Anaplastic large cell lymphoma, CD30/Ki-1 positive, expressing the CD15/Leu-M1 antigen: Immunohistochemical and morphological relationships to Hodgkin's disease. Virchows Arch A Pathol Anat Histopathol 1990;416:229–235.

135. Perkins PL, Ross CW, Schnitzer B. CD30-positive, anaplastic large-cell lymphomas that express CD15 but lack CD45: A possible diagnostic pitfall. Arch Pathol Lab Med 1992; 116:1192–1196.

136. Hasui K. Paraffin-immunohistochemical analysis of 226 non-Hodgkin's malignant lymphomas in the endemic area of human T-cell leukemia virus type 1. Acta Pathol Jpn 1991;41:350–362.

137. Ordonez NG. Role of immunohistochemistry in distinguishing epithelial peritoneal mesotheliomas from peritoneal and ovarian serous carcinomas. Am J Surg Pathol 1998;22:1203–1214.

138. Goldblum J, Hart WR. Localized and diffuse mesotheliomas of the genital tract and peritoneum in women: A clinicopathologic study of nineteen true mesothelial neoplasms, other than adenomatoid tumors, multicystic mesotheliomas, and localized fibrous tumors. [see comments] Am J Surg Pathol 1995;19:1124–1137.

139. Andrion A, Feyles E, Zai G, et al. Malignant peritoneal mesothelioma mimicking mesenteric inflammatory disease. Pathol Res Pract 1994;190:615–622; discussion 623–626.

140. Weidner N. Malignant mesothelioma of peritoneum. Ultrastruct Pathol 1991;15:515–520.

141. Khoury N, Raju U, Crissman JD, et al. A comparative immunohistochemical study of peritoneal and ovarian serous tumors, and mesotheliomas. Hum Pathol 1990;21:811–819.

142. O'Hara CJ, Corson JM, Pinkus GS, et al. ME1: A monoclonal antibody that distinguishes epithelial-type malignant mesothelioma from pulmonary adenocarcinoma and extrapulmonary malignancies. Am J Pathol 1990;136:421–428.

143. Truong LD, Maccato ML, Awalt H, et al. Serous surface carcinoma of the peritoneum: A clinicopathologic study of 22 cases. Hum Pathol 1990;21:99–110.

144. Wick MR, Mills SE, Dehner LP, et al. Serous papillary carcinomas arising from the peritoneum and ovaries: A clinicopathologic and immunohistochemical comparison. Int J Gynecol Pathol 1989;8:179–188.

145. Eyden BP, Banik S, Harris M. Malignant epithelial mesothelioma of the peritoneum: Observations on a problem case. Ultrastruct Pathol 1996;20:337–344.

146. Shah IA, Salvatore JR, Kummet T, et al. Pseudomesotheliomatous carcinoma involving pleura and peritoneum: A clinicopathologic and immunohistochemical study of three cases. Ann Diagn Pathol 1999;3:148–159.

147. Rothacker D, Mobius G. Varieties of serous surface papillary carcinoma of the peritoneum in northern Germany: A thirty-year autopsy study. Int J Gynecol Pathol 1995;14: 310–318.

148. Zhou C, Gilks CB, Hayes M, et al. Papillary serous carcinoma of the uterine cervix: A clinicopathologic study of 17 cases. Am J Surg Pathol 1998;22:113–120.

149. Riva C, Fabbri A, Facco C, et al. Primary serous papillary adenocarcinoma of the vagina: A case report. Int J Gynecol Pathol 1997;16:286–290.

150. Mezger J, Lamerz R, Permanetter W. Diagnostic significance of carcinoembryonic antigen in the differential diagnosis of malignant mesothelioma. J Thorac Cardiovasc Surg 1990;100:860–866.

151. Mainguene C, Aillet G, Kremer M, et al. Immunohistochemical study of ovarian tumors using the OC 125 monoclonal antibody as a basis for potential in vivo and in vitro applications. J Nucl Med Allied Sci 1986;30:19–22.

152. Scharl A, Crombach G, Vierbuchen M, et al. CA 125 in normal tissues and carcinomas of the uterine cervix, endometrium and fallopian tube. I: Immunohistochemical detection. Arch Gynecol Obstet 1989;244:103–112.

153. van Niekerk CC, Jap PH, Thomas CM, et al. Marker profile of mesothelial cells versus ovarian carcinoma cells. Int J Cancer 1989;43:1065–1071.

154. Leake J, Woolas RP, Daniel J, et al. Immunocytochemical and serological expression of CA 125: A clinicopathological study of 40 malignant ovarian epithelial tumours. Histopathology 1994;24:57–64.

155. Loy TS, Quesenberry JT, Sharp SC. Distribution of CA 125 in adenocarcinomas: An immunohistochemical study of 481 cases. Am J Clin Pathol 1992;98:175–179.

156. Gotzos V, Vogt P, Celio MR. The calcium binding protein calretinin is a selective marker for malignant pleural mesotheliomas of the epithelial type. [published erratum appears in Pathol Res Pract 1996;192:646] Pathol Res Pract 1996;192:137–147.

157. Riera JR, Astengo-Osuna C, Longmate JA, et al. The immunohistochemical diagnostic panel for epithelial mesothelioma: A reevaluation after heat-induced epitope retrieval. [see comments] Am J Surg Pathol 1997;21:1409–1419.

158. Nagel H, Hemmerlein B, Ruschenburg I, et al. The value of anti-calretinin antibody in the differential diagnosis of normal and reactive mesothelia versus metastatic tumors in effusion cytology. Pathol Res Pract 1998;194: 759–764.

159. Gotzos V, Wintergerst ES, Musy JP, et al. Selective distribution of calretinin in adenocarcinomas of the human co-

lon and adjacent tissues. Am J Surg Pathol 1999;23:701–711.

160. Clover J, Oates J, Edwards C. Anti-cytokeratin 5/6: A positive marker for epithelioid mesothelioma. Histopathology 1997;31:140–143.

161. Suo Z, Holm R, Nesland JM. Squamous cell carcinomas: An immunohistochemical study of cytokeratins and involucrin in primary and metastatic tumours. Histopathology 1993;23:45–54.

162. Schwerer MJ, Baczako K. Expression of cytokeratins typical for ductal and squamous differentiation in the human stomach: An immunohistochemical study of normal foveolar epithelium, *Helicobacter pylori* gastritis and intestinal metaplasia. Histopathology 1996;29:131–137.

163. Kupryjanczyk J. Neuroendocrine tumors of the ovary—a review. Verh Dtsch Ges Pathol 1997;81:253–259.

164. Chou YY, Shun CT, Huang SC, et al. Primary ovarian carcinoid tumor. J Formos Med Assoc 1996;95:148–152.

165. Ueda G, Shimizu C, Saito J, et al. An immunohistochemical study of neuroendocrine cells in gynecologic tumors. Int J Gynaecol Obstet 1989;29:165–172.

166. Stagno PA, Petras RE, Hart WR. Strumal carcinoids of the ovary: An immunohistologic and ultrastructural study. Arch Pathol Lab Med 1987;111:440–446.

167. Eichhorn JH, Young RH, Scully RE. Primary ovarian small cell carcinoma of pulmonary type: A clinicopathologic, immunohistologic, and flow cytometric analysis of 11 cases. Am J Surg Pathol 1992;16:926–938.

168. Fukunaga M, Endo Y, Miyazawa Y, et al. Small cell neuroendocrine carcinoma of the ovary. Virchows Arch 1997;430:343–348.

169. Kleinman GM, Young RH, Scully RE. Primary neuroectodermal tumors of the ovary: A report of 25 cases. Am J Surg Pathol 1993;17:764–778.

170. Carlsson B, Havel G, Kindblom LG, et al. Ependymoma of the ovary: A clinico-pathologic, ultrastructural and immunohistochemical investigation: A case report. Apmis 1989;97:1007–1012.

171. Guerrieri C, Jarlsfelt I. Ependymoma of the ovary: A case report with immunohistochemical, ultrastructural, and DNA cytometric findings, as well as histogenetic considerations. Am J Surg Pathol 1993;17:623–632.

172. Kurman RJ, Norris HJ. Endodermal sinus tumor of the ovary: A clinical and pathologic analysis of 71 cases. Cancer 1976;38:2404–2419.

173. Prat J, Bhan AK, Dickersin GR, et al. Hepatoid yolk sac tumor of the ovary (endodermal sinus tumor with hepatoid differentiation): A light microscopic, ultrastructural and immunohistochemical study of seven cases. Cancer 1982;50:2355–2368.

174. Clement PB, Young RH, Scully RE. Endometrioid-like variant of ovarian yolk sac tumor: A clinicopathological analysis of eight cases. Am J Surg Pathol 1987;11:767–778.

175. Okamoto T, Hirabayashi K, Ishiguro T. Immunohistochemical type distinction of alpha-fetoprotein in various alpha-fetoprotein-secreting tumors. Jpn J Cancer Res 1993;84:360–364.

176. Nogales FF, Bergeron C, Carvia RE, et al. Ovarian endometrioid tumors with yolk sac tumor component, an unusual form of ovarian neoplasm: Analysis of six cases. Am J Surg Pathol 1996;20:1056–1066.

177. Young RH. New and unusual aspects of ovarian germ cell tumors. Am J Surg Pathol 1993;17:1210–1224.

178. Ishikura H, Scully RE. Hepatoid carcinoma of the ovary: A newly described tumor. Cancer 1987;60:2775–2784.

179. Khunamornpong S, Siriaunkgul S, Chunduan A. Metastatic hepatocellular carcinoma of the ovary. Int J Gynaecol Obstet 1999;64:189–191.

180. Oortman EH, Elliott JP. Hepatocellular carcinoma metastatic to the ovary: A case report. Am J Obstet Gynecol 1983;146:715–717.

181. Young RH, Gersell DJ, Clement PB, et al. Hepatocellular carcinoma metastatic to the ovary: A report of three cases discovered during life with discussion of the differential diagnosis of hepatoid tumors of the ovary. Hum Pathol 1992;23:574–580.

182. Zirker TA, Silva EG, Morris M, et al. Immunohistochemical differentiation of clear-cell carcinoma of the female genital tract and endodermal sinus tumor with the use of alpha-fetoprotein and Leu-M1. Am J Clin Pathol 1989;91:511–514.

183. Berger G, Verbaere J, Feroldi J. Placental site trophoblastic tumor of the uterus: An ultrastructural and immunohistochemical study. Ultrastruct Pathol 1984;6:319–329.

184. Jacobsen GK, Jacobsen M. Alpha-fetoprotein (AFP) and human chorionic gonadotropin (HCG) in testicular germ cell tumours: A prospective immunohistochemical study. Acta Pathol Microbiol Immunol Scand [A] 1983;91:165–176.

185. Bhalang K, Kafrawy AH, Miles DA. Immunohistochemical study of the expression of human chorionic gonadotropin-beta in oral squamous cell carcinoma. Cancer 1999;85:757–762.

186. Hishima T, Fukayama M, Hayashi Y, et al. Neuroendocrine differentiation in thymic epithelial tumors with special reference to thymic carcinoma and atypical thymoma. Hum Pathol 1998;29:330–338.

187. Trias I, Campo E, Benasco C, et al. Human chorionic gonadotropin in esophageal carcinomas: An immunohistochemical study. Pathol Res Pract 1991;187:503–507.

188. Caruso RA. Hepatoid gastric adenocarcinoma: A histological and immunohistochemical study of a case. Eur J Basic Appl Histochem 1991;35:203–209.

189. Boucher LD, Yoneda K. The expression of trophoblastic cell markers by lung carcinomas. Hum Pathol 1995;26:1201–1206.

190. Wachner R, Wittekind C, von Kleist S. Immunohistological localization of beta-HCG in breast carcinomas. Eur J Cancer Clin Oncol 1984;20:679–684.

191. Yamase HT, Wurzel RS, Nieh PT, et al. Immunohistochemical demonstration of human chorionic gonadotropin in tumors of the urinary bladder. Ann Clin Lab Sci 1985;15:414–417.

192. Mohabeer J, Buckley CH, Fox H. An immunohistochemical study of the incidence and significance of human chorionic gonadotrophin synthesis by epithelial ovarian neoplasms. Gynecol Oncol 1983;16:78–84.

193. Wilson TS, McDowell EM, McIntire KR, et al. Elaboration of human chorionic gonadotropin by lung tumors: An immunocytochemical study. Arch Pathol Lab Med 1981;105:169–173.

194. Kuida CA, Braunstein GD, Shintaku P, et al. Human chorionic gonadotropin expression in lung, breast, and renal carcinomas. Arch Pathol Lab Med 1988;112:282–285.

195. Campo E, Palacin A, Benasco C, et al. Human chorionic gonadotropin in colorectal carcinoma: An immunohistochemical study. Cancer 1987;59:1611–1616.

196. Matias-Guiu X, Prat J. Ovarian tumors with functioning stroma: An immunohistochemical study of 100 cases with human chorionic gonadotropin monoclonal and polyclonal antibodies. Cancer 1990;65:2001–2005.

197. Watanabe S, Watanabe T, Li WB, et al. Expression of the germ cell alkaline phosphatase gene in human choriocarcinoma cells. J Biol Chem 1989;264:12611–12619.

198. Moch H, Oberholzer M, Dalquen P, et al. Diagnostic tools for differentiating between pleural mesothelioma and lung adenocarcinoma in paraffin embedded tissue. Part I: Immunohistochemical findings. Virchows Arch A Pathol Anat Histopathol 1993;423:19–27.

199. Nouwen EJ, Hendrix PG, Dauwe S, et al. Tumor markers in the human ovary and its neoplasms: A comparative immunohistochemical study. Am J Pathol 1987;126:230–242.

200. Hamilton-Dutoit SJ, Lou H, Pallesen G. The expression of placental alkaline phosphatase (PLAP) and PLAP-like enzymes in normal and neoplastic human tissues: An immunohistological survey using monoclonal antibodies. Apmis 1990;98:797–811.

201. Matias-Guiu X, Pons C, Prat J. Mullerian inhibiting substance, alpha-inhibin, and CD99 expression in sex cord–stromal tumors and endometrioid ovarian carcinomas resembling sex cord–stromal tumors. Hum Pathol 1998;29:840–845.

202. Pelkey TJ, Frierson HF Jr, Mills SE, et al. The diagnostic utility of inhibin staining in ovarian neoplasms. Int J Gynecol Pathol 1998;17:97–105.

203. Stewart CJ, Jeffers MD, Kennedy A. Diagnostic value of inhibin immunoreactivity in ovarian gonadal stromal tumours and their histological mimics. Histopathology 1997; 31:67–74.

204. Rishi M, Howard LN, Bratthauer GL, et al. Use of monoclonal antibody against human inhibin as a marker for sex cord–stromal tumors of the ovary. Am J Surg Pathol 1997; 21:583–589.

205. Arora DS, Cooke IE, Ganesan TS, et al. Immunohistochemical expression of inhibin/activin subunits in epithelial and granulosa cell tumours of the ovary. J Pathol 1997; 181:413–418.

206. McCluggage WG, Sloan JM, Murnaghan M, et al. Gynandroblastoma of ovary with juvenile granulosa cell component and heterologous intestinal type glands. Histopathology 1996;29:253–257.

207. Gurusinghe CJ, Healy DL, Jobling T, et al. Inhibin and activin are demonstrable by immunohistochemistry in ovarian tumor tissue. Gynecol Oncol 1995;57:27–32.

208. Goodfellow PN, Pym B, Pritchard C, et al. MIC2: A human pseudoautosomal gene. Philos Trans R Soc Lond B Biol Sci 1988;322:145–154.

209. Hildebrandt RH, Rouse RV, Longacre TA. Value of inhibin in the identification of granulosa cell tumors of the ovary. Hum Pathol 1997;28:1387–1395.

210. Barzilay J, Rakowsky E, Rahima M, et al. Malignant lymphoma of the ovary: Report of a case and review of the literature. Obstet Gynecol 1984;64:93S–94S.

211. Lawlor ER, Murphy JI, Sorensen PH, et al. Metastatic primitive neuroectodermal tumour of the ovary: Successful treatment with mega-dose chemotherapy followed by peripheral blood progenitor cell rescue. Med Pediatr Oncol 1997;29:308–312.

212. Aguirre P, Scully RE. Malignant neuroectodermal tumor of the ovary, a distinctive form of monodermal teratoma: Report of five cases. Am J Surg Pathol 1982;6:283–292.

213. Burke M, Beilby JO. Unusual malignant neuroectodermal tumours of the ovary—case report and literature review. Histopathology 1984;8:1059–1067.

214. Hittmair A, Rogatsch H, Hobisch A, et al. CD30 expression in seminoma. Hum Pathol 1996;27:1166–1171.

215. Pallesen G, Hamilton-Dutoit SJ. Ki-1 (CD30) antigen is regularly expressed by tumor cells of embryonal carcinoma. Am J Pathol 1988;133:446–450.

216. Latza U, Foss HD, Durkop H, et al. CD30 antigen in embryonal carcinoma and embryogenesis and release of the soluble molecule. Am J Pathol 1995;146:463–471.

217. Zaloudek C, Norris HJ. Granulosa tumors of the ovary in children: A clinical and pathologic study of 32 cases. Am J Surg Pathol 1982;6:503–512.

218. Young RH, Dickersin GR, Scully RE. Juvenile granulosa cell tumor of the ovary: A clinicopathological analysis of 125 cases. Am J Surg Pathol 1984;8:575–596.

219. Young RH, Kozakewich HP, Scully RE. Metastatic ovarian tumors in children: A report of 14 cases and review of the literature. Int J Gynecol Pathol 1993;12:8–19.

220. Scully RE, Dickersin GR. Small cell carcinoma of the ovary that is commonly associated with hypercalcemia is a neuroendocrine tumor on the basis of presently available evidence. [letter; comment] Int J Gynecol Pathol 1989;8: 296–297.

221. Scully RE. Small cell carcinoma of hypercalcemic type. Int J Gynecol Pathol 1993;12:148–152.

222. Young RH, Oliva E, Scully RE. Small cell carcinoma of the hypercalcemic type in the ovary. [editorial] Gynecol Oncol 1995;57:7–8.

223. Young RH, Oliva E, Scully RE. Small cell carcinoma of the ovary, hypercalcemic type: A clinicopathological analysis of 150 cases. Am J Surg Pathol 1994;18:1102–1116.

224. Dickersin GR, Kline IW, Scully RE. Small cell carcinoma of the ovary with hypercalcemia: A report of eleven cases. Cancer 1982;49:188–197.

225. Dickersin GR, Scully RE. Ovarian small cell tumors: An electron microscopic review. Ultrastruct Pathol 1998;22: 199–226.

226. Aguirre P, Thor AD, Scully RE. Ovarian small cell carcinoma: Histogenetic considerations based on immunohistochemical and other findings. Am J Clin Pathol 1989;92: 140–149.

227. Jungbluth AA, Busam KJ, Gerald WL, et al. A103: An anti-melan—a monoclonal antibody for the detection of malignant melanoma in paraffin-embedded tissues. [see comments] Am J Surg Pathol 1998;22:595–602.

228. Busam KJ, Iversen K, Coplan KA, et al. Immunoreactivity for A103, an antibody to melan-A (Mart-1), in adrenocortical and other steroid tumors. [see comments] Am J Surg Pathol 1998;22:57–63.

229. Hoon V, Thung SN, Kaneko M, et al. HMB-45 reactivity in renal angiomyolipoma and lymphangioleiomyomatosis. Arch Pathol Lab Med 1994;118:732–734.

230. Eble JN. Angiomyolipoma of kidney. Semin Diagn Pathol 1998;15:21–40.

231. Gyure KA, Hart WR, Kennedy AW. Lymphangiomyomatosis of the uterus associated with tuberous sclerosis and malignant neoplasia of the female genital tract: A report of two cases. Int J Gynecol Pathol 1995;14:344–351.

232. Longacre TA, Hendrickson MR, Kapp DS, et al. Lymphangioleiomyomatosis of the uterus simulating high-stage endometrial stromal sarcoma. Gynecol Oncol 1996;63:404–410.

233. Kretschmar CS, Colbach C, Bhan I, et al. Desmoplastic small cell tumor: A report of three cases and a review of the literature. J Pediatr Hematol Oncol 1996;18:293–298.

234. Backer A, Mount SL, Zarka MA, et al. Desmoplastic small round cell tumour of unknown primary origin with lymph node and lung metastases: Histological, cytological, ultrastructural, cytogenetic and molecular findings. Virchows Arch 1998;432:135–141.

235. Young RH, Eichhorn JH, Dickersin GR, et al. Ovarian involvement by the intra-abdominal desmoplastic small round cell tumor with divergent differentiation: A report of three cases. Hum Pathol 1992;23:454–464.

236. Slomowitz BM, Girota M, Aledo A, et al. Desmoplastic small round cell tumor with primary ovarian involvement: Case report and review. Gynecol Oncol 2000;79:124–128.

237. Young RH, Scully RE. Alveolar rhabdomyosarcoma metastatic to the ovary: A report of two cases and a discussion of the differential diagnosis of small cell malignant tumors of the ovary. Cancer 1989;64:899–904.

238. Nielsen GP, Oliva E, Young RH, et al. Primary ovarian rhabdomyosarcoma: A report of 13 cases. Int J Gynecol Pathol 1998;17:113–119.

239. Young RH, Prat J, Scully RE. Ovarian Sertoli-Leydig cell tumors with heterologous elements. I: Gastrointestinal epithelium and carcinoid: A clinicopathologic analysis of thirty-six cases. Cancer 1982;50:2448–2456.

240. Young RH, Perez-Atayde AR, Scully RE. Ovarian Sertoli-Leydig cell tumor with retiform and heterologous components: Report of a case with hepatocytic differentiation and elevated serum alpha-fetoprotein. Am J Surg Pathol 1984;8:709–718.

241. Young RH, Scully RE. Ovarian Sertoli-Leydig cell tumors: A clinicopathological analysis of 207 cases. Am J Surg Pathol 1985;9:543–569.

242. Young RH. Sertoli-Leydig cell tumors of the ovary: Review with emphasis on historical aspects and unusual variants. Int J Gynecol Pathol 1993;12:141–147.

243. Zaloudek C, Norris HJ. Sertoli-Leydig tumors of the ovary: A clinicopathologic study of 64 intermediate and poorly differentiated neoplasms. Am J Surg Pathol 1984;8:405–418.

244. Prat J, Young RH, Scully RE. Ovarian Sertoli-Leydig cell tumors with heterologous elements. II: Cartilage and skeletal muscle: A clinicopathologic analysis of twelve cases. Cancer 1982;50:2465–2475.

245. Roth LM, Anderson MC, Govan AD, et al. Sertoli-Leydig cell tumors: A clinicopathologic study of 34 cases. Cancer 1981;48:187–197.

246. Jones PA, Wolkowicz MJ, Harrington MA, et al. Methylation and expression of the Myo D1 determination gene. Philos Trans R Soc Lond B Biol Sci 1990;326:277–284.

247. Menesce LP, Eyden BP, Edmondson D, et al. Immunophenotype and ultrastructure of alveolar soft part sarcoma. J Submicrosc Cytol Pathol 1993;25:377–387.

248. Tonin PN, Scrable H, Shimada H, et al. Muscle-specific gene expression in rhabdomyosarcomas and stages of human fetal skeletal muscle development. Cancer Res 1991; 51:5100–5106.

249. Prayson RA, Hart WR, Petras RE. Pseudomyxoma peritonei: A clinicopathologic study of 19 cases with emphasis on site of origin and nature of associated ovarian tumors. Am J Surg Pathol 1994;18:591–603.

250. Ronnett BM, Kurman RJ, Zahn CM, et al. Pseudomyxoma peritonei in women: A clinicopathologic analysis of 30 cases with emphasis on site of origin, prognosis, and relationship to ovarian mucinous tumors of low malignant potential. Hum Pathol 1995;26:509–524.

251. Guerrieri C, Franlund B, Fristedt S, et al. Mucinous tumors of the vermiform appendix and ovary, and pseudomyxoma peritonei: Histogenetic implications of cytokeratin 7 expression. Hum Pathol 1997;28:1039–1045.

252. Young RH, Gilks CB, Scully RE. Mucinous tumors of the appendix associated with mucinous tumors of the ovary and pseudomyxoma peritonei: A clinicopathological analysis of 22 cases supporting an origin in the appendix. Am J Surg Pathol 1991;15:415–429.

253. Cuatrecasas M, Matias-Guiu X, Prat J. Synchronous mucinous tumors of the appendix and the ovary associated with pseudomyxoma peritonei: A clinicopathologic study of six cases with comparative analysis of c-Ki-ras mutations. Am J Surg Pathol 1996;20:739–746.

254. Prat J. Ovarian tumors of borderline malignancy (tumors of low malignant potential): A critical appraisal. Adv Anat Pathol 1999;6:247–274.

255. Snyder RR, Norris HJ, Tavassoli F. Endometrioid proliferative and low malignant potential tumors of the ovary: A clinicopathologic study of 46 cases. Am J Surg Pathol 1988;12:661–671.

256. Young RH, Hart WR. Metastases from carcinomas of the pancreas simulating primary mucinous tumors of the ovary: A report of seven cases. Am J Surg Pathol 1989;13:748–756.

257. Young RH, Scully RE. Ovarian metastases from carcinoma of the gallbladder and extrahepatic bile ducts simulating primary tumors of the ovary: A report of six cases. Int J Gynecol Pathol 1990;9:60–72.

258. Kommoss F, Oliva E, Bhan AK, et al. Inhibin expression in ovarian tumors and tumor-like lesions: An immunohistochemical study. Mod Pathol 1998;11:656–664.

259. Devouassoux-Shisheboran M, Silver SA, Tavassoli FA. Wolffian adnexal tumor, so-called female adnexal tumor of probable wolffian origin (FATWO): Immunohistochemical evidence in support of a wolffian origin. Hum Pathol 1999; 30:856–863.

260. Kariminejad MH, Scully RE. Female adnexal tumor of probable wolffian origin: A distinctive pathologic entity. Cancer 1973;31:671–677.

261. Daya D, Young RH, Scully RE. Endometrioid carcinoma of the fallopian tube resembling an adnexal tumor of probable wolffian origin: A report of six cases. Int J Gynecol Pathol 1992;11:122–130.

262. Zhang J, Young RH, Arseneau J, et al. Ovarian stromal tumors containing lutein or Leydig cells (luteinized thecomas and stromal Leydig cell tumors)—a clinicopathological analysis of fifty cases. Int J Gynecol Pathol 1982;1:270–285.

263. Seidman JD, Abbondanzo SL, Bratthauer GL. Lipid cell (steroid cell) tumor of the ovary: Immunophenotype with analysis of potential pitfall due to endogenous biotin-like activity. Int J Gynecol Pathol 1995;14:331–338.

264. Young RH, Scully RE. Oxyphilic tumors of the female and male genital tracts. Semin Diagn Pathol 1999;16:146–161.

265. Abeler V, Kjorstad KE, Nesland JM. Small cell carcinoma of the ovary. A report of six cases. [see comments] Int J Gynecol Pathol 1988;7:315–329.

CHAPTER 16

Diagnostic Immunohistochemistry of Pediatric Small Round Cell Tumors

Deborah Belchis, M.D.

Pediatric small round cell tumors comprise a group of diverse, diagnostically challenging primitive or undifferentiated neoplasms. Immunohistochemistry and molecular diagnostics have greatly improved our ability to separate and classify some of these tumors. The use of these ancillary tools has become important in confirming or even diagnosing challenging cases.[1] However, the more we use these tools diagnostically, the more it becomes apparent that these special techniques have pitfalls of their own.[2] The importance of good communication between clinicians, radiologists, and pathologists cannot be overstated. In addition, these ancillary tools are always to be interpreted after a careful evaluation of the light microscopic findings.[3] Finally, additional techniques such as flow cytometry for leukemias,[4] electron microscopy,[5] and molecular analysis[6] may be required for final confirmation of the diagnosis or to provide prognostic information.[7-9] Therefore, with all these tumors, protocols for handling the specimen and for tissue procurement should be standardized and routinely followed. Protocols for handling these tumors have been published.[10-13] These protocols should be reviewed with all involved personnel, from cancer group managers who may be better versed with the requirements of clinical trial protocols, to the surgeons who need to be guided regarding the amount of tissue required so that all the needed studies can be performed.

The tumors included in this category of neoplasms encompass neuroblastoma, desmoplastic small round cell tumor (DSRCT), Ewing's sarcoma (ES), primitive neuroectodermal tumor (PNET), Wilms' tumor, lymphomas and leukemias, malignant rhabdoid tumors, epithelioid sarcoma with rhabdoid phenotype, myxoid chondrosarcoma, rhabdomyosarcoma, malignant ectomesenchymoma, poorly differentiated synovial sarcoma, and small cell osteosarcoma. In many instances, the combination of the clinical presentation and the light microscopic appearance is sufficient to make a diagnosis. For example, a tumor in a baby with an adrenal mass and elevated catecholamine levels, which micro-scopically reveals neuroblasts, background neuropil, calcifications, and thin fibrovascular septa, can be comfortably diagnosed as a neuroblastoma (Fig. 16-1). However, an undifferentiated rhabdomyosarcoma may require immunohistochemistry or molecular analysis to confirm the skeletal muscle differentiation of the tumor. The decision about when to order these special studies depends on both the complexity of the tumor and the pathologist's experience with these neoplasms. Usually, the pathologist has formulated a differential diagnosis based on the light microscopic findings and the clinical data. An initial limited panel is often the first step toward refining or confirming the diagnosis. If this results in unexpected findings, a second, more comprehensive panel may then be used. In both cases, however, a multiple antibody panel is usually used, as reliance on one antibody can be misleading.[14, 15] For example, desmin-positive PNETs[16] and CD99+ synovial sarcomas[17] are known to occur.

ANTIBODIES

The following antibodies are most helpful in distinguishing these tumors (Table 16-1).

Vimentin. Vimentin is an intermediate filament of approximately 57,000 kd[18] that is consistently expressed by rhabdomyosarcoma, ES, PNETs, DSRCT, malignant rhabdoid tumors, malignant ectomesenchymomas, and mesenchymal chondrosarcomas.[19] According to some authors, 100% of PNETs express vimentin with either a diffuse pattern or a focal dot-like positivity (Fig. 16-2).[20] Neuroblastomas and T-cell acute lymphoblastic leukemias do not express vimentin.[20]

CD99 (p30/32MIC2). This group of antibodies detects a transmembrane 30,000- to 32,000-kd glycoprotein that is the product of the MIC2 gene. The MIC2 gene is a pseudoautosomal gene and is expressed independent of sex. It has been mapped to the terminal region of the short arm of the X chromosome Xp22.32pter and to the euchromatin

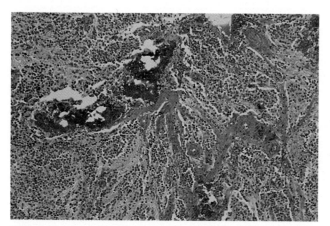

Figure 16–1. Differentiating neuroblastoma. Note the neuropil and the schwannian stroma. (H&E, ×200)

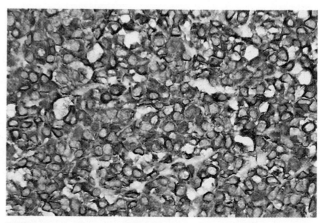

Figure 16–2. Dot-like pattern of vimentin in a peripheral neuroectodermal tumor. (Immunoperoxidase, vimentin, ×400)

region of the Y chromosome Yq11-pter. The gene has been cloned and has been shown to be virtually identical in both the X and Y chromosomes.[21, 22]

CD99 is a reliable and useful marker for the PNET and Ewing's family of tumors in which it demonstrates uniform and strong membranous staining[23–26, 27] (Fig. 16–3). It is consistently expressed by 85 to 95% of ES/PNETs.[26, 28] Lack of staining with any of the three antibody preparations on the market (O13, 12E7, HBA-71; see Table 16–1) is unusual and may be an indication to perform additional studies, such as molecular analysis or electron microscopy, to support the diagnosis of ES/PNET.[29] CD99 is also positive in T-cell acute

lymphoblastic leukemia and lymphoblastic lymphoma (ALL) (Fig. 16–4),[25, 30] acute myelogenous leukemia (AML) or chloroma,[31] the small blue cell component of mesenchymal chondrosarcoma,[32] and synovial sarcoma.[33] It stains cortical thymocytes, and expression has been demonstrated in thymomas.[34] Because ALL and PNETs are histologically similar-appearing tumors, the positive expression exhibited by both neoplasms can lead to misdiagnosis,[35] especially with unusual clinical presentations. In a study by Ramani and associates,[25] immunoreactivity for 12E7 was identified in 13 of 15 cases of ES, 14 of 15 PNETs, 4 of 14 embryonal rhabdomyosarcomas, 7 of 11 T-lympho-

Table 16–1. Antibodies

Antibody	Source	Dilution*	Antigen Retrieval	Staining Pattern
Vimentin	BioGenex	1:6000	Yes	Cytoplasmic or dot-like
CD99-013,	Signet	1:25	Yes	Membranous
HBA-71	Signet			
12E7	DAKO			
Neuron-specific enolase (NSE)	DAKO	1:400	Yes	Cytoplasmic
CAM5.2	Becton, Dickinson and Co.	1:4	Enzyme	Cytoplasmic or dot-like
Cytokeratin AE1/AE3	Boehringer Mannheim	1:800	Yes	Cytoplasmic
Leu7 (CD57)	Immunotech	1:50	Yes	Cytoplasmic
Epithelial membrane antigen (EMA)	DAKO	1:400	No	Cytoplasmic
Synaptophysin	BioGenex	1:200	Yes	Cytoplasmic
Muscle-specific actin (MSA) (HHF-35)	Biomeda	No dilution	No	Cytoplasmic
Desmin	DAKO	1:200	Yes	Cytoplasmic or dot-like
CD45 (leukocyte common antigen [LCA])	DAKO	1:200	Yes	Cytoplasmic
Terminal deoxynucleotidyl transferase (TdT)	DAKO	1:20 (2-hr incubation)	Yes	Nuclear
S-100 protein	BioGenex	1:200	Yes	Nuclear and cytoplasmic
TrkA	McGill Cancer Center	1:1000–1:4000	No	Membranous
MyoD1-clone 5.8A	Novacastra		Yes	Nuclear stain
Myogenin	Imgenex		Yes	Nuclear stain

*Dilutions refer to ones used in the immunoperoxidase laboratory at Hershey Medical Center.

blastic lymphomas, and 1 T-cell ALL. The ES, PNETs, and lymphoid tumors all showed membranous staining, whereas the rhabdomyosarcomas exhibited cytoplasmic staining. More recently, MIC2 expression was documented in 6 of 11 chloromas and 13 of 30 AMLs.[31] According to this study, MIC2 was more commonly detected in M1-, M3-, HLA-Dr− AML than in HLA-Dr+ AML. Continuing experience with CD99 has demonstrated expression of this antibody in a greater variety of tumors, such as lymphomas and synovial sarcomas, decreasing its specificity for PNETs. It has been speculated that its detection is related to the more widespread use of antigen retrieval techniques such as heat-induced epitope retrieval.[33] Whatever the reason, this emphasizes the importance of using a panel of antibodies, paying attention to the pattern of staining, and correlating the findings with the clinical presentation.

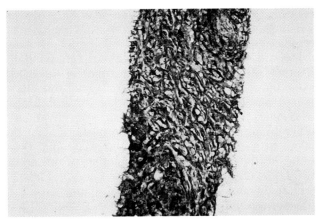

Figure 16–4. Lymphoblastic lymphoma demonstrating strong membranous staining for CD99. (Immunoperoxidase, CD99, ×400)

Neuron-Specific Enolase. Enolase exists as three distinct immunologic subtypes: alpha, beta, and gamma. Neuron-specific enolase (NSE) refers to the gamma subunit. Although originally noted to be present in high concentrations in the brain, subsequent studies have shown the subunit to be ubiquitously present. It is most useful in identifying neuroblastic and neuroendocrine tumors.[19] The polyclonal antibody is expressed in neuroblastoma, ES/PNETs,[36] DSRCTs, and sporadically in rhabdomyosarcomas.[10, 37, 38] Intense cytoplasmic positivity can be found in alveolar rhabdomyosarcomas. In conjunction with other antibodies such as CD99, this can be a useful marker in the diagnosis of PNETs.[39] However, as it is relatively nonspecific, NSE should not be used and interpreted alone.[14, 40–42]

Cytokeratin. The cytokeratins are a class of intermediate filaments. They comprise a group of 19 separate polypeptides ranging from low to high molecular weight. Both monoclonal preparations and polyclonal cocktails of cytokeratins are available. Different tumors can be distinguished by the different cytokeratins they express. For example,

mesothelioma can be separated from a variety of adenocarcinomas by using a panel of cytokeratins.[19] Using a cocktail, cytokeratin is present in DSRCT[43] and malignant rhabdoid tumors.[18, 44] It is focally and less consistently positive in alveolar and embryonal rhabdomyosarcomas[18] and in ES/PNET.[10] In one study of 50 well-established cases of ES/PNET, 20% of cases were immunoreactive to cytokeratin using antigen retrieval—five diffusely and five focally positive.[45] Cytokeratin is negative in neuroblastoma and most lymphomas and leukemias, although immunoblastic or anaplastic lymphomas may be cytokeratin-positive and EMA+ (see further on), causing confusion.

Leu7 (CD57). This is a monoclonal antibody that recognizes a myelin-associated glycoprotein in the central and peripheral nervous systems and in tumors originating from these locations.[46, 47] Like NSE, Leu7 is not specific for neural differentiation. It is present in neuroblastomas, PNETs, myxoid chondrosarcoma, DSRCT, and malignant ectomesenchymoma. It is absent in ES.[20, 39] It is inconsistently found in malignant rhabdoid tumors.[48]

Synaptophysin. Synaptophysin is a 38-kd transmembrane glycoprotein originally isolated from presynaptic vesicles of neurons. It is a highly specific marker for neuroendocrine differentiation.[49] Neuroblastomas and DSRCTs express synaptophysin.[50] PNETs and malignant ectomesenchymomas are variably positive.[10, 20] ES and rhabdomyosarcomas are negative in general.[20] Malignant rhabdoid tumors show inconsistent results,[51–54] with some studies showing greater than 50% of cases to express synaptophysin,[48] as well as other markers typically associated with neural origin.

Muscle-Specific Actin (MSA or HHF-35). The actins are a family of contractile proteins found ubiquitously in all cells. They are separated on their electrophoretic mobility into alpha, beta, and gamma. HHF-35 is an antibody recognizing the alpha and gamma smooth muscle actins.[19] It is a useful marker for rhabdomyosarcoma, especially in

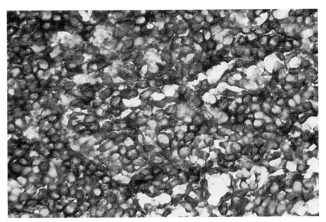

Figure 16–3. Strong, diffuse membranous staining for CD99 in a case of Ewing's sarcoma. (Immunoperoxidase, CD99, ×200)

combination with desmin,[18, 55] and can help distinguish rhabdomyosarcoma from DSRCT, which is typically negative for HHF-35.[43]

Desmin. Desmin is a 52- to 55-kd intermediate filament and serves as an integral part of the cytoskeleton of cardiac, smooth, and skeletal muscle.[19] It is a particularly sensitive marker for rhabdomyosarcomas.[55] However, it is also seen in many other tumors, and its sole presence should not be taken to be diagnostic of rhabdomyosarcoma. Desmin positivity is also a characteristic finding in DSRCT, being found in 90% of cases.[43] PNET[16] and malignant ectomesenchymomas may also express desmin.[20] Malignant rhabdoid tumors are typically negative, with rare cases found to express desmin.[44, 48, 56] Antigen retrieval is an important technique in identifying desmin expression.

CD45 (Leukocyte Common Antigen). Leukocyte common antigen (LCA) is commonly used to detect leukemias and lymphomas. Misdiagnoses associated with this antibody typically arise when a hematologic malignancy lacks expression. Rhabdomyosarcoma, malignant rhabdoid tumor, ES, PNET, DSRCT, and neuroblastoma are all negative for CD45, as is expected. However, LCA− lymphoblastic lymphomas-leukemias and granulocytic sarcoma are well described and can easily be misinterpreted as ES or other round cell tumor.[35] Therefore, using this as the sole antibody to exclude a hematologic process is risky. The addition of terminal deoxynucleotidyl transferase (TdT), which is almost uniformly positive in LCA− lymphoblastic lymphoma, and CD43, which stains most granulocytic sarcomas, can help avoid some of these pitfalls.[35, 57, 58]

Epithelial Membrane Antigen. Epithelial membrane antigen (EMA) is an antibody to milk fat globule membranes and is characteristically positive in epithelial malignancies. However, it is also positive in some soft tissue tumors.[19] Synovial sarcoma,[59–62] epithelioid sarcoma,[63] DSRCT,[43] and malignant rhabdoid tumors[44] express EMA. PNET, ES, rhabdomyosarcoma, and neuroblastomas are typically EMA−. Lymphomas can express EMA, and this is seen more typically in immunoblastic or anaplastic lymphomas.[64]

S-100 Protein. S-100 is a dimeric calcium-binding acidic protein that is present in central and peripheral nervous systems. S-100 positivity can be seen in PNET, neuroblastomas, DSRCT, malignant ectomesenchymoma, and mesenchymal chondrosarcoma.[19]

New Antibodies Under Investigation

Nerve Growth Factor Family, Trk Receptors, and Neuroblastoma. The pattern of expression of neurotrophic factors and their tyrosine kinase receptors, TrkA, TrkB, and TrkC, appears to be a marker for the biologic behavior of neuroblastomas.[65–68] TrkA is a high-affinity receptor for nerve growth factor, TrkB encodes a receptor of brain-derived neurotrophic factor and neurotrophic growth factor 4/5, and TrkC encodes a receptor for neurotrophic-3.[69] Nerve growth factor is responsible for the growth and differentiation of neural crest–derived cells.[70] The expression of TrkA in neuroblastomas has been evaluated both by identification of mRNA in frozen tissue and by immunohistochemical detection of the protein. Both techniques have demonstrated a strong correlation between the expression of TrkA and localized or regional or stage 4s disease.[71] Localized stage 4s disease had strong or mixed reactivity in 92% of tumors versus stage 4 metastatic tumors, in which only 34% expressed high or mixed immunoreactivity, and most were negative.[72]

The immunohistochemical assay was found to be superior to mRNA detection, presumably because the sensitivity of detecting mRNA was too great.[72] Correlating TrkA expression with N-myc amplification revealed the two to be inversely related in the majority of cases, as would be anticipated.[71] In one study, 46 stage I, stage II, and stage IV-S tumors lacking N-myc amplification demonstrated a high level of TrkA expression.[73] One stage 4s tumor with high N-myc also had high TrkA expression and was regressing at the time of surgery. Comparing the subset of patients whose neuroblastomas had no amplification of N-myc and low levels of TrkA, these patients showed a much worse prognosis than patients with no N-myc amplification and high TrkA expression. Therefore, the NGF/TRK-A pathway may be a fundamental factor in the ability of neuroblastic tumors to differentiate and regress.

TrkA was specific for neuroblastomas, with reactivity absent in concomitantly tested PNETs, ES, DSRCTs, rhabdomyosarcomas, and osteosarcomas.[70] A potential pitfall in its use is its lack of staining in undifferentiated neuroblastoma, the histologic appearance most likely to cause diagnostic confusion. Therefore, its use as a marker for neuroblastoma may be limited.[70]

TrkB and brain-derived neurotrophic factor are often expressed in dopaminergic neurons of normal lineage. Aggressive neuroblastomas often demonstrate dopaminergic characteristics. TrkB can be found in its full length or its truncated form in neuroblastic tumors. The truncated form is associated with maturing tumors, whereas N-myc−amplified tumors are more likely to express full-length TrkB receptors.[68] TrkB in its full-length form may therefore be an unfavorable prognostic factor related to N-myc amplification, although the data are only preliminary.

CD44. CD44, a cell surface glycoprotein, is a polymorphic molecule with different isoforms. The CD44 molecules act as receptors for hyaluronate and are involved in cell-to-cell interaction or cell-to-extracellular matrix interaction, lymphocyte activation, and the induction of homotypic cell aggregation. CD44 overexpression has been shown to correlate with enhanced tumorigenicity and metastatic ability in some tumors, including breast and colon carcinoma and non-Hodgkin's lymphoma. Evaluation of CD44 in neuroblastoma has demonstrated an opposite effect, with 100% of favorable tumors expressing CD44 and only 50% of advanced-stage neuroblastoma immunoreactive for CD44. In addition, progression-free survival was also significantly higher in CD44+ patients within the high-risk group.[74]

Myogenic Regulatory Proteins. MyoD1, myogenin, myf-5, and MRF4-herculin/myf-6 compose a family of myogenic regulatory factors that are involved in skeletal muscle differentiation. These regulatory factors are expressed much earlier than are structural proteins such as desmin or actin. MyoD1 (clone 5.8A, Novacastra Laboratories, Newcastle upon Tyne, UK) and myogenin (Imgenex, San Diego, CA) are expressed in less differentiated forms of rhabdomyosarcoma that lack morphologic evidence of rhabdomyogenous differentiation, such as strap cells.[75] MyoD1 in particular is expressed in primitive cells and is absent from cells exhibiting morphologic features of differentiation.[76] Several studies have demonstrated the specificity of MyoD1 as a marker for rhabdomyosarcoma.[75–77] This is in contrast to desmin, which has shown immunoreactivity in PNETs and congenital rhabdoid tumors. The latter in particular indicates that desmin is not as specific for muscle as previously assumed. Because the 5.8A MyoD1 antibody can exhibit strong cytoplasmic staining in nonrhabdomyogenous tumors such as neuroblastoma, strict adherence to the requirement for nuclear staining is necessary to obtain this high specificity. However, expression of MyoD1 is not restricted to rhabdomyosarcomas, as occasional positivity has been noted in Wilms' tumors and an ectomesenchymoma, both of which are known to contain rhabdomyogenous differentiation.[78] Subsequent studies have indicated that myogenin may stain alveolar rhabdomyosarcomas more diffusely and strongly, providing a means of immunohistochemically distinguishing embryonal and alveolar subsets.[79]

Choosing a Panel of Antibodies

As indicated earlier, when confronted with a small round cell tumor, the pathologist needs to amass as much clinical information as possible to help focus the differential diagnosis. Given the overlap of staining of some of these tumors and the variability that might be encountered because of fixation or preservation artifact, a "shotgun" approach to immunohistochemical analysis is not usually ideal or cost-effective. Beginning with a limited panel helps refine the differential diagnosis and allows a more systematic use of financial and tissue resources. To a certain extent, the panel used depends on the laboratory's resources and capabilities. Therefore, it is best to start with antibodies that are readily available. An initial panel might reasonably consist of CD99, vimentin, desmin, muscle-specific actin, cytokeratin, synaptophysin, LCA, and TDT. If TDT is not available, CD43 may be useful.[35] This battery of stains would help differentiate among DSRCTs, neuroblastoma, lymphoblastic lymphoma, PNETs, and ES, rhabdomyosarcoma, and malignant rhabdoid tumor.

SPECIFIC TUMORS

A brief mention of the most common small round cell tumors and their staining patterns follows. This highlights some of the most helpful stains to be used for these tumors (Table 16–2) and also hopefully provides insight into some of the pitfalls of these stains. Finally, it also serves to illustrate the growing utility of molecular analysis

Table 16–2. Profile of Immunostaining of the Common Pediatric Small Round Cell Tumors

Tumor	Vimentin	Cytokeratin	Epithelial Membrane Antigen	Neuron-Specific Enolase	Myogenin	Desmin	MyoD1	Muscle-Specific Actin	CD99	Terminal Deoxynucleotidyl Transferase
Neuroblastoma	N	N	N	+	N	N	N	N	N	N
ES/PNET	+	N	N	−/+	N	N	N	N	+	N
Rhabdomyosarcoma	+	N	N	N	+	+	+	+	N	N
DSRCT	+	+	+	+	N	+		N	N	N
Congenital rhabdoid tumor	+	+	+	+		+/−		N	N	N
Lymphoblastic lymphoma	+	N	N	N	N	N	N	N	+	+
Synovial sarcoma	+	+	+	N	N	N	N	N	+/−	N

The panel indicates the most common staining patterns of the tumors. Aberrant staining occurs and can cause diagnostic difficulties.
+, positive staining; N, no staining; a blank space indicates no studies have been done; +/−, mostly positive; −/+, mostly negative.
ES/PNET, Ewing's sarcoma/primitive neuroectodermal tumor; DSRCT, desmoplastic small round cell tumor.

in confirming and even diagnosing the most challenging of cases (Table 16–3).

Neuroblastic Tumors

Neuroblastic tumors encompass a group of tumors derived from the neural crest and that demonstrate varying degrees of neural and schwannian differentiation.[80, 81] It is one of the most common extracranial malignancies in childhood, with only leukemias and brain tumors being more frequent. The most common locations for these tumors are the adrenal medulla, extra-adrenal retroperitoneum, paravertebrally from the neck to the pelvis, and the posterior mediastinum. They are a neoplasm of the autonomic nervous system and arise in any location in which autonomic ganglia and paraganglia are located.[1, 15, 20, 80–88] Additional, less common locations include paratesticular or paraovarian tumors, kidney, or as either part of or as the sole component of a teratoma.[84] In its most undifferentiated form, neuroblastoma can be extremely difficult to distinguish from peripheral neuroectodermal tumors, malignant rhabdoid tumors, and lymphomas or leukemias (Fig. 16–5). As with other small round cell tumors, crush artifact, which is especially problematic in small biopsies, can add to the diagnostic difficulty. Immunohistochemically, the primitive neuroblasts are positive for NSE, synaptophysin, Leu7, chromogranin A (Fig. 16–6), protein gene product 9.5, GD2 (a ganglioside on human neuroblastoma cell membranes), and NB84[89] and are negative for actin, desmin, and low molecular weight cytokeratin.[37, 87] However, a neuroblastoma with rhabdomyogenous differentiation has been described, illustrating the ability of these tumors to show divergent differen-

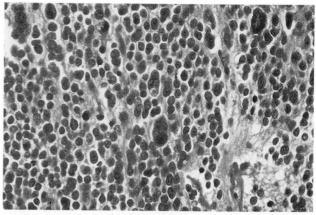

Figure 16–5. Undifferentiated neurobastoma easily confused with other small round cell tumors. (H&E, ×400)

tiation.[90] None of these antibodies is specific for neuroblastoma. NSE will stain up to 25% of rhabdomyosarcomas[84] and Leu7 will stain leukemias and some rhabdomyosarcomas.[19] Judicious use of other antibodies such as actin and other lymphoma-leukemia markers prevents confusion with those entities. Neuroblastomas are notably negative for vimentin and CD99, both of which help to distinguish this entity from the Ewing's family of tumors.[20, 89] Malignant rhabdoid tumors, which may be confused with neuroblastoma clinically and microscopically, can also be differentiated based on their staining pattern, with rhabdoid tumors exhibiting strong expression of vimentin, cytokeratins, and EMA.[44]

There is no molecular marker specific for neuroblastoma. Deletion or rearrangement of the short arm of chromosome 1 is the most common karyotypic abnormality.[39] The consistent finding of dele-

Table 16–3. Useful Molecular Markers in Pediatric Small Round Cell Tumors

Tumors	Translocation	Fusion Gene
Neuroblastoma	t(1p36;17q)	Unknown
ES/PNET	t(11;22)(q24;q12)	EWS/FLI-1
	t(21;22)(q22;q12)	EWS/ER6
	t(7;22)(p22;q12)	EWS/ETV1
	t(17;22)(q21;q22)	EWS/EIA-F
	t(2;22)(q33;q12)	EWS/FEV
Desmoplastic small round cell tumor	t(11;22)(q13;q12)	EWS/WT1
Alveolar rhabdomyosarcoma	t(2;13)(q35;q14)	PAX3/FKHR
	t(1;13)(q36;q14)	PAX7/FKHR
Synovial sarcoma	t(X,18)(p11;q11)	SYT/SSX1
		SYT/SSX2
Congenital rhabdoid tumor	22q11 abnormalities	
B-cell ALL	t(8;14)(q24;q32)	cmyc/Ig heavy chain
	t(8;22)(q24)	
	t(2;8)(q24)	
Early B-cell ALL or pre–pre-B-cell ALL	t(4;11)(q21;q23)	

ES/PNET, Ewing's sarcoma/primitive neuroectodermal tumor; ALL, acute lymphoblastic lymphoma.
    Data from: Thorner PS, Squire JA. Molecular genetics in the diagnosis and prognosis of solid pediatric tumors. Pediatr Dev Pathol 1998; 1:337–365; Kushner BH, LaQuaglia MP, Cheung NKV, et al. Clinically critical impact of molecular genetic studies in pediatric solid tumors. Med Pediatr Oncol 1999; 33:530–535; and Zutter MM, Hess JL. Guidelines for the diagnosis of leukemia or lymphoma in children. Am J Clin Pathol 1998; 109:S9–S22.

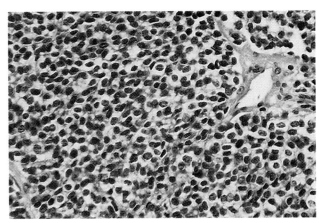

▧▧ *Figure 16–6.* Chromogranin positivity in neuroblastoma. (Immunoperoxidase, ×200)

▧▧ *Figure 16–7.* Sea of small round cells is the characteristic appearance of Ewing's sarcoma. (H&E, ×400)

tions of 1p suggests the presence of a tumor suppressor gene at that location.[9, 91] Anomalies in this region may have prognostic significance.[7–9, 91–93] Homogeneously staining regions and double-minute chromosomes are also found in about half of tumors.[39, 84] A notable molecular finding in neuroblastoma is N-myc amplification, which has been found to be an unfavorable feature.[65, 66]

KEY DIAGNOSTIC POINTS

- Neuroblastic tumors express neural crest markers: NSE, chromogranin, synaptophysin, Leu7, protein product 9.5, and GD2.
- Neuroblastic tumors typically show lack of expression of actin, desmin, cytokeratin, vimentin, and CD99.
- TrkA expression correlates with good prognostic categories and shows an inverse correlation with N-myc.
- There is no specific molecular marker for this tumor.

Peripheral Neuroectodermal Tumors/ Ewing's Tumor

Originally considered separate neoplasms, ES and PNETs are now assumed to represent a family of tumors of presumed neuroectodermal origin that share similar histologic, immunohistochemical, and molecular features.[1, 84, 85, 94–96] Although ES is most commonly found in bone, extraosseous ES occurs and can be difficult to separate by light microscopy alone. PNETs most commonly occur on the chest wall, but involvement of the retroperitoneal and paravertebral soft tissues, head, and neck, and soft tissue tumors of the lower and upper extremities are well described.[85, 97–101] ES/ PNETs can occur from infancy to old age.[1, 20, 85] Histologically, ES is classically described as "a sea of primitive uniform cells with round to oval

nuclei and scant cytoplasm (Fig. 16–7) with little to no evidence of neural differentiation," whereas PNETs can exhibit neural differentiation with both pseudo and true rosette formation (Fig. 16–8).[1, 102] Some tumors have a background fibrillary stroma. PNET is often distinguished from ES by evidence of neural differentiation, either in the form of rosette formation or immunoreactivity with neurofilament, S-100, or Leu7. Given the wide age range, locations, and the histologic variability associated with these tumors, the differential diagnosis is slightly broader than that of neuroblastoma and includes neuroblastoma, malignant rhabdoid tumor, DSRCT, lymphoma-leukemia, rhabdomyosarcoma, and monophasic synovial sarcoma. Rare examples of PNETs arising in the kidneys have also been described,[103] and these need to be distinguished from a Wilms' tumor.

Immunohistochemical confirmation of the diagnosis of ES/PNET is considered by many to be essential,[20] with useful antibodies including CD99, vimentin, NSE, Leu7, desmin, MSA, and cytokeratin.[22, 24, 34, 104] Both ES and PNETs stain for vimentin and CD99. Up to 95% of PNETs and ES exhibit

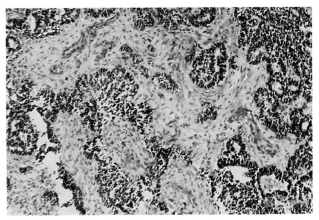

▧▧ *Figure 16–8.* Neural differentiation in primitive neuroectodermal tumor (PNET). (H&E, ×200)

strong membranous staining for CD99 (see Fig. 16–4). This can be helpful in ruling out a blastemal Wilms' tumor (Fig. 16–9).[25] Almost 100% of ES/PNETs are either focally or diffusely positive for vimentin in a dot-like or perinuclear pattern, and 30 to 40% of tumors express Leu7. NSE is a nonspecific antibody, but diffuse and strong positivity can be supportive of the diagnosis of PNET,[39] although neuroblastomas are also strongly and diffusely positive for NSE, and therefore this would not exclude this diagnosis. PNETs also show variable staining for S-100 (40%), synaptophysin (40 to 50% of cases), chromogranin (20%), neurofilament (40%), and glial acid fibrillary protein (<10%).[20, 39] Less than 10% of PNETs demonstrate cytokeratin, EMA, and desmin positivity. In the majority of cases, the combination of vimentin and CD99 and NSE positivity with concomitant negative expression for cytokeratins, muscle, and hematologic antibodies would argue against a diagnosis of neuroblastoma, rhabdomyosarcoma, desmoplastic round cell tumor, and leukemia-lymphoma. In the most diagnostically challenging cases or when the clinical presentation is unusual, molecular analysis is extremely useful and can now be performed on formalin-fixed, paraffin-embedded tissue.[18, 39, 95, 105, 106] Both ES and PNET share the same cytogenetic abnormalities. Two predominant translocations have been identified: t(11;22)(q24;q12), occurring in 85 to 90% of cases, and translocation t(21;22)(q22;q12), occurring in 5 to 10% of cases.[107, 108] The translocations result in the fusion of the ES gene in 22q12 with the FLI-1 gene in 11q24 for the former and ERG, a transcription factor closely related to FLI-1, for the latter.[109] The FLI-1 gene is a member of the Ets proto-oncogene family of transcription factors. An additional, rare translocation reported in ES/PNETs is t(7;22)(p22;q12) involving the EWS gene on 22q12 and the ETV1 gene on 7p22, yielding a chimeric transcript with a fusion protein containing the N-terminal domain of EWS and C-terminal DNA binding domain of ETV1. The identification of the chimeric EWS/FLI-1, EWS/ERG, or EWS/ETV1 transcripts by either Northern blot analysis or by reverse transcriptase polymerase chain reaction (PCR) provides strong support for the diagnosis of ES/PNET[18, 39]

KEY DIAGNOSTIC POINTS

- Immunohistochemical analysis of these tumors is considered by many to be essential.
- The combination of vimentin, CD99, and NSE positivity with negative expression of cytokeratins, muscle, and hematologic markers helps establish the diagnosis.
- Rare cases can exhibit cytokeratin and desmin positivity.
- Atypical ES can mimic DSRCTs, and molecular markers may be helpful in differentiating the two entities.
- Tumors negative for CD99 expression using all three antibodies on the market are rare, and this finding should stimulate either molecular or electron microscopic confirmation of the diagnosis.
- The identification of the chimeric EWS/FLI-1, EWS/ERG, or EWS/ETV1 transcripts by either Northern blot analysis or reverse transcriptase PCR provides strong support for the diagnosis of ES/PNET.

Desmoplastic Small Round Cell Tumor

DSRCT is a relatively recently described tumor occurring predominantly in children and young adults, with an age range of 6 to 49 years.[110–113] The typical presentation is that of a young adolescent male with abdominal distension and widespread tumor implants throughout the pelvis and abdomen. Grossly, the tumor forms bulky multinodular masses with smooth bosselated surfaces.[43, 114] The microscopic pattern of the tumor can vary, as found in a study of 109 cases by Gerald and coworkers.[43] The classic appearance is characterized by small round tumor cells arranged in nests and aggregates separated by a dense to fibromyxoid stroma (Fig. 16–10). The tumor cells can vary in appearance from round to rhabdoid to clear cell phenotypes (Fig. 16–11). Rosette formation can be seen. Intermediate filaments in varying amounts are seen by electron microscopy and correspond to the rhabdoid phenotype exhibited by some tumor cells. Immunohistochemically, the tumor cells demonstrate a distinct phenotype, with coexpression of epithelial, neural, and muscle markers. Diagnostic confusion with this tumor tends to arise when the clinical presentation is atypical, that is, extra-abdominal location, such as pleura,[115] central nervous system,[116] and lymph node.[117] The immunohistochemical coexpression of desmin, cytokeratin, vimentin, and NSE helps confirm a diagnosis of DSRCT in these instances (Fig. 16–12). Desmin,

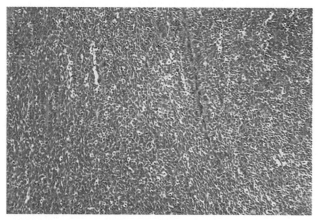

Figure 16–9. Blastemal Wilms' tumor characterized by undifferentiated primitive cells. (H&E, ×200)

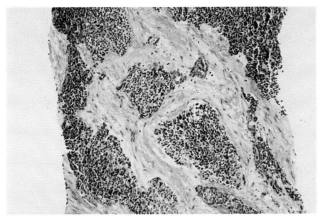

Figure 16-10. Classic appearance of desmoplastic small round cell tumor with nests of small tumor cells separated by a fibromyxoid stroma. (H&E, ×100)

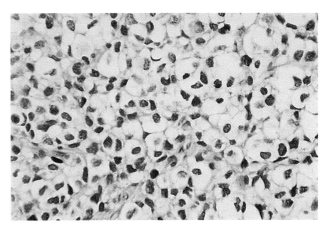

Figure 16-11. High-power view of DSRCT demonstrating tumor cells with clear cytoplasm. (H&E, ×400)

cytokeratin, and vimentin are the antibodies most commonly expressed in DSRCT. Combining the studies by Gerald and associates[43] and Ordonez,[118] 89.7 to 100% of tumors stain with desmin, and in Ordonez' study the staining was strong and diffuse in 75% of cases. In both studies, the staining was often globoid or dot-like in appearance. A similar pattern was noted with other intermediate filaments as well. A mixture of CAM5.2 and AE1/AE3 cytokeratins stained 85.9 to 95% of cases. The tumors did not express CK5/CK6 or CK20.[118] Vimentin was expressed in 81 to 97% of cases, EMA in 92.6 to 96% with cytoplasmic staining, MOC31 in 90% with a membranous staining pattern, and NSE in 72 to 81% with cytoplasmic staining. Leu7 was expressed in 67% of cases in a cytoplasmic pattern. Twenty to 35% of cases stained with CD99.

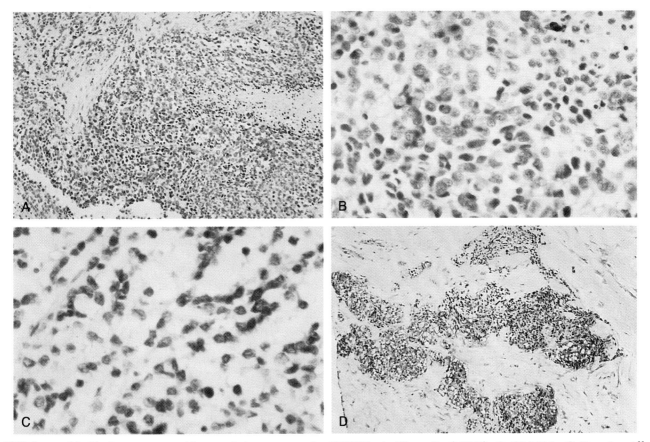

Figure 16-12. Immunoperoxidase staining pattern for DSRCT. *A*, Vimentin (×200). *B*, CAM5.2. *C*, Desmin. All antibodies displayed a dot-like or globoid positive staining pattern. *D*, Neuron-specific enolase (NSE).

Gerald and colleagues[43] found cytoplasmic reactivity with CD99, but Ordonez[118] found predominantly membranous staining, with a cytoplasmic pattern less common. MSA was positive in 16% of cases, smooth muscle actin in 19%, and chromogranin in 5%. Although DSRCT is positive for desmin, it is not positive for MyoD1, myogenin, and myoglobin, suggesting that the desmin expression is not an indication of true muscle differentiation. The MSA is also positive much less commonly than desmin (16% versus 100%).[118] This can be a useful discriminating point between rhabdomyosarcoma and DSRCT.

Although immunohistochemistry can be helpful in confirming a diagnosis of DSRCT, there is no panel of antibodies specific for this entity. ES/PNET, Wilms' tumor, synovial sarcoma, and DSRCT overlap. Cytokeratin can be found in both DSRCT and PNET. Both DSRCT and PNET can be positive for NSE and synaptophysin. Rhabdomyosarcoma can sometimes be excluded by lack of staining by the tumor with muscle markers, other than desmin, such as MSA, myoglobin, and MyoD1. In diagnostically difficult cases or unusual clinical settings, molecular confirmation of the diagnosis may be essential. DSRCT is now recognized to have a novel t(11;22)(p13;q12) translocation, which creates the chimeric fusion product EWS-WT1, joining the EWS gene to the WT1 gene.[119-127]

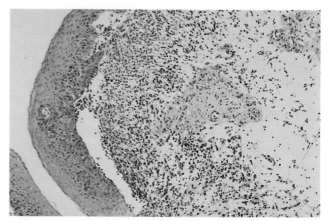

Figure 16-13. Botryoid rhabdomyosarcoma with cambium layer and immature cells in a myxoid stroma. (H&E, ×100)

KEY DIAGNOSTIC POINTS

- Coexpression of desmin, cytokeratin, and vimentin, especially with a dot-like positivity, helps confirm the diagnosis of DSRCT.
- Lack of membranous staining for CD99 supports a diagnosis of DSRCT over PNET.
- Lack of expression of muscle-specific actin in the face of desmin positivity supports a diagnosis of DSRCT over rhabdomyosarcoma.
- Molecular identification of the chimeric fusion product EWS-WT1 provides strong support for the diagnosis in atypical cases.

Rhabdomyosarcoma

Rhabdomyosarcoma is the most common soft tissue sarcoma in childhood, composing 5 to 8% of childhood cancers.[128] Although rhabdomyosarcoma is by definition a tumor of skeletal muscle differentiation, it often occurs in areas where skeletal muscle is absent. Different histologic subtypes of rhabdomyosarcoma are recognized and have been delineated by the Intergroup Rhabdomyosarcoma Group.[55] These subtypes correspond to different prognostic groups. The botryoid and spindle cell variants of embryonal rhabdomyosarcoma correspond to a superior prognosis (Fig. 16-13), the embryonal form shows an intermediate prognosis,

and the alveolar subtype and undifferentiated sarcomas are found to have the worst prognosis.[55, 101, 129, 130] Clinically, rhabdomyosarcoma shows a bimodal distribution, with more than 50% of cases occurring in the first decade of life and being predominantly of the embryonal subtype. A second peak occurs in adolescence, and these tumors are predominantly of alveolar histology. As advances in therapy have led to longer survival for some subtypes of rhabdomyosarcoma, accurate identification of the tumor and the subtype has become increasingly important. The Intergroup Rhabdomyosarcoma Group found immunohistochemistry pivotal in making or confirming the diagnosis of rhabdomyosarcoma in 20% of cases. Using a comprehensive battery of commercially available antibodies, the group studied 228 tumors encompassing all subtypes.[55] Ninety-nine percent of the tumors expressed immunoreactivity for polyclonal desmin (DAKO, dilution 1:500), 62% for monoclonal desmin (clone DE-R-11, DAKO 1:25), and 94% for muscle-specific actin (HHF-35, Enzo Diagnostics, Farmingdale, NY). Alpha smooth muscle actin, however, demonstrated positivity in only 4% of cases. Myoglobin was noted in only 78% of cases and was seen predominantly in the more differentiated tumors and was negative in the less differentiated tumors. Although expression of a muscle antigen is not diagnostic for rhabdomyosarcoma in the absence of staining by the other antibodies in the panel, it is strongly supportive of that diagnosis.[130] However, the same study of 288 cases also demonstrated that 14% of tumors were positive for CD99, 2% were positive for epithelial membrane antigen, 19% were positive for S-100 protein, and 6% were positive for NSE. Others have described similar results.[130] None of the tumors was positive for LCA, and almost all the tumors were uniformly positive for vimentin. Antigen retrieval was found to be essential for identification of vimentin, monoclonal desmin, and CD99 expression. The Intergroup Rhabdomy-

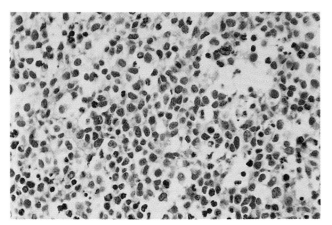

Figure 16–14. Solid variant of alveolar rhabdomyosarcoma. (H&E, ×200)

osarcoma Group found that coexpression of polyclonal desmin and MSA was strongly supportive of the diagnosis of rhabdomyosarcoma. In an article, they recommended a panel of three antibodies when the diagnosis was uncertain: polyclonal desmin, MSA, and CD99.[55] CD99 is added to exclude ES/PNET, which is a common differential diagnostic dilemma. In the rare cases that are CD99+, the Intergroup Rhabdomyosarcoma Group found positivity of both MSA and polyclonal desmin to be the discriminating factor. In addition, the pattern of staining of CD99 differed in the rhabdomyosarcomas in that it produces weak and granular cytoplasmic staining as opposed to the strong membranous staining seen in ES/PNET tumors. It is important to remember when using these panels that other tumors, such as neuroblastoma, can show myogenous differentiation and desmin positivity.[90] The addition of a more specific skeletal muscle marker, such as MyoD1 or myogenin, or molecular analysis may be helpful in these situations.

The diagnostic difficulty with rhabdomyosarcoma is not limited to making the diagnosis of rhabdomyosarcoma but also includes rendering the correct subtype.[128–134] New immunohistochemical stains and molecular analysis may be critical components in the diagnosis, subtyping, and prognostication of these tumors. The histologic subtypes that most commonly cause diagnostic confusion are the solid variant of alveolar rhabdomyosarcoma[130, 135–137] (Fig. 16–14) and the most undifferentiated form of embryonal rhabdomyosarcoma (Fig. 16–15). Cases of the former have been misdiagnosed as embryonal rhabdomyosarcoma before molecular analysis revealed the characteristic t(2;13)(q35;q14) translocation.[106] The importance of this distinction lies with the much more aggressive behavior and worse prognosis associated with alveolar rhabdomyosarcoma compared with the embryonal subtype.[138] Studies of the myogenic regulatory genes and their protein expression suggest that myogenin protein expression may correlate with the alveolar subtype (see earlier discussion). Because these proteins are markers of skeletal muscle differentiation, they appear to be more restricted in their expression to tumors with true skeletal muscle differentiation. Desmin, by contrast, marks tumors of both skeletal muscle origin and nonskeletal muscle origin; therefore, it is not as helpful as markers that are more lineage-specific.

Characteristic cytogenetic and molecular abnormalities are associated with alveolar and embryonal rhabdomyosarcoma.[139–141] Alveolar rhabdomyosarcoma is consistently associated with either of two translocations involving the PAX genes: t(2;13)(q35;q14) or t(1;13)(p36;q14).[135] The first is the more common translocation and creates a PAX3-FKHR fusion protein that is a more potent transcriptional activator than PAX3 by itself.[106] Clinically, patients with this translocation are typically older and present with metastases in multiple sites. The second translocation is less common and creates a PAX7-FKHR fusion product.[105] These tumors are more often localized and when metastases are present at diagnosis, they tend to be limited to bone or distant lymph nodes. Both these fusion transcripts can be identified by reverse tran-

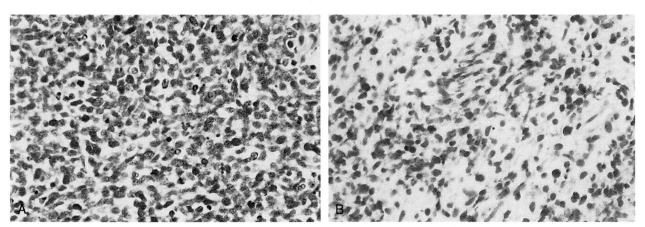

Figure 16–15. Undifferentiated embryonal rhabdomyosarcoma. *A,* H&E (×400). *B,* Desmin with staining of cytoplasmic processes. (×400)

scriptase PCR (RT-PCR) or by fluorescence in situ hybridization (FISH), which are relatively easy and rapid techniques. Embryonal rhabdomyosarcomas are associated with loss of heterozygosity on the short arm of chromosome 11 at 11p15.5.[106] Molecular analysis should be performed on any tumor exhibiting either an unusual staining profile or an atypical clinical presentation or course. Desmin-negative rhabdomyosarcomas occur and can easily be misdiagnosed as neuroblastoma or PNET.[105] In addition, the type of translocation present may, in the future, provide prognostic information that can be used to guide therapy.

KEY DIAGNOSTIC POINTS

* Most cases can be diagnosed by light microscopy alone, with up to 20% of cases causing diagnostic confusion.
* An initial panel consisting of desmin, MSA (HHF-35), CD99 (to exclude ES/PNET), LCA, vimentin, and a pan-cytokeratin is usually adequate. Positive staining with desmin and MSA and negative staining with the rest provide strong support for the diagnosis of rhabdomyosarcoma.
* Beware the rare cytokeratin-positive, desmin-negative, and CD99+ tumors.
* MyoD1 and myogenin are newly developed antibodies that show high specificity and sensitivity for rhabdomyosarcomas and can be useful either up front or as a back-up if not routinely available. Both require antigen retrieval and are nuclear stains.
* Alveolar rhabdomyosarcoma has characteristic translocations and fusion products that should be looked for if immunohistochemistry is nondiagnostic or if the clinical setting is unusual.

Congenital Rhabdoid Tumor

Congenital rhabdoid tumor is an uncommon, recently described distinct tumor presenting at birth or in the neonatal period with widespread metastatic disease.[51, 53] Clinically, the tumor is easily confused with other small blue cell tumors of infancy, including neuroblastoma, ES/PNET, and rhabdomyosarcoma. Pathologically, they are easily confused with embryonal rhabdomyosarcoma, epithelioid sarcoma, neuroblastoma, PNET/ES, synovial sarcoma, and lymphoma.[56] Congenital rhabdoid tumors are primitive tumors without evidence of differentiation whose name is derived from the rhabdoid appearance of some the tumors cells.[44, 48, 54, 142] The histologic appearance can vary from epithelioid to spindled. Immunohistochemically, these tumors demonstrate polyphenotypic expression with diffuse prominent paranuclear reactivity for vimentin (100% of cases), focal or diffuse expression of

cytokeratin (CAM5.2 or AE1/AE3) (100%), focal or diffuse membranous or paranuclear reactivity for EMA (89%), and variable expression of desmin, NSE, MSA, and CD99 (Fig. 16–16).[44] The strong vimentin and cytokeratin expression helps distinguish these tumors from neuroblastomas, negative CD99 and positive cytokeratin expression argue against a diagnosis of PNET, and negative LCA or TdT helps rule out lymphoma or leukemia. However, given the polyphenotypic nature of these tumors, immunohistochemical overlap with other small blue cell tumors occurs. In addition, aberrant expression of cytokeratin can make it difficult to distinguish PNETs, congenital rhabdoid tumors, and DSRCTs. Rare positivity with CD99 and desmin can make it difficult to distinguish congenital rhabdoid tumors from PNETs and rhabdomyosarcomas, respectively.

Molecular analysis of renal and extrarenal malignant rhabdoid tumors has revealed chromosomal abnormalities involving chromosome 22q11.[44] Subsequent studies have identified a putative tumor suppressor gene, hSNF5/INI1, at this locus.[143–147] Mutations in this gene are believed to be responsible for a variety of tumors, some of which exhibit rhabdoid features, including malignant rhabdoid tumor, chorioid plexus carcinomas, central PNET, and medulloblastoma.[146]

KEY DIAGNOSTIC POINTS

* Congenital rhabdoid tumors are highly aggressive tumors of infancy and are often widely disseminated at initial presentation.
* Tumor cells with rhabdoid features are always present but may make up a variable percentage of the tumor population. Often, the majority of the cells are primitive and undifferentiated and difficult to distinguish histologically from PNETs, rhabdomyosarcomas, or DSRCTs.
* These tumors characteristically show diffuse reactivity for vimentin and at least focal reactivity for cytokeratin and EMA.
* Congenital rhabdoid tumors can show variable expression for desmin and CD99, making distinction from rhabdomyosarcomas, which can also aberrantly express cytokeratin, and DSRCTs difficult.
* In difficult cases, molecular analysis to identify monosomy or deletion of chromosome 22q11 may provide support for the diagnosis.

Lymphoma-Leukemia

Lymphomas and leukemias are an important group of malignant tumors belonging to the category of small round cell tumors of childhood. The most difficult of these lesions to separate from other small round cell tumors is lymphoblastic

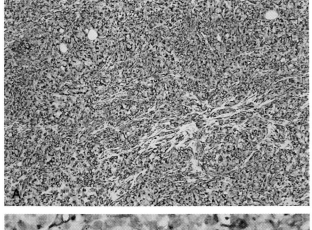

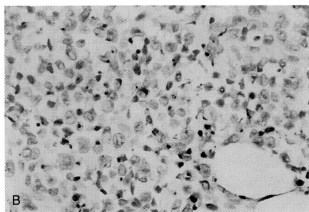

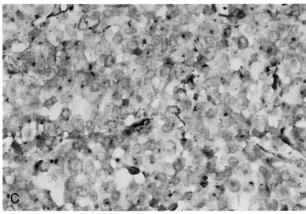

Figure 16–16. Congenital rhabdoid tumor. *A,* Vimentin showing diffuse strong expression. *B,* Cytokeratin CAM5.2 with dot-like positivity. *C,* CD99 with both cytoplasmic and membrane staining.

lymphoma. Using hematoxylin and eosin (H&E) alone, it can be impossible to distinguish lymphoblastic lymphoma from ES, PNET, neuroblastoma, and rhabdomyosarcoma (Fig. 16–17).[4] Often, the discohesiveness of the cells can be diagnostic; however, scrape preparations of PNETs and ES can also exhibit discohesion and a fine nuclear chromatin pattern (Fig. 16–18). TdT, CD34, and HLA-DR positivity can be helpful in identifying the lymphoid nature of the cells. Pre–pre-B-cell ALL and pre–B-cell ALL express TdT and early B-cell antigens such as HLA-DR, CD34, CD19, and CD10. B-cell ALL demonstrates surface Ig HLA-DR and CD19 and CD10.[4] LCA is typically expressed by T cells, B cells, myeloid cells, and macrophages. However, there are examples of LCA− lymphoblastic lymphomas, leading to their misdiagnosis as ES.[35] Because of the importance of making the correct diagnosis, adding TdT to the initial immunohistochemical panel may be appropriate. A second alternative is to include it as part of a second panel, which would then be run in any atypical clinical scenario or if the first immunohistochemical panel leads to unusual results. As indicated earlier, CD99 is frequently positive in lymphoblastic lymphoma and therefore cannot by itself be used to distinguish it from ES/PNET. Cytokeratin is also typically negative in both tumors, demonstrating again the importance of reliable hematologic markers to confirm the diagnosis. B- and

T-cell markers can also be important in these cases. Negative expression for desmin and actin would help rule out a rhabdomyosarcoma.

It is important to realize that the immunohistochemical and cytogenetic profile of hematologic malignancies is also important for therapeutic and prognostic implications. For example, the diagnosis of pre–pre-B-cell ALL with expression of CD19, CD10, HLA-DR, and TdT corresponds to a tumor that will respond well to therapy with a potential cure in 85% of cases. The identification of the

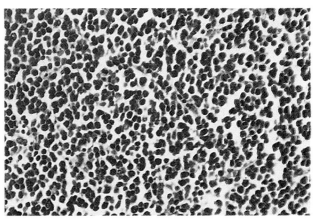

Figure 16–17. Diffuse small round cell appearance of lymphoblastic lymphoma. (H&E, ×400)

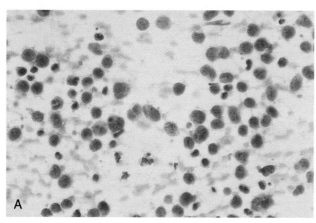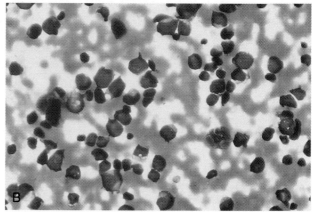

Figure 16–18. Alcohol-fixed (*A*) and air-dried touch (*B*) preparations of Ewing's sarcoma showing small cells easily confused with lymphoblastic lymphoma.

Philadelphia chromosome in a morphologically similar tumor carries a dismal prognosis and calls for more aggressive therapy.[4]

KEY DIAGNOSTIC POINTS

- Because of its uniform small blue cell appearance, lymphoblastic lymphoma is the most difficult hematologic malignancy to distinguish from other small round cell tumors.
- TdT, CD43, and LCA expression are important in confirming the hematologic origin of these tumors.
- Negative desmin and actin expression argue against a diagnosis of rhabdomyosarcoma.
- CD99 is routinely positive in lymphoblastic lymphoma and is therefore not helpful in distinguishing this tumor from ES/PNET.
- Immunohistochemical and cytogenetic analyses are essential components of the work-up of lymphomas and leukemias.

Wilms' Tumor

Wilms' tumor is the most common pediatric renal neoplasm, composing approximately 80% of primary renal tumors. It can exhibit a wide range of histologic appearances that can make its distinction from other pediatric renal neoplasms difficult. The pattern most likely to cause confusion with other small round cell neoplasms is the blastemal histologic appearance. Monomorphous sheets of small blue cells characterize this histologic subtype. The cells can appear discohesive. The differential diagnosis usually includes lymphoma, PNET, neuroblastoma, DSRCT, and rhabdomyosarcoma. Wilms' tumors do not exhibit any specific immunophenotype.[148] The tumors are positive for cytokeratin and lack expression of CD99, a feature that helps distinguish them from ES/PNET. One study has suggested that the blastemal component of Wilms' tumor is commonly desmin-positive but

negative for myogenin and MyoD1, which are more specific markers of rhabdomyogenous differentiation.[149] Other studies have not found desmin to be positive in Wilms' tumors. In general, the most important clue to the correct diagnosis in these cases is the clinical history, indicating the kidney as the origin of the tumor.

KEY DIAGNOSTIC POINTS

- The blastemal Wilms' tumor is the histologic pattern most likely to be confused with other small round cell tumors.
- A positive cytokeratin and negative CD99 profile is helpful in excluding a diagnosis of ES/PNET.
- Clinical information identifying the kidney as the source of the tumor can be the most important aid in arriving at the correct diagnosis.

Poorly Differentiated Synovial Sarcoma

Synovial sarcoma is the fourth most common soft tissue sarcoma in adults[19, 33] and the second most common soft tissue sarcoma in children, surpassed only by rhabdomyosarcoma.[150] In one large series, it composed 17 to 29% of cases.[151] Classically, synovial sarcoma presents as a para-articular soft tissue mass with a biphasic histologic appearance. However, its occurrence in other sites is well described, including neck,[152] heart,[153] lung and pleura,[150, 154–157] and prostate.[158] Synovial sarcoma may be classified as biphasic, monophasic spindle, poorly differentiated, or epithelial.[159] The monophasic spindle morphologic appearance and the poorly differentiated subtype can be confused with other small round cell tumors.[33] Immunohistochemical expression of cytokeratin and vimentin and lack of expression of CD99 and neural markers can help confirm the diagnosis of synovial sarcoma. However, the monophasic variant can be negative for cytokeratin.[33, 160] In addition, as with DSRCT, the poorly differentiated subtype can express CD99.[17, 33] Synovial sarcomas have a characteristic (X,18)(p11;q11) translocation, creating the chimeric product SYT/SSX1 or SYT/SSX2 in more than 90% of cases.[106, 161] The ability to use formalin-fixed, paraffin-embedded tissue makes molecular confirmation of the diagnosis possible on any atypical case.[162] The specificity of the SYT/SSX RT-PCR assay for synovial sarcoma has been demonstrated in a large series of sarcomas.[163]

KEY DIAGNOSTIC POINTS

- The monophasic or poorly differentiated subtypes of synovial sarcoma are the ones most commonly confused with other small round cell tumors.
- Synovial sarcomas can occur in locations other than the extremities.
- Immunoreactivity for cytokeratin and vimentin with lack of expression of CD99 and neural markers can help confirm the diagnosis.
- Cytokeratin-negative and CD99+ cases of synovial sarcoma have been described.
- Synovial sarcoma is associated with a specific translocation and fusion product that can be assayed in diagnostically confusing cases.

In conclusion, the availability of more specific and more sensitive immunohistochemical markers has enabled pathologists to categorize undifferentiated small blue cell tumors more accurately. As treatment for these tumors improves, accurate and specific diagnoses are required. Immunohistochemistry is only one of the tools available to the pathologist to categorize this group of tumors correctly, with electron microscopy and molecular analysis also of great use. However, the ease of use and the ready availability of immunohistochemistry make it the first choice of most pathologists. Therefore, awareness of its strengths and pitfalls is essential.

References

1. Dehner LP. Primitive neuroectodermal tumor and Ewing's sarcoma. Am J Surg Pathol 1993;17:1–13.
2. Parham DM. Immunohistochemistry of childhood sarcomas: Old and new markers. Mod Pathol 1993;6:133–138.
3. Carbone A, Gloghini A, Volpe R. The value of immunohistochemistry in the diagnosis of soft tissue sarcomas. Ann Oncol 1992;3 Suppl 2:S51–S54.
4. Zutter MM, Hess JL. Guidelines for the diagnosis of leukemia or lymphoma in children. Am J Clin Pathol 1998;109(4 Suppl 1):S9–S22.
5. Mierau GW, Berry PJ, Malott RL, Weeks DA. Appraisal of the comparative utility of immunohistochemistry and electron microscopy in the diagnosis of childhood round cell tumors. Ultrastruct Pathol 1996;20:507–517.
6. Mierau GW, Weeks DA, Hicks MJ. Role of electron microscopy and other special techniques in the diagnosis of childhood round cell tumors. Hum Pathol 1998;29:1347–1355.
7. Rubie H, Delattre O, Hartmann O, et al. Loss of chromosome 1p may have a prognostic value in localised neuroblastoma: Results of the French NBL 90 Study: Neuroblastoma Study Group of the Societe Francaise d'Oncologie Pediatrique (SFOP). Eur J Cancer 1997;33:1917–1922.
8. Schleiermacher G, Delattre O, Peter M, et al. Clinical relevance of loss heterozygosity of the short arm of chromosome 1 in neuroblastoma: A single-institution study. Int J Cancer 1996;69:73–78.
9. Schleiermacher G, Peter M, Michon J, et al. Two distinct deleted regions on the short arm of chromosome 1 in neuroblastoma. Genes Chromosomes Cancer 1994;10:275–281.
10. Askin FB, Perlman EJ. Neuroblastoma and peripheral neuroectodermal tumors. Am J Clin Pathol 1998;109(4 Suppl 1):S23–S30.
11. Stocker JT. An approach to handling pediatric liver tumors. Am J Clin Pathol 1998;109(4 Suppl 1):S67–S72.
12. Stocker JT, Mosijczuk AD. Handling the pediatric tumor. [editorial] Am J Clin Pathol 1998;109(4 Suppl 1):S1–S3.
13. Zuppan CW. Handling and evaluation of pediatric renal tumors. Am J Clin Pathol 1998;109(4 Suppl 1):S31–S37.
14. Tsokos M, Linnoila RI, Chandra RS, Triche TJ. Neuron-specific enolase in the diagnosis of neuroblastoma and other small, round-cell tumors in children. Hum Pathol 1984;15:575–584.
15. Dehner L. Pathologic anatomy of classic neuroblastoma: Including prognostic features and differential diagnosis. In: Pochedly D, ed. Neuroblastoma: Tumor Biology and Therapy. Boca Raton: CRC Press, 1990:111–143.
16. Parham DM, Dias P, Kelly DR, et al. Desmin positivity in primitive neuroectodermal tumors of childhood. Am J Surg Pathol 1992;16:483–492.
17. DeiTos A, Wadden C, Calonje E, et al. Immunohistochemical demonstration of glycoprotein p30/32MIC2 (CD99) in synovial sarcoma: A potential cause of diagnostic confusion. Appl Immunohistochem 1995;3:168–173.
18. Hibshoosh H, Lattes R. Immunohistochemical and molecular genetic approaches to soft tissue tumor diagnosis: A primer. Semin Oncol 1997;24:515–525.
19. Enzinger F, Weiss S. Soft Tissue Tumors. 3rd ed. St. Louis: CV Mosby, 1995.
20. Coffin C, Dehner L. Neurogenic tumors of soft tissue. In: Coffin C, Dehner L, O'Shea P, eds. Pediatric Soft Tissue Tumors: A clinical, pathological, and therapeutic approach. Baltimore: Williams & Wilkins, 1997:80–132.
21. Levy R, Dilley J, Fox RI, Warnke R. A human thymus-leukemia antigen defined by hybridoma monoclonal antibodies. Proc Natl Acad Sci U S A 1979;76:6552–6556.
22. Stevenson AJ, Chatten J, Bertoni F, Miettinen M. CD99 (p30/32MIC2) neuroectodermal/Ewing's sarcoma antigen as an immunohistochemical marker: Review of more than 600 tumors and the literature experience. Appl Immunohistochem 1994;2:231–240.
23. Kovar H, Dworzak M, Strehl S, et al. Overexpression of the pseudoautosomal gene MIC2 in Ewing's sarcoma and peripheral primitive neuroectodermal tumor. Oncogene 1990;5:1067–1070.
24. Halliday BE, Slagel DD, Elsheikh TE, Silverman JF. Diagnostic utility of MIC-2 immunocytochemical staining in the differential diagnosis of small blue cell tumors. Diagn Cytopathol 1998;19:410–416.
25. Ramani P, Rampling D, Link M. Immunocytochemical study of 12E7 in small round-cell tumours of childhood: An assessment of its sensitivity and specificity. Histopathology 1993;23:557–561.
26. Perlman EJ, Dickman PS, Askin FB, et al. Ewing's sarcoma—routine diagnostic utilization of MIC2 analysis: A Pediatric Oncology Group/Children's Cancer Group Intergroup Study. Hum Pathol 1994;25:304–307.
27. Weidner N, Tjoe J. Immunohistochemical profile of monoclonal antibody O13: Antibody that recognizes glycoprotein p30/32MIC2 and is useful in diagnosing Ewing's sarcoma and peripheral neuroepithelioma. [see comments] Am J Surg Pathol 1994;18:486–494.
28. Ambros IM, Ambros PF, Strehl S, et al. MIC2 is a specific

marker for Ewing's sarcoma and peripheral primitive neuroectodermal tumors: Evidence for a common histogenesis of Ewing's sarcoma and peripheral primitive neuroectodermal tumors from MIC2 expression and specific chromosome aberration. Cancer 1991;67:1886–1893.

29. Dehner LP. On trial: A malignant small cell tumor in a child: Four wrongs do not make a right. Am J Clin Pathol 1998;109:662–668.

30. Riopel M, Dickman PS, Link MP, Perlman EJ. MIC2 analysis in pediatric lymphomas and leukemias. Hum Pathol 1994;25:396–399.

31. Zhang P, Barcos M, Stewart C, et al. Immunoreactivity of MIC2 (CD99) in acute myelogenous leukemia and related diseases. Modern Pathology 2000;13:452–458.

32. Granter SR, Renshaw AA, Fletcher CD, et al. CD99 reactivity in mesenchymal chondrosarcoma. Hum Pathol 1996;27:1273–1276.

33. Folpe AL, Schmidt RA, Chapman D, Gown AM. Poorly differentiated synovial sarcoma: Immunohistochemical distinction from primitive neuroectodermal tumors and high-grade malignant peripheral nerve sheath tumors. Am J Surg Pathol 1998;22:673–682.

34. Fellinger EJ, Garin-Chesa P, Triche TJ, et al. Immunohistochemical analysis of Ewing's sarcoma cell surface antigen p30/32MIC2. Am J Pathol 1991;139:317–325.

35. Ozdemirli M, Fanburg-Smith JC, et al. Precursor B-lymphoblastic lymphoma presenting as a solitary bone tumor and mimicking Ewing's sarcoma: A report of four cases and review of the literature. Am J Surg Pathol 1998;22:795–804.

36. Kawaguchi K, Koike M. Neuron-specific enolase and Leu-7 immunoreactive small round-cell neoplasm. The relationship to Ewing's sarcoma in bone and soft tissue. Am J Clin Pathol 1986;86:79–83.

37. Carter RL, al-Sams SZ, Corbett RP, Clinton S. A comparative study of immunohistochemical staining for neuron-specific enolase, protein gene product 9.5 and S-100 protein in neuroblastoma, Ewing's sarcoma and other round cell tumours in children. Histopathology 1990;16:461–467.

38. Schmidt D, Harms D. The applicability of immunohistochemistry in the diagnosis and differential diagnosis of malignant soft tissue tumors: A reevaluation based on the material of the Kiel Pediatric Tumor Registry. Klin Padiatr 1990;202:224–229.

39. Meis-Kindblom JM, Stenman G, Kindblom LG. Differential diagnosis of small round cell tumors. Semin Diagn Pathol 1996;13:213–241.

40. Triche TJ, Tsokos M, Linnoila RI, et al. NSE in neuroblastoma and other round cell tumors of childhood. Prog Clin Biol Res 1985;175:295–317.

41. Pahlman S, Esscher T, Nilsson K. Expression of gamma-subunit of enolase, neuron-specific enolase, in human non-neuroendocrine tumors and derived cell lines. Lab Invest 1986;54:554–560.

42. Haimoto H, Takahashi Y, Koshikawa T, et al. Immunohistochemical localization of gamma-enolase in normal human tissues other than nervous and neuroendocrine tissues. Lab Invest 1985;52:257–263.

43. Gerald WL, Ladanyi M, de Alava E, et al. Clinical, pathologic, and molecular spectrum of tumors associated with t(11;22)(p13;q12): Desmoplastic small round-cell tumor and its variants. J Clin Oncol 1998;16:3028–3036.

44. White FV, Dehner LP, Belchis DA, et al. Congenital disseminated malignant rhabdoid tumor: A distinct clinicopathologic entity demonstrating abnormalities of chromosome 22q11. Am J Surg Pathol 1999;23:249–256.

45. Mai G, Antonescu C, Huvos A, et al. Cytokeratin Immunoreactivity in Ewing's sarcoma: Prevalence in 50 cases confirmed by molecular diagnostic studies. Am J Surg Pathol 2000;24:410–416.

46. Michels S, Swanson PE, Robb JA, Wick MR. Leu-7 in small cell neoplasms: An immunohistochemical study with ultrastructural correlations. Cancer 1987;60:2958–2964.

47. Arbor D, Weiss L. CD57: A review. Appl Immunohistochem 1995;3:137–152.

48. Fanburg-Smith JC, Hengge M, Hengge UR, et al. Extrarenal rhabdoid tumors of soft tissue: A clinicopathologic and immunohistochemical study of 18 cases. Ann Diagn Pathol 1998;2:351–362.

49. Miettinen M. Synaptophysin and neurofilament proteins as markers for neuroendocrine tumors. Arch Pathol Lab Med 1987;111:813–818.

50. Miettinen M, Rapola J. Synaptophysin—an immuno-histochemical marker for childhood neuroblastoma. Acta Pathol Microbiol Immunol Scand [A] 1987;95:167–170.

51. Kodet R, Newton WA Jr, Sachs N, et al. Rhabdoid tumors of soft tissues: A clinicopathologic study of 26 cases enrolled on the Intergroup Rhabdomyosarcoma Study. Hum Pathol 1991;22:674–684.

52. Tsokos M, Kouraklis G, Chandra RS, et al. Malignant rhabdoid tumor of the kidney and soft tissues: Evidence for a diverse morphological and immunocytochemical phenotype. Arch Pathol Lab Med 1989;113:115–120.

53. Tsuneyoshi M, Daimaru Y, Hashimoto H, Enjoji M. Malignant soft tissue neoplasms with the histologic features of renal rhabdoid tumors: An ultrastructural and immunohistochemical study. Hum Pathol 1985;16:1235–1242.

54. Parham DM, Weeks DA, Beckwith JB. The clinicopathologic spectrum of putative extrarenal rhabdoid tumors: An analysis of 42 cases studied with immunohistochemistry or electron microscopy. Am J Surg Pathol 1994;18:1010–1029.

55. Qualman SJ, Coffin CM, Newton WA, et al. Intergroup Rhabdomyosarcoma Study: Update for pathologists. Pediatr Dev Pathol 1998;1:550–561.

56. Coffin C, Dehner L. Soft tissue tumors of nosologic uncertainty. In: Coffin C, Dehner L, O'Shea P, eds. Pediatric Soft Tissue Tumors. Baltimore: Williams & Wilkins, 1997.

57. Soslow RA, Bhargava V, Warnke RA. MIC2, TdT, bcl-2, and CD34 expression in paraffin-embedded high-grade lymphoma/acute lymphoblastic leukemia distinguishes between distinct clinicopathologic entities. Hum Pathol 1997;28:1158–1165.

58. Suzumiya J, Ohshima K, Kikuchi M, et al. Terminal deoxynucleotidyl transferase staining of malignant lymphomas in paraffin sections: A useful method for the diagnosis of lymphoblastic lymphoma. J Pathol 1997;182:86–91.

59. Lopes JM, Bjerkehagen B, Holm R, et al. Immunohistochemical profile of synovial sarcoma with emphasis on the epithelial-type differentiation: A study of 49 primary tumours, recurrences and metastases. Pathol Res Pract 1994;190:168–177.

60. Miettinen M. Keratin subsets in spindle cell sarcomas: Keratins are widespread but synovial sarcoma contains a distinctive keratin polypeptide pattern and desmoplakins. Am J Pathol 1991;138:505–513.

61. Ordonez NG, Mahfouz SM, Mackay B. Synovial sarcoma: An immunohistochemical and ultrastructural study. Hum Pathol 1990;21:733–749.

62. Tsujimoto M, Ueda T, Nakashima H, et al. Monophasic and biphasic synovial sarcoma: An immunohistochemical study. Acta Pathol Jpn 1987;37:597–604.

63. Miettinen M, Fanburg-Smith JC, Virolainen M, et al. Epithelioid sarcoma: An immunohistochemical analysis of 112 classical and variant cases and a discussion of the differential diagnosis. Hum Pathol 1999;30:934–942.

64. Kagami Y, Suzuki R, Taji H, et al. Nodal cytotoxic lymphoma spectrum: A clinicopathologic study of 66 patients. Am J Surg Pathol 1999;23:1184–1200.

65. Brodeur GM. Molecular pathology of human neuroblastomas. Semin Diagn Pathol 1994;11:118–125.

66. Brodeur GM. Molecular basis for heterogeneity in human neuroblastomas. Eur J Cancer 1995;4:505–510.

67. Brodeur GM, Nakagawara A, Yamashiro DJ, et al. Expression of TrkA, TrkB and TrkC in human neuroblastomas. J Neurooncol 1997;31(1–2):49–55.

68. Brodeur GM, Maris JM, Yamashiro DJ, et al. Biology and

genetics of human neuroblastomas. J Pediatr Hematol Oncol 1997;19:93–101.

69. Nakagawara A, Liu XG, Ikegaki N, et al. Cloning and chromosomal localization of the human TRK-B tyrosine kinase receptor gene (NTRK2). Genomics 1995;25:538–546.

70. Kramer K, Gerald W, LeSauteur L, et al. Monoclonal antibody to human Trk-A: Diagnostic and therapeutic potential in neuroblastoma. Eur J Cancer 1997;33:2090–2091.

71. Nakagawara A, Arima-Nakagawara M, Scavarda NJ, et al. Association between high levels of expression of the TRK gene and favorable outcome in human neuroblastoma. N Engl J Med 1993;328:847–854.

72. Kramer K, Gerald W, LeSauteur L, et al. Prognostic value of TrkA protein detection by monoclonal antibody 5C3 in neuroblastoma. Clin Cancer Res 1996;2:1361–1367.

73. Tanaka T, Hiyama E, Sugimoto T, et al. Trk A gene expression in neuroblastoma: The clinical significance of an immunohistochemical study. Cancer 1995;76:1086–1095.

74. Combaret V, Lasset C, Frappaz D, et al. Evaluation of CD44 prognostic value in neuroblastoma: Comparison with the other prognostic factors. Eur J Cancer 1995;31A:545–549.

75. Wang NP, Marx J, McNutt MA, et al. Expression of myogenic regulatory proteins (myogenin and MyoD1) in small blue round cell tumors of childhood. Am J Pathol 1995;147:1799–1810.

76. Cui S, Hano H, Harada T, et al. Evaluation of new monoclonal anti-MyoD1 and anti-myogenin antibodies for the diagnosis of rhabdomyosarcoma. Pathol Int 1999;49:62–68.

77. Dias P, Parham DM, Shapiro DN, et al. Myogenic regulatory protein (MyoD1) expression in childhood solid tumors: Diagnostic utility in rhabdomyosarcoma. Am J Pathol 1990;137:1283–1291.

78. Dias P, Parham DM, Shapiro DN, et al. Monoclonal antibodies to the myogenic regulatory protein MyoD1: Epitope mapping and diagnostic utility. Cancer Res 1992;52:6431–6439.

79. Dias P, Chen B, Dilday B, et al. Strong immunostaining for myogenin in rhabdomyosarcoma is significantly associated with tumors of the alveolar subclass. Am J Pathol 2000;156:399–408.

80. Shimada H. Tumors of the neuroblastoma group. In: Williams R, ed. Topics in Pediatric Pathology. Philadelphia: Hanley & Belfus, 1993L:43–59.

81. Joshi VV, Silverman JF. Pathology of neuroblastic tumors. Semin Diagn Pathol 1994;11:107–117.

82. Ambros IM, Ambros PF. Schwann cells in neuroblastoma. Eur J Cancer 1995;4:429–434.

83. Ambros PF, Ambros IM, Strehl S, et al. Regression and progression in neuroblastoma: Does genetics predict tumour behaviour? Eur J Cancer 1995;4:510–515.

84. Askin F. Neuroblastoma and peripheral neuroectodermal tumors: A clinicopathologic review. In: Stocker J, Askin F, eds. Pathology of Solid Tumors in Children. London: Chapman & Hall, 1998:25–50.

85. Coffin CM, Dehner LP. Peripheral neurogenic tumors of the soft tissues in children and adolescents: A clinicopathologic study of 139 cases. Pediatr Pathol 1989;9:387–407.

86. d'Amore ES, Ninfo V. Soft tissue small round cell tumors: Morphological parameters. Semin Diagn Pathol 1996;13:184–203.

87. Shimada H, Ambros IM, Dehner LP, et al. Terminology and morphologic criteria of neuroblastic tumors: Recommendations by the International Neuroblastoma Pathology Committee. Cancer 1999;86:349–363.

88. Shimada H, Ambros IM, Dehner LP, et al. The International Neuroblastoma Pathology Classification (the Shimada system). Cancer 1999;86:364–372.

89. Miettinen M, Chatten J, Paetau A, Stevenson A. Monoclonal antibody NB84 in the differential diagnosis of neuroblastoma and other small round cell tumors. Am J Surg Pathol 1998;22:327–332.

90. Layfield LJ, Glasgow BJ. Rhabdomyosarcomatous differentiation in a neuroblastoma: A potential pitfall in the cyto-

logic diagnosis of small round-cell tumors of childhood. Diagn Cytopathol 1991;7:193–197.

91. Takeda O, Homma C, Maseki N, et al. There may be two tumor suppressor genes on chromosome arm 1p closely associated with biologically distinct subtypes of neuroblastoma. Genes Chromosomes Cancer 1994;10:30–39.

92. Rubie H, Hartmann O, Michon J, et al. N-Myc gene amplification is a major prognostic factor in localized neuroblastoma: Results of the French NBL 90 study: Neuroblastoma Study Group of the Société Française d'Oncologie Pédiatrique. J Clin Oncol 1997;15:1171–1182.

93. Stock C, Ambros IM, Mann G, et al. Detection of Ip36 deletions in paraffin sections of neuroblastoma tissues. Genes Chromosomes Cancer 1993;6:1–9.

94. Pagani A, Macri L, Rosolen A, et al. Neuroendocrine differentiation in Ewing's sarcomas and primitive neuroectodermal tumors revealed by reverse transcriptase-polymerase chain reaction of chromogranin mRNA. Diagn Mol Pathol 1998;7:36–43.

95. de Alava E, Gerald WL. Molecular biology of the Ewing's sarcoma/primitive neuroectodermal tumor family. J Clin Oncol 2000;18:204.

96. Dehner LP. Neuroepithelioma (primitive neuroectodermal tumor) and Ewing's sarcoma. At least a partial consensus. [editorial; comment] Arch Pathol Lab Med 1994;118:606–607.

97. Kawauchi S, Fukuda T, Miyamoto S, et al. Peripheral primitive neuroectodermal tumor of the ovary confirmed by CD99 immunostaining, karyotypic analysis, and RT-PCR for EWS/FLI-1 chimeric mRNA. Am J Surg Pathol 1998;22:1417–1422.

98. Jurgens H, Bier V, Harms D, et al. Malignant peripheral neuroectodermal tumors: A retrospective analysis of 42 patients. Cancer 1988;61:349–357.

99. Hasegawa SL, Davison JM, Rutten A, et al. Primary cutaneous Ewing's sarcoma: Immunophenotypic and molecular cytogenetic evaluation of five cases. Am J Surg Pathol 1998;22:310–318.

100. Lawlor ER, Mathers JA, Bainbridge T, et al. Peripheral primitive neuroectodermal tumors in adults: Documentation by molecular analysis. J Clin Oncol 1998;16:1150–1157.

101. Tsokos M. Peripheral primitive neuroectodermal tumors: Diagnosis, classification, and prognosis. Perspect Pediatr Pathol 1992;16:27–98.

102. Schmidt D, Herrmann C, Jurgens H, Harms D. Malignant peripheral neuroectodermal tumor and its necessary distinction from Ewing's sarcoma: A report from the Kiel Pediatric Tumor Registry. Cancer 1991;68:2251–2259.

103. Marley EF, Liapis H, Humphrey PA, et al. Primitive neuroectodermal tumor of the kidney—another enigma: A pathologic, immunohistochemical, and molecular diagnostic study. Am J Surg Pathol 1997;21:354–359.

104. Fellinger EJ, Garin-Chesa P, Glasser DB, et al. Comparison of cell surface antigen HBA71 (p30/32MIC2), neuron-specific enolase, and vimentin in the immunohistochemical analysis of Ewing's sarcoma of bone. Am J Surg Pathol 1992;16:746–755.

105. Kushner BH, LaQuaglia MP, Cheung NK, et al. Clinically critical impact of molecular genetic studies in pediatric solid tumors. Med Pediatr Oncol 1999;33:530–535.

106. McManus AP, Gusterson BA, Pinkerton CR, Shipley JM. The molecular pathology of small round-cell tumours—relevance to diagnosis, prognosis, and classification. J Pathol 1996;178:116–121.

107. Ladanyi M, Lewis R, Garin-Chesa P, et al. EWS rearrangement in Ewing's sarcoma and peripheral neuroectodermal tumor: Molecular detection and correlation with cytogenetic analysis and MIC2 expression. Diagn Mol Pathol 1993;2:141–146.

108. Ladanyi M, Heinemann FS, Huvos AG, et al. Neural differentiation in small round cell tumors of bone and soft tissue with the translocation t(11;22)(q24;q12): An immunohistochemical study of 11 cases. Hum Pathol 1990;21:1245–1251.

109. Delattre O, Zucman J, Melot T, et al. The Ewing family of tumors—a subgroup of small-round-cell tumors defined by specific chimeric transcripts. [see comments] N Engl J Med 1994;331:294–299.

110. Variend S, Gerrard M, Norris PD, Goepel JR. Intra-abdominal neuroectodermal tumour of childhood with divergent differentiation. [see comments] Histopathology 1991;18:45–51.

111. Ordonez NG, Zirkin R, Bloom RE. Malignant small-cell epithelial tumor of the peritoneum coexpressing mesenchymal-type intermediate filaments. Am J Surg Pathol 1989;13:413–421.

112. Gerald WL, Miller HK, Battifora H, et al. Intra-abdominal desmoplastic small round-cell tumor: Report of 19 cases of a distinctive type of high-grade polyphenotypic malignancy affecting young individuals. [see comments] Am J Surg Pathol 1991;15:499–513.

113. Gonzalez-Crussi F, Crawford SE, Sun CC. Intraabdominal desmoplastic small-cell tumors with divergent differentiation: Observations on three cases of childhood. Am J Surg Pathol 1990;14:633–642.

114. Ordonez NG. Desmoplastic small round cell tumor. I: A histopathologic study of 39 cases with emphasis on unusual histological patterns. Am J Surg Pathol 1998;22:1303–1313.

115. Parkash V, Gerald WL, Parma A, et al. Desmoplastic small round cell tumor of the pleura. Am J Surg Pathol 1995;19:659–665.

116. Tison V, Cerasoli S, Morigi F, et al. Intracranial desmoplastic small-cell tumor: Report of a case. Am J Surg Pathol 1996;20:112–117.

117. Backer A, Mount SL, Zarka MA, et al. Desmoplastic small round cell tumour of unknown primary origin with lymph node and lung metastases: Histological, cytological, ultrastructural, cytogenetic and molecular findings. Virchows Arch 1998;432:135–141.

118. Ordonez NG. Desmoplastic small round cell tumor. II: An ultrastructural and immunohistochemical study with emphasis on new immunohistochemical markers. Am J Surg Pathol 1998;22:1314–1327.

119. Antonescu CR, Gerald WL, Magid MS, Ladanyi M. Molecular variants of the EWS-WT1 gene fusion in desmoplastic small round cell tumor. Diagn Mol Pathol 1998;7:24–28.

120. Barnoud R, Delattre O, Peoc'h M, et al. Desmoplastic small round cell tumor: RT-PCR analysis and immunohistochemical detection of the Wilm's tumor gene WT1. Pathol Res Pract 1998;194:693–700.

121. de Alava E, Ladanyi M, Rosai J, Gerald WL. Detection of chimeric transcripts in desmoplastic small round cell tumor and related developmental tumors by reverse transcriptase polymerase chain reaction: A specific diagnostic assay. Am J Pathol 1995;147:1584–1591.

122. Gerald WL, Rosai J, Ladanyi M. Characterization of the genomic breakpoint and chimeric transcripts in the EWS-WT1 gene fusion of desmoplastic small round cell tumor. Proc Natl Acad Sci U S A 1995;92:1028–1032.

123. Ladanyi M, Gerald WL. Specificity of the EWS/WT1 gene fusion for desmoplastic small round cell tumour. [letter] J Pathol 1996;180:462.

124. Ladanyi M, Gerald W. Fusion of the EWS and WT1 genes in the desmoplastic small round cell tumor. Cancer Res 1994;54:2837–2840.

125. Ladanyi M. The emerging molecular genetics of sarcoma translocations. Diagn Mol Pathol 1995;4:162–173.

126. Ladanyi M. Diagnosis and classification of small round-cell tumors of childhood. [letter; comment] Am J Pathol 1999;155:2181–2182.

127. Leuschner I, Radig K, Harms D. Desmoplastic small round cell tumor. Semin Diagn Pathol 1996;13:204–212.

128. O'Shea P. Myogenic tumors of soft tissue. In: Coffin C, Dehner L, O'Shea P, eds. Pediatric Soft Tissue Tumors: A Clinical, Pathologic, And Therapeutic Approach. Baltimore: Williams & Wilkins, 1997:214–253.

129. Tsokos M, Webber BL, Parham DM, et al. Rhabdomyosarcoma: A new classification scheme related to prognosis. [see comments] Arch Pathol Lab Med 1992;116:847–855.

130. Tsokos M. The diagnosis and classification of childhood rhabdomyosarcoma. Semin Diagn Pathol 1994;11:26–38.

131. Cavazzana AO, Schmidt D, Ninfo V, et al. Spindle cell rhabdomyosarcoma: A prognostically favorable variant of rhabdomyosarcoma. Am J Surg Pathol 1992;16:229–235.

132. Kraus DH, Saenz NC, Gollamudi S, et al. Pediatric rhabdomyosarcoma of the head and neck. Am J Surg 1997;174:556–560.

133. Leuschner I, Newton WA Jr, Schmidt D, et al. Spindle cell variants of embryonal rhabdomyosarcoma in the paratesticular region: A report of the Intergroup Rhabdomyosarcoma Study. [published erratum appears in Am J Surg Pathol 1993;17:858] Am J Surg Pathol 1993;17:221–230.

134. Leuschner I. Spindle cell rhabdomyosarcoma: Histologic variant of embryonal rhabdomyosarcoma with association to favorable prognosis. Curr Top Pathol 1995;89:261–272.

135. Douglass EC, Rowe ST, Valentine M, et al. Variant translocations of chromosome 13 in alveolar rhabdomyosarcoma. Genes Chromosomes Cancer 1991;3:480–482.

136. Douglass EC, Shapiro DN, Valentine M, et al. Alveolar rhabdomyosarcoma with the t(2;13): Cytogenetic findings and clinicopathologic correlations. Med Pediatr Oncol 1993;21:83–87.

137. Parham DM, Shapiro DN, Downing JR, et al. Solid alveolar rhabdomyosarcomas with the t(2;13): Report of two cases with diagnostic implications. Am J Surg Pathol 1994;18:474–478.

138. Harms D. Alveolar rhabdomyosarcoma: A prognostically unfavorable rhabdomyosarcoma type and its necessary distinction from embryonal rhabdomyosarcoma. Curr Top Pathol 1995;89:273–296.

139. Biegel JA, Meek RS, Parmiter AH, et al. Chromosomal translocation t(1;13)(p36;q14) in a case of rhabdomyosarcoma. Genes Chromosomes Cancer 1991;3:483–484.

140. Douglass EC, Valentine M, Etcubanas E, et al. A specific chromosomal abnormality in rhabdomyosarcoma. [published erratum appears in Cytogenet Cell Genet 1988;47(4): following 232] Cytogenet Cell Genet 1987;45(3–4):148–155.

141. Valentine M, Douglass EC, Look AT. Closely linked loci on the long arm of chromosome 13 flank a specific 2;13 translocation breakpoint in childhood rhabdomyosarcoma. Cytogenet Cell Genet 1989;52(3–4):128–132.

142. Dominey A, Paller AS, Gonzalez-Crussi F. Congenital rhabdoid sarcoma with cutaneous metastases. J Am Acad Dermatol 1990;22(5 Pt 2):969–974.

143. Versteege I, Sevenet N, Lange J, et al. Truncating mutations of hSNF5/INI1 in aggressive paediatric cancer. Nature 1998;394:203–206.

144. Simons J, Teshima I, Zielenska M, et al. Analysis of chromosome 22q as an aid to the diagnosis of rhabdoid tumor: A case report. Am J Surg Pathol 1999;23:982–988.

145. Sevenet N, Lellouch-Tubiana A, Schofield D, et al. Spectrum of hSNF5/INI1 somatic mutations in human cancer and genotype-phenotype correlations. Hum Mol Genet 1999;8:2359–2368.

146. Sevenet N, Sheridan E, Amram D, et al. Constitutional mutations of the hSNF5/INI1 gene predispose to a variety of cancers. Am J Hum Genet 1999;65:1342–1348.

147. Rousseau-Merck MF, Versteege I, Legrand I, et al. hSNF5/INI1 inactivation is mainly associated with homozygous deletions and mitotic recombinations in rhabdoid tumors. Cancer Res 1999;59:3152–3156.

148. Beckwith B. Renal tumors. In: Stocker J, Askin F, eds. Pathology of Solid Tumors in Children. London: Chapman & Hall, 1998:1–23.

149. Folpe AL, Patterson K, Gown AM. Antibodies to desmin identify the blastemal component of nephroblastoma. Mod Pathol 1997;10:895–900.

150. Argani P, Askin FB, Colombani P, Perlman EJ. Occult pulmonary synovial sarcoma confirmed by molecular techniques. Pediatr Dev Pathol 2000;3:87–90.

151. Miser J, Triche T, Kinsella T, Pritchard D. Other soft tissue sarcomas of childhood. In: Pizzo P, Poplack D, eds. Principles and Practices of Pediatric Oncology. 3rd ed. Philadelphia: Lippincott-Raven, 1997:878–879.

152. Pai S, Chinoy RF, Pradhan SA, et al. Head and neck synovial sarcomas. J Surg Oncol 1993;54:82–86.

153. Casselman FP, Gillinov AM, Kasirajan V, et al. Primary synovial sarcoma of the left heart. Ann Thorac Surg 1999; 68:2329–2331.

154. Keel SB, Bacha E, Mark EJ, et al. Primary pulmonary sarcoma: A clinicopathologic study of 26 cases. Mod Pathol 1999;12:1124–1131.

155. Gaertner E, Zeren EH, Fleming MV, et al. Biphasic synovial sarcomas arising in the pleural cavity: A clinicopathologic study of five cases. Am J Surg Pathol 1996;20: 36–45.

156. Zeren H, Moran CA, Suster S, et al. Primary pulmonary sarcomas with features of monophasic synovial sarcoma: A clinicopathological, immunohistochemical, and ultrastructural study of 25 cases. Hum Pathol 1995;26:474–480.

157. Nicholson AG, Goldstraw P, Fisher C. Synovial sarcoma of the pleura and its differentiation from other primary pleural tumours: A clinicopathological and immunohistochemical review of three cases. Histopathology 1998;33:508–513.

158. Fritsch M, Epstein JI, Perlman EJ, et al. Molecularly confirmed primary prostatic synovial sarcoma. Hum Pathol 2000;31:246–250.

159. Fisher C. Synovial sarcoma. Ann Diagn Pathol 1998;2:401–421.

160. Fisher C. Synovial sarcoma: Ultrastructural and immunohistochemical features of epithelial differentiation in monophasic and biphasic tumors. Hum Pathol 1986;17:996–1008.

161. Fligman I, Lonardo F, Jhanwar SC, et al. Molecular diagnosis of synovial sarcoma and characterization of a variant SYT-SSX2 fusion transcript. Am J Pathol 1995;147:1592–1599.

162. Argani P, Zakowski MF, Klimstra DS, et al. Detection of the SYT-SSX chimeric RNA of synovial sarcoma in paraffin-embedded tissue and its application in problematic cases. [published erratum appears in Mod Pathol 1998;11: 592] Mod Pathol 1998;11:65–71.

163. Hiraga H, Nojima T, Abe S, et al. Diagnosis of synovial sarcoma with the reverse transcriptase-polymerase chain reaction: Analyses of 84 soft tissue and bone tumors. Diagn Mol Pathol 1998;7:102–110.

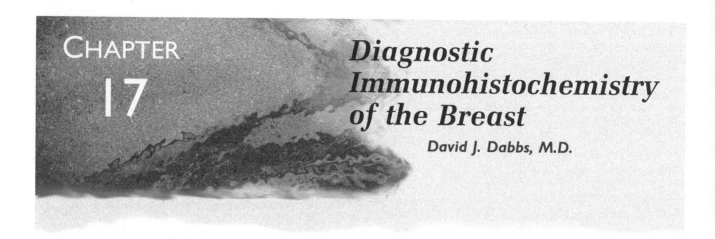

CHAPTER 17

Diagnostic Immunohistochemistry of the Breast

David J. Dabbs, M.D.

IMMUNOHISTOCHEMISTRY IN THE DIFFERENTIAL DIAGNOSIS OF EPITHELIAL LESIONS

Myoepithelial Cells

Epithelial lesions of the breast are not only the most frequent lesions encountered by the surgical pathologist but also the largest source of anguish in the differential diagnosis of benign versus malignant lesions. Some of the sources of angst for the surgical pathologist are severalfold:[1, 2]

- Distinguishing benign non-neoplastic proliferative lesions from malignant conditions, such as the various forms of adenosis
- Distinguishing in situ carcinoma from invasive malignancy
- Distinguishing pseudoinvasive lesions from invasive malignancies, such as in situ carcinoma involving various forms of adenosis
- Distinguishing neoplastic proliferative lesions from in situ or invasive carcinoma, such as radial scar, atypical ductal hyperplasia, and tubular carcinoma (TC)
- Distinguishing atypical papilloma from papillary carcinoma in situ
- Determining microinvasion (MIC) in intraductal carcinoma

In all these diagnostic situations, it is the presence of the myoepithelial cell (MEC) in intimate relationship with the epithelial cells of the lesion that determines the difference between in situ and invasive disease and between benign pseudoinvasive lesions and invasive carcinoma. Microglandular adenosis, a distinct nonorganoid benign form of adenosis, is the only known exception to this statement (see further on).

The presence of MECs that envelop ductal-lobular epithelium, situated on the epithelial basal lamina, has always been considered to be the important criterion that separates invasive from noninvasive neoplasms.[3–8]

Myoepithelial cells can be visualized rather easily in normal breast ductules and acini, but when these structures dilate and fill with proliferating cells, or are compressed, it is virtually impossible to visualize them. In recent years, there have been claims that several antibodies are able to identify MECs, including antibodies to S-100 protein, cytokeratins, smooth muscle actins, muscle-specific actins, calponin, and smooth muscle myosin heavy chain (SMMHC).

Antibodies to S-100 protein are not sensitive or specific for MEC and decorate MEC in an erratic manner.[9–13] Cytokeratin cocktail antibodies, in addition to CK14 and CK17 identify MEC,[14, 15] but they also immunostain acinar cells, which makes it difficult to differentiate MECs because of their proximity to the acinar cells. Anti–smooth muscle actins react with stromal myofibroblasts in addition to MECs[16–20] and thus are not specific for MECs. The cross-reaction with myofibroblasts makes it difficult to identify MECs specifically, especially in ductal carcinoma in situ (DCIS), in which there may be periductal stromal desmoplasia.

Nayar and associates and Bose and colleagues found that although anti–smooth muscle actin (DAKO, Carpinteria, CA) and muscle-specific actin HHF-35 (Enzo, Farmingdale, NY) decorated MECs in the majority of benign breast lesions, occasional benign lesions were negative for these antibodies, and there was a substantial cross-reaction with stromal myofibroblasts, especially with anti–smooth muscle actin, with up to 36% of cases showing ductal cell decoration with HHF-35 (Table 17–1).[13, 21]

Wang and coworkers surveyed antibodies to calponin and SMMHC in a variety of benign lesions and carcinomas of the breast.[22]

SMMHC is a structural component (200 kd) unique to smooth muscle cells, which functions within the hexagonal array of the thick-thin filament contractile apparatus.[23]

Calponin, a 34-kd polypeptide, modulates actomyosin adenosine triphosphatase (ATPase) activity in the smooth muscle contractile apparatus and is unique to smooth muscle.[24, 25]

In their analysis of 70 carcinomas and a variety of benign sclerosing and papillary lesions, Wang

Table 17–1. Immunostaining of Tumor Cells in Breast Carcinoma[13]		
S-100 Protein (%)	HHF-35 (%)	Smooth Muscle Actin (%)
46	62	12

and colleagues found that (1) calponin and SMMHC always detected MEC in the benign lesions and (2) compared with smooth muscle actin antibody 1A4, calponin and SMMHC rarely reacted with desmoplastic stromal myofibroblasts, allowing for a more decisive interpretation of the lesion.[22] There was no immunostaining of tumor cells.

My experience has been similar with calponin and SMMHC (Figs. 17–1 to 17–6). Benign proliferative or sclerosing lesions of the breast invariably demonstrate crisp immunostaining for MECs with little or no immunostaining of stromal myofibroblasts, enabling the pathologist to distinguish decisively the following conditions from invasive carcinoma: ductal or lobular in situ carcinoma, even in the presence of periductal stromal desmoplasia or heavy lymphoid infiltrates; sclerosing adenosis (SA) (with or without DCIS involvement); cancerization of lobules; radial scars with stromal elastosis-desmoplasia; TC;

and intracystic papillary carcinoma. My colleagues and I have also demonstrated the utility of these antibodies to define invasive carcinoma with core needle biopsies of the breast in problem cases in which the diagnosis of invasive carcinoma is difficult to make.[26] In core biopsies of the breast, calponin and SMMHC can help discriminate invasion from DCIS when lesions are low grade and lobular in configuration, are heavily infiltrated by lymphoid aggregates or cancerizing lobules, or have an abundant pericellular desmoplastic stromal response that simulates jagged stromal infiltration.[26]

Immunohistochemistry is useful to help discriminate the three dominant benign lesions of the breast—SA, microglandular adenosis (MGA), and TC (Table 17–2; Figs. 17–7 to 17–10), but a detailed morphologic study of the lesion is essential.[27]

The MECs are seen by immunohistochemistry (IHC) in all forms of adenosis except the microglandular form, the only benign lesion that is known not to contain MECs.[28] In addition to the distinct nonorganoid morphology of MGA, tubular adenosis, described by Lee and colleagues, may mimic both MGA and carcinoma but differs from MGA by containing MECs.[29] Microglandular adenosis is positive with S-100 protein, whereas SA and TC are S-100−.

It is not uncommon for apocrine change,[28] or in

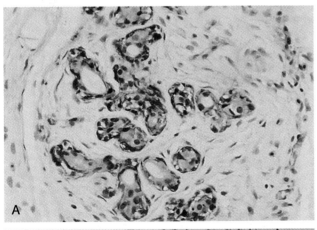

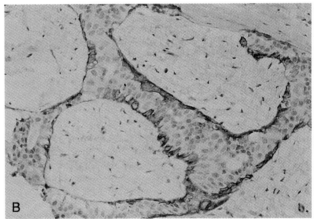

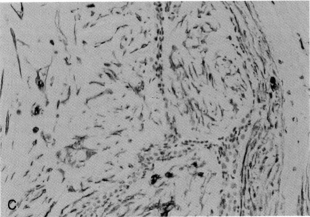

Figure 17–1. Smooth muscle myosin heavy chain (SMMHC) decorates the myoepithelial cells (MEC) of a breast lobule (*A*) and identifies the MEC in a fibroadenoma (*B*), whereas vimentin immunostains the stromal cells of a fibroadenoma (*C*).

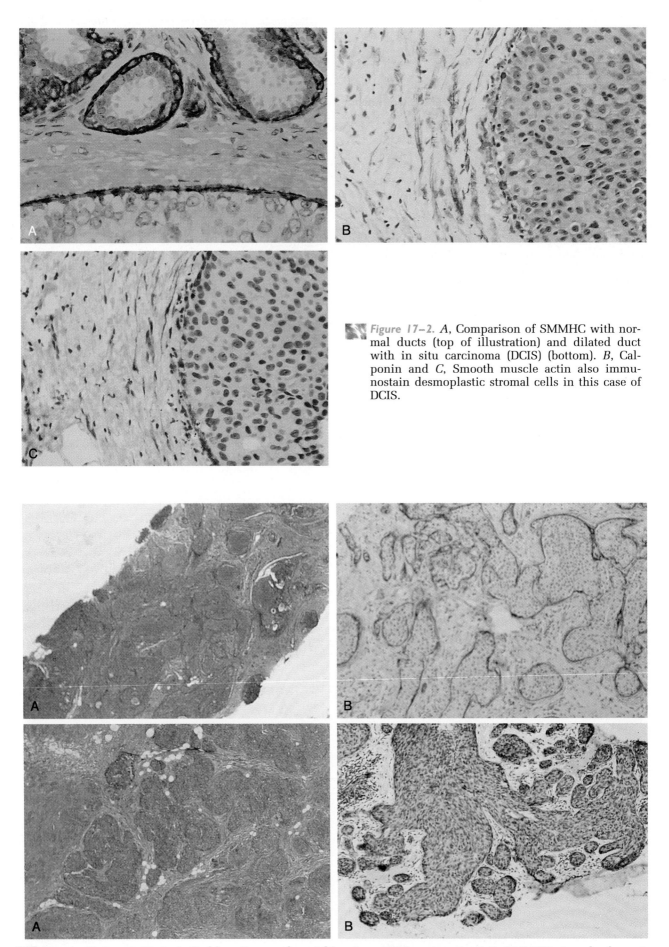

Figure 17–2. A, Comparison of SMMHC with normal ducts (top of illustration) and dilated duct with in situ carcinoma (DCIS) (bottom). B, Calponin and C, Smooth muscle actin also immunostain desmoplastic stromal cells in this case of DCIS.

Figures 17–3 and 17–4. A, Problematic core breast biopsies—DCIS or invasion? B, SMMHC strongly decorates MEC along tongues of neoplastic cords in both cases, clearly indicative of DCIS.

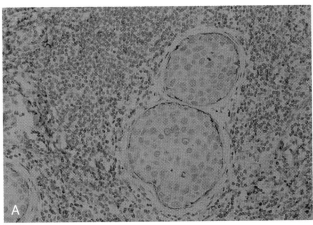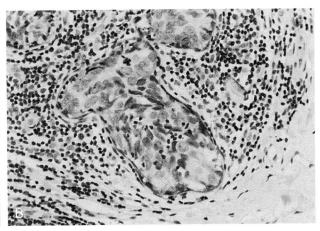

Figure 17–5. *A* and *B*, These cases of DCIS are heavily obscured with lymphocytes, yet clearly reflect the presence of MEC with SMMHC.

situ carcinoma, to involve adenosis[30, 31] and as stated, the identification of MECs effectively rules out an invasive process.

The MEC is also characteristically prominent in papillomas of the breast, and antibodies to MECs can help discriminate papillomas from intraductal papillary carcinoma in difficult cases,[32] because pure papillary carcinoma lacks the MEC and is not demonstrable with MEC antibodies.[12, 33] Some papillomas show the features of an "atypical papilloma," areas in which there is atypical ductal hyperplasia that overgrows the papilloma.[34] These atypical areas lack MECs by immunoperoxidase examination.[35]

Type IV collagen is an integral component of the basal lamina (BL) that envelops normal and proliferative benign cells,[36] but it appears to be less useful to discriminate for invasive carcinoma.[20, 37] Type IV collagen may be detected in the majority of benign conditions but is discontinuous and erratically detected in practice, especially in DCIS and radial scars.[21] In most instances, discontinuous type IV collagen is not synonymous with microscopic invasion.

The MEC also is an intimate partner with the neoplastic proliferation of epithelial cells seen in adenoid cystic carcinoma (ACC) (Fig. 17–6 *C* and *D*). In ACC, the MEC are seen within the arches of the pseudocribriform architecture, whereas in cribriform DCIS, the MEC are confined to the duct periphery. In adenomyoepitheliomas, MEC proliferate in a haphazard fashion, mostly as stromal cells within the stroma, or admixed with the epithelial proliferation.

MYOEPITHELIAL CELL TUMORS VERSUS PRIMARY SARCOMAS

Tumors of the breast in which MECs predominate include adenomyoepithelioma and myoepithelial cell carcinoma (MECC).[38–41] Although the majority of adenomyoepitheliomas are benign, occasional tumors may exhibit aggressive behavior in the form of carcinoma or myoepithelial carcinoma.[42–45]

The typical immunostaining pattern of the myoepithelial components of these tumors is strong cytoplasmic staining for simple keratins (CAM5.2) and broad spectrum cocktails such as AE1/AE3. Tumor cells are typically positive with S-100 protein and muscle markers such as SMMHC, calponin, muscle-specific actin, and alpha-smooth muscle actin.[39, 41] Occasional cells exhibit immunostaining with glial fibrillary acidic protein (GFAP).[39, 41] This combination of smooth muscle and keratin markers distinguishes the myoepithelial tumors from sarcomatoid carcinomas, which typically coexpress only keratin and vimentin. Malignant myoepithelial tumors may also show divergent heterologous differentiation.[38]

Myoepithelial tumors and sarcomatoid carcinomas need to be separated from the rare primary spindle cell sarcoma of the breast, which may include fibrosarcoma (vimentin-positive) leiomyosarcoma and rhabdomyosarcoma (positive with muscle markers), synovial sarcoma (positive with CK7 and CK19),[46] malignant nerve sheath tumors (S-100+ and vimentin-positive) and malignant fibrous histiocytomas (vimentin-positive). Although each of these tumors may have characteristic light microscopic features, immunostaining patterns may be useful in the diagnostic distinction (Table 17–3).

The rare myofibroblastoma of the breast is distinguished immunohistochemically from myoepithelial tumors by lack of immunostaining for keratins, S-100 protein, and SMMHC.[47–49] The myofibroblastoma may also demonstrate CD34+ cells (Fig. 17–11).[50]

MICROINVASIVE CARCINOMA OF THE BREAST

The concept of MIC in breast carcinoma evolved in the context of early microscopic invasion arising from intraductal carcinomas, most of which were of the high-grade (comedo) type.[51, 52]

Early ultrastructural studies on MIC demon-

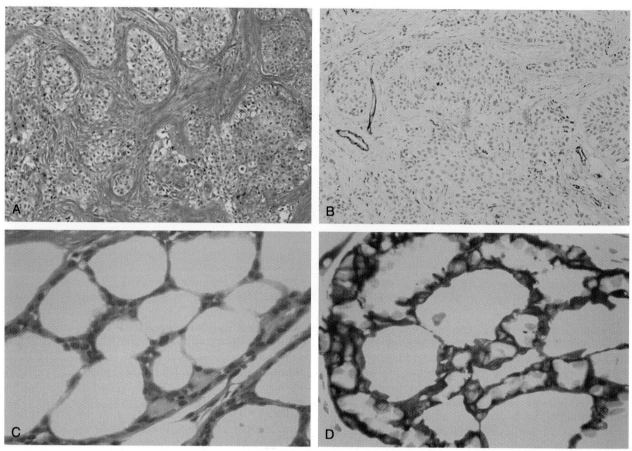

Figure 17–6. A, This infiltrative-appearing breast core biopsy is clearly invasive carcinoma, as seen in *B* with complete lack of SMMHC. A blood vessel serves as positive internal control. Histologic section of adenoid cystic carcinoma (*C*), showing intimate MEC relation with epithelial cells (*D*) with smooth muscle myosin heavy chain (SMMHC).

strated tumor cells protruding through gaps in BL and discontinuities of MECs, but these changes were not synonymous with invasion at the level of the light microscope.[53] Indeed, there have been a variety of definitions of microinvasive carcinoma over the years, with no clear consensus on the definition.[51, 52, 54–59]

Rosen prefers to use the term *microinvasive car-*

Table 17–2. Differential Diagnosis: Tubular Carcinoma, Microglandular Adenosis, Tubular Adenosis, Sclerosing Adenosis

	Histology	Myoepithelial Cells	S-100 Protein	Type IV Collagen
Tubular carcinoma	Random invasion, fat invasion Tear-drop–shaped open tubules Apical snouts Stromal desmoplasia	No	No	No
Microglandular adenosis	Random nonorganoid pattern Round, open tubules No fat invasion No stromal desmoplasia	No	Yes	Yes
Tubular adenosis	Vague lobular pattern possible Elongated, narrow branching tubules Luminal secretion Fat infiltration possible Stromal sclerosis Apocrine change or DCIS can involve it	Yes	No	No
Sclerosing adenosis	Lobular pattern Often compressed, no glandular lumina Stromal sclerosis Apocrine change or DCIS can involve it	Yes	No	No

DCIS, ductal carcinoma in situ.

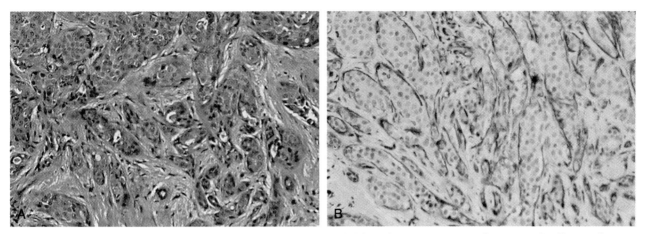

Figure 17–7. Sclerosing adenosis may simulate carcinoma (*A*) but demonstrates envelopment of cell nests by MEC with SMMHC immunostaining (*B*).

cinoma for tumors with no single invasive focus of "1.0 mm or greater in diameter."[60] Crucial in this definition is that the invasive focus consists of a jagged infiltrative nest with stromal-lymphocytic response or single infiltrative cells (Fig. 17–12). It is only with these morphologic features that MEC antibodies may be useful in confirming the suspi-

cions of invasion. The latter is necessary because of the vagaries of tangential sectioning of lobules involved by DCIS.

Prasad and associates used the technique of simultaneous immunostaining for smooth muscle actin and cytokeratin to confirm microinvasive breast carcinoma.[61]

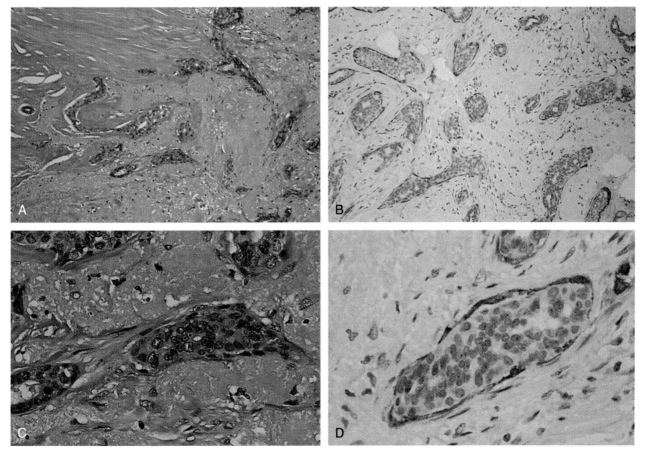

Figure 17–8. Simulating cancer, this case of radial scar shows prominent elastosis (*A* and *C*), but strong SMMHC decoration of MEC is seen, indicative of a benign process (*B* and *D*).

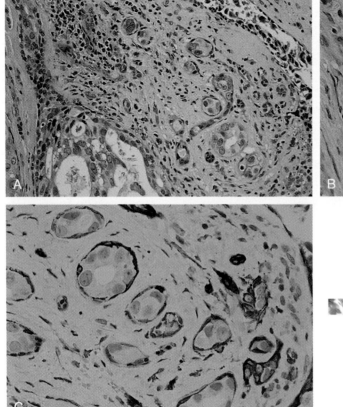

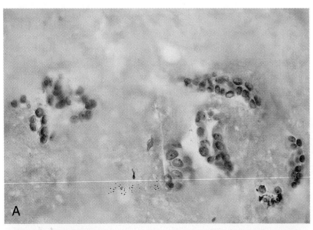

Figure 17-9. A and B, Carcinoma in situ involving sclerosing adenosis is always frightful to look at, but the diagnosis is confirmed (C) with SMMHC documenting the presence of MEC.

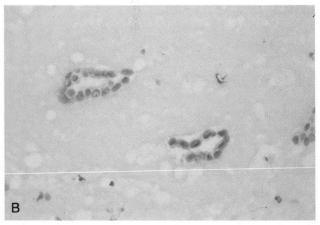

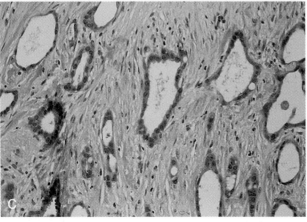

Figure 17-10. A, Cell block of breast aspirate showing abnormal tubules. B, No smooth muscle myosin heavy chain (SMMHC) immunostaining, consistent with tubular carcinoma, which is confirmed in tissue excision specimen (C).

Table 17–3. Myoepithelial Tumors Versus Spindle Cell Sarcomas of the Breast

	CK14	CK7	CK19	Glial Fibrillary Acidic Protein	S-100 Protein	HHF-35
Myoepithelial carcinoma	+	+	N	+/−	+	+
Sarcomatoid carcinoma	N	−/+	N	N	N	N
Fibrosarcoma	N	N	N	N	N	N
Leiomyosarcoma, rhabdomyosarcoma	N	N	R-N	N	N	+
Nerve sheath sarcoma	N	N	N	N	−/+	N
Synovial sarcoma	N	+	+	N	R-N	N
Malignant fibrous histiocytoma	N	N	N	N	N	N

Key +, almost always positive; +/−, most cases are positive; −/+, most cases are negative; R, rare; N, negative.

KEY DIAGNOSTIC POINTS: MYOEPITHELIAL CELL ANTIBODIES

- The presence of MEC enveloping proliferating-sclerosing breast lesions is indicative of a benign or noninvasive process.
- MECs are uniformly present in breast papillomas and may progressively disappear with carcinomatous architecture or overgrowth of atypical ductal hyperplasia.
- SMMHC and calponin antibodies are the cleanest discriminators for the presence of MEC, especially in desmoplastic-sclerotic proliferations.
- Muscle-specific actin (HHF-35), followed by smooth muscle actin, is useful to detect MECs and has lesser sensitivity and specificity (versus positive immunostaining of desmoplastic myofibroblasts).
- Intraductal carcinoma rarely lacks MECs, especially when using SMMHC and calponin antibodies.
- MEC antibodies may be confirmatory for diagnosing microinvasive carcinoma provided that the lesion is no greater than 1 mm and has jagged invasive configuration, stromal response, single invasive cells, or a combination of the three.
- **Tubular Carcinoma:** SMMHC(−), type IV collagen(−), S-100(−)

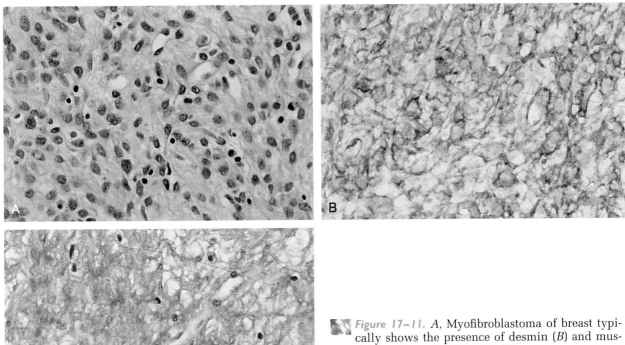

Figure 17–11. A, Myofibroblastoma of breast typically shows the presence of desmin (*B*) and muscle-specific actin (HHF-35) (*C*).

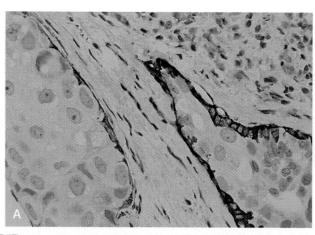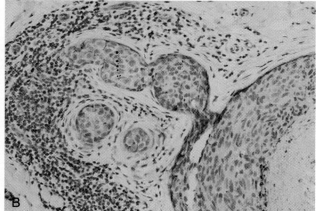

Figure 17–12. A and *B,* The differential diagnosis in these jagged foci includes invasive carcinoma; the presence of myoepithelial cells (MECs) with SMMHC staining rules out invasive carcinoma.

- **Tubular Adenosis:** SMMHC+, type IV collagen–positive, S-100(−)
- **Microglandular Adenosis:** SMMHC(−), type IV collagen(−), S-100+
- **Sclerosing Adenosis:** SMMHC+, type IV collagen–positive, S-100(−)

PROLIFERATIVE DUCTAL LESIONS AND DUCTAL CARCINOMA IN SITU

Immunohistochemical studies of ductal hyperplasia, atypical hyperplasia, and duct carcinoma in situ have revealed some interesting biologic differences in expression of a variety of cell components.

Differences in cytokeratin expression have been described between hyperplasia and duct carcinoma in situ.[17, 62–65] The antibody 34βE12 recognizes CK1, CK5, CK10, and CK14, and these keratins are typically found in duct-derived epithelium and squamous epithelium. Normal breast MECs and luminal cells express 34βE12, as does proliferative duct epithelium and, to a lesser extent, atypical ductal hyperplasia. DCIS is largely negative for 34βE12 (Figs. 17–13 and 17–14) but may show some positive cells.[62, 63, 65] Most DCIS is uniformly positive for CAM5.2, reflecting a shift away from high molecular weight keratins. The 34βE12 immunostaining profile for DCIS and atypical ductal hyperplasia (ADH) is very similar and cannot be used to distinguish DCIS from ADH[65] but can be an aid to histomorphology in separating DCIS from florid hyperplasia in difficult cases.[65]

KEY DIAGNOSTIC POINTS: 34βE12 AND DUCTAL CARCINOMA IN SITU VERSUS ATYPICAL DUCTAL HYPERPLASIA

- Cytokeratin antibody 34βE12 routinely decorates florid ductal hyperplasia of breast intensely.

- DCIS of all types is largely negative with 34βE12 but may show rare immunostaining.
- In conjunction with histomorphology, 34βE12 may help distinguish DCIS from florid hyperplasia.

PAGET'S DISEASE OF THE BREAST

Paget's disease occurs as a mammary form and extramammary (EM) form. Paget's disease of the breast is almost always indicative of an underlying breast carcinoma, which may be in situ or invasive,[66–68] whereas EM Paget's disease may be an indicator of metastatic carcinoma.

Paget's disease of the breast is manifested as CK7+ malignant cells infiltrating the epidermis of the nipple. Tumor cells are conspicuous by their infiltrative "shotgun" pattern, large size, abundant cytoplasm, signet ring forms, and, sometimes, mucin positivity. Epidermal keratinocytes are negative with CK7. Most Paget's cases are CK7+, gross cystic disease fluid protein-15 (GCDFP-15+), and polyclonal carcinoembryonic antigen (pCEA)+, which is characteristic of breast, but occasional cases may be CK7−. The monoclonal antibody clone CEAD-14 is largely negative in Paget's cells, as it is for ductal cancers in general. Toker cells are CK7+ and may be present in the skin of the normal nipple, but generally they are inconspicuous compared with Paget's cells[69] and do not cause diagnostic problems.

In cases of florid papillomatosis of the nipple, some CK7+ cells may be found in the epidermis, a pitfall to be aware of in diagnosing Paget's disease of the nipple.[70]

Malignant melanoma is distinguished by the lack of any type of keratin staining and presence of HMB-45 positivity, but it should be noted that malignant melanoma on the nipple is extraordinarily rare.

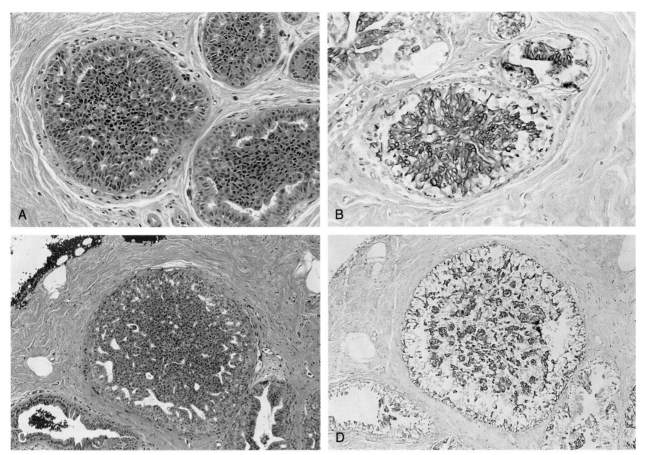

Figure 17–13. These cases of florid duct hyperplasia (*A* and *C*) are typically strongly positive for keratin 903 (34βE12) (*B* and *D*).

The Paget's cells may be assessed for estrogen receptor[71] or the neu-oncoprotein.[72]

KEY DIAGNOSTIC POINTS OF MAMMARY PAGET'S DISEASE

- CK7+, GCDFP-15+, pCEA+, CEAD-14 (rare to negative)
- Pitfall: CK7+ cells in the epidermis in cases of florid nipple duct papillomatosis

MICROMETASTATIC DISEASE IN AXILLARY LYMPH NODES

The excision of sentinel axillary lymph nodes (SLNs) is the newest investigative tool to promise new directions in the treatment of breast cancer patients.

Historically, complete axillary cleanouts have been performed with lumpectomy or mastectomy specimens primarily for staging purposes, providing information that is used to determine adjuvant

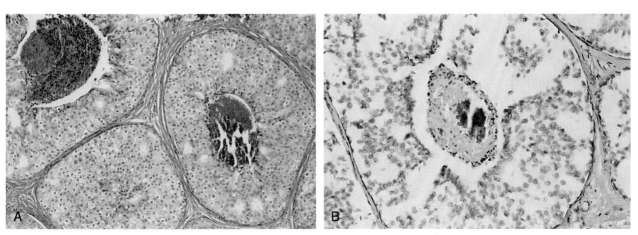

Figure 17–14. Ductal carcinoma in situ (*A*) is usually negative with keratin 903 (*B*).

chemotherapy. The complete axillary lymph node dissection (ALND) does not change the course of the disease, although with removal of involved axillary nodes, the control of local recurrence in the axilla is easier. The morbidity associated with this procedure is substantial in terms of limitation of arm motion, arm pain, and chronic lymphedema.

The concept of an SLN was spawned by Cabanas[73] in his study of penile carcinoma.

The pioneering studies of sentinel lymph node metastasis (SLNM) originated with the study of melanoma patients; the goal was to spare these patients the morbidity of large regional lymph node dissections. Patients with melanomas who had SLN surgery were found to have a relatively orderly progression of lymph node metastases, with the sentinel lymph node receiving the initial deposits of metastatic cells, followed by metastases in more distal lymph node groups.[74]

The same rationale is now being used for breast cancer patients. The SLN is identified by injecting a radioisotope and blue dye before planned surgical excision. The SLN, identified by a combination of visual inspection for blue dye and intraoperative scanning for radioactivity, is harvested and submitted for pathologic study. The rationale is that for patients who are SLN-negative, a further morbid procedure of axillary cleanout is unnecessary, but for SLN-positive patients, an axillary cleanout is indicated to provide better control for possible local recurrence. The controversy in this approach arises from several valid questions:

1. What is the natural history of micrometastatic (MM) disease in the axilla?
2. Is MM SLN disease an obligate pathway to clinically manifested local recurrence in the axilla?
3. Is MM SLN disease an indication for adjuvant chemotherapy?
4. How should the excised SLN be examined pathologically?
5. Does MM SLN disease affect overall survival?
6. What are the biologic parameters of MM disease that can predict the behavior of the disease in an individual patient?

These are interesting and provocative questions for the care of the breast cancer patient. The American Joint Commission on Cancer defines micrometastasis as a cluster of cells that are no larger than 2 mm. Recent studies with more than 10 years of follow-up conclude that micrometastases are associated with a small but statistically significant decrease in tumor-free survival and overall survival when compared with truly node-negative cases,[75] but they are not an independent prognostic factor.[76] The size of the metastatic deposit, taken together with tumor size and other factors, may additionally stratify patients at risk for further disease.[77]

Currently, lumpectomy or mastectomy followed by complete ALND is the standard of care,[78] and SLN is still considered an investigative tool until more of the preceding questions can be answered.

For the surgical pathologist, the appropriate triage and examination of the SLN is of utmost importance, but even here some controversy exists.

Current standards for lymph node handling[79] call for gross-serial 2-mm sectioning of the lymph node with two hematoxylin and eosin (H&E)-stained sections and one section immunostained with keratin. Although this technique is performed in most laboratories, exhaustive sectioning of the entire SLN has demonstrated a dramatic increase in micrometastasis detection, with as many as 46% of patients with T1 lesions having MM SLN disease.[80, 81] Using this procedure, Dowlatshahi and colleagues[81] sectioned the SLN at 2-mm intervals perpendicular to the long axis, examined an H&E-stained segment, then sectioned through the block, examining H&E-stained and keratin-immunostained segments at 0.25-mm intervals. Examining the lymph node at levels of 0.25 mm appears to be practical and should detect all micrometastases present that are 0.25 mm.[82]

Currently, there is no consensus as to the "appropriate" way to process and examine an SLN. The data do seem to suggest, however, that exhaustive, complete examination of an SLN would be the most efficient and efficacious way of serving the patient.

Cytokeratin immunostaining of SLNs should involve the use of the AE1/AE3 cocktail; CAM5.2 is less desirable because of the manner in which it decorates dendritic cells in the lymph node.[82a] Other keratin cocktails also work well.[83] Micrometastatic cells occur in small clusters less than 2 mm in diameter within the lymph node or subcapsular sinus (Fig. 17–15), and they need to be distinguished from the dendritic appearance of the interstitial reticulum cells of the lymph node, which are also keratin-positive.[84, 85] Studies with larger numbers of patients are needed to discern if the site of lymph node micrometastasis (peripheral sinus versus parenchyma of lymph node) is clinically significant.

Aggregates of breast epithelial cells in the subcapsular sinus of axillary lymph nodes have been described by Carter and associates[86] as occurring as a result of "mechanical transport" after a breast biopsy. The key histologic feature to recognize to make this diagnosis is the association of these cells with altered red blood cells and hemosiderin macrophages.

KEY DIAGNOSTIC POINTS: SENTINEL LYMPH NODE MICROMETASTATIC DISEASE

- Section lymph node at 2-mm intervals, examine with H&E and antibodies to CK8 and CK18.
- There is a trend toward examining the entire lymph node at 0.25-mm intervals with keratin.
- The SLN procedure is still investigative but will probably be adapted in some form as the

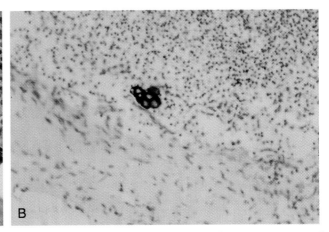

Figure 17-15. Atypical cell in subcapsular lymph node sinus (*A*) is keratin-positive (*B*), which is consistent with micrometastatic disease.

standard of care in the future to reduce cost and patient morbidity while enhancing patient outcomes.

SYSTEMIC METASTASIS OF BREAST CARCINOMA

Gross Cystic Disease Fluid Protein

Originally described by Pearlman and colleagues[87] and Haagensen and associates,[88] the prolactin-inducing protein identified by Murphy and coworkers[89] has the same amino acid sequence as gross cystic disease fluid protein fraction-15 (GCDFP-15) and is found in abundance in breast cystic fluid and any cell type that has apocrine features.[90-92] The latter, in addition to breast, includes acinar structures in salivary glands, apocrine glands, and sweat glands, and in Paget's disease of skin, vulva, and prostate.[93-97]

Homologous-appearing carcinomas of the breast, skin adnexa, and salivary glands demonstrate a great deal of overlap immunostaining with GCDFP-15.[98] Aside from these immunoreactivities, most other carcinomas show no appreciable immunostaining.[93] Breast carcinoma metastatic to the skin (or locally recurrent) may be difficult to distinguish from skin adnexal tumors.[99] Wick and associates, in a study of the overlapping morphologic features of breast, salivary gland, and skin adnexal tumors, found that GCDFP-15 was infrequently found in eccrine sweat gland carcinomas, a paucity of CEA was found in breast carcinomas, and estrogen receptors were largely absent in salivary duct carcinomas.[98]

The positive predictive value and specificity for detection of breast carcinoma with GCDFP-15 are both 99%.[93] The sensitivity for the monoclonal antibody clone D6 (Cambridge Research Laboratories, Cambridge, MA) has been reported to be as high as 74%,[93] but the experience of others has been closer to 50%.[100]

Since the specificity of GCDFP antibodies for breast carcinoma is so high, this antibody is often used in a screening panel in the appropriate clinical situation, which often turns out to be the presentation of a woman with metastasis of unknown primary or a new lung mass in a patient with a history of breast cancer. Others have demonstrated the utility and specificity of GCDFP-15 antibodies in the distinction of breast carcinoma metastatic in the lung.[101, 102]

Fiel and colleagues, in a study of the utility of GCDFP-15 on cytologic specimens, found positive immunostaining for 56.5% of recurrent or metastatic breast carcinoma and observed that GCDFP-15 must be performed on formalin-fixed or Bouin's solution–fixed slides because alcohol fixation nullifies the antibody to GCDFP-15.[103]

Carcinoembryonic Antigen

CEA is a 180-kd glycoprotein that is 50% carbohydrate.[104] There are many CEA antibodies available to a variety of CEA epitopes. The polyclonal antibodies commonly cross-react with tissue-nonspecific cross-reacting antigen and biliary glycoprotein I.[105, 106] This older CD66e series of CEA antibodies typically reacts strongly and diffusely with ductal carcinomas of the breast in addition to lung and colorectal carcinomas. However, the CEAD-14 clone (Enteric Products, Stoney Brook, NY)[107, 108] reacts with only a small subset of carcinomas of the breast (mostly high grade), which is a very useful diagnostic point of distinction for breast carcinomas[109] that are metastatic to lung, liver, lymph node, or brain. Breast carcinomas are rarely (13% of cases) positive with CEAD-14, and when they are, the positivity is usually focal, but it may be diffuse in a high-grade carcinoma.[109] A new lung mass in a breast cancer patient whose tumor is CEAD-14− is strong evidence against a lung primary,[109] and this result can be confirmed by the use of nuclear staining for thyroid transcription factor-1 (TTF-1), which is positive in lung carcinoma.[110]

Cytokeratins and Cadherins

The vast majority of ductal and lobular breast carcinomas express CK7 but may demonstrate few positive cells with CK20.[111] Cytokeratins are of little use for distinguishing breast carcinoma from other carcinomas because of the large number of carcinomas that are positive for CK7. However, a carcinoma that is strongly and diffusely positive for CK20 is solid evidence against a breast carcinoma, as most carcinomas with this profile are derived from the gastrointestinal tract.[112]

CK19 was initially believed to be absent in medullary breast carcinomas, a feature that was to distinguish medullary and poorly differentiated ductal carcinomas.[113] Subsequent studies showed great overlap, however, with Jensen and colleagues and Dalal and coworkers concluding that CK19 was present in both medullary and poorly differentiated ductal carcinomas.[114, 115]

Lehr and colleagues[115a] have described the usefulness of CK8, detected with CAM5.2, to distinguish ductal from lobular carcinoma. The pattern of CK8 immunostaining for ductal carcinoma is a peripheral cytoplasmic accentuation with cells appearing to "mold to each other." Lobular carcinomas tend to show a distinct perinuclear cytoplasmic decoration, creating a "bag of marbles" appearance with neighboring tumor cells.

Several authors[115b-115e] have described the presence of E-cadherin in ductal carcinomas, whereas lobular carcinomas lack this substance. Using antibody to E-cadherin 67A4 (Zymed, South San Francisco, CA) Lehr and coworkers found a peripheral cytoplasmic pattern of immunostaining in ductal carcinomas.[115a] Testing for the presence of E-cadherin has utility in distinguishing ductal carcinoma in situ from lobular carcinoma in situ, and this is important for therapeutic reasons.[115e]

Estrogen Receptor

Intuitively, it would seem as though the estrogen receptors/progesterone receptors (ERs/PRs) would be confined to hormone-responsive tissues such as breast, but even the literature of the late 1990s on this topic is controversial. Although some authors conclude that ERs/PRs are found only in subsets of breast carcinomas and carcinomas of the ovary and endometrium,[102, 116, 117] others have observed mostly ERs, rarely PRs, in carcinomas of the lung, stomach, and thyroid.[118-122]

Vargas and colleagues[118] demonstrated the estrogen-related protein p29 in 98% of non–small cell lung cancers by IHC, suggesting that the estrogen axis may be important in this group of malignancies. This same group of tumors were all negative with the commercially available antibody ER1D5 (DAKO, Carpenteria, CA). Survival of this group of patients differed for men versus women, suggesting some gender-specific p29 associated–factor influence.

In a study by myself and my colleagues,[122a] ERs were observed using antibody 6F11 (Ventana, Tuc-

son, AZ) with heat-induced epitope retrieval (HIER) in 67% of lung adenocarcinomas, but no immunostaining of the same carcinomas was seen with ER1D5 (DAKO, Carpinteria, CA). As a result of these findings, we are reluctant to use the presence of ERs in an adenocarcinoma of lung as definitive evidence of a metastatic breast carcinoma with antibody ER 6F11. Other investigators have arrived at the same conclusion regarding the low specificity of ER in carcinomas of unknown primary.[117]

KEY DIFFERENTIAL DIAGNOSTIC POINTS OF METASTATIC BREAST CARCINOMA

- GCDFP-15 has 99% specificity and 50% sensitivity for breast carcinoma.
- Salivary gland carcinomas and skin adnexal carcinomas have overlap staining with GCDFP-15.
- Formalin- or Bouin's solution–fixed preparations are ideal for cytologic specimens; alcohol fixation ruins antibody immunoreactivity.
- Metastatic breast carcinoma in lung:
  Breast: GCDFP-15+/−, TTF-1(−), CEAD-14 (R-N)
  Lung carcinoma: GCDFP-15(−), TTF-1+, CEAD-14+
- Estrogen receptor alone is not a sensitive or specific test to detect metastatic breast carcinoma.

PROGNOSTIC FACTORS FOR BREAST CANCER BY IMMUNOHISTOCHEMISTRY

Paraffin-embedded tissue, used for the primary morphologic diagnosis of breast carcinoma, also lends itself to a variety of antibody tests that not only shed a great deal of light on the biology of the disease but also serves as a cutting edge medium for the development of tests that may have an impact on how the disease is treated.

Pathologic features of breast carcinoma that have prognostic value include:
- Tumor size
- Lymph node status
- Histologic type of tumor
- Nuclear grade
- Mitotic activity
- Estrogen and progesterone receptors

These parameters, which should be included in each pathologist's surgical pathology report, have been thoroughly studied and been found to have significant predictive value for the patient's clinical course and response to therapy. Most of these parameters have been tried and tested as the Scarff-Bloom-Richardson or Nottingham Index.[123]

ER and PR ligand binding assays have been validated by long-term follow-up for clinical use, with established cutoffs for positive results.

Of all of the previously mentioned factors, the ER/PR immunohistochemical test has been controversial, because there was no agreed upon standard of what constitutes a positive immunohistochemical test for ER/PR.[124] The same principle holds true for the dizzying array of "new" immunohistochemically derived prognostic factors listed in Table 17–4. Most of the studies behind these newer prognostic factors have technical limitations, have not been standardized, have been derived from small data bases, and have been performed in nonrandomized clinical trials in which treatment arms have been nonuniform with inadequate follow-up. All these tests are available, and virtually any laboratory will perform them on request. In our laboratory, such requests often come from clinicians or patients who have been "targeted" by today's mass media. Our laboratory currently performs the HER-2 test by IHC on every new breast cancer case, the demand driven purely by the clinician. Ravdin[125] asks the question, "Should HER-2 status be determined on all new breast cancer patients?" His answer is no—the test should be reserved for patients with metastases who need to know if they are HER-2+ so that they can be treated with trastuzumab (Herceptin).

Recent data from several publications[126, 127] indicate that HER-2/neu+ patients are more responsive to doxorubicin chemotherapy, and at my institution, clinicians use these data to customize their treatment regimens.

In this section, we discuss the IHC tests that are performed (somewhat) routinely, in that they may have direct, immediate therapeutic implications. There is no doubt that many of the putative prognostic factors in Table 17–4 will, one day soon, be incorporated into a "high-tech" prognostic-therapeutic decision tree based on outcomes analysis.

For an exhaustive current update on new, putative prognostic factors, the reader is referred to Bowcock.[128]

Needle biopsy of the breast and fine needle aspiration (FNA) cytologic techniques are the most common methods of making the diagnosis of breast carcinoma. All the diagnostic and prognostic tests

Table 17–4. Additional Immunohistochemical Prognostic Markers to Be Validated

p53
Nm23
EGFR
Cathepsin D
MIB-1
Microvascular density
PS2
p-Glycoprotein
bcl-2
Fibroblast growth factor
Transforming growth factor-beta
Insulin-like growth factor network
Matrix metalloproteinases

EGFR, epidermal growth factor receptor.

(SMMHC, muscle-specific actin, ER, PR, MIB-1, p53, HER-2/neu, and so on) can be applied to these small biopsies and yield reliable results.[26, 129–136] Of all these tests on core biopsy specimens, only progesterone gives a substantial number of false-negative results because of the wide heterogeneity of immunoperoxidase staining in tissue.[135]

Hormone Receptors

Recognition that estrogen ablation had an impact on groups of patients with breast cancer[137] and that clinical responsiveness correlated with the expression of the estrogen receptor were seminal events in the treatment of patients with breast cancer.[138]

ERs/PRs bind hormones that exert their effects in the nucleus. Nuclear immunostaining for both receptor proteins can be demonstrated in normal breast acini, which serve as internal controls for the testing procedure. Nuclear staining in normal breast tissue is heterogeneous and varies with the menstrual cycle.[139]

One of the effects of estrogen is to induce the PR, and thus the coordinate expression of both hormones in the same cell reflects the fidelity of the ER/PR axis in the cell. In carcinomas of the breast, most PR+ tumors are also ER+, and only 10% of PR+ tumors are ER−.[140, 141] Patients with positive PRs have a significantly longer disease-free survival than patients who are PR−.[142–147]

Since the early 1990s, the immunohistochemical assay (ICA) determination of ER/PR levels has replaced the dextran-coated charcoal (DCC) method. The DCC method, the gold standard for many years, suffers significant drawbacks, namely, (1) tumor sampling error; (2) heavy reliance on obtaining tissue immediately on termination of the blood supply to the tumor, usually in the operating room; (3) normal tissue contamination; and (4) analytic error.

Some of the advantages of the ICA method include (1) histologic documentation of the tumor tissue to be assayed; (2) appreciation of the heterogeneity of ERs/PRs in tumor cell nuclei; (3) rapid assessment of the tissue for ERs/PRs by direct visualization or semiquantitative methods, or both; (4) rapid turnaround time; (5) lower cost; and (6) ability to use minute quantities of tissue.

Some of the first ICA antibodies to be used would work well only on frozen tumor samples. The H222 (Abbot Laboratories, Abbot Park, IL) antibody functioned well on frozen tissue, but subsequent studies on formalin-fixed, paraffin-embedded tissues stressed the importance of short (<24 hr) formalin fixation times for optimal results. Longer fixation times extinguished immunoreactivity,[148] necessitating special attention to the presence of a positive internal control on the section of tumor.[149, 150]

Detailed studies by Frigo and colleagues with the H222 antibody showed that a variety of fixatives had no advantage over formalin fixation when used with the labeled streptavidin method.[151]

Battifora and coworkers did a comparative analysis between DCC and IHC in 166 patients with 6-year follow-up and concluded that there was 94% agreement between the methods when the DCC threshold of 20 fmol/mg was used with the H222 antibody.[152] Several studies subsequently confirmed that the results obtained with the H222 antibody gave results comparable to results from frozen section studies.[148, 153–159]

The appearance of second-generation ER antibodies (ER1D5, DAKO, Carpinteria, CA) combined with newer antigen retrieval methods[160–162] has rendered the DCC method obsolete.[163]

Early concordance studies with ER ICA and the DCC method showed good correlation and high sensitivity and specificity in terms of correlation with H222 results,[164] overall survival, or disease-free survival.[165–169]

Quantitation of results of the ICA is an issue of some controversy. A survey of the literature reveals that some authors set a "positive" ER result at greater than or equal to 5% nuclear staining, whereas others set a "positive" result at a minimum of 10% nuclear staining. Still others rely on the "H score," which includes measures of percent positive nuclei with intensity of nuclear staining.

Pertschuk and colleagues and Taylor and associates argued that using a percentage of nuclear staining of 10% as a minimum for a positive result was reproducible and correlated well clinically.[167, 170, 171] Ferno and associates also found correlation with clinical response with the value of 10% nuclear staining, finding no additional value in the nuclear staining intensity.[172]

Schultz and coworkers and Remmele and associates compared visual subjective immunoscoring with image analysis; both groups concluded that image analysis quantitation was no better than visual semiquantitation, which is cheaper and simple and rapid.[173, 174]

In a review of the topic, Barnes and colleagues used a triad of staining intensity, percent positive cells, and degree of heterogeneity of staining to arrive at an index number that is predictive of endocrine response.[175] These investigators set their cutoff points for a positive result based on the results of DCC-associated endocrine response, with a sensitivity of 71% and a specificity of 62%.[175]

Clark and associates concluded that even patients with 1% positive staining for ERs/PRs benefited with adjuvant endocrine treatment.[176]

Reproducibility studies of scoring the ICA for ERs/PRs are few. van Diest and associates observed that scoring at the extremes (zero versus strongly positive) gave the best reproducibility, whereas intermediate scores were more difficult to agree on, yielding an overall agreement of 61%.[177]

A high concordance rate has been reported between measurements made by the DCC and by IHC on formalin-fixed, paraffin-embedded tissues.[178, 179]

Quantitative results of the ICC method correlate closely with biochemical results and are predictive of prognosis.[180–184] Few studies have examined whether the presence of ER predicts an endocrine response, and of the studies that have, the numbers of patients in the study have been small.[185] Veronese and colleagues, in a study using ER1D5, found that ER1D5 staining was predictive of response to tamoxifen in 65 homogeneously treated patients, and was a discriminator for relapse-free and overall survival.[186] Barnes and coworkers and Goulding and colleagues confirmed that the ER by IHC correlated better than the DCC method, and the results were strongly related to patient outcome, regardless of the method of immunoscoring.[187, 188]

In one of the largest studies with long follow-up, Harvey and associates studied the correlation with DCC and the response to endocrine therapy in 1982 patients and found that the ER IHC assay correlated well with DCC, predicted therapeutic response groups, and had distinct advantages over the DCC method.

All the controversy regarding the interpretation of what constitutes positive ER by IHC has been laid to rest by a statement issued in the November 1–3, 2000 National Institutes of Health (NIH) Consensus Statement on Adjuvant Therapy for Breast Cancer: Any positive nuclear ER immunostaining is considered to be a positive result and should be a definitive reason for instituting antiestrogen therapy for a patient.

The fact that ER/PR by IHC can be performed on minute quantities of tissue is a distinct advantage, especially for patients with a diagnosis of carcinoma made by FNA.[182] Several studies demonstrate the high sensitivity and specificity and correlation with DCC for ER/PR determination in FNA specimens.[131, 189]

The ER/PR IHC methods can also be applied to ThinPrep techniques, and they work well in the proprietary fixative PreservCyt (Cytyc, Boxborough, MA).[190, 191]

Rosen was the first to describe tumor histopathologic correlations with ER/PR expression.[192] Tumor types that tend to be ER+ include tubular, mucinous, and papillary carcinomas, along with ductal carcinomas of good (low) nuclear grade.[140, 141]

Progesterone nuclear staining by the IHC method is more heterogeneous than ER,[193] and may be a cause of false-negative results, especially in core biopsies[135] or needle aspirates. My institution has seen similar results on some core biopsies; as a result, if we obtain a negative PR or ER result on a core biopsy specimen, we repeat the test on the excisional breast lumpectomy specimen.

The sensitivity, specificity, and concordance studies for PR using antibody 1A6 have all been comparable to the study results of ER.[194–197]

Much remains to be learned about the biology of sex steroid receptors and their significance in the management of patients with breast cancer. The discovery of an additional form of ER (ER beta)[198–200] may shed light on some of the paradoxical data that we have been trying to explain.

KEY DIAGNOSTIC POINTS OF HORMONE RECEPTORS

- ER/PR false-negative results increase in core biopsies using FNA: It may be necessary to repeat immunostains on excisional biopsy specimens.
- There are at least seven described methodologies for determination of cutoff values for a positive and negative ER/PR result. The current NIH consensus statement considers any positive nuclear ER immunostaining a positive ER result.
- ER/PR values are best used with the patient's clinical condition to help predict endocrine response.

HER-2/neu Oncoprotein

The 185-kd oncoprotein HER-2/neu is a member of the tyrosine kinase receptor family, is a growth factor receptor with 50% homology to the epidermal growth factor receptor, and has surface membrane, transmembrane, and cytoplasmic domains.[201–203] Produced as a product of the c-*erb*-B2 gene located on chromosome 17q12-21.32,[204, 205] it is the cytoplasmic domain that has activating phosphorylation and transcription initiating functions, and it is the domain to which antibodies for immunohistochemical studies have been derived. The activating ligand for the HER-2 receptor is unknown.

Since the initial report describing the association of HER-2 amplification with poor clinical outcome,[206] the gene product has been the subject of at least 48 prognostic studies involving 15,000 patients with breast cancer.[207] For lymph node–negative patients, the relationship of HER-2/neu and outcome seems to be weak,[208, 209] with most studies showing no relationship between the two.[210–219] Original studies on this topic were conflicting and controversial, probably because of the wide variation of antibodies in use, the use of archived specimens without HIER, and confounding influences of patients who had been treated with adjuvant chemotherapy.[220]

The results for lymph node–positive disease seems to be more clear cut, with the vast majority of studies showing a poorer prognosis with overexpression of HER-2/neu.[127, 207, 211, 213, 214, 216, 219, 221–230]

The current clinical use for the HER-2/neu status of the breast cancer patient is twofold: (1) as a predictor of response to therapy, especially for doxorubicin, and (2) to determine which patients would respond to monoclonal antibody therapy.

Muss and colleagues[127] studied chemotherapy response in 1572 women divided on the basis of HER-2 overexpression and concluded that high-dose chemotherapy with doxorubicin, cyclophosphamide, and fluorouracil in HER-2+ patients resulted in significantly better response than in patients who were HER-2−.

Paik and associates, using archival paraffin material from the National Surgical Adjuvant Breast Project (NSABP) and an antibody cocktail composed of the CB11 clone antibody (Ventana, Tucson, AZ) and polyclonal rabbit antibody (Zymed, South San Francisco, CA), concluded that patients who were HER-2+ obtained a preferential benefit from doxorubicin therapy.[126]

In 1998, clinical trials proved the efficacy of trastuzumab as an effective monoclonal antibody treatment to blockade the HER-2 receptor, resulting in substantial response of tumor shrinkage when used in combination with chemotherapy.[231, 232]

The immunohistochemical method of determining a positive HER-2 test result (oncoprotein overexpression) has evolved since the early 1990s as a variety of different antibodies have been studied.[220] More recently, fluorescence in situ hybridization (FISH) has been advocated as a new gold standard for HER-2 analysis, because it has the distinct advantage of detection of gene amplification. The advantages and limitations of both these procedures are listed in Table 17–5. Frozen and formalin-fixed tissues, as well as cytologic preparations, can be used for both IHC and FISH.[233, 234] There is a better than 90% concordance between the FISH and IHC methods.

Concordance between the two methods is best when membrane immunostaining is recorded, while cytoplasmic staining is disregarded.[235] The scoring method follows from the Food and Drug Administration (FDA)-approved HercepTest Kit (DAKO, Carpinteria, CA). Positive results are interpreted as 3+, which is characterized by strong, diffuse membrane ("chicken wire") staining (Fig. 17–16), and 2+, which is characterized by at least 10% of tumor cells showing complete membrane staining. Such staining in this instance is often weak. All other results—less than 10% of cells

Table 17–5. Benefits and Limitations of Immunohistochemistry Versus Fluorescence In Situ Hybridization for HER-2/neu

Immunohistochemistry	Fluorescence In Situ Hybridization
Formalin-fixed or frozen tissue, alcohol-fixed cytologic preparations	Formalin-fixed and cytologic preparations
Performed easily in most laboratories	Requires special training to perform and interpret
Inexpensive	Currently expensive
Quick turnaround time, easy to interpret	Rare cases with gene amplification have no immunohistochemical overexpression
Rare positive cases may not be gene-amplified	More accurate
Comparable results on current reliable antibodies	May be difficult to interpret Signal heterogeneity may be a problem

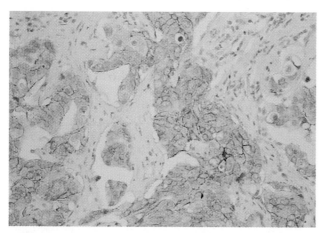

Figure 17–16. Typical strong positive circumferential cell membrane immunostaining ("chicken wire") with HER-2/neu.

- Overexpression correlates with response to doxorubicin.
- Overexpression correlates with response to monoclonal antibody therapy.
- There are comparable IHC results with monoclonal or polyclonal antibodies from DAKO, Ventana (CB11), and Zymed (TAB250).
- FISH detects gene amplification, and IHC detects gene product overexpression.
- FISH and IHC can be performed on paraffin sections and cytologic needle aspirates.
- There is controversy regarding the number of false-positive HER-2 results by IHC.
- There is no agreement as to which method should be used.
- The use of FISH for HER-2-neu is advocated in cases that are 2+ by IHC or in the gray zone between 2+ and 3+.

staining and often incomplete membrane staining—are interpreted as negative.

At my institution, we examined 87 archival cases of breast carcinoma with anti-p185 antibodies from DAKO (polyclonal), Zymed (TAB250 and polyclonal), and Ventana (CB11 clone). The results from all the antibodies were comparable in sensitivity and specificity (Table 17–6). The DAKO antibody had 19 to 26% more positive cases compared with the other antibodies. The number of positive cases in this study were not as great as the 60% of positive cases that Roche and Ingle described.[236]

Jacobs and associates found good interlaboratory agreement for HER-2 by IHC, with both laboratories using the same primary antibody but different methodologies and scoring methods.[237]

Roche and Ingle, in studying several groups of patients, concluded that the DAKO antibody with the HercepTest yields an unacceptable number of false-positive HER-2 results.[236] This problem has not yet been addressed and, as a result, standardization of reporting is nonuniform.

Allred and Swanson reviewed the topic of IHC HER-2/neu and concluded that clinical validation of the IHC procedure has not yet been completed.[238]

Prostate Specific Antigen

Prostate specific antigen (PSA) is present in 30 to 40% of female breast carcinomas[239–242] and has been described in male breast carcinomas.[243] The importance of PSA immunoreactive breast carcinoma lies in the pitfall of the diagnosis of metastatic prostate carcinoma[243] especially in a male with a breast mass. Prostate carcinoma may be distinguished from male breast carcinoma, as breast carcinomas tend to be strongly, diffusely positive for CK7 and polyclonal CEA, whereas prostate carcinoma staining is largely negative with both antibodies. In the two patients described by Gupta,[243] serum PSA was not elevated.

References

1. Joshi MG, Lee AKC, Pederson CA, et al. The role of immunocytochemical markers in the differential diagnosis of proliferative and neoplastic lesions of the breast. Mod Pathol 1996;9:57–62.
2. Rudland PS, Leinster SJ, Winstanley J, et al. Immunocytochemical identification of cell types in benign and malignant breast diseases: Variations in cell markers accompany the malignant state. J Histochem Cytochem 1993;41:543–553.
3. Gusterson BA, Warburton MJ, Mitchell D, et al. Distribution of myoepithelial cells and basement membrane proteins in the normal breast and in benign and malignant breast diseases. Cancer Res 1982;42:4763–4770.
4. Bussolati G, Botta G, Gugliotta P. Actin-rich (myoepithelial cells) in ductal carcinoma in situ of the breast. Virchows Arch B 1980;34:251–259.
5. Bussolati G. Actin-rich (myoepithelial) cells in lobular carcinoma in situ of the breast. Virchows Arch B 1980;32:165–176.
6. Bussolati G, Botto-Micca FB, Eusebi V, et al. Myoepithelial cells in lobular carcinoma in situ of the breast. Ultrastruct Pathol 1981;2:219–230.
7. Ahmed A. The myoepithelium in human breast carcinoma. J Pathol 1974;113:129–135.
8. Gould VE, Jao W, Battifora H. Ultrastructural analysis in the differential diagnosis of breast tumors: The signifi-

Table 17–6. HER-2 Immunostaining Comparison of Four Antibodies

Antibody	Positive Results	Cytoplasm	Sensitivity (%)	Specificity (%)
DAKO	21/87	4/87		
CB11	23/87	7/87	81	97*
TAB250	22/87	0/87	74	97†
ZYMED-R	23/87	49/87	78	98‡

* Ventana, Tucson, AZ.
† Zymed monoclonal (Zymed Laboratories; South San Francisco, CA).
‡ Zymed polyclonal rabbit.

cance of myoepithelial cells, basal lamina, intracyto-plasmic lumina and secretory granules. Pathol Res Pract 1980;167:45–70.

9. Hijazi YM, Lessard JL, Weiss MA, et al. Use of anti-actin and S-100 protein antibodies in differentiating benign and malignant sclerosing breast lesions. Surg Pathol 1989;2:125–135.

10. Dwarakanath S, Lee AK, Dellilis RA, et al. S-100 protein positivity in breast carcinomas: A potential pitfall in diagnostic immunohistochemistry. Hum Pathol 1987;18:1144–1148.

11. Egan MJ, Newman J, Crocker J, et al. Immunohistochemical localization of S-100 in benign and malignant conditions of the breast. Arch Pathol Lab Med 1987;111:28–31.

12. Raju U, Lee MW, Zarbo RJ, et al. Papillary neoplasia of the breast: Immunohistochemically defined myoepithelial cells in the diagnosis of benign and malignant papillary breast neoplasms. Mod Pathol 1989;2:569–576.

13. Nayar R, Brelund C, Bedrossian U, et al. Immunoreactivity of ductal cells with putative myoepithelial markers: A potential pitfall in breast carcinoma. Ann Diagn Pathol 1999;3:165–173.

14. Nagle RB, Bocker W, Davis JR, et al. Characterization of breast carcinomas by two monoclonal antibodies distinguishing myoepithelial from luminal epithelial cells. J Histochem Cytochem 1986;34:869–881.

15. Jarasch ED, Nagle RB, Kaufman M, et al. Differential diagnosis of benign epithelial proliferations and carcinomas of the breast using antibodies to cytokeratins. Hum Pathol 1988;19:276–289.

16. Bocker W, Bier B, Freytag G, et al. An immunohistochemical study of the breast using antibodies to basal and luminal keratins, alpha-smooth muscle actin, vimentin, collagen IV and laminin. Part II. Virchows Arch A Pathol Anat Histopathol 1992;421:323–330.

17. Bocker W, Bier B, Freytag G, et al. An immunohistochemical study of the breast using antibodies to basal and luminal keratins, alpha-smooth muscle actin, vimentin, collagen IV and laminin. Part I. Virchows Arch A Pathol Anat Histopathol 1992;421:315–322.

18. Gottlieb C, Raju U, Greenwald, KA. Myoepithelial cells in the differential diagnosis of complex benign and malignant breast lesions: An immunohistochemical study. Mod Pathol 1990;3:135–140.

19. Gugliotta P, Sapino A, Macri L, et al. Specific demonstration of myoepithelial cells by anti–alpha smooth muscle actin antibody. J Histochem Cytochem 1993;36:659–663.

20. Raymond WA, Leong AS. Assessment of invasion in breast lesions using antibodies to basement membrane components and myoepithelial cells. Pathology 1991;23:291–297.

21. Bose S, DeRosa CM, Ozzello L. Immunostaining of type IV collagen and smooth muscle actin as an aid in the diagnosis of breast lesions. Breast J 1999;5:194–201.

22. Wang NP, Wan BC, Skelly M, et al. Antibodies to novel myoepithelium-associated proteins distinguish benign lesions and carcinoma in situ from invasive carcinoma of the breast. Appl Immunohistochem 1997;5:141–151.

23. Titus MA. Myosins. Curr Opin Cell Biol 1993;5:77–81.

24. Winder SJ, Walsh MP. Calponin: Thin filament–linked regulation of smooth muscle contraction. Cell Signal 1993;5:677–686.

25. Gimoa M, Herzog M, Vancekerckhove J, et al. Smooth muscle specific expression of calponin. FEBS Lett 1990;274:159–162.

26. Dabbs DJ, Pickeral J, Tung MY, et al. Predicting invasion in stereotactic core biopsies of breast: Qualitative differences of antibodies that detect myoepithelial cells. Mod Pathol, in press.

27. Someren A, Sewell CW. Differential Diagnosis in Pathology: Breast Disorders. New York: Igaku-Shoin, 1997.

28. Eusebi V, Foschini MP, Betts CM, et al. Microglandular adenosis, apocrine adenosis, and tubular carcinoma of the breast: An immunohistochemical comparison. Am J Surg Pathol 1993;17:99–109.

29. Lee KC, Chan JK, Gwi E. Tubular adenosis of the breast: A distinct benign lesion mimicking invasive carcinoma. Am J Surg Pathol 1996;20:46–54.

30. Eusebi V, Collina G, Bussolati G. Carcinoma in situ in sclerosing adenosis of the breast: An immunohistochemical study. Semin Diagn Pathol 1989;6:146–152.

31. Rasbridge SA. Carcinoma in situ involving sclerosing adenosis: A mimic of invasive breast carcinoma. Histopathology 1995;27:269–273.

32. Papotti M, Gugliotta P, Eusebi V, et al. Immunohistochemical analysis of benign and malignant papillary lesions of the breast. Am J Surg Pathol 1983;7:451–461.

33. Purcell CA, Norris HJ. Intraductal proliferations of the breast: A review of histologic criteria for atypical ductal hyperplasia and ductal carcinoma in situ, including apocrine and papillary lesions. Ann Diagn Pathol 1998;2:135–145.

34. McKinney CD, Fechner RE. Papillomas of the breast: A histologic spectrum including atypical hyperplasia and duct carcinoma in situ. Pathol Annu 1995;30:137–178.

35. Raju U, Vertes D. Breast papillomas with atypical ductal hyperplasia. Hum Pathol 1996;27:1231–1238.

36. Barsky SH, Siegal GP, Jannota F, et al. Loss of basement membrane components by invasive tumors but not their benign counterparts. Lab Invest 1983;49:140–147.

37. Chomette G, Auriol M, Tranbaloc P, et al. Stromal changes in early invasive breast carcinoma: An immunohistochemical, histoenzymological and ultrastructural study. Pathol Res Pract 1990;186:70–79.

38. Simpson RH, Cope N, Skalova A, et al. Malignant adenomyoepithelioma of the breast with mixed osteogenic, spindle cell and carcinomatous differentiation. Am J Surg Pathol 1998;22:631–636.

39. Maiorano E, Ricco R, Virgintino D, et al. Infiltrating myoepithelioma of the breast. Appl Immunohistochem 1994;2:130–136.

40. Foschini MP, Eusebi V. Carcinomas of the breast showing myoepithelial cell differentiation: A review of the literature. Virchows Arch 1998;432:303–310.

41. Chen PC, Chen CK, Nicastri AD, et al. Myoepithelial carcinoma of the breast with distant metastasis and accompanied by adenomyoepitheliomas. Histopathology 1994;24:543–548.

42. Young RH. Adenomyoepithelioma of the breast: A report of three cases and review of the literature. Am J Clin Pathol 1988;89:308–314.

43. Thorner PS, Kahn HJ, Baumal R, et al. Malignant myoepithelioma of the breast: An immunohistochemical study by light and electron microscopy. Cancer 1986;57:745–750.

44. Tavassoli FA. Myoepithelial lesions of the breast: Myoepitheliosis, adenomyoepithelioma and myoepithelial carcinoma. Am J Surg Pathol 1991;15:554–568.

45. Schurch W, Potvin C, Seemayer TA. Malignant myoepithelioma (myoepithelial carcinoma) of the breast: An ultrastructural and immunohistochemical study. Ultrastruct Pathol 1985;8:1–11.

46. Smith TA, Machen K, Fisher C, et al. Usefulness of cytokeratin subsets for distinguishing monophasic synovial sarcoma from malignant peripheral nerve sheath tumors. Am J Clin Pathol 1999;112:641–648.

47. Deligeorgi-Politi H, Kontozoglou T, Joseph M, et al. Myofibroblastoma of the breast: Cytologic, histologic, immunohistochemical and ultrastructural findings in two cases with differing cellularity. Breast J 1997;3:365–371.

48. Julien M, Trojani M, Coindre JM. Myofibroblastoma of the breast: Report of 8 cases. Ann Pathol 1994;14:143–147.

49. Wargotz ES, Weiss SW, Norris HJ. Myofibroblastoma of the breast: Sixteen cases of a distinctive benign mesenchymal tumor. Am J Surg Pathol 1987;11:493–502.

50. Damiani S, Miettinin M, Peterse JL, et al. Solitary fibrous tumor (myofibroblastoma) of the breast. Virchows Arch 1994;425:89–92.

51. Schwartz GF, Patchefsky AS, Finkelstein SD, et al. Nonpalpable in situ ductal carcinoma of the breast: Predictors of multicentricity and microinvasion and implications for treatment. Arch Surg 1989;124:29–32.

52. Patchefsky AS, Schwartz GF, Finkelstein SD, et al. Heterogeneity of intraductal carcinoma of the breast. Cancer 1989;63:731–741.

53. Tamimi SO, Ahmed A. Stromal changes in early invasive and non-invasive breast carcinoma: An ultrastructural study. J Pathol 1986;150:43–49.

54. Silverstein MJ, Waisman JR, Gamagami P, et al. Intraductal carcinoma of the breast (208 cases): Clinical factors influencing treatment choice. Cancer 1990;66:102–108.

55. Schuh ME, Nemoto T, Penetrante RB, et al. Intraductal carcinoma: Analysis of presentation, pathologic findings and outcome of disease. Arch Surg 1986;121:1303–1307.

56. Wong JH, Kopald KH, Morton DL. The impact of microinvasion on axillary node metastases and survival in patients with intraductal breast cancer. Arch Surg 1990;125:1298–1302.

57. Solin LJ, Fowble BL, Yeh I-T, et al. Microinvasive ductal carcinoma of the breast treated with breast conserving surgery and definitive radiation. Int J Radiat Oncol Biol Phys 1992;23:961–968.

58. Rosner D, Lane WW, Penetrante R. Duct carcinoma in situ with microinvasion: A curable entity using surgery alone without need for adjuvant therapy. Cancer 1991;67:1498–1503.

59. Force PW. Standardized management of breast cancer specimens. Am J Clin Pathol 1973;60:789–798.

60. Rosen PP. Intraductal carcinoma. In: Breast Pathology. Philadelphia: Lippincott-Raven, 1997:264–265.

61. Prasad ML, Hyjek E, Giri DD, et al. Double immunolabeling with cytokeratin and smooth-muscle actin in confirming early invasive carcinoma of breast. Am J Surg Pathol 1999;23:176–181.

62. Masood S, Sim SJ, Lu L. Immunohistochemical differentiation of atypical hyperplasia vs. carcinoma in situ. Cancer Detect Prev 1992;16:225–235.

63. Raju U, Crissman JD, Zarbo RJ, et al. Epitheliosis of the breast: An immunohistochemical characterization and comparison to malignant intraductal proliferation of the breast. Am J Surg Pathol 1990;14:939–947.

64. Soini Y, Miettinin M. Immunohistochemical evaluation of the cytoarchitecture of benign and malignant breast lesions. APMIS 1993;100:901–907.

65. Monifar F, Man YG, Lininger RA, et al. Use of keratin 34βE12 as an adjunct in the diagnosis of mammary intraepithelial neoplasia-ductal type-benign and malignant intraductal proliferations. Am J Surg Pathol 1999;23:1048–1058.

66. Ashikari R, Park K, Huvos A, et al. Paget's disease of the breast. Cancer 1970;26:680–685.

67. Kister SJ, Haagensen CD. Paget's disease of the breast. Am J Surg 1977;119:606–609.

68. Salvadori B, Fariselli G, Saccozzi R. Analysis of 100 cases of Paget's disease of the breast. Tumori 1976;62:529–536.

69. Lundquist K, Kohler S, Rouse RV. Intraepidermal cytokeratin 7 expression is not restricted to Paget cells but is also seen in Toker cells and Merkel cells. Am J Surg Pathol 1999;23:212–219.

70. Zeng Z, Melamed J, Symmans P, et al. Benign proliferative nipple duct lesions frequently contain CAM5.2 and anti-cytokeratin 7 immunoreactive cells in the overlying epidermis. Am J Surg Pathol 1999;23:1349–1355.

71. Tani E, Skoog L. Immunocytochemical detection of estrogen receptors in mammary Paget cells. Acta Cytol 1988;23:825–828.

72. Meissner K, Riviere A, Haupt G, et al. Study of neu-protein expression in mammary Paget's disease with and without underlying breast carcinoma and in extramammary Paget's disease. Am J Pathol 1990;137:1305–1309.

73. Cabanas RM. An approach for the treatment of penile carcinoma. Cancer 1977;39:456–466.

74. Reintgen D, Cruse CW, Wells K, et al. The orderly progression of melanoma lymph node metastasis. Ann Surg 1994;220:759–767.

75. Steinhoff MM. Axillary node micrometastases: Detection and biologic significance. Breast J 1999;5:325–329.

76. Mansi JL, Gogas H, Bliss JM, et al. Outcome of primary breast cancer patients with micrometastases: A long term follow-up study. Lancet 1999;354:197–202.

77. Nasser IA, Lee AK, Bosari S, et al. Occult axillary lymph node metastases in "node negative" breast carcinoma. Hum Pathol 1993;24:950–957.

78. Bass SS, Lyman GH, McCann CR, et al. Lymphatic mapping and sentinel lymph node biopsy. Breast J 1999;5:288–295.

79. Association of Directors of Anatomic and Surgical Pathology Annual Meeting, Chicago, 1998.

80. Allred DC, Elledge RM. Caution concerning micrometastatic breast carcinoma in sentinel lymph nodes. [editorial] Cancer 1999;86:905–907.

81. Dowlatshahi K, Fan M, Bloom KJ, et al. Occult metastases in the sentinel lymph nodes of patients with early stage breast carcinoma. Cancer 1999;86:990–996.

82. Meyer J. Sentinel lymph node biopsy: Strategies for pathologic examination of the specimen. J Surg Oncol 1998;69:212–218.

82a. Xu X, Roberts SA, Pasha TL, Zhang PJ. Undesirable cytokeratin immunoreactivity of native nonepithelial cells in sentinel lymph nodes from patients with breast carcinoma. Arch Pathol Lab Med 2000;124:1310–1313.

83. Czerniecki BJ, Scheff AM, Callans LS, et al. Immunohistochemistry with pancytokeratins improves sensitivity of sentinel lymph node biopsy in patients with breast carcinoma. Cancer 1999;85:1098–1103.

84. Doglioni C, Dell'Orto P, Zanetti G, et al. Cytokeratin immunoreactive cells of lymph nodes and spleen in normal and pathologic conditions. Virchow's Arch A Pathol Anat Histopathol 1990;416:479–490.

85. Iuzzolino P, Bontempini L, Doglioni C, et al. Keratin immunoreactivity in extrafollicular reticular cells of the lymph node. Am J Clin Pathol 1989;91:239–240.

86. Carter BA, Jensen RA, Simpson JF, et al. Benign transport of breast epithelium into axillary lymph nodes after biopsy. Am J Clin Pathol 2000;113:259–265.

87. Pearlman WH, Giueriguian JD, Sawyer ME, et al. A specific progesterone binding component of human breast fluid. J Biol Chem 1973;248:5736–5741.

88. Haagensen DEJ, Mazoujian G, Holder WDJ, et al. Evaluation of a breast cyst fluid protein detectable in the plasma of breast carcinoma patients. Ann Surg 1977;185:279–285.

89. Murphy LC, Lee-Wing M, Goldenberg GJ, et al. Expression of the gene encoding a prolactin-inducible protein by human breast cancers in vivo. Cancer Res 1987;47:4160–4164.

90. Losi L, Lorenzini R, Eusebi V, et al. Apocrine differentiation in invasive carcinoma of the breast: Comparison of monoclonal and polyclonal gross cystic disease fluid protein-15 antibodies with prolactin-inducible protein mRNA expression. Appl Immunohistochem 1995;3:91–98.

91. Mazoujian G, Parish TH, Haagensen DEJ, et al. Immunoperoxidase localization of GCDFP-15 with mouse monoclonal antibodies versus rabbit antiserum. J Histochem Cytochem 1988;36:377–382.

92. Eusebi V, Magalhaes F, Azzopardi JG, et al. Pleomorphic lobular carcinoma of the breast: An aggressive tumor showing apocrine differentiation. Hum Pathol 1992;23:655–662.

93. Wick MR, Lillemoe TJ, Copland GT, et al. Gross cystic disease fluid protein-15 as a marker for breast cancer: Immunohistochemical analysis of 690 human neoplasms and comparison with alpha-lactalbumin. Hum Pathol 1989;20:281–287.

94. Viacava P, Naccarato AG, Bevilacqua G. Spectrum of GCDFP-15 expression in human fetal and adult normal tissues. Virchows Arch 1998;432:255–260.

95. Mazoujian G, Margolis R. Immunohistochemistry of gross cystic disease fluid protein (GCDFP-15) in 65 benign sweat gland tumors of the skin. Am J Dermatopathol 1988;10:28–35.

96. Mazoujian G, Pinkus GS, David S, et al. Immunohistochemistry of a breast gross cystic disease fluid protein (GCDFP-15): A marker of apocrine epithelium and breast

carcinomas with apocrine features. Am J Pathol 1983;110: 105–112.

97. Swanson PE, Pettinato G, Lillemoe TJ, et al. Gross cystic disease fluid protein-15 in salivary gland tumors. Arch Pathol Lab Med 1991;115:158–163.

98. Wick MR, Ockner DM, Mills SE, et al. Homologous carcinomas of the breasts, skin and salivary glands: A histologic and immunohistochemical comparison of ductal mammary carcinoma, ductal sweat gland carcinoma and salivary duct carcinoma. Am J Clin Pathol 1998;109:75–84.

99. Ormsby AH, Snow JL, Su WPD, et al. Diagnostic immuno-histochemistry of cutaneous metastatic breast carcinoma: A statistical analysis of the utility of gross cystic disease fluid protein-15 and estrogen receptor protein. J Am Acad Dermatol 1995;32:711–716.

100. Mazoujian G, Bodian C, Haagensen DEJ, et al. Expression of GCDFP-15 in breast carcinomas: Relationship to pathologic and clinical factors. Cancer 1989;63:2156–2161.

101. Kaufman O, Deidesheimer T, Muehlenberg M, et al. Immunohistochemical differentiation of metastatic breast carcinomas from metastatic adenocarcinomas of other common sites. Histopathology 1996;29:233–240.

102. Raab SS, Berg SC, Swanson PE, et al. Adenocarcinoma in the lung in patients with breast cancer: A prospective analysis of the discriminatory value of immunohistology. Am J Clin Pathol 1993;100:27–35.

103. Fiel MI, Cernaianu G, Burstein DE, et al. Value of GCDFP-15 (BRST-2) as a specific immunocytochemical marker for breast carcinoma in cytologic specimens. Acta Cytol 1996; 40:637–641.

104. Pritchard DG, Todd CW, Egan ML. Chemistry of carcino-embryonic antigen. Methods Cancer Res 1978;14:55–85.

105. Svenberg T. Carcinoembryonic antigen–like substances of human bile: Isolation and partial characterization. Int J Cancer 1976;17:588–596.

106. Nach-J Pusztaszeri G. Demonstration of a partial identity between CEA and a normal glycoprotein. Immunochemistry 1972;9:1031–1033.

107. Pavelic ZP, Pavelic L, Pavelic K, et al. Utility of anti-carcinoembryonic antigen monoclonal antibodies for differentiating ovarian adenocarcinomas from gastrointestinal metastases to the ovary. Gynecol Oncol 1991;40:112–117.

108. Pavelic ZP, Petrelli NJ, Herrera L, et al. D-14 monoclonal antibody to carcinoembryonic antigen: Immunohistochemical analysis of formalin-fixed, paraffin-embedded human colorectal carcinoma, tumors of non-colorectal origin and normal tissues. J Cancer Res Clin Oncol 1990;116:112–117.

109. Fabian C, Dabbs DJ. The immunohistochemical discrimination of breast carcinoma metastatic in lung. Breast J 1997;3:135–141.

110. Harlamert HA, Mira J, Bejarno PA, et al. Thyroid transcription factor-1 and cytokeratin 7 and 20 in pulmonary and breast carcinomas. Acta Cytol 1998;42:1382–1388.

111. Wang MP, Zee S, Zarbo RJ, et al. Coordinate expression of cytokeratins 7 and 20 defines unique subsets of carcinomas. Appl Immunohistochem 1995;3:99–107.

112. Moll R, Lowe A, Laufer J, et al. Cytokeratin 20 in human carcinomas: A new histodiagnostic marker detected by monoclonal antibodies. Am J Pathol 1992;140:427–447.

113. Larsimont D, Lespagnard L, Degeyten M, et al. Medullary carcinoma of the breast: A tumor lacking keratin 19. Histopathology 1994;24:549–552.

114. Dalal P, Shousha S. Keratin 19 in paraffin sections of medullary carcinoma and other benign and malignant breast lesions. Mod Pathol 1995;8:413–416.

115. Jensen ML, Kiaer H, Melsen F. Medullary carcinoma versus poorly differentiated ductal carcinoma: An immuno-histochemical study with keratin 19 and estrogen receptor staining. Histopathology 1996;29:241–245.

115a. Lehr HA, Folpe A, Yaziji H, et al. Cytokeratin 8 immuno-staining pattern and E-cadherin expression distinguish lobular from ductal breast carcinoma. Am J Clin Pathol 2000; 114:190–196.

115b. Moll R, Mitze M, Frixen UH, et al. Differential loss of E-cadherin expression in infiltrating ductal and lobular carcinomas. Am J Pathol 1993;143:1731–1742.

115c. Rasbridge SA, Gillett CE, Sampson SA, et al. Epithelial (E-) and placental (P-) cadherin cell adhesion molecule expression in breast carcinoma. J Pathol 1993;169:245–250.

115d. Siitonen SM, Kononen JT, Helin HJ, et al. Reduced E-cadherin expression is associated with invasiveness and unfavorable prognosis in breast cancer. Am J Clin Pathol 1996;105:394–402.

115e. Acs G, Lawton TJ, Rebbeck TR, et al. Differential expression of E-cadherin in lobular and ductal neoplasms of the breast and its biologic and diagnostic implications. Am J Clin Pathol 2001;115:85–98.

116. Bacchi CE, Garcia RL, Gown AM. Immunolocalization of estrogen and progesterone receptors in neuroendocrine tumors of the lung, skin, gastrointestinal and female genital tracts. Appl Immunohistochem 1997;5:17–22.

117. Deamant FT, Pombo MT, Battifora H. Estrogen receptor immunohistochemistry as a predictor of site of origin in metastatic breast cancer. Appl Immunohistochem 1993;1: 188–192.

118. Vargas SO, Leslie KO, Vacek PM, et al. Estrogen receptor related protein 29 in primary non-small cell carcinoma: Pathologic and prognostic correlations. Cancer 1998;82: 1495–1500.

119. Beattie CW, Hansen NW, Thomas PA. Steroid receptors in human lung cancer. Cancer Res 1985;45:4206–4214.

120. Kaiser U, Hofmann J, Schilli M, et al. Steroid hormone receptors in cell lines and tumor biopsies of human lung cancer. Int J Cancer 1996;67:357–364.

121. Su JM, Shu HK, Chang H, et al. Expression of estrogen and progesterone receptors in non-small cell lung cancer: Immunohistochemical study. Anticancer Res 1996;16:3803–3806.

122. Cagle PT, Mody DR, Schwartz MR. Estrogen and progesterone receptors in bronchogenic carcinoma. Cancer Res 1990;50:6632–6635.

122a. Dabbs DJ, Liu Y, Raab SS et al. Immunohistochemical detection of estrogen receptor in pulmonary adenocarcinomas is dependent upon the antibody used. Mod Pathol 2000;13:208A.

123. Genestie C, Zafrani B, Asselain B. Comparison of the prognostic value of Scarff-Bloom-Richardson and Nottingham histological grades in a series of 825 cases of breast cancer: Major importance of the mitotic count as a component of both grading systems. Anticancer Res 1998;18:571–576.

124. Allred, C, Harvey JM, Berado M, et al. Prognostic and predictive factors in breast cancer by immunohistochemical analysis. Mod Pathol 1999;11:155–168.

125. Ravdin PM. Should HER-2 status be routinely measured for all breast cancer patients? Semin Oncol 1999;26:117–123.

126. Paik S, Bryant J, Park C, et al. ErbB-2 and response to doxorubicin in patients with axillary lymph node-positive, hormone receptor negative breast cancer. J Natl Cancer Inst 1998;90:1361–1370.

127. Muss HB, Thor AD, Berry DA, et al. C-erbB-2 expression and response to adjuvant therapy in women with node-positive early breast cancer. N Engl J Med 1994;330:1260–1266.

128. Bowcock AM, ed. Breast Cancer Molecular Genetics, Pathogenesis and Therapeutics. Totowa, NJ: Humana Press, 1999.

129. Masood S. Estrogen and progesterone receptors in cytology. Diagn Cytopathol 1992;8:475–491.

130. Masood S, Dee S, Goldstein JD. Immunocytochemical analysis of progesterone receptors in breast cancer. Am J Clin Pathol 1991;96:59–63.

131. Marrazzo A, Taormina P, Leonardi P, et al. Immunocyto-chemical determination of estrogen and progesterone receptors on 219 fine-needle aspirates of breast cancer: A prospective study. Anticancer Res 1995;15:521–526.

132. Keshgegian AA, Inverso K, Kline TS. Determination of estrogen receptor by monoclonal antireceptor antibody in

aspiration biopsy cytology from breast carcinoma. Am J Clin Pathol 1988;89:24–29.

133. Keunen-Boumeester V, Van der Kwast TH, Van Laarhoven HA, Henzen-Logmans SC. Ki-67 staining in histological subtypes of breast carcinoma and fine needle aspiration smears. J Clin Pathol 1989;134:733.

134. Jacobs TW, Sisiopikou KP, Prioleau JE, et al. Do prognostic marker studies on core needle biopsy specimens of breast carcinoma accurately reflect the marker status of the tumor? Mod Pathol 1998;11:259–264.

135. Zidan A, Christie Brown JS, Peston D, et al. Estrogen and progesterone receptor assessment in core biopsy specimens of breast carcinoma. J Clin Pathol 1997;50:27–29.

136. Puglisi F, Scalone PF, Bazzocchi M, et al. Image guided core breast biopsy: A suitable method for preoperative biological characterization of small (pT1) breast carcinomas. Cancer Lett 1998;133:223–229.

137. Beatson GT. On the treatment of inoperable cases of carcinoma of the mamma: Suggestions for a new method of treatment, with illustrative cases. Lancet 1896;2:104–107.

138. McGuire W, Carbone P, Vollmer E. Estrogen Receptors in Human Breast Cancer. New York: Raven Press, 1975.

139. Jacquemier JD, Hassoun J, Torrente M, et al. Distribution of estrogen and progesterone receptors in healthy tissue adjacent to breast lesions at various stages of the menstrual cycle-immunocytochemical study of 107 cases. Breast Cancer Res Treat 1990;15:109–117.

140. Reiner A, Reiner G, Spona J, et al. Histopathologic characterization of human breast cancer in correlation with estrogen receptor status: A comparison of immunocytochemical and biochemical analysis. Cancer 1988;64:1149–1154.

141. Lesser ML, Rosen PP, Seine RT, et al. Estrogen and progesterone receptors in breast carcinoma: Correlations with epidemiology and pathology. Cancer 1981;48:299–309.

142. Clark GM, McGuire WL. Steroid receptors and other prognostic factors in primary breast cancer. Semin Oncol 1988;15:20–25.

143. Castagnetta L, Traina A, Carruba G, et al. The prognosis of breast cancer patients in relation to the estrogen receptor status of both primary disease and involved nodes. Br J Cancer 1992;66:167–170.

144. Brdar B, Graf D, Padovan R, et al. Estrogen and progesterone receptors as prognostic factors in breast cancer. Tumori 1988;74:45–52.

145. Crowe JP, Hubay CA, Pearson OH, et al. Estrogen receptor status as a prognostic indicator for stage I breast cancer patients. Breast Cancer Res Treat 1982;2:171–176.

146. Clark GM, McGuire WL, Hubay CA, et al. Progesterone receptors as a prognostic factor in stage II breast cancer. N Engl J Med 1983;309:1343–1347.

147. Pichon MF, Pallud C, Hacene K, et al. Prognostic value of progesterone receptor after long-term follow-up in primary breast cancer. Eur J Cancer 1992;28:1676–1680.

148. Shintaku A, Said JW. Detection of estrogen receptors in routinely processed formalin-fixed paraffin sections of breast carcinoma: Use of DNAase pretreatment to enhance sensitivity of the reaction. Am J Clin Pathol 1987;87:161–167.

149. Esteban JM, Battifora H, Warsi Z, et al. Quantification of estrogen receptors on paraffin embedded tumors by image analysis. Mod Pathol 1991;4:53–57.

150. Cohen C, Unger ER, Sgoutas D, et al. Automated immunohistochemical estrogen receptor in fixed embedded breast carcinoma. Am J Clin Pathol 1991;95:335–339.

151. Frigo B, Scopsi L, Faber M, et al. Application of an estrogen receptor–immunocytochemical assay primary monoclonal antibody to paraffin-embedded human breast tumor tissue: Personal experience and review of the literature. Appl Immunohistochem 1993;1:136–142.

152. Battifora H, Mehta P, Ahn C, et al. Estrogen receptor immunohistochemical assay in paraffin-embedded tissue: A better gold standard? Appl Immunohistochem 1993;1:39–45.

153. Styliandu A, Papadimitriou CS. Immunohistochemical demonstration of estrogen receptors on routine paraffin sections of breast carcinomas: A comparison with frozen sections and an enzyme immunoassay. Oncology (Basel) 1992;49:15–21.

154. Katz RL, Patel S, Sneige N, et al. Comparison of immunocytochemical and biochemical assays for estrogen receptor in fine needle aspirates and histologic sections from breast carcinomas. Breast Cancer Res Treat 1990;15:191–203.

155. Cowen PN, Teasdale J, Jackson P, et al. Estrogen receptor in breast cancer: Prognostic studies using a new immunohistochemical assay. Histopathology 1990;17:319–325.

156. Cheng L, Binder SW, Fu YS. Methods in laboratory investigation: Demonstration of estrogen receptors by monoclonal antibody in formalin-fixed breast tumors. Lab Invest 1988;58:346–353.

157. Giri DD, Dangerfield VJM, Lonsdale R, et al. Immunohistology of estrogen receptor content of adjacent cryostat sections of breast carcinoma by radioligand binding and enzyme assay. J Clin Pathol 1987;40:734–740.

158. Jackson P, Teasdale J, Cowen PN, et al. Development and validation of a sensitive immunohistochemical estrogen receptor assay for use on archival breast cancer tissue. Histochemistry 1989;92:149–152.

159. Graham DM, Jin L, Lloyd RV. Detection of estrogen receptor in paraffin-embedded sections of breast carcinoma by immunohistochemistry and in situ hybridization. Am J Surg Pathol 1991;15:475–485.

160. Leong A-Y, Milios J. Comparison of antibodies to estrogen and progesterone receptors and the influence of microwave antigen retrieval. Appl Immunohistochem 1993;1:282–288.

161. Kell DL, Kamel O, Rouse RV. Immunohistochemical analysis of breast carcinoma estrogen and progesterone receptors in paraffin-embedded tissue: Correlation of clones ER1D5 and 1A6 with a cytosol based hormone receptor assay. Appl Immunohistochem 1993;1:275–281.

162. Cattoretti G, Pileri S, Parravicini C, et al. Antigen unmasking on formalin-fixed, paraffin-embedded tissue sections. J Pathol 1993;171:83–98.

163. Battifora H. Immunocytochemistry of hormone receptors in routinely processed tissue: The new gold standard. [editorial] Appl Immunohistochem 1994;2:143–145.

164. Mauri FA, Veronese S, Frigo B, et al. ER1D5 and H222 (ER-ICA) antibodies to human estrogen receptor protein in breast carcinomas: Results of a multicentric comparative study. Appl Immunohistochem 1994;2:157–163.

165. DeSombre ER, Thorpe SM, Rose C, et al. Prognostic usefulness of estrogen receptor immunocytochemical assays for human breast cancer. Cancer Res 1986;46:4256s–4264s.

166. Kinsel LB, Szabo E, Greene GL, et al. Immunocytochemical analysis of estrogen receptors as a predictor of prognosis in breast cancer patients: Comparison with quantitative biochemical methods. Cancer Res 1989;49:1052–1056.

167. Pertschuk LP, Kim DS, Nayer K, et al. Immunocytochemical estrogen and progestin receptor assays in breast cancer with monoclonal antibodies: Histopathologic, demographic and biochemical correlations and relationship to endocrine response and survival. Cancer 1990;66:1663–1670.

168. Pertschuk LP, Eisenberg KB, Carter AC, et al. Immunohistologic localization of estrogen receptors in breast cancer with monoclonal anitbodies. Cancer 1985;55:1513–1518.

169. McGuire WL, DeLaGarza M. Improved sensitivity in the measurement of estrogen receptors in human breast cancer. J Clin Endocrinol Metab 1973;37:986–989.

170. Taylor CR. Paraffin section immunocytochemistry for estrogen receptor: The time has come. Cancer 1996;77:2419–2422.

171. Pertschuk L, Feldman J, Eisenberg K, et al. Immunohistochemical detection of progesterone receptor in breast cancer with monoclonal antibody: Relation to biochemical assay, disease-free survival, and clinical endocrine response. Cancer 1988;62:342–349.

172. Ferno M, Andersson C, Fallenius G, et al. Estrogen receptor analysis of paraffin sections and cytosol samples of primary breast cancer in relation to outcome after adjuvant tamoxifen treatment: The South Sweden Breast Cancer Group. Acta Oncol 1996;35:17–22.

173. Remmele W, Schicketanz KH. Immunohistochemical determination of estrogen and progesterone receptor content in human breast cancer: Computer-assisted image analysis. Pathol Res Pract 1993;189:862–866.

174. Schultz DS, Katz RL, Patel S, et al. Comparison of visual and CAS-200 quantitation of immunocytochemical staining in breast carcinoma samples. Anal Quant Cytol Histol 1992;14:35–40.

175. Barnes DM, Millis RR, Beex LVAM, et al. Increased use of immunohistochemistry for estrogen receptor measurement in mammary carcinoma: The need for quality assurance. Eur J Cancer 1998;34:1677–1682.

176. Clark GM, Harvey JM, Osborne CK, et al. Estrogen receptor status determined by immunohistochemistry is superior to biochemical ligand-binding (LB) assay for evaluating breast cancer patients. Proc Am Soc Clin Oncol 1997;16:29A.

177. van Diest PJ, Weger DR, Lindholm J, et al. Reproducibility of subjective immunoscoring of steroid receptors in breast cancer. Anal Quant Cytol Histol 1996;18:351–354.

178. Wilbur DC, Willis J, Mooney RA, et al. Estrogen and progesterone detection in archival formalin-fixed, paraffin-embedded tissue from breast carcinoma: A comparison in immunohistochemistry with the dextran-coated charcoal assay. Mod Pathol 1992;5:79–84.

179. Tesch M, Shawwa A, Henderson R. Immunohistochemical determination of estrogen and progesterone receptor status in breast cancer. Am J Clin Pathol 1993;99:8–12.

180. McClelland RA, Finlay P, Walker KJ, et al. Automated quantitation of immunohistochemical localized estrogen receptors in human breast cancer. Cancer Res 1990;50:3545–3550.

181. Esteban JM, Kandalaft PI, Mehta P. Improvement of the quantification of estrogen and progesterone receptors in paraffin-embedded tumors by image analysis. Am J Clin Pathol 1993;99:32–38.

182. Charpin C, Andrac L, Habib M-C, et al. Immunodetection in fine-needle aspirates and multiparametric (SAMBA) image analysis: Receptors (monoclonal antiestrogen and antiprogesterone) and growth fraction (monoclonal Ki-67) evaluation in breast carcinomas. Cancer 1989;63:863–872.

183. Layfield L, Saria EA, Conlon DH, et al. Estrogen and progesterone receptor status determined by the Ventana ES 320 automated immunohistochemical stainer and the CAS 200 image analyzer in 236 early-stage breast carcinomas: Prognostic significance. J Surg Oncol 1996;61:177–184.

184. de Mascarel I, Soubeyran G, MacGrogan J, et al. Immunohistochemical analysis of estrogen receptors in 938 breast carcinomas. Appl Immunohistochem 1995;3:222–231.

185. Pertschuk LP, Feldman JG, Kim YD, et al. Estrogen receptor immunocytochemistry in paraffin-embedded tissues with ER1D5 predicts breast cancer endocrine response more accurately than H222Sp gamma in frozen sections or cytosol-based ligand-binding assays. Cancer 1996;77:2514–2519.

186. Veronese SM, Barbareschi M, Morelli L. Predictive value of ER1D5 antibody immunostaining in breast cancer: A paraffin-based retrospective study of 257 cases. Appl Immunohistochem 1995;3:85–90.

187. Barnes DM, Harris WH, Smith P, et al. Immunohistochemical determination of estrogen receptor: Comparison of different methods of assessment of staining and correlation with clinical outcome of breast cancer patients. Br J Cancer 1996;74:1445–1451.

188. Goulding H, Pinder S, Cannon P, et al. A new immunohistochemical antibody for the assessment of estrogen receptor status on routine formalin-fixed tissue samples. Hum Pathol 1995;26:291–294.

189. Marcot I, Migeon C, Parache RM, et al. A comparative study of hormone receptors in breast cancer with quantitative immunocytochemistry and biochemistry. Bull Cancer 1997;84:613–618.

190. Tabbarra SO, Sidaway MK, Frost A, et al. The stability of estrogen and progesterone receptor expression on breast carcinoma cells stored as PreservCyt suspensions and as ThinPrep slides. Cancer 1998;84:355–360.

191. Leung SW, Bedard YC, Estrogen and progesterone receptor contents in ThinPrep processed fine needle aspirates of breast. Am J Clin Pathol 1999;112:50–56.

192. Rosen PP, Menendez-Botet CJ, Nisselbaum JS, et al. Pathological review of breast lesions analyzed for estrogen receptor protein. Cancer Res 1975;35:3187–3194.

193. Layfield L, Saria E, Mooney EE, et al. Tissue heterogeneity of immunohistochemically detected estrogen receptor: Implications for image analysis quantification. Am J Clin Pathol 1998;110:758–764.

194. MacGrogan G, Soubeyran I, DeMascarel I, et al. Immunohistochemical detection of progesterone receptors in breast invasive ductal carcinomas: A correlative study of 942 cases. Appl Immunohistochem 1996;4:219–227.

195. Gibney EM, Lawson D, DeRose PB, et al. Image cytometric progesterone quantitation: Comparison with visual semiquantitation and cytosolic assay. Appl Immunohistochem 1998;6:62–68.

196. Elias JM, Margiotta M, Sexton TR, et al. Immunohistochemical detection of sex steroid receptors in breast carcinoma using routine paraffin sections: Comparison with frozen sections and enzyme immunoassay. J Cell Biochem Suppl 1994;19:126–133.

197. Soomo S, Shousa S, Sinnet HD. Estrogen and progesterone receptors in scree-detected carcinoma: An immunohistological study using paraffin sections. Histopathology 1992;21:543–547.

198. Pennsi E. Differing roles found for estrogen's two receptors. Science 1997;277:1439.

199. Kuiper GGJM, Enmark E, Pelto-Huikko M, et al. Cloning of a novel receptor expressed in rat prostate and ovary. Proc Natl Acad Sci U S A 1996;93:5925–5930.

200. Paech K, Webb P, Kuiper GGJM, et al. Differential ligand activation of estrogen receptor alpha and ER beta at AP1 sites. Science 1997;277:1508–1510.

201. Bargmann C, Hung MC, Weinber RA. The neu oncogene encodes an epidermal growth factor receptor-related protein. Nature 1986;319:226–230.

202. Schecter A, Stern DF, Vaidyanathan L, et al. The neu oncogene: An erb-B–related gene encoding an 185,000 Mr tumor antigen. Nature 1984;312:513–516.

203. King CR, Kraus MH, Aaronson SA. Amplification of a novel V-erbB–related gene in a human mammary carcinoma. Science 1985;229:974–976.

204. Popescu NC, King CR, Kraus MH. Location of the human erbB-2 gene on normal and rearranged chromosomes 17 to bands q12-21.32. Genomics 1989;4:362–366.

205. Shih C, Padhy LC, Murray M, et al. Transforming genes of carcinomas and neuroblastomas introduced into mouse fibroblasts. Nature 1981;290:261–264.

206. Slamon DJ, Clark GM, Wong SG, et al. Human breast cancer: Correlation of relapse and survival with amplification of Her-2/neu oncogene. Science 1987;235:177–182.

207. Hanna W, Kahn HJ, Trudeau M. Evaluation of Her-2/neu (erbB-2) status in breast cancer: From bench to bedside. Mod Pathol 1999;12:827–834.

208. Clark G. Should selection of adjuvant chemotherapy for patients with breast cancer be based on erb-2 status? J Natl Cancer Inst 1998;90:1320–1321.

209. Andrulis IL, Bull SB, Blackstein ME, et al. Neu/erbB-2 amplification identifies a poor prognosis group of women with node-negative breast cancer. J Clin Oncol 1998;16:1340–1349.

210. Bianchi S, Paglierani M, Zampi G, et al. Prognostic significance of cerbB-2 expression in node negative breast cancer. Br J Cancer 1993;67:625–629.

211. Borg A, Tandon AK, Sigurdsson H, et al. HER-2/neu amplification predicts poor survival in node positive breast cancer. Cancer Res 1990;50:4332–4337.

212. Clark GM, McGuire WL. Follow-up study of HER-2/neu amplification in primary breast cancer. Cancer Res 1991;51:944–948.

213. Lovekin C, Ellis IO, Locker A, et al. C-erb-2 oncoprotein expression in primary and advanced breast cancer. Br J Cancer 1991;63:439–443.

214. McCann AH, Dervan PA, O'Reagan M, et al. Prognostic significance of c-erbB-2 and estrogen receptor status in human breast cancer. Cancer Res 1991;51:3296–3303.

215. Noguchi M, Koyasaki N, Ohta N, et al. C-erbB-2 oncoprotein expression versus internal mammary lymph node metastases as additional prognostic factors in patients with axillary lymph node positive breast cancer. Cancer 1992; 69:2953–2960.

216. O'Reilly SM, Barnes DM, Camplejohn RS, et al. The relationship between c-erbB-2 expression, SS-phase fraction, and prognosis in breast cancer. Br J Cancer 1991;63:444–446.

217. Paterson MC, Dietrich KD, Kanylik J, et al. Correlation between c-erbB-2 amplification and risk of recurrent disease in lymph node negative breast cancer. Cancer Res 1991;54:556–567.

218. Rosen PP, Lesser ML, Arroyo CD, et al. Immunohistochemical detection of HER-2/neu in patients with axillary lymph node-negative breast carcinoma. Cancer 1995;75: 1320–1326.

219. Toikkanen S, Helin H, Isola J, et al. Prognostic significance of HER-2 oncoprotein expression in breast cancer: A 20-year follow-up. J Clin Oncol 1992;10:1044–1048.

220. Pres MF, Hung G, Godolphin GW, et al. Sensitivity of ER-2/neu antibodies in archival tissue samples: Potential source of error in immunohistochemical studies of oncogene expression. Cancer Res 1994;54:2771–2777.

221. Anbazhagan R, Gelber RD, Bettelheim R, et al. Association of c-erbB-2 expression and S phase fraction in the prognosis of node-positive breast cancer. Ann Oncol 1991;2:47–53.

222. Borresen AL, Ottestad L, Gaustad A, et al. Amplification and protein overexpression of the neu/HER-2/c-erbB-2 proto-oncogene in human breast carcinomas: Relationship to loss of gene sequences on chromosome 17, family history and prognosis. Br J Cancer 1990;62:585–590.

223. Gusterson BA, Gelber RD, Goldhirsch A, et al. Prognostic importance of c-erbB-2 expression in breast cancer. J Clin Oncol 1992;10:1049–1056.

224. Marks JR, Humphrey PA, Wu K, et al. Overexpression of p53 and Her-2/neu proteins as prognostic markers in early-stage breast cancer. Ann Surg 1994;219:332–341.

225. Quenel N, Wafflart J, Bonichon F, et al. The prognostic value of c-erB-2 in primary breast carcinomas: A study of 942 cases. Breast Cancer Res Treat 1995;35:283–291.

226. Rilke F, Colnaghi MI, Cascinelli N, et al. Prognostic significance of Her-2/neu expression in breast cancer and its relationship to other prognostic factors. Int J Cancer 1991; 49:44–49.

227. Winstanley J, Cooke T, Murray GD, et al. The long term prognostic significance of c-erbB-2 in primary breast cancer. Br J Cancer 1991;63:447–450.

228. Schonborn I, Zschiesche W, Spitzer E, et al. C-erbB-2 overexpression in primary breast cancer: Independent prognostic factor in patients at high risk. Breast Cancer Res Treat 1994;29:287–295.

229. Tetu B, Brisson J. Prognostic significance of HER-2/neu oncoprotein expression in node-positive breast cancer: The influence of the pattern of immunostaining and adjuvant therapy. Cancer 1994;73:2359–2365.

230. Kallioniemmi OP, Holli K, Visakorpi T, et al. Association of c-erbB-2 protein overexpression with high rate of cell proliferation, increased risk of visceral metastasis, and poor long-term survival in breast cancer. Int J Cancer 1991; 49:650–655.

231. Slamon D, Leyland-Jones B, Shak S, et al. Addition of Herceptin (humanized anti-Her-2 antibody) to first line chemotherapy for (Her-2+/MBC) markedly increases anticancer activity: A randomized, multinational controlled phase III trial. Proc ASCO 1998;17:98a.

232. Pegram MD, Lipton A, Hayes DF, et al. Phase II study of receptor-enhanced chemosensitivity using recombinant humanized anti-p185 Her-2/neu monoclonal antibody plus cisplatin in patients with Her-2/neu–overexpressing metastatic breast cancer refractory to chemotherapy treatment. J Clin Oncol 1998;16:2659–2671.

233. Persons DL, Borrelli KA, Hsu PH. Quantitation of Her-2/neu and c-myc gene amplification in breast carcinoma using fluoresence in situ hybridization. Mod Pathol 1997;10: 720–727.

234. Mezzelani A, Alasio L, Bartoli C, et al. C-erbB2/neu gene and chromosome 17 analysis in breast cancer by FISH on archival cytological fine needle aspirates. Br J Cancer 1999;80:519–525.

235. Pauletti G, Godolphin W, Press M, et al. Detection and quantification of HER-2/neu gene amplification in human breast cancer archival material using fluoresence in situ hybridization. Oncogene 1996;13:63–72.

236. Roche PC, Ingle JN. Increased HER2 with U.S. Food and Drug Administration–approved antibody. J Clin Oncol 1999;17:434.

237. Jacobs TW, Gown AM, Yazdii H, et al. Her-2/neu protein expression in breast cancer evaluated by immunohistochemistry. Am J Clin Pathol 2000;113:251–258.

238. Allred DC, Swanson PE. Testing for erbB-2 by immunohistochemistry in breast cancer. Am J Clin Pathol 2000;113: 171–175.

239. Diamandis EP, Yu H, Lopez-Otin C. Prostate specific antigen—a new constituent of breast fluid. Breast Cancer Res Treat 1996;38:259–264.

240. Melegos DN, Diamandis EP. Diagnostic value of molecular forms of prostate specific antigen for female breast cancer. Clin Biochem 1996;29:193–200.

241. Yu H, Diamandis EP, Sutherland DJ. Immunoreactive prostate specific antigen levels in female and male breast tumors and its association with steroid hormone receptors and patient age. Clin Biochem 1994;27:75–79.

242. Yu H, Diamandis EP, Levesque M, Giai M, et al. Prostate specific antigen in breast cancer, benign breast disease and normal breast tissue. Breast Cancer Res Treat 1996;40:171–178.

243. Gupta RK. Immunoreactivity of prostate specific antigen in male breast carcinomas: Two examples of a diagnostic pitfall in discriminating a primary breast cancer from metastatic prostate carcinoma. Diagn Cytopathol 1999;21:167–169.

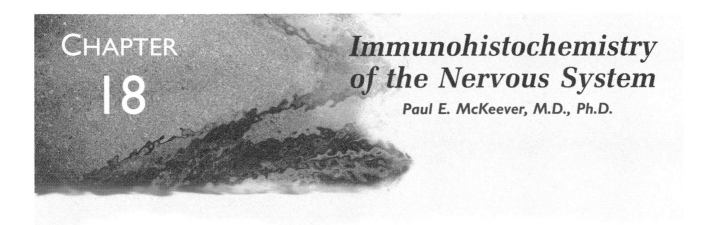

CHAPTER 18

Immunohistochemistry of the Nervous System

Paul E. McKeever, M.D., Ph.D.

This chapter focuses on the diagnostic immunohistochemistry (IHC) of nervous system diseases. Summaries in Tables 18–2 through 18–11, algorithms shown in Boxes 1 and 2, and histograms in some of the figures provide information about pathologic entities to assist in reading the text and establishing diagnoses. Suspected specific disease can be checked directly in the individual table in which its structural, immunohistochemical, and topographic features are listed, or on the algorithms. The text and figures elaborate on these features.

Features of unknown diseases may be found in individual algorithms and tables. These and the text assist diagnosis. For example, for diagnosis of a nervous system mass, specific tables in the chapter summarize differential features according to the composition of the mass, as follows:

- Fibrillar cells: Table 18–5; Figs. 18–7 to 18–9
- Epithelioid cells: Table 18–6; Figs. 18–1, 18–17, 18–31A
- More than one type of cell: Table 18–7; Fig. 18–26
- Small anaplastic cells: Table 18–8; Figs. 18–33 to 18–37
- "Syncytial" cells: Table 18–9; Fig. 18–39

Box 1 focuses on a difficult problem in diagnostic neuropathology that is virtually solved with IHC: the differential diagnosis of clear cell lesions. Box 2 displays differential immunohistochemical staining characteristics of epithelioid tumors.

Immunohistochemical stains most used for diagnosis of nervous system diseases are listed in alphabetical order in Table 18–1. Immunohistochemical staining of brain lesions should always be controlled. It is best if the tissue specimen itself is selected to have not only the lesion of interest but also tissue with regions that react positively and negatively to the stain being used, to serve as internal standard tissue controls.[1, 2] For example, a specimen being stained with glial fibrillary acidic protein (GFAP) could contain regions of gliosis ("positive" control) and meninges ("negative" control). A distant second best is a separate tissue control that contains regions both positive and negative for the immunohistochemical marker being evaluated in the specimen. A section of this tissue control can be included with each batch of diagnostic slides to gauge the intensity of background and positive staining responses. One should remember, however, that the separate tissue control will not have been fixed just as long or heated just the same as the one in question.

Individual neoplasms may lack a marker generally representative of their type. Others may respond to different markers as they progress to higher grades of malignancy.[3, 4] Because these characteristics may cause individual neoplasms not to stain for a marker, a positive immunostaining result is more meaningful than a negative result. For this reason, positive rather than negative features are emphasized in the discussion of each entity in this chapter.

If a lesion is not identified immediately, a differential diagnosis may be constructed, for which a group of appropriate immunohistochemical stains is described in the text, algorithms, and tables. The following example describes the application of this approach to an actual case.

Figure 18–1 shows cerebral tumor from the lumbosacral region of a middle-aged woman. Its H&E-stained slide reveals a neoplasm with uncommon clear cells and mainly epithelioid cells, and abundant round to oval nuclei with fine chromatin (Fig. 18–1A). Its IHC is focally positive to epithelial membrane antigen (EMA) (see Fig. 18–1B). Boxes 1 and 2 have columns showing carcinoma, chordoma, craniopharyngioma, pituitary adenoma, and meningioma to be EMA+. This tumor is negative for cytokeratin (CK) CAM5.2 (see Fig. 18–1C), so it does not fit the immunohistochemical profile of carcinoma, chordoma, or craniopharyngioma. It is negative for chromogranin A (see Fig. 18–1D) and hormones of pituitary adenomas. (It was also

The work described in this chapter is supported in part by NIH CA68545 and CA47558 grants awarded by the U.S. Public Health Service.

Box 1. Differential Diagnoses of Clear Cell Lesions*

Immunohistochemical Stain Response				Margin	Entity
GFAP+	EMA−			Diffuse	Oligodendroglioma
				Diffuse	PXA
		Syn−	KP1−	Sharp	Clear Cell Ependymoma
				Sharp	DNT
		Syn+		Sharp	Central Neurocytoma
		Syn−	KP1+		Demyelination
			KP1+		Infarct
GFAP−	EMA+		KP1−	Sharp	Clear Cell Meningioma
				Sharp	Renal Cell Carcinoma
	EMA−				Hemangioblastoma

*Unmarked boxes reflect neoplasms for which the feature or the immunohistochemical stain response is not decisive.

DNT, dysembryoplastic neuroepithelial tumor; EMA, epithelial membrane antigen; GFAP, glial fibrillary acidic protein; PXA, pleomorphic xanthoastrocytoma; Syn, synaptophysin.

Modified from Gokden M, Roth KA, Carroll SL, et al. Clear cell neoplasms and pseudoneoplastic lesions of the central nervous system. Semin Diagn Pathol 1997;14:253−269.

found to be negative for GFAP, synaptophysin, and HMB-45.) Table 18−6, which summarizes the differential diagnosis for epithelioid cells, confirms the immunohistochemical profile for meningioma and notes common features and locations. The tumor in the example was observed to have rare whorls and to involve the spinal meninges. In comparison with descriptions of meningiomas in the text, the example tumor's cells were epithelioid and focally syncytial. Its clear cells were not prominent, and it lacked cytoplasmic glycogen found in the clear cell variant. The tumor was interpreted as a meningothelial meningioma with prominent epithelioid appearance.

CLINICAL AND RADIOGRAPHIC PERSPECTIVE OF LESIONS

Major categories of lesions of the brain, spinal cord, and meninges, such as solitary and multiple masses, cysts, vascular malformations, and abscesses, are likely to be recognized clinically through the use of computed tomography (CT), magnetic resonance imaging (MRI), or angiography or on viewing of a gross specimen.

Multiple lesions can be produced by neoplasms or by degenerative, vascular, and infectious diseases. The *M-rule* for differential diagnosis of common multiple central nervous system (CNS) neo-

Box 2. Differential Diagnoses of a Mass of Epithelioid Cells*

Immunohistochemical Stain Response						Neoplasm
GFAP+	CAM5.2−	EMA−	S-100+	CgA−		Oligodendroglioma
					Syn−	Ependymoma
					Syn+	Choroid Plexus Papilloma
GFAP−	CAM5.2+	EMA+	S-100−	CgA−	Syn−	Chordoma
					Syn−	Craniopharyngioma
						Carcinoma
						Pituitary Adenoma
		EMA−		CgA+	Syn+	Paraganglioma
		EMA+			Syn−	Meningioma
	CAM5.2−	EMA−	S-100+	CgA−		Melanoma
						Hemangioblastoma

*Unmarked boxes reflect neoplasms for which the immunohistochemical stain response is not decisive.

CgA, chromogranin A; EMA, epithelial membrane antigen; GFAP, glial fibrillary acidic protein; Syn, synaptophysin.

Modified from McKeever PE. New methods of brain tumor analysis. In: Mena H, ed. Dr. Kenneth M. Earle Memorial Neuropathology Review, Washington, D.C.: Armed Forces Institute of Pathology, Feb 24, 2000.

Table 18–1. Immunohistochemical Stains Particularly Useful for Nervous Tissue

Primary Antibody/Source/Dilution*	Principal Lesions and Tissue Components	Antigen Rescue*
A6 (CD45RO)/Zymed/1:50	T lymphocytes	Mw 15 min in citrate, pH 6.0
Chromogranin A/Dr. Lloyd/1:160	Pituitary adenoma; paraganglioma; neuroendocrine tumors	Mw 15 min in citrate, pH 6.0
Collagen type IV/DAKO/1:8	Fibrosis; abscess; sarcoma; teratoma; fibrous cyst and vessel walls; dura	Ventana protease 1, 16 min
CAM5.2 cytokeratin/BD/1:10	Carcinoma; craniopharyngioma; chordoma; epithelia	Ventana protease 2, 16 min
EMA/DAKO/1:50	Carcinoma; meningioma; craniopharyngioma; chordoma; epithelia	Mw 15 min in citrate, pH 6.0
GFAP/DAKO/1:6400	Gliosis; gliomas; CNS parenchyma	Ventana protease 2, 16 min
HV antigen/DAKO/1:1000	Herpes simplex encephalitis; CMV; herpes zoster	None
JCV/SV40 viral antigen/Lee Biomolecular/ 1:500	PML	None
KP-1 (CD68)/DAKO/1:1600	Macrophages	Mw 15 min in citrate, pH 6.0
L26 (CD20)/DAKO/1:500	B lymphocytes; B lymphoma	Mw 15 min in citrate, pH 6.0
MIB-1/Immunotech/1:25	Proliferating cells	Mw 15 min in citrate, pH 6.0
NF/DAKO/1:50	Ganglion cell tumors; neurofibroma; PNET; Alzheimer's disease; CNS parenchyma	Mw 15 min in citrate, pH 6.0
Prealbumin/DAKO/1:500	Choroid plexus tumors	None
S-100 protein/DAKO/1:500	Gliomas; PNET; melanoma; schwannoma; neurofibroma and chondroid tumors; chordoma; CNS; PNS	None
Synaptophysin/BioGenex/1:600	Neuronal and pineal tumors; PNET; medulloblastoma	Mw 10 min in citrate, pH 6.0
Toxoplasma/BioGenex/neat	Toxoplasmosis	None
Vimentin/DAKO/1:800	Many cells; excessive in meningiomas	Mw 15 min in citrate, pH 6.0

* Modified from McKeever PE. New methods of brain tumor analysis. In: Mena H, ed. Dr. Kenneth M. Earle Memorial Neuropathology Review. Washington, D.C.: Armed Forces Institute of Pathology, Feb 24, 2000, with the expert advice and careful assistance of the immunohistology staff of the Immunoperoxidase Laboratory, Department of Pathology, University of Michigan Medical School.

CMV, cytomegalovirus; CNS, central nervous system; EMA, epithelial membrane antigen; GFAP, glial fibrillary acidic protein; HV, herpesvirus; NF, neurofilament; PML, progressive multifocal leukoencephalopathy; PNET, primitive neuroectodermal tumor; PNS, peripheral nervous system; Mw, microwave starting in cold buffer for time noted.

Table modified from McKeever PE, Blaivas M. The brain, spinal cord, and meninges. In: Sternberg SS, ed. Diagnostic Surgical Pathology. 2nd ed. New York: Raven Press, 1994:409–492.

plasms includes metastases, malignant lymphoma, melanoma, and (late stages only) medulloblastoma.

The tomographic density of hemorrhage is sufficiently unique to identify hemorrhage as a major component of a lesion. Calcifications and relationships with the skull are resolved well on CT, and gray and white matter, edema, and melanin on MRI. Vascular abnormalities are frequently defined angiographically.

Non-neoplastic lesions are often evaluated by a neurologist. Thus, a major neurologic symptom (e.g., dementia, weakness, or visual loss) or category of neurologic disease (e.g., demyelination) may focus the differential diagnosis (see Table 18–3).

NON-NEOPLASTIC BRAIN LESIONS

Reactive Changes

GLIOSIS

Gliosis is a reaction of the CNS to injury of the brain or spinal cord. Although subtle changes occur earlier, gliosis is usually appreciated by 2 to 3 weeks after an injury. Nearly any injury of the CNS can cause gliosis, so its presence is not diagnostic of a specific pathologic entity (Table 18–2).[5]

Anti-GFAP immunostain (Fig. 18–2) highlights the dark brown intense immunoreactivity, relatively low nuclear to cytoplasmic ratio, and the separation of astrocytes in gliosis. When identification of gliosis is critical, an age-matched autopsy control slide containing tissue from the same region of normal CNS can be stained concurrently. Both the number and the density of GFAP+ cells and cellular processes should be greater in the specimen than in the normal control.

The GFAP stain helps distinguish gliosis from glioma (see Table 18–2). GFAP+ cells are uniformly spaced apart in gliosis (see Fig. 18–2). This spacing of individual reactive astrocytes is more uniform than that found in the margin of an infiltrative glioma (see section on Tumor and Tumor Margin). The nuclear to cytoplasmic ratio of gliosis is less than that of a glioma seen with a GFAP stain.[6] Gliosis does not expand the brain like a glioma.

MACROPHAGES

Phagocytic cells may be seen in any condition that involves parenchymal destruction or irritation (Table 18–3; Fig. 18–3A; see Table 18–2). Macrophages are rich in enzymes like alpha-antichymo-

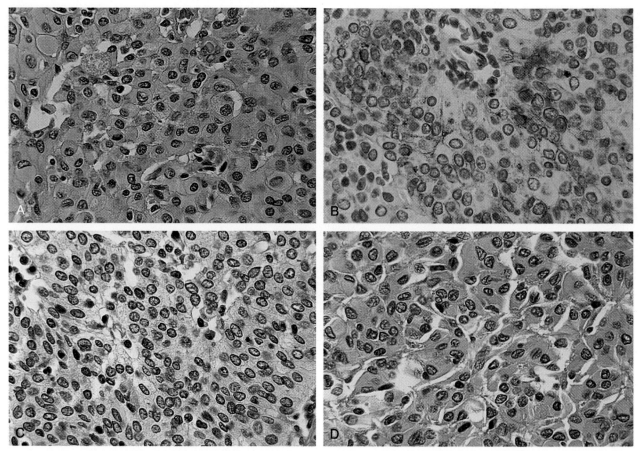

Figure 18–1. This actual case illustrates how the algorithms (see Boxes 1 and 2), tables, and text assist interpretation from initial impression to final diagnosis (see text). Large mass is from the lumbosacral region of a middle-aged woman. (H&E) It is focally epithelial membrane antigen (EMA)+ (*B*), CAM5.2− (*C*), and chromogranin A (CgA) negative (*D*). It also reacted positively to vimentin and negatively to glial fibrillary acidic protein (GFAP) and synaptophysin (*not shown*). This tumor is a meningothelial meningioma with prominent epithelioid cells. (From McKeever PE. New methods of brain tumor analysis. In: Mena H, ed. Dr. Kenneth M. Earle Memorial Neuropathology Review. Washington, D.C.: Armed Forces Institute of Pathology, February 24, 2000.)

Table 18–2. Differential Diagnosis of Cells Infiltrating Central Nervous System Parenchyma

Diagnosis	Differential Features		
	Structures	*Antibody*	*Locations**
Gliosis†	Cells fibrillar; uncrowded; round/oval nuclei	GFAP in stellate glial processes	CNS
Macrophages	Cells and nuclei round to elongated; cell content reflects injury	KP-1; α-ACT	CNS; meninges
Encephalitis/cerebritis	Perivascular mixture of inflammatory cells	LCA; L26; A6; κ and λ Ig; α-ACT; KP-1; microorganism	CNS gray matter/CNS
Hemorrhage	RBCs or macrophages with hemosiderin	Fibrin; KP-1	Deep cerebrum; cerebellum; CNS
Margin of gliomas‡	Cells fibrillar; angular nuclei indent each other; (mitoses)‡§	GFAP	CNS
Lymphoma	Perivascular noncohesive small round cells	LCA; L26; A6; κ and λ Ig	Deep cerebrum; CNS; meninges

* Most common or most specific location is listed first.
† Nonspecific reaction to injury.
‡ Suspicion of margin of glioma on frozen section should be followed by a request for another, more central biopsy. Mitoses suggest margin of a high-grade glioma.
§ Parentheses around a differential feature indicate an uncommon feature that is very useful in differential diagnosis when found.
CNS, central nervous system; GFAP, glial fibrillary acid protein; α-ACT, alpha-antichymotrypsin; Ig, immunoglobulin; LCA, leukocyte common antigen; RBC, red blood cell.
Modified from McKeever PE, Blaivas M. The brain, spinal cord, and meninges. In: Sternberg SS, ed. Diagnostic Surgical Pathology. 2nd ed. New York: Raven Press, 1994:409–492.

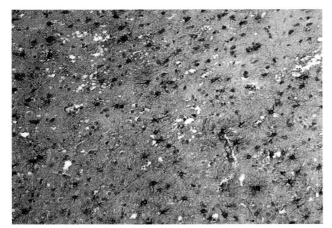

Figure 18-2. GFAP stain of gliosis. This gliosis is in the cerebral cortex from a patient with Creutzfeldt-Jakob disease (CJD). The glia are reactive and stellate with abundant brown cytoplasmic GFAP, quite different from the remote gliosis illustrated in the case of long-standing seizures (see Fig. 18-31*B*). The coalescing vacuoles are a feature of CJD but not of gliosis in general. (Anti-GFAP with H&E)

trypsin and muramidase and possess markers of mononuclear phagocytic cells, reacting with antibodies KP-1 and MAC387. All these features can be stained using IHC. Around hemorrhages or traumatic lesions, macrophages contain hemosiderin. In cerebritis, meningitis, or encephalitis, the macrophages are pleomorphic cells, some loaded with cellular debris (see Fig. 18-3). They may contain yeast and other organisms. Macrophages swollen plump by phagocytosis within the CNS are called

granular or *Gitter cells*. They are large and round with a foamy cytoplasm filled with lipid droplets (Fig. 18-4; see Fig. 18-3*A*). Macrophages that are small cells with scant cytoplasm participate in the chronic inflammatory infiltrate centered on blood vessels in encephalitides, in glial nodules, around dying neurons (neuronophagia), and in other inflammatory, demyelinating, and degenerative processes.[7, 8] KP-1 stains them well (see Fig. 18-3*A*).

PERIVASCULAR INFLAMMATION

Perivascular inflammation is usually evident without IHC. However, the small round cells with high nuclear to cytoplasmic ratios can be easily mistaken for neuroectodermal clusters that are particularly common in brains of children. Leukocyte common antigen (LCA), L26, A6, and UCHL1 markers distinguish the inflammation by highlighting lymphocytes (see Fig. 18-3*B* and *C*).

Irritation of the CNS elicits inflammation around blood vessels. This process includes surgical wounds and implants.[9] KP-1+ macrophages ingest the irritant or injured cellular constituents and move them to the perivascular space.[7] In the absence of classic lymph nodes in the brain, this perivascular region is where cells that respond to antigen intermingle. Depending on the severity and duration of illness, the perivascular inflammation varies substantially.[10] Old hemorrhage exemplifies a minimal response characterized mainly by perivascular macrophages laden with hemosiderin (see Table 18-2). Viral or allergic encephalitis produces a maximal response with abundant perivas-

Table 18-3. Biopsies Directed Toward a Neurologic Symptom or Specific Disease

| Symptom/Suspected Disease* | Confirmatory Features of Suspected Disease | | |
	Structures	*Antibody*	*Locations†*
Herpes simplex encephalitis	Encephalitis (Table 18-2); Cowdry A amphophilic nuclear inclusions of 90-100-nm "target" capsids	HSV	Temporal or basilar frontal lobe(s); CNS; frequently bilateral
Toxoplasmosis	Necrosis containing 3-5-nm tachyzoites; (cysts); (inflammation)‡	Toxoplasma	CNS; frequent multiple lesions
Progressive multifocal leukoencephalopathy	Demyelination; bizarre glia; amphophilic nuclear inclusions of 15-25-nm or 30-40-nm diameter	JCV/SV40; myelin; neurofilament; KP-1	Cerebral white matter; CNS
Dementia/Creutzfeldt-Jakob disease	Cytoplasmic vacuoles indenting nuclei; gliosis	PrPres; GFAP	Bilateral cerebral cortex; gray matter
Small vessel disease	Vasculitis or arterial sclerosis or congophilic angiopathy	A6; L26; CD31; amyloid; muscle actin; elastin	Cerebrum; CNS; frequent multiple lesions
Dementia/Alzheimer's disease	Argyrophilic plaques; neurofibrillary tangles of bihelical filaments	Neurofilament; tau; ubiquitin; Alz-50	Bilateral cerebral cortex
Demyelination	Loss of myelin; gliosis; Gitter cells; with or without axonal preservation	Myelin; neurofilament; KP-1	Cerebral white matter; CNS
Epilepsy	Low-grade glioma or ganglioglioma; or gliosis; or vascular malformation	GFAP; neurofilament; elastin	Cerebral cortex

* The order of tabulated lesions follows the order of discussion in text.
† Most common or most specific location is listed first.
‡ Parentheses around a differential feature indicate an uncommon feature that is very useful in differential diagnosis when found.
CNS, central nervous system; GFAP, glial fibrillary acid protein; HSV, herpes simplex virus.
Modified from McKeever PE, Blaivas M. The brain, spinal cord, and meninges. In: Sternberg SS, ed. Diagnostic Surgical Pathology. 2nd ed. New York: Raven Press, 1994:409-492.

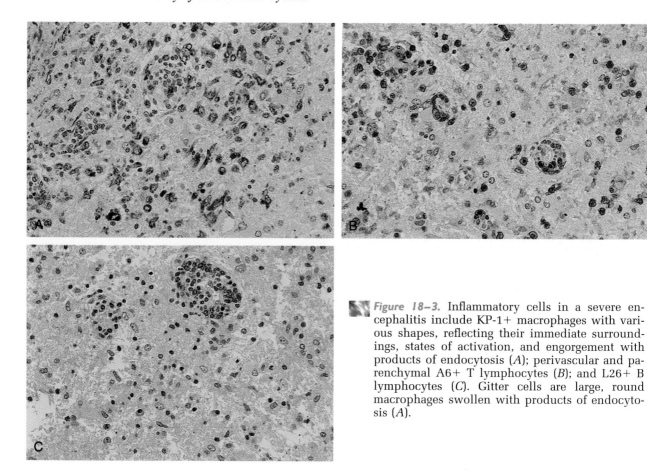

Figure 18–3. Inflammatory cells in a severe encephalitis include KP-1+ macrophages with various shapes, reflecting their immediate surroundings, states of activation, and engorgement with products of endocytosis (*A*); perivascular and parenchymal A6+ T lymphocytes (*B*); and L26+ B lymphocytes (*C*). Gitter cells are large, round macrophages swollen with products of endocytosis (*A*).

cular macrophages and many A6+ T lymphocytes. Some diseases affect mainly veins, like perivenous encephalitis, or small arteries, like CADASIL (cerebral autosomal dominant arteriopathy with subcortical infarcts and leukoencephalopathy). Affected vessels may be distinguished with anti–smooth muscle actin or myosin, because cerebral arteries have a thicker circumferential layer of spindle-shaped smooth muscle cells than cerebral veins.[105, 106]

FIBROSIS

Fibrosis is rare in brain tissue. It occurs around abscesses (see Fig. 18–4), in granulomas, and in desmoplastic and sarcomatous tumors. Fibrosis is more common in meninges. Meningeal fibrosis develops after traumatic injuries, meningitis, vasculitis involving meningeal vessels, and radiation therapy, and as a desmoplastic response to a tumor.

Various constituents of fibrosis can be detected with immunohistochemical stains: collagen, fibronectin, tenascin, and laminin.[11–16] Some of these markers require light fixation or special antigen rescue, which can be difficult to obtain.[13] At present, type IV collagen works best for most brain and meningeal tissues.[17] For routine identification of fibrosis, standard tinctorial stains rival immunohistochemical stains (see Fig. 18–4).

Infectious Diseases

Infections may produce meningitis, cerebritis, abscess, encephalitis, or encephalopathy. Except for encephalopathy, inflammation is a prominent

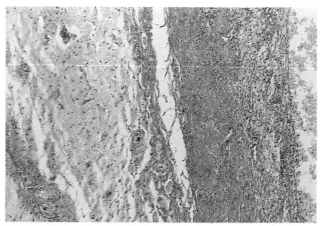

Figure 18–4. This specimen from a brain abscess shows an inflammatory lesion with a distinctive wall of collagen stained cyan with Masson's trichrome stain. Brain around this wall (orange side) contains highly reactive (gemistocytic) astrocytes. Toward the center of the abscess (gray side) are leukocytes and swollen macrophages.

feature. It proceeds from acute to chronic phases much like a systemic infection, and these phases usually do not require immunohistochemical evaluation. Exceptions occur in distinguishing infection from lymphoma. Infections cause polyclonal inflammation and often show a prominent T-cell component that stains with immunohistochemical markers, including A6 and UCHL1 (see Table 18–1). Mature, EMA+ plasma cells signify inflammation when present. On the other hand, large neoplastic cells in primary brain lymphomas are usually B cells that stain with L26, even when they are accompanied by smaller polyclonal reactive lymphocytes. Each histopathologic type of infection is briefly described here, followed by discussions of the organisms that cause it.

Histopathology

Meningitis is inflammation of the meninges that cover the brain and spinal cord. Leptomeningitis affects the thin meninges: the pia and arachnoid. Pachymeningitis affects the thick dura and is less common than leptomeningitis in nonsurgical cases. Organisms (usually, but not always, bacteria) access the meninges by local extension from sinuses or from the blood stream. The perivascular space in the CNS is an extension of the subarachnoid space, so persistent meningitis may progress to cerebritis or to an abscess.

Cerebritis is focal inflammation of brain parenchyma (*myelitis* in the spinal cord). Cerebritis precedes abscess formation but requires an early biopsy to be seen (see Tables 18–2 and 18–10). The inflammatory infiltrate is composed of neutrophils, macrophages, lymphocytes, and plasma cells, with or without parenchymal necrosis. Septic cerebritis is usually caused by bacterial agents, most often streptococci or staphylococci, and less commonly by gram-negative organisms, such as *Escherichia coli, Pseudomonas,* and *Haemophilus influenzae.* Cerebritis also occurs around neoplasms, ruptured vascular malformations, infarcts, and traumatic lesions.

Granulomatous forms of meningitis and cerebritis are seen in:
- Tuberculosis and other mycobacterial infections
- Fungal, parasitic, or spirochetal infections
- Idiopathic conditions, such as sarcoidosis, Crohn's disease, systemic lupus erythematosus, Wegener's and lymphomatoid granulomatoses, histiocytosis X, acquired immunodeficiency syndrome (AIDS), and Whipple's disease

Frequently, the only way to establish a definitive diagnosis is through biopsy and culture.[18–29]

An *abscess* combines features of inflammation and fibrosis in response to a suppurative microorganism, often bacterial or fungal.[30] A mixture of polymorphonuclear leukocytes, polyclonal T and B lymphocytes, macrophages, and plasma cells (with or without necrosis) confirms inflammation. Poly-

morphism of inflammatory components can be verified in difficult cases with A6 (CD45RO) and L26 (CD20) immunohistochemical stains for polyclonal T and B lymphocytes, KP-1 (CD68) for macrophages, and EMA for plasma cells (see Tables 18–1 and 18–10).

The wall of a brain abscess consists of a lining of CD31+ and CD34+ vascular tissue and collagen surrounded by highly GFAP+ reactive gliosis. Adjacent brain is edematous. Because collagen is rare within the CNS, its presence is an important diagnostic feature of an abscess (see Table 18–10). Collagen may be difficult to distinguish from fibrillary gliosis on a slide stained with H&E. It can be confirmed histochemically with Masson's trichrome stain or immunohistochemically with staining for collagen or fibronectin (see Fig. 18–4 and Table 18–1).

Encephalitis is inflammation of brain tissue (see Fig. 18–3). It is usually caused by viral or rickettsial organisms that produce brain inflammation more diffuse than cerebritis.[30, 31] Most viral infections are self-limited and cause only meningitis or mild meningoencephalitis. The entities emphasized here require surgical attention and are more serious.[32]

Encephalopathy (which translates as "brain suffering") that is caused by infection may show little or no inflammation. This is especially true for the spongiform encephalopathies caused by prions, such as Creutzfeldt-Jakob disease (CJD). Brain cell death followed by gliosis is the common feature of the encephalopathies. A *leukoencephalopathy* ("white brain suffering") targets white matter. A *myelopathy* (cord-medulla suffering) generally targets the spinal cord.

Organisms

Every brain biopsy specimen should be handled in such a way that if inflammation is found at surgery, it will be possible to culture the tissue for aerobic or anaerobic bacteria and fungi and to use special stains, immunostaining techniques, and electron microscopy. For most organisms today that grow in vitro, microbiologic culture is preferable to IHC or polymerase chain reaction (PCR) assay.

This chapter emphasizes organisms refractory to culture that can be identified with good immunohistochemical markers. Molecular pathology offers probes for the rapid diagnosis of diseases caused by a number of viruses, rickettsia, bacteria, fungi, and other infectious agents.[19–21]

Fungal and parasitic infections are increasingly common in immunocompromised hosts. The common organisms are *Cryptococcus neoformans, Listeria monocytogenes, Aspergillus fumigatus,* and conventional bacteria such as *H. influenzae, Streptococcus pneumoniae, Staphylococcus epidermidis,* and *Pseudomonas.*[21] Cryptococcal meningitis is the most common form of fungal meningitis, but in its presence, brain inflammation may be minimal. Chronic infections with these organisms produce granulomas. The organisms can be cultured or found with special stains, such as periodic acid–Schiff (PAS) and Gomori's methenamine silver (GMS), but immunohistochemical analysis with specific reagents is an option for organisms refractory to culture.[23-26] Species identification can be accomplished with immunostaining.[27]

Tuberculosis can involve any region of the CNS and its coverings. The disease usually causes granulomatous inflammation with or without caseating necrosis, meningitis, or arteritis. The extensive time required to grow mycobacteria invites preliminary testing with IHC, PCR assay, or acid-fast stains.[28, 29] Cases of sarcoidosis have been shown to contain mycobacterial antigens.[29]

Syphilis is rising in incidence, predominantly among immunocompromised patients, and contributing to the differential diagnosis of granulomatous inflammation.[33] The responsible organism, *Treponema pallidum*, is refractory to culture, and silver stains for it also stain brain, producing background staining that confounds detection. IHC offers an alternative and more specific test.[34]

A patient history of travel around the world opens possibilities for parasitic infections. The most common parasitic infection of the CNS is *neurocysticercosis*, which prevails in developing countries.[35] If a brain cyst contains a typical cysticercus with a characteristic invaginated scolex, the disorder can be identified without IHC. Immunohistochemical analysis using cerebrospinal fluid (CSF) from proven cases as the source of primary antibody is available for mangled or degenerated organisms in cases for which the glycocalyx remains to be found.[36] *Schistosomiasis* infects the brain and spinal cord.[37] It can be highlighted with the immunohistochemical stain for standard high molecular weight CK.[38] This stain is readily available. Because there is little CK in brain, bits of organism stand out. If a thorough search fails to show the various organisms described in granulomatous disease, neurosarcoidosis should be considered.[39]

Whipple's disease is more often anticipated than diagnosed in the brain. Rarely, it manifests as a primary brain disease without gastrointestinal symptoms.[40] The causative bacillus is *Tropheryma whippelii*.[41] The diagnosis can be made on brain biopsy specimen evaluated by light microscopy with immunoperoxidase staining for group B streptococci.[42] Histologic features include PAS+, diastase-resistant rods in macrophages, microgranulomas, perivascular A6+ and L26+ lymphocytes, and microglia reactive for KP-1 or *Ricinus communis* (RCA). Biopsy of the central cingulate gyrus, mediobasal temporal region, and insular cortex yields the most diagnostic tissue.

Caused by a tick-borne spirochete, *Borrelia burgdorferi*, Lyme disease is now the most common tick-transmitted disease in the United States. It has acute as well as chronic CNS involvement.[43, 44] Detection of *B. burgdorferi* by measurement of *Borrelia*-specific DNA using the PCR assay is the best technique available.[45, 46]

The most common cause of nonepidemic encephalitis, and the most often found on biopsy, is *herpes simplex virus (HSV)* (see Table 18–3). The process is usually but not always localized to the temporal and frontal lobes.[31] The earliest lesion is an area of vascular engorgement with ischemic changes in neurons, positive for HSV on immunoperoxidase technique performed on routine paraffin-embedded tissue. Perivascular inflammation is characteristic, composed predominantly of A6+ and L26+ lymphocytes mixed with KP-1+ macrophages and accompanied by varying degrees of focal necrosis and hemorrhage. Cowdry type A inclusion bodies in neurons and oligodendrocytes, evidence of HSV, are not easy to demonstrate in small brain biopsy specimens. This fact is a strong argument for sensitive and specific methods of identification, such as in situ hybridization (ISH) and IHC.[47, 48] PCR assay is also used.[49] Electron microscopy may demonstrate viral particles within the nuclei or cytoplasm but is less sensitive and less specific. Culture and sequential serologic CSF evaluations are slow but are still the most accurate methods of diagnosis for many viral CNS infections, including HSV. Intranuclear inclusion bodies are consistent with HSV but may be produced by many viruses, such as cytomegalovirus, varicella-zoster, JC virus (JCV), and simian virus 40 (SV40).[50]

Rabies produces round to oval, eosinophilic, 1- to 7-μm cytoplasmic inclusions.[51] Immunostains and PCR assay are available for diagnosis.[52]

Subacute sclerosing panencephalitis and milder encephalitis are caused by measles virus. Focal lymphocytic inflammation in the leptomeninges and perivascular spaces, with many CD4+ cells, patchy GFAP+ fibrillary astrocytosis, and occasional microglial nodules, involve the cerebral cortex.[53] Diffuse mononuclear inflammation, gliosis, and loss of myelin occur in subcortical white matter. Inclusion bodies are Cowdry type A and may be seen on H&E-stained slides; their specific identification requires IHC.[54]

Acquired Immunodeficiency Syndrome

CNS lesions in AIDS reflect the entire spectrum of neuropathologic disease, beginning with cerebritis, meningitis, encephalitis, and vascular disease and ending with degenerative-metabolic changes and neoplasia. The lesions have been summarized in several detailed reviews.[55-57]

PRIMARY MANIFESTATIONS OF HUMAN IMMUNODEFICIENCY VIRUS

Human immunodeficiency virus (HIV) encephalitis can be reliably diagnosed by histologic evaluation. The hallmark of HIV encephalitis is multinucleated giant cells. They are mixed with macrophages and microglia, and they form multiple foci of various sizes within the white matter, deep gray matter, and cortex. Multinucleated giant cells contain virions detectable by electron microscopy.[58] Immunohistochemical detection of HIV p24 antigen and ISH are useful in subtle cases.[59, 60] Primary dendritic damage in HIV encephalitis can be detected by synaptophysin immunoperoxidase and a modified Golgi impregnation technique.[61] Immunohistochemical identification of serum proteins in neurons and glia suggest that blood-brain barrier alterations contribute to AIDS dementia.[62]

HIV leukoencephalopathy, another form of CNS HIV infection, is characterized by diffuse damage to the white matter with loss of myelin, reactive astrogliosis, multinucleated cells, macrophages, and virtually no inflammation. IHC or ISH helps confirm the association of HIV with the process. Rarely, acute fulminating fatal leukoencephalopathy can be the only manifestation of HIV infection.[63] Leukoencephalopathy occasionally manifests as marked vacuolar myelin swelling.[60] This finding is more common in the spinal cord, however, where it forms multiple foci of vacuolar myelopathy that resemble combined systems degeneration without pernicious anemia.

Still another manifestation of HIV infection, lymphocytic meningitis is remarkable for heavy lymphocytic infiltrates within the leptomeninges and perivascular spaces. HIV cerebral vasculitis and granulomatous angiitis may occur with lymphocytic or lymphoplasmahistiocytic-multinucleated giant cell infiltration of cerebral vessel walls, occasionally accompanied by necrosis.[64]

INFECTIONS SECONDARY TO AIDS

Opportunistic infections are common in patients with AIDS but may also be found in other immunodeficient patients. *Toxoplasmosis* is the most common of these infections.[65, 66] It manifests as a necrotizing encephalomyelitis characterized by discrete lesions that contain free trophozoites or cysts filled with parasites at the periphery of the necrotic foci. Immunoperoxidase or immunofluorescence stains pinpoint the organism that is not easily found on routine H&E-stained sections.[18, 66, 67]

Cytomegalovirus (CMV) infection follows toxoplasmosis in frequency and varies from virtually no associated inflammation to severe necrotizing meningoencephalitis and ependymitis.[68, 69] Immunohistochemistry, ISH, and PCR assay are useful for detecting the virus in paraffin-embedded tissue if bizarre giant cells with nuclear inclusions are not evident.[70]

Severe encephalitis results from coinfection with HIV and JCV.[71] Tuberculosis and neurosyphilis affect patients with AIDS.[72, 73] Microscopic examination reveals focal lymphoplasmacytic inflammatory infiltrates in a predominantly perivascular arrangement.[74] Exotic CNS infections in patients with AIDS include amebic encephalitis,[75] trypanosomiasis,[76] and strongyloidiasis.[77]

PROGRESSIVE MULTIFOCAL LEUKOENCEPHALOPATHY

Progressive multifocal leukoencephalopathy (PML) is a disease manifested as multiple discrete foci of destruction of myelin with relative preservation of axons, often with no other evidence of inflammation. Radiographically, it may simulate multiple sclerosis or a mass. It is caused by DNA papovavirus, predominantly JCV (rarely SV40 virus) in immunodeficient patients (see Table 18–3). JC papovavirus has nothing in common with prions. Common underlying diseases are leukemia and AIDS.[78] PML also occurs in patients with various types of carcinoma, tuberculosis, systemic lupus erythematosus, and sarcoidosis or after the immunosuppression associated with organ transplantation.

Brain biopsy may show a destructive process within the white matter, with multiple lipid-laden macrophages, frequent large glial nuclei with a ground-glass appearance, and many large, unusual glia with pleomorphic and hyperchromatic nuclei. Perivascular infiltrates of mature lymphocytes are prominent in some cases. The pathology of JCV infection is similar in patients with and without AIDS, although bizarre astrocytes are less common, and perivascular inflammatory cells more common, in patients with AIDS.[78]

Glial nuclei are filled with virions in this disease. PML should be differentiated from multiple sclerosis, other demyelinating disorders, and astrocytic neoplasia. Random distribution of rather uniformly distorted astrocytes among multiple lipid-laden macrophages is helpful in differentiating this lesion from an astrocytic neoplasm. Bizarre astrocytes and abnormal oligodendrocytes with large nuclei containing inclusion bodies are characteristic. Diagnosis of PML is confirmed by electron microscopy, ISH, immunostaining (Fig. 18–5), or PCR assay for JCV, SV40, and BK virus.[79–81] In one study, CSF was positive for JC viral DNA sequences on PCR assay in one fourth of patients with PML.[81]

Spongiform Encephalopathies

Spongiform encephalopathies are characterized by vacuoles (spongiform change) in the gray matter.[82, 83] Vacuoles vary in size up to 30 μm in diameter and larger (Fig. 18–6). They are in the neuropil and cellular perikaryon. Their neuroanatomic distribution varies among specific diseases and in individual cases. Lack of inflammation is usual. Specimens in which a spongiform encephalopathy is suspected should be processed as described in the section on Dementias.

The spongiform encephalopathies include Creutzfeldt-Jakob disease (CJD), the much-publicized "mad cow" disease, scrapie, kuru, Gerstmann-Sträussler-Scheinker (GSS) syndrome, and fatal familial insomnia.[84-88] They are transmitted by infectious proteins called *prions*, modified forms of normal counterpart proteins. Hereditary prion diseases, such as familial fatal insomnia, GSS syndrome, and familial CJD, have germline mutations that produce prions. Infectious prion diseases, such as "mad cow" disease, scrapie, kuru, and spontaneous CJD, are transmitted by intimate contact with prions. Like catalysts, these pathogenic prions propagate by inducing their ubiquitous normal counterparts to refold in the pathogenic conformation. As this cycle continues, a growing percentage of normal counterpart proteins is converted to the pathogenic configuration.

Prions are very difficult to inactivate. Agents that completely denature protein, like bleach and strong alkali or acid (see section on Dementias) are effective, but ultraviolet light, routine formalin fixative, and standard disinfectants fail to eradicate prions.

CJD was a common diagnosis in one evaluation of cerebral biopsy specimens for dementia.[83] Vacuoles in the neuropil and perikaryon of neurons are regionally and temporally variable in CJD (see Figs. 18–2 and 18–6). Spongiform changes usually diminish in late-stage disease (see Table 18–3). In contrast, GFAP+ gliosis gradually increases (see Fig. 18–2). Immunostaining with anti–prion protein (PrP) antiserum is a useful tool in the identification of isoforms of this protein for the rapid diagnosis of CJD.[88, 89] Definitive diagnosis can be

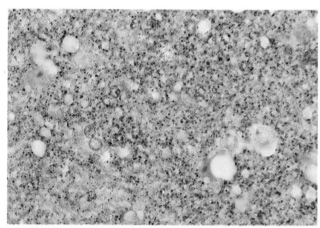

Figure 18–6. Creutzfeldt-Jakob disease (CJD). Biopsy specimen from the cerebral frontal lobe of an elderly man who had displayed progressive behavioral and memory changes for a few weeks. Patches of vacuoles and synaptic depletion can be seen in the cortical gray matter. Each tiny brown dot is a synapse in the neuropil stained with synaptophysin. Vacuoles in neuronal cytoplasm indent their nuclei. (Anti-synaptophysin with hematoxylin counterstain)

achieved by Western blot analysis for prion proteins resistant to digestion by proteinase K enzyme.[84]

In 1996, the European Union banned imports of British beef following the mysterious deaths of young "fast food" enthusiasts in 1995 from an atypical variant of CJD. These deaths and the deaths of cattlemen with bovine spongiform encephalopathy (BSE) in their herds were highly publicized.[90-92] Thus emerged the epidemic of "mad cow" disease. Microscopic plaques that stain immunohistochemically for prion protein are the most striking and consistent neuropathologic features of this atypical variant of CJD.[93] They are even more distinctive when surrounded by spongiform change.

The lack of inflammatory response in hereditary prion disorders such as GSS syndrome, fatal familial insomnia, and familial CJD is similar to that seen in sporadic CJD and kuru.[86, 94] In one study, cerebral biopsy specimens from three patients with GSS syndrome demonstrated multicentric amyloid plaques.[95] Immunostaining with PrP antiserum is a useful tool in detecting the amyloid plaques in GSS syndrome and the isoforms of this protein.[94]

Cerebrovascular Diseases

Hemorrhage into brain tissue has many causes and often accompanies other lesions within the CNS. The major role of IHC is to identify certain causes of hemorrhage, like amyloid and neoplasm. *Amyloid angiopathy* is a common cause of spontaneous intracerebral hemorrhage in the elderly (see Table 18–3).[96] Immunohistochemical staining with an antibody to β/A4 protein is more sensitive than

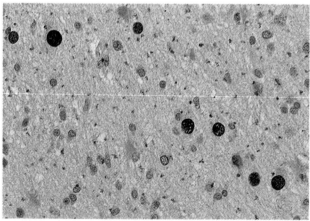

Figure 18–5. Progressive multifocal leukoencephalopathy (PML). The patient, a young woman, had systemic lupus erythematosus, which was treated with high-dose anti-inflammatory and cytotoxic agents. Immunohistochemical detection of JC viral antigen in swollen oligodendroglial nuclei stained brown. Negative smaller round oligodendroglial and elongated astrocytic nuclei counterstained purple with hematoxylin. (Courtesy of Dr. Riccardo Valdez, University of Michigan, Ann Arbor, MI.)

Congo red stain in demonstrating the extent of vascular amyloid.[97, 98]

Most neoplasms that cause brain hemorrhages are metastatic renal cell carcinoma, choriocarcinoma, melanoma (see Chapters 6, 7, 15, and 16), leukemia (see Chapters 4 and 20), and glioblastoma. Glioblastoma contains GFAP+ cellular processes, vimentin-positive vascular proliferations, and an MIB-1 proliferation index (see later) high among gliomas.

Hemorrhages in persons with *hypertension* often occur within the cerebral hemispheres, especially in the lateral areas of the basal ganglia.[99] Coagulopathy is an important cause of intracerebral hemorrhage, including drug-induced coagulopathy. Saccular aneurysms occasionally rupture into the brain, but radiography reveals their nature. Embolism is an important cause of hemorrhagic cerebral infarcts.[100] Sinus thrombosis followed by venous infarction may occur, usually as a complication of a pre-existing infectious or inflammatory disease.[101]

Nontraumatic *subarachnoid hemorrhages* are usually due to rupture of a saccular aneurysm, most often located at a branch of a major artery or the circle of Willis. Their source is radiographically apparent.

A *subdural hematoma* may follow a traumatic event and is seen in elderly patients as well as in patients with systemic cancer and brain tumors.[102–104] Membranes are formed on both sides of the hematoma, and membrane formation requires several weeks to complete. The membrane on the dural side is usually two to five vimentin-positive fibroblasts thick in a 5-day-old subdural hematoma. It eventually becomes as thick as normal dura with new collagen that reacts with immunohistochemical stains for type IV collagen and fibronectin.

SMALL VESSEL DISEASE

Brain biopsy specimens obtained in search of "small vessel disease" may require sectioning through the entire block of tissue to yield diagnostic material. Excessively involved vessels may not be recognizable, but CD31 shows them by high-

lighting their endothelial cells (see Table 18–3); it is the endothelial marker of choice for its sensitivity and specificity.[103] Involvement of small cerebral veins that have few spindle-shaped smooth muscle cells compared with arteries of the same diameter can be assessed with anti–smooth muscle actin or myosin.[105, 106] Causes are often cryptogenic in isolated angiitis of the CNS.[107] Systemic vasculitides that may affect brain are associated with (1) lupus erythematosus, (2) drugs, including cocaine, heroine, and amphetamines, (3) infection, including zoster-varicella virus and meningovascular syphilis, (4) toxins, (5) granulomatous disease, (6) Wegener's disease, (7) relapsing polychondritis, and (8) Behçet's disease.[108–116] IHC aids identification of microorganisms and classification of inflammatory cell types.

VASCULAR MALFORMATION

Five types of vascular malformations are recognized[118–120]:
- Capillary telangiectasia
- Cavernous angioma
- Arteriovenous malformation (AVM)
- Venous malformation
- Sturge-Weber disease (cerebrofacial or cerebrotrigeminal angiomatosis)

Although they may occur anywhere in the CNS, AVMs have a predilection for the cerebral hemispheres (Table 18–4). Elastic stains identify medium to large arteries and their abnormal counterparts. In AVMs, these stains often show abnormal vessels with focal loss or duplication of elastin. There is a monoclonal anti-elastin antibody, but special stains like Movat's pentachrome stain are usually used.[64, 117]

Abnormal smooth muscle layers can be highlighted with muscle actin. Cerebral veins are reported to lack the continuous circumferential layer of spindle-shaped smooth muscle cells present in cerebral arteries,[105, 106] but these differential features have not yet been convincingly shown to exist in vascular malformations. IHC can be used to identify and localize vascular collagen, fibronectin,

Table 18–4. Vascular Malformation

Type	Location	Histology
AVM	Cerebral hemispheres; brain stem; cerebellum	Veins and arteries with often poorly formed elastic membrane; gliotic brain tissue
Venous malformation	CNS; spinal leptomeninges	Veins and gliotic or normal brain tissue; no arteries
Capillary telangiectasia	Pons; brainstem; CNS	Thin-walled dilated capillaries within brain parenchyma
Cavernous angioma	CNS	Clusters of abnormal, often fibrotic or hyalinized vessels with elastic lamina and without intervening brain tissue

AVM, arteriovenous malformation; CNS, central nervous system.
Modified from McKeever PE, Blaivas M. The brain, spinal cord, and meninges. In: Sternberg SS, ed. Diagnostic Surgical Pathology. 2nd ed. New York: Raven Press, 1994:409–492.

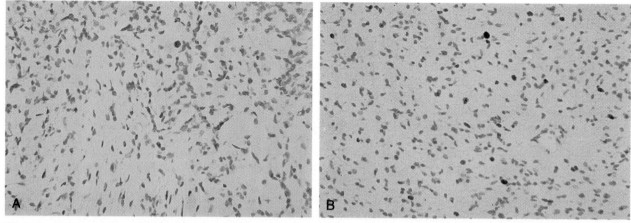

Figure 18–7. Diffuse fibrillary astrocytomas, grade II. MIB-1 antibody distinguishes long and short survivals in patients with grade II astrocytoma. *A,* Specimen with few brown MIB-1+ nuclei was taken from a patient who survived more than 8 years. *B,* Specimen with many MIB-1+ nuclei was taken from a patient who survived less than 6 months. Hematoxylin counterstain colors MIB-1− nuclei purple. (From McKeever PE, Strawderman MY, Yamini B, et al. MIB-1 proliferation index predicts survival among patients with grade II astrocytomas. J Neuropathol Exp Neurol 1998;57:931–936.)

myofibroblasts (vimentin and muscle actin), and endothelial cells (CD31).

TUMORS

Different neoplasms of brain predominate in adults and in children. More pediatric neoplasms occur in the posterior fossa than in the anterior fossa, and the opposite is true of adult neoplasms.

Grading Malignant Potential of Tumors

The World Health Organization (WHO) has established uniform terminology and grading of brain tumors according to histologic criteria.[120] Starting with the most "benign" as grade I, numerical grades II, III, and IV represent increasing malignancy. The numerical grades assigned by the WHO classification are included in parentheses after the tumor names in headings in this section of the chapter. The most important aids to assessing grade of malignancy provided by IHC are as follows[121, 122]:

- Cell type identification
- Identification of vascular proliferations with vimentin; CD31, CD34, *Ulex europaeus* (Ulex), and factor VIII endothelial markers; and smooth muscle actin
- Proliferation markers such as MIB-1 and proliferating cell nuclear antigen (PCNA) to supplement mitotic activity in assessing the growth potential of gliomas (Fig. 18–7)

A rule of thumb for grading is that primary brain tumors without mitotic activity and with a distinct margin tend to be grade I, whereas infiltrating tumors tend to be grade II and higher. Neurofilament and synaptophysin stains aid assessment of tumor infiltration by staining pre-existing axons, especially in white matter, and pre-existing synapses in gray matter. With a good nuclear counterstain, infiltrating neoplastic cells are evident with these stains.[123]

Proliferation antigens, such as MIB-1 and PCNA, are nuclear antigens that appear during one or more proliferative phases of the cell cycle. A labeling index (*LI*; also called *PI* for proliferation index) can be derived from them.[124–127] The LI of any of the proliferation antigens is the number of antigen-positive cells divided by the total number of cells in sampled microscopic areas of the tumor. Histologic grading of astrocytomas correlates with LI.[125]

MIB-1 is an antibody that detects proliferating cells in various phases of the cell cycle. MIB-1 LI differentiates between grade II and grade III gliomas.[128] Tests of the prognostic value of MIB-1 LI are promising.[125, 129–132] In one analysis, MIB-1 LI was the only independent predictor of survival. Among groups of patients with low-grade astrocytomas, MIB-1 distinguishes tumors with good prognosis by means of a low LI (see Fig. 18–7A).[133, 134]

PCNA is an auxiliary protein to DNA polymerase.[135] It is synthesized in late G_1 and S phases of the cell cycle and is associated with DNA repair enzymes.[136] One study of many variables among 45 patients with glioma showed only PCNA and histopathologic diagnosis to be independently predictive of survival.[137] Other studies have shown PCNA to be predictive to a limited extent but not independent of other factors.[138] More studies of PCNA with better antibodies that distinguish proliferation from DNA repair and yield distinct staining are needed.[136]

Apoptosis is the programmed death of cells. An apoptotic index, analogous to the LI for proliferation mentioned previously, can be determined from cytologic and cytochemical assays. The balance between cell proliferation and cell death affects tumor growth.[139]

Tumor progression in gliomas is associated with an increase in the grade of malignancy, resulting in a poorer prognosis. Cyclin-dependent kinase 4 inhibitor (CDKN2/p16) is a cell cycle regulatory protein that has been demonstrated to be inactivated by mutations, deletions, or transcriptional silencing during pathogenesis of a variety of human malignancies. CDKN2/p16 immunocytochemistry may identify those low-grade gliomas that are likely to progress and to have poor outcome and that thus would need more aggressive therapy.[140] Various other genes and their immunoreactive proteins are altered during glioma tumor progression; they have been reviewed elsewhere.[141]

Gliomas

Glioma is a term that describes astrocytoma, glioblastoma, ependymoma, oligodendroglioma, and their various subtypes and combinations. An important general rule is that gliomas tend to contain GFAP and to lack collagen, reticulin, and fibronectin in their parenchyma, distinguishing them from nonglial neoplasms[142, 143] (see Boxes 1 and 2). However, oligodendroglioma cells are more variable in their GFAP expression. Like other gliomas, they contain less specific glial proteins, such as Leu7 and S-100 protein.[144] Uncommon variants like xanthoastrocytomas may have parenchymal reticulin (see Tables 18–1 and 18-5). Gliomas lack widespread CK in their parenchyma but have been misinterpreted because of cross-reactivity between some anti-CK antibodies and GFAP (Fig. 18–8).

Clinical needs are expanding the pathologist's role in the interpretation of gliomas. For example, the effectiveness of procarbazine-CCNU-vincristine (PCV) chemotherapy for gliomas with an oligodendroglial component, especially malignant gliomas with 1p or 19q chromosomal deletions,[145] has increased the value of recognizing these tumors. Also, postoperative systemic thromboses are a ma-

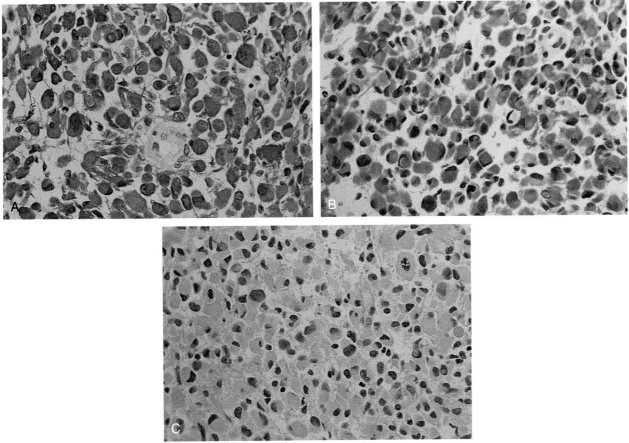

Figure 18–8. *A* to *C*, Three sections of an anaplastic astrocytoma. *A* is stained for GFAP. *B* is stained with a monoclonal antibody "cocktail" for cytokeratin that contains AE1/AE3, demonstrating the known cross-reactivity of AE1/AE3 with GFAP. *C* is stained with CAM5.2 monoclonal antibody to cytokeratin, showing that this glioma is actually negative for cytokeratin. This malignant astrocytoma demonstrates high-grade cytologic features, including mitotic activity (*C*), anaplastic nuclei, and pleomorphic cells ranging from gemistocytes to nuclei nearly devoid of cytoplasm. Vascular features and the degree of anaplasia were insufficient to confirm grade IV (glioblastoma), and there was no coagulation necrosis (compare with Fig. 18–9). (Hematoxylin counterstains) (From McKeever PE. New methods of brain tumor analysis. In: Mena H, ed. Dr. Kenneth M. Earle Memorial Neuropathology Review. Washington, D.C.: Armed Forces Institute of Pathology, February 24, 2000.)

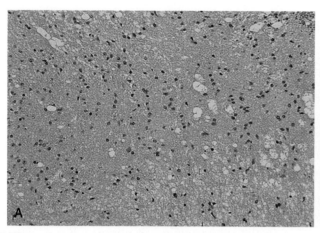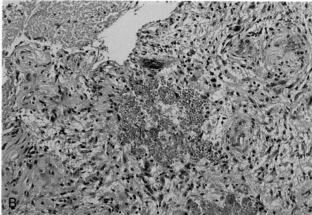

Figure 18–9. Stereotactic biopsy specimens of a left temporoparietal mass in an elderly woman. *A,* The first specimen shows gliosis and rare neoplastic glia, classification and grade uncertain. *B,* The last of several more specimens shows glioblastoma with highly pleomorphic fibrillar cells, mitotic spindles, vascular proliferation, and necrosis. (From McKeever PE. New methods of brain tumor analysis. In: Mena H, ed. Dr. Kenneth M. Earle Memorial Neuropathology Review. Washington, D.C.: Armed Forces Institute of Pathology, February 24, 2000.)

jor complication of brain tumor surgery. The pathologist may be able to identify patients likely to encounter this difficulty by reporting the tumors (usually malignant gliomas) that contain thrombosed vessels.[146]

The histologic term *low-grade* as applied to astrocytomas and other gliomas does not necessarily imply a benign neoplasm or even a favorable prognosis. The designation *benign,* implying that once removed the glioma will not recur, is frequently encountered only among WHO grade I astrocytomas, gangliogliomas, and ependymomas. Even these tumors need to be in favorable locations where they can be completely resected, thus giving the patient a good chance for cure.[147]

TUMOR AND TUMOR MARGIN

It is important to recognize two types of specimens of glioma (Fig. 18–9). The first type is the *tumor* itself (see Tables 18-5 to 18–8), which has cellular density exceeding that of surrounding brain (Fig. 18–9B). This tumor nidus is optimal for histopathologic classification.[148, 149]

The second type of specimen is brain tissue infiltrated by the *margin* of the glioma and is a product of the infiltrative nature of many gliomas.[150] Immunohistochemical stains for brain neuroanatomic components are very helpful in identifying this brain tissue. Neurofilament protein localizes axons in white matter, where axons are neuroanatomically oriented in parallel, and in gray matter.[123] The extent that glioma cells infiltrate this axonal meshwork in brain tissue is evident from the hematoxylin counterstain in immunohistochemical preparations (Fig. 18–10). Synaptophysin stains a finely pixelated "carpet" of synapses in gray matter; glioma cells disrupt this carpet.

If only the margin is available for examination, it is often impossible to determine the histologic grade and type of glioma giving rise to an infiltrative margin of neoplastic glia. Further from the glioma itself, neoplastic glia in CNS parenchyma are difficult to distinguish from gliosis (Fig. 18–11; see Fig. 18–9A). Nonetheless, GFAP can help identify gliosis by showing excess cytoplasmic GFAP and regular spacing between cells in gliosis (see Fig. 18–2).

ASTROCYTOMAS

Astrocytomas are among the most fibrillar of CNS neoplasms, more fibrillar than other gliomas except tanycytic ependymomas and subependymomas (Table 18–5). Astrocytomas nearly always contain GFAP (Fig. 18–12A; see Fig. 18–8A), although the amount is variable.[151] GFAP is the single most important immunohistochemical marker distinguishing astrocytomas from nearly all nonglial neoplasms.[144, 151, 152] Nerve sheath tumors occasionally show focal GFAP, in substantially lesser amounts than fibrillary astrocytomas that resemble them.[152] Many astrocytomas express vimentin, and when they do, this feature distinguishes them from vimentin-negative oligodendrogliomas.[153, 154]

Pilocytic Astrocytoma (WHO Grade I)

Pilocytic means "composed of hair cells," one of the major features of the pilocytic astrocytoma. Parallel bundles of elongated, fibrillar, cytoplasmic processes resemble mats of hair (see Fig. 18–12A).[155] These hair-like processes contain large amounts of glial fibrils, which stain well with immunoperoxidase for GFAP (see Table 18–5).

A diagnosis of pilocytic astrocytoma is about the

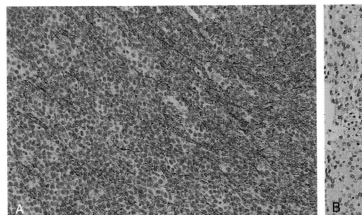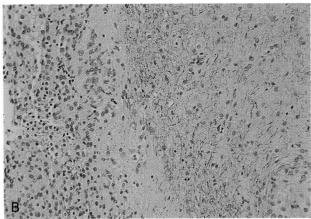

Figure 18–10. *A,* The neurofilament (NF) immunohistochemical stain highlights axons in brain, facilitating evaluation of glioma infiltration into brain tissue. Crowded round and elongated nuclei of a grade II oligoastrocytoma (stained purple with hematoxylin) diffusely infiltrate between long brown axonal constituents of the underlying brain tissue. *B,* In contrast, this pleomorphic xanthoastrocytoma (PXA) does not infiltrate between individual brown axons, and its margin with cerebral cortex is distinct. Other features of the PXA, its pleomorphic cells and nuclei and its lipid vacuoles, may be seen without IHC (see Fig. 18–16). (From McKeever PE. New methods of brain tumor analysis. In: Mena H, ed. Dr. Kenneth M. Earle Memorial Neuropathology Review. Washington, D.C.: Armed Forces Institute of Pathology, February 24, 2000.)

only "good news" within the group of astrocytomas. This tumor has a better prognosis than its diffuse counterparts, especially when it occurs in the cerebellum.[156] It is critical to distinguish pilocytic astrocytoma from fibrillary grade II astrocytoma, which has a poorer prognosis. Even the better prognosis is tempered by the facts that (1) adequate surgical removal of a pilocytic astrocytoma depends on its location and (2) some pilocytic astrocytomas develop as multicentric disease.[157] The 10-year survival of patients with supratentorial tumors is 100% after gross total resection and 74% after subtotal resection or biopsy.[158] Pilocytic astrocytomas rarely manifest malignant degeneration, which is indicated by hypercellularity, mitoses, and necrosis.

Some pilocytic astrocytomas have surprisingly discrete margins, but others show local microscopic infiltration despite a well-demarcated MRI appearance.[159] The extent of microscopic infiltration can be evaluated by combining GFAP staining to identify the edge of the highly GFAP+ tumor and neurofilament protein (NF) staining to identify axons in white matter at the edge of the tumor in serial sections. Comparing these sections facilitates interpretation of infiltration.

Most, but not all, pilocytic astrocytomas occur in children or young adults. They are most abundant

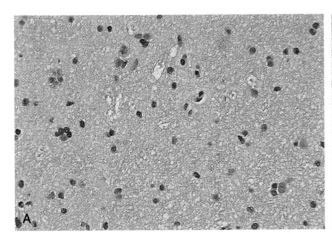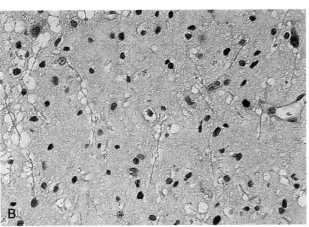

Figure 18–11. Gliosis and non-neoplastic perineuronal oligodendroglia (*A*) near a metastatic carcinoma (*not shown*) appear similar to the margin of a grade II fibrillary astrocytoma (*B*) distant from its nidus. Nuclei are more pleomorphic and hyperchromatic in *B* (compare with lighter nuclei in capillary endothelium at sides of panels). (H&E) (From McKeever PE. New methods of brain tumor analysis. In: Mena H, ed. Dr. Kenneth M. Earle Memorial Neuropathology Review. Washington, D.C.: Armed Forces Institute of Pathology, February 24, 2000.)

Table 18–5. Differential Diagnosis of a Mass of Fibrillar Cells

Diagnosis*	Differential Features		
	Structures	*Antibody†*	*Locations‡*
Fibrosis	Spindle cells of meningeal or perivascular origin	Type IV collagen (+); vimentin (+)	Meninges; CNS
Granuloma	Like fibrosis with "whorls" and inflammation	Microorganisms (see Table 18–1)	Basal meninges; CNS
Pilocytic astrocytoma	Hypercellularity; hair-like fibrillarity; Rosenthal fibers; microcysts	GFAP (+); S-100; alpha B-crystalline	Cerebellum; thalamus/hypothalamus; optic nerve; CNS
Astrocytoma	Hypercellularity; angular nuclei cluster and indent one another; infiltrates CNS	GFAP (+/−); S-100	Cerebrum; brain stem; spinal cord; CNS
Anaplastic astrocytoma	Increase in above features; mitoses	GFAP (+/−); S-100	Cerebrum; brainstem; CNS
Gemistocytic astrocytoma	Hypercellularity; cells swollen with hyaline pink cytoplasm and eccentric pleomorphic nuclei; infiltrates CNS	GFAP (+/−)	Cerebrum
Giant cell astrocytoma	Giant astrocytes with thick fibrils; large round/oval nuclei	GFAP (+/−)	Lateral ventricle; subependymal
Astroblastoma	Perivascular rosettes with expanded glial cell processes	Nonfibrillar GFAP (+/−)	Cerebrum; CNS
Pleomorphic xanthoastrocytoma	Pleomorphic cells are often vacuolated	GFAP (+/−); type IV collagen (+/−)	Leptomeninges; cerebral cortex
Ependymoma	Hypercellularity; ependymal or perivascular rosettes, or both; round/oval nuclei; cilia; and basal bodies	GFAP (+/−)	Cerebrum; cerebellum; spinal cord; CNS
Tanycytic ependymoma/subependymoma	Combination of astrocytoma and ependymoma; round/oval nuclei cluster among fibrillar mats	GFAP (+)	Spinal cord; fourth ventricle; subependymal; CNS
Anaplastic ependymoma	Preceding features with mitoses; necrosis	GFAP (+/−); S-100	Cerebrum; cerebellum
Glioblastoma multiforme	Regions of coagulation necrosis; mitoses; pleomorphism; endothelial proliferation	GFAP (+/−); S-100	Cerebrum; CNS
Gliosarcoma	Glioblastoma plus fibrosarcoma intermixed	GFAP (+/−); fibronectin; type IV collagen (+/−); laminin; vimentin (+/−)	Cerebrum
Ganglion cell tumors	Binucleated and pleomorphic neurons; diagnosis depends on gliomatous and neuroblastic elements	GFAP (+/−); synaptophysin (+/−); PGP9.5; neurofilament (+/−); type IV collagen	Cerebrum; CNS
Central neurocytoma	Round cells and nuclei; thin fibrils near vessels	Synaptophysin (+/−); neurofilament (R)	Septum pellucidum; lateral ventricles
Pineocytoma	Normal pineal structures	Synaptophysin (+/−); neurofilament (R)	Pineal
Polar spongioblastoma	Rhythmic palisades of fibrillary cells		Cerebrum; CNS
Fibroblastic meningioma	Spindle cells; interdigitating cell processes and desmosomes; (thick collagen) (whorls)§	Vimentin (+); EMA (+/−); S-100 (R)	Falx, tentorium; meninges; choroid plexus
Fibrosarcoma/malignant fibrous histiocytoma	Hypercellular; pleomorphic spindle cells and nuclei; mitoses; necrosis	Vimentin; collagen	Meninges; CNS
Schwannoma	Verocay bodies; Antoni A and B; thin pericellular basement membrane	S-100 (+); Leu7; type IV collagen	Eighth cranial nerve; spinal roots; PNS
Neurofibroma	Multiple cell types spread axons	Neurofilament (R); EMA; S-100 (+); Leu7	Spinal root; PNS; cranial nerve
Histiocytosis	Sheet-like pattern of macrophages, fibroblasts, and leukocytes	α-ACT; S-100 (+/−)	Parasellar; CNS; systemic
Melanoma	Anaplasia, mitoses, necrosis	HMB-45 (+/−); S-100 (+)	CNS/meninges; frequent multiple metastases; systemic

* The order of tabulated lesions follows the order of discussion in text.
† Key to staining results:
  (+) = Almost always strong, diffuse positivity
  (+/−) = Variable, many positive
  R = Rare cells may be positive
‡ Most common or most specific location is listed first.
§ Parentheses around a differential feature indicate an uncommon feature that is very useful in differential diagnosis when found.
α-ACT, alpha-antichymotrypsin; CNS, central nervous system; EMA, epithelial membrane antigen; GFAP, glial fibrillary acid protein; PNS, peripheral nervous system.
Modified from McKeever PE, Blaivas M. The brain, spinal cord, and meninges. In: Sternberg SS, ed. Diagnostic Surgical Pathology. 2nd ed. New York: Raven Press, 1994:409–492.

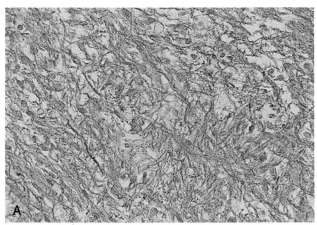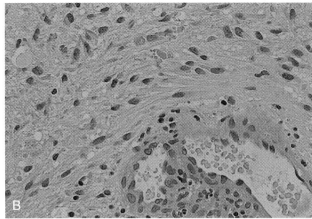

Figure 18–12. This tumor was in the cerebellar midline of a young man with headaches and vomiting. *A*, Pilocytic astrocytoma features numerous brown GFAP+ cytoplasmic processes. Pale gray, refractile globules, some with brown GFAP+ rims, are Rosenthal fibers. The GFAP– Rosenthal fiber resides in astrocytic processes. *B*, Pale gray Rosenthal fibers in this tumor mingle with pink, periodic acid-Schiff (PAS)+ protein droplets. (PAS with diastase) Both are less uniform in diameter than the light brown intravascular erythrocytes. (From McKeever PE. New methods of brain tumor analysis. In: Mena H, ed. Dr. Kenneth M. Earle Memorial Neuropathology Review. Washington, D.C.: Armed Forces Institute of Pathology, February 24, 2000.)

in the posterior fossa and around the third ventricle, thalamus, hypothalamus, neurohypophysis, and optic nerve. Cerebral hemispheric pilocytic astrocytomas are less common, but it is important to recognize them to ensure appropriate treatment.[160]

Rosenthal fibers are highly eosinophilic, hyaline structures. They are round, oval, or beaded with slightly irregular margins.[64, 160] Their beaded appearance results from their formation within glial processes. In comparison with erythrocytes, they are pink rather than orange and have greater variation in size and shape.[64] IHC reveals that they contain beta-crystalline and are GFAP– (see Fig. 18–12A). Although Rosenthal fibers assist in distinguishing the pilocytic astrocytoma from other variants, they are of no value in differentiating astrocytomas from gliosis because they occur in both abnormalities.

Eosinophilic droplets of protein are often found in pilocytic astrocytomas. These protein droplets are usually smaller and more aggregated than Rosenthal fibers. They are usually intracellular but occasionally are extracellular and up to 40 μm in diameter.[149, 161] They are PAS+ (see Fig. 18–12B). Both eosinophilic protein droplets and Rosenthal fibers are immunoreactive with alpha B-crystalline, a lens protein in the small heat shock protein family.[161, 162] Alpha B-crystalline also stains cortical Lewy bodies, other astrocytomas, schwannomas, hemangioblastomas, and chordomas.[162, 163]

Observations of the levels of subtypes of S-100 protein suggest that modifications in the level of expression of S-100A3 protein distinguish pilocytic astrocytomas from WHO grade II to IV astrocytomas.[164] These subtypes may have future diagnostic use.

Cystic cerebellar pilocytic astrocytomas resemble hemangioblastomas, which may have focally

GFAP+ cells and a GFAP+ cyst wall. Unlike in hemangioblastoma, the mural nodule of a pilocytic astrocytoma contains highly fibrillar and abundantly GFAP+ neoplastic astrocytes without clear vacuoles from lipids.[165] CD31 and other endothelial cell markers show less abundant capillaries in the astrocytoma than in the hemangioblastoma.

Diffuse Astrocytoma (Low-Grade Astrocytoma) (WHO Grade II)

The *fibrillary astrocytoma* is more common than the protoplasmic astrocytoma.[149] Fibrillary astrocytomas are a mixture of cellular processes (fibrils) and nuclei of greater angularity and density than normal or reactive astrocytes (Fig. 18–13; see Fig. 18-11B). They contain more intracytoplasmic fibrils, and their cellular processes are longer than those in protoplasmic astrocytomas. Thus, only the fibrillary astrocytoma stains well with phosphotungstic acid hematoxylin (PTAH), which stains fibrillar protein arrays, whereas both astrocytomas contain GFAP that can be stained immunohistochemically.[120] Prognostic implications of these two categories of low-grade astrocytoma are unclear.

The term *diffuse* appropriately describes an astrocytoma whose margin gradually diminishes in cellularity. Within the extensive margin, neoplastic cells intermingle with brain parenchyma (see Fig. 18–13).[64] NF immunohistochemical staining highlights parallel axons of white matter infiltrated by neoplastic astrocytes, and MIB-1 reveals a low LI in these neoplastic astrocytes because they have been diluted by normal and reactive glia. Diffuse invasion of brain may also be evident as formation of secondary structures of Scherer, described in the section on Gliomas.

The diffuse nature of the growth and infiltration

of "low-grade" astrocytomas demonstrates why they are so seldom cured despite their relatively benign histologic features. Postoperative survival is highly variable but usually 3 to 10 years. The extreme variation in prognosis among grade II diffuse astrocytomas places a premium on better measures of outcome for individual patients. A low MIB-1 LI identifies patients with good prognosis (Fig. 18–14; see Fig. 18–7).[134]

Astrocytomas are worse in the brainstem, especially those unassociated with neurofibromatosis type 1 (NF-1).[166] A study of 25 well-differentiated adult cerebral astrocytomas suggests dedifferentiation to a more malignant astrocytoma to be a more common cause of death than growth of the original low-grade tumor.[167] The variety of chromosomal abnormalities in astrocytomas includes losses in chromosomes 13, 22, X, and Y and gains in chromosome 7.[1] These changes can be detected with fluorescent and immunohistochemically enhanced ISH procedures.[168]

Anaplastic Astrocytoma (WHO Grade III)

The designation *anaplastic* emphasizes the high grade of malignancy of the anaplastic astrocytoma. Features shared by high-grade gliomas are mitotic activity as well as increases in cellular density, nuclear pleomorphism (see Fig. 18–8), and nuclear hyperchromatism. Anaplastic astrocytomas retain GFAP+ cellular processes and GFAP reactivity around their anaplastic nuclei (see Fig. 18–8A)[64]; this important feature distinguishes them from re-

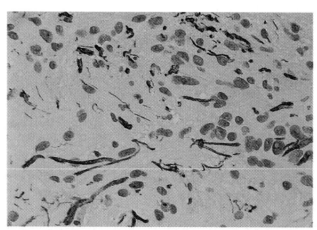

Figure 18–13. Pleomorphism of blue nuclei as well as crowding, touching, and indentation occurs in this diffuse grade II astrocytoma. These nuclei infiltrate between pre-existing axons stained brown with anti–NF protein stain. Diffuse infiltration of brain distinguishes most grade II and higher astrocytomas from grade I tumors. (Immunoperoxidase anti–NF protein with hematoxylin) (From McKeever PE. Neurofilament (NF) and synaptophysin stains reveal diagnostic and prognostic patterns of interaction between normal and neoplastic tissues. Presented at the annual meeting of the Histochemical Society, Bethesda, MD, March 24, 2000.)

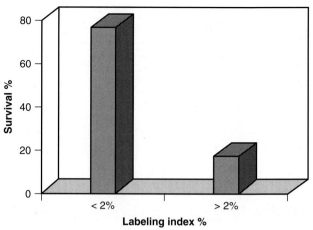

Figure 18–14. Probabilities of survival of patients with grade II astrocytomas in which MIB-1 labeling indices were ≤2% and >2%. *Bars* represent data from McKeever PE, Strawderman MY, Yamini B, et al. MIB-1 proliferation index predicts survival among patients with grade II astrocytomas. J Neuropathol Exp Neurol 1998;57:931–936.

active astrocytes trapped in other tumors. Their MIB-1 LIs are intermediate among gliomas.[125]

The lack of foci of coagulation necrosis and lack of conspicuous vascular proliferation in an astrocytic glioma distinguishes anaplastic astrocytomas from glioblastomas (see Table 18–5).[120] Average survival of patients with anaplastic astrocytoma is slightly more than 2 years. In pediatric patients, a low MIB-1 L1 identifies a group of patients who have a better prognosis.[169]

Gemistocytic Astrocytoma (WHO Grade II or III)

Gemistocytes are cells swollen with hyaline, pink cytoplasm that is reactive for GFAP (see Table 18–5 and Fig. 18–8A).[64] Their hyperchromatic and angulated nuclei are at the rim of the cells, producing a bizarre caricature of a reactive astrocyte. Perivascular cuffs of lymphocytes, a mixture of T and B cells positive for A6 and L26, are common in these tumors. Krouwer and associates[170] studied gemistocytic astrocytomas, which they separated into group A (>60% gemistocytes) and group B (20–60% gemistocytes), along with other astrocytomas. Because both groups with gemistocytes were associated with shorter average 5-year survival than other types of grade II astrocytomas, these researchers suggested that gemistocytic astrocytomas be considered anaplastic astrocytomas.

Gemistocytic astrocytomas are distinguished from oligodendrogliomas with microgemistocytes by their more angulated and pleomorphic nuclei and their longer GFAP+ cellular processes; from gangliogliomas by their lack of synaptophysin-positive neoplastic neurons; and from subependymal giant cell tumors by their smaller and more angulated nuclei and greater tendency to infiltrate brain.

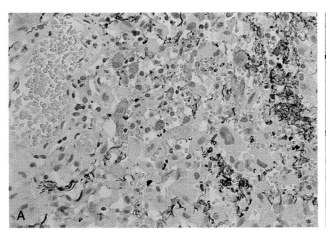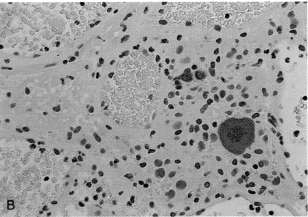

▓ ▓ *Figure 18–15.* Giant cell astrocytoma. *A,* Huge cells with large nuclei and nucleoli and abundant, finely granular cytoplasm variably reactive for GFAP mingle with bundles of thick, dark brown GFAP+ cellular processes that are part of the tumor. Despite their size, most nuclei and nucleoli lack sharp edges. *B,* Nuclei have delicately stippled chromatin and rare mitoses. There are a few NF+ and many NF− cells in this subependymal giant cell astrocytoma. One neoplastic cell has a mitosis and shows NF reactivity. This is a rare indication of the neoplastic nature of this cell type. This tumor grew from the septum pellucidum of a 20-year-old woman with tuberous sclerosis. (Immunoperoxidase anti-GFAP with hematoxylin) (From McKeever PE. New methods of brain tumor analysis. In: Mena H, ed. Dr. Kenneth M. Earle Memorial Neuropathology Review. Washington, D.C.: Armed Forces Institute of Pathology, February 24, 2000.)

Other Variants of Astrocytoma

The *subependymal giant cell astrocytoma (GCA)* has a distinctive location, histology, and association with tuberous sclerosis (TS).[171] The suppressor gene product associated with TS, tuberin, is predictably lost in GCA associated with TS.[172] The tumor arises from the medial portion of the floor of the lateral ventricle in the region where the subependymal nodules of giant astrocytes in TS, called "candle gutterings," are frequently found (see Table 18–5). It is composed of giant "astrocytes" with large nuclei and prominent nucleoli (Fig. 18–15). Although these tumors are pleomorphic, most nuclei lack sharp angulations and the giant cells are not crowded. These cells may contain glial filaments variably positive for GFAP (see Fig. 18–15*A*).

IHC has revealed partial neuronal differentiation in some GCAs (see Fig. 18–15*B*), complicating their classification as astrocytomas (versus gangliogliomas).[173] These giant astrocytes and their characteristically thick cytoplasmic processes have a tendency to form disoriented fascicles. It is very important to recognize this histologic entity, because (1) their pleomorphism is at variance with their relatively benign behavior and WHO grade I and (2) many GCAs are associated with TS.[120]

The existence of *astroblastoma* as a pure pathologic entity is debated.[204, 228] Its WHO grade is estimated to be II or IV.[120] Astroblastic "rosettes" resemble perivascular pseudorosettes of ependymomas, except that the astroblastic processes remain thick the entire distance from cell body to adventitia of the vessel.[173] Foot processes may even thicken near the adventitia. Immunohistochemical stains used in conjunction with routine neurohistochemical stains define this neoplasm: Although astroblastomas express focal GFAP, they do not stain with PTAH. This dichotomy may be due to expression of a nonfibrillar form of the GFAP molecule different from the fibrils of ependymoma and astrocytoma that stain for both.

The *pleomorphic xanthoastrocytoma* is a supratentorial astrocytoma that often involves both the leptomeninges and cerebral cortex (see Table 18–5).[174] It has a more distinct margin with brain than most astrocytomas (see Fig. 18–10*B*). Its fibrillarity and its pleomorphic, hyaline, lipid-laden, and multinucleated cells are clues to its diagnosis (Fig. 18–16). Intracellular lipid content and protein

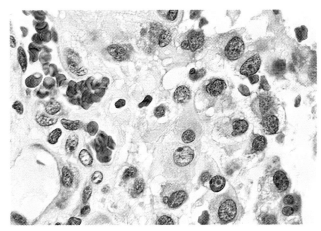

▓ ▓ *Figure 18–16.* Pleomorphic xanthoastrocytoma. Round lipid vacuoles are visible in pleomorphic astrocytes with H&E in this particular specimen. Note that nuclear to cytoplasmic ratios are low, chromatin is finely granular, and nuclear membranes have gentle curves despite the large pleomorphic nuclei and nucleoli.

granular degeneration vary from abundant to absent in individual tumors.

Pleomorphic xanthoastrocytoma may assume a clear cell appearance, requiring identification by a panel of immunohistochemical reagents (see Box 1).[175] Astrocytes are identified from their characteristic strongly GFAP+ cells, often with coexpression of alpha-1-antitrypsin.[176] Sparse lipid droplets are conspicuously negative for GFAP. These cells may be surrounded by reticulin fibers and basement membranes positive for type IV collagen, breaking a general rule that glioma cells lack reticulin.[177, 178] Neuronal elements occur in some tumors, suggesting that a pleomorphic xanthoastrocytoma may be the glial portion of a ganglioglioma.[179]

The *granular cell astrocytoma* must be recognized because its granular cytoplasm simulates infarct and demyelinating disease. Its granules react with EMA, but there is no EMA surface staining of its cells.[180] Continued growth over time and, in some cases, focal GFAP staining distinguish granular cell astrocytoma from infarct and demyelination.[181] The tumor is rare.

EPENDYMOMAS

Ependymomas are an excellent example of how IHC highlights structural features important to their interpretation.

The cellular conformations of ependymomas vary between fibrillar and epithelial, posing special problems of differentiation not only from other gliomas but also from carcinomas and meningiomas (Table 18–6; see Table 18–5). These latter differentiations are facilitated if one recalls that even epithelioid ependymomas frequently stain

---

Table 18–6. Differential Diagnosis of a Mass of Epithelioid Cells

Diagnosis*	Differential Features		
	Structures	*Antibody†*	*Locations‡*
Gitter cells/xanthogranuloma	Crowded macrophages engorged with lipid vacuoles; eccentric nucleus; noncohesive cells	α-ACT (+/−); KP-1 (+); muramidase (+/−)	CNS
Ependymoma/malignant ependymoma	Structures of ependymoma or malignant ependymoma plus epithelioid cells	GFAP (+/−); cytokeratin (R); EMA (R)	Cerebellum; cerebrum; spinal cord; CNS
Myxopapillary ependymoma	Cuboidal/columnar epithelium on hyaline fibrovascular papillae; variable fibrillarity	GFAP (+/−)	Regions of the filum terminale
Oligodendroglioma	Round cells and nuclei with prominent perinuclear halos; nests of cells between delicate vessels	Leu7 (+); S-100 (+)	Cerebrum; CNS
Anaplastic oligodendroglioma	Above features with mitoses and pleomorphism	Leu7 (+/−); S-100 (+/−)	Cerebrum; CNS
Choroid plexus papilloma	Large mass with structure of choroid plexus	Laminin (+); cytokeratin (+); transthyretin (+/−); synaptophysin; IGF-II	Fourth ventricle; lateral ventricle; CP angle; choroid plexus
Choroid plexus carcinoma	Above features with anaplasia and mitoses; (necrosis)§	Cytokeratin (+); CD44; synaptophysin; transthyretin (R)	Preceding lesions
Medulloepithelioma	Columnar epithelium with "basement membrane" on both surfaces; fibrovascular base for papillae and tubules		Deep cerebrum; cauda equina; CNS
Meningioma	Whorls; psammoma bodies; interdigitating cell processes and desmosomes; (thick collagen)§	Vimentin (+); EMA (+/−); S-100 (R)	Falx, tentorium; meninges; choroid plexus; (extracranial)§
Chordoma	Masses or cords of physaliphorous cells	Cytokeratin (+); S-100 (+); EMA (+); vimentin (+)	Cauda equina; clivus; spinal canal
Craniopharyngioma	Squamous; adamantinomatous	Cytokeratin (+)	Suprasellar; sellar
Carcinoma	Distinct margin with CNS; anaplasia; mitoses; necrosis	Cytokeratin (+); EMA (+/−)	Cerebrum; cerebellum; meninges; CNS; frequent multiple masses; systemic
Melanoma	Anaplasia; mitoses, necrosis	HMB-45 (+/−); S-100 (+)	Preceding locations

* The order of tabulated lesions follows the order of discussion in text.
† Key to staining results:
   (+) = Almost always strong, diffuse positivity
   (+/−) = Variable, many positive
   R = Rare cells may be positive
‡ Most common or most specific location is listed first.
§ Parentheses around a differential feature indicate an uncommon feature that is very useful in differential diagnosis when found.
α-ACT, alpha-antichymotrypsin; CNS, central nervous system; CP; cerebellopontine; EMA, epithelial membrane antigen; GFAP, glial fibrillary acidic protein; IGF-II, insulin-like growth factor II.
Modified from McKeever PE, Blaivas M. The brain, spinal cord, and meninges. In: Sternberg SS, ed. Diagnostic Surgical Pathology. 2nd ed. New York: Raven Press, 1994:409–492.

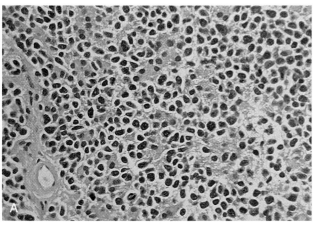

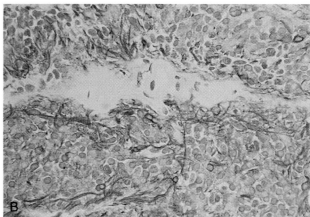

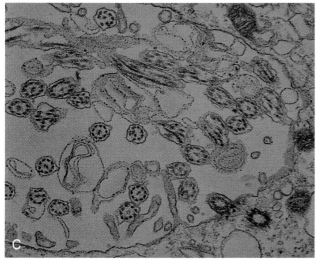

Figure 18–17. *A* and *B,* Sections of a tumor. *A,* This tumor is composed of epithelioid cells. (H&E) *B,* The tumor is GFAP+, and this stain highlights slight fibrillarity near the appropriately GFAP− vessels. *C,* Electron microscopy reveals cilia and basal bodies of ependymoma. This clear cell ependymoma mimics oligodendroglioma. (From McKeever PE. New methods of brain tumor analysis. In: Mena H, ed. Dr. Kenneth M. Earle Memorial Neuropathology Review. Washington, D.C.: Armed Forces Institute of Pathology, February 24, 2000.)

with anti-GFAP, have distinctive ultrastructure, and often contain at least a few cells with fibrillar processes (Fig. 18–17; see Boxes 1 and 2). The anti-GFAP stain highlights these fibrillar processes, greatly facilitating their identification (see Fig. 18–17*A* and *B*). A good place to look for these fibrillar processes is around vessels.

In contrast to nonglial neoplasms, aggregated ependymoma cells lack a basement membrane. Immunostaining shows no collagen or fibronectin in these aggregates, in contrast to the positive vascular adventitia.[64, 142]

One should look for rosettes to confirm suspicion of an ependymoma (see Tables 18–5 and 18–6). *Perivascular rosettes* are most useful because they occur in nearly all ependymomas.[64] They have a fibrillar zone that is at least three erythrocyte diameters wide around central vessels. Anti-GFAP stains the fibrillar zone, making a subtle zone easier to find (see Fig. 18–17*B*). The processes taper to become very thin as they radiate from the cells to the vascular adventitia, distinguishing them from the thick processes of astroblastic formations. True *ependymal rosettes* are characteristic, but some samples of ependymoma lack them. The ependymal rosette consists of ependymal cells spaced around a lumen (Fig. 18–18).

Cilia often protrude into the lumen from the ependymal lining. Some tumors show expanded ependymal rosettes, and others have long ependymal linings that do not close into rosettes.

Many ependymomas have a relatively discrete margin with brain compared with other gliomas.[64] This margin is revealed best in white matter with the NF immunohistochemical stain, which shows an abrupt border between the NF+ axons abundant in white matter and the NF− ependymoma. Synaptophysin shows a corresponding distinct border between positively reacting neuropil and negatively reacting tumor.[123]

Electron microscopy is a useful adjunct to IHC for difficult ependymomas (see Fig. 18–17*C*). It shows cilia, basal bodies, cytoplasmic inclusions of microvilli, and elongated intercellular junctions.

Rare ependymomas have sparse CK or EMA immunoreactivity on their most differentiated epithelium. They have much less CAM5.2 low molecular weight CK than choroid plexus papillomas and carcinomas. CAM5.2 is recommended to distinguish them.

The general features of ependymoma just described are useful in identifying the variants of ependymoma discussed in this section, except where specifically excluded.

Low-Grade Ependymoma

The designation *low-grade* is often dropped from the name for this group of tumors, which are referred to simply as "ependymomas." The features just described and the nuclear features of low-grade ependymomas distinguish them from other tumors. Nuclei of ependymomas are typically round or oval with prominent light and dark regions stained with hematoxylin (see Figs. 18–17A and 18–18). In the parenchyma away from rosettes, nuclei tend to be more uniformly crowded than nuclei in low-grade astrocytomas and less crowded than in medulloblastomas and primitive neuroectodermal tumors (see Figs. 18–7, 18–11, 18–17, and 18–34).

Epithelioid ependymomas occasionally have remarkably distinct margins with brain that imitate margins of nonglial neoplasms (see Box 2). Anti-GFAP stain for glial filaments is extremely helpful in differentiating these ependymomas from carcinomas, pituitary adenomas, craniopharyngiomas, and meningiomas (see Fig. 18–17B and Table 18–6). The stain accentuates fibrillar cellular processes, which distinguish the ependymoma.[64]

Papillary ependymomas closely resemble choroid plexus papillomas. Solid regions of ependymoma parenchyma where GFAP+ neoplastic cells grow on one another rather than on fibrovascular stroma can be appreciated from their lack of collagen and fibronectin with immunohistochemical staining.[64] Histologic grade is less predictive of survival in ependymoma than in astrocytoma.[182, 183] Radiographic evidence of residual disease after surgery predicts markedly reduced survival, putting a premium on correct intraoperative diagnosis

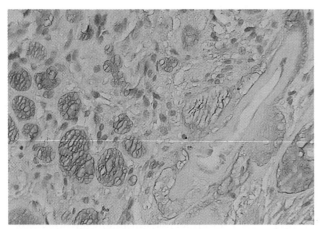

Figure 18–18. Myxopapillary ependymoma. This tumor originated in the cauda equina of a middle-aged woman who had experienced knee pains for several years. It has epithelioid cells and blue-tinged mucin both in the center of vague ependymal rosettes and in the perivascular space. (Alcian blue and nuclear fast red) (From McKeever PE, Blaivas M. The brain, spinal cord, and meninges. In: Sternberg SS, ed. Diagnostic Surgical Pathology. 2nd ed. New York: Raven Press, 1994:409–492.)

and grossly total removal of the tumor. In infratentorial ependymomas, expression of large amounts of GFAP is associated with better prognosis.[184]

Clear Cell Ependymoma

Clear cell ependymoma resembles oligodendroglioma and central neurocytoma (Fig. 18–19A; see Figs. 18–17A and 18–29A). It is an epithelioid ependymoma that also has clear perinuclear halos. Immunohistochemical staining for GFAP may reveal ependymal features such as perivascular fibrils (see Fig. 18–17B). The clear cell appearance of these ependymomas requires a panel of immunohistochemical reagents or, often, electron microscopy to differentiate them from other clear cell tumors (see Fig. 18–17C and Box 1).[175, 185, 186]

Tanycytic Ependymoma

Tanycytic ependymomas are found within the brain and particularly the spinal cord.[64] Their round to oval nuclei with distinctly light and dark regions of chromatin resemble those of ependymoma. Their abundant GFAP+ cellular processes resemble astrocytomas. They form structures replete with nuclei next to zones of fibrillar cellular processes. These structures are distinguished from Verocay bodies by their diffuse, extensive GFAP positivity and their lack of type IV collagen. They are not limited to surrounding GFAP– vessels like the perivascular rosettes of other ependymomas. The margins of tanycytic ependymomas with surrounding parenchyma tend to be discrete, to exclude NF+ axons of spinal cord tracts, and to be potentially resectable, the last being a good reason to distinguish them from diffuse astrocytomas. Diffuse astrocytoma cells infiltrate between NF+ axons.

Subependymoma (WHO Grade I)

The subependymoma protrudes from the wall of a ventricle into the ventricular space.[64, 155] Its histologic and immunohistochemical features closely resemble those of tanycytic ependymoma (see Table 18–5). It is usually benign.

Myxopapillary Ependymoma (WHO Grade I; Rarely Grade II)

The myxopapillary ependymoma (MXPE) appears the least glial in H&E-stained slides. It is nearly always found in the region of the filum terminale, cauda equina, sacrum, and adjacent extravertebral soft tissues (see Fig. 18–18 and Table 18–6). This ependymoma differs from others in its amount of mucin production. Its hallmark is parenchymal and perivascular mucin produced by ependymal cells (Fig. 18–18). MXPE is often papillary but may be solid.

Although the differential features described in the general discussion of ependymomas can be useful, the peculiar morphology and growth of MXPEs pose unique problems. Individual tumors vary dramatically between epithelial and fibrillar cells. The most difficult variants of MXPE to recognize are those that are nearly all myxoid or all epithelial. The highly myxoid variety may produce cords of cells in a mucoid matrix resembling chordoma, a neoplasm found in the same location. Presence of GFAP is the key immunohistochemical feature distinguishing MXPE from chordoma.

Fibrillary MXPE may be confused with fibrous meningioma and schwannoma. The epithelial and papillary variants may resemble carcinoma or meningioma.[64] A positive GFAP stain response differentiates the MXPE from GFAP− carcinoma and meningioma. MXPE lacks type IV collagen and fibronectin-positive basement membranes around each cell, a feature of schwannoma (see Fig. 18–47A).

In contrast to metastatic carcinoma, MXPEs lack malignant cytology, have a lower MIB-1 LI, and are focally fibrillar.[187, 188] Paragangliomas may mimic MXPEs, but MXPEs lack chromogranin A and express GFAP.[64]

Anaplastic Ependymoma (Malignant Ependymoma) (WHO Grade III or IV)

Anaplastic ependymomas are ependymomas with malignant features, including conspicuous mitotic activity, nuclear and cellular pleomorphism, multinucleated and giant cells, high cellular density, necrosis, and vascular proliferation (see Tables 18–5 and 18–6).

Histopathologic features of malignancy do not accurately predict poor survival.[189] This problem may eventually be solved by IHC. The combination of increased vimentin expression and decreased GFAP expression may predict poor survival in infratentorial anaplastic ependymomas.[184]

OLIGODENDROGLIOMA (WHO GRADE II)

The oligodendroglioma and particularly its anaplastic counterpart have been found to respond to PCV chemotherapy.[145, 190] This feature has put a premium on the recognition of both tumors. Chromosomal deletions in 1p and 19q are associated with favorable prognosis, and many such deletions occur in these tumors.[145, 191] The pure oligodendroglioma differs from other gliomas, except for a few ependymomas, in having an epithelioid rather than a fibrillar appearance (see Table 18–6). This appearance is most evident within the central portion of the neoplasm, which is most crowded with neoplastic cells.[64] *Perinuclear halos* are an important feature of formalin-fixed paraffin sections of oligo-

dendroglioma (Fig. 18–19). Well-differentiated oligodendrogliomas have remarkably round and regular nuclei centrally placed within cells, which thereby resemble fried eggs. Their vessels are usually numerous, fine, CD31+ capillaries that sometimes segregate the parenchyma into small lobules.[192]

The category of oligodendroglioma was broadened in the late 1990s to include some tumors formerly considered astrocytomas or mixed gliomas, but it is now being narrowed again. Microgemistocytes have been considered oligodendroglial and are distinguished by their round nuclei and short processes from gemistocytic astrocytoma cells.[193] Microgemistocytes have a ball of cytoplasmic GFAP immunoreactivity near their nucleus and shorter cellular processes than gemistocytic astrocytes and astrocytomas (see Fig. 18–19B).

The epithelioid appearance of pure oligodendrogliomas imitates that of true epithelial neoplasms (see Fig. 18–19C and Table 18–6). Suprasellar oligodendrogliomas may be mistaken for pituitary adenomas (see Box 2). Oligodendrogliomas may be confused with meningotheliomatous meningiomas or with lipoid metaplasia in meningiomas. Anaplastic oligodendrogliomas simulate metastatic carcinoma, particularly renal cell carcinoma. GFAP+ tumor cells (see Fig. 18–19B) distinguish the oligodendroglioma from these other tumors, but not all oligodendrogliomas have GFAP+ neoplastic cells. In their absence, the tumor margin with brain is key (see Box 1). All types of oligodendroglioma, including oligoastrocytoma, have diffuse margins (see Fig. 18–10A). It is also helpful to find reactive astrocytes widely dispersed within an oligodendroglioma (see Fig. 18–19A), a pattern not seen in meningioma.

Even macroscopically discrete oligodendrogliomas show a more diffuse margin with brain than adenomas, carcinomas, and meningiomas. Either NF or synaptophysin used as a brain tissue marker[123] or the presence of GFAP+ gliosis delineates a sharp margin with brain in these other tumors, even carcinomas that engulf chunks of brain (see Figs. 18–22 and 18–23B). Among these tumors, secondary structures are seen only with the oligodendroglioma (see sections on Astrocytomas and Gliomas). Precise localization of the biopsy specimens is helpful, because oligodendrogliomas do not originate from the adenohypophysis or dura and rarely invade them. A panel of immunostains for chromogranin and pituitary hormones can identify adenomas, but there is no specific marker for oligodendroglia that withstands paraffin embedding. The discovery of such a marker would be a major contribution to neuropathology.

The broad specificity of Leu7 and S-100 limit their use for immunohistochemical analysis of oligodendroglioma. However, an oligodendroglioma invading the meninges can be differentiated from a syncytial meningioma by its positivity with the Leu7 monoclonal antibody, because meningiomas

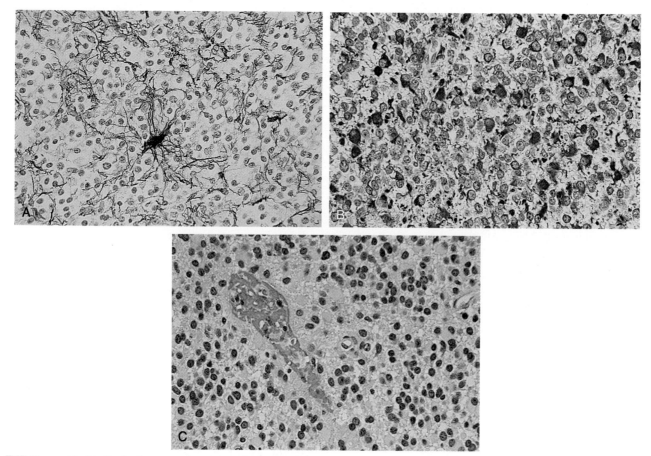

![figure marker] *Figure 18–19.* Both these tumors are considered oligodendrogliomas according to current criteria, primarily on the basis of the roundness of their nuclei and also of their perinuclear halos. *A,* The first tumor has GFAP– neoplastic cells with interlaced GFAP+ processes from intermingling of reactive astrocytes with smaller nuclei. *B,* The second tumor contains numerous GFAP+ "microgemistocytes" with brown balls of cytoplasmic GFAP and relatively short processes. *C,* The H&E preparation of the second tumor shows perinuclear halos in many cells better than GFAP. (Reproduced, with permission, from McKeever PE. Insights about brain tumors gained through immunohistochemistry and in situ hybridization of nuclear and phenotypic markers. The Journal of Histochemistry and Cytochemistry 46:585–594, 1998.)

are typically Leu7–. The expression of synaptophysin by up to 18% of oligodendrogliomas[194] should be kept in mind so that they are not confused with central neurocytomas (CNs) and dysembryoplastic neuroepithelial tumors (DNTs). Both CN and DNT have distinct margins with brain, in contrast to the diffuse margin of oligodendroglioma.

MIB-1 may be useful in predicting good outcome among patients with oligodendrogliomas. MIB-1 LIs less than or equal to 5% have been found to correlate with better survival.[195] Vimentin expression correlates with poor prognosis.[194] Some of this vimentin expression may be due to astrocytic differentiation.[154]

Oligoastrocytoma (Mixed Oligodendroglioma-Astrocytoma) (WHO Grade II)

The oligoastrocytoma is a mixed glioma composed of both astrocytoma and oligodendroglioma,

as described in the respective sections on these tumors (see Fig. 18–10*A*). The problem of distinguishing these pure entities from the mixed oligoastrocytoma has been addressed elsewhere.[196] A solution to this problem awaits a good marker for neoplastic oligodendroglia. Much less common than oligoastrocytoma, mixed gliomas may have a component of ependymoma.[173]

Difficulties are encountered in the attempt to determine whether individual tumors contain a mixture of both oligodendroglial and astrocytic elements and whether both elements are neoplastic. Each element must be conspicuous for this diagnosis. Oligodendroglioma cells must be distinguished from infiltrating macrophages with lipid. The former have neoplastic nuclei and lack immunohistochemical macrophage markers like KP-1 (see Figs. 18–3*A* and 18–19*A*).

The astrocytic component can be assessed for neoplastic cells with hematoxylin, if necessary, after an adjustment to light GFAP staining that does not hide the nuclei. For automatic stainers, the primary anti-GFAP antibody can be titrated to a dilution that shows a discernible light brown. In manual staining, either this titrating can be done or the diaminobenzidine (DAB) substrate can be used for less than half the usual time. Regular-strength hematoxylin counterstain then reveals nuclear details without interference from a dark brown immunohistochemical reaction product, which somehow obscures nuclei even though glial fibrils are cytoplasmic. A good nuclear counterstain should always be used with immunohistochemical analysis of brain lesions. Indistinct cell borders and infiltrations in brain require the counterstain for orientation. The counterstain provides important information about cell type and reactive versus neoplastic cells.

Oligoastrocytomas can undergo anaplastic transformation to grade III neoplasms. A frequent problem is overgrowth of the oligodendroglial component by fibrillar, GFAP+ neoplastic astrocytes. This tumor progression may ultimately result in a glioblastoma.

Anaplastic Oligodendroglioma (Malignant Oligodendroglioma) (WHO Grade III)

The features of anaplastic transformation in oligodendroglioma are similar to those in anaplastic ependymoma (Fig. 18–20).[120] However, limited amounts of vascular proliferation are frequently present in oligodendroglioma, and in isolation, they cannot be considered evidence of malignant transformation (see Table 18–6). Vascular proliferation is highlighted by vimentin and CD31 stains. Alvord[196] has discussed the prognostic importance and difficulty of distinguishing malignant-appear-

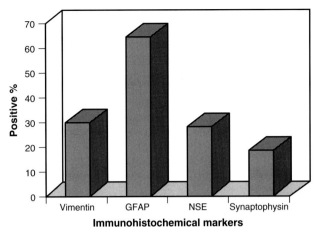

Figure 18–21. Immunohistochemical staining responses among more than 80 cases of oligodendrogliomas (grades II and III). GFAP, glial fibrillary acidic protein; NSE, neuron-specific enolase. *Bars* represent percentages of cases positive for these four markers. (Data from Dehghani F, Schachenmayr W, Laun A, et al. Prognostic implication of histopathological, immunohistochemical and clinical features of oligodendrogliomas: A study of 89 cases. Acta Neuropathol 1998;95:493–504.)

ing oligodendrogliomas from glioblastomas, which are associated with poorer survival.

Partial losses in chromosomes 1 and 19 in anaplastic oligodendrogliomas correspond with particularly good response to PCV chemotherapy.[145] Both ISH enhanced by immunostaining and PCR assay methods detect these chromosomal abnormalities.[191] Although these losses are common in anaplastic oligodendrogliomas, their presence is not restricted to this glioma.

Anaplastic and low-grade oligodendrogliomas may express neuronal markers and vimentin (Fig. 18–21). Synaptophysin-positive cells are scattered sparsely when present.

GLIOBLASTOMA MULTIFORME (GLIOBLASTOMA) (WHO GRADE IV)

In large part resulting from revelations of its frequent expression of GFAP+ fibrillar cellular processes, glioblastoma is now considered the most malignant of astrocytomas rather than an embryonal neuroglial malignancy. It often contains focal astrocytoma, less often oligodendroglioma, and rarely ependymoma.[120] A lower grade astrocytoma may progress to glioblastoma over time, and many of these progressions are associated with loss of genetic material in chromosome 10.[197, 198] These losses can be observed with comparative genomic hybridization[197] or ISH enhanced with immunostaining[199] or by PCR assay. Amplifications of chromosome 7 DNA are also demonstrated by these techniques.[200]

The diagnostic criteria for glioblastoma were relaxed in the 1990s.[120] Formerly, the cytologic cri-

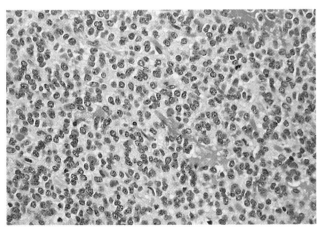

Figure 18–20. This anaplastic oligodendroglioma, grade III, is more crowded with more pleomorphic nuclei than the grade II oligodendrogliomas shown in Fig. 18–19. Mitotic figures are numerous. (H&E) (From McKeever PE. New methods of brain tumor analysis. In: Mena H, ed. Dr. Kenneth M. Earle Memorial Neuropathology Review. Washington, D.C.: Armed Forces Institute of Pathology, February 24, 2000.)

teria of anaplastic astrocytoma (mitotic activity, hypercellularity, pleomorphic, nuclear hyperchromasia) plus both vascular proliferation and spontaneous necrosis were required (see Fig. 18–9*B*). Now, either vascular proliferation *or* spontaneous coagulation necrosis is sufficient addition to anaplasia for the diagnosis of glioblastoma.

If necrosis is absent, *vascular proliferation* (increased density of cells in vascular walls) should be unequivocal; it can be highlighted with vascular endothelial growth factor (VEGF),[201] vimentin, collagen type IV, or fibronectin stain. Other malignant features of glioblastomas are bizarre nuclei, multinucleated cells, and extreme pleomorphism (see Figs. 18–9*B*, 18–23*A*, and 18–24). Unfortunately, the heterogeneity of glioblastomas for these histologic features compromises diagnoses obtained on small specimens, such as those obtained with stereotactic needle biopsy, and jeopardizes accurate grading (see Fig. 18–9).[201, 202]

Most confusion arises in distinguishing glioblastoma from malignant meningioma and from carcinoma. Unlike carcinoma and meningioma, glioblastomas contain fibrillar neoplastic cells that express GFAP in their cellular processes (Figs. 18–22 to 18–24; see Tables 18–5 to 18–7 and 18–9; see Figs. 18–1 and 18–9*B*). The cytologic features of the GFAP+ cells should be checked for anaplasia to confirm glioblastoma, because either carcinoma or malignant melanoma may trap islands of CNS parenchyma and stimulate gliosis (see Figs. 18–22 and 18–23). Sarcoma is easily confused with glioblastoma on H&E staining, but GFAP reveals the glioblastoma (see Fig. 18–24). Although the rapid growth of a glioblastoma may produce a "pseudocapsule," neoplastic glia are evident beyond this margin within brain tissue (Fig. 18–25).

Two varieties of glioblastomas are those that arise de novo and those that arise by progression from lower grade gliomas. The former are often associated with CDKN2A deletions, PTEN altera-

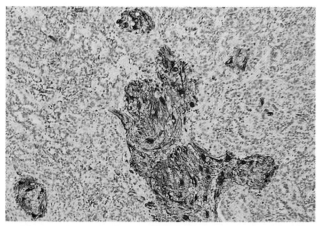

Figure 18–22. This metastatic carcinoma in an elderly man was clinically judged to be a glioma because of its solitary nature and no known primary. Its clear cells and crowded, anaplastic nuclei resemble those of an anaplastic oligodendroglioma. Here at the margin, however, it engulfs brain, excluding rather than intermingling with the resulting islands of brown, GFAP+ gliosis. Subsequent clinical evaluation revealed the primary CK+ and GFAP– carcinoma in his left lung base. (From McKeever PE. New methods of brain tumor analysis. In: Mena H, ed. Dr. Kenneth M. Earle Memorial Neuropathology Review. Washington, D.C.: Armed Forces Institute of Pathology, February 24, 2000.)

tions, and epidermal growth factor receptor (EGFR) amplification, the latter with p53 mutations.[203] EGFR and some p53 alterations can be defined immunohistochemically.

Gliosarcoma (WHO Grade IV)

A gliosarcoma is a mixture of glioblastoma and sarcoma (Fig. 18–26). Regions of collagen-positive and GFAP– sarcoma cells bridge the glioblastoma

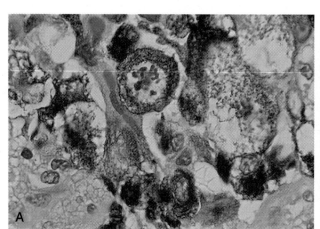
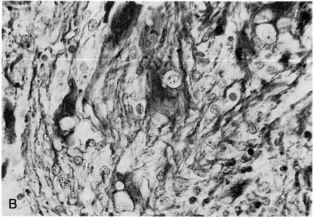

Figure 18–23. Glioblastoma versus trapped gliosis. The importance of examining the perikaryon (cytoplasm around the nucleus) for the marker is shown in these two different tumors stained for GFAP. *A,* GFAP surrounds and touches neoplastic nuclei and a mitosis in the glioblastoma. *B,* GFAP intimately contacts only reactive astrocytic nuclei in this gliosis trapped by metastatic carcinoma. The carcinoma was CK+ (not shown). See also Figure 18–22. (From McKeever PE. New methods of brain tumor analysis. In: Mena H, ed. Dr. Kenneth M. Earle Memorial Neuropathology Review. Washington, D.C.: Armed Forces Institute of Pathology, February 24, 2000.)

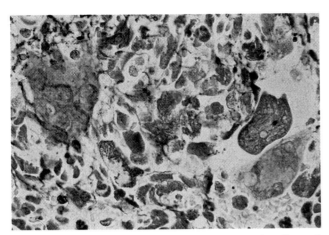

Figure 18-24. Extreme pleomorphism of cells and nuclei in a glioblastoma includes a huge brown, GFAP+ cell with multiple nuclei. Giant cell glioblastomas were called *monstrocellular sarcomas* prior to recognition of their GFAP reactivity. (From McKeever PE. New methods of brain tumor analysis. In: Mena H, ed. Dr. Kenneth M. Earle Memorial Neuropathology Review. Washington, D.C.: Armed Forces Institute of Pathology, February 24, 2000.)

in a marbled configuration (see Table 18-5). Differences in collagen messenger RNA and cellular DNA content indicate the extent of variation between these regions.[204, 205] Despite the fact that gliosarcomas often seem more circumscribed than the glioblastoma, gliosarcoma can metastasize.[150, 206] Tumor progression from gliosarcoma to pure sarcoma lacking GFAP+ cells can occur.[206, 207] The glial and mesenchymal elements have similar genetic alterations.[199, 208]

Glioblastoma and Gliosarcoma with Epithelial Metaplasia (WHO Grade IV)

Rarely, gliosarcomas and glioblastomas produce adenoid formations or epithelial foci with squamous differentiation and keratin pearls.[209, 210] These regions stain immunohistochemically for CK and EMA (Table 18-7; see Fig. 18-26D). Adequate sampling and the awareness that these regions are focal and that other regions of these gliomas will show the familiar fibrillar, GFAP+ neoplastic cells of a glioblastoma are necessary to avoid confusion of this tumor with carcinoma. It is important to remember that carcinoma cells are GFAP-.

Glioblastomas manifest other peculiar features. Rare glioblastomas occur with granular cell tumors.[211] Some epithelioid glioblastomas contain diffuse cytoplasmic lipid.[212]

Neuronal Tumors

Neuronal tumors contain an abnormal proliferation of neurons. They range from the most benign gangliocytoma to the rare anaplastic ganglioglioma,

ganglioneuroblastoma, and CNS neuroblastoma[120] (see Tables 18-5, 18-7, and 18-8). Most low-grade ganglion cell neoplasms have a better prognosis than gliomas found in the same location, and their proper identification is important.

The identification and evaluation of ganglion cell neoplasms has four important stages:
1. Recognition of neurons (Fig. 18-27).
2. Confirmation that neurons are neoplastic
3. Determination of whether glia are present
4. Evaluation of any glia for neoplasia

Many neoplastic cells, particularly cells of glioblastomas, melanomas and astrocytomas, resemble neurons because of their large size or prominent nucleoli.[151, 213, 214] These cells lack NF and synaptophysin markers of neurons (see Figs. 18-25 and 18-37D). The most important step in using NF or synaptophysin to identify a neuron is to trace the marker back to the cell body (perikaryon). Synaptophysin is present in the neuropil, making evaluation of cellular surface staining difficult. Commercial anti-NF and anti-synaptophysin immunoperoxidase markers of neurons must be chosen carefully, and their use must be controlled by staining of normal brain specimens in the same batch of slides and preferably in the same slide as the unknown tumor (see Box 2). In cases refractory to immunohistochemical stains, electron microscopy positively identifies Nissl substance, neurofilaments, neurosecretory granules, and synapses in neoplastic cells.[215] Future immunohistochemical stains may identify neurons by showing their "on target" nuclear features rather than their cytoplasmic or confusing surface features.[216]

A common error in determining whether identified neurons are neoplastic is to interpret a field of normal neurons infiltrated by glioma cells as a ganglioglioma. Nevertheless, many neoplastic neurons show either synaptophysin or NF in their cytoplasm (see Fig. 18-27B). As previously described, the synaptophysin or NF should be traced

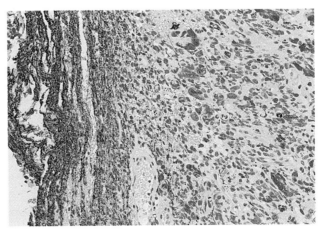

Figure 18-25. This giant cell glioblastoma has a relatively abrupt margin with brown NF+ cerebral white matter. However, near the appropriately NF- vessel and large abnormal mitotic spindle, the tumor infiltrates between brown long axons.

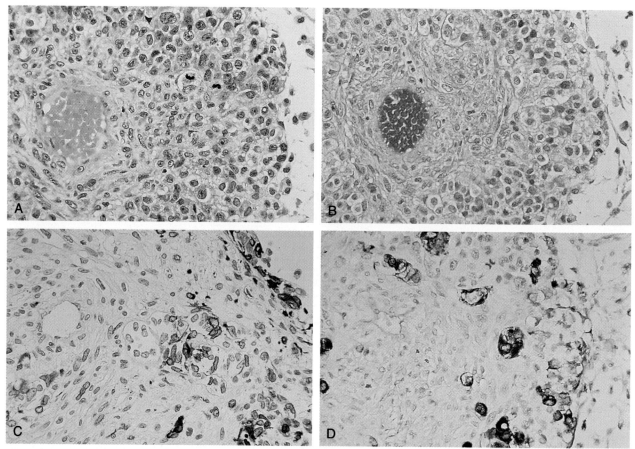

Figure 18-26. This gliosarcoma, shown in *A* with H&E staining, had regions and bands of collagen-positive, GFAP− sarcoma cells and other regions of GFAP+, collagen-negative malignant astrocytes. *B,* Shown under high magnification here, sarcoma cells produce cyan collagen as they wander away from a vessel into tumor parenchyma. (Masson's trichrome stain) *C,* A nearby section shows most collagen-associated cells to be GFAP−, whereas malignant astrocytes further from the vessel are GFAP+. *D,* Epithelial metaplasia of brown CAM5.2+ cells was present in small foci in other regions of this gliosarcoma. (From McKeever PE. New methods of brain tumor analysis. In: Mena H, ed. Dr. Kenneth M. Earle Memorial Neuropathology Review. Washington, D.C.: Armed Forces Institute of Pathology, February 24, 2000.)

back to a cell body, and hematoxylin-stained nuclear features should be used to determine whether the cell is neoplastic according to standard criteria for pleomorphism and atypia. Evidence of neuronal neoplasia includes hypercellularity and disarray of neurons, binucleated neurons, and pleomorphism in cells that respond positively to staining for synaptophysin or NF (see Fig. 18–27*B*). Degenerative changes in such neoplastic neurons may occur.[213] Ganglion cell tumors may show heavy bands of collagen and fibronectin-positive fibrous tissue, or they may show perivascular round cells, but neither of these is invariably present.

Gangliocytoma (WHO Grade I), Ganglioglioma (WHO Grade I or II), and Anaplastic Ganglioglioma (WHO Grade III or IV)

Gangliocytoma, ganglioglioma, and anaplastic ganglioglioma may arise anywhere[217] but are most common in the cerebrum, particularly the temporal lobe.

Once a ganglion cell neoplasm has been identified, the glial element must be evaluated (see Table 18–5). A section lightly stained for GFAP with immunoperoxidase (either with less than half the usual time in DAB substrate in manual staining, or with use of a lower primary antibody titer in an automatic stainer) and fully counterstained with hematoxylin facilitates this determination by providing a better view of glial nuclei. If the light brown cells appear reactive, cluster near the margin of the neoplasm, and do not meet the criteria for neoplasia described in the section on Diffuse Astrocytoma, the tumor is a gangliocytoma or central neurocytoma (see later). If the GFAP+ cells are neoplastic but not anaplastic, the neoplasm is a ganglioglioma (see Fig. 18–30*B*). If these glial elements are anaplastic (see sections on Anaplastic Astrocytoma and Glioblastoma), the neoplasm is an anaplastic ganglioglioma.[64] The proliferative capacity of the GFAP+ glial component of gan-

Table 18–7. Differential Diagnosis of a Mass of Conspicuously Different Cells

Diagnosis*	Structures	Antibody†	Locations‡
		Differential Features	
Oligoastrocytoma	Mixture of astrocytoma (Table 18–5) and oligodendroglioma (Table 18–6)	GFAP (+/−); Leu7 (+); S-100 (+)	Cerebrum; CNS
Anaplastic oligoastrocytoma	Above features with mitoses and pleomorphism	GFAP (+/−); Leu7 (+/−); S-100 (+/−)	Cerebrum; CNS
Glioblastoma/gliosarcoma with epithelial metaplasia	Structures of glioblastoma/gliosarcoma (Table 18–5) plus epithelial regions	GFAP (+/−); S-100 (+/−); cytokeratin (+/−); EMA (+/−)	Cerebrum; CNS
Ganglion cell tumors	Binucleated and pleomorphic neurons plus glioma (Table 18–5) plus fibrosis plus inflammation	GFAP (+/−); synaptophysin (+/−); PGP9.5; neurofilament (R); type IV collagen (R)	Cerebrum, CNS
Desmoplastic medulloblastoma	Regions of medulloblastoma and fibrosis	Synaptophysin; S-100; type IV collagen; neurofilament (R); GFAP (R)	Lateral cerebellum; CNS; meninges; (extra-axial)§
Transitional meningioma	Regions of fibrous (Table 18–5) and syncytial (Table 18–9) meningioma	Vimentin (+); EMA (+/−); S-100 (R)	Falx; tentorium; meninges; choroid plexus
Hemangioblastoma	Multivacuolated stromal cells between many capillaries; hypervascularity; (fibrillarity is frozen section artifact)§	CD31 (+/−); factor VIII (+/−); NSE (+/−)	Cerebellum; spinal cord; CNS
Desmoplastic carcinoma	Regions of carcinoma (Table 18–6) and fibrosis (Table 18–5); occasional inflammation	Cytokeratin (+/−); EMA (+/−)	Cerebrum; cerebellum; meninges; CNS; frequent multiple masses; systemic
Melanoma	Regions of fibrillar and epithelioid melanoma (Tables 18–5 and 18–6)	HMB-45 (+/−); S-100 (+)	Cerebrum; cerebellum; meninges; CNS; frequently multiple masses; systemic

* The order of tabulated lesions follows the order of discussion in text.
† Key to staining results:
  (+) = Almost always strong, diffuse positivity
  (+/−) = Variable, many positive; or mixed cell populations
  R = Rare cells may be positive
‡ Most common or most specific location is listed first.
§ Parentheses around a differential feature indicate an uncommon feature that is very useful in differential diagnosis when found.
CNS, central nervous system; EMA, epithelial membrane antigen; GFAP, glial fibrillary acidic protein; NSE, neuron-specific enolase.
Modified from McKeever PE, Blaivas M. The brain, spinal cord, and meninges. In: Sternberg SS, ed. Diagnostic Surgical Pathology. 2nd ed. New York: Raven Press, 1994:409–492.

glion cell tumors is critical to their histologic grade and can be assessed immunohistochemically with MIB-1 or PCNA. Only the astrocytic component has immunoreactivity for such proliferation markers, and it is usually low.[218]

If the GFAP stain response is negative and no neoplastic glia are found, the tumor is purely neuronal. Gangliocytomas tend to be benign. They often contain immunocytochemical positivity for at least one neurotransmitter peptide or amine, including somatostatin, corticotropin-releasing hormone, beta-endorphin, galanin, vasoactive intesti-

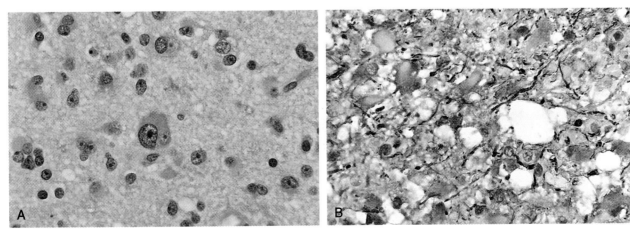

Figure 18–27. Ganglioglioma from the parietal lobe of a middle-aged man with progressive unilateral loss of coordination exhibits binucleated ganglion cells with large nucleoli and Nissl substance on H&E (*A*) and NF staining (*B*). This specimen was prepared with immunoperoxidase anti-NF protein with hematoxylin.

nal peptide, calcitonin, serotonin, catecholamines, and met-enkephalin.[219]

Dysplastic Gangliocytoma of the Cerebellum

An unusual variant of a gangliocytoma, dysplastic gangliocytoma of the cerebellum (DGC) is also known as Lhermitte-Duclos disease.[171] Hyperplastic and disordered, synaptophysin-positive granular cell neurons enlarge a part of the cerebellum into bizarre "megafolia." This rare tumor looks dysplastic but has recurred after surgery. The growth potential of individual tumors can be monitored by staining for MIB-1. Some DGCs are familial, and some are associated with Cowden's syndrome or with multiple hamartoma-neoplasia syndrome.[220]

Dysembryoplastic Neuroepithelial Tumor

DNT may be the hamartomatous counterpart of a ganglioglioma.[221] It is multinodular within the cerebral cortex, most often in the temporal lobe cortex. Some DNTs are cystic (Fig. 18–28A). Some are incidental findings, but many others are associated with long-standing partial complex seizure disorders in children and young adults.[222]

The DNT has prominent cells that resemble oligodendroglia and NF+ neurons or synaptophysin-positive neurons or both that often appear to float within Alcian blue–positive acid mucopolysaccharide.[155, 222] These are called "floating neurons" (see Fig. 18–28B). Other large neurons lack their normal spacing (see Fig. 18–28C). GFAP+ astrocytes are variably present within the tumor and often surround it. This tumor's low MIB-1 LI, mature histotopographic appearance, and association with cortical dysplasia suggest a maldevelopmental origin.[223]

Oligodendrogliomas can produce mucopolysaccharide and can even "float" an occasional normal neuron. Lack of mass effect, discrete cortical location, low MIB-1 LI, and lack of brain infiltration typify DNTs and distinguish them from oligodendrogliomas.[224] Evaluating the tumor margin with serial sections evaluated immunohistochemically for NF, MIB-1, and synaptophysin shows these features.[123] Neuronal nuclear antigen, if present, may also identify a DNT.[225]

Central Neurocytoma

Recognized fairly recently, CN has stimulated much interest because of its structural beauty, hid-

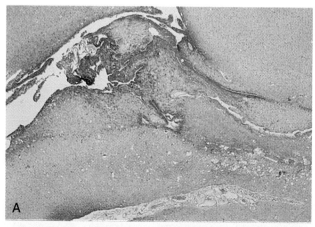

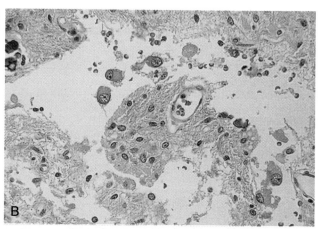

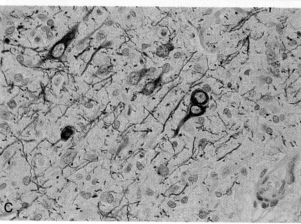

Figure 18–28. Dysembryoplastic neuroepithelial tumor (DNT). *A,* This cystic tumor has multiple cortical nodules surrounded by brown GFAP+ astrocytes near a collapsed cyst. *B,* Neurons float in cystic spaces. *C,* Brown, large, NF+ "kissing neurons" compress and mold into one another. This specimen is from a 40-year-old man who had long-standing, medically refractory epilepsy and a right frontal multinodular cortical tumor. (From McKeever PE. New methods of brain tumor analysis. In: Mena H, ed. Dr. Kenneth M. Earle Memorial Neuropathology Review. Washington, D.C.: Armed Forces Institute of Pathology, February 24, 2000.)

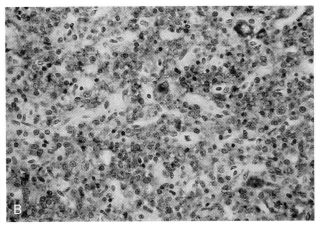

Figure 18–29. Central neurocytoma. *A,* The fibrillar perivascular zone and round cells with halos around round nuclei imitate features of ependymoma and oligodendroglioma. (H&E) *B,* Neoplastic cells ubiquitously express synaptophysin. (Reproduced with permission from McKeever PE. Insights about brain tumors gained through immunohistochemistry and in situ hybridization of nuclear and phenotypic markers. The Journal of Histochemistry and Cytochemistry 46:585–594, 1998.)

den identity, and benign prognosis (Fig. 18–29*A*).[226, 227] It is the most common neoplasm involving the septum pellucidum in young adults.[227] Although it often has slightly more fibrillarity, CN resembles oligodendroglioma (see Tables 18–5 and 18–6; see Box 1). Careful application of immunohistochemical markers facilitates proper identification of the tumor, which for years had been mistaken for a glioma (Fig. 18–29). CNs express synaptophysin (see Fig. 18–29*B*), the specificity and immunoreactivity of which have improved.[228–230] They are usually GFAP− but many contain reactive astrocytes. If the synaptophysin stain response is equivocal, electron microscopy is recommended to distinguish central neurocytoma from oligodendroglioma and ependymoma.[231] Microtubules, 100- to 200-nm dense-core vesicles, and clear vesicles identify its true neuronal lineage. Although radiotherapy has been used to treat CNs, a good prognosis usually follows total surgical excision.[229]

DESMOPLASTIC INFANTILE GANGLIOGLIOMA

Desmoplastic infantile gangliogliomas (DIGs) often attain considerable size and resemble very fibrous gangliogliomas (Fig. 18–30*A*). These neoplasms are found in patients younger than 3 years, are frequently cystic, and often involve the meninges.[64, 232] Their substantial differentiation produces a mixture of GFAP+ glial cell (Fig. 18–30*B*), NF+ and synaptophysin-positive neurons, and vimentin-positive fibrovascular cells.[233]

GANGLIONEUROBLASTOMA (WHO GRADE III) AND NEUROBLASTOMA (WHO GRADE IV)

Neuroblasts are rare in both gangliocytomas and gangliogliomas. Neuroblasts are identified from their spherical nuclei, prominent central nucleoli,

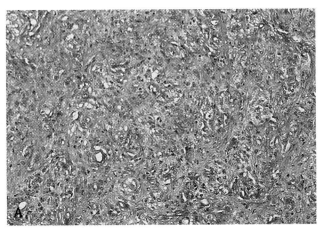
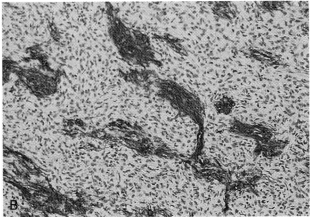

Figure 18–30. Desmoplastic infantile ganglioglioma (DIG). *A,* This massive tumor of the left cerebral hemisphere of a male infant contains red-stained abnormal binucleated neurons and glia mixed within a complex network of blue desmoplasia. (trichrome) *B,* GFAP highlights islands of brown astrocytes.

synaptophysin immunoreactivity, and negativity for lymphocyte markers such as LCA, A6, and L26 (Table 18–8). They may show transitional forms that are mature and recognizable ganglion cells. If more than half of a tumor's neoplastic cells are neuroblasts but it still contains mature neoplastic ganglion cells, the neoplasm is a ganglioneuroblastoma.

Fields of primitive neuroblasts with a tendency to form rosettes having fibrillary cores and no lumen (Homer Wright rosettes) are features of neuroblastoma in the cerebrum. The differentiation of this rare entity from a primitive neuroectodermal tumor is controversial.[173, 234]

Choroid Plexus Epithelial Tumors

Most choroid plexus neoplasms appear in childhood. They can occur in any portion of choroid plexus (see Table 18–6) but are more common in the lateral ventricles of children and the fourth ventricle of adults.[64]

CHOROID PLEXUS PAPILLOMA (WHO GRADE I)

In contrast to papillary ependymoma, the choroid plexus papilloma contains a layer of columnar to cuboidal epithelial cells over a basement membrane and fibrovascular stroma. The type IV collagen and laminin in this stroma contrast with ependymomas, which have solid parenchyma without collagen or laminin (see Tables 18–5 and 18–6; see section on Ependymomas). Focal GFAP reactivity in certain choroid plexus papillomas suggests focal ependymal differentiation.[235, 236] This overlap in immunostaining responses includes other markers, although choroid plexus papillomas express substantially more CAM5.2 cytokeratin and EMA than ependymomas.[235, 236] The CAM5.2 response is often particularly robust (Fig. 18–31*A*). Transthyretin is a potential marker of this papilloma (see Fig. 18–31*B*), but its spectrum of reactivity is broad.[237, 238]

Newer potential markers of choroid plexus papillomas include insulin-like growth factor II (IGF-II) and synaptophysin. IGF-II is found in papillomas but not in normal choroid plexus.[239] Synaptophysin is present in normal choroid plexus, choroid plexus papilloma, and choroid plexus carcinoma but not in metastatic papillary carcinoma.[240] Both markers may assist in the differential diagnoses. CD44 is preferentially expressed on atypical papilloma and choroid plexus carcinoma and may be a marker of aggressive choroid plexus tumors.[241] Aggressive tumors have higher mean MIB-1 LIs of 6%.[242] These new stains are promising, and their results should be verified with larger series of cases.

An epithelial lining of CAM5.2 cytokeratin–positive cells in the choroid plexus papilloma, lack of whorls, and lack of syncytial foci distinguish it from papillary meningioma. Secretory meningioma has focal CK response but not in an epithelial lining with a fibrovascular core. The choroid plexus

Table 18–8. Differential Diagnosis of a Mass of Small, Crowded, Anaplastic Cells

Diagnosis	Differential Features		
	Structures	*Antibody**	*Locations†*
Ependymoblastoma	Like PNET; ribbons/cords of cells; true ependymal rosettes	Vimentin (+/−); GFAP (R)	Cerebrum; cerebellum
Medulloblastoma/pineoblastoma/neuroblastoma/PNET	Slight fibrillarity; (Homer Wright rosettes); (palisades); "carrot" nuclei; (neural or glial foci)‡	Synaptophysin (+/−); PGP9.5; S-100 (R); neurofilament (R); GFAP (R)	Cerebellum; brainstem; pineal; CNS; (extra-axial)‡
Rhabdomyosarcoma/medullomyoblastoma	Like PNET; muscle striations	Desmin (+/−); muscle-specific actin	Pineal; cerebellum; CNS
Atypical teratoid/rhabdoid tumor	Like PNET; more cytoplasm	Vimentin (+); GFAP (+/−); cytokeratin (+/−); EMA (R); synaptophysin (R); chromogranin (R)	Cerebellum; brain
Hemangiopericytoma	Hypercellularity; thick pericellular matrix; mitoses	Vimentin (+)	Falx, tentorium meninges; (extracranial)‡
Lymphoma	Noncohesive round cells; vascular wall invasion	L26 (+); LCA (+/−); monoclonal κ and λ Ig	Deep cerebrum; CNS; meninges; may be multiple
Small cell carcinoma	Cohesive cells; (epithelioid); (desmosomes)‡	Cytokeratin (+); EMA; synaptophysin (+/−)	CNS; meninges; frequent multiple masses; systemic

* Key to staining results:
  (+) = Almost always strong, diffuse positivity
  (+/−) = Variable, many positive
  R = Rare cells may be positive
† Most common or most specific location is listed first.
‡ Parentheses around a differential feature indicate an uncommon feature that is very useful in differential diagnosis when found.
CNS, central nervous system; EMA, epithelial membrane antigen; GFAP, glial fibrillary acidic protein; Ig, immunoglobulin; LCA, leukocyte common antigen; PNET, primitive neuroectodermal tumor.
Modified from McKeever PE, Blaivas M. The brain, spinal cord, and meninges. In: Sternberg SS, ed. Diagnostic Surgical Pathology. 2nd ed. New York: Raven Press, 1994:409–492.

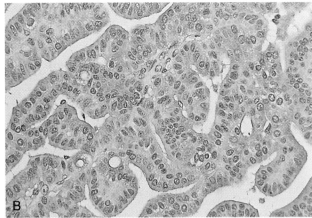

Figure 18–31. Choroid plexus papilloma. This choroid plexus papilloma from the lateral ventricle of a child is composed of well-differentiated columnar epithelium resting upon a fibrovascular stroma. It expresses CAM5.2 low molecular weight cytokeratin (*A*) and transthyretin (*B*). The fibrovascular stroma is easily identified from its negativity for cytokeratin. (Immunoperoxidase anti-CAM5.2 and anti-prealbumin) (From McKeever PE, Blaivas M. The brain, spinal cord, and meninges. In: Sternberg SS, Diagnostic Surgical Pathology. 2nd ed. New York: Raven Press, 1994;409–492.)

papilloma lacks the necrosis and anaplasia seen in metastatic papillary carcinoma.

CHOROID PLEXUS CARCINOMA (WHO GRADE III OR IV)

The choroid plexus carcinoma (anaplastic choroid plexus papilloma) is a rare neoplasm that is most difficult to distinguish from metastatic carcinoma (see Table 18–6).[243] Each of these tumors produces CK, and each may produce transthyretin. If found, a transitional zone between papilloma and carcinoma of the choroid plexus confirms choroid plexus carcinoma. Primary carcinoma of the choroid plexus so closely resembles metastatic carcinoma that the latter must be carefully excluded before the diagnosis of primary choroid plexus carcinoma can be made.[120, 173] Occult pulmonary or gastrointestinal primary tumors are common sources. The paucity of these primary systemic carcinomas in children facilitates diagnosis of choroid plexus carcinoma in a patient in this age group. Some choroid plexus carcinomas express CD44 cell adhesion molecule not seen in the most benign papillomas.[242] The mean MIB-1 LI of choroid plexus carcinomas is 14%, higher than that of papillomas.[242]

Pineal Cell Tumors

Tumors described in this section arise from pineal cells or their precursors.[244] Because tumors that arise from pineal cells are neurons, synaptophysin immunoreactivity is common. Some tumors also react for retinal-S antigen (Fig. 18–32).[245] Many other tumors, including gliomas, meningiomas, and germ cell tumors, occur in the pineal region. They are described in their respective sections in this chapter.

PINEOCYTOMA (WHO GRADE II)

Pineocytoma simulates the normal pineal gland (see Table 18–5). Synaptophysin-positive cells with round nuclei are divided by fibrovascular stroma into lobules. Other cells surround fibrillary centers.[171] The cells are fibrillar and often radiate toward the vessels.[244] Immunohistochemical stains for NFs may reveal expansions at the tips of these processes resembling clubs,[173] and electron microscopy shows their similarity to neurons.[64] These neural features distinguish pineocytoma from gliomas. The major source of confusion with this histologic picture is with normal pineal gland. An MIB-1 LI higher than normal pineal gland, a specimen larger than the 0.5-cm diameter of the normal pineal gland, or invasion beyond the pineal gland confirms the diagnosis of pineocytoma.

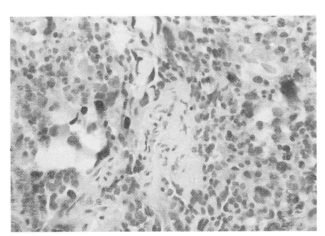

Figure 18–32. Pineocytoma. Neoplastic cells with round nuclei include some that express retinal-S antigen. (Courtesy of Dr. Hernando Mena, Chairman, Department of Neuropathology, Armed Forces Institute of Pathology, Washington, D.C.)

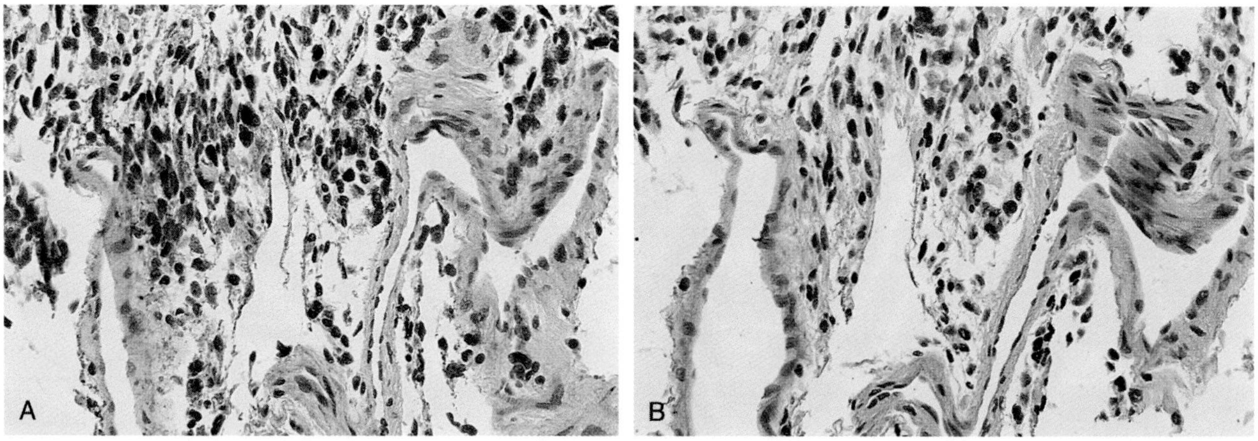

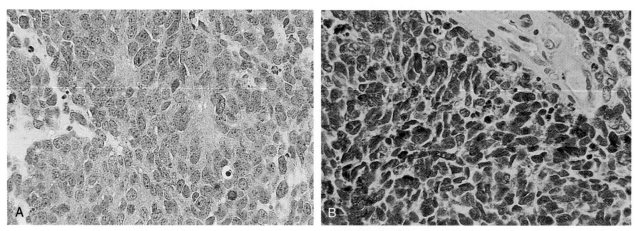

Figure 18–33. Crowded malignant cells with pleomorphic and hyperchromatic nuclei in this pineal tumor express synaptophysin (*A*) but not GFAP (*B*) in serial sections of this pineoblastoma.

PINEAL CELL TUMOR OF INTERMEDIATE GRADE (WHO GRADE III)

Primary pineal cell tumors are less differentiated than pineocytomas and more differentiated than pineoblastomas. They show mitotic activity and moderate crowding of their synaptophysin-positive cells. They may contain regions that resemble pineocytoma near regions like pineoblastoma. Their proliferation is regionally variable, with "hot spots" of proliferation higher than that of pineocytoma.

PINEOBLASTOMA (GRADE IV)

Pineoblastoma resembles medulloblastoma (Figs. 18–33 and 18–34) except for its origin in the pineal gland (see Table 18–8). Fibrillary rosettes may be evident and are more common than Flexner-Wintersteiner rosettes. Synaptophysin is most use-

ful in identifying neuronal differentiation in these tumors (see Fig. 18–33*A*), because NF immunoreactivity is often negative. Both pineoblastoma and medulloblastoma have been classified as primitive neuroectodermal tumors (PNETs).[234] Some tumors express retinal-S antigen.[245] It would be interesting to know whether this "sight"-specific marker is any more common in pineoblastomas than in other PNETs.

Undifferentiated and Multipotential Tumors (All WHO Grade IV)

MEDULLOBLASTOMA

The medulloblastoma is a PNET that arises in the cerebellum or in the roof of the fourth ventricle (see Fig. 18–34 and Table 18–8). It is most

Figure 18–34. One medulloblastoma with well-differentiated Homer Wright rosettes, from the posterior fossa of a girl of elementary school age, was positive for both NF (*A*) and synaptophysin (*not shown*). Another, less well differentiated medulloblastoma, from the posterior fossa of boy of the same age, was synaptophysin-positive (*B*) and NF– (*not shown*). Synaptophysin highlights the sparse fibrillar cellular processes. (From McKeever PE. New methods of brain tumor analysis. In: Mena H, ed. Dr. Kenneth M. Earle Memorial Neuropathology Review. Washington, D.C.: Armed Forces Institute of Pathology, February 24, 2000.)

common in children but also occurs among young adults[246] and rarely in patients older than 35 years.[149] It is often associated with isochromosome 17q (one chromosome composed of two long arms of chromosome 17), which can be detected by ISH enhanced by immunostaining.[121, 247] Because medulloblastomas commonly spread along CSF pathways, treatment should be directed at the entire neuraxis. About 5% of medulloblastomas metastasize to a systemic location,[248] particularly to bone marrow, where synaptophysin staining aids their recognition.

Nuclear crowding and high nuclear to cytoplasmic ratio impart a distinctly *blue* macroscopic appearance to the medulloblastoma on H&E staining. This collection of small malignant cells must be distinguished from small cell undifferentiated carcinoma and lymphoma (see Table 18–8). The examiner should look for cellular processes. To indicate medulloblastoma, the fibrillar cellular processes must come directly from the neoplastic cells. Synaptophysin, S-100 protein, and, less often, NF protein stains highlight these processes. Rosettes with cores filled with fibrils (Homer Wright rosettes) in the CNS are characteristic of medulloblastomas (see Fig. 18–34A); however, in many biopsy samples of medulloblastoma, rosettes are only vague to nonexistent.

Virtually all medulloblastomas express synaptophysin, a marker of neuronal differentiation unseen in lymphoma and uncommon in carcinoma (Fig. 18–34B). Although this valuable marker is best seen on frozen sections,[249] it is more often evident after routine paraffin-formalin processing than NF epitopes. Protein gene product 9.5 (PGP9.5) is another marker of neuronal differentiation of these tumors. S-100 protein may be found in medulloblastomas, but its finding must be carefully interpreted because of its presence in other neoplasms in the differential diagnosis, including most gliomas and some carcinomas.[64, 250] Staining for synaptophysin and the presence of fibrillar cellular processes works best, in my experience (see Fig. 18–34B). Difficult cases can be examined for their ultrastructure.

Although confirmation by larger studies would be appropriate, evidence suggests that GFAP reactivity is associated with longer survival with medulloblastoma than nonreactivity.[251–253]

DESMOPLASTIC MEDULLOBLASTOMA

Regions, and sometimes whole specimens, of medulloblastomas may contain excessive fibrous tissue that can be demonstrated by type IV collagen or Masson's trichrome staining (Fig. 18–35; see Table 18–7). These neoplasms are often located more laterally in the cerebellum than other medulloblastomas and typically occur in young adults. The argument that desmoplastic medulloblastoma is an entity distinct from classic medullo-

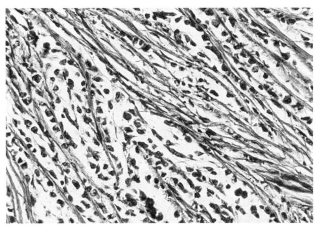

Figure 18–35. This desmoplastic medulloblastoma infiltrates between cyan-colored collagen fibers. (Masson's trichrome) (From McKeever PE. New methods of brain tumor analysis. In: Mena H, ed. Dr. Kenneth M. Earle Memorial Neuropathology Review. Washington, D.C.: Armed Forces Institute of Pathology, February 24, 2000.)

blastoma is supported by observations of differences in DNA content of these two types of tumor.[254]

The desmoplastic reaction is believed to be due to a fibrous connective tissue proliferation on the part of the leptomeningeal cells in the arachnoid space as a result of focal invasion by medulloblastoma cells.[255] These malignant neoplasms sometimes have a remarkable resemblance to the single-file patterns of small cell carcinoma, but the neoplastic cells express synaptophysin and occasionally NF protein in their fibrillar processes (see Table 18–7). Pale islands of cells with perinuclear halos are often neuroblastic and react positively to staining for synaptophysin.[256]

Desmoplasia in some medulloblastomas must be distinguished from infiltrations of vascular walls by CNS lymphomas. Lymphoma cells are the same whether they are in vascular walls or tumor parenchyma. In contrast, the cells of the parenchyma in medulloblastomas have darker, more angulated nuclei than the vascular cells.

PRIMITIVE NEUROECTODERMAL TUMOR

The features and differential diagnosis of PNET can be found in the section on Medulloblastoma. Hart and Earle[257] described PNET. Rorke and colleagues,[234] observing that PNET, medulloblastoma, and pineoblastoma are indistinguishable by histology alone if their location is unknown, named all of these neoplasms PNETs (see Table 18–8). Thus, when one compares nomenclatures, medulloblastoma and pineoblastoma are subsets of central nervous system PNETs (cPNETs) that happen to occur in specific neuroanatomic locations. From H&E staining, immunohistochemical, and ultrastructural features, Rorke and colleagues[234] recognized the following entities:

- PNET not otherwise specified
- PNET with astrocytes
- PNET with oligodendroglia
- PNET with ependymal cells
- PNET with neuronal cells
- PNET with other cells
- PNET with mixed cellular elements

Markers of neuronal differentiation such as synaptophysin and PGP9.5, which are more sensitive than the first generation of anti-NF antibodies, are expanding the numbers of PNETs with neuronal differentiation.[230, 249, 258] Expression of a variety of other ectodermal and neuroectodermal antigens and association with neural tube defects reflects the embryonal nature of these neoplasms.[259–262]

In contrast to the cPNET, the peripheral PNET (pPNET) is defined by its t(11,22q24;q12) chromosomal translocation.[263] Peripheral PNETs are intensely immunoreactive with MIC2 (Fig. 18–36) and neuron-specific enolase (NSE).[264] Sites of occurrence of pPNET include neural crest derivatives, gonads, chest wall, bone including vertebral column, cranial vault, and cauda equina.[265, 266] Peripheral PNETs are highly aggressive. They recur locally and metastasize to specific organs.[267]

MEDULLOMYOBLASTOMA

Medullomyoblastomas occur in the midline posterior fossa of children and contain smooth or striated muscle fibers.[149] They are mixtures of stainable muscle cells and small neuroectodermal cells resembling medulloblastoma, in contrast to pure primary intracranial rhabdomyosarcomas, which do not contain cells derived from neuroectoderm.[155, 268] Synaptophysin and retinal-S antigen markers facilitate detection of these neuroectodermal cells.[269] Immunoperoxidase stains for desmin and muscle-specific actin markers confirm muscular differentiation (see Table 18–8).[270, 271] Mesodermal elements other than muscle are occasionally found in medulloblastomas and medullomyoblastomas.[268, 270] The lipomatous medulloblastoma has been described as a distinct entity with a better prognosis.[270]

ATYPICAL TERATOID-RHABDOID TUMOR

Atypical teratoid-rhabdoid tumor has been defined relatively recently (see Table 18–8). Infants and young children suffer from this highly malignant tumor.[272] It occurs in the posterior fossa and metastasizes early through the CSF. Malignant cells have more pink cytoplasm and are more epithelial than those in medulloblastoma. The plethora of immunohistochemical markers that these express contributes significantly to the definition of this tumor (Fig. 18–37). Atypical teratoid-rhabdoid

tumor contains multiple intermediate filament (IF) types: always vimentin, and often focal GFAP, CK, or other IF types. EMA, synaptophysin, and chromogranin may be present. Atypical teratoid-rhabdoid tumors have abnormalities of chromosome 22 that help to distinguish them from other PNETs, including medulloblastoma.[272]

RARE EMBRYONAL TUMORS

The *primitive polar spongioblastoma* is a pediatric tumor with rhythmic palisades of delicate cellular processes and nuclei (see Table 18–5). The unipolar and bipolar cells are immunoreactive for NSE, but not for GFAP.[273]

The *medulloepithelioma* looks like carcinoma but occurs in childhood, an unlikely age for carcinoma. The pseudostratified columnar epithelium of medulloepithelioma is crowded with cells that resemble those lining the embryonic neural tube. It rests on a type IV collagen basement membrane and fibrous stroma. The basal layer of the epithelium expresses nestin, vimentin, and microtubule-associated protein type 5 immunoreactivity.[274] Focal differentiation and expression of either GFAP, S-100 protein, NSE (Fig. 18–38), NF protein, CK, or EMA immunoreactivity frequently occur.[274, 275]

The *ependymoblastoma* usually occurs in the cerebrum of a child (see Table 18–8).[276] It resembles a PNET decorated with very well formed rosettes lined by mitotically active epithelioid cells. Unlike in medulloepithelioma, the rosettes in ependymoblastoma merge into densely cellular malignant cells without a collagenous stroma. Ependymoblastomas contain vimentin. Their GFAP− rosettes stain differently from GFAP+ rosettes in ependymomas.[155] Ependymoblastoma is more cellular than anaplastic ependymoma and has less vascular proliferation.

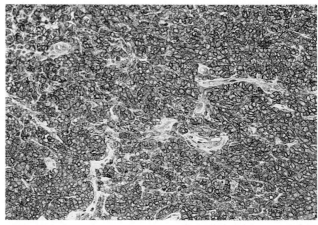

Figure 18–36. This peripheral primitive neuroectodermal tumor (pNET) is diffusely and intensely positive for MIC2.

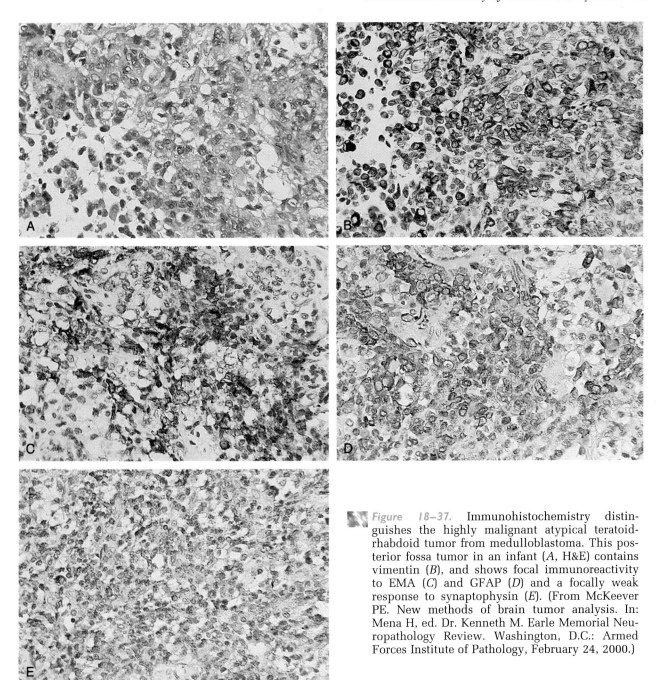

Figure 18-37. Immunohistochemistry distinguishes the highly malignant atypical teratoid-rhabdoid tumor from medulloblastoma. This posterior fossa tumor in an infant (*A*, H&E) contains vimentin (*B*), and shows focal immunoreactivity to EMA (*C*) and GFAP (*D*) and a focally weak response to synaptophysin (*E*). (From McKeever PE. New methods of brain tumor analysis. In: Mena H, ed. Dr. Kenneth M. Earle Memorial Neuropathology Review. Washington, D.C.: Armed Forces Institute of Pathology, February 24, 2000.)

Meningeal and Related Tumors

MENINGIOMAS

Meningeal location is a major discriminator of meningioma from other primary intracranial neoplasms (Table 18–9; see Tables 18–5 to 18–7). Most meningiomas are attached to dura or falx, facilitating their recognition. Meningiomas arise less commonly from the choroid plexus and very rarely within the CNS parenchyma itself.[277]

The classic genetic abnormality in meningioma is partial or complete loss of chromosome 22.[1] This loss can be detected by chromosomal ISH visualized by immunostaining.

Certain features provide evidence of meningioma. A *syncytial* appearance is a distinctive feature of meningothelial meningiomas and a focal feature of other subtypes of meningioma (Fig. 18–39; see Table 18–9). The structural bases of this syncytial appearance are numerous tightly interdigitating cellular processes held together by desmosomes rather than a true syncytium. Meningothelial whorls and psammoma bodies typify meningiomas. The presence of these features on H&E-stained slides diminishes the need for immunohistochemical analysis.[171] Psammoma bodies are concentrically laminated calcifications.

Most meningiomas contain EMA,[278] although it

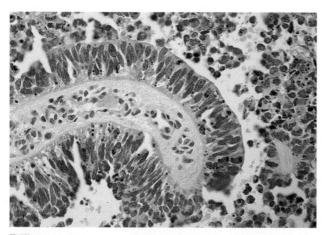

Figure 18–38. Medulloepithelioma. Anaplastic cells of this papillary neoplasm are weakly positive for gamma-enolase (neuron-specific enolase [NSE]). They form a pseudostratified epithelium with dense material on its surface. (From McKeever PE. New methods of brain tumor analysis. In: Mena H, ed. Dr. Kenneth M. Earle Memorial Neuropathology Review. Washington, D.C.: Armed Forces Institute of Pathology, February 24, 2000.)

is often expressed focally and can be missed in small specimens. EMA positivity plus lack of GFAP distinguishes meningiomas from gliomas (Fig. 18–40; see Fig. 18–1*B*).[279] Expression of S-100 protein by meningiomas is variable. The intensity of vimentin expression by meningiomas has stimulated its use in these tumors. Vimentin markers should be used only in combination with other markers, because many other tumors express vimentin. Meningiomas are variable in these three markers, but they often have more reticulin, fibronectin, and collagen in their parenchyma than low-grade gliomas.

There are reasons to assess the progesterone and estrogen receptors of meningiomas, particularly those that have not been totally removed surgically. Receptor-positive meningiomas may respond to therapy that blocks the hormone in question. Hormone receptor status may affect decisions about pregnancy (see Fig. 18–39).

FIBROUS MENINGIOMA (FIBROBLASTIC MENINGIOMA) (WHO GRADE I)

Fibrous meningiomas are firm tumors composed of spindle cells (see Table 18–5).[280] They resemble schwannomas, solitary fibrous tumors, fibrillary astrocytomas, and pilocytic astrocytomas.[64, 281] Fibrous meningiomas contain parenchymal collagen, often in large, pink bundles on H&E staining that distinguish them from astrocytomas.[64]

The similarity of fibrous meningiomas to schwannomas poses a particular diagnostic problem with tumors in the cerebellopontine angle and around spinal nerve roots.[280] Structures that identify meningiomas in this context include whorls, psammoma bodies, and very thick bundles of collagen. Fibrous meningiomas express EMA, which schwannomas lack. The former also usually show more vimentin and less S-100 protein than schwannomas.

Fibrous meningiomas can be distinguished from solitary fibrous tumors (SFTs) by their immunohistochemical profiles.[281, 282] Fibrous meningiomas express more EMA, S-100 protein, and glycogen, and less CD34 than SFTs (Fig. 18–41; see Fig. 18–45).[281]

MENINGOTHELIOMATOUS MENINGIOMA (SYNCYTIAL MENINGIOMA) (WHO GRADE I)

Meningotheliomatous meningioma is the classic "syncytial" meningioma (see Fig. 18–39) that re-

Table 18–9. Differential Diagnosis of a Mass That Includes "Syncytial" Cells

	Differential Features		
Diagnosis	*Structures*	*Antibody**	*Locations†*
Meningiomas	Whorls; psammoma bodies; interdigitating cell processes and desmosomes; (thick collagen)‡	Vimentin (+); EMA (+/−); S-100 (R)	Falx, tentorium; meninges; choroid plexus; (extracranial)‡
Anaplastic meningioma	Decrease in preceding features; mitoses; necrosis; CNS invasion	Vimentin (+); EMA (R); S-100 (R)	Same as above
Hemangiopericytic meningioma	Hypercellularity; thick pericellular matrix; mitoses	Vimentin (+)	Same as above

* Key to staining results:
(+) = Almost always strong, diffuse positivity
(+/−) = Variable, many positive
R = Rare cells may be positive
† Most common or most specific location is listed first.
‡ Parentheses around a differential feature indicate an uncommon feature that is very useful in differential diagnosis when found.
CNS, central nervous system; EMA, epithelial membrane antigen
Modified from McKeever PE, Blaivas M. The brain, spinal cord, and meninges. In: Sternberg SS, ed. Diagnostic Surgical Pathology. 2nd ed. New York: Raven Press, 1994:409–492.

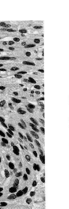

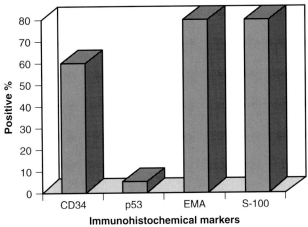

Figure 18-39. Meningotheliomatous meningioma. This meningioma could not be totally resected because of its location. It has a syncytial appearance and rounded nuclei. When the patient contemplated pregnancy, the tumor's hormonal receptors were assessed. It is positive for progesterone receptors (dark brown nuclei).

Figure 18-41. Bar graph of immunostaining characteristics of 20 fibrous meningiomas. Percentages positive are as reported in Perry A, Scheithauer BW, Nascimento AG. The immunophenotypic spectrum of meningeal hemangiopericytoma: A comparison with fibrous meningioma and solitary fibrous tumor of meninges. Am J Surg Pathol 1997;21:1354–1360.

sembles the small clusters of meningeal cells found normally in the meninges and choroid plexus. Whorls and psammoma bodies are often sparse (see Table 18-9). Some meningothelial meningiomas are divided into lobules by their fibrovascular stroma.

Meningothelial meningioma occasionally appears fibrillar or epithelioid (see Fig. 18-1*A*) and simulates ependymoma,[280] but it lacks GFAP and usually contains enough stromal type IV collagen, reticulin, or EMA (see Fig. 18-1*B*) to be distinctive.

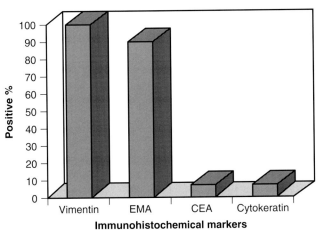

Figure 18-40. Immunohistochemical staining results in 29 cases of meningioma stained with broad-spectrum antibodies to epithelial membrane antigen (EMA), carcinoembryonic antigen (CEA), and cytokeratin (AE1/AE3). Percentages positive for all antibodies except for vimentin are as reported in Ng HK, Tse CC, Lo ST. Meningiomas and arachnoid cells: An immunohistochemical study of epithelial markers. Pathology 1987;19:253–257.

Confusion with myxopapillary ependymoma can be a problem, although this tumor usually shows at least focal GFAP.

Intraparenchymal meningiomas can be confused with oligodendrogliomas (see Box 2). EMA reactivity identifies most meningiomas. The margin of meningiomas with CNS parenchyma evaluated with synaptophysin and NF CNS markers is more discrete than that of gliomas. Some meningothelial meningiomas lack the classic whorls and psammoma bodies, whereas others show distinct epithelioid cellular margins (see Fig. 18-1*A*). These tumors may be confused with carcinoma and adenoma. Intraparenchymal meningiomas express little or no CAM5.2 cytokeratin and no pituitary peptides or chromogranin A (see Figs. 18-3 to 18-5).

TRANSITIONAL MENINGIOMA (MIXED MENINGIOMA) (WHO GRADE I)

Transitional meningiomas are composed of syncytial and fibroblastic components, as described previously. The presence of cells intermediate in type between syncytial and fibroblastic justifies their designation.[283] Prominent whorls, psammoma bodies, and clusters of "syncytial" cells make these very common meningiomas among the easiest to identify. IHC is usually not necessary for their identification (see Table 18-7).

PSAMMOMATOUS MENINGIOMA (WHO GRADE I)

Psammomatous meningiomas are crowded with psammoma bodies.[64] They are often spinal in location. This benign variant is recognized as meningioma from the finding of syncytial vimentin and EMA+ cells between the conspicuous, concentrically laminated psammoma bodies.

HIGHLY VASCULAR MENINGIOMAS (WHO GRADE I)

Hemangioblastic meningioma, angioblastic meningioma, and angiomatous meningioma are all highly vascular meningiomas.[64, 120, 283] Their vessels can be highlighted with CD31, CD34, factor VIII, and *Ulex* endothelial markers, vimentin, and muscle actin. For these meningiomas, CD34 causes less background staining than the other markers.

OTHER MENINGIOMAS

Recognizing the other meningioma variants is more critical than some claim. It helps to avoid mistaking them for other entities, including tumors with different treatments. Meningioma variants include choroid,[64] lipoblastic,[284] arachnoid trabecular,[285] microcystic,[286] glycogen-rich,[287] lymphoplasmacyte-rich,[120] osteogenic,[288] cartilaginous,[288] and secretory[289–291] (Fig. 18–42) meningiomas. Positive responses for vimentin and focal EMA help identify these tumors.[292]

Keys to distinguishing these variants of menin-

gioma from carcinoma and sarcoma are finely granular chromatin, few mitoses, and meningeal features (see Table 18–9). Meningiomas generally express more vimentin and less CAM5.2 cytokeratin than carcinomas. *Chordoid meningioma* has less CAM5.2 cytokeratin than chordoma and the typical ultrastructural features of meningiomas.[293, 294]

The *secretory meningioma* is spectacular (see Fig. 18–42). It displays focal CAM5.2 reactivity in cells immediately surrounding its secretory granules, which are positive for carcinoembryonic antigen (CEA), carbohydrate antigen 19-9, and PAS.[295] Properly stained, this tumor can be nothing other than secretory meningoma.

AGGRESSIVE OR MALIGNANT MENINGIOMAS

Clear Cell Meningioma

One of the many reasons to subclassify meningiomas is to identify more aggressive variants. The subtype clear cell meningioma is exemplary (Fig. 18–43). Although they look benign, many clear cell meningiomas are biologically aggressive.[296, 297] Their clear cells resemble those in oligodendroglioma and clear cell ependymoma (see Box 1).[175] A mixture of clear cells and meningothelial features

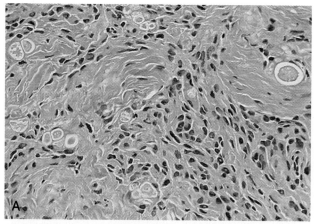

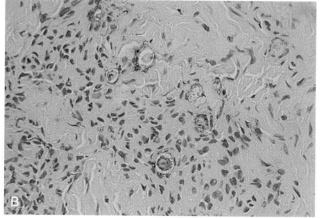

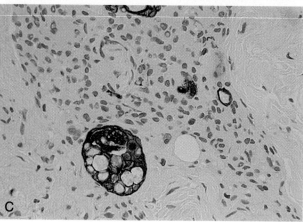

Figure 18–42. Secretory meningioma. Strikingly cytokeratin-positive structures that resemble acini suggest carcinoma, but the cytologic features are meningothelial. The secretory meningioma contains pink globules (*A*, H&E) that are oddly reactive for carcinoembryonic antigen (*B*) and are surrounded by cytokeratin-positive cells (*C*). (From McKeever PE. New methods of brain tumor analysis. In: Mena H, ed. Dr. Kenneth M. Earle Memorial Neuropathology Review. Washington, D.C.: Armed Forces Institute of Pathology, February 24, 2000.)

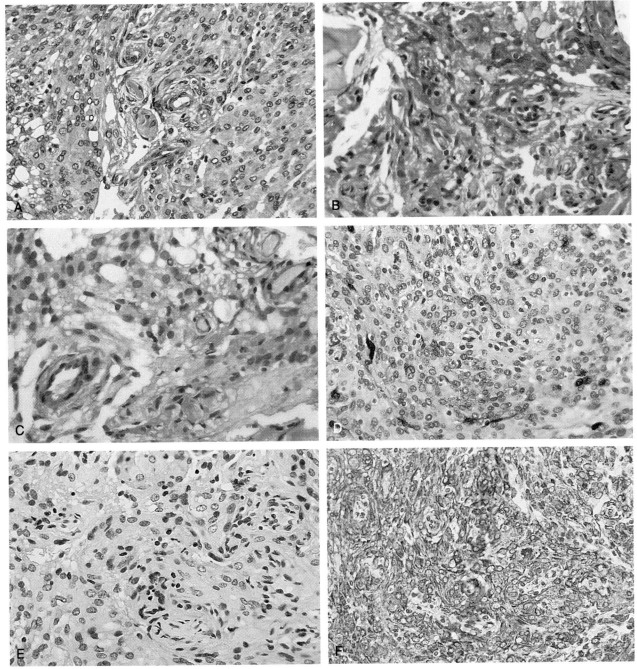

Figure 18–43. Clear cell meningioma. This tumor has recurred several times. The clear cell meningioma (*A*, H&E) contains red PAS+ glycogen (*B*) eliminated by enzymes that digest glycogen (*C*). This one contained scattered S-100 protein–positive cells (*D*) and no CK+ cells (*E*). The clear cell meningioma tends to be aggressive and difficult to manage surgically. Like most meningiomas, it is abundantly vimentin-positive (*F*). (From McKeever PE. New methods of brain tumor analysis. In: Mena H, ed. Dr. Kenneth M. Earle Memorial Neuropathology Review. Washington, D.C.: Armed Forces Institute of Pathology, February 24, 2000.)

is a key to its diagnosis.[175, 298] Cytoplasmic glycogen helps to confirm the diagnosis (see Fig. 18–43*B* and *C*).[296] Diffusely positive vimentin and focally positive EMA aid identification of its meningothelial origin (see Fig. 18–43*F* and Table 18–9).[299] This variant is particularly common in the lumbar and cerebellopontine angle regions.[297]

Rhabdoid Meningioma

A highly aggressive tumor, rhabdoid meningioma contains barely cohesive cells that are filled with abundant whorls of filaments that show immunocytochemical reactivity for vimentin.[3, 300] These filaments push the meningothelial nuclei to the side of the cell.

Entirely rhabdoid tumors are difficult to distinguish from gemistocytic gliomas. In such cases, vimentin predominance, EMA reactivity, and lack of GFAP reveal their true identity.

Atypical Meningioma (WHO Grade II)

Atypical meningiomas show more cellularity and mitotic activity than benign meningiomas. They have larger nucleoli, patternless sheet-like growth, and foci of necrosis.[120] Although the diagnostic criteria for this meningioma are subjective, the tumor is recognized as a distinct diagnostic entity with histopathologic features between those of benign and malignant meningiomas. Atypical meningiomas usually retain vimentin and at least slight, focal EMA immunoreactivity. They tend to be aggressive and to recur locally. Chromosomal abnormalities in addition to standard loss of 22 and increased MIB-1 LI may forecast greater aggressiveness.[301]

Anaplastic Meningioma (Malignant Meningioma) (WHO Grade III)

Anaplastic meningiomas are meningiomas with obviously malignant cytologic features, high mitotic index, spontaneous tumor *necrosis,* and brain *invasion.*[302, 303] Brain invasion through the pia is a particularly significant finding that can be confirmed with vimentin staining to identify meningioma cells in brain. Invasion of adjacent cerebral parenchyma or of small blood vessels within the tumor is more ominous than the dural invasion common in lower grade meningiomas (see Table 18–9). Nuclear staining for p53 tumor suppressor gene product is evident in 10% of malignant meningiomas. The mean MIB-1 LI among 20 tumors in one series was 11.7%, with a wide range between 1% and 24% in individual tumors.[304]

Papillary Meningioma (WHO Grade II or III)

Papillary configurations in meningiomas are associated with high rates of local recurrence and metastases. The papillae have a CD31+ vascular core. Meningioma cells produce rosettes around these vessels, and in addition to expected vimentin and S-100 protein, they may express CK.[303]

The recognition of a papillary meningioma in other than the dural locations characteristic of meningioma is difficult. Papillary meningiomas resemble papillary ependymomas, choroid plexus papillomas, and carcinomas.[283] One should look for a high ratio of vimentin to CK and absence of GFAP to identify the meningioma.

Other Meningeal Tumors

HEMANGIOPERICYTOMA (HEMANGIOPERICYTIC MENINGIOMA) (WHO GRADE II)

A highly cellular and mitotically active neoplasm, hemangiopericytoma is rich in pericellular reticulin stainable with anti–type IV collagen. Eighty percent of these tumors recur, and 23% metastasize.[305, 306]

Hemangiopericytomas are distinguished from benign meningiomas by their hypercellularity, higher mitotic index, and microscopic tendency to bulge into vascular lumens without bursting through the endothelium (see Table 18–8). Although there are exceptions, these tumors tend to lack markers other than the relatively ubiquitous factor XIIIa, mesenchymal markers, and Leu7.[290, 307]

The spectrum of immunohistochemical markers for hemangiopericytoma overlaps with that for fibrous meningioma, but lack of EMA and S-100 is distinctive for the former (Fig. 18–44).[281] The hemangiopericytoma is distinguished from malignant glioma and metastatic carcinoma by foci of extensive reticulin around individual neoplastic cells. Also, hemangiopericytoma lacks the GFAP found in glioma, and its nuclei are less pleomorphic and less spindled than those of fibrosarcoma.

SOLITARY FIBROUS TUMOR

The solitary fibrous tumor resembles fibrous meningioma but has a different immunohistochemical profile (Fig. 18–45; see Fig. 18–41).[281] It is more common in pleura than dura. Malignant

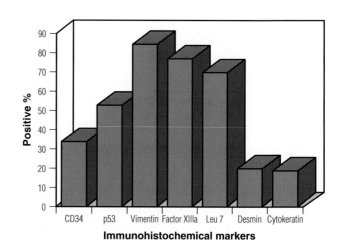

Figure 18–44. Immunochemical staining results of 27 meningeal hemangiopericytomas. Percentages positive are as reported in Perry A, Scheithauer BW, Nascimento AG. The immunophenotypic spectrum of meningeal hemangiopericytoma: A comparison with fibrous meningioma and solitary fibrous tumor of meninges. Am J Surg Pathol 1997;21:1354–1360.

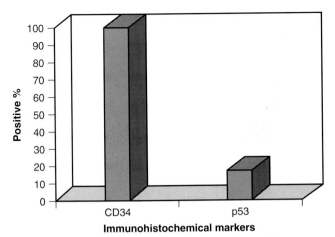

Figure 18–45. Bar graph of eight solitary fibrous tumors. Percentages positive are as reported in Perry A, Scheithauer BW, Nascimento AG. The immunophenotypic spectrum of meningeal hemangiopericytoma: A comparison with fibrous meningioma and solitary fibrous tumor of meninges. Am J Surg Pathol 1997;21:1354–1360.

transformation of the solitary fibrous tumor may be associated with trisomy 8.[308]

Chordoma and Sarcomas

CHORDOMA

Approximately 40% of chordomas arise in the clivus, and 10% along cervical, 2% along thoracic, 2% along lumbar, and more than 45% in the sacral portions of the spinal canal.[64]

Physaliphorous cells of chordomas contain large, characteristic intracytoplasmic vacuoles (Fig. 18–46; see Table 18–6). Because the cells frequently grow in cords, these vacuoles occasionally line up like beads on a string, distinguishing chordoma

from chondroid neoplasms, which have individual cells embedded in cartilage.[309] Chordomas contain CK (see Fig. 18–46A), EMA, 5′-nucleotidase, and desmosomes, whereas chondrosarcomas lack these features.[310, 311] Presence of CK is the standard discriminator of chordoma from CK-negative chondrosarcoma.

Chordoma cells are exuberantly bifilamentous (see Fig. 18–46), containing vimentin and CK in the same cell.[312] The vacuoles of physaliphorous cells contain mucin and glycogen.[313] Their structure is distinct from that of watery perinuclear oligodendroglial halos and the multiplicity of smaller lipid vacuoles of hemangioblastomas (see Figs. 18–19, 18–46, and 18–51B).

Malignant histologic transformation of chordoma is uncommon.[314] Nevertheless, relentless local invasion of clinically sensitive regions results in a poor long-term prognosis.

Chondroid chordomas contain regions of classic chordoma that are positive for EMA, CK, and S-100 as well as chondroid regions that are S-100+ and lack EMA and CK.[315] The existence of chondroid chordoma has been challenged by some researchers, who prefer to interpret such tumors as either chordomas or low-grade chondrosarcomas.

SARCOMAS (WHO GRADE III OR IV)

Sarcomas are rare among brain tumors. Reported incidences of primary intracranial sarcomas vary from 0.08% to 4.3%, the former percentage being more contemporary.[316] GFAP immunohistochemical analysis has demonstrated that tumors formerly considered sarcomas are actually primary brain tumors, particularly glioblastomas, medulloblastomas, and primary lymphomas.[317]

Causes of some sarcomas are known or suspected.[318, 319] Intracranial radiation is a surprisingly common cause of sarcoma.[4, 319] Intracranial Ka-

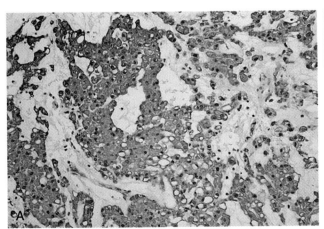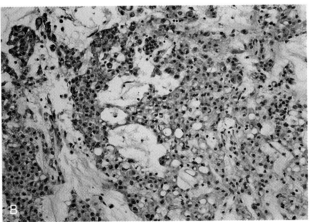

Figure 18–46. Chordoma. *A,* Cords of physaliphorous cells are positive for CK, a most important immunohistochemical feature in distinguishing chordoma from CK− chondrosarcoma. *B,* The tumor also was positive for vimentin. This specimen demonstrates the propensity of chordomas to express more than one intermediate filament.

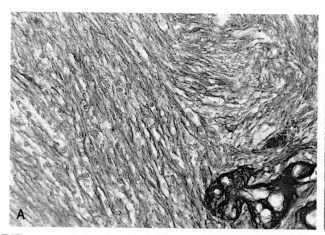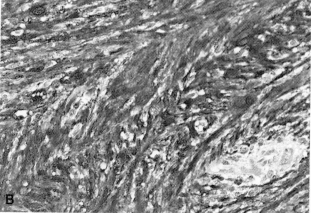

Figure 18–47. Schwannoma of a peripheral nerve in the brachial plexus of a young man. *A,* Type IV collagen–positive basement membranes surround each tumor cell in compact Antoni A tissue. Darker brown vessel in corner of figure has more collagen. *B,* Nuclei and cytoplasm are abundantly immunoreactive for S-100 protein, but vessel in corner is not.

posi's sarcoma is rare,[318] most cases being associated with immunodeficiency.

The mesenchymal chondrosarcoma is rare. It originates in the intracranial and spinal meninges and cauda equina in childhood and young adulthood.[320] It resembles hemangiopericytoma except for islands of cartilage.[120]

Poorly differentiated chondrosarcomas are rare and usually involve the meninges. A key feature is evidence of cartilage production, which is often sparse. Presence of S-100 protein as evidence of chondroid differentiation must be interpreted cautiously in meningeal and CNS neoplasms, because most gliomas, chordoma, melanoma, nerve sheath tumors, and an occasional meningioma contain this protein (see Figs. 18–43*D*, 18–47*B*, and 18–54*C*).[144, 279, 309]

Primary cerebral rhabdomyosarcomas are rare.[321] Synaptophysin-negative staining differentiates them from synaptophysin-positive medullomyoblastomas.[269]

Lack of GFAP+ neoplastic glia distinguishes fibrosarcoma from glioblastoma invading the meninges and from gliosarcoma.[4] For specific features that differentiate sarcomas, see Chapter 3.

Nerve Sheath Tumors

Benign nerve sheath tumors (WHO grade I) can be subclassified as either schwannoma or neurofibroma, as described in the discussions of these tumors (see Table 18–5). Malignant nerve sheath tumors (WHO grade III or IV) are much more difficult to subclassify when they lose the characteristics of their benign counterparts. Leu7 and S-100 protein markers differentiate nerve sheath tumors from other tumors known to lack these markers.[322–324]

SCHWANNOMA (NEURILEMOMA, NEURINOMA) (WHO GRADE I)

The presence of a noninvasive tumor next to a peripheral nerve suggests the diagnosis of schwannoma. Verocay bodies are more distinctive of schwannomas than the Antoni A and Antoni B patterns but are not seen in all schwannomas.

Bilateral eighth nerve schwannomas indicate neurofibromatosis of NF-2 type. Unusual locations and associations with meningeal proliferation are also seen with NF-2.[325] Both NF-2 and schwannomas are associated with abnormalities in chromosome 22.[1]

The histologic appearance of schwannoma is similar to that of fibrous meningioma, tanycytic ependymoma, subependymoma, and astrocytoma. Schwannoma is distinguished from astrocytoma and ependymoma by its abundant parenchymal reticulin, which is positive for type IV collagen (Fig. 18–47*A*). Schwannomas have continuous basement membranes all along the exterior surfaces of their cells (see Table 18–5). Focal reactivity of some schwannomas with anti-GFAP requires care in the use of these antisera to distinguish the tumors from astrocytomas.[326] However, a negative GFAP response supports the diagnosis of schwannoma.

When they lack the characteristic features of meningioma, like meningeal whorls and psammoma bodies, fibrous meningiomas are more difficult than gliomas to distinguish from schwannomas. Antoni A and Antoni B growth patterns in schwannomas resemble those seen in fibrous meningiomas. Schwannomas contain Leu7 and S-100 protein[144, 323] and lack EMA. Reactivity of meningiomas for EMA is therefore a useful discriminator. Both tumors contain S-100 protein, but S-100 is more ubiquitous and abundant in schwannomas (Fig. 18–47*B*).[64, 279] There is evidence that sole expression of the beta subunit of S-100 may distinguish eighth nerve schwannomas from some men-

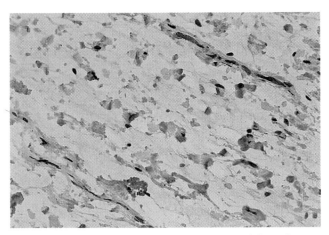

Figure 18–48. Neurofibroma. Occasional long brown axons within the tumor are dispersed among proliferating cells. (Anti-NF stain with hematoxylin counterstain) (Courtesy of Drs. Andrew Flint and Victor Elner, University of Michigan, Ann Arbor, MI.)

ingiomas.[327] If present, GFAP+ foci distinguish schwannoma from meningioma. Meningioma cells are GFAP−.

NEUROFIBROMA (WHO GRADE I)

The key to recognition of neurofibromas is their involvement within peripheral nerve rather than next to it (see Table 18–5). Neurofibroma differs from schwannoma in having stainable NF+ axons running through the tumor itself rather than confined to the periphery.[64] The larger the neurofibroma, the more the axons are "diluted" with neoplastic cells. Fortunately, today's anti-NF antibodies can detect individual axons in a "haystack" of tumor tissue (Fig. 18–48). This is because the neurofibroma is a swelling of the nerve itself, with a mixture of Schwann cells, fibroblasts, collagen, and mucoid material enclosed in a weakly EMA+ perineurium. In contrast, schwannomas grow next to and compress the nerve, so that neurofilaments are not evident within the central tumor nidus.

Plexiform neurofibromas are multiple swollen fascicles. They are associated with von Recklinghausen's disease (NF-1).[1]

MALIGNANT NERVE SHEATH TUMOR

See Chapter 3.

Neuroendocrine Tumors

See Chapter 9.

Germ Cell Tumors

Within the cranial vault, 95% of primary germ cell tumors are found along the midline in the pineal and suprasellar regions, especially the former.[328] About one tenth involve both regions, and one fourth arise in the suprasellar cistern.[328, 329] Germ cell tumors rarely involve spinal cord[330] or peripheral nerve.

Germinomas are the most common intracranial germ cell neoplasm. There are few differences between intracranial and gonadal germinomas.[331] For details about germ cell tumors, see Chapters 14 and 15.

Hematopoietic and Lymphoid Neoplasms

LYMPHOMA (WHO GRADE III OR IV)

Primary CNS lymphomas grow within the CNS parenchyma (see Table 18–8). They have a diffuse invasive margin. These lymphomas are nearly always of B-cell origin (Fig. 18–49).[1, 332–334] The incidence of this B-cell neoplasm is increasing only partly because of its occurrence in immunosuppressed patients and in patients with AIDS and other immunocompromised conditions.[335–337] With few exceptions, AIDS-related lymphomas have poor outcomes.[337–339] Primary CNS lymphomas of T-cell origin are rare.[340]

In paraffin sections, L26 B-cell and A6 T-cell markers should be used along with LCA.[335, 341, 342] Because primary CNS lymphoma invades CNS parenchyma, responses to CNS markers like GFAP must be interpreted with extreme caution. The nuclear counterstain identifies the non-neoplastic nuclei of gliosis in GFAP+ cells intermixed among lymphoma cells.[64] Monoclonal staining for B-cell (or, rarely, T-cell) markers helps distinguish lymphoma from CNS inflammation, which is polyclonal (see Fig. 18–3B and C), and from nonlymphoid neoplasms.[343] However, many lymphomas contain polyclonal reactive lymphoid elements, which may be recognized from their smaller size and benign nuclei.[342]

The aforementioned markers are sufficient for most primary CNS lymphomas (see Box 1). For details about subclassifying these and other lymphomas, see Chapter 4.

LEUKEMIA

The diagnosis of leukemia within the craniospinal vault is usually established by cytologic examination of CSF.[344, 345, 429] Terminal intraparenchymal CNS hemorrhages reflect blast crises leading to leukocyte counts greater than 300,000/mm³, resulting in intravascular leukostasis.[149] Cerebral vasculitis is rarely associated with leukemia.[346] Focal masses of leukemic cells (chloromas) in the meninges may be heralded by peripheral eosinophilia.[347]

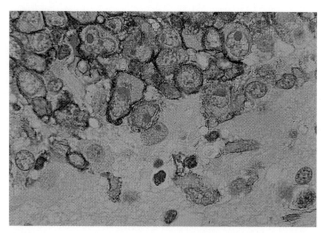

Figure 18–49. Primary brain lymphoma. Hematoxylin nuclear counterstain reveals malignant lymphocytes with clumped chromatin and huge nucleoli. The immunohistochemical stain is L26, a B-lymphocyte marker. Malignant lymphocytes were negative for T-cell and macrophage markers (*not shown*). (From McKeever PE. New methods of brain tumor analysis. In: Mena H, ed. Dr. Kenneth M. Earle Memorial Neuropathology Review. Washington, D.C.: Armed Forces Institute of Pathology, February 24, 2000.)

HISTIOCYTOSIS

Histiocytosis occurs predominantly in children and young adults (see Table 18–5).[64] The CNS is often involved secondary to bony involvement or to systemic involvement, often by Langerhans' histiocytosis. Non-Langerhans' types of histiocytosis also occur (Fig. 18–50).[348–350] Although any region of brain or meninges may be affected, the parasellar region is particularly susceptible.[351–353] A typical lesion is firm because of the collagen fibers mixed with histiocytes and inflammatory cells. New lesions are less fibrotic than old. Langhans cells are S-100 protein–positive. The literature suggests that CD1a has good sensitivity in this disease. However, a colleague and I have seen cases that appear to be Langerhans cell histiocytosis but were CD1a– in paraffin preparations. This finding may simply be due to different antibodies or staining protocols. Lack of structural GFAP in cellular fibrils distinguishes histiocytes from astrocytes and from ependymal and subependymal cells. Electron microscopy identifies the Birbeck granules of Langerhans cell histiocytosis.[351]

Miscellaneous Intracranial or Spinal Masses

HEMANGIOBLASTOMA (CAPILLARY HEMANGIOBLASTOMA) (WHO GRADE I)

The capillary hemangioblastoma resembles an endocrine neoplasm (Fig. 18–51). It has close juxtaposition of capillary and stromal cells (see Table 18–7) and occasionally shows secretory granules or expresses erythropoietin.[354] Its pink, vacuolated stromal cells often contain NSE, present in neuroendocrine cells.[355]

Some hemangioblastomas are associated with the von Hippel–Lindau complex.[356] This complex should be considered in patients with more than one tumor or a hemangioblastoma in an unusual location.[357]

Because the hemangioblastoma is nonfibrillar, it should not resemble an astrocytoma. However, the resemblance may occur for two reasons, sampling and artifact. Cerebellar hemangioblastomas are often cystic, with the actual neoplasm embedded somewhere in the wall of the cyst as a mural nodule. Biopsy specimens of the cyst wall may show conspicuously GFAP+ gliosis. One should look for regular spacing between cells and reactive nuclear features in these gliotic cells to distinguish them from gliomas.

Sampling a hemangioblastoma can reveal scattered GFAP+ cells.[358–360] Some of these cells are reactive astrocytes, common near the periphery of the tumor. However, others are stromal cells, most common in the cellular and angioglioma variants of hemangioblastoma, which either take up GFAP from adjacent reactive astrocytes or express their own GFAP.[360, 361] To minimize confusion, the central portion of the solid tumor should be sampled.

Epithelioid hemangioblastoma can resemble paraganglioma[362] or renal cell carcinoma.[280] Hemangioblastomas have more capillaries and much less chromogranin A than paragangliomas.[363] Compared with renal cell carcinoma, hemangioblastoma has more uniform distribution of nuclear chromatin, absence of necrosis, small nucleoli, and intimate arrangement of capillaries and stromal cells (see Fig. 18–51*A*). This arrangement is accentuated by staining with CD31, CD34, anti–factor

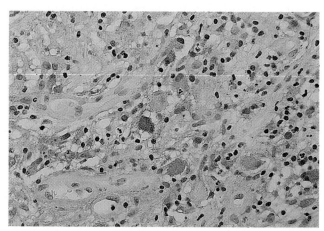

Figure 18–50. Histiocytosis. This specimen, from a mass within the brain parenchyma, contains S-100+ cells. The immunohistochemical stain highlights intracellular leukocytes seen in Rosai-Dorfman disease.

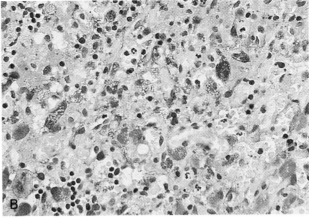

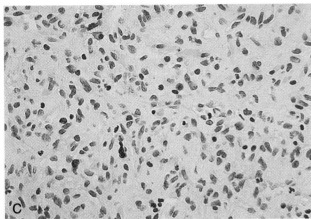

Figure 18–51. Cerebellar hemangioblastoma. *A,* Contrast-enhanced tumor in the right cerebellar hemisphere of an elderly woman contains a mixture of many capillaries and vacuolated cells. (H&E) *B,* The cerebellar hemangioblastoma was positive for NSE. The anti-NSE stains stromal cells and highlights their clear, round lipid vacuoles. *C,* The specimen is negative for EMA. A single brown EMA+ plasma cell confirms the integrity of this stain. (From McKeever PE. New methods of brain tumor analysis. In: Mena H, ed. Dr. Kenneth M. Earle Memorial Neuropathology Review. Washington, D.C.: Armed Forces Institute of Pathology, February 24, 2000. Courtesy of Dr. Roger A. Hawkins, Greenville, PA.)

VIII, or anti–gamma enolase (NSE).[355, 364] In contrast to renal cell carcinoma, hemangioblastomas tend to stain for NSE, and they do not stain for EMA (Fig. 18–51B and C).

CRANIOPHARYNGIOMA (WHO GRADE I)

The epithelial appearance of craniopharyngioma is distinctive. A properly sampled craniopharyngioma, including a sample of the solid mass associated with cystic craniopharyngiomas,[365, 366] is difficult to confuse with other brain tumors because of its characteristic epithelium, which may be adamantinomatous, keratinizing, or both (see Tables 18–6 and 18–11). Three of four craniopharyngiomas calcify, a feature helping to distinguish them from metastatic carcinoma, which rarely calcifies in brain and is rarely as differentiated as craniopharyngioma.[148, 365] Craniopharyngiomas express more high molecular weight keratin than most carcinomas metastatic to brain (Fig. 18–52).

Confusion can arise from sampling of only the intensely GFAP+ gliotic margin of a craniopharyngioma, which may closely resemble a pilocytic astrocytoma. The highly reactive and fibrillar gliosis surrounding a craniopharyngioma may be distinguished from that of pilocytic astrocytoma on the basis of the even spacing between GFAP+ cells,

the lower cellularity, and the lack of microcysts in the former (see section on Gliosis). If a craniopharyngioma nearby is suspected, keratin immunohistochemical analysis may reveal epithelial cells in the gliosis.[367]

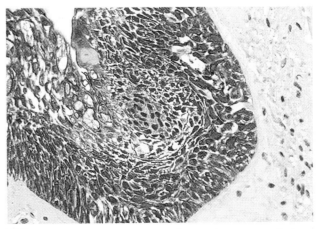

Figure 18–52. Most craniopharyngiomas are obvious from their structural features, as was this adamantinomatous craniopharyngioma. Nonetheless, its immunoreactivity for high molecular weight keratin 903 distinguishes it even further and emphasizes the presence of cytoplasm of shrunken epithelial cells ("stellate reticulum").

Metastatic Tumors (All Tumors WHO Grade IV)

CARCINOMA

Important characteristics of carcinoma as it relates to the CNS and meninges are its distinctively epithelial structure (Fig. 18–53A; see Table 18–6) and the overwhelming predominance of metastatic over primary carcinomas. Metastatic carcinomas are described in detail in Chapter 7. Rare primary brain carcinomas occur in the choroid plexus, from germ cell tumors of the pineal and suprasellar regions, and from cysts.[64, 173, 368] This section emphasizes how to distinguish between carcinomas (Fig. 18–53B to D) and primary intracranial tumors (see Box 2).

Metastatic carcinoma uncommonly produces neoplastic meningitis. Although its clinical features resemble those of inflammatory meningitis, cytologic examination of the CSF distinguishes the two.[344, 345, 369, 429]

Many carcinomas metastatic to the CNS and me-ninges are adenocarcinomas that form acini and produce mucin. Others are small cell or undifferentiated carcinoma. The histologic hallmarks of carcinoma metastatic to the CNS are an epithelial appearance and a *distinct tumor margin* with CNS parenchyma. *Distinct epithelial borders* and lack of fibrillar cytoplasmic processes contrast with the pattern of glioblastoma. Within CNS parenchyma, few neoplasms other than glioblastoma or anaplastic glioma show the intensity of nuclear pleomorphism, profuse mitotic abnormalities, or spontaneous tumor necrosis present in metastatic carcinomas. Carcinomas metastatic to the CNS stain abundantly for CAM5.2 cytokeratin (see Fig. 18–53C) and, less commonly, for K903 keratin, and often for EMA. These features and the lack of GFAP (see Fig. 18–53B) together distinguish carcinomas from gliomas.[210, 212, 370] In distinguishing carcinomas from gliomas, one should avoid the use of AE1/AE3 anti-CK, which cross-reacts with GFAP (see Fig. 18–8). Another common mistake is to interpret gliosis trapped by advancing

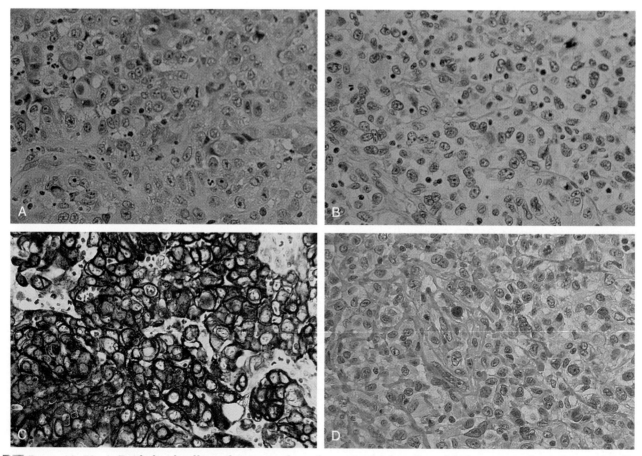

Figure 18–53. A, Epithelioid cells in this tumor from the parietal lobe of an elderly woman show distinct borders between cells. (H&E) These particular epithelioid cells are pleomorphic and contain malignant nuclear features. The algorithm in Box 2 offers a way to dissect the differential diagnosis of a brain tumor composed of epithelioid cells. Nearby sections of the tumor shown in A are negative for GFAP (B), highly positive for CAM5.2 cytokeratin (C), and negative for S-100 protein (D). It was also positive for EMA and negative for chromogranin A (*not shown*). The diagnostic path in Box 2 leads to carcinoma. (From McKeever PE. New methods of brain tumor analysis. In: Mena H, ed. Dr. Kenneth M. Earle Memorial Neuropathology Review. Washington, D.C.: Armed Forces Institute of Pathology, February 24, 2000.)

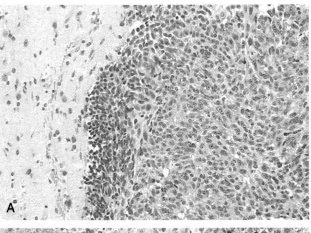

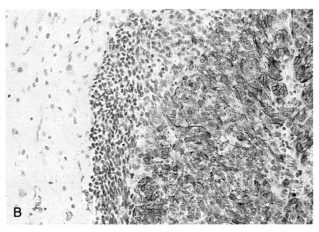

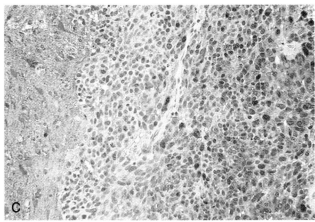

Figure 18–54. Decisive and supplemental markers of a melanoma with rare pigmented cells. All sections are of the edge of this melanoma in brain (*A*, H&E). *B*, The melanoma only is positive for HMB-45, a decisive marker of the melanocytic cells. *C*, Both the melanoma and brain are positive for S-100 protein. S-100 is best for screening but does not distinguish melanoma from primary brain tumors, such as glioma. (From McKeever PE. New methods of brain tumor analysis. In: Mena H, ed. Dr. Kenneth M. Earle Memorial Neuropathology Review. Washington, D.C.: Armed Forces Institute of Pathology, February 24, 2000.)

carcinoma as GFAP+ neoplasm (see Figs. 18–22 and 18–23*B*).

Meningiomas usually contain focal EMA, but so do many carcinomas. Meningiomas may contain CK, especially secretory meningiomas in proximity to their secretory globules. These tumors can often be distinguished from carcinoma on the basis of their focal CK staining (see Fig. 18–42*C*).[64] Most meningiomas have more diffuse and more intense vimentin staining than carcinomas, and their CK to vimentin ratio is lower than that of carcinomas. Importantly, all but the most malignant meningiomas lack the abnormal and abundant mitotic spindles found in metastatic carcinomas. Malignant meningiomas generally lack CAM5.2 cytokeratin.

Metastatic *renal cell carcinoma* must be distinguished from hemangioblastoma and oligodendroglioma. These neoplasms contain clear cytoplasm and distinct cell borders[175] (see Box 1). Presence of EMA and CK distinguish renal cell carcinoma from cerebellar hemangioblastoma and oligodendroglioma.[371]

Small cell carcinoma can be very difficult to distinguish from lymphoma and medulloblastoma (PNET). EMA or CK is expressed abundantly by small cell carcinoma, infrequently and focally by medulloblastoma, and not by brain lymphoma.[144] Although either small cell carcinoma or medullo-

blastoma may express synaptophysin, S-100 protein, or NSE, stains for these substances are valuable discriminators for the trained eye; they accentuate the fibrillarity of medulloblastoma, in contrast to the epithelioid cells of small cell carcinoma.

MELANOCYTIC NEOPLASMS

Metastatic melanoma is the most common melanocytic tumor encountered in the nervous system (Fig. 18–54). Its histologic features are variable (see Tables 18–5 to 18–7). Melanomas are described in Chapter 6. Melanomas are often strongly S-100 protein positive (see Fig. 18–54*C*), a marker of low specificity in brain because it is also seen in many CNS tumors.[144, 372] HMB-45 is the marker recommended as most likely to discriminate melanoma from other brain tumors (see Fig. 18–54*B*).

Rare meningiomas, schwannomas, ependymomas, neuroblastomas, and PNETs contain melanin.[173] They can be identified from their individually described features.

Primary melanomas confined to the craniospinal vault are rare. Most arise from meningeal melanocytes. They are often found in the meninges, where they may infiltrate the CNS via the perivascular space.[173] Primary melanocytomas are less malignant.[64, 120] They occur in Meckel's cave and elsewhere.

CYSTS

Cysts differ from tumors in their lack of a solid nodule of tissue.[64] This simple fact is critical to distinguishing glial cysts from gliomas and epithelial cysts from cystic craniopharyngiomas. Cysts specific to nervous tissue are emphasized here. Others are described in their primary chapters.

Glial Cyst, Simple Cyst, Pineal Cyst, and Wall of Syrinx

The common denominator of four cysts of various locations and obscure etiologies—glial cyst, simple cyst, pineal cyst, and wall of syrinx—is that the wall is lined only by gliosis (Table 18–10). Histologic characteristics of these cysts are those of gliosis: Highly GFAP+ stellate cells are uniformly spaced, with vast tangles of GFAP+ astrocytic processes between them.[373] It is sometimes only with the passage of time that such cysts are proven not to be associated with low-grade astrocytomas.[64]

Neuroepithelial Cyst and Ependymal Cyst

Both the neuroepithelial cyst and ependymal cyst have an epithelioid surface that is positive for S-100 protein and GFAP, resting on a fibrillary glial base that is also positive for these two antibodies.[374] These cysts often occur near a ventricle (Table 18–11). They rarely cause aseptic meningitis.[375]

Colloid Cyst

Location is a key feature of colloid cyst, which is more precisely called colloid cyst of the third ventricle (see Table 18–11). Its location in the third ventricle, usually near the choroid plexus and foramen of Monro, helps distinguish the colloid cyst from other cysts that superficially resemble it but that occur in different locations. This cyst's simple columnar and cuboidal epithelium, which may be flattened to squamous epithelium, often contains a mixture of ciliated and nonciliated cells.[376] Motile and sensory cilia suggest olfactory and respiratory epithelium.[377] These cells are positive for CK or EMA.[374] The cyst contents are predominantly carboxymucins, rendering them positive for PAS and Alcian blue.[378]

Dermoid Cyst

Dermoid cysts are frequently midline cysts, possibly arising from embryonic inclusions of skin at the time of closure of the neural groove (see Table 18–11). They occur between the cerebellar hemispheres, in the fourth ventricle, in the lumbosacral region of the cord, and in the skull. These cysts may involve CNS, meninges, or both.[149, 155] Rup-

Table 18-10. Differential Diagnosis of a Cyst with Wall of Fibrillar Cells

Diagnosis	Differential Features		
	Structures	*Antibody**	*Locations†*
Cavitary gliosis	Wall of gliosis	GFAP in glial filaments (+); S-100 (+)	Cerebrum; CNS
Abscess	Wall of granulation tissue; fibrosis (Table 18–5); inflammation and gliosis; purulent contents	Collagen (+); reticulin (+); L26 (+/−); A6 (+/−); LCA; κ and λ Ig; α-ACT; KP-1 (+/−); microorganisms	Basal frontal and temporal lobes; CNS
Cystic astrocytoma	Wall of pilocytic astrocytoma	GFAP (+); S-100 (+)	Cerebellum; CNS
Hemangioblastoma	Wall of gliosis; mural nodule of hemangioblastoma (Table 18–7)	Factor VIII (+/−); CD31 (+/−); NSE (+/−); Wall: GFAP (+)	Cerebellum; CNS
Glial cyst, simple cyst, pineal cyst, wall of syrinx	Wall of gliosis; Rosenthal fibers	GFAP in glial filaments (+); S-100 (+); alpha B-crystalline	Pineal, cerebellum, spinal cord; brainstem
Meningeal cyst	Wall of dura, arachnoid; "syncytial" cells	Collagen (+/−); EMA (+/−)	Spinal epidural surface

* Key to staining results:
   (+) = Almost always strong, diffuse positivity
   (+/−) = Variable, many positive
   R = Rare cells may be positive
† Most common or most specific location is listed first.

α-ACT, alpha-antichymotrypsin; CNS, central nervous system; EMA, epithelial membrane antigen; GFAP, glial fibrillary acidic protein; Ig, immunoglobulin; LCA, leukocyte common antigen; NSE, neuron-specific enolase.

Modified from McKeever PE, Blaivas M. The brain, spinal cord, and meninges. In: Sternberg SS, ed. Diagnostic Surgical Pathology. 2nd ed. New York: Raven Press, 1994:409–492.

Differential Diagnosis of a Cyst with Wall Lined by Epithelium

		Differential Features	
Diagnosis	Structures	Antibody*	Locations†
Cystic craniopharyngioma	Wall of adamantinomatous or incompletely keratinized squamous epithelium; cyst contains "motor oil"	Cytokeratin (+)	Suprasellar; sella
Ependymal cyst	Columnar epithelium usually ciliated	GFAP (+)	Spinal cord; brain
Colloid cyst	Fibrous wall lined by inner ciliated and/or nonciliated simple columnar epithelium; cyst contains colloid and cell ghosts	Cytokeratin (+); EMA	Third ventricle
Dermoid cyst	Epidermoid cyst features plus adnexa of skin; cyst contains sebum, squames, and hair	Keratin (+)	Midline cerebellum; fourth ventricle; skull; spinal dura; cauda equina
Epidermoid cyst	Fibrous wall lined by inner keratinizing stratified squamous epithelium; cyst contains waxy squames	Keratin (+)	CP angle; temporal lobe; spinal dura; pineal; sella; brainstem; CNS
Enterogenous cyst	Lining as above; cyst contains mucin; rests on collagen	Cytokeratin (+); EMA	Spinal cord

* Key to staining results:
 (+) = Almost always strong, diffuse positivity
† Most common or most specific location is listed first.
CNS, central nervous system; CP, cerebellopontine; EMA, epithelial membrane antigen; GFAP, glial fibrillary acidic protein.
Modified from McKeever PE, Blaivas M. The brain, spinal cord, and meninges. In: Sternberg SS, ed. Diagnostic Surgical Pathology. 2nd ed. New York: Raven Press, 1994:409–492.

tured dermoid cysts can cause sterile meningitis and inflammation resembling an abscess. Identification of squamous epithelial cells with CK or cholesterol clefts within the inflammation are clues to its true cause.

Epidermoid Cyst

Epidermoid cysts are more common in lateral than midline sites, but they have been found in many different locations (see Table 18–11). Common locations are the cerebellopontine angle, around the pons, near the sella, within the temporal lobe, in the diploë, and in the spinal canal.[149] Rarely, carcinoma arises within an epidermoid cyst.[368]

Enterogenous Cyst

Enterogenous cysts occur throughout the craniospinal vault. Such a cyst is lined by columnar epithelium, which secretes mucus (see Table 18–11). The epithelium resembles intestinal epithelium or, more rarely, bronchial epithelium.[379] It is immunoreactive for keratin and EMA. Some reactivity for CEA and S-100 protein has been noted.[379, 380]

Meningeal Cyst

A cyst that is located in the posterior or lateral epidural space in the spinal canal and that is lined only by fibrous tissue resembling dura and lacking arachnoid membrane is a meningeal cyst or diverticulum (see Table 18–10). A subdural or subarachnoid cyst that has a thinner wall than the epidural cyst and that protrudes toward brain or spinal cord is an arachnoid cyst. Reactivity for vimentin, progesterone receptors, and EMA is common. This immunoreactivity resembles that of arachnoid granulations and meningiomas.[381] Other cysts have variable thickness and are more difficult to categorize.

DEMENTIAS

Dementia has numerous causes.[382] Biopsy specimens intended to determine the etiology of dementia may be submitted along with note of the clinical suspicion of Alzheimer's disease or CJD. Any biopsy specimen being evaluated for the etiology of dementia, however, should be processed as if it were CJD until proven otherwise. The processing is as follows: The specimen is fixed in 10% formalin. Then a third of the specimen, which must include a portion of cerebral cortex, is fixed in either neat formic acid or 10% formalin plus 20% bleach for primary processing, and the major portion is held in 10% formalin without formic acid or bleach. One should avoid placing any portion of the fresh specimen in bleach without formalin, which would dissolve the tissue. A small portion of cortex is held in glutaraldehyde, in case electron microscopy is needed later.

The neat formic acid or *formalin-bleach* solution inactivates the infective agent and provides tissue preservation adequate to screen for CJD with H&E and GFAP. GFAP is a very stable antigen that resists oxidation. One should look for vacuoles in neurons and gray matter on H&E-stained specimens and for substantial stellate gliosis on GFAP-stained specimens. If these features are not present, the remaining portions of the specimen fixed optimally without bleach can then be processed and stained as needed to investigate other diagnostic possibilities (see Table 18–3).

Neurons are lost in all dementias. Neuronal loss is more difficult to assess than other findings in most biopsy specimens. The assessment requires quantitation more suited to morphometry than to the interpretative eye, and there is anatomic variation in neuronal density. Neuronal loss causes *gliosis,* which is easier to appreciate than loss of neurons after staining.

Control tissue, consisting of age- and location-matched cerebral cortex tissue obtained from autopsy specimens, provides a valuable baseline for assessing various abnormalities peculiar to dementias. This control is particularly important for assessing cytoplasmic vacuoles, minimal gliosis, and numbers of neurons.

Alzheimer's Disease

Minimal criteria necessary to diagnose Alzheimer's disease in autopsy brain specimens have been established.[383–386] These criteria refer to counts of argyrophilic plaques (and neurofibrillary tangles) in microscopic fields under a 10× or 20× objective. Powers[385] has commented that the vast majority of Alzheimer's cases are straightforward and a simple silver stain is sufficient for establishing a neuropathologic diagnosis. The diagnosis of Alzheimer's disease requires clinical input, and it should not be attempted on biopsy material without the clinical certainty of dementia.

Chief among the microscopic criteria for Alzheimer's disease is the number of argyrophilic plaques (see Table 18–3). Initial classification schemes emphasized precise numbers of plaques adjusted for different age groups.[383] Subsequent assessments have been semiquantitative (none, sparse, moderate, and frequent).[384]

Argyrophilic plaques are not adequately demonstrated for enumeration by H&E stains. Bielschowsky's silver stain is recommended for staining both argyrophilic plaques and neurofibrillary tangles (Fig. 18–55).[143, 383] Thioflavin S, excited by blue light suitable for fluorescein fluorescence, also reveals these structures.[213, 387, 388] Neurofibrillary tangles are located in neurons and are composed of bihelical filaments.[188, 213] These filaments are now being detected immunohistochemically by staining of their protein constituents, tau and ubiquitin.[389, 390] Neurofibrillary tangles are also intensely stained by Alz-50, a monoclonal antibody raised against a brain with Alzheimer's disease.[391, 392] Antisera to amyloid detects amorphous plaques seen in silver stains.[393–395] A Lewy body variant of Alzheimer's disease has been described.[396, 397]

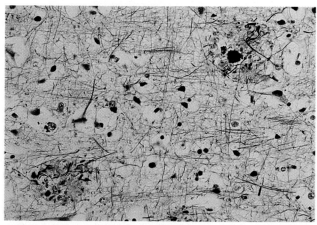

Figure 18–55. Alzheimer's disease. Two plaques at opposite corners of this specimen contain dark, twisted neurites. Although argyrophilic plaques key to the diagnosis stain with ubiquitin and other immunohistochemical stains, the Bielschowsky silver stain is still the "gold standard," as it were, for this disease. The patient, a middle-aged woman, had displayed progressive dementia for at least 3 years and satisfied the CERAD criteria[384] for diagnosis of Alzheimer's disease.

Multi-Infarct Vascular Dementia

Cerebral ischemic injury is a common cause of dementia in the elderly. Combination cases of vascular dementia and Alzheimer's disease are also quite frequent. Vascular causes of dementia include subcortical vascular dementia, multi-infarct dementia, ischemic dementia, cerebral autosomal dominant arteriopathy with subcortical infarcts and leukoencephalopathy (CADASIL), and "leuko-araiosis."[398, 399]

Other Dementias

The definition of various other causes of dementia has improved.[398] The most common among these is dementia with Lewy bodies. Assessment and enumeration of cerebral Lewy bodies in cortical neurons can be made with the aid of anti-ubiquitin and alpha-synuclein immunocytochemical analysis.[398, 400]

So-called dementia lacking distinctive histology is a member of the frontal lobe dementia group of diseases.[401] Pick's disease is quite rare. Specimens mainly are derived from material obtained at autopsy.[402] Additional causes of dementia are Lafora's disease, neuronal ceroid lipofuscinosis, adrenoleukodystrophy, and others reviewed elsewhere.[403–405]

DEMYELINATION

Unless progressive multifocal leukoencephalopathy is found in a biopsy specimen, demyelinating diseases are usually investigated clinically and at autopsy (see Table 18–3).

Primary demyelination affects only the myelin, in contrast to loss of myelin *secondary* to loss of axons. Primary demyelinating lesions are characterized histologically by destruction of myelin and abundant foamy KP-1+ macrophages containing myelin debris and lipid droplets. Within the lesion, NF+ axons are spared (Fig. 18–56). If the lesion was induced by a virus, amphophilic inclusions may be found, particularly at the periphery of the lesion. Viral disorders known to cause demyelination are HIV, JCV, SV40, cytomegalovirus, Epstein-Barr virus, and varicella-zoster. Immunohistochemical analysis, ISH, and PCR assay are available for detecting many of these viruses.[59, 60, 79–81, 406, 407]

The major demyelinating disorder is multiple sclerosis (MS). MS should be differentiated from other disorders in which the histologic appearance of the lesions and the relapsing and remitting clinical course are similar.[408] Acute MS lesions, in addition to plentiful foamy macrophages with increased proteases,[409] have perivascular LCA+ lymphocytes, EMA+ and immunoglobulin-positive plasma cells, variable GFAP+ gliosis, and less endothelial CD34 immunostaining.[410] The macrophages stain positively for class II major histocompatibility complex antigens (HLA-DR; Ia).[411] They contain myelin debris related to phagocytosis. Oligodendroglia are usually seen only at the periphery of the lesions.[412] Acute plaques can show blood-brain barrier leakage from vessel wall damage with intramural complement on smooth muscle cells and infiltration by HLA-DR–positive macrophages.[413]

Macrophages can accumulate in an active region of white matter demyelination to the extent that they mimic oligodendroglioma and hemangioblastoma (see Box 1).[175, 414] KP-1 is used to confirm the presence of macrophages. Oligodendrogliomas have fewer cytoplasmic vacuoles, more central nuclei, and Leu7 and S-100 protein immunoreactivity, fea-

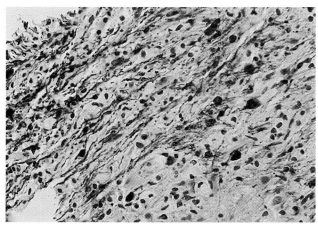

Figure 18–56. Primary demyelination with preservation of brown NF+ axons. Some axons are swollen and are called spheroids. Lipid-laden macrophages and gliosis are not stained brown in this section of this brain biopsy specimen, but their pale gray features are still evident.

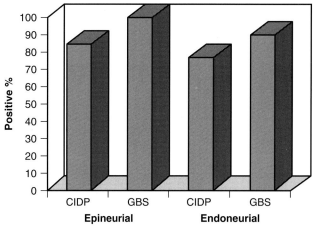

Figure 18–57. Locations of T lymphocytes among sural nerve biopsy specimens from 13 cases of chronic inflammatory demyelinating polyneuropathy (CIDP) and 22 cases of Guillain-Barré syndrome (GBS). Percentages positive are as reported in Schmidt B, Toyka KV, Keifer R, et al. Inflammatory infiltrates in sural nerve biopsies in Guillain-Barré syndrome and chronic inflammatory demyelinating neuropathy. Muscle Nerve 1996;19:474–487.

tures that distinguish them from lipid-laden macrophages. Hemangioblastomas have more factor VIII and CD31 reactive capillaries and less Leu7 (CD57) than oligodendrogliomas. Lipid-laden macrophages in a region of demyelination can be distinguished from neoplasia on the basis of the histochemical or electron microscopic demonstration of small, round globules of phagocytosed myelin.[143, 415]

In peripheral nerve, KP-1 (CD68)–positive macrophages engulf myelin and cluster around endoneurial vessels.[416] T lymphocytes that are immunoreactive with CD3, CD4, and CD8 are abundant in the endoneurium, and B lymphocytes are virtually absent, in chronic inflammatory demyelinating polyneuropathy (CIDP).[417] T lymphocytes are prominent in both CIDP and Guillain-Barré syndrome (Fig. 18–57).[416]

EPILEPSY

Complex partial epilepsy (previously called "temporal lobe epilepsy") may involve the temporal, frontal, parietal, or occipital lobe. About 80% of complex partial seizures originate in the temporal lobe, and thus, the most common surgical procedure for intractable epilepsy is temporal lobectomy.[418–420] Immunostaining for GFAP, with the use of age-matched temporal lobe autopsy control tissue, is recommended for detection and neuroanatomic localization of the most common abnormality, gliosis (Fig. 18–58; see Table 18–3).[64]

Other changes are frequently observed, such as loss of pyramidal neurons in the hippocampus, large numbers of corpora amylacea (see Fig. 18–58), deposits of hemosiderin pigment in perivascular macrophages, and focal meningeal fibrosis. Occasionally, calcification and ferrugination of large

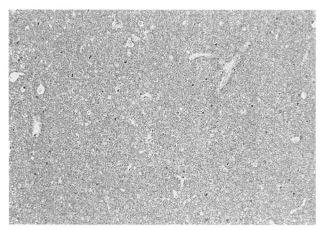

Figure 18–58. Pyramidal cell layer of cornu Ammonis region 1 of hippocampus in a patient with decades of partial complex seizures. Two large, clear, GFAP− neurons can be seen near a vessel at one side of the field. Other neurons have died. Although there are numerous brown GFAP+ fibrils of gliosis, the astrocytes are quiescent and have little brown cytoplasm around their nuclei. Round, fuzzy, light purple bodies the size of nuclei are *corpora amylacea*, common in such specimens. This neuronal loss and gliosis happened many years ago.

pyramidal neurons can be seen in the hippocampus.[421, 422] Cytoarchitectural studies of gray and white matter in resected temporal neocortex may reveal features of neuronal dysgenesis, such as neuronal ectopia, neuronal clustering, and subpial gliosis.[423]

Deep or surface electrodes are occasionally placed within the region of the future surgical resection in order to monitor and evaluate the seizure activity. The surgeon should inform the pathologist if such electrodes have been used. The electrodes leave a tract of encephalomalacia with chronic inflammation of A6+ and L26+ T and B lymphocytes, KP-1+ macrophages, and hemorrhage in the surgical specimen.[426] Surface electrodes cause focal meningitis.

A variety of clinically unsuspected pathologic entities are found in individual specimens. Stereotactic resection of cerebral lesions in partial epilepsy often yields vascular malformations and glial neoplasms.[425] Primary intracerebral tumors manifesting as medically refractory epilepsy are usually low-grade gliomas, mixed tumors with glial or neuronal components or both, hamartomas, or dysembryoplastic neuroepithelial tumors (see Figs. 18–12*A*, 18–19*A*, and 18–27).[426, 427]

PITFALLS IN DIAGNOSIS

Is It Really Negative?

The simple question whether a specimen is really "negative" for the marker in question must be asked to avoid misinterpretation. Whenever possible, one should include a positive control for the marker, as described earlier, within the *same block* as the lesion to be identified (Fig. 18–59). A positive control from a different block does not work as well. If this control tissue does not stain, then the lesion cannot be evaluated with the immunohistochemical stain.

Are the Cells of Interest Positive?

A good nuclear counterstain is essential to correct interpretation of immunohistochemical stain

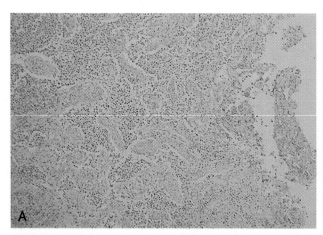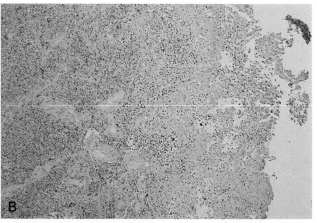

Figure 18–59. Importance of internal tissue control for immunohistochemistry. Tiny tissue fragment at the edge of two sections of this tumor specimen and corners of the two illustrations is brain. Brain tissue, which always makes S-100 protein, is the internal positive control. Two procedures were used to test for S-100 protein. *A,* One procedure for S-100 protein does not stain the tumor, but neither does it stain the brain. *B,* The second procedure stains the brain fragment dark brown and also stains the tumor. Only the second procedure is a reliable stain for S-100, and it reveals the tumor to be S-100+. Subsequent HMB-45 staining suggested metastatic melanoma, and ultimately, the cutaneous primary tumor was found. (From McKeever PE. New methods of brain tumor analysis. In: Mena H, ed. Dr. Kenneth M. Earle Memorial Neuropathology Review. Washington, D.C.: Armed Forces Institute of Pathology, February 24, 2000.)

responses. The counterstain distinguishes reactive, neoplastic, and necrotic cells as well as neuroanatomic relationships. Necrotic cells have nuclear pyknosis, karyorrhexis, and karyolysis. Necrotic regions generate false-positive response to immunohistochemical staining. Both features need to be recognized to avoid misinterpretation.

Reactive astrocytosis is associated with many brain tumors. Nuclear features of GFAP+ cells must be examined to distinguish reactive from neoplastic astrocytes (see Fig. 18−23). The immunoreactivity in closest proximity to the definitive nuclei should be checked for correct identification of these cells. This rule has general application to other markers (see Figs. 18−15*B* and 18−49).

Neoplastic cells have atypical or pleomorphic nuclei. Their chromatin patterns are often distinctive (see Fig. 18−11*B*). Glioma nuclei are crowded. WHO grade III and higher gliomas and other malignancies show mitoses (see Figs. 18−8*A*, 18−8*C*, and 18−23*A*).

Demyelination versus Neoplasm

Demyelination may be confused with neoplastic disease because it produces abundant gliosis.[428] Large cells with short chromosomes spread apart in their cytoplasm mimic mitotic activity in a glioma.[414] If numerous lipid-laden KP-1+ macrophages are encountered within parenchyma and around vessels, demyelinating disease should be considered. Appropriate stains for myelin, NF stain for axons (see Box 2), and features described in the following section on Gliosis versus Glioma should be considered in the interpretation (see Figs. 18−3*A*, 18−11*A* and *B*, and 18−56).

Gliosis versus Glioma

Distinguishing gliosis from glioma can be most difficult (see Fig. 18−9*A*).[64] Diffuse gliomas infiltrate brain tissue and stimulate their own gliosis, compounding the problem. Features that distinguish glioma cells from gliosis and normal parenchyma include individual cell variation in GFAP staining, nuclear hyperchromasia (Fig. 18−11*B*), nuclear cluster formation, nuclear molding (Fig. 18−13), mitoses, and calcifications. Mitoses suggest not only that the tumor is a glioma but also that it has a high grade of malignancy. Abnormal variations in size and shape of glial nuclei are common in margins of gliomas.

In astrocytomas, ependymomas, and astrocytic gliomas, GFAP stain is ideal for highlighting glioma cells. GFAP stain delineates the cytoplasm in both gliosis and glioma, facilitating interpretation of these cells. High nuclear to low brown cytoplasmic ratios typify gliomas. Mitotic spindles with chromosomes near each other and surrounded by little cytoplasm (see Fig. 18−23*A*) are exceptionally rare in gliosis (Fig. 18−23*B*). Reac-

tive astrocytes have much lower nuclear to cytoplasmic ratios, abundant dark brown stellate processes, and spaces between them so that they resemble trees in an apple orchard (see Fig. 18−2). There is a possibility that immunohistochemical markers of proliferation, like PCNA and MIB-1, will help distinguish neoplastic glia from gliosis at these margins.

Gliomas expand but gliosis contracts. This important feature is difficult to confirm without serial radiographs and in situ observation of the confluence of the actual mass and its margin to exclude the possibility of gliosis around another tumor.

Granular *calcifications* scattered among hypercellular glia distinguish glioma from gliosis and normal white matter.[148, 150] Caution is required not to overinterpret calcifications associated with neurons and neuropil within 0.5 cm of a large mass. Although microcysts, calcifications, and mitoses are important diagnostic features of gliomas, they are not seen in every case and are uncommon within the margins of gliomas invading CNS parenchyma.

Another important feature distinguishing the margin of a glioma from gliosis is *cellular density* (see Table 18−2). Some gliomas exhibit *uneven distribution* of cellular density (see Fig. 18−10). Others obscure the junction between gray matter and white matter. Still others spawn *secondary structures of Scherer*, the most distinctive being subpial and perineuronal gliomatosis; these secondary structures are collections of neoplastic glia beneath the pia or around neurons.[64] GFAP stain highlights secondary structures from astrocytomas. Secondary structures of oligodendrogliomas show much less synaptophysin than the neuropil of gray matter and are highlighted as lightly staining clusters of cells around neurons or vessels.[123]

Glioma nuclei frequently touch and even indent one another (see Fig. 18−13), even among scattered clusters of cells in the diffuse margins of gliomas. Gliosis, however, consists of evenly spaced astrocytes with high GFAP immunoreactivity (see Fig. 18−2). This even spacing is best seen with anti-GFAP staining at low magnification. The low nuclear to cytoplasmic ratio of gliosis is seen at high magnification. Because the nuclei of gliomas are more pleomorphic than normal or gliotic CNS parenchyma, nuclear *pleomorphism* and *hyperchromasia* (seen best with a good nuclear counterstain like hematoxylin) help identify a glioma (see Figs. 18−7 to 18−9, 18−11, and 18−13).[1]

Infiltrating versus Noninfiltrating Cells

Noninfiltrating gliomas are often surgically resectable, a characteristic that places a premium on distinguishing them from infiltrating gliomas. This distinction can be difficult in fragmented or incomplete specimens.

After the possibility of neoplastic neurons has

been ruled out (see section on Neuronal Tumors), neuroanatomic brain tissue constituents are useful markers for distinguishing noninfiltrating from infiltrating gliomas. Axons run close together in parallel in white matter tracts and are identifiable in gray matter also. Noninfiltrating gliomas leave these axons unmolested (see Fig. 18–10*B*), whereas infiltrating gliomas spread them apart (see Fig. 18–10*A*) and cause some to swell. Synaptophysin carpets the neuropil of gray matter with tiny brown dots. Synaptophysin-negative glioma cells either stop abruptly or infiltrate this fine carpet.[123]

In specimens that lack discernible brain tissue, information is still available after the tumor has been stained. If axons of non-neoplastic origin are found in the glioma, it is an infiltrative glioma (see Fig. 18–13). This feature distinguishes infiltrating gliomas from noninfiltrating gliomas, which have more discrete margins with brain tissue.

Abscess versus Neoplasm

Entities that produce collagen within the CNS may be confused with the wall of an abscess (see Fig. 18–4; see Tables 18–5, 18–7, 18–10, and 18–11). Sarcomatous and desmoplastic neoplasms and various cysts with collagenous walls may simulate abscesses (see Figs. 18–26*B*, 18–30*A*, and 18–35). These tumors may be distinguished by the lack of an inflammatory component and the presence of a neoplastic component. More problematic are cysts that have ruptured and exuded material foreign to the CNS, such as colloid or squamous epithelial cells. If this material is not detectable on H&E staining within the inflammatory reaction, immunohistochemical stains for cyst wall material, such as CK stains for epithelial cells, assist the interpretation.[367] These other lesions are sterile in situ and do not stain for microorganisms as would an abscess (see Box 2).

ACKNOWLEDGMENTS

The following colleagues provided particularly valuable assistance. Drs. Mila Blaivas, Jeanne Bell, Larry Junck, and Ricardo Lloyd provided key citations. I thank Ms. Dianna Banka and Ms. Peggy Otto for their skill and patience in preparing this chapter. Mr. Mark Deming carefully prepared the illustrations. Immunohistologists and histopathologists in the University of Michigan Medical Center Pathology Laboratories prepared fine microscopic slides.

References

1. McKeever PE. New methods of brain tumor analysis. In: Mena H, ed. Dr. Kenneth M. Earle Memorial Neuropathology Review. Washington, D.C., Armed Forces Institute of Pathology, Feb 24, 2000.
2. Finley JL, Silverman JF, Dickens MA. Immunocytochemical evaluation of central nervous system tumors obtained by the Cavitron ultrasonic surgical aspirator. Diagn Cytopathol 1990;6:308–312.
3. Kepes JJ, Moral LA, Wilkinson SB, et al. Rhabdoid transformation of tumor cells in meningiomas: A histologic indication of increased proliferative activity: Report of four cases. Am J Surg Pathol 1998;22:231–238.
4. McKeever PE, Wichman A, Chronwall BM, et al. Sarcoma arising from a gliosarcoma. South Med J 1984;77:1027–1325.
5. Silverberg GD. Simple cysts of the cerebellum. J Neurosurg 1971;35:320–327.
6. Daumas-Duport C, Scheithauer B, O'Fallon J, Kelly P. Grading of astrocytomas: A simple and reproducible method. Cancer 1988;62:2152–2165.
7. McKeever PE, Balentine JD. Macrophage migration through the brain parenchyma to the perivascular space following particle ingestion. Am J Pathol 1978;93:153–164.
8. Graeber MB, Wolfgang JS. Microglia: Immune network in the CNS. Brain Pathol 1991;1:2–5.
9. Del Bigio MR. Biologic reactions to cerebrospinal fluid shunt devices: A review of the cellular pathology. Neurosurgery 1998;42:319–325.
10. Caplan R, Curtiss S, Chugani HT, Vinters HV. Pediatric Rasmussen encephalitis: Social communication, language, PET and pathology before and after hemispherectomy. Brain Cogn 1996;32:45–66.
11. Lowry A, Wilcox D, Masson EA, Williams PE. Immunohistochemical methods for semiquantitative analysis of collagen content in human peripheral nerve. J Anat 1997;191:367–374.
12. Kubota T, Sato K, Kabuto M, et al. Clear cell (glycogen-rich) meningioma with special reference to spherical collagen deposits. Noshuyo Byori 1995;12:53–60.
13. Mighell AJ, Robinson PA, Hume WJ. Patterns of immunoreactivity to an anti-fibronectin polyclonal antibody in formalin-fixed, paraffin-embedded oral tissues are dependent on methods of antigen retrieval. J Histochem Cytochem 1995;43:1107–1114.
14. McKeever PE, Fligiel SEG, Varani J, et al. Products of cells cultured from gliomas. IV: Extracellular matrix proteins of gliomas. Int J Cancer 1986;37:867–874.
15. Vitolo D, Paradiso P, Uccini S, et al. Expression of adhesion molecules and extracellular matrix proteins in glioblastomas: Relation to angiogenesis and spread. Histopathology 1996;28:521–528.
16. Higuchi M, Ohnishi T, Arita N, et al. Expression of tenascin in human gliomas: Its relation to histological malignancy, tumor dedifferentiation and angiogenesis. Acta Neuropathol 1993;85:481–487.
17. Ogawa K, Oguchi M, Nakashima Y, et al. Distribution of collagen type IV in brain tumors: An immunohistochemical study. J Neurooncol 1989;7:357–366.
18. Sun T, Greenspan J, Tenenbaum M, et al. Diagnosis of cerebral toxoplasmosis using fluorescein-labeled antitoxoplasma monoclonal antibodies. Am J Surg Pathol 1986;10:312–316.
19. Kaneko K, Onodera O, Miyatake T, Tsuji S. Rapid diagnosis of tuberculous meningitis by polymerase chain reaction (PCR). Neurology 1990;40:1617–1618.
20. Kristiansen BE, Ask E, Jenkins A, et al. Rapid diagnosis of meningococcal meningitis by polymerase chain reaction. Lancet 1991;337:1568–1569.
21. Figueroa ME, Rasheed S. Molecular pathology and diagnosis of infectious diseases. Am J Clin Pathol 1991;95:S8–S21.
22. Skolnik PR, Davis KR, Cohen ME, et al. Cerebral mucormycosis. Case records of the Massachusetts General Hospital. Weekly clinicopathological exercises. Case 52-1990. A 31-year-old HIV-seropositive woman with a cerebral lesion seven years after treatment of carcinoma of the cervix. N Engl J Med 1990;323:1823–1833.
23. Philips P, Weiner MH. Invasive aspergillosis diagnosed by immunohistochemistry with monoclonal and polyclonal reagents. Hum Pathol 1987;18:1015–1024.

24. Monteagudo C, Marcilla A, Mormeneo S, et al. Specific immunohistochemical identification of *Candida albicans* in paraffin-embedded tissue with a new monoclonal antibody (1B12). Am J Clin Pathol 1995;103:130–135.

25. Kleinman GM, Zagzag D, Miller DC. Diagnostic use of immunohistochemistry in neuropathology. Neurosurg Clin N Am 1994;5:97–126.

26. Reed JA, Hemann BA, Alexander JL, Brigati DJ. Immunomycology: Rapid and specific immunocytochemical identification of fungi in formalin-fixed, paraffin-embedded material. J Histochem Cytochem 1993;41:1217–1221.

27. Kaufman L, Standard PG, Jalbert M, Kraft DE. Immunohistologic identification of *Aspergillus* spp. and other hyaline fungi by using polyclonal fluorescent antibodies. J Clin Microbiol 1997;35:2206–2209.

28. Luo D. Immunohistochemical demonstration of mycobacterial antigen. Chin J Tuberc Respir Dis 1990;13:360–362, 381–382.

29. Ang SC, Moscovic EA. Cross-reactive and species specific *Mycobacterium tuberculosis* antigens in the immunoprofile of Schaumann bodies: A major clue to the etiology of sarcoidosis. Histol Histopathol 1996;11:125–134.

30. Parker JC, Dyer ML. Neurologic infections due to bacteria, fungi, and parasites. In: Davis RL, Robertson DM, eds. Textbook of Neuropathology. New York: Williams & Wilkins, 1985:632–703.

31. Latronico N, Candiani A. Brainstem herpes virus encephalitis. Lancet 1987;8520:690–691.

32. Whitley RJ. Viral encephalitis. N Engl J Med 1990;323:242–248.

33. Edmonds LC, Stubbs SE, Ryu JH. Syphilis: A disease to exclude in diagnosing sarcoidosis. Mayo Clin Proc 1992;67:37–41.

34. Guarner J, Greer PW, Bartlett J, et al. Congenital syphilis in a newborn: An immunopathologic study. Mod Pathol 1999;12:82–87.

35. Garcia HH, Martinez M, Gilman R, et al. The Cysticercosis Working Group in Peru: Diagnosis of cysticercosis in endemic regions. Lancet 1991;338:549–551.

36. Shankar SK, Ravi V, Suryanarayana V, et al. Immunoreactive antigenic sites of *Cysticercus cellulosae* relevant to human neurocysticercosis—immunocytochemical localization using human CSF as source of antibody. Clin Neuropathol 1995;14:33–36.

37. Selwa LM, Brunberg JA, Mandell SH, Garofalo EA. Spinal cord schistosomiasis: A pediatric case mimicking intrinsic cord neoplasm. Neurology 1991;41:755–757.

38. Diogo CM, Mendonca MC, Savino W, et al. Immunoreactivity of a cytokeratin-related polypeptide from adult *Schistosoma mansoni*. Int J Parasitol 1994;24:727–732.

39. Sauter MK, Panitch HS, Kristt DA. Myelopathic neurosarcoidosis: Diagnostic value of enhanced MRI. Neurology 1991;41:150–151.

40. Fleming JL, Wiesner RH, Shorter RG. Whipple's disease: Clinical, biochemical, and histopathologic features and assessment of treatment in 29 patients. Mayo Clin Proc 1988;63:539–551.

41. Relman DA, Schmidt TM, MacDermot RP, Falkow S. Identification of the uncultured bacillus of Whipple's disease. N Engl J Med 1992;327:293–301.

42. Schwartz MA, Selhorts JB, Ochs AL, et al. Oculomasticatory myorrhythmia: A unique movement disorder occurring in Whipple's disease. Ann Neurol 1986;20:677–683.

43. Cadavid D, Barbour AG. Neuroborreliosis during relapsing fever: Review of the clinical manifestations, pathology, and treatment of infections in humans and experimental animals. Clin Infect Dis 1998;26:151–164.

44. Halperin J, Volkman DJ, Wu P. Central nervous system abnormalities in Lyme neuroborreliosis. Neurology 1991;41:1571–1582.

45. Magnarelli LA, Anderson JF, Johnson RC. Cross-reactivity in serological tests for Lyme disease and other spirochetal infections. J Infect Dis 1987;156:183–188.

46. Keller TL, Halperin JJ, Whitman M. PCR detection of *Borrelia burgdorferi* DNA in cerebrospinal fluid of Lyme neuroborreliosis patients. Neurology 1992;42:32–42.

47. White CL, Taxy JB. Early morphologic diagnosis of herpes simplex encephalitis: Advantages of electron microscopy and immunoperoxidase staining. Hum Pathol 1983;14:135–139.

48. Fleming KA. Analysis of viral pathogenesis by in situ hybridization. J Pathol 1992;166:95–96.

49. Rogers BB, Josephson SL, Mak SK. Detection of herpes simplex virus using the polymerase chain reaction followed by endonuclease cleavage. Am J Pathol 1991;139:1–6.

50. Morgello S, Block GA, Price RW, Petito CK. Varicella-zoster virus leukoencephalitis and cerebral vasculopathy. Arch Pathol Lab Med 1988;112:173–177.

51. Mrak RE, Young L. Rabies encephalitis in humans: Pathology, pathogenesis and pathophysiology. J Neuropathol Exp Neurol 1994;53:1–10.

52. Jackson AC, Ye H, Phelan CC, et al. Extraneural organ involvement in human rabies. Lab Invest 1999;79:945–951.

53. Nagano I, Nakamura S, Toshioka M, Kogure K. Immunocytochemical analysis of the cellular infiltrate in brain lesions in subacute sclerosing panencephalitis. Neurology 1991;41:1639–1642.

54. McQuaid S, Cosby SL, Koffi K, et al. Distribution of measles virus in the central nervous system of HIV-seropositive children. Acta Neuropathol 1998;96:637–642.

55. An SF, Scaravilli F. Early HIV-1 infection of the central nervous system. Arch Anat Cytol Pathol 1997;45:94–105.

56. Budka H. Neuropathology of myelitis, myelopathy, and spinal infections in AIDS. Neuroimaging Clin N Am 1997;7:639–650.

57. Wiley CA. Pathology of neurologic disease in AIDS. Psychiatr Clin North Am 1994;17:1–15.

58. Mirra SS, de Rio C. The fine structure of acquired immunodeficiency syndrome encephalopathy. Arch Pathol Lab Med 1989;113:858–865.

59. Shapshak P, Sun NCJ, Resnick L, et al. The detection of HIV by in situ hybridization. Mod Pathol 1990;3:146–153.

60. Tan SV, Guiloff RJ, Scaravilli F. AIDS-associated vacuolar myelopathy: A morphometric study. Brain 1995;118:1247–1261.

61. Mashliah E, Ge N, Morey M, et al. Cortical dendritic pathology in human immunodeficiency virus encephalitis. Lab Invest 1992;3:285–291.

62. Power C, Kong PA, Crawford TO, et al. Cerebral white matter changes in acquired immunodeficiency syndrome dementia: Alterations of the blood-brain barrier. Ann Neurol 1993;34:339–350.

63. Jones H Jr, Ho DD, Forgacs P, et al. Acute fulminating fetal leukoencephalopathy as the only manifestation of human immunodeficiency virus infection. Ann Neurol 1988;23:519–522.

64. McKeever PE. The brain, spinal cord and meninges. In: Sternberg SS, Antonioli DA, Mills SE, et al, eds. Diagnostic Surgical Pathology, vol. 1. 3rd ed. Philadelphia: Lippincott Williams & Wilkins, 1999:389–482.

65. Bertoli F, Espino M, Arosemena JR 5th, et al. A spectrum in the pathology of toxoplasmosis in patients with acquired immunodeficiency syndrome. Arch Pathol Lab Med 1995;119:214–224.

66. Arnold SJ, Kinney MC, McCormick MS, et al. Disseminated toxoplasmosis: Unusual presentations in the immunocompromised host. Arch Pathol Lab Med 1997;121:869–873.

67. Zimmer C, Daeschlein G, Patt S, Weigel K. Strategy for diagnosis of *Toxoplasma gondii* in stereotactic brain biopsies. Stereotact Funct Neurosurg 1991;56:66–75.

68. Rhodes RH. Histopathology of the central nervous system in the acquired immunodeficiency syndrome. Hum Pathol 1987;18:636–643.

69. Vinters HV, Kowk MK, Ho HW, et al. Cytomegalovirus in the nervous system of patients with the acquired immune deficiency syndrome. Brain 1989;112:245–268.

70. Persons DL, Moore JA, Fishback JL. Comparison of polymerase chain reaction, DNA hybridization, and histology with viral culture to detect cytomegalovirus in immunosuppressed patients. Mod Pathol 1991;4:149–152.

71. Vazeux R, Cumont M, Girard PM, et al. Severe encephalitis resulting from coinfections with HIV and JC virus. Neurology 1990;40:944–948.
72. Daley CL, Small PM, Schecter GF, et al. An outbreak of the tuberculosis with accelerated progression among persons infected with the human immunodeficiency virus. N Engl J Med 1992;4:231–235.
73. Feraru ER, Aronow HA, Lipton RB. Neurosyphilis in AIDS patients: Initial CSF VDRL may be negative. Neurology 1990;40:541–543.
74. Fleet WS, Watson RT, Ballinger WE. Resolution of a gumma with steroid therapy. Neurology 1986;36:1104–1107.
75. Martinez AJ, Visvesvara GS. Free-living, amphizoic and opportunistic amebas. Brain Pathol 1997;7:583–598.
76. Oddó D, Casanova M, Acuña G, et al. Acute Chagas' disease (Trypanosomiasis americana) in acquired immunodeficiency syndrome: Report of two cases. Hum Pathol 1992;23:41–44.
77. Dutcher JP, Marcus SL, Tanowitz HB, et al. Disseminated strongyloidiasis within central nervous system involvement diagnosed antemortem in a patient with acquired immunodeficiency syndrome and Burkitt's lymphoma. Cancer 1990;66:2417–2420.
78. Aksamit AJ, Gendelman HE, Orenstein JM, Pezeshkpour GH. AIDS-associated progressive multifocal leukoencephalopathy (PML): Comparison to non-AIDS PML with in situ hybridization and immunohistochemistry. Neurology 1990;40:1073–1078.
79. Prayson RA, Estes ML. Stereotactic brain biopsy for diagnosis of progressive multifocal leukoencephalopathy. South Med J 1993;86:1381–1394.
80. Hulette CM, Downey BT, Burger PC. Progressive multifocal leukoencephalopathy: Diagnosis by in situ hybridization with a biotinylated JC virus DNA probe using an automated histomatic code-on slide stainer. Am J Surg Pathol 1991;15:791–797.
81. Stoner GL, Ryschkewitsch CF. Capsid protein VP1 deletions in JC virus from two AIDS patients with progressive multifocal leukoencephalopathy. J Neurovirol 1995;1:189–194.
82. Manetto V, Medori R, Cortelli P, et al. Fatal familial insomnia: Clinical and pathologic study of five new cases. Neurology 1992;42:312–319.
83. Hulette CM, Earl NL, Crain BJ. Evaluation of cerebral biopsies for the diagnosis of dementia. Arch Neurol 1992;49:28–31.
84. Castellani RJ, Parchi P, Madoff L, et al. Biopsy diagnosis of Creutzfeldt-Jakob disease by Western blot: A case report. Hum Pathol 1997;28:623–626.
85. Richardson EP Jr, Masters CL. The nosology of Creutzfeldt-Jakob disease and conditions related to the accumulation of PrPCJD in the nervous system. [review] Brain Pathol 1995;5:33–41.
86. Capellari S, Vital C, Parchi P, et al. Familial prion disease with a novel 144-bp insertion in the prion protein gene in a Basque family. Neurology 1997;49:133–141.
87. Bruce ME, Will RG, Ironside JW, et al. Transmissions to mice indicate that "new variant" CJD is caused by the BSE agent. Nature 1997;389:498–501.
88. Grigoriev V, Escaig-Haye F, Streichenberger N, et al. Submicroscopic immunodetection of PrP in the brain of a patient with a new variant of Creutzfeldt-Jakob disease. Neurosci Lett 1999;264:57–60.
89. Serban D, Taraboulos A, DeArmond J, Prusiner SB. Rapid detection of Creutzfeldt-Jakob disease and scrapie prion proteins. Neurology 1990;40:110–117.
90. Smith PEM, Zeidler M, Ironside JW, et al. Creutzfeldt-Jakob disease in a dairy farmer. [letter] Lancet 1995;346:898.
91. Britton TC, al-Sarraj S, Shaw C, et al. Sporadic Creutzfeldt-Jakob disease in a 16-year-old in the UK. [letter] Lancet 1995;346:1155.
92. Bateman D, Hilton D, Love S, et al. Sporadic Creutzfeldt-Jakob disease in an 18-year-old in the UK. [letter] Lancet 1995;346:1155–1156.

93. Ironside JW, Sutherland K, Bell JE, et al. A new variant of Creutzfeldt-Jakob disease: Neuropathological and clinical features. Cold Spring Harb Symp Quant Biol 1996;50:523–527.
94. Kitamoto T, Yamaguchi K, Doh-ura K, Tateishi J. A prion protein missense variant is integrated in kuru plaque cores in patients with Gerstmann-Sträussler syndrome. Neurology 1991;41:306–310.
95. Tateishi J, Kitamoto T, Doh-ura K, et al. Immunochemical, molecular genetic, and transmission studies on a case of Gerstmann-Sträussler-Scheinker syndrome. Neurology 1990;40:1578–1581.
96. Gilbert JJ, Vinters HV. Cerebral amyloid angiopathy: Incidence and complications in the aging brain. I: Cerebral hemorrhage. Stroke 1983;14:915–923.
97. Ishihara T, Takahashi M, Yokota T, et al. The significance of cerebrovascular amyloid in the aetiology of superficial (lobar) cerebral haemorrhage and its incidence in the elderly population. J Pathol 1991;165:229–234.
98. Vinters HV, Secor DL, Pardridge WM, Gray F. Immunohistochemical study of cerebral amyloid angiopathy. III: Widespread Alzheimer A4 peptide in cerebral microvessel walls colocalizes with gamma trace in patients with leukoencephalopathy. Ann Neurol 1990;28:34–42.
99. Chen ST, Chen SD, Hsu CY, Hogan EL. Progression of hypertensive intracerebral hemorrhage. Neurology 1989;39:1509–1514.
100. Kittner SJ, Sharkness CM, Sloan MA, et al. Infarcts with a cardiac source of embolism in the NINDS stroke data bank: Neurologic examination. Neurology 1992;42:299–302.
101. García-Moncó J, Beldarrain G. Superior sagittal sinus thrombosis complicating Crohn's disease. Neurology 1991;41:1324–1325.
102. Minette SE, Kimmel DW. Subdural hematoma in patients with systemic cancer. Mayo Clin Proc 1989;64:637–642.
103. Miettinen M, Lindenmayer AE, Chaubal A. Endothelial cell markers CD31, CD34, and BNH9 antibody to H- and Y-antigens—evaluation of their specificity and sensitivity in the diagnosis of vascular tumors and comparison with von Willebrand factor. Mod Pathol 1994;7:82–90.
104. Allen JC, Miller DC, Budzilovich GN, Epstein FJ. Brain and spinal cord hemorrhage in long-term survivors of malignant pediatric brain tumors: A possible late effect of therapy. Neurology 1991;41:148–150.
105. Takahashi A, Ushiki T, Abe K, et al. Cytoarchitecture of periendothelial cells in human cerebral venous vessels as compared with the scalp vein: A scanning electron microscopic study. Arch Histol Cytol 1994;57:331–339.
106. Malandrini A, Carrera P, Palmeri S, et al. Clinicopathological and genetic studies of two further Italian families with cerebral autosomal dominant arteriopathy. Acta Neuropathol 1996;92:115–122.
107. Moore PM. Diagnosis and management of isolated angiitis of the central nervous system. Neurology 1989;39:167–173.
108. Blue MC, Rosenblum WI. Granulomatous angiitis of the brain with herpes zoster and varicella encephalitis. Arch Pathol Lab Med 1983;107:126–128.
109. Hook EW III, Marra CM. Acquired syphilis in adults. N Engl J Med 1992;326:1060–1069.
110. Levine SR, Brust JCM, Futrell N, et al. A comparative study of the cerebrovascular complications of cocaine: Alkaloidal versus hydrochloride—a review. Neurology 1991;41:1173–1177.
111. Sloan MA, Kittner SJ, Rigamonti D, Price TR. Occurrence of stroke associated with use/abuse of drugs. Neurology 1991;41:1358–1364.
112. Serena M, Biscaro R, Moretto G, Recchia E. Peripheral and central nervous system involvement in essential mixed cryoglobulinemia: A case report. Clin Neuropathol 1991;10:177–180.
113. Levine DN, David KR, Richardson EP, Pomerantz RJ. A 46-year-old woman with progressive dementia. N Engl J Med 1989;320:514–524.
114. Stewart SS, Ashizawa T, Dudley AW Jr, et al. Cerebral vasculitis in relapsing polychondritis. Neurology 1988;38:150–152.

115. Wechsler B, Vidaihet M, Piette JC, et al. Cerebral venous thrombosis in Behçet's disease: Clinical study and long-term follow-up of 25 cases. Neurology 1992;42:614–618.

116. Phanthumchinda K, Intragumtornchai T, Kasantikul V. Stroke-like syndrome, mineralizing microangiopathy, and neuroaxonal dystrophy following intrathecal methotrexate therapy. Neurology 1991;41:1847–1848.

117. Mighell AJ, Robinson PA, Hume WJ. Histochemical and immunohistochemical localization of elastic system fibers in focal reactive overgrowths of oral mucosa. J Oral Pathol Med 1997;26:153–158.

118. Gueguen B, Merland JJ, Riche MC, Rey A. Vascular malformations of the spinal cord: Intrathecal perimedullary arteriovenous fistulas fed by medullary arteries. Neurology 1987;37:969–979.

119. Farmer J-P, Cosgrove GR, Villemure J-G, et al. Intracerebral cavernous angiomas. Neurology 1988;38:1699–1704.

120. Kleihues P, Burger PC, Scheithauer BW. International Histological Classification of Tumours (Histological Typing of Tumours of the Central Nervous System.). vol. 21. 2nd ed. Berlin: Springer-Verlag, 1993.

121. McKeever PE, Burger PC, Nelson JS: Introduction to neurooncology. In: Nelson JS, Parisi JF, Schochet SS Jr, eds: Principles and Practice of Neuropathology. St. Louis: CV Mosby, 1993;109–122.

122. McKeever PE. Molecular neuropathology in brain tumor diagnosis. In: Kornblith PL, Walker MD, eds. Advances in Neuro-oncology II. Armonk, New York, Futura, 1997:139–178.

123. McKeever PE. Neurofilament (NF) and synaptophysin stains reveal diagnostic and prognostic patterns of interaction between normal and neoplastic tissues. Presented at the annual meeting of the Histochemical Society, Bethesda, MD, March 24, 2000.

124. Shi S-R, Cote RJ, Taylor CR. Antigen retrieval immunohistochemistry: Past, present, and future. J Histochem Cytochem 1997;45:327–343.

125. McKeever PE, Ross DA, Strawderman MS, et al. A comparison of the predictive power for survival in gliomas provided by MIB-1, bromodeoxyuridine and proliferating cell nuclear antigen with histopathologic and clinical parameters. J Neuropathol Exp Neurol 1997;7:798–805.

126. Mukhopadhyay SK, McKeever PE, Greenberg HS, et al. Random sampling by glitter drop method. Life Sci 1990;46:507–512.

127. Gerdes J, Schwab U, Lemke H, Stein H. Production of a mouse monoclonal antibody reactive with a human nuclear antigen associated with cell proliferation. Int J Cancer 1983;31:13–20.

128. Hsu DW, Louis DN, Efird JT, et al. Use of MIB-1 (Ki-67) immunoreactivity in differentiating grade II and grade III gliomas. J Neuropathol Exp Neurol 1997;56:857–865.

129. Montine TJ, Vandersteenhoven JJ, Aguzzi A, et al. Prognostic significance of Ki-67 proliferation index in supratentorial fibrillary astrocytic neoplasms. Neurosurgery 1994;34:674–678.

130. Karamitopoulou E, Perentes E, Diamantis I, Maraziotis T. Ki-67 immunoreactivity in human central nervous system tumors: A study with MIB 1 monoclonal antibody on archival material. Acta Neuropathol (Berlin) 1994;87:47–54.

131. Prayson RA, Khajavi K, Comair YG. Cortical architectural abnormalities and MIB1 immunoreactivity in gangliogliomas: A study of 60 patients with intracranial tumors. J Neuropathol Exp Neurol 1995;54:513–520.

132. Sallinen PK, Haapasalo HK, Visakorpi T, et al. Prognostication of astrocytoma patient survival by Ki67 (MIB-1), PCNA, and S-phase fraction using archival paraffin-embedded samples. J Pathol 1994;174:275–282.

133. Giannini C, Scheithauer BW, Burger PC. Cellular proliferation in pilocytic and diffuse astrocytomas. J Neuropathol Exp Neurol 1999;58:46–53.

134. McKeever PE, Strawderman MS, Yamini B, et al. MIB-1 proliferation index predicts survival among patients with grade II astrocytoma. J Neuropathol Exp Neurol 1998;57:931–936.

135. Prelich G, Tan C-K, Kostura M, et al. Functional identity of proliferating cell nuclear antigen and a DNA polymerase-S auxiliary protein. Nature 1987;326:517–519.

136. Aboussekhra A, Wood RD. Detection of nucleotide excision repair incisions in human fibroblasts by immunostaining for PCNA. Exp Cell Res 1995;221:326–332.

137. Korkolopoulou P, Christodoulou P, Lekka-Katsouli I, et al. Prognostic significance of proliferating cell nuclear antigen (PCNA) expression in gliomas. Histopathology 1994;25:349–355.

138. Ang LC, Plewes M, Tan L, et al. Proliferating cell nuclear antigen expression in the survival of astrocytoma patients. Can J Neurol Sci 1994;21:306–310.

139. Schiffer D, Cavalla P, Migheli A, et al. Apoptosis and cell proliferation in human neuroepithelial tumors. Neurosci Lett 1995;195:81–84.

140. Taniguchi K, Wakabayashi T, Yoshida T, et al. Immunohistochemical staining of DNA topoisomerase II alpha in human gliomas. J Neurosurg 1999;91:477–482.

141. Sehgal A. Molecular changes during the genesis of human gliomas. Semin Surg Oncol 1998;14:3–12.

142. Chronwall BM, McKeever PE, Kornblith PL. Glial and nonglial neoplasms evaluated on frozen section by double immunofluorescence for fibronectin and glial fibrillary acidic protein. Acta Neuropathol (Berl) 1983;59:283–287.

143. McKeever PE, Balentine JD. Histochemistry of the nervous system. In: Spicer SS, ed. Histochemistry in Pathologic Diagnosis. New York: Marcel-Dekker, 1987:871–957.

144. Cáccamo DV, Rubinstein LJ. Tumors: Applications of immunocytochemical methods. In: Garcia JH, Budka H, McKeever PE, et al, eds. Neuropathology: The Diagnostic Approach. Philadelphia: CV Mosby, 1997:193–218.

145. Cairncross JG, Ueki K, Zlatescu MC, et al. Specific genetic predictors of chemotherapeutic response and survival in patients with anaplastic oligodendrogliomas. J Natl Cancer Inst 1998;90:1473–1479.

146. Rodas RA, Fenstermaker RA, McKeever PE, et al. Correlation of intraluminal thrombosis in brain tumor vessels with postoperative thrombotic complications: A preliminary report. J Neurosurg 1998;89:200–205.

147. Cohen ME, Duffner PK, Heffner RR, et al. Prognostic factors in brainstem gliomas. Neurology 1986;36:602–605.

148. Martin F Jr, Lemmen LJ. Calcification in intracranial neoplasms. Am J Pathol 1952;28:1107–1129.

149. Rubinstein LJ. Tumors of the Central Nervous System. Washington, D.C.: Armed Forces Institute of Pathology, 1972.

150. Burger PC, Scheithauer BW, Vogel FS. Surgical Pathology of the Nervous System and Its Coverings, 3rd ed. New York: Churchill Livingstone, 1991.

151. Trojanowski JQ, Lee VMY, Schlaepfer WW. An immunohistochemical study of human central and peripheral nervous system tumors, using monoclonal antibodies against neurofilaments and glial filaments. Hum Pathol 1984;15:248–257.

152. Stanton C, Perentes E, Collins VP, Rubinstein LJ. GFA protein reactivity in nerve sheath tumors: A polyvalent and monoclonal antibody study. J Neuropathol Exp Neurol 1987;46:634–643.

153. Nakopoulou L, Kerezoudi E, Thomaides T, et al. An immunocytochemical comparison of glial fibrillary acidic protein, S-100p and vimentin in human glial tumors. J Neurooncol 1990;8:33–40.

154. Yung WK, Luna M, Borit A. Vimentin and glial fibrillary acidic protein in human brain tumors. Neurooncol 1985;3:35–38.

155. Burger PC, Scheithauer BW. Atlas of Tumor Pathology: Tumors of the Central Nervous System. Washington, D.C.: Armed Forces Institute of Pathology, 1994.

156. Hayostek C, Shaw EG, Scheithauer BW, et al. Astrocytomas of the cerebellum: A comparative clinicopathologic study of pilocytic and diffuse astrocytomas. Cancer 1993;72:856–869.

157. Mamelak AN, Prados MD, Obana WG, et al. Treatment options and prognosis for multicentric juvenile pilocytic astrocytoma. J Neurosurg 1994;81:24–30.

158. Forsyth PA, Shaw EG, Scheithauer BW, et al. 51 cases of supratentorial pilocytic astrocytomas: A clinicopathologic, prognostic, and flow cytometric study. Cancer 1993;72:1335–1342.
159. Coakley KJ, Huston J, Scheithauer BW, et al. Pilocytic astrocytomas: Well-demarcated magnetic resonance appearance despite frequent infiltration histologically. Mayo Clin Proc 1995;70:747–751.
160. Clark GB, Henry JM, McKeever PE. Cerebral pilocytic astrocytoma. Cancer 1985;56:1128–1133.
161. Murayama S, Bouldin TW, Suzuki K. Immunocytochemical and ultrastructural studies of eosinophilic granular bodies in astrocytic tumors. Acta Neuropathol 1992;83:408–414.
162. Lowe J, McDermott H, Pike I, et al. Alpha B crystallin expression in non-lenticular tissues and selective presence in ubiquitinated inclusion bodies in human disease. J Pathol 1992;166:61–68.
163. Hitotsumatsu T, Iwaki T, Fukui M, Tateishi J. Distinctive immunohistochemical profiles of small heat shock proteins (heat shock protein 27 and alpha B-crystallin) in human brain tumors. Cancer 1996;77:352–361.
164. Camby I, Nagy N, Lopes MB, et al. Supratentorial pilocytic astrocytomas, astrocytomas, anaplastic astrocytomas and glioblastomas are characterized by a differential expression of S100 proteins. Brain Pathol 1999;9:1–19.
165. Schneider JH Jr, Raffel C, McComb JG. Benign cerebellar astrocytomas of childhood. Neurosurgery 1992;30:58–62.
166. Molloy PT, Bilaniuk LT, Vaughan SN, et al. Brainstem tumors in patients with neurofibromatosis type 1. Neurology 1995;1897–1902.
167. Vertosick FT Jr, Selker RG, Arena VC. Survival of patients with well-differentiated astrocytomas diagnosed in the era of computed tomography. Neurosurgery 1991;28:496–501.
168. Bigner SH, Schrock E. Molecular cytogenetics of brain tumors. J Neuropathol Exp Neurol 1997;56:1173–1181.
169. Ho DM, Wong TT, Hsu CY, et al. MIB-1 labeling index in nonpilocytic astrocytoma of childhood: A study of 101 cases. Cancer 1998;82:2459–2466.
170. Krouwer HGJ, Davis RL, Silver P, Prados M. Gemistocytic astrocytomas: A reappraisal. J Neurosurg 1991;74:399–406.
171. McKeever PE, Blaivas M, Nelson JS. Diagnosis of nervous system tumors by light microscopic methods. In: Garcia JH, Budka H, McKeever PE, et al, eds. Neuropathology: The Diagnostic Approach. Philadelphia: CV Mosby, 1997:193–218.
172. Kimura N, Watanabe M, Date F, et al. HMB-45 and tuberin in hamartomas associated with tuberous sclerosis. Mod Pathol 1997;10:952–959.
173. Russell DS, Rubinstein LJ. Pathology of Tumours of the Nervous System. Baltimore: Williams & Wilkins, 1989.
174. Levy RA, Allen R, McKeever P. Pleomorphic xanthoastrocytoma presenting with massive intracranial hemorrhage. AJNR 1996;17:154–156.
175. Gokden M, Roth KA, Carroll SL, et al. Clear cell neoplasms and pseudoneoplastic lesions of the central nervous system. Semin Diagn Pathol 1997;14:253–269.
176. Kros JM, Vecht CJ, Stefanko SZ. The pleomorphic xanthoastrocytoma and its differential diagnosis: A study of five cases. Hum Pathol 1991;22:1128–1135.
177. Kepes JJ, Rubinstein LJ, Eng LF. Pleomorphic xanthoastrocytoma: A distinctive meningocerebral glioma of young subjects with relatively favorable prognosis: A study of 12 cases. Cancer 1979;44:1839–1852.
178. Grant JW, Gallagher PJ. Pleomorphic xanthoastrocytoma: Immunohistochemical methods for differentiation from fibrous histiocytomas with similar morphology. Am J Surg Pathol 1986;10:336–341.
179. Powell SZ, Yachnis AT, Rorke LB, et al. Divergent differentiation in pleomorphic xanthoastrocytoma: Evidence for a neuronal element and possible relationship to ganglion cell tumors. Am J Surg Pathol 1996;20:80–85.
180. Geddes JF, Thom M, Robinson SF, et al. Granular cell change in astrocytic tumors. Am J Surg Pathol 1996;20:55–63.
181. Dickson DW, Suzuki KI, Kanner R, et al. Cerebral granular cell tumor: Immunohistochemical and electron microscopy study. J Neuropathol Exp Neurol 1996;45:304–314.
182. Healey EA, Barnes PD, Kupsky WJ, et al. The prognostic significance of postoperative residual tumor in ependymoma. Neurosurgery 1991;28:666–671.
183. Schiffer D, Chio A, Giordana MT, et al. Histologic prognostic factors in ependymoma. Child Nerv Syst 1991;7:177–182.
184. Figarella-Branger D, Gambarelli D, Dollo C, et al. Infratentorial ependymomas of childhood: Correlation between histologic features, immunohistological phenotype, silver nucleolar organizer region staining values and post-operative survival in 16 cases. Acta Neuropathol (Berl) 1991;82:208–216.
185. Kawano N, Yada K, Aihara M, Yagishita S: Oligodendroglioma-like cells (clear cells) in ependymoma. Acta Neuropathol (Berl) 1984;3:122–127.
186. Kakita A, Takahashi H, Fusejima T, et al. Clear cell variants of intracranial tumors: Meningioma and ependymoma. Noshuyo Byori 1995;12:111–126.
187. Kindblom LG, Lodding P, Hagmar B, Stenman G. Metastasizing myxopapillary ependymoma of the sacrococcygeal region: A clinicopathologic, light- and electron microscopic, immunohistochemical, tissue culture, and cytogenetic analysis of a case. Acta Pathol Microbiol Immunol Scand [A] 1986;94:79–90.
188. Graham DI, Lantos PL. Greenfield's Neuropathology, 6th ed. New York: Oxford University Press, 1997.
189. Ross GW, Rubinstein LJ. Lack of histopathological correlation of malignant ependymomas with postoperative survival. J Neurosurg 1989;70:31–36.
190. Mason WP, Krol GS, DeAngelis LM. Low-grade oligodendroglioma responds to chemotherapy. Neurology 1996;46:203–207.
191. Yong WH, Chou D, Ueki K, et al. Chromosome 19q deletions in human gliomas overlap telomeric to D19S219 and may target a 425 kb region centromeric to D19S112. J Neuropathol Exp Neurol 1995;54:622–626.
192. Bruner JM. Oligodendroglioma: Diagnosis and prognosis. Semin Diagn Pathol 1987;4:251–261.
193. Kros JM, de Jong AA, van der Kwast TH. Ultrastructural characterization of transitional cells in oligodendrogliomas. J Neuropathol Exp Neurol 1992;51:186–193.
194. Dehghani F, Schachenmayr W, Laun A, et al. Prognostic implication of histopathological, immunohistochemical and clinical features of oligodendrogliomas: A study of 89 cases. Acta Neuropathol 1998;95:493–504.
195. Coons SW, Johnson PC, Pearl DK. The prognostic significance of Ki-67 labeling indices for oligodendrogliomas. Neurosurgery 1997;41:878–884.
196. Alvord EC. Is necrosis helpful in the grading of gliomas? [editorial opinion] J Neuropathol Exp Neurol 1992;51:127–132.
197. Schröck E, Thiel G, Lozanova T, et al. Comparative hybridization of human malignant gliomas reveals multiple amplification sites and nonrandom chromosomal gains and losses. Am J Pathol 1994;144:1203–1218.
198. McKeever PE, Dennis TR, Burgess AC, et al. Chromosomal breakpoint at 17q11.2 and insertion of DNA from three different chromosomes in a glioblastoma with exceptional glial fibrillary acidic protein expression. Cancer Genet Cytogenet 1996;87:41–47.
199. Horiguchi H, Hirose T, Kannuki S, et al. Gliosarcoma: An immunohistochemical, ultrastructural and fluorescence in situ hybridization study. Pathol Int 1998;48:595–602.
200. Liu L, Ichimura K, Pettersson EH, et al. Chromosome 7 rearrangements in glioblastomas: Loci adjacent to EGFR are independently amplified. J Neuropathol Exp Neurol 1998;57:1138–1145.
201. Takekawa Y, Sawada T. Vascular endothelial growth factor and neovascularization in astrocytic tumors. Pathol Int 1998;48:109–114.
202. Paulus W, Peiffer J. Intratumoral histologic heterogeneity of gliomas: A quantitative study. Cancer 1989;64:442–447.
203. Rasheed BK, Wiltshire RN, Bigner SH, Bigner DD. Molecu-

lar pathogenesis of malignant gliomas. Curr Opin Oncol 1999;11:162–167.

204. Davenport RD, McKeever PE. Ploidy of endothelium in high grade astrocytomas. Anal Quant Cytol Histol 1987;9: 25–29.

205. McKeever PE, Zhang K, Nelson JS, Phan SH. Type IV collagen messenger RNA localizes within cells of abnormal vascular proliferations of glioblastoma and sarcomatous regions of gliosarcoma. J Histochem Cytochem 1993; 41:1124.

206. Vandenberg SR, Herman MM, Rubinstein LJ. Embryonal central neuroepithelial tumors: Current concepts and future challenges. Cancer Metastasis Rev 1987;5:343–365.

207. McKeever PE, Davenport RD, Shakui P. Patterns of antigenic expression in cultured glioma cells. Crit Rev Neurobiol 1991;6:119–147.

208. Boerman RH, Anderl K, Herath J, et al. The glial and mesenchymal elements of gliosarcomas share similar genetic alterations. J Neuropathol Exp Neurol 1996;55:973–981.

209. Kepes JJ, Sher J, Oliver MG. Light and electron microscopic study of "adenoid" components in gliomas: Fibroblastic activity of neoplastic astrocytes. J Neuropathol Exp Neurol 1985;44:359.

210. Mörk SJ, Rubinstein LJ, Kepes JJ, et al. Patterns of epithelial metaplasia in malignant gliomas. II: Squamous differentiation of epithelial like formations in gliosarcomas and glioblastomas. J Neuropathol Exp Neurol 1988;47:101–118.

211. Harris CP, Townsend JJ, Brockmeyer DL, Heilbrun MP. Cerebral granular cell tumor occurring with glioblastoma multiforme: Case report. Surg Neurol 1991;36:202–206.

212. Rosenblum MK, Erlandson RA, Budzilovich GN. The lipidrich epithelioid glioblastoma. Am J Surg Pathol 1991;15: 925–934.

213. Oberc-Greenwood MA, McKeever PE, Kornblith PL, Smith BH. A human ganglioglioma containing paired helical filaments. Hum Pathol 1984;15:834–838.

214. Wirnsberg GH, Becker H, Ziervogel K, Hofler H. Diagnostic immunohistochemistry of neuroblastic tumors. Am J Surg Pathol 1992;15:49–57.

215. Biggs PJ, Powers JM. Neuroblastic medulloblastoma with abundant cytoplasmic actin filaments. Arch Pathol Lab Med 1984;108:326–329.

216. Laeng RH, Scheithauer BW, Altermatt HJ. Anti-neuronal nuclear autoantibodies, types 1 and 2: Their utility in the study of tumors of the nervous system. Acta Neuropathol 1998;96:329–339.

217. Karamitopoulou E, Perentes E, Probst A, et al: Ganglioglioma of the brain stem: Neurological dysfunction of 16-year duration. Clin Neuropathol 1995;14:162–168.

218. Wolf HK, Muller MB, Spanle M, et al. Ganglioglioma: A detailed histopathological and immunohistochemical analysis of 61 cases. Acta Neuropathol 1994;88:166–173.

219. Felix I, Bilbao JM, Asa SL, et al. Cerebral and cerebellar gangliocytomas: A morphological study of nine cases. Acta Neuropathol 1994;88:246–251.

220. Lindboe CF, Helseth E, Myhr G. Lhermitte-Duclos disease and giant meningioma as manifestations of Cowden's disease. Clin Neuropathol 1995;14:327–330.

221. Daumas-Duport C, Scheithauer BW, Chodkiewicz JP, et al. Dysembryoplastic neuroepithelial tumors of young patients with intractable partial seizures: Report of 39 cases. Neurosurgery 1988;23:545–556.

222. Daumas-Duport C: Dysembryoplastic neuroepithelial tumors. Brain Pathol 1993;3:283–295.

223. Prayson RA, Morris HH, Estes ML, et al. Dysembryoplastic neuroepithelial tumor: A clinicopathologic and immunohistochemical study of 11 tumors including MIB1 immunoreactivity. Clin Neuropathol 1996;15:47–53.

224. Daumas-Duport C, Varlet P, Bacha S, et al. Dysembryoplastic neuroepithelial tumors: Nonspecific histological forms —a study of 40 cases. J Neurooncol 1999;41:267–280.

225. Wolf HK, Buslei R, Blumcke I, et al. Neural antigens in oligodendrogliomas and dysembryoplastic neuroepithelial tumors. Acta Neuropathol 1997;94:436–443.

226. Yasargil MG, von Ammon K, von Deimling A, et al. Central neurocytoma: Histopathological variants and therapeutic approaches. J Neurosurg 1992;76:32–37.

227. Nishio S, Fujiwara S, Tashima T, et al. Tumors of the lateral ventricular wall, especially the septum pellucidum: Clinical presentation and variations in pathological features. Neurosurgery 1990;27:224–230.

228. von Deimling A, Kleihues P, Saremaslani P, et al. Histogenesis and differentiation potential of central neurocytomas. Lab Invest 1991;64:585–591.

229. Figarella-Branger D, Pellissier JF, Daumas-Duport C, et al. Central neurocytomas: Critical evaluation of a small-cell neuronal tumor. Am J Surg Pathol 1992;16:97–109.

230. Miller DC, Koslow M, Budzilovich GN, Burstein DE. Synaptophysin: A sensitive and specific marker for ganglion cells in central nervous system neoplasms. Hum Pathol 1990;21:271–276.

231. Barbosa MD, Balsitis M, Jaspan T, Lowe J. Intraventricular neurocytoma: A clinical and pathological study of three cases and review of the literature. Neurosurgery 1990;26: 1045–1054.

232. VandenBerg SR, May EE, Rubinstein LJ, et al. Desmoplastic supratentorial neuroepithelial tumors of infancy with divergent differentiation potential ("desmoplastic infantile gangliogliomas"): Report on 11 cases of a distinctive embryonal tumor with favorable prognosis. J Neurosurg 1987; 66:58–71.

233. Sperner J, Gottschalk J, Neumann K, et al. Clinical, radiological and histological findings in desmoplastic infantile ganglioglioma. Childs Nerv Syst 1994;10:458–463.

234. Rorke LB, Gilles FH, Davis RL, Becker LE. Revision of the World Health Organization classification of brain tumors for childhood brain tumors. Cancer 1985;56:1869–1886.

235. Mannoji H, Becker LE. Ependymal and choroid plexus tumors: Cytokeratin and GFAP expression. Cancer 1988;61: 1377–1385.

236. Furness PN, Lowe J, Tarrant GS. Subepithelial basement membrane deposition and intermediate filament expression in choroid plexus neoplasms and ependymomas. Histopathology 1990;16:251–255.

237. Herbert J, Cavallaro T, Dwork AJ. A marker for primary choroid plexus neoplasms. Am J Pathol 1990;136:1317–1325.

238. Albrecht S, Rouah E, Becker LE, Bruner J. Transthyretin immunoreactivity in choroid plexus neoplasms and brain metastases. Mod Pathol 1991;4:610–614.

239. Kubo S, Ogino S, Fukushima T, et al. Immunocytochemical detection of insulin-like growth factor II (IGF-II) in choroid plexus papilloma: A possible marker for differential diagnosis. Clin Neuropathol 1999;18:74–79.

240. Kepes JJ, Collins J. Choroid plexus epithelium (normal and neoplastic) expresses synaptophysin: A potentially useful aid in differentiating carcinoma of the choroid plexus from metastatic papillary carcinomas. J Neuropathol Exp Neurol 1999;58:398–401.

241. Varga Z, Vajtai I, Aguzzi A. The standard isoform of CD44 is preferentially expressed in atypical papillomas and carcinomas of the choroid plexus. Pathol Res Pract 1996;192: 1225–1231.

242. Varga Z, Vajtai I. Prognostic markers in the histopathological diagnosis of tumors of the choroid plexus. Orv Hetil 1998;139:761–765.

243. Imaya H, Kudo M. Malignant choroid plexus papilloma of the IV ventricle. Childs Nerv Syst 1991;7:109–111.

244. D'Andrea AD, Packer RJ, Rorke LB, et al. Pineocytomas of childhood: A reappraisal of natural history and response to therapy. Cancer 1987;59:1353–1357.

245. Mena H, Rushing EJ, Ribas JL, et al. Tumors of pineal parenchymal cells: A correlation of histological features, including nucleolar organizer regions, with survival in 35 cases. Hum Pathol 1995;26:20–30.

246. Roberts RO, Lynch CF, Jones MP, Hart MN. Medulloblastoma: A population-based study of 532 cases. J Neuropathol Exp Neurol 1991;50:134–144.

247. Giordana MT, Migheli A, Pavanelli E. Interphase cytogenetics of medulloblastoma: Isochromosome 17q is a constant finding. J Neuropathol Exp Neurol 1997;56:609.

248. Farwell JR, Dohrmann GJ, Flannery JT. Medulloblastoma in childhood: An epidemiological study. J Neurosurg 1984; 61:657–664.

249. Gould VE, Jansson DS, Molenaar WM, et al. Primitive neuroectodermal tumors of the central nervous system: Patterns of expression of neuroendocrine markers, and all classes of intermediate filament proteins. Lab Invest 1990; 62:498–509.

250. Budka H. Pathology of midline brain tumors: Immunocytochemical tumor markers and classificatory aspects. Acta Neurochir Suppl (Wien) 1985;35:23–30.

251. Goldberg-Stern H, Gadoth N, Stern S, et al. The prognostic significance of glial fibrillary acidic protein staining in medulloblastoma. Cancer 1991;68:568–573.

252. Caputy AJ, McCullough DC, Manz HJ, et al. A review of the factors influencing the prognosis of medulloblastoma: The importance of cell differentiation. J Neurosurg 1987; 66:80–87.

253. Packer RJ, Sutton LN, Rorke LB, et al. Prognostic importance of cellular differentiation in medulloblastoma of childhood. J Neurosurg 1984;61:296–301.

254. Giangaspero F, Chieco P, Ceccarelli C, et al. "Desmoplastic" versus "classic" medulloblastoma: Comparison of DNA content, histopathology and differentiation. Virchows Arch A Pathol Anat Histopathol 1991;418:207–214.

255. Rubinstein LJ, Northfield DWC. The medulloblastoma and the so-called "arachnoidal cerebellar sarcoma": A critical re-examination of a nosological problem. Brain 1964;87: 379–412.

256. Katsetos CD, Herman MM, Frankfurter A, et al. Cerebellar desmoplastic medulloblastomas: A further immunohistochemical characterization of the reticulin-free pale islands. Arch Pathol Lab Med 1989;113:1019–1029.

257. Hart MN, Earle KM. Primitive neuroectodermal tumors of the brain in children. Cancer 1973;32:890–897.

258. Harris MD, Moore IE, Steart PV, Weller RO. Protein gene product (PGP) 9.5 as a reliable marker in primitive neuroectodermal tumours—an immunohistochemical study of 21 childhood cases. Histopathology 1990;16:271–277.

259. Gould VE, Rorke LB, Jansson DS, et al. Primitive neuroectodermal tumors of the central nervous system express neuroendocrine markers and may express all classes of intermediate filaments. Hum Pathol 1990;21:245–252.

260. Freyer DR, Hutchinson RJ, McKeever PE. Primary primitive neuroectodermal tumor of the spinal cord associated with neural tube defect. Pediatr Neurosci 1989;15:181–187.

261. Fellinger EJ, Garin-Chesa P, Triche TJ, et al. Immunohistochemical analysis of Ewing's sarcoma cell surface antigen p30/32MIC2. Am J Pathol 1991;139:317–325.

262. Kramm CM, Korf HW, Czerwionka M, et al. Photoreceptor differentiation in cerebellar medulloblastoma: Evidence for a functional photopigment and authentic S-antigen (arrestin). Acta Neuropathol (Berl) 1991;81:296–302.

263. Dehner LP. Primitive neuroectodermal tumor and Ewing's sarcoma. Am J Surg Pathol 1993;17:1–13.

264. Tsuji S, Hisaoka M, Morimitsu Y, et al. Peripheral primitive neuroectodermal tumour of the lung: Report of two cases. Histopathology 1998;33:369–374.

265. Auge B, Kantelip B, Chataigner H, et al. Peripheral primitive neuroectodermal tumors of bone: A review of three cases. Rev Rhum Engl Ed 1999;66:92–96.

266. Katayama Y, Kimura S, Watanabe T, et al. Peripheral-type primitive neuroectodermal tumor arising in the tentorium: Case report. J Neurosurg 1999;90:141–144.

267. Pappo AS, Cheah MSC, Saldivar VA, et al. Disseminated primitive neuroectodermal tumor: Diagnosis using immunocytochemistry, electron microscopy, and molecular probes. Cancer 1989;63:2515–2521.

268. Anwer UE, Smith TW, DeGirolami U, Wilkinson HA. Medulloblastoma with cartilaginous differentiation. Arch Pathol Lab Med 1989;113:84–88.

269. Holl T, Kleihues P, Yasargil MG, Wiestler OD. Cerebellar medullomyoblastoma with advanced neuronal differentia-

270. Soylemezoglu F, Soffer D, Onol B, et al: Lipomatous medulloblastoma in adults: A distinct clinicopathological entity. Am J Surg Path 1996;20:413–418.

271. Chowdhury C, Roy S, Mahapatra AK, Bhatia R. Medullomyoblastoma: A teratoma. Cancer 1985;55:1495–1500.

272. Rorke LB, Packer R, Biegel J. Central nervous system atypical teratoid/rhabdoid tumors of infancy and childhood. J Neurooncol 1995;24:21–28.

273. Jansen GH, Troost D, Dingemans KP. Polar spongioblastoma: An immunohistochemical and electron microscopical study. Acta Neuropathol (Berl) 1990;81:228–232.

274. Khoddami M, Becker LE. Immunohistochemistry of medulloepithelioma and neural tube. Pediatr Pathol Lab Med 1997;17:913–925.

275. Figarella-Branger D, Gambarelli D, Perez-Castillo M, et al. Ectopic intrapelvic medulloepithelioma: Case report. Neuropathol Appl Neurobiol 1992;18:408–414.

276. Mork SJ, Rubinstein LJ. Ependymoblastoma: A reappraisal of a rare embryonal tumor. Cancer 1985;55:1536–1542.

277. Salvati M, Artico M, Lunardi P, Gagliardi FM. Intramedullary meningioma: Case report and review of the literature. Surg Neurol 1992;37:42–45.

278. Ng HK, Tse CC, Lo ST. Meningiomas and arachnoid cells: An immunohistochemical study of epithelial markers. Pathology 1987;19:253–257.

279. Meis JM, Ordonez NG, Bruner JM. Meningiomas: An immunohistochemical study of 50 cases. Arch Pathol Lab Med 1986;110:934–937.

280. Kepes JJ. Differential diagnostic problems in brain tumors. In: Minckler J, ed. Pathology of the Nervous System, vol. 2. New York: McGraw-Hill Blakiston, 1971:2219–2240.

281. Perry A, Scheithauer BW, Nascimento AG. The immunophenotypic spectrum of meningeal hemangiopericytoma: A comparison with fibrous meningioma and solitary fibrous tumor of meninges. Am J Surg Pathol 1997;21:1354–1360.

282. Carneiro SS, Scheithauer BW, Nascimento AG, et al. Solitary fibrous tumor of the meninges: A lesion distinct from fibrous meningioma: A clinicopathologic and immunohistochemical study. Am J Clin Pathol 1996;106:217–224.

283. Kepes JJ. Meningiomas: Biology, Pathology, and Differential Diagnosis. Chicago: Year Book Medical, 1982.

284. Lattes R, Bigotti G. Lipoblastic meningioma: "Vacuolated meningioma." Hum Pathol 1991;22:164–171.

285. Ito H, Kawano N, Yada K, Kameya T. Meningiomas differentiating to arachnoid trabecular cells: A proposal for histological subtype "arachnoid trabecular cell meningioma." Acta Neuropathol (Berl) 1991;82:327–330.

286. Kulah A, Ilcayto R, Fiskeci C. Cystic meningiomas. Acta Neurochir (Wien) 1991;111:108–113.

287. Shiraishi K. Glycogen-rich meningioma: Case report and short review. Neurosurg Rev 1991;14:61–64.

288. Kepes JJ. Presidential address: The histopathology of meningiomas: A reflection of origins and expected behavior. J Neuropathol Exp Neurol 1986;45:95–107.

289. Louis DN, Hamilton AJ, Sobel RA, Ojemann RG. Pseudopsammomatous meningioma with elevated serum carcinoembryonic antigen: A true secretory meningioma: Case report. J Neurosurg 1991;74:129–132.

290. Winek RR, Scheithauer BW, Wick MR. Meningioma, meningeal hemangiopericytoma (angioblastic meningioma), peripheral hemangiopericytoma, and acoustic schwannoma: A comparative immunohistochemical study. Am J Surg Pathol 1989;13:251–261.

291. Chen WYK, Kepes JJ. Extensive intracellular mucoid changes in meningiomas: A manifestation of polyvinylpyrrolidone (PVP) effect on tissues with mesenchymal characteristics. J Neuropathol Exp Neurol 1985;44:360.

292. Kobata H, Kondo A, Iwasaki K, et al. Chordoid meningioma in a child: Case report. J Neurosurg 1998;88:319–323.

293. Kobata H, Kondo A, Iwasaki K, et al. Chordoid menin-

gioma in a child: Case report. J Neurosurg 1998;88:319–323.

294. Zuppan CW, Liwnicz BH, Weeks DA. Meningioma with chordoid features. Ultrastruct Pathol 1994;18:29–32.

295. Probst-Cousin S, Villagran-Lillo R, Lahl R, et al. Secretory meningioma: Clinical, histologic, and immunohistochemical findings in 31 cases. Cancer 1997;79:2003–2015.

296. Prinz M, Patt S, Mitrovics T, Cervos-Navarro J. Clear cell meningioma: Report of a spinal case. Gen Diagn Pathol 1996;141:261–267.

297. Zorludemir S, Scheithauer BW, Hirose T, et al. Clear cell meningioma: A clinicopathologic study of a potentially aggressive variant of meningioma. Am J Surg Pathol 1995;19:493–505.

298. Imlay SP, Snider TE, Raab SS. Clear-cell meningioma: Diagnosis by fine-needle aspiration biopsy. Diagn Cytopathol 1998;18:131–136.

299. Alameda F, Lloreta J, Ferrer MD, et al. Clear cell meningioma of the lumbo-sacral spine with chordoid features. Ultrastruct Pathol 1999;23:51–58.

300. Perry A, Scheithauer BW, Stafford SL, et al. "Rhabdoid" meningioma: An aggressive variant. Am J Surg Pathol 1998;22:1482–1490.

301. Cerdá-Nicolás M, López-Ginés C, Peydró-Olaya A, et al. Histologic and cytogenetic patterns in benign, atypical, and malignant meningiomas: Does correlation with recurrence exist? Int J Surg Pathol 1995;2:301–310.

302. De la Monte SM, Flickinger J, Linggood RM. Histopathologic features predicting recurrence of meningiomas following subtotal resection. Am J Surg Pathol 1986;10:836–843.

303. Kobayashi S, Haba R, Hirakawa E, et al. Cytology and immunohistochemistry of anaplastic meningiomas in squash preparations: A report of two cases. Acta Cytol 1995;39:118–124.

304. Prayson RA. Malignant meningioma: A clinicopathologic study of 23 patients including MIB-1 and p53 immunohistochemistry. Am J Clin Pathol 1996;105:719–726.

305. Jellinger K, Slowik F. Histological subtypes and prognostic problems in meningiomas. J Neurol 1975;208:279–298.

306. Hart LL, Weinberg JB. Metastatic hemangiopericytoma with prolonged survival. Cancer 1987;60:916–920.

307. Probst-Cousin S, Rickert CH, Gullotta F. Factor XIIIa-immunoreactivity in tumors of the central nervous system. Clin Neuropathol 1998;17:79–84.

308. Miettinen MM, el-Rifai W, Sarlomo-Rikala M, et al. Tumor size-related DNA copy number changes occur in solitary fibrous tumors but not in hemangiopericytomas. Mod Pathol 1997;10:1194–1200.

309. Nakamura Y, Becker LE, Marks A. Distribution of immunoreactive S100 protein in pediatric brain tumors. J Neuropathol Exp Neurol 1983;42:136–145.

310. Miettinen M, Lehto VP, Dahl D, Virtanen I. Differential diagnosis of chordoma, chondroid, and ependymal tumors as aided by anti-intermediate filament antibodies. Am J Pathol 1983;112:160–169.

311. Walker WP, Landas SK, Bromley CM, Sturm MT. Immunohistochemical distinction of classic and chondroid chordomas. Mod Pathol 1991;4:661–666.

312. Abenoza P, Sibley K. Chordoma: An immunohistologic study. Hum Pathol 1986;17:744–747.

313. Lam R. The nature of cytoplasmic vacuoles in chordoma cells: A correlative enzyme and electron microscopic histochemical study. Pathol Res Pract 1990;186:642–650.

314. Nanda A, Hirsh LF, Antoiniades K. Malignant fibrous histiocytoma in a recurrent thoracic chordoma: Case report and literature review. Neurosurgery 1991;28:588–592.

315. Persson S, Kindblom LG, Angervall L. Classical and chondroid chordoma: A light-microscopic, histochemical, ultrastructural and immunohistochemical analysis of the various cell types. Pathol Res Pract 1991;187:828–838.

316. Paulus W, Slowik F, Jellinger K. Primary intracranial sarcomas: Histopathological features of 19 cases. Histopathology 1991;18:395–402.

317. McKeever PE. Insights about brain tumors gained through immunohistochemistry and in situ hybridization of nuclear and phenotypic markers. J Histochem Cytochem 1998;46:585–594.

318. Ariza A, Kim JH. Kaposi's sarcoma of the dura mater. Hum Pathol 1988;19:1461–1463.

319. Powell HC, Marshall LF, Igneizi RJ. Post-irradiation pituitary sarcoma. Acta Neuropathol (Berl) 1977;39:165–167.

320. Rushing EJ, Mena H, Smirniotopoulos JG. Mesenchymal chondrosarcoma of the cauda equina. Clin Neuropathol 1995;14:150–153.

321. Matsukado Y, Yokota A, Marubayashi T. Rhabdomyosarcoma of the brain. J Neurosurg 1975;43:215–221.

322. Weiss SW, Langloss JM, Enzinger FM. Value of S-100 protein in the diagnosis of soft tissue tumors with particular reference to benign and malignant Schwann cell tumors. Lab Invest 1983;49:299–315.

323. Perentes E, Rubinstein LJ. Immunohistochemical recognition of human nerve sheath tumors by anti-Leu 7 monoclonal antibody. Acta Neuropathol 1985;68:319–324.

324. Wick MR, Swanson PE, Scheithauer BW, Manivel JC. Malignant peripheral nerve sheath tumor: An immunohistochemical study of 62 cases. Am J Clin Pathol 1987;87:425–433.

325. Geddes JF, Sutcliffe JC, King TT. Mixed cranial nerve tumors in neurofibromatosis type 2. Clin Neuropathol 1995;14:310–313.

326. Gould VE, Moll R, Moll I, et al. The intermediate filament complement of the spectrum of nerve sheath neoplasms. Lab Invest 1986;55:463–474.

327. Hayashi K, Hoshida Y, Horie Y, et al. Immunohistochemical study on the distribution of alpha and beta subunits of S-100 protein in brain tumors. Acta Neuropathol (Berl) 1991;81:657–663.

328. Jennings MT, Gelman R, Hochberg F. Intracranial germ-cell tumors: Natural history and pathogenesis. J Neurosurg 1985;63:155–167.

329. Inoue HK, Haganuma H, Ono N. Pathobiology of intracranial germ-cell tumors: Immunochemical, immunohistochemical, and electron microscopic investigations. J Neurooncol 1987;5:105–115.

330. Gonzalez-Crussi F, Winkler RF, Mirkin DL. Sacrococcygeal teratomas in infants and children: Relationship of histology and prognosis in 40 cases. Arch Pathol Lab Med 1978;102:420–425.

331. Nakagawa Y, Perentes E, Ross GW, et al. Immunohistochemical differences between intracranial germinomas and their gonadal equivalents: An immunoperoxidase study of germ cell tumours with epithelial membrane antigen, cytokeratin, and vimentin. J Pathol 1988;156:67–72.

332. Henry JM, Heffner RR Jr, Dillard SH, et al. Primary malignant lymphomas of the central nervous system. Cancer 1974;34:1293–1302.

333. Garvin AJ, Spicer SS, McKeever PE. The cytochemical demonstration of intracellular immunoglobulin: In neoplasms of lymphoreticular tissue. Am J Pathol 1976;82:457–478.

334. O'Neill BP, Kelly PJ, Earle JD, et al. Computer assisted stereotaxic biopsy for the diagnosis of primary central nervous system lymphoma. Neurology 1987;37:1160–1164.

335. Davenport RD, O'Donnell LJ, Schnitzer B, McKeever PE. Non-Hodgkin's lymphoma of the brain following Hodgkin's disease: An immunohistochemical study. Cancer 1991;67:440–443.

336. Hayakawa T, Takakura K, Abe H, et al. Primary central nervous system lymphoma in Japan: A retrospective, cooperative study by CNS-Lymphoma Study Group in Japan. J Neurooncol 1994;19:197–215.

337. Morgello S. Pathogenesis and classification of primary central nervous system lymphoma: An update. Brain Pathol 1995;5:383–393.

338. Forsyth P, Yahalom J, DeAngelis L. Combined-modality therapy in the treatment of primary central nervous system lymphoma in AIDS. Neurology 1994;44:1473–1479.

339. Chamberlain M. Long survival in patients with acquired

immune deficiency syndrome–related primary central system lymphoma. Cancer 1994;73:1728–1730.

340. Ferracini R, Bergmann M, Pileri S, et al. Primary T-cell lymphoma of the central nervous system. Clin Neuropathol 1995;14:125–129.

341. Nakamine H, Yokote H, Itakura T, et al. Non-Hodgkin's lymphoma involving the brain: Diagnostic usefulness of stereotactic needle biopsy in combination with paraffin-section immunohistochemistry. Acta Neuropathol (Berl) 1989;78:462–471.

342. Nishiyama A, Saito T, Abe S, Kumanishi T. An immunohistochemical analysis of T cells in primary B cell malignant lymphoma of the brain. Acta Neuropathol (Berl) 1989;79:27–29.

343. Stewart CJ, Farquharson MA, Kerr T, McCorriston J. Immunoglobulin light chain mRNA detected by in situ hybridization in diagnostic fine needle aspiration cytology specimens. J Clin Pathol 1996;49:749–754.

344. Bigner SH, Johnston WW. The cytopathology of cerebrospinal fluid. I: Nonneoplastic conditions, lymphoma and leukemia. Acta Cytol (Baltimore) 1981;25:345–353.

345. An-Foraker SH. Cytodiagnosis of malignant lesions in cerebrospinal fluid. Review and cytohistologic correlation. Acta Cytol (Baltimore) 1985;29:286–290.

346. Lowe J, Russel NH. Cerebral vasculitis associated with hairy cell leukemia. Cancer 1987;60:3025–3028.

347. Henson JW, Wiley RG. CNS chloromas in patients presenting with eosinophilia. Neurology 1989;39:1386–1388.

348. Huang HY, Huang CC, Lui CC, et al. Isolated intracranial Rosai-Dorfman disease: Case report and literature review. Pathol Int 1998;48:396–402.

349. Deodhare SS, Ang LC, Bilbao JM. Isolated intracranial involvement in Rosai-Dorfman disease: A report of two cases and review of the literature. Arch Pathol Lab Med 1998; 122:161–165.

350. Adle-Biassette H, Chetritt J, Bergemer-Fouquet AM, et al. Pathology of the central nervous system in Chester-Erdheim disease: Report of three cases. J Neuropathol Exp Neurol 1997;56:1207–1216.

351. Mrak RE. Tumors: Applications of ultrastructural methods. In: Garcia JH, Budka H, McKeever PE, et al, eds. Neuropathology: The Diagnostic Approach. Philadelphia: CV Mosby, 1997:96–192.

352. Eriksen B, Janinis J, Variakojis D, et al. Primary histiocytosis X of the parieto-occipital lobe. Hum Pathol 1988;19: 611–614.

353. McKeever PE, Lloyd RV. Tumors of the pituitary region. In: Garcia JH, Budka H, McKeever PE, et al, eds. Neuropathology: The Diagnostic Approach. Philadelphia: CV Mosby, 1997:219–262.

354. Tachibana O, Yamashima T, Yamashita J. Immunohistochemical study of erythropoietin in cerebellar hemangioblastomas associated with secondary polycythemia. Neurosurgery 1991;28:24–26.

355. Feldenzer JA, McKeever PE. Selective localization of gamma-enolase in stromal cells of cerebellar hemangioblastomas. Acta Neuropathol (Berl) 1987;72:281–285.

356. Jeffreys R. Pathological and haematological aspects of posterior fossa haemangioblastomata. J Neurol Neurosurg Psychiatry 1975;38:112–129.

357. Rubio A, Meyers SP, Powers JM, et al. Hemangioblastoma of the optic nerve. Hum Pathol 1994;25:1249–1251.

358. Kepes JJ, Rengachary SS, Lee SH. Astrocytes in the hemangioblastomas of the central nervous system and their relationship to stromal cells. Acta Neuropathol (Berl) 1979;47:99–104.

359. McComb RD, Eastman PJ, Hahn FJ, Bennett DR. Cerebellar hemangioblastoma with prominent stromal astrocytosis: Diagnostic and histogenetic considerations. Clin Neuropathol 1987;6:149–154.

360. Deck JHN, Rubinstein LJ. Glial fibrillary acidic protein in stromal cells of some capillary hemangioblastomas: Significance and possible implications of an immunoperoxidase study. Acta Neuropathol (Berl) 1981;54:173–181.

361. McComb RD, Eastman PJ, Hahn FJ, et al. Cerebellar hem-angioblastoma with prominent stromal astrocytosis: Diagnostic and histogenetic considerations. Clin Neuropathol 1987;6:149–154.

362. Silverstein AM, Quint DJ, McKeever PE. Intraductal paraganglioma of the thoracic spine. Am J Neuroradiol 1990; 11:614–616.

363. Lloyd RV. Immunohistochemical localization of chromogranin in polypeptide hormone producing cells and tumors. In: Lechago J, Kameya T, eds. Endocrine Pathology Update. Philadelphia: Field and Wood Publisher, 1990.

364. McComb RD, Jones RT, Pizzo SV, Bigner DD. Localization of factor VIII/von Willebrand factor and glial fibrillary acidic protein in the hemangioblastoma: Implications for stromal cell histogenesis. Acta Neuropathol (Berl) 1982;56: 207–213.

365. Petito CK, DeGirolami U, Earle KM. Craniopharyngiomas: A clinical and pathological review. Cancer 1976;37:1944–1952.

366. Smith AR, Elsheikh TM, Silverman JF. Intraoperative cytologic diagnosis of suprasellar and sellar cystic lesions. Diagn Cytopathol 1999;20:137–147.

367. McKeever PE, Spicer SS. Pituitary histochemistry. In: Spicer SS, ed. Histochemistry in Pathologic Diagnosis. New York: Marcel-Dekker, 1987:603–645.

368. Wong SW, Ducker TB, Powers JM. Fulminating parapontine epidermoid carcinoma in a four-year-old boy. Cancer 1976;37:1525–1531.

369. Weller M, Stevens A, Sommer N, et al. Tumor cell dissemination triggers an intrathecal immune response in neoplastic meningitis. Cancer 1992;69:1475–1480.

370. Thomas P, Battifora H. Keratins versus epithelial membrane antigen in tumor diagnosis: An immunohistochemical comparison of five monoclonal antibodies. Hum Pathol 1987;18:128–134.

371. Andrew SM, Gradwell E. Immunoperoxidase labelled antibody staining in differential diagnosis of central nervous system haemangioblastomas and central nervous system metastases of renal carcinomas. J Clin Pathol 1986;39:917–919.

372. Cochran AJ, Wen DR. S-100 protein as a marker for melanocytic and other tumors. Pathology 1985;17:340–345.

373. Rushing EJ, Mena J, Ribas JL. Primary pineal parenchymal lesions: A review of 53 cases. J Neuropathol Exp Neurol 1991;50:364.

374. Coca S, Martinez A, Vaquero J, et al. Immunohistochemical study of intracranial cysts. Histol Histopathol 1993;8: 651–654.

375. Kuroda Y, Abe M, Nagumo F, et al. Neuroepithelial cyst presenting as recurrent aseptic meningitis. Neurology 1991;41:1834–1835.

376. Ho KL, Garcia JH. Colloid cysts of the third ventricle: Ultrastructural features are compatible with endodermal derivation. Acta Neuropathol 1992;83:605–612.

377. McKeever PE, Brissie NT. Scanning electron microscopy of neoplasms removed at surgery: Surface topography and comparison of meningioma, colloid cyst, ependymoma, pituitary adenoma, schwannoma and astrocytoma. J Neuropathol Exp Neurol 1977;36:875–896.

378. McKeever PE, Hall BJ, Spicer SS. The origin of colloid cysts of the third ventricle. J Neuropathol Exp Neurol 1978;37:658.

379. Bejjani GK, Wright DC, Schessel D, et al. Endodermal cysts of the posterior fossa: Report of three cases and review of the literature. J Neurosurg 1998;89:326–335.

380. Fujita T, Kayama T, Saito S, et al. Immunohistochemical detection of tumor marker in recurrent clivus enterogenous cyst—case report. Neurol Med Chir (Tokyo) 1997;37: 479–482.

381. Go KG, Blankenstein MA, Vroom TM, et al. Progesterone receptors in arachnoid cysts: An immunocytochemical study in 2 cases. Acta Neurochirurg 1997;139:349–354.

382. Whetsell WO Jr. Considering dementia. Hum Pathol 1989; 20:1–2.

383. Khachaturian ZS. Diagnosis of Alzheimer's disease. Arch Neurol 1985;42:1097−1104.

384. Mirra SS, Heyman A, McKeel D, et al. The Consortium to Establish a Registry for Alzheimer's Disease (CERAD). Part II: Standardization of the neuropathologic assessment of Alzheimer's disease. Neurology 1991;41:479−486.

385. Powers JM. Diagnostic criteria for the neuropathologic assessment of Alzheimer's disease. Neurobiol Aging 1997; 18,S4:S53−S54.

386. National Institute on Aging, and Reagan Institute Working Group on Diagnostic Criteria of the Neuropathological Assessment of Alzheimer's Disease: Consensus recommendations for the postmortem diagnosis of Alzheimer's disease. Neurobiol Aging 1997;18:S1−S2.

387. Terry RD, Hansen LA, DeTeresa R, et al. Senile dementia of the Alzheimer type without neocortical neurofibrillary tangles. Neuropathol Exper Neurol 1987;46:262−268.

388. Mirra SS, Gearing M, Hughes J, et al. Interlaboratory comparison of neuropathology assessments in Alzheimer's disease: A study of the Consortium to Establish a Registry for Alzheimer's Disease (CERAD). J Neuropathol Exp Neurol 1994;53:303−315.

389. Spillantini MG, Crowther RA, Goedert M. Comparison of the neurofibrillary pathology in Alzheimer's disease and familial presenile dementia with tangles. Acta Neuropathol 1996;92:42−48.

390. Feany MB, Dickson DW. Neurodegenerative disorders with extensive tau pathology: A comparative study and review. Ann Neurol 1996;40:139−148.

391. Wolozin B, Davies P. Alzheimer-related neuronal protein A68: Specificity and distribution. Ann Neurol 1987;22: 521−526.

392. Dwork AJ, Liu D, Kaufman MA, et al. Archival, formalin-fixed tissue: Its use in the study of Alzheimer's type changes. Clin Neuropathol 1998;17:45−49.

393. Barger SW, Harmon AD. Microglial activation by Alzheimer amyloid precursor protein and modulation by apolipoprotein E. Nature 1997;388:878−881.

394. Lue LF, Brachova L, Civin WH, Rogers J. Inflammation, A beta deposition, and neurofibrillary tangle formation as correlates of Alzheimer's disease neurodegeneration. J Neuropathol Exp Neurol 1996;55:1083−1088.

395. Yankner BA, Mesulam M-M. β-Amyloid and the pathogenesis of Alzheimer's disease. N Engl J Med 1991;325:1849−1857.

396. Hansen L, Salmon D, Galasko D, et al. The Lewy body variant in Alzheimer's disease: A clinical and pathologic entity. Neurology 1990;40:1−8.

397. Armstrong TP, Hansen LA, Salmon DP, et al. Rapidly progressive dementia in a patient with the Lewy body variant of Alzheimer's disease. Neurology 1991;41:1178−1180.

398. Garcia JH, Budka H, McKeever PE, et al, eds. Neuropathology: The Diagnostic Approach. Philadelphia: CV Mosby, 1997.

399. Chui HC, Victoroff JI, Margolin D, et al. Criteria for the diagnosis of ischemic vascular dementia proposed by the State of California Alzheimer's Disease Diagnostic and Treatment Centers. Neurology 1992;42:473−480.

400. Spillantini MG, Crowther RA, Jakes R, et al. Filamentous alpha-synuclein inclusions link multiple system atrophy with Parkinson's disease and dementia with Lewy bodies. Neurosci Lett 1998;251:205−208.

401. Knopman DS, Mastri AR, Frey WH II, et al. Dementia lacking distinctive histologic features: A common non-Alzheimer degenerative dementia. Neurology 1990;40:251−256.

402. Rasool CG, Selkoe DJ. Sharing of specific antigens by degenerating neurons in Pick's disease and Alzheimer's disease. N Engl J Med 1985;312:700−705.

403. Drury I, Blaivas M, Abou-Khalil BW, Beydoun A. Biopsy results in a kindred with Lafora disease. Arch Neurol 1993;50:102−105.

404. Coker SB. The diagnosis of childhood neurodegenerative disorders presenting as dementia in adults. Neurology 1991;41:794−798.

405. Yoneda M, Tanno Y, Nonaka I, et al. Simple detection of tRNA^{Lys} mutation in myoclonus epilepsy associated with ragged-red fibers (MERRF) by polymerase chain reaction with a mismatched primer. Neurology 1991;41:1838−1840.

406. Wanschitz J, Hainfellner JA, Simonitsch I, et al. Non-HTLV-I associated pleomorphic T-cell lymphoma of the brain mimicking post-vaccinal acute inflammatory demyelination. Neuropathol Appl Neurobiol 1997;23: 43−49.

407. Tachikawa N, Goto M, Hoshino Y, et al. Detection of *Toxoplasma gondii*, Epstein-Barr virus, and JC virus DNAs in the cerebrospinal fluid in acquired immunodeficiency syndrome patients with focal central nervous system complications. Intern Med 1999;38:556−562.

408. Swanson JW. Multiple sclerosis: Update in diagnosis and review of prognostic factors. Mayo Clin Proc 1989;64:577−586.

409. Cossins JA, Clements JM, Ford J, et al. Enhanced expression of MMP-7 and MMP-9 in demyelinating multiple sclerosis lesions. Acta Neuropathol 1997;94:590−598.

410. Allen IV, McQuaid S, McMahon J, et al. The expression of the endothelial cell antigen CD34 in demyelinating disease. Neuropathol Appl Neurobiol 1996;22:101−107.

411. Lee SC, Moore GRW, Golenwsky G, Raine CS. Multiple sclerosis: A role for astroglia in active demyelination suggested by class II MHC expression and ultrastructural study. J Neuropathol Exp Neurol 1990;49:122−136.

412. Rodriguez M. Multiple sclerosis: Basic concepts and hypothesis. Mayo Clin Proc 1989;64:570−576.

413. Gay D, Esiri M. Blood-brain barrier damage in acute multiple sclerosis plaques: An immunocytological study. Brain 1991;114:557−572.

414. Zagzag D, Miller DC, Kleinman GM, et al. Demyelinating disease versus tumor in surgical neuropathology: Clues to a correct pathologic diagnosis. Am J Surg Pathol 1993;17: 537−545.

415. Hunter SB, Ballinger WE, Rubin JJ. Multiple sclerosis mimicking primary brain tumor. Arch Pathol Lab Med 1987;111:464−468.

416. Schmidt B, Toyka KV, Kiefer R, et al. Inflammatory infiltrates in sural nerve biopsies in Guillain-Barré syndrome and chronic inflammatory demyelinating neuropathy. Muscle Nerve 1996;19:474−487.

417. Matsumuro K, Izumo S, Umehara F, et al. Chronic inflammatory demyelinating polyneuropathy: Histological and immunopathological studies on biopsied sural nerves. J Neurol Sci 1994;127:170−178.

418. Mathieson G. Pathologic aspects of epilepsy with special reference to the surgical pathology of focal cerebral seizures. Adv Neurol 1975;8:107−136.

419. Armstrong DD, Bruton CJ. Postscript: What terminology is appropriate for tissue pathology? How does it predict outcome? In: Engel J, ed. Surgical Treatment of the Epilepsies. New York: Raven Press, 1987:541−552.

420. Babb TL, Brown WJ. Pathological findings in epilepsy. In: Engel J, ed. Surgical Treatment of the Epilepsies. New York: Raven Press, 1987:511−540.

421. Theodore WH, Katz D, Kufta C, et al. Pathology of temporal lobe foci: Correlation with CT, MRI, and PNET. Neurology 1990;40:797−803.

422. Sackellares JC, Siegel GJ, Abou-Khalil BW, et al. Differences between lateral and mesial temporal metabolism interictally in epilepsy of mesial temporal origin. Neurology 1990;40:1420−1426.

423. Hardiman O, Burke T, Phillips J, et al. Microdysgenesis in resected temporal neocortex: Incidence and clinical significance in focal epilepsy. Neurology 1988;38:1041−1047.

424. Walczak TS, Radtke RA, McNamara JO, et al. Anterior temporal lobectomy for complex partial seizures: Evaluation, results, and long-term follow-up in 100 cases. Neurology 1990;40:413−418.

425. Cascino GD, Kelly PJ, Hirschorn KA, et al. Stereotactic resection of intra-axial cerebral lesions in partial epilepsy. Mayo Clin Proc 1990;65:1053−1060.

426. Volk EE, Prayson RA. Hamartomas in the setting of chronic epilepsy: A clinicopathologic study of 13 cases. Hum Pathol 1997;28:227–232.

427. Smith DF, Hutton JL, Sandemann D, et al. The prognosis of primary intracerebral tumours presenting with epilepsy: The outcome of medical and surgical management. J Neurol Neurosurg Psychiatry 1991;54:915–920.

428. Reith KG, Di Chiro G, Cromwell LD, et al. Primary demyelinating disease simulating glioma of the corpus callosum. J Neurosurg 1981;55:620–624.

429. Bigner SH, Johnston WW. The cytopathology of cerebrospinal fluid. II: Metastatic cancer, meningeal carcinomatosis and primary central nervous system neoplasms. Acta Cytol (Baltimore) 1981;25:461–479.

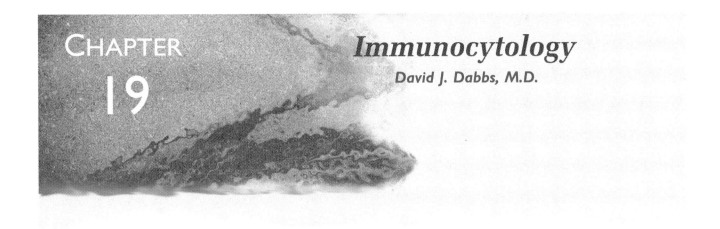

CHAPTER 19

Immunocytology

David J. Dabbs, M.D.

The application of immunostaining procedures in the work-up of difficult diagnostic cases in cytopathology has paralleled the progress that we have experienced in surgical pathology. There is substantial literature that attests to the usefulness, effectiveness, and cost efficiencies of immunocytochemistry (ICC) in cytology.[1-9] The immunoperoxidase method for immunohistochemistry has withstood the test of time in surgical pathology, with movement toward more standard methodology, antigen retrieval, antibody use, and reporting. Similar standards have been accumulating rapidly for ICC techniques in cytology.

Antibodies for use in immunocytologic study include polyclonal and monoclonal antibodies to oncofetal antigens, mucosubstances, carbohydrates, glycoproteins, intermediate filaments, and cell-specific antigens.

In this first section, practical techniques in immunocytology are reviewed.

IMMUNOCYTOLOGY TECHNIQUES

The Specimen

SPECIMEN COLLECTION

The gamut of specimens that can be used for ICC includes exfoliative cell preparations, effusions, direct imprints, fine needle aspirates, and thin-layer collection samples. These specimens can be processed through air drying or immediate fixation in alcohol or can be processed as cytocentrifuge or cell block preparations.

The most important initial task of the cytopathologist is to ensure that the conventional Romanowsky or Papanicolaou stains have been examined, that a differential diagnosis is generated, and that the appropriate question to be answered by ICC is formulated. It is of equal importance to be certain that the sample to be used for ICC contains the cells in question. A critical task of the cytopathologist is to confirm that the immunoperoxi-

dase-stained slides that are being examined do, in fact, contain the abnormal cells in question, because even normal cells in the sample may have the capability to react with the same immunostains that decorate tumor cells.

FIXATION

Prerequisites for adequate ICC studies[1] are a well-spread film of cells on a glass slide,[2] adequate fixation[3] removal of blood and proteinaceous material, and a sensitive, reproducible method of ICC.[4]

Wet fixation into alcohol must be performed without delay, because partial air drying may result in false-positive results. Air-dried smears are often more cellular than alcohol-fixed slides because some material often floats off the slide when it is alcohol-fixed. Air-dried slides minimize cell loss and result in a more even film of cells. Such slides must be fixed immediately before performance of ICC, and the types of preferred fixatives vary among cytopathologists. Cold acetone and 95% alcohol[10] are common fixatives, and B5 may be used for lymphoid markers and neuroendocrine antibodies.[11] Leong and colleagues advocate the use of initial fixation in 0.1% formol-saline solution, followed by fixation in 95% ethanol for 10 minutes.[12, 13] Postfixation enhances cell morphologic features and is not required for immunostaining. The antibodies used with the 0.1% formol-saline solution are listed in Table 19–1. I experienced similar results with preparations that were relatively free of background blood and mucus.[14]

An important point to keep in mind is that the antibodies to S-100 protein and gross cystic disease fluid protein-15 (GCDFP-15) do not work well in primary alcohol fixatives because of cytoplasmic antigen leaching. Consequently, false-negative results abound for these antibodies in alcohol fixatives. This can be overcome by triaging air-dried slides and fixing in 0.1% formol-saline.

Table 19–1. Antibodies Used in Immunocytology with Formol-Saline Fixation

Antibody	Clone	Dilution	Source
Keratin	AE1/AE3	2000	Boehringer-Mannheim
Keratin	CAM5.2	30	Becton, Dickinson
Vimentin	V9	1000	DAKO
Desmin	D33	150	DAKO
Smooth muscle actin	1A4	30,000	Sigma
S-100 protein	Polyclonal	30,000	DAKO
Chromogranin A	A11	5000	BioGenex
Thyroglobulin	DAK-Tg6	4000	DAKO
Calcitonin	CAL-3-F5	2000	DAKO
Neurofilament	2F11	150	DAKO
CD57	HNK-1	50	Becton, Dickinson
Prostate-specific antigen	ER-PR8	150	DAKO
Prostate acid phosphatase	PASE/4LJ	3000	DAKO
Neuron-specific enolase	BBS/NC/VI-H14	1000	DAKO
Leukocyte common antigen	T29/33	60	DAKO
CD20	L26	300	DAKO
CD45RO	UCHL1	400	DAKO

REHYDRATION AND STORAGE

Air-dried slides and partially fixed air-dried slides can be rehydrated in normal saline to optimize immunoreactivity as well as cytomorphology.[15–17] Chan and Kung found the optimal time for rehydration to be less than 1 minute, provided that the air-drying time did not exceed 30 minutes.[17] This procedure may be used when cytomorphology is critically important, since air-dried slides can sit for up to 1 week at room temperature and still be used for ICC provided that they are fixed immediately before use as already described.[12]

Slides for ICC, whether air-dried or fixed, can be stored at −70°C for at least 1 month and still maintain immunoreactivity.[13]

ANTIGEN RETRIEVAL

Antigen retrieval is an essential component of the immunocytology staining procedure and imparts consistency to the quality of staining. Heat-induced epitope retrieval (HIER) is the most consistent technique, the most common of which is microwaving in 10 mmol citrate buffer for 10 minutes to boiling.[18–20] This technique must be investigated with each antibody to determine optimal microwaving time and subsequent antibody titer.

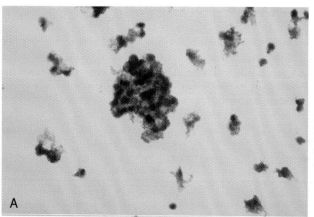
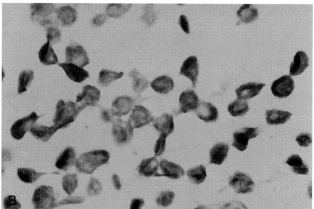
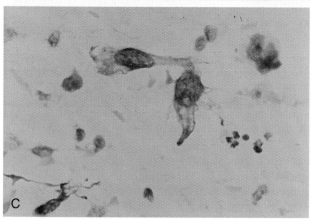

Figure 19–1. *A–C*, Immunocytologic ThinPrep preparation showing results with chromogranin *(A)*, cytokeratin CAM5.2 *(B)*, and muscle actin *(C)*. Note the exceptionally clean background.

FIXATION OF HORMONE RECEPTORS

Although the ER1D5 (DAKO, Carpinteria, CA) antibody can be used on alcohol-fixed smears of breast tumors, formalin fixation of these smears yields a superior stained product.[21] Formalin fixation (10%) may be accomplished on air-dried smears (up to 14 hours) for hormone receptors[12] or the 0.1% formol-saline may be used. Breast prognostic markers, including c-*erb*-B2 and MIB-1 proliferation marker, work well in formalin fixation.

PreservCyt (Cytyc Corporation, Boxborough, MA), a preservative used with the ThinPrep processor (Cytyc Corporation), stabilizes estrogen receptors/progesterone receptors (ERs/PRs) for up to 56 days of storage.[22] The obvious convenience here is for collection of specimens from clinicians at remote sites. This is especially valuable for needle aspiration specimens that are submitted from physicians' offices and radiology and operating room suites.[23]

THIN-LAYER TECHNIQUE

ICC using the proprietary solutions Cytolyt and PreservCyt, with or without processing on the ThinPrep processor provides excellent immunostaining results (Fig. 19–1).[24–27] In my experience, lower antibody concentrations can be used, the background was cleaner, immunostaining was crisp,[24] and immunoreactivity was stable even with long-term storage in Preservcyt.[22] The antibodies that were investigated with this technique are listed in Table 19–2.

CELL BLOCKS

Cell blocks are a luxury to have when studying a cytologic specimen because of their versatility. In addition to the obvious advantage for studying tissue architecture, 10 to 12 additional sections can be cut for ICC (Fig. 19–2). Ten percent buffered formalin is used for fixation for tissue fragments, and the block is processed analogous to any surgical specimen. Storage of the specimen is easier with unlimited antigen preservation. For these reasons, cell blocks are the superior method for ICC for any cytologic specimen.

Suspensions or bloody specimens may be fixed in formol-saline to lyse red cells, or the specimen may be collected in RPMI salt solution, treated with a commercial thrombin-plasma agent to organize a clot, and then fixed in 10% formalin and processed like a surgical specimen.[28]

CONTROLS

Positive and negative controls should be performed with each test sample. Tissue controls are typically used in most laboratories for convenience, but the ideal control should be a cytology sample. If tissue controls are used, caution must be exercised in interpretation, because a different set of artifacts is present in tissue compared with cytology samples. Cytologic controls can be obtained on a daily basis from the surgical pathology bench, with the use of aspirates or direct imprints. These preparations can be air dried and fixed in formol-saline just before use. It is more practical to use cells on the cytology slide as a positive-negative internal control, depending on the antibody and cells that are present.

Specimens of Limited Quantity

Almost any source of cytology specimen is at risk of being of limited quantity by virtue of a limited number of cells spread over several slides. This is a drawback when the cytopathologist must rely on immunocytology studies to arrive at a de-

Table 19–2. Antibodies Used with Cytolyt and PreservCyt (ThinPrep Slides)

Antibody	Dilution	Source
mCEA	PD	Biomeda (Foster City, CA)
pCEA	PD	Biomeda
CEAD-14	PD	Enteric Products (Stony Brook, NY)
CD 43	40	DAKO (Carpinteria, CA)
CD 68	150	DAKO
Chromogranin	PD	Biomeda
Collagen IV	25	DAKO
Desmin	75	DAKO
EMA	100	DAKO
Estrogen receptor	50	DAKO
Progesterone receptor	20	BioGenex (San Ramon, CA)
GCDFP-15	25	Signet (Dedham, MA)
HAM-56	6000	Enzo (Farmingdale, NY)
hCG	1000	DAKO
Insulin	1000	DAKO
AE1/AE3	200	Boehringer-Mannheim (Indianapolis, IN)
K903	50	Enzo
CAM5.2	PD	Becton, Dickinson (Franklin Lakes, NJ)
CD30	100	DAKO
CD20	40	DAKO
Laminin	5	DAKO
MAC387	75	DAKO
HHF-35	PD	Biomeda
NSE	400	DAKO
PLAP	20	DAKO
PSA	10	DAKO
PAP	PD	Biomeda
CD34	800	BioGenex
Synaptophysin	30	BioGenex
Thyroglobulin	PD	DAKO
UCHL1	200	DAKO
Vimentin	PD	DAKO
HMB-45	PD	Enzo
O13	800	Signet
Lambda	40,000	DAKO
Alpha fetoprotein	PD	Immunstain

mCEA, monoclonal carcinoembryonic antigen; pCEA, polyclonal carcinoembryonic antigen; EMA, epithelial membrane antigen; GCDFP-15, gross cystic disease fluid protein-15; hCG, human chorionic gonadotropin; NSE, neuron-specific enolase; PLAP, placenta-like alkaline phosphatase; PSA, prostate-specific antigen; PAP, prostatic acid phosphatase.

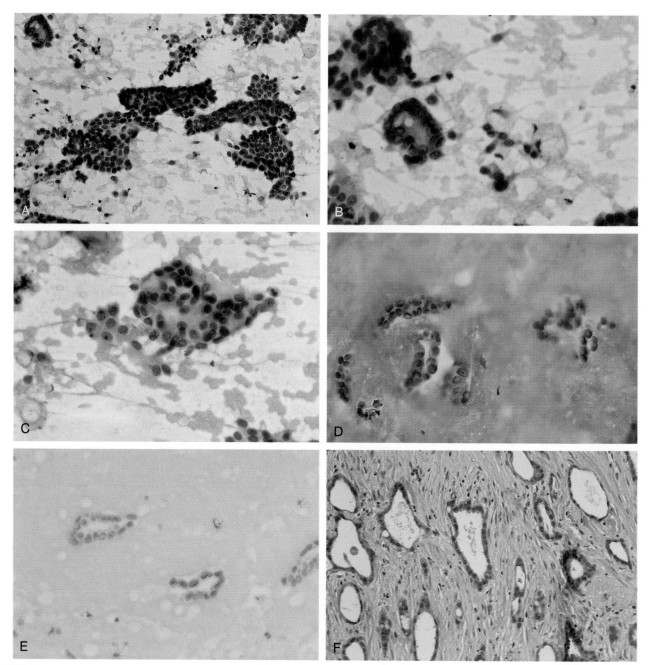

Figure 19–2. *A–C*, Papanicolaou-stained breast aspirate of tubular carcinoma, illustrating whole tubules en face *(A)*, tubular lumens *(B)*, and comma-shaped glands *(C)*. *D and E*, Cell block of tubular carcinoma *(D)* shows angular glands that are negative for smooth muscle myosin heavy chain *(E)*, confirming the diagnostic impression. *F*, Tissue from resection of tubular carcinoma.

finitive diagnosis. It must be emphasized that the cytopathologist must be satisfied with the nature of the specimen under study, without forcing a diagnosis based on a compromised limited sample.

Since most cytopathologists use both alcohol-fixed and air-dried smears/cytospins for interpretation, these same slides can be harvested for further immunostaining using the standard immunostaining techniques. Travis and Wold,[29] and Abendroth and Dabbs[14] studied the procedure of immunostaining previously stained air-dried or alcohol-fixed slides. The slides had been recently prepared or archived and stained with either a Romanowsky

stain or a Papanicolaou stain. Immunostaining was performed on these slides with and without a preceding decolorization step. The results with both types of stains, with or without prior decolorization, were similar—immunostaining worked well. Background staining was more of a problem on the air-dried unfixed cases.[14] Thus, recently stained or archived cytology slides can be used for immunoperoxidase studies, which include commonly used antibodies such as CAM5.2, AE1/AE3, K903, carcinoembryonic antigen (CEA), desmin, HHF-35 (muscle-specific actin), vimentin, CD20, and CD45RO.[14]

Cytologic material can also be used in a variation of the dual immunolabeling technique.[30] With this method, cytology slides that were subjected to an immunoperoxidase test and produced a negative result can be subjected to another immunoperoxidase test using a different antibody (Fig. 19–3).[30] It is imperative to use positive and negative controls with both test runs. For example, a poorly differentiated tumor that is tested with leukocyte common antigen and found to be negative may be found to be positive with keratin, confirming the carcinomatous nature of the specimen. Antibodies that have been used with this method include CAM5.2, AE1/AE3, K903, GCDFP-15, vimentin, CD20, CD45RO, muscle-specific actin (HHF-35), desmin, CEA, and S-100.[30]

Sherman and associates[31] described the cell transfer technique for use with limited cytologic samples. In this technique, cells are lifted off of a slide by redissolving them in a new mounting medium. The medium can be removed from the slide, cut into pieces, and restuck to slides for individual antibody studies (Fig. 19–4). The results of immunostains are generally good, although Hunt and colleagues have described some decreased staining with this method.[32]

Interpretation and Limitations of Immunocytochemistry

As in surgical pathology, the morphologic study of the specimen in concert with the clinicopatho-

logic correlations is of paramount importance in arriving at a correct diagnosis. No amount of immunostaining will afford a correct diagnosis without a thorough patient work-up or tissue examination. Only when immunostaining findings are combined with clinical and other ancillary data is a patient work-up considered complete.

There is a plethora of antibodies that are available for use in cytology, and none of them is specific for its intended target. Antibodies may be polyclonal or monoclonal, vary in sensitivity and specificity, or may be dependent on certain types of fixative for proper immunoreactivity. In addition, the differentiation of many tumors exhibits a wide spectrum. For these reasons, it is important to use known positive and negative controls with a panel of multiple antibodies that are known to be positive and negative in the cytologic study. A negative result by itself is of lesser value than a positive result, unless the cytology specimen itself contains known positive and negative control cells.

The pattern of immunostaining will depend on the presence of neoplastic cells, the location of (e.g., cell membrane, cytoplasm, or nucleus), proper fixation, background staining, and antibody concentration. Immunostaining for any antigen is rarely uniform in nature. Heterogeneity of immunostaining is the rule rather than the exception, and it is proper to state the pattern, cell localization, and distribution of positive and negative immunostaining relative to normal cells that may be present in the sample.

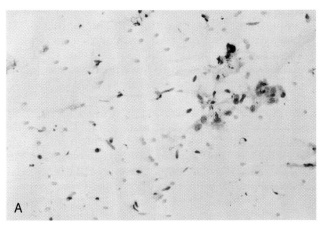
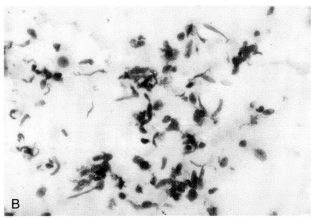
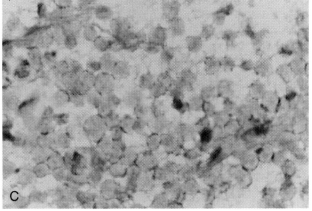

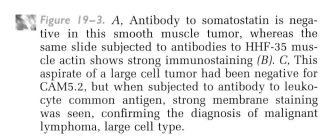

Figure 19–3. A, Antibody to somatostatin is negative in this smooth muscle tumor, whereas the same slide subjected to antibodies to HHF-35 muscle actin shows strong immunostaining *(B). C,* This aspirate of a large cell tumor had been negative for CAM5.2, but when subjected to antibody to leukocyte common antigen, strong membrane staining was seen, confirming the diagnosis of malignant lymphoma, large cell type.

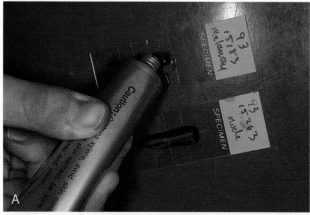

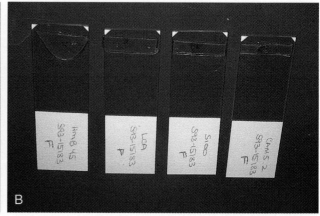

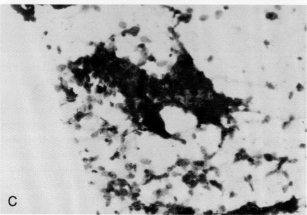

Figure 19–4. Illustration of the cell transfer method. *A,* Quick Mount is added to the slide in order to peel off the cells after baking in an oven. The cells, now suspended in Quick Mount, are then cut into four pieces and baked to adhere the cells onto slides *(B). C,* Keratin AE1/AE3 is strongly positive on the sample that was transferred.

False-positive immunostaining results can be a result of a multitude of factors. First and foremost, the cytopathologist must not mistake normal cellular elements for neoplastic cells, especially in samples in which neoplastic cells are few and far between. The same caution applies to reactive cells in the sample. Drying the slide during any step in the immunoperoxidase procedure results in nonspecific antibody binding that can be misinterpreted as positive findings. Necrotic, poorly preserved, and crushed cells must be avoided because nonspecific binding may yield a false-positive result. Care must be taken not to overinterpret the higher background that is generally seen with polyclonal antibodies. This nonspecific binding to stromal elements can be avoided by carefully assessing the patterns of staining of normal, neoplastic, and stromal elements. Antibodies may cross-react with non–target cell components, or the antibody used may not be as specific as advertised. Only experience and comfort with the antibody in use will satisfy the observer's interpretation in these situations. Improper fixation and incomplete blocking of endogenous peroxidase or biotin activity are well-known sources of false-positive results. Proper blocking with commercial blocking products should eliminate this problem.

False-negative interpretations are also potentially multifactorial in nature. Improper fixation resulting in denaturation or masking of antigen may com-
pletely escape the observer. Only by ascertaining the working dilution of each antibody and ensuring quality fixation can this problem be eliminated. Antibody concentration is a critical determinant, as concentrations that are too low or too high can cause false-negative and false-positive results, respectively. Insufficient antigen retrieval or even decolorization of specimens can cause false-negative results. The type of fixation is critical for antibody performance, and the best example of false-negative results is that antibodies to S-100 protein and GCDFP-15 do not work in primary alcohol fixatives.

The common causes of false-positive and false-negative findings in immunocytology are given in Tables 19–3 and 19–4.

Table 19–3. Immunocytology: Common Causes of False-Positive Results

Antibody is not specific as advertised
Misinterpretation of neoplastic population
Insufficient peroxidase-biotin clocking
Necrotic cells
Dried preparation
Reactive cells misinterpreted
Antibody cross-reactivity
Nonspecific antibody binding
Inappropriate fixation
Antigen diffusion
Antibody concentration too high

Table 19–4. Immunocytology: Common Causes of False-Negative Results

Sample lacks a neoplastic population
Antigen expression is below sensitivity of antibody
Antibody concentration is too low
Poor antigen preservation (fixation)
Antigen diffusion (S-100 protein and GCDFP-15)
Denaturation, prolonged fixation
Insufficient antigen retrieval
Papanicolaou decolorization

GCDFP-15, gross cystic disease fluid protein-15.

DIAGNOSTIC EFFUSION IMMUNOCYTOLOGY

The pleural, pericardial, and abdominal cavities are lined by mesothelial cells, a specialized form of epithelial cell that provides a barrier between the vascular-connective tissue space and cavitary space. Injury to the mesothelial cell results in exposure or disruption of the mesothelial cell basement membrane, which then becomes covered by a fibrinous exudate. Mesothelial repair is heralded by the proliferation of the spindled submesothelial reserve cells, which are rich in vimentin, low molecular weight keratins 8 and 18, and desmin (Fig. 19–5).[33–36] The spindle cell proliferation gradually acquires high molecular weight keratins that are recognized ultrastructurally by the appearance of cytoplasmic tonofilaments. Once the surface cuboidal mesothelial cells are re-established, the cells lose or reduce vimentin expression. This cycle of events explains the keratin-vimentin coexpression that we commonly see in mesothelial cells and demonstrates that a spindle cell population of mesothelial cells exists in the reparative state, similar qualitatively to the spindle cell population witnessed in sarcomatoid mesotheliomas.[37]

Desmin is also commonly found in mesothelial cells of effusions.[38] Using commercially available antibodies to cytokeratin, vimentin, and desmin, Ferrandez-Izquierdo and coworkers found triple coexpression of all mesothelial cells in effusions and in one mesothelioma.[38] The authors concluded that desmin was regularly expressed in mesothelial cells in effusions and was a useful diagnostic feature.

Since the pleural, pericardial, and abdominal cavities provide such a huge surface area, it is not surprising that neoplastic cells invade this surface with great frequency. The challenge of the cytopathologist is to be able to distinguish a neoplastic from a reactive process in serous effusions[1] and be able to provide the site of origin of the neoplastic process if it is unknown at the time that the patient presents with the effusion (Table 19–5).[2]

Monte and colleagues in a 1987 study of 1548 effusions provided an appropriate perspective of

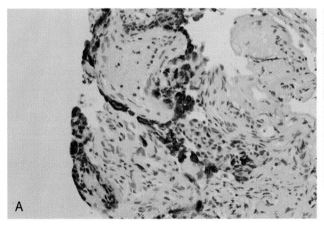

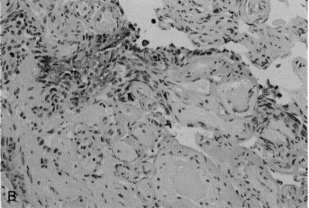

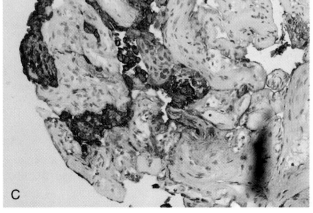

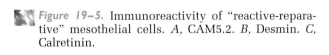

Figure 19–5. Immunoreactivity of "reactive-reparative" mesothelial cells. *A,* CAM5.2. *B,* Desmin. *C,* Calretinin.

Table 19–5. Antibody Panels in the Study of Body Cavity Effusions

	Carcinoem-bryonic Antigen	Epithelial Membrane Antigen	BerEP4	B72.3	LeuM1	Thyroid Trans-cription Factor-1	Ca 15.3	Gross Cystic Disease Fluid Protein-15	CK5/CK6	Calret-inin	Desmin
Reactive meso-thelial cells	N	R-N	N	N	N	N	N	N	+	+	+
Mesothelioma	N	+	N	N	N	N	N	N	+	+	+
Lung adenocar-cinoma	+	+	+	+	+	+	+	N	R-N	R	N
Breast adeno-carcinoma	+/−	+	+	+	+/−	N	+	+	N	N	N
Ovarian serous carcinoma	−/+	+	+	+	+/−	N	+	N	−/+	N	N

+, almost always positive; N, negative; R-N, rarely positive with focal staining; +/−, mostly positive, majority of cells positive; −/+, mostly negative.

the challenge of malignant effusions.[39] Of the 1548 effusions, 154 of 641 ascitic fluids were malignant, with 86% being adenocarcinoma, and most were of ovarian origin. Pleural effusions accounted for 860 cases; 174 of 860 were malignant, and 78% of these were adenocarcinoma, the majority from lung primaries. The second most common site of origin was breast carcinoma. In 7 patients with ascites and 18 patients with pleural effusions, a primary malignancy was not initially apparent. Of the 47 patients with pericardial effusions, 10 were positive for adenocarcinoma, and none had an unknown primary. An initial manifestation of malignancy as a pericardial effusion is distinctly rare. Patients with malignant effusions do poorly as a group and have a poor prognosis.[39, 40]

The majority of malignant effusions thus appear to arise in clinical settings in which patients have an existing documented malignancy. The clinical relevancy to the study of effusions with immunocytology thus appears to exist for patients who do not have a diagnosed malignancy, patients who are suspected of having a secondary malignancy, and patients whose cytologic diagnosis of their effusions lies within the differential diagnosis of reactive versus neoplastic versus malignant mesothelioma.

Diagnostic Approach to the Study of Effusions

Effusions as fluid specimens can be processed as direct smears, as cytospins, and as cell blocks. A combination of these preparations studied together is more efficient at detecting malignancy than is a single preparation alone. Fixation should include ethanol- and air-dried smears that are fixed in 0.1% formol-saline to provide optimal fixation for the entire spectrum of antibodies that may be used, including antibodies to S-100 protein and GCDFP-15, which do not work in primary ethanol fixation.[41] Cell blocks are preferred for study because of their formalin fixation and source of multiple sections for immunostudies.

It is essential to know the patient's clinical history, site of effusion, and the clinical questions that need to be answered. Along with the observed cytomorphologic features, this is the starting point for addressing the patient's problem.

The clue to the process origin in the effusion begins with cytomorphology. Benign mesothelial cells occur in small clusters and exhibit small N/C ratios. There is almost always a background of inflammatory cells and fibrin. Reactive mesothelial cells have a broader spectrum of appearances, with prominent anisocytosis and anisonucleosis. Cells may be arranged into tridimensional clusters mimicking "cell balls" of adenocarcinoma. Cells may be vacuolated and simulate signet ring cells of adenocarcinoma. Nuclei may be hyperchromatic or exhibit prominent nucleoli. Commonly, mesothelial cells have an exocytoplasmic-endocytoplasmic demarcation in which the cytoplasm proximal to the nucleus appears more dense than the peripheral cytoplasm. This feature is particularly useful for the identification of mesothelial cells in general. These cytoplasmic features are recapitulated in the majority of epithelial mesotheliomas. These mesotheliomas present as highly cellular specimens with very large masses of tumor cells. Intercellular "windows," caused by the long microvilli along cell membranes, are a clue to their mesothelial nature. Although cytomorphologic features alone can yield a definitive diagnosis in up to 90% of cases, immunocytochemical studies may be required for other cases in which malignant cells are bland or are obscured by inflammation or inflammation-related mesothelial hyperplasia (Fig. 19–6).

Electron microscopy has been considered the gold standard for the diagnosis of epithelial mesothelioma, but in less differentiated epithelial types in which long microvilli are absent, and when the effusion specimen is not suitable for electron microscopy, ICC using the panel approach has been found useful for arriving at a correct diagnosis.

Antibody Panels Approach

Since the differential diagnosis of effusions almost always includes (reactive) mesothelial cells, malignant mesothelioma, and metastatic carci-

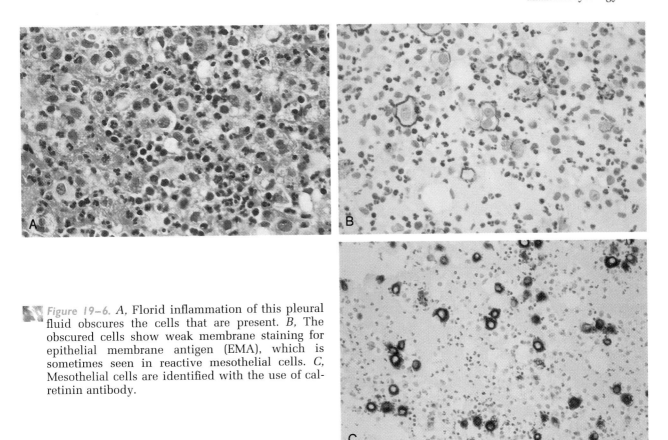

Figure 19–6. *A,* Florid inflammation of this pleural fluid obscures the cells that are present. *B,* The obscured cells show weak membrane staining for epithelial membrane antigen (EMA), which is sometimes seen in reactive mesothelial cells. *C,* Mesothelial cells are identified with the use of calretinin antibody.

noma, it is essential to use a panel of antibodies that have appropriate sensitivity and specificity for distinguishing the entities under study. Recall from the previous discussion that lung and breast carcinomas are the most common tumors found in pleural effusions, whereas ovarian carcinomas and carcinomas of gastrointestinal origin are most commonly found in abdominal effusions.

THYROID TRANSCRIPTION FACTOR-1: LUNG CARCINOMA IN EFFUSIONS

Lung carcinomas, both non–small cell and small cell can be distinguished from mesothelioma and other adenocarcinomas by virtue of strong immunostaining for polyclonal or monoclonal antibodies to CEA, along with strong nuclear immunostaining for thyroid transcription factor-1 (TTF-1).[42] The TTF-1 antibody[43] works in cytologic preparations, including the pulmonary wash, lavage, effusion, and fine needle aspirate.[42] The TTF-1 antibody is highly specific for pulmonary carcinomas, with a sensitivity range of 10 to 30% for squamous carcinoma, 66% for non–small cell carcinomas, and 90% for small cell carcinomas (Fig. 19–7).[44-46] This antibody is especially useful because it is negative in breast carcinomas.[45] In addition, Anwar and Schmidt did not find TTF-1 immunostaining in 37 mesotheliomas.[47]

Unfortunately, there are no other antibodies cur-

rently available for effusion studies by ICC that are as specific as antibodies to TTF-1, thyroglobulin, or prostate-specific antigen. The ICC diagnosis of metastatic carcinoma in malignant effusions typically follows an antibody panel approach, analogous to the work-up of metastatic carcinomas of unknown primary.

EPITHELIAL MEMBRANE ANTIGEN

Epithelial membrane antigen (EMA) typically decorates most carcinomas in a diffuse cytoplasmic fashion but may also impart a diagnostic, thick, crisp membrane pattern of staining on some cases of epithelial mesothelioma.[48] This membranous pattern of staining correlates with the presence of long, bushy microvilli on the cell. Normal or reactive mesothelial cells rarely react with EMA.[11, 48–58] Usually, it is the reactive mesothelial cells that may show a weak to moderate membranous staining pattern in 3 to 4% of cases (see Fig. 19–6).[55]

Frisman and colleagues, using logistic regression analysis, included EMA in a panel of CEA and B72.3 to best discriminate the presence of carcinoma in effusions.[50]

EMA was positive in 97% of carcinomas studied by Singh and coworkers.[56]

Therefore, EMA cannot blindly separate carcinoma from mesothelioma, and it is usually negative to weak in reactive-atypical mesothelial cells.

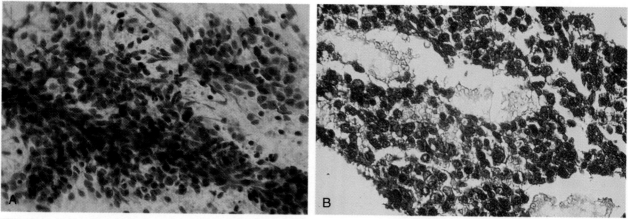

Figure 19–7. This tumor, cytomorphologically a small cell "oat cell" carcinoma *(A)*, is seen to be positive for nuclear thyroid transcription factor-1 (TTF-1) *(B)*, indicative of a lung origin.

CARCINOEMBRYONIC ANTIGEN

Polyclonal or monoclonal antibody for CEA is useful in the study of malignant effusions, because many types of carcinomas are positive for CEA, whereas mesothelial cells and malignant mesothelioma are negative.[59–62] A few investigators found some CEA immunostaining of mesotheliomas, but most of these studies were performed with polyclonal antibody.[63, 64]

Mason and associates found a 90% sensitivity for monoclonal CEA in effusions from a variety of sites.[49] Others have experienced CEA sensitivities for detection of adenocarcinoma of 50 to 80%.[7, 65–67] These differences in sensitivities likely reflect the types of adenocarcinomas in the effusions that were studied. Most lung carcinomas and gastrointestinal carcinomas, along with many breast carcinomas, are positive for CEA, whereas most female genital, renal, and prostate carcinomas are negative.[68–70] High concentrations of CEA in pleural effusions by enzyme immunoassay are virtually diagnostic of metastatic carcinoma,[68] although there is a false-positive rate of 9%.[71]

In immunohistochemical studies, the best sensitivities and specificities for CEA have been found with clones CEJ065 and A5B7.[72, 73] CEA is one of the best discriminating markers for mesothelioma versus lung adenocarcinoma in pleural effusions. CEA is not particularly useful in abdominal effusions to discriminate abdominal papillary mesothelioma from papillary serous ovarian carcinomas, as 0 to 35% of ovarian carcinomas are reported as positive.[74–77]

BerEP4

The BerEP4 antibody is directed against 34- and 39-kd glycoproteins that are present on the cell membranes of most epithelial cells but are absent from mesothelial cells. Developed by Latza and associates[78] in 1990, multiple studies of malignant effusions have shown a sensitivity of 60 to 100% for the detection of adenocarcinomas.[78–88] These same studies underscore the fact that BerEP4 immunostaining of mesothelioma or mesothelial cells is rare, on the order of 4% or less, and that the staining is always very weak and focal.[79, 81, 89–92]

Ordonez[93] observed BerEP4 in 26% of mesotheliomas (focal, few cells), 100% (20 of 20) of pulmonary adenocarcinomas, and 83 to 93% of nonpulmonary adenocarcinomas. All adenocarcinomas stained diffusely.

Specificity of BerEP4 for adenocarcinoma is 90 to 100%, with positive predictive and negative predictive values of 96% and 70%.[81]

TUMOR-ASSOCIATED GLYCOPROTEIN (TAG-72, B72.3)

TAG-72 has been recognized by a multitude of investigators as having a high specificity for the detection of adenocarcinoma in effusions.[11, 67, 94–96] It is commonly found on adenocarcinomas of lung, gastrointestinal tract, breast, ovary, endometrium, and pancreas.[97, 98]

Ordonez[99] and Riera and colleagues[73] reported positive B72.3 on 80% of lung adenocarcinomas and 2 to 5% of mesotheliomas. Sporadic staining of mesothelial cells in effusions was observed by Esteban and colleagues.[100] Most authors report the absence of immunostaining of B72.3 on reactive mesothelial cells.[66, 79, 89, 94, 95, 101, 102] Sensitivity for adenocarcinoma detection is in the range of 60%,[67] but this number improves when B72.3 is combined with other antibodies (see further on).

Papillary serous carcinomas involving the abdomen are commonly positive with B72.3, in contrast to mostly negative results with CEA, and therefore B72.3 is useful to discriminate these carcinomas from mesothelioma.[89, 91, 92, 94–96]

CD15 (LeuM1)

In 1986, Sheibani and colleagues were the first to describe results with LeuM1 antibody to CD15 for distinguishing pulmonary adenocarcinoma from mesothelioma.[103] Subsequent investigators similarly found 70 to 100% of pulmonary adenocarcinomas positive for LeuM1, with only 2 to 10% of mesotheliomas staining.[73, 104–106] LeuM1 has a high specificity for distinguishing mesothelioma from pulmonary adenocarcinoma, but its sensitivity is poor when compared with CEA.[107]

MOC31

MOC31 reacts with a 38-kd membrane glycoprotein of epithelial cells.[108] Since 1994, a host of investigators has concluded that there is a very high specificity for adenocarcinomas, with only rare mesothelioma staining.[109–112]

Ordonez[109] found strong immunostaining in 89% of adenocarcinomas from various sites, with only focal decoration of 5% of mesotheliomas.

New Diagnostic Antibodies Under Development

There are several antibodies that show promise in the study of effusion specimens, but additional studies would be useful to confirm their utility.

CA 15-3

The Ca 15-3 antigen, expressed on the luminal cytoplasm of benign and malignant breast epithelium, was studied for its ability to detect breast carcinoma in tissue[113] and in effusions.[114] Zimmerman and colleagues,[115] using a second-generation clone (Zymed, South San Francisco, CA) of Ca 15-3 in cell block material from effusions, found that the sensitivity for all types of adenocarcinoma was 91%, with a specificity of 95%. The sensitivity for breast carcinoma alone was 97%.

SIALOSYL-TN

Sialosyl-Tn is an abnormally glycosylated MN blood group precursor that appears on malignant and dysplastic epithelium. Using cell block material from body cavity fluids, Zimmerman and associates[116] demonstrated 100% specificity for adenocarcinomas (40 malignant effusions), 78% sensitivity, a positive predictive value of 100%, and a negative predictive value of 76%. With these results, the antibody may be useful or confirmatory when used with an antibody panel.

Affirmative Identification of Mesothelial Differentiation

Up to this point, all the previously described immunoreagents identify mesothelial cells by a default negative stain result. This type of result is less than optimal, although still valuable. Several antibodies have been studied that are able to identify mesothelial cells by virtue of a positive immunostaining result. Some of these valuable antibodies include calretinin and CK5/CK6.

CALRETININ

The 29-kd calcium-binding protein was used by Doglioni and coworkers[117] to study pleural fluids and tissues. They observed calretinin immunostaining in all 44 mesotheliomas, but only rare focal decoration of a variety of adenocarcinomas, and focal staining of 23% of lung adenocarcinomas. Additional investigators reported similar findings,[86, 118–120] but it was the study of Ordonez that showed the difference of sensitivities of the antibodies from Chemicon and Zymed.[121] The Zymed antibody sensitivity was 100% compared with a Chemicon sensitivity of 74%. Focal, weak staining of adenocarcinomas was seen in 9% and 4%, respectively.

Nagel and colleagues[122] had a similar experience with the study of cytospins, finding a sensitivity for mesothelial cells of 93%, with 5% of tumor cells immunostaining.

CK5/CK6

The 1989 immunohistochemical study of Moll and colleagues[123] confirmed the biochemical study of Blobel and colleagues,[124] in which keratin 5 was found to be a constituent of mesothelioma but not lung adenocarcinoma. Clover and associates[125] found rare, weak staining for CK5/CK6 in 4 of 27 lung adenocarcinomas with the D5/16B4 antibody clone, whereas Ordonez[126] found focal staining in 6.5% of nonpulmonary adenocarcinomas and diffuse staining in all mesotheliomas and squamous cell carcinomas. Given these data, CK5/CK6 is a useful way to identify epithelial mesothelioma and reactive mesothelial cells.

Coordinate Expression of CK7/CK20

Since the initial studies that demonstrated the utility of coordinate expression of CK7/CK20 for identifying subsets of carcinomas in tissues,[127, 128] several investigators have demonstrated the utility of these antibodies in Papanicolaou-stained specimens, effusions, fine needle aspirates, and cell blocks.[127–132] The reader is referred to Chapter 7 for an exhaustive survey of the use of the CK7/CK20 panel.

Antibody Panels for the Study of Malignant Effusions

From the foregoing discussions, it is apparent that the antibodies that are optimal to use as part of a panel in the study of malignant effusions should include those that have the highest sensitivity and specificity for the antigen under study. These recommended panels have changed significantly over the years as a result of clinical efficacy studies, and undoubtedly they will continue to evolve. Frisman and coworkers,[50] using logistic regression analysis, concluded that an abbreviated panel using antibodies to CEA, EMA, and B72.3 was sufficient to characterize adequately 95% of the 100 effusions that they studied. Unfortunately, there have been no other studies in which logistic regression analysis was used.

Combinations of antibodies in a panel to study effusions add statistical power to the study process. Antibodies to CEA (monoclonal), EMA, and B72.3 may dispense with up to 95% of effusions, but there remains the other problematic 5% of cases. If the goal of the observer is to identify only adenocarcinoma, BerEP4, LeuM1, and MOC31, along with calretinin and CK5/CK6, should be added to the panel. Specific antibodies to cell lineage should be used when appropriate, depending on the site of effusion, and so on—for example, TTF-1 should be used to distinguish lung carcinoma in a pleural effusion.

References

1. Chess Q, Hajdu S. The role of immunoperoxidase staining in diagnostic cytology. Acta Cytol 1986;30:1–7.
2. Flens MJ, Valk PVD, Tadema TM, et al. The contribution of immunocytochemistry in diagnostic cytology, comparison and evaluation with immunohistology. Cancer 1990;65:2704–2711.
3. Johnston WW, Szpak CA, Thor A, et al. Techniques in immunocytochemistry, application to diagnostic pathology. Arch Pathol Lab Med 1989;113:641–644.
4. Lai C-R, Pan C-C, Tsay S-H. Contribution of immunocytochemistry in routine diagnostic cytology. Diagn Cytopathol 1996;14:221–225.
5. Leong A-Y, Wannakrairot P. A retrospective analysis of immunohistochemical staining in identifying poorly differentiated round cell and spindle cell tumors: Results, reagents and costs. Pathology 1992;24:254–260.
6. Nadji M. The potential value of immunoperoxidase techniques in diagnostic cytology. Acta Cytol 1980;24:442–447.
7. Shield PW, Perkins G, Wright RG. Immunocytochemical staining of cytology specimens. How helpful is it? Am J Clin Pathol 1996;105:157–162.
8. Wazir JF, Martin-Bates E, Woodward G, et al. Evaluation of immunocytochemical staining as a method of improving diagnostic accuracy in a routine cytopathology laboratory. Cytopathology 1991;2:75–82.
9. Weintraub J, Redard M, Vassilakos P. The application of immunocytochemical techniques to routinely fixed and stained cytologic specimens. Pathol Res Pract 1990;186:658–665.
10. Schofield J, Krausz T. Metastatic disease and lymphomas. In: Gray W, ed. Serous Cavities. London: Churchill-Livingstone, 1995.
11. Nance K, Silverman JF. Immunocytochemical panel for the identification of malignant cells in serous effusions. Am J Clin Pathol 1993;95:867–874.
12. Leong A-Y, Suthipintawong C, Vinyuvat S. Immunostaining of cytologic preparations: A review of technical problems. Appl Immunohistochem 1999;7:214–220.
13. Suthipintawong C, Leong A-Y, Vinyuvat S. Immunostaining of cell preparations: A comparative evaluation of common fixatives and protocols. Diagn Cytopathol 1996;15:167–174.
14. Abendroth CS, Dabbs DJ. Immunocytochemical staining of unstained versus previously stained cytologic preparations. Acta Cytol 1995;39:379–386.
15. Randall B, van Amerongen L. Commercial laboratory practice evaluation of air-dried/rehydrated cervico-vaginal smears vs traditionally-fixed smears. Diagn Cytopathol 1997;16:174–176.
16. Ng WF, Choi FB, Cheung LLH, et al. Rehydration of air-dried smears with normal saline: Application in fluid cytology. Acta Cytol 1994;38:56–64.
17. Chan JKC, Kung ITM. Rehydration of air-dried smears with normal saline: Application in fine-needle aspiration cytologic examination. Am J Clin Pathol 1988;89:30–34.
18. Leong A-Y, Milios J. An assessment of the efficacy of the microwave antigen-retrieval procedure on a range of tissue antigens. Appl Immunohistochem 1993;1:267–274.
19. Gown AM, deWever N, Battifora H. Microwave-based antigen unmasking: A revolutionary new technique for routine immunohistochemistry. Appl Immunohistochem 1993;1:256–266.
20. Shi S, Key ME, Kalara KL. Antigen-retrieval in formalin-fixed paraffin-embedded tissues: An enhancement method for immunohistochemical staining based on microwave oven heating of tissue sections. J Histochem Cytochem 1991;39:741–748.
21. Suthipintawong C, Leong A-Y, Chan KW, et al. Immunostaining of estrogen receptor, progesterone receptor, MIB-1 antigen and c-erbB-2 in cytologic specimens: A simplified method with formalin fixation. Diagn Cytopathol 1997;17:127–133.
22. Tabbara SO, Sidaway M, Frost AR, et al. The stability of estrogen and progesterone receptor expression on breast carcinoma cells stored as PreservCyt suspensions and as ThinPrep slides. Cancer Cytopathol 1998;84:355–360.
23. Ducatman B, Hogan CL, Wang HH. A triage system for processing fine needle aspiration cytology specimens. Acta Cytol 1989;33:797–799.
24. Dabbs DJ, Abendroth CS, Grenko RT, et al. Immunocytochemistry on the ThinPrep processor. Diagn Cytopathol 1997;17:388–392.
25. Guiter GE, Gatscha RM, Zakowski MF. ThinPrep vs conventional aspirations of sarcomas: A morphological and immunocytochemical study. Diagn Cytopathol 1999;21:351–354.
26. Leung SW, Bedard YC. Immunocytochemical staining on ThinPrep processed smears. Mod Pathol 1996;9:304–306.
27. Kaplan MA, Segura AM, Wang HH, et al. Evaluation of Cytolyt and PreservCyt as preservatives for immunocytochemistry for cytokeratin in fine needle aspiration. Appl Immunohistochem 1998;6:23–29.
28. Fowler LJ, Valente PT. Cell block techniques and immunocytochemistry. Diagn Cytopathol 1996;14:281.
29. Travis WD, Wold LE. Immunoperoxidase staining of fine needle aspiration specimens previously stained by the Papanicolaou technique. Acta Cytol 1987;31:517–520.
30. Dabbs DJ, Wang X. Immunocytochemistry on cytologic specimens of limited quantity. Diagn Cytopathol 1998;18:166–169.
31. Sherman ME, Jimenez-Joseph D, Gangi MD, et al. Immunostaining of small cytologic specimens. Facilitation with cell transfer. Acta Cytol 1994;38:18–22.
32. Hunt JL, van de Rijn M, Gupta PK. Immunohistochemical analysis of gel-transferred cells in cytologic preparations following smear division. Diagn Cytopathol 1998;18:377–380.
33. Carter D, Otis CN. Three types of spindle cell tumor of the pleura: Fibroma, sarcoma and sarcomatoid mesothelioma. Am J Surg Pathol 1988;12:747–753.
34. Truong LD, Rangdaeng S, Cagle P, et al. The diagnostic utility of desmin: A study of 584 cases and review of the literature. Am J Clin Pathol 1990;93:305–314.

35. Van Muijen GNP, Ruiter DJ, Warnaar SD. Coexpression of intermediate filament polypeptides in human fetal and adult tissues. Lab Invest 1987;57:359–369.

36. Potzsch B, Grulich-Henn J, Rossing R, et al. Identification of endothelial and mesothelial cells in human omental tissue and in omentum-derived cultured cells by specific cell markers. Lab Invest 1990;6:841–852.

37. Bolen JW, Hammar SP, McNutt MA. Serosal tissue: Reactive tissue as a model for understanding mesotheliomas. Ultrastruct Pathol 1987;11:251–262.

38. Ferrandez-Izquierdo A, Navarro-Fos S, Gonzalez-Devesa M, et al. Immunocytochemical typification of mesothelial cells in effusions: In vivo and in vitro models. Diagn Cytopathol 1994;10:256–262.

39. Monte SA, Ehya H, Lang WR. Positive effusion cytology as the initial presentation of malignancy. Acta Cytol 1987;31:448–452.

40. Bonnefoi H, Smith IE. How should cancer presenting as a malignant pleural effusion be managed? Br J Cancer 1996;74:832–835.

41. Fiel M, Cernaaianu G, Burstein DE. Value of GCDFP-15 (BRST-2) as a specific immunocytochemical marker for breast carcinoma in cytologic specimens. Acta Cytol 1996;40:637–641.

42. Harlamert HA, Mira J, Bejarano PA, et al. Thyroid transcription factor-1 and cytokeratins 7 and 20 in pulmonary and breast carcinoma. Acta Cytol 1998;42:1382–1388.

43. Holzinger A, Dingle S, Bejarano PA, et al. Monoclonal antibody to thyroid transcription factor-1: Production, characterization and usefulness in tumor diagnosis. Hybridoma 1996;15:49–53.

44. Fabbro D, DiLoreto C, Stamerra O, et al. TTF-1 gene expression in human lung tumors. Eur J Cancer 1996;32:512–517.

45. Bejarano PA, Baughman RP, Biddinger PW, et al. Surfactant proteins and thyroid transcription factor-1 in pulmonary and breast carcinomas. Mod Pathol 1996;9:445–452.

46. DiLoreto C, DiLauro V, Puglisi F, et al. Immunocytochemical expression of tissue specific transcription factor-1 in lung carcinomas. J Clin Pathol 1997;50:30–32.

47. Anwar F, Schmidt RA. Thyroid transcription factor-1 distinguishes mesothelioma from pulmonary adenocarcinoma. Lab Invest 1999;79:181A.

48. Leong A-Y, Parkinson R, Milios J. "Thick" cell membranes revealed by immunocytochemical staining: A clue to the diagnosis of mesothelioma. Diagn Cytopathol 1990;6:9–13.

49. Mason MR, Bedrossian CWM, Fahey CA, et al. Value of immunocytochemistry in the study of malignant effusions. Diagn Cytopathol 1987;3:215–221.

50. Frisman DM, McCarthy WF, Schleiff P, et al. Immunocytochemistry in the differential diagnosis of effusions: Use of logistic regression to select a panel of antibodies to distinguish adenocarcinomas from mesothelial proliferations. Mod Pathol 1993;6:179–184.

51. Ghosh AK, Spriggs AI, Taylor-Papadimitriou J, et al. Immunocytochemical staining of cells in pleural and peritoneal effusions with a panel of monoclonal antibodies. J Clin Pathol 1983;36:1154–1164.

52. Cibas EM, Corson JM, Pinkus GS. The distinction of adenocarcinoma from malignant mesothelioma in cell blocks of effusions: The role of routine histochemistry and immunohistochemical assessment of carcinoembryonic antigen, keratin proteins, epithelial membrane antigen and milk-fat globule-derived antigen. Hum Pathol 1987;18:67–74.

53. Brown RW, Clark GM, Tandon AK, et al. Multiple-marker immunohistochemical phenotypes distinguishing malignant pleural mesothelioma from pulmonary adenocarcinoma. Hum Pathol 1993;24:345–354.

54. Al-Nafussi A, Carder PJ. Monoclonal antibodies in the cytodiagnosis of serous effusions. Cytopathology 1990;1:119–128.

55. Silverman JF, Nance K, Phillips B, et al. The use of immunoperoxidase panels for the cytologic diagnosis of malignancy in serous effusions. Diagn Cytopathol 1987;3:134–140.

56. Singh HK, Silverman JF, Berns L, et al. Significance of epithelial membrane antigen in the work-up of problematic serous effusions. Diagn Cytopathol 1995;13:3–7.

57. To A, Dearnaley DP, Omerod MG, et al. Epithelial membrane antigen: Its use in the cytodiagnosis of malignancy. Am J Clin Pathol 1982;78:214–219.

58. Walts AE, Said JW, Shintaku IP. Epithelial membrane antigen in the cytodiagnosis of effusions and aspirates: Immunocytochemical and ultrastructural localization in benign and malignant cells. Diagn Cytopathol 1987;3:41–49.

59. Sehested M, Ralfkjaer E, Rasmussen J. Immunoperoxidase demonstration of carcinoembryonic antigen in pleural and peritoneal effusions. Acta Cytol 1983;27:124–127.

60. O'Brien JM, Kirkham SE, Burke B, et al. CEA, ZGM and EMA: Localization in cells of pleural and peritoneal effusion: Preliminary study. Invest Cell Pathol 1980;3:251–258.

61. Walts AE, Johnathan WS, Banks-Schlegel S. Keratin and carcinoembryonic antigen in exfoliated mesothelial and malignant cells: An immunoperoxidase study. Am J Clin Pathol 1983;80:671–676.

62. Orell SR, Dowling KD. Oncofetal antigens as tumor markers in the cytologic diagnosis of effusions. Acta Cytol 1983;27:625–629.

63. Ghosh AK, Butler EB. Immunocytochemical staining reactions of anti-carcinoembryonic antigen, Ca and anti-human milk fat globule monoclonal antibodies on benign and malignant exfoliated cells. J Clin Pathol 1987;40:1424–1427.

64. Guzman J, Bross KJ, Wurtzemberger G, et al. Immunocytology in malignant pleural mesothelioma: Expression of tumor markers and distribution of lymphocyte subsets. Chest 1989;95:590–595.

65. Pinto MM. CA-15.3 assay in effusions: Comparison with carcinoembryonic antigen and CA-125 assay and cytologic diagnosis. Acta Cytol 1996;40:437–442.

66. Delahaye M, van der Ham F, van der Kwast TH. Complementary value of five carcinoma markers for the diagnosis of malignant mesothelioma, adenocarcinoma metastasis, and reactive mesothelium in serous effusions. Diagn Cytopathol 1997;17:115–120.

67. Mezger J, Stotzer O, Schilli G, et al. Identification of carcinoma cells in ascitic and pleural fluid: Comparison of four pan-epithelial antigens with carcinoembryonic antigen. Acta Cytol 1992;36:75–81.

68. Pinto MM, Bernstein LH, Brogan DA, et al. Carcinoembryonic antigen in effusions: A diagnostic adjunct to cytology. Acta Cytol 1987;31:113–118.

69. Lee JS, Nam JH, Lee MC, et al. Immunohistochemical panel for distinguishing between carcinoma and reactive mesothelial cells in serous effusions. Acta Cytol 1996;40:631–636.

70. Athanassiadou P, Athanassiades P, Lazaris D, et al. Immunocytochemical differentiation of reactive mesothelial cells and adenocarcinoma cells in serous effusions with the use of carcinoembryonic antigen. Acta Cytol 1994;38:718–722.

71. Garcia-Pachon E, Padilla-Navias I, Dosda MD, et al. Elevated level of carcinoembryonic antigen in nonmalignant pleural effusions. Chest 1998;113:1143–1144.

72. Ordonez NG. The immunohistochemical diagnosis of mesothelioma: Differentiation of mesothelioma and lung adenocarcinoma. Am J Surg Pathol 1989;13:276–291.

73. Riera JR, Astengo-Osuna C, Longmate JA, et al. The immunohistochemical diagnostic panel for epithelial mesothelioma: A reevaluation after heat induced epitope retrieval. Am J Surg Pathol 1997;21:1409–1419.

74. Sheahan K, O'Brien MJ, Burke B, et al. Differential reactivities of carcinoembryonic antigen (CEA) and CEA-related monoclonal and polyclonal antibodies in common epithelial malignancies. Am J Clin Pathol 1990;94:157–164.

75. Ordonez NG. Role of immunohistochemistry in distinguishing epithelial peritoneal mesotheliomas from peritoneal and ovarian serous carcinomas. Am J Surg Pathol 1998;22:1203–1214.

76. Khoury N, Raju U, Crissman JD, et al. A comparative immunohistochemical study of peritoneal and ovarian serous tumors, and mesotheliomas. Hum Pathol 1990;21:811–819.

77. Bollinger DJ, Wick MR, Dehner LP, et al. Peritoneal malignant mesothelioma versus serous papillary adenocarcinoma: A histochemical and immunohistochemical comparison. Am J Surg Pathol 1989;13:659–670.

78. Latza U, Niedobitek G, Schwarting R, et al. Ber-EP4: New monoclonal antibody which distinguishes epithelia from mesothelia. J Clin Pathol 1990;43:213–219.

79. Shield PW, Callan JJ, Devine PL. Markers for metastatic adenocarcinoma in serous effusion specimens. Diagn Cytopathol 1995;11:1–9.

80. Lidang JM, Johansen P. Immunocytochemical staining of serous effusions: An additional method in the routine cytology practice? Cytopathology 1994;5:93–103.

81. Maguire B, Whitaker D, Carallo S, et al. Monoclonal antibody Ber-EP4: Its use in the differential diagnosis of malignant mesothelioma and carcinoma in cell blocks of malignant effusions and FNA specimens. Diagn Cytopathol 1994;10:130–134.

82. Flynn MK, Johnston W, Bigner S. Carcinoma of ovarian and other origins in effusions: Immunocytochemical study with a panel of antibodies. Acta Cytol 1993;37:439–447.

83. Diaz-Arias A, Loy TS, Bickel JT, et al. Utility of Ber-EP4 in the diagnosis of adenocarcinoma in effusions: An immunocytochemical study of 232 cases. Diagn Cytopathol 1993;9:516–521.

84. Stoop JA, Hendriks JGM, Berends D. Identification of malignant cells in serous effusions using a panel of monoclonal antibodies Ber-EP4, MCA-b-12 and EMA. Cytopathology 1992;3:297–302.

85. De Angelis M, Buley ID, Heryet A, et al. Immunocytochemical staining of serous effusions with monoclonal antibody Ber-EP4. Cytopathology 1992;3:111–117.

86. Bailey ME, Brown RW, Mody DR, et al. Ber-EP4 for differentiating adenocarcinoma from reactive and neoplastic mesothelial cells in serous effusions: Comparison with carcinoembryonic antigen, B72.3 and LeuM1. Acta Cytol 1996;40:1212–1216.

87. Illingworth AL, Young JA, Johnson GD. Immunofluorescent staining of metastatic carcinoma cells in serous fluid with carcinoembryonic antibody, epithelial membrane antibody, AUA-1 and Ber-EP4. Cytopathology 1994;5:270–281.

88. Matter-Walstra KW, Kraft R. Atypical cells in effusions: Diagnostic value of cell image analysis combined with immunocytochemistry. Diagn Cytopathol 1996;15:263–269.

89. Kuhlmann L, Berghauser KH, Schaffer R. Distinction of mesothelioma from carcinoma in pleural effusions: An immunocytochemical study on routinely processed cytoblock preparations. Pathol Res Pract 1991;187:467–471.

90. Sheibani K, Shin SS, Kezirian J, et al. Ber-EP4 antibody as a discriminant in the differential diagnosis of malignant mesothelioma versus adenocarcinoma. Am J Surg Pathol 1991;15:779–784.

91. Dejmek A, Hjerpe A. Immunohistochemical reactivity in mesothelioma and adenocarcinoma: A stepwise logistic regression analysis. APMIS 1994;102:255–264.

92. Gaffey MJ, Mills SE, Swanson PE, et al. Immunoreactivity for Ber-EP4 in adenocarcinomas, adenomatoid tumors and malignant mesotheliomas. Am J Surg Pathol 1992;16:3–9.

93. Ordonez NG. Value of the Ber-EP4 antibody in differentiating pleural mesothelioma from adenocarcinoma: The M.D. Anderson experience and a critical review of the literature. Am J Clin Pathol 1998;109:85–89.

94. Martin SE, Moshiri S, Thor A, et al. Identification of adenocarcinoma in cytospin preparations of effusions using monoclonal antibody B72.3. Am J Clin Pathol 1986;86:10–18.

95. Johnston WW, Szpak CA, Lottich SC, et al. Use of a monoclonal antibody (B72.3) as an immunocytochemistry adjunct to diagnosis of adenocarcinoma in human effusions. Cancer Res 1985;45:1984–1990.

96. Szpak C, Johnston W, Lottich A, et al. Patterns of reactivity of four novel monoclonal antibodies (B72.3, DF3, B1.1, B6.2) with cells in human malignant and benign effusions. Acta Cytol 1984;28:356–357.

97. Johnston WW. Applications of monoclonal antibodies in clinical cytology as exemplified by studies with monoclonal antibody B72.3. Acta Cytol 1987;31:537–556.

98. Johnson VG, Schlom J, Paterson AJ, et al. Analysis of human tumor associated glycoprotein (TAG-72) identified by monoclonal antibody B72.3. Cancer Res 1986;46:850–857.

99. Ordonez NG. The immunohistochemical diagnosis of epithelial pleural mesothelioma. Pathol Case Rev 1999;4:234–241.

100. Esteban JM, Yokata S, Husain S, et al. Immunocytochemical profile of benign and carcinomatous effusions—a practical approach to difficult diagnosis. Am J Clin Pathol 1990;94:698–705.

101. Tickman RJ, Cohen C, Varma VA, et al. Distinction between carcinoma cells and mesothelial cells in serous effusions: Usefulness of immunohistochemistry. Acta Cytol 1990;34:491–496.

102. Lauritzen AF. Diagnostic value of monoclonal antibody B72.3 in detecting adenocarcinoma cells in serous effusions. APMIS 1989;97:761–766.

103. Sheibani K, Battifora H, Burke JS. Antigenic phenotype of malignant mesotheliomas and pulmonary adenocarcinomas: An immunohistologic analysis demonstrating the value of Leu M1 antigen. Am J Pathol 1986;123:212–219.

104. Garcia-Prats MD, Ballesttttin C, Sotelo T, et al. A comparative evaluation of immunohistochemical markers for the differential diagnosis of malignant pleural tumors. Histopathology 1998;32:462–472.

105. Brown RW, Clark GM, Tandon AK, et al. Multiple marker immunohistochemical phenotypes distinguishing malignant pleural mesothelioma from pulmonary adenocarcinoma. Hum Pathol 1993;24:347–354.

106. Wirth PR, Legier J, Wright GLJ. Immunohistochemical evaluation of seven antibodies for differentiation of pleural mesothelioma from lung adenocarcinoma. Cancer 1991;67:655–662.

107. Ordonez NG. Value of antibodies 44-A36, SM3, HBME-1 and thrombomodulin in differentiating epithelial pleural mesothelioma from lung adenocarcinoma: A comparative study with other commonly used antibodies. Am J Surg Pathol 1997;21:1399–1408.

108. DeLeij L, Helrich W, Stein R, et al. SCLC-cluster-2 antibodies detect the pancarcinoma/epithelial glycoprotein EGP-2. Int J Cancer 1994;8:60–63.

109. Ordonez NG. Value of the MOC-31 monoclonal antibody in differentiating epithelial pleural mesothelioma from lung adenocarcinoma. Hum Pathol 1998;29:166–169.

110. Sosolik RC, McGaughy VR, DeYound BR. A potential addition to the pulmonary adenocarcinoma versus mesothelioma immunohistochemistry panel. Mod Pathol 1997;10:716–719.

111. Edwards C, Oates J. OV 632 and MOC-31 in the diagnosis of mesothelioma and adenocarcinoma: An assessment of their use in formalin-fixed and paraffin wax embedded material. J Clin Pathol 1995;48:626–630.

112. Ruitenbeek T, Gouw AS, Poppema S. Immunocytology of body cavity fluids: MOC-31, a monoclonal antibody discriminating between mesothelial and epithelial cells. Arch Pathol Lab Med 1994;118:265–269.

113. Brown RW, Campagna LB, Dunn JK, et al. Immunohistochemical identification of tumor markers in metastatic adenocarcinoma: A diagnostic adjunct in the determination of primary site. Am J Clin Pathol 1997;107:12–19.

114. Szpak CA, Johnston WW, Lottich SC, et al. Patterns of reactivity of four novel monoclonal antibodies (B72.3, DF3, B1.1, B6.2) with cells in malignant and benign effusions. Acta Cytol 1984;28:356–367.

115. Zimmerman RL, Fogt F, Goonewardene S. Diagnostic value of a second generation Ca 15-3 antibody to detect adenocarcinoma in body cavity effusions. Cancer 2000;90:230–234.

116. Zimmerman RL, Fogt F, Bibbo M. Diagnostic utility of sialosyl-Tn in discriminating carcinomatous cells from benign mesothelium in body cavity effusions. Acta Cytol 1999;43:1079–1084.

117. Doglioni C, Dei Tos AP, Laurino L, et al. A novel immuno-

cytochemical marker for mesothelioma. Am J Surg Pathol 1996;20:1037–1046.

118. Gotzos V, Vogt P, Celio MR. The calcium binding protein calretinin is a selective marker for malignant pleural mesothelioma of the epithelial type. Pathol Res Pract 1996; 192:137–147.

119. Simsir A, Fetsch P, Mehta D, et al. E-cadherin, N-cadherin and calretinin in pleural effusions: The good, the bad and the worthless. Diagn Cytopathol 1999;20:125–130.

120. Leers MPG, Aarts MMJ, Theunissen PHMH. E-cadherin and calretinin: A useful combination of immunochemical markers for differentiation between mesothelioma and metastatic adenocarcinoma. Histopathology 1998;32:209–216.

121. Ordonez NG. Value of calretinin immunostaining in differentiating epithelial mesothelioma from lung adenocarcinoma. Mod Pathol 1998;11:929–933.

122. Nagel H, Hemmerlein B, Ruschenberg I, et al. The value of anti-calretinin antibody in the differential diagnosis of normal and reactive mesothelia versus metastatic tumors in effusion cytology. Pathol Res Pract 1998;194:759–764.

123. Moll R, Dhouailly D, Sun T-T. Expression of keratin 5 as a distinctive feature of epithelial and biphasic mesotheliomas. An immunohistochemical study using monoclonal antibody. Virchows Arch B Cell Pathol 1989;58:129–145.

124. Blobel GA, Moll R, Franke RR, et al. The intermediate cytoskeleton of malignant mesotheliomas and its diagnostic significance. Am J Pathol 1985;121:235–247.

125. Clover J, Oates J, Edwards C. Anti-cytokeratin 5/6: A positive marker for mesothelioma. Histopathology 1997;31:140–143

126. Ordonez NG. Value of cytokeratin 5/6 immunostaining in distinguishing epithelial mesothelioma of the pleura from lung adenocarcinoma. Am J Surg Pathol 1998;22:1215-1221.

127. Wang NP, Zee S, Zarbo RJ, et al. Coordinate expression of cytokeratins 7 and 20 defines unique subsets of carcinomas. Appl Immunohistochem 1995;3:99–107.

128. Zee S, Wang NP, Bacchi CE, et al. Cytokeratin (CK) 7 and CK 20 immunophenotyping can distinguish among carcinomas of different primary sites: An immunohistochemical study. Mod Pathol 1995;8:142A.

129. Blumenfeld W, Turi GK, Harrison G, et al. Utility of cytokeratin 7 and 20 subset analysis as an aid in the identification of primary site of origin of malignancy in cytologic specimens. Diagn Cytopathol 1999;20:63–66.

130. Sack MJ, Roberts SA. Cytokeratins 20 and 7 in the differential diagnosis of metastatic carcinomas in cytologic specimens. Cytopathology 1997;16:132–136.

131. Ascoli V, Taccogna S, Scalzo CC, et al. Utility of cytokeratin 20 in identifying the origin of metastatic carcinomas in effusions. Diagn Cytopathol 1995;12:303–308.

132. Baars JH, De Ruijter JLM, Smedts F, et al. The applicability of keratin 7 monoclonal antibody in routinely Papanicolaou stained cytologic specimens for the differential diagnosis of carcinomas. Am J Clin Pathol 1994;101:257–261.

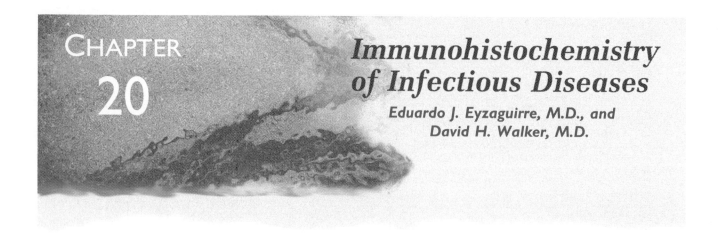

CHAPTER 20

Immunohistochemistry of Infectious Diseases

Eduardo J. Eyzaguirre, M.D., and
David H. Walker, M.D.

Since the 1980s, surgical pathologists in general and infectious disease pathologists in particular have dealt with an increasing number of surgical specimens from patients in whom one or multiple infectious agents may be responsible for disease.[1] In this context, pathologists have played an important role in recognizing infectious agents. In many cases, when fresh tissue is not available for culture, pathologists can provide a rapid morphologic diagnosis and facilitate clinical decisions in patient treatment.[2] In addition, pathologists have played a central role in the identification of emerging and re-emerging infectious agents and describing the pathogenetic processes of emerging diseases, such as *Hantavirus* pulmonary syndrome and other viral hemorrhagic fevers, leptospirosis, and rickettsial and ehrlichial infections.[3–5]

Conventionally, microbial identification in infectious diseases has been made primarily by using serologic assays and culture techniques. However, serologic results can be difficult to interpret in the setting of immunosuppression or when only a single sample is available for evaluation. In addition, fresh tissue is not always available for culture, and culture of fastidious pathogens can be difficult and may take weeks or months to yield results. Some microorganisms have distinctive morphologic characteristics that allow their identification in formalin-fixed tissues using routine and special stains. Nevertheless, in several instances it is difficult or even impossible to identify an infectious agent specifically by conventional morphologic methods.

Immunohistochemistry is one of the most powerful techniques in surgical pathology. There has been an increasing interest in the use of specific antibodies to viral, bacterial, fungal, and parasitic antigens in the detection and identification of the causative agents in many infectious diseases. The use of a specific antibody to detect a microbial antigen was first performed by Coons and associates[6] to detect pneumococcal antigen in tissues. The advantages of immunohistochemistry over conventional methods are listed in Table 20–1, and Table 20–2 shows the contributions of immu-

nohistochemistry in infectious diseases. It is important to emphasize that both monoclonal and polyclonal antibodies must be tested for possible cross-reactivities with other organisms. The widespread occurrence of common antigens among bacteria and pathogenic fungi is well established.[1, 7] Finally, it is important to understand that the only limitations are the availability of specific antibodies and the preservation of epitopes.[1, 8] It is well known that for larger microorganisms, such as protozoa, fungi, and some bacteria, pretreatment of formalin-fixed, paraffin-embedded tissue is not required. In contrast, for smaller infectious agents, for example, microorganisms such as viruses and chlamydiae, pretreatment of the tissue with proteolytic enzymes or heat-induced epitope retrieval is necessary in order to enhance immunoreactivity.

VIRAL INFECTIONS

Immunohistochemistry has played an important role not only in the diagnosis of a large number of viral infections but also in the study of their pathogenesis and epidemiology. Traditionally, the diagnosis of viral infections has relied on cytopathic changes observed on routine histopathologic examination. Several viral pathogens produce characteristic intracellular inclusions, which allow pathologists to make a presumptive diagnosis of viral infection. However, only 50% of the known viral diseases are associated with characteristic intracellular inclusions.[9] In addition, formalin, which is the most commonly used fixative in histopathology, is a poor fixative for demonstrating the morphologic and tinctorial features of viral inclusions.[9] When viral inclusions are not detected in hematoxylin and eosin–stained sections, or when the viral inclusions present cannot be differentiated from those of other viral diseases, immunohistochemical techniques offer a more reliable alternative to reach a specific diagnosis.

Table 20–1. Advantages of Immunohistochemistry for the Diagnosis of Infectious Diseases

Allows rapid results

Can be performed on formalin-fixed, paraffin-embedded tissue, reducing the risk of exposure to serious infectious diseases

High sensitivity, allowing identification of infectious agents even before morphologic changes occur

Useful for retrospective diagnosis of individual patients and for in-depth study of the disease

Specificity: monoclonal antibodies and some polyclonal antibodies allow for specific identification of infectious agents

Hepatitis B Virus

In many instances, the morphologic changes induced by hepatitis B virus in hepatocytes are not typical enough to render a presumptive diagnosis of hepatitis B viral infection. In other instances, there may be so little hepatitis B surface antigen (HBsAg) that it cannot be demonstrated by techniques such as orcein staining. In these cases, immunohistochemical techniques to detect HBsAg are more sensitive than histochemical methods and are helpful in reaching the diagnosis.[10] Immunostaining for HBsAg has been used in the diagnosis of hepatitis B and in the study of carrier states.[11, 12] Eighty percent or more of cases with positive serologic results for HBsAg demonstrate cytoplasmic HBsAg using immunohistochemistry[13] (Fig. 20–1). By immunoperoxidase localization, hepatitis B core antigen (HBcAg) can be demonstrated within the nuclei or the cytoplasm, of hepatocytes, or both (Fig. 20–2). A study demonstrated that predominantly cytoplasmic expression of HBcAg was associated with a higher grade of hepatitis activity.[14]

Cytomegalovirus

Cytomegalovirus (CMV) is an important opportunistic pathogen in immunocompromised patients. Histologic diagnosis of CMV in fixed tissues usually rests on the identification of characteristic cytopathic effects, including intranuclear or cytoplasmic inclusions, or both. However, histologic examination lacks sensitivity, and in some cases atypical cytopathic features can be confused with reactive or degenerative changes.[15] In these cases,

Table 20–2. Contributions of Immunohistochemistry to the Diagnosis of Infectious Diseases

Allows identification of new human pathogens

Allows microbiologic-morphologic correlation, establishing the pathogenic significance of microbiologic results

Provides a rapid morphologic diagnosis, allowing early treatment of serious infectious diseases

Contributes to understanding of the pathogenesis of infectious diseases and provides a diagnosis when fresh tissue is not available or when culture methods do not exist

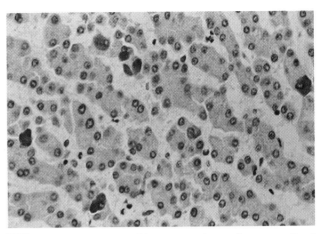

Figure 20–1. Liver biopsy specimen from a patient with chronic hepatitis B. Scattered hepatocytes show cytoplasmic reactivity with monoclonal antibody to HBsAg. (Immunoperoxidase staining with diaminobenzidine [DAB] and hematoxylin counterstain, ×400)

immunohistochemistry using monoclonal antibodies against early and late CMV antigens allows the detection of CMV antigens in the nucleus and cytoplasm of infected cells (Fig. 20–3). In addition, immunohistochemistry may allow detection of CMV antigens early in the course of the disease when cytopathic changes have not yet developed.[16–21] The sensitivity of immunohistochemistry is better than light microscopic identification of viral inclusions and compares favorably with culture and in situ hybridization.[16, 18, 19, 21, 22] Additionally, immunohistochemical assays can be completed faster than the shell vial technique, with immunofluorescence or culture allowing for rapid results that are important for early anti-CMV therapy.[21]

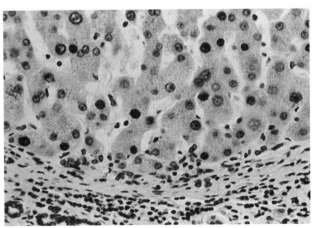

Figure 20–2. Chronic active hepatitis B. Numerous hepatocytes display intranuclear reactivity with polyclonal antibody to hepatitis B core antigen (HBcAg). (Immunoperoxidase staining with DAB and hematoxylin counterstain, ×400)

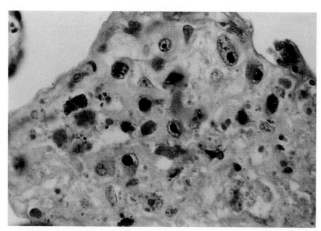

Figure 20–3. Cytomegalovirus (CMV) villitis in a case of congenital CMV infection. Stromal cells and Hofbauer cells show intranuclear and cytoplasmic CMV antigen. (Immunoperoxidase staining with diaminobenzidine [DAB] and hematoxylin counterstain, ×400)

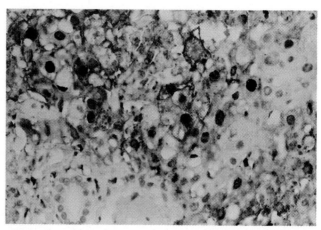

Figure 20–4. Herpes simplex hepatitis. The nuclei and cytoplasm of many hepatocytes and Kupffer cells are strongly immunostained for herpes simplex antigen. (Immunoperoxidase staining with DAB and hematoxylin counterstain, ×400)

Herpesviruses

Histologically, the diagnosis of herpes simplex virus (HSV) infection involves the detection of multinucleated giant cells containing characteristic molded, ground glass–appearing nuclei and Cowdry's type A intranuclear inclusions. When there are abundant viral inclusions within infected cells, the diagnosis is usually straightforward. However, the diagnosis of HSV infection can be difficult when the characteristic intranuclear inclusions or multinucleated cells, or both, are absent.[23] In these cases, the use of immunohistochemistry to detect HSV antigens is necessary.[24, 25] Immunohistochemistry using either polyclonal or monoclonal antibodies against HSV antigens has proved to be a sensitive and specific technique to detect HSV infections[26, 27] (Fig. 20–4). Although polyclonal antibodies against the major HSV glycoprotein antigens are sensitive, they do not allow distinction between HSV-1 and HSV-2 because these two viruses are antigenically similar.[28] In addition, the histologic features of HSV infection are not specific and can also occur in patients with varicella zoster virus (VZV) infection. Monoclonal antibodies against the VZV envelope glycoprotein gp1 are sufficiently sensitive and specific to allow a clear-cut distinction between HSV and VZV infections.[24, 29, 30]

Immunohistochemistry has also been useful in demonstrating the association of human herpes virus type 8 (HHV-8) with Kaposi's sarcoma, primary effusion lymphoma, and multicentric Castleman's disease.[31–35]

Adenoviruses

Adenovirus is increasingly recognized as a cause of morbidity and mortality among immunocompromised patients secondary to transplant and con-genital immunodeficiency.[36, 37] Rarely, adenovirus infection has been described in HIV-infected patients.[38–40] Characteristic adenovirus inclusions are amphophilic, intranuclear, homogeneous, and glassy. However, in some cases, the infection may contain only rare cells showing the characteristic cytopathic effects.[39] In addition, other viral inclusions, including CMV, human papillomavirus, HSV, and VZV, can be mistaken for adenovirus inclusions and vice versa. A monoclonal antibody that is reactive with all 41 serotypes of adenovirus has been used in an immunohistochemical technique to demonstrate intranuclear adenoviral antigen in immunocompromised patients (Fig. 20–5).[39–43]

Parvovirus B19

Parvovirus B19 has been associated with asymptomatic infections, erythema infectiosum, acute

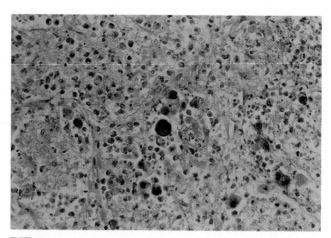

Figure 20–5. Adenovirus pneumonia. Infected cells within a necrotizing exudate show intranuclear reactivity with antibody to adenovirus antigen. (Immunoperoxidase staining with aminoethylcarbazole [AEC] and hematoxylin counterstain, ×400)

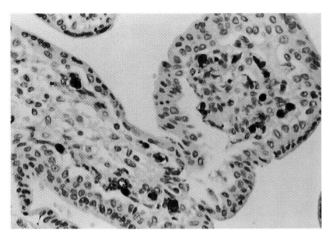

Figure 20–6. Hydrops fetalis caused by parvovirus B19 infection. Normoblasts within the villous capillaries show intranuclear viral antigen. (Immunoperoxidase staining with DAB and hematoxylin counterstain, ×600)

arthropathy, aplastic crisis, hydrops fetalis, and chronic anemia and red cell aplasia. The diagnosis of parvovirus infection can be achieved by identifying typical findings in bone marrow specimens, including decreased or absent red cell precursors, giant pronormoblasts, and eosinophilic or amphophilic intranuclear inclusions in erythroid cells.[44, 45] Because effective intravenous immunoglobulin therapy is available, a rapid and accurate diagnostic method is important. Immunohistochemistry with a monoclonal antibody against VP1 and VP2 capsid proteins has been used as a rapid and sensitive method to establish the diagnosis of parvovirus B19 infection in formalin-fixed, paraffin-embedded tissues.[46–49] Immunohistochemistry is of particular help in detecting parvovirus B19 antigen in cases with sparse inclusions, to study cases not initially identified by examination of routinely stained tissue sections, or in cases of hydrops fetalis in which there is advanced cytolysis[46, 50, 51] (Fig. 20–6). Several studies have found a good correlation between morphologic, immunohistochemical, in situ hybridization and polymerase chain reaction (PCR) studies.[45, 46, 49, 51]

Viral Hemorrhagic Fevers

Since the 1980s, numerous emerging and re-emerging agents of viral hemorrhagic fevers have attracted the attention of pathologists.[3–5] These investigators have played an important role in the identification of these agents and supporting epidemiologic, clinical, and pathogenetic studies of the emerging viral hemorrhagic fevers.[4, 5] Immunohistochemistry has improved the ability of pathologists to diagnose and study the pathogenesis of these diseases.

In 1993, several previously healthy individuals died of rapidly progressive pulmonary edema, respiratory insufficiency, and shock in the southwestern United States.[52, 53] Immunohistochemistry was central in the identification of viral antigens of a previously unknown *Hantavirus*.[54, 55] Immunohistochemical analysis was also important in identifying the occurrence of unrecognized cases of *Hantavirus* pulmonary syndrome prior to 1993 and in showing the distribution of viral antigen in endothelial cells of the microvasculature, particularly the lung.[54–56] The utility of immunohistochemistry as a sensitive and rapid diagnostic method has also been established for the diagnosis of other viral hemorrhagic fevers such as yellow fever (Fig. 20–7),[57–59] dengue hemorrhagic fever,[59, 60] Crimean-Congo hemorrhagic fever,[61] and Ebola hemorrhagic fever.[62–64]

Other Viruses

Immunohistochemistry has also proved useful in the detection of human papillomavirus (HPV) in formalin-fixed tissue using polyclonal antibodies against the viral capsid, which are highly conserved from species to species and from type to type (Fig. 20–8).[65–67] One disadvantage of immunohistochemistry is that this technique detects only productive and not latent infections and cannot be used to determine the type of virus present. In addition, immunohistochemistry has been shown to be less sensitive than in situ hybridization in detecting HPV in tissue.[65, 68, 69]

BK virus infections are frequent during infancy; in immunocompetent individuals, the virus remains latent in the kidneys, central nervous system, and B lymphocytes. In immunocompromised patients, the infection reactivates and spreads to other organs. In the kidney, the infection is associated with mononuclear interstitial inflammatory infiltrates and tubular atrophy, findings that can be difficult to distinguish from acute transplant rejection. In this setting, immunohistochemistry has

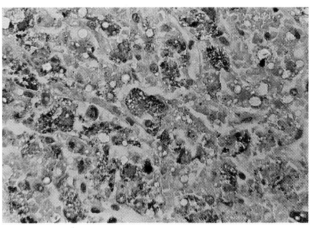

Figure 20–7. Yellow fever. Abundant yellow fever viral antigen is seen within hepatocytes and Kupffer cells. (Immunoperoxidase staining with AEC and hematoxylin counterstain, ×400) (Courtesy of Dr. JF Aronson, University of Texas Medical Branch.)

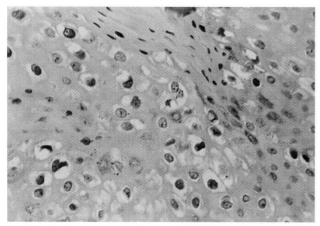

Figure 20–8. Immunoperoxidase staining for human papillomavirus (HPV) in a patient with mild squamous dysplasia. HPV viral antigen localizes within the nuclei of koilocytotic cells. (DAB with hematoxylin counterstain, ×600)

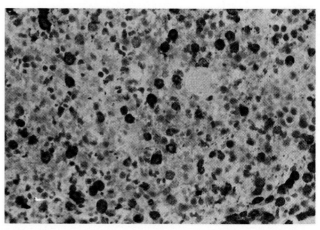

Figure 20–9. Renal transplant patient with post-transplant lymphoproliferative disorder. Immunoperoxidase staining for Epstein-Barr virus (EBV) latent membrane protein shows strong cytoplasmic immunoreactivity within several lymphocytes. (DAB with hematoxylin counterstain, ×400)

been useful to demonstrate BK virus infection.[70, 71] The human polyomavirus JC is a double-stranded DNA virus that causes progressive multifocal leukoencephalopathy (PML). Immunohistochemical technique using a polyclonal rabbit antiserum against the protein VP1 is a specific, sensitive, and rapid method for confirming the diagnosis of PML.[72–75] Immunohistochemistry has been also used to confirm the diagnosis of respiratory viral diseases such as influenza A virus and respiratory syncytial virus infections when cultures were not available.[72, 75–78] Other viral infections that can be demonstrated using immunohistochemical methods include Epstein-Barr virus (Fig. 20–9),[79] rabies virus,[5, 80, 81] enterovirus and in particular enterovirus 71,[82–86] and newer viral agents such as *Hendra* virus,[5, 87, 88] and *Nipah* virus,[5] and the emerging pathogen West Nile virus.[89, 90]

BACTERIAL INFECTIONS

Among bacterial infections, the greatest number of immunohistochemical studies have been performed in the investigation of *Helicobacter pylori*. A few studies have evaluated the use of immunohistochemistry in other bacterial, mycobacterial, rickettsial, and spirochetal infections.

Antigen retrieval is generally not required for the immunohistochemical demonstration of bacteria in fixed tissue. However, interpretation of the results can be complicated by the fact that many of these antibodies will cross-react with other bacteria. Moreover, antibodies may react with only portions of the bacteria, and they may label remnants of bacteria or spirochetes when viable organisms are no longer present.

Although *H. pylori* can be identified in gastric biopsies using hematoxylin and eosin, the detection rate is only 66%, with many false-positive and false-negative results.[91] Conventional histochemical methods such as silver stains are more sensitive than hematoxylin and eosin alone in detecting *H. pylori*. However, for the detection of scant numbers of organisms, immunohistochemistry has proved to be highly specific and sensitive, less expensive when all factors are considered, and superior to conventional histochemical methods (Fig. 20–10).[92, 93] Immunohistochemistry for detection of *H. pylori* in gastric biopsies has also been shown to improve

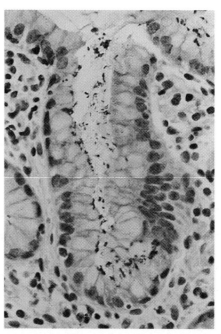

Figure 20–10. Numerous curved *Helicobacter pylori* in the superficial mucus are clearly demonstrated by immunoperoxidase staining in this patient with chronic active gastritis. (DAB with hematoxylin counterstain, ×600)

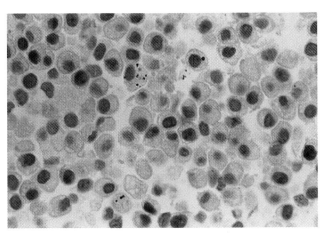

Figure 20–11. Immunoperoxidase staining of *Chlamydia pneumoniae* using a monoclonal antibody to detect elementary bodies within HeLa 229 cells. (DAB with hematoxylin counterstain, ×600)

the rate of identification of the organism after treatment even when histologic examination and cultures were falsely negative.[94-96]

In addition to *H. pylori*, other bacteria can be identified by immunohistochemistry in formalin-fixed tissue. Immunohistochemistry is useful in identifying *Haemophilus influenzae*,[97-99] *Chlamydia* species (Fig. 20–11),[100-102] *Yersinia pestis* infections,[103-105] *Legionella pneumophila* and *L. dumoffii*,[106, 107] *Listeria monocytogenes*,[108-110] *Salmonella*,[111, 112] mycobacteria,[113, 114] rickettsial infections, including life-threatening Rocky Mountain spotted fever (Fig. 20–12), boutonneuse fever, and typhus fever as well as rickettsial pox and African tick bite fever, ehrlichial infections,[115-119] and spirochetal infections, including syphilis, leptospirosis, and borreliosis.[120-124]

FUNGAL INFECTIONS

The great majority of fungi are readily identified by hematoxylin and eosin staining alone or in combination with histochemical stains (periodic acid–Schiff [PAS], Gomori's methenamine silver [GMS]) by routine histopathology. However, these stains cannot distinguish morphologically similar fungi with potentially different resistance to antimycotic drugs. In addition, fungal elements may appear atypical in tissue sections because of several factors, including steric orientation, age of the fungal lesion, effects of antifungal chemotherapy, type of infected tissue, and host immune response.[125, 126] Currently, the final identification of fungi relies on culture techniques; however, culture may take several days or longer to give a definitive result, and many times surgical pathologists have no access to fresh tissue.

In past years, immunohistochemistry has been used to identify various fungal elements in paraffin-embedded, formalin-fixed tissue.[127-129] Immu-

nohistochemical methods have the advantage of providing a rapid and specific identification of several fungi and allowing pathologists to be able to identify unusual filamentous fungal and yeast infections and accurately distinguish them from confounding artifacts.[128, 130] In addition, immunohistochemistry can allow pathologists to correlate microbiologic and histologic findings of fungal infections and distinguish them from harmless colonization. An important limitation of immunohistochemistry in the identification of fungi is the well-known, widespread occurrence of common antigens among pathogenic fungi that frequently results in cross-reactivity with the use of polyclonal antibodies and even with some monoclonal antibodies.[128, 130-132] Therefore, assessment of cross-reactivity using a panel of fungi is an important step in the evaluation of immunohistochemical methods.[128, 129]

Candida species are often stained weakly with hematoxylin and eosin, and sometimes the yeast form may be difficult to differentiate from *Histoplasma capsulatum, Cryptococcus neoformans,* and even *Pneumocystis carinii.* Polyclonal and monoclonal antibodies against *Candida* genus antigens are sensitive and strongly reactive and do not show cross-reactivity with other fungi tested.[128, 129, 133, 134]

Identification of *Cryptococcus neoformans* usually is not a problem when the fungus produces a mucicarmine-positive capsule. However, infections by capsule-negative strains are more difficult to diagnose. Polyclonal antibodies raised against *C. neoformans* yeast cells are sensitive and specific.[128, 129]

Sporothrix schenckii may be confused in tissue sections with *Blastomyces dermatitidis* and fungal agents of phaeohyphomycosis. In addition, yeast cells of *Sporothrix schenckii* may be sparsely present in tissues. Specific antibodies raised

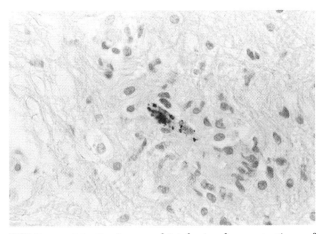

Figure 20–12. Immunohistologic demonstration of *Rickettsia rickettsii* within endothelial cells surrounded by a small glial nodule in the brainstem of this patient with fatal Rocky Mountain spotted fever. (Immunoperoxidase staining with AEC and hematoxylin counterstain, ×600)

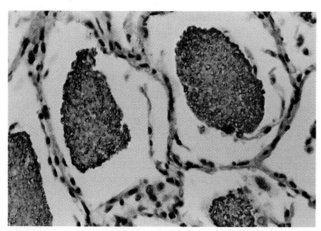

Figure 20–13. Human immunodeficiency virus (HIV)-infected immunodeficient patient with *Pneumocystis carinii* pneumonia. Cohesive aggregates of cyst forms and trophozoites within alveolar spaces are demonstrated with a monoclonal antibody against *Pneumocystis carinii* in an immunoperoxidase technique. (DAB with hematoxylin counterstain, ×400)

against yeast cells of *S. schenckii* are sensitive but demonstrate cross-reactivity with *Candida* species; however, after specific adsorption of the antibody with *Candida* yeast cells, the cross-reactivity is eliminated.[128, 129]

Polyclonal and monoclonal antibodies have been produced for the identification of *Aspergillus* species.[128, 132, 135, 136] However, in most cases, these antibodies have been found to cross-react with other fungi. Two monoclonal antibodies (164G and 611F) have been produced that react only with specifically recognized *Aspergillus fumigatus, Aspergillus flavus,* and *Aspergillus niger.*[137]

Cysts and trophozoites of *Pneumocystis carinii* can be detected in bronchoalveolar lavage specimens using monoclonal antibodies that yield results that are slightly more sensitive than GMS, Giemsa, or Papanicolaou staining for detecting cysts (Fig. 20–13).[129, 138, 139]

Immunohistochemistry has also been used to detect *Blastomyces, Coccidioides, Histoplasma*, and *Penicillium.*[128–130, 140] However, the antibodies used showed significant cross-reactivity with several other fungi.

PROTOZOAL INFECTIONS

Protozoa usually can be identified in tissue sections stained with hematoxylin and eosin or Giemsa stains; however, because of the small size of the organisms and the subtle distinguishing features, an unequivocal diagnosis cannot always be made. The role of immunohistochemistry in the detection of protozoal infections has been limited to cases in which morphology of the parasite is distorted by tissue necrosis or autolysis. In addition, in immunocompromised patients, toxo-

plasmosis can have an unusual disseminated presentation, with numerous tachyzoites without bradyzoites.[141] Immunohistochemistry has been used to identify *Cryptosporidium,*[142] *Entamoeba histolytica,*[143] *Leishmania,*[144–146] *Toxoplasma* (Fig. 20–14),[141, 147] and *Trypanosoma cruzi.*[148, 149]

PATHOLOGISTS, IMMUNOHISTOCHEMISTRY, AND BIOTERRORISM

Currently, there is an increasing concern about the use of infectious agents as potential biologic weapons. Biologic warfare agents may vary from rare exotic viruses to common bacterial agents. The Centers for Disease Control (CDC) has issued the recommendations for a complete public health response to a biologic attack.[150–152] Two important components of this response plan include the rapid detection, diagnosis, and characterization of biologic agents. Pathologists using newer diagnostic techniques such as immunohistochemistry, in situ hybridization, and PCR will have a direct impact on the rapid detection and control of emerging infectious diseases from natural or intentional causes. Currently, the CDC has developed immunohistochemical methods using polyclonal or monoclonal antibodies for most of the potential biologic warfare agents, including antibodies to the causative agents of anthrax,[5, 153] brucellosis,[5] plague,[5, 103–105] Q fever,[5, 115, 154, 155] tularemia,[5] viral encephalitides,[5, 156, 157] and viral hemorrhagic fevers.[5] Immunohistochemistry provides a simple, sensitive, and specific method for the rapid detection, either at the time of investigation or retrospectively, of biologic threats, facilitating the rapid implementation of effective public health responses.

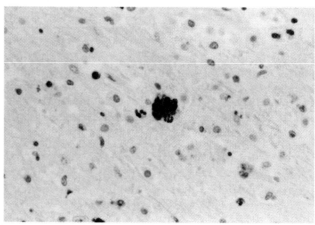

Figure 20–14. HIV-infected patient with toxoplasmic encephalitis. Immunoperoxidase highlights pseudocysts and scattered tachyzoites. (DAB with hematoxylin counterstain, ×400).

References

1. Cartun RW. Use of immunohistochemistry in the surgical pathology laboratory for the diagnosis of infectious diseases. Pathol Case Rev 1999;4:260–265.
2. Watts JC. Surgical pathology in the diagnosis of infectious diseases. [editorial] Am J Clin Pathol 1994;102:711–712.
3. Schwartz DA, Bryan RT. Infectious disease pathology and emerging infections: Are we prepared? Arch Pathol Lab Med 1996;120:117–124.
4. Schwartz DA. Emerging and reemerging infections: Progress and challenges in the subspecialty of infectious disease pathology. Arch Pathol Lab Med 1997;121:776–784.
5. Zaki SR, Paddock CD. The emerging role of pathology in infectious diseases. In: Scheld WM, Armonstrong D, Hughes JM, eds. Emerging Infections vol. 3. Washington, DC: ASM Press, 1999:181–200.
6. Coons AH, Creech HJ, Jone RN, et al. The demonstration of pneumococcal antigen in tissues by use of fluorescent antibodies. J Immunol 1942;45:159–170.
7. Jeavons L, Hunt L, Hamilton A. Immunochemical studies of heat-shock protein 80 of *Histoplasma capsulatum*. J Med Vet Mycol 1994;32:47–57.
8. Werner M, Chott A, Fabiano A, Battifora H. Effect of formalin tissue fixation and processing on immunohistochemistry. Am J Surg Pathol 2000;24:1016–1019.
9. Chandler FW. Invasive microorganisms. In: Spicer SS (ed). Histochemistry in Pathology Diagnosis. New York: Marcel Dekker, 1987:77–101.
10. Clausen PP, Thomsen P. Demonstration of hepatitis B surface antigen in liver biopsies: A comparative investigation of immunoperoxidase and orcein staining on identical sections on formalin-fixed, paraffin-embedded tissue. Acta Pathol Microbiol Scand [A] 1978;86A:383.
11. Thomsen P, Clausen PP. Occurrence of Hepatitis B surface antigen in a consecutive material of 1539 liver biopsies. Acta Pathol Microbiol Immunol Scand [A] 1983;91:71.
12. Al Adnani MS, Ali SM. Patterns of chronic liver disease in Kuwait with special reference to localization of hepatitis B surface antigen. J Clin Pathol 1984;37:549.
13. Taylor CR. Lung, pancreas, colon and rectum, stomach, liver. In: Taylor CR, Cote RJ, eds. Immunomicroscopy: A Diagnostic Tool for the Surgical Pathologist. Philadelphia: WB Saunders, 1994.
14. Park YN, Han KH, Kim KS, et al. Cytoplasmic expression of hepatitis B core antigen in chronic hepatitis B virus infection: Role of precore stop mutants. Liver 1999;19:199–205.
15. Anwar F, Erice A, Jessurun J. Are there cytopathic features associated with cytomegalovirus infection predictive of resistance to antiviral therapy? Ann Diagn Pathol 1999;3:19–22.
16. Sheehan MM, Coker R, Coleman DV. Detection of cytomegalovirus (CMV) in HIV+ patients: Comparison of cytomorphology, immunohistochemistry and in situ hybridization. Cytopathalogy 1998;9:29–37.
17. Kutza AS, Muhl E, Hackstein H, et al. High incidence of active cytomegalovirus infection among septic patients. Clin Infect Dis 1998;26:1076–1082.
18. Saetta A, Agapitos E, Davaris PS. Determination of CMV placentitis: Diagnostic application of the polymerase chain reaction. Virchows Arch 1998;432:159–162.
19. Solans EP, Yong S, Husain AN, et al. Bronchioalveolar lavage in the diagnosis of CMV pneumonitis in lung transplant recipients: An immunocytochemical study. Diagn Cytopathol 1997;16:350–352.
20. Nebuloni M, Pellegrinelli A, Ferri A, et al. Etiology of microglial nodules in brains of patients with acquired immunodeficiency syndrome. J Neurovirol 2000;6:46–50.
21. Rimsza LM, Vela EE, Frutiger YM, et al. Rapid automated combined in situ hybridization and immunohistochemistry for sensitive detection of cytomegalovirus in paraffin-embedded tissue biopsies. Am J Clin Pathol 1996;106:544–548.
22. Colina F, Juca NT, Moreno E, et al. Histological diagnosis of cytomegalovirus hepatitis in liver allografts. J Clin Pathol 1995;48:351–357.
23. Feiden W, Borchard F, Burrig KF, et al. Herpes esophagitis. I: Light microscopical immunohistochemical investigations. Virchows Arch A Pathol Anat Histopathol 1984;404:167–176.
24. Nikkels AF, Delvenne P, Sadzot-Delvaux C, et al. Distribution of varicella zoster virus and herpes simplex virus in disseminated fatal infections. J Clin Pathol 1996;49:243–248.
25. Greenson JK, Beschorner WE, Boitnott JK, et al. Prominent mononuclear cell infiltrate is characteristic of herpes esophagitis. Hum Pathol 1991;22:541–549.
26. Wang JY, Montone KT. A rapid simple in situ hybridization method for herpes simplex virus employing a synthetic biotin-labeled oligonucleotid probe: A comparison with immunohistochemical methods for HSV detection. J Clin Lab Anal 1994;8:105–115.
27. Kobayashi TK, Ueda M, Nishino T, et al. Brush cytology of herpes simplex virus infection in oral mucosa: Use of the ThinPrep processor. Diagn Cytopathol 1998;18:71–75.
28. Nicoll JAR, Love S, Burton PA, et al. Autopsy findings in two cases of neonatal herpes simplex virus infection: Detection of virus by immunohistochemistry, in situ hybridization and the polymerase chain reaction. Histopathology 1994;24:257–264.
29. Nikkels AF, Debrus S, Sadzot-Delvaux C, et al. Comparative immunohistochemical study of herpes simplex and varicella zoster infections. Virchows Arch A Pathol Anat Histopathol 1993;422:121–126.
30. Cohen PR. Tests for detecting herpes simplex virus and varicella zoster virus infections. Dermatol Clin 1994;12:51–68.
31. Katano H, Sato Y, Kurata T, et al. Expression and localization of human herpesvirus 8–encoded proteins in primary effusion lymphoma, Kaposi's sarcoma, and multicentric Castleman's disease. Virology 2000;269:335–344.
32. Katano H, Suda T, Morishita Y, et al. Human herpesvirus 8–associated solid lymphomas that occur in AIDS patients takes anaplastic large cell morphology. Mod Pathol 2000;13:77–85.
33. Ely SA, Powers J, Lewis D, et al. Kaposi's sarcoma–associated herpesvirus-positive primary effusion lymphoma arising in the subarachnoid space. Hum Pathol 1999;30:981–984.
34. Katano H, Sato Y, Kurata T, et al. High expression of HHV-8–encoded ORF73 protein in spindle-shaped cells of Kaposi's sarcoma. Am J Pathol 1999;155:47–52.
35. Said JW, Shintaku IP, Asou H, et al. Herpesvirus 8 inclusions in primary effusion lymphoma: Report of a unique case with T-cell phenotype. Arch Pathol Lab Med 1999;123:257–260.
36. Flomenberg P, Babbitt J, Drobyski WR, et al. Increasing incidence of adenovirus disease in bone marrow transplant recipients. J Infect Dis 1994;169:775–781.
37. Strickler JG, Singleton TP, Copenhaver GM, et al. Adenovirus in the gastrointestinal tracts of immunosuppressed patients. Am J Clin Pathol 1992;97:555–558.
38. Yi ES, Powell HC. Adenovirus infection of the duodenum in an AIDS patient: An ultrastructural study. Ultrastruct Pathol 1994;18:549–551.
39. Yan Z, Nguyen S, Poles M, et al. Adenovirus colitis in human immunodeficiency virus infection: An underdiagnosed entity. Am J Surg Pathol 1998;22:1101–1106.
40. Dombrowski F, Eis-Hubinger AM, Ackermann T, et al. Adenovirus-induced liver necrosis in a case of AIDS. Virchows Arch 1997;431:469–472.
41. Simsir A, Greenebaum E, Nuovo G, et al. Late fatal adenovirus pneumonitis in a lung transplant recipient. Transplantation 1998;65:592–594.
42. Saad RS, Demetris AJ, Lee RG, et al. Adenovirus hepatitis in the adult allograft liver. Transplantation 1997;64:1483–1485.
43. Ohori NP, Michaels MG, Jaffe R, et al. Adenovirus pneu-

monia in lung transplant recipients. Hum Pathol 1995;26: 1073–1079.

44. Brown KE, Young NS. Parvovirus B19 infection and hematopoiesis. Blood Rev 1995;9:176–182.

45. Jordan JA, Penchansky L. Diagnosis of human parvovirus B19–induced anemia: Correlation of bone marrow morphology with molecular diagnosis using PCR and immunohistochemistry. Cell Vision 1995;2:279–282.

46. Morey AL, O'Neil HJ, Coyle PV, et al. Immunohistological detection of human parvovirus B19 in formalin-fixed, paraffin-embedded tissues. J Pathol 1992;166:108.

47. Puvion-Dutilleul F, Puvion E. Human parvovirus B19 as a causative agent for rheumatoid arthritis. Proc Nat Acad Sci U S A 1998;95:8227–8232.

48. Yufu Y, Matsumoto M, Miyamura T, et al. Parvovirus B19–associated haemophagocytic syndrome with lymphadenopathy resembling histiocytic necrotizing lymphadenitis (Kikuchi's disease). Br J Haematol 1997;96:868–871.

49. Vadlamudi G, Rezuke N, Ross JW, et al. The use of monoclonal antibody R92F6 and polymerase chain reaction to confirm the presence of parvovirus B19 in bone marrow specimens of patients with acquired immunodeficiency syndrome. Arch Pathol Lab Med 1999;123:768–773.

50. Wright C, Hinchliffe SA, Taylor C. Fetal pathology in intrauterine death due to parvovirus B19 infection. Br J Obstet Gynaecol 1996;103:133–136.

51. Essary LR, Vnencak-Jones CL, Manning SS, et al. Frequency of parvovirus B19 infection in nonimmune hydrops fetalis and utility of three diagnostic methods. Hum Pathol 1998;29:696–701.

52. Khan AS, Khabbaz RF, Armstrong RC, et al. Hantavirus pulmonary syndrome: The first 100 US cases. J Infect Dis 1996;173:1297–1303.

53. Moolenaar RL, Dalton C, Lipman HB, et al. Clinical features that differentiate hantavirus pulmonary syndrome from three other acute respiratory illnesses. Clin Infect Dis 1995;21:643–649.

54. Nolte KB, Feddersen RM, Foucar K, et al. Hantavirus pulmonary syndrome in the United States: A pathological description of a disease caused by a new agent. Hum Pathol 1995;26:110–120.

55. Zaki SR, Greer PW, Coffield LM, et al. Hantavirus pulmonary syndrome: Pathogenesis of an emerging infectious disease. Am J Pathol 1995;146:552–579.

56. Zaki SR, Khan AS, Goodman RA, et al. Retrospective diagnosis of hantavirus pulmonary syndrome, 1978–1993: Implications for emerging infectious diseases. Arch Pathol Lab Med 1996;120:134–139.

57. Monath TP, Ballinger ME, Miller BR, et al. Detection of yellow fever viral RNA by nucleic acid hybridization and viral antigen by immunohistochemistry in fixed human liver. Am J Trop Med Hyg 1989;40:663–668.

58. De Brito T, Siqueira SA, Santos RT, et al. Human fatal yellow fever: Immunohistochemical detection of viral antigens in the liver, kidney, and heart. Pathol Res Pract 1992; 188:177–181.

59. Hall WC, Crowell TP, Watts DM, et al. Demonstration of yellow fever and dengue antigens in formalin-fixed paraffin-embedded human liver by immunohistochemical analysis. Am J Trop Med Hyg 1991;45:408–417.

60. Ramos C, Sanchez G, Pando RH, et al. Dengue virus in the brain of a fatal case of hemorrhagic dengue fever. J Neurovirol 1998;4:465–468.

61. Burt FJ, Swanepoel R, Shieh W-J, et al. Immunohistochemical and in situ localization of Crimea-Congo hemorrhagic fever (CCHF) virus in human tissues and implications for CCHF pathogenesis. Arch Pathol Lab Med 1997;121:839–846.

62. Ksiazek TG, Rollin PE, Williams AJ, et al. Clinical virology of Ebola hemorrhagic fever (EHF): Virus, virus antigen, and IgG and IgM antibody findings among EHF patients in Kikwit, Democratic Republic of Congo. J Infect Dis 1999; 179:S177–S187.

63. Wyers M, Formenty P, Cherel Y, et al. Histopathological and immunohistochemical studies of lesions associated with Ebola virus in a naturally infected chimpanzee. J Infect Dis 1999;179:S54–S59.

64. Zaki SR, Shieh W-J, Greer PW, et al. A novel immunohistochemical assay for the detection of Ebola virus in skin: Implications for diagnosis, spread, and surveillance of Ebola hemorrhagic fever. J Infect Dis 1999;179:S36–S37.

65. Delvenne P, Fontaine M-A, Delvenne C, et al. Detection of human papillomaviruses in paraffin-embedded biopsies of cervical intraepithelial lesions: Analysis by immunohistochemistry, in situ hybridization, and the polymerase chain reaction. Mod Pathol 1994;7:113–119.

66. Lopez-Beltran A, Escudero AL, Carrasco-Aznar JC, et al. Human papillomavirus infection and transitional cell carcinoma of the bladder: Immunohistochemistry and in situ hybridization. Pathol Res Pract 1996;192:154–159.

67. Wools K, Bryan JT, Katz BP, et al. Detection of human papillomavirus L1 protein in condylomata acuminata from various anatomical sites. Sex Transm Dis 1994;21:103–106.

68. Meyer MP, Markiw CA, Matuscak RR, et al. Detection of human papillomavirus DNA in genital lesions by using a modified commercially available in situ hybridization assay. J Clin Microbiol 1991;29:1308.

69. Wilbur DC, Reichman RC, Stoler MH. Detection of infection by human papillomavirus in genital condyloma: A comparison study using immunohistochemistry and in situ nucleic acid hybridization. Am J Clin Pathol 1988;89:505.

70. Pappo O, Demetris AI, Raikow RB, et al. Human polyomavirus infection of renal allografts: Histopathologic diagnosis, clinical significance and literature review. Mod Pathol 1996;9:105–109.

71. Nebuloni M, Tosoni A, Boldorini R, et al. BK virus renal infection in a patient with the acquired immunodeficiency syndrome. Arch Pathol Lab Med 1999;123:807–811.

72. Jochum W, Weber T, Frye S, et al. Detection of JC virus by anti-VP1 immunohistochemistry in brains with progressive multifocal leukoencephalopathy. Acta Neuropathol 1997; 94:226–231.

73. Aoki N, Mori M, Kato K, et al. Antibody against synthetic multiple antigen peptides (MAP) of JC virus capsid protein (VP1) without cross reaction to BK virus: A diagnostic tool for progressive multifocal leukoencephalopathy. Neuroscience Lett 1996;205:111–114.

74. Silver SA, Arthur RR, Rozan YS, et al. Diagnosis of progressive multifocal leukoencephalopathy by stereotactic brain biopsy utilizing immunohistochemistry and the polymerase chain reaction. Acta Cytol 1995;39:35–44.

75. Guarner J, Shieh W-J, Dawson J, et al. Immunohistochemical and in situ hybridization studies of influenza A virus infection in human lungs. Am J Clin Pathol 2000;114:227–233.

76. Cartun RW, Tahhan HR, Knibbs DR, et al. Immunocytochemical identification of respiratory syncytial virus (RSV) in formalin-fixed, paraffin-embedded tissue from immunocompromised hosts. Mod Pathol 1989;2:15.

77. Nielson KA, Yunis EJ. Demonstration of respiratory syncytial virus in an autopsy series. Pediatr Pathol 1990;10:491–502.

78. Wright C, Oliver KC, Fenwick FI, et al. A monoclonal antibody pool for routine immunohistochemical detection of human respiratory syncytial virus antigens in formalin-fixed, paraffin-embedded tissue. J Pathol 1997;182:238–244.

79. Lones MA, Shintaku IP, Weiss LM, et al. Posttransplant lymphoproliferative disorder in liver allograft biopsies: A comparison of three methods for the demonstration of Epstein-Barr virus. Hum Pathol 1997;28:533–539.

80. Sinchaisri TA, Nagata T, Yoshikawa Y, et al. Immunohistochemical and histopathological study of experimental rabies infection in mice. J Vet Med Sci 1992;54:409–416.

81. Jackson AC, Ye H, Phelan CC, et al. Extraneural organ involvement in human rabies. Lab Invest 1999;79:945–951.

82. Yousef GE, Mann GF, Brown IN, et al. Clinical and re-

search application of an enterovirus group—reactive monoclonal antibody. Intervirology 1987;28:199—205.

83. Hohenadl C, Klingel K, Rieger P, et al. Investigation of the coxsackievirus B3 nonstructural proteins 2B, 2C, and 3AB: A generation of specific polyclonal antisera and detection of replicating virus in infected tissue. J Virol Methods 1994;47:279—295.

84. Zhang H, Li Y, Peng T, et al. Localization of enteroviral antigen in myocardium and other tissues from patients with heart muscle disease by an improved immunohistochemical technique. J Histochem Cytochem 2000;48:579—584.

85. Li Y, Bourlet T, Andreoletti L, et al. Enteroviral capsid protein VP1 is present in myocardial tissues from some patients with myocarditis or dilated cardiomyopathy. Circulation 2000;101:231—234.

86. Wong KT, Chua KB, Lam SK. Immunohistochemical detection of infected neurons as a rapid diagnosis of enterovirus 71 encephalomyelitis. Ann Neurol 1999;45:271—272.

87. Hooper PT, Russell GM, Selleck PW, et al. Immunohistochemistry in the identification of a number of new diseases in Australia. Vet Microbiol 1999;68:89—93.

88. Williamson MM, Hooper PT, Selleck PW, et al. Experimental hendra virus infection in pregnant guinea-pigs and fruit bats *(Pteropus poliocephalus)*. J Comp Pathol 2000; 122:201—207.

89. Sampson BA, Ambrosi C, Charlot A, et al. The pathology of human West Nile virus infection. Hum Pathol 2000;31: 527—531.

90. Steele KE, Linn MJ, Schoepp RJ, et al. Pathology of fatal West Nile virus infections in native and exotic birds during the 1999 outbreak in New York City, New York. Vet Pathol 2000;37:208—224.

91. El-Zimaity HMT, Graham DY, Al-Assis MT, et al. Interobserver variation in the histopathological assessment of *Helicobacter pylori* gastritis. Hum Pathol 1996;27:35—41.

92. Barbosa AJ, Queiros DMM, Mendes EN, et al. Immunocytochemical identification of *Campylobacter pylori* in gastritis and correlation with culture. Arch Pathol Lab Med 1988;11:288—291.

93. Toulaymant M, Marconi S, Garb J, et al. Endoscopic biopsy pathology of *Helicobacter pylori* gastritis. Arch Pathol Lab Med 1999;123:778—781.

94. Marcio L, Angelucci D, Grossi L, et al. Anti—*Helicobacter pylori*—specific antibody immunohistochemistry improves the diagnostic accuracy of *Helicobacter pylori* in biopsy specimens from patients treated with triple therapy. Am J Gastroenterol 1998;93:223—226.

95. Tokunaga Y, Shirahase H, Yamamoto E, et al. Semiquantitative evaluation for diagnosis of *Helicobacter pylori* infection in relation to histological changes. Am J Gastroenterol 1998;93:26—29.

96. Chan WY, Hui PK, Leung KM, et al. Coccoid forms of *Helicobacter pylori* in the human stomach. Am J Clin Pathol 1994;102:503—507.

97. Terpstra WJ, Groeneveld K, Eijk PP, et al. Comparison of two nonculture techniques for detection of *Hemophilus influenzae* in sputum: In situ hybridization and immunoperoxidase staining with monoclonal antibodies. Chest 1988;94:126S.

98. Groeneveld K, van Alphen L, van Ketel RJ, et al. Nonculture detection of *Haemophilus influenzae* in sputum with monoclonal antibodies specific for outer membrane lipoprotein P6. J Clin Microbiol 1989;27:2263.

99. Forsgren J, Samuelson A, Borrelli S, et al. Persistence of nontypeable *Haemophilus influenzae* in adenoid macrophages: A putative colonization mechanism. Acta Otolaryngol 1996;116:766—773.

100. Shurbaji MS, Dumler JS, Gage WR, et al. Immunohistochemical detection of chlamydial antigens in association with cystitis. Am J Pathol 1990;93:363.

101. Paukku M, Puolakkainen M, Paavonen T, et al. Plasma cell endometritis is associated with *Chlamydia trachomatis* infection. Am J Clin Pathol 1999;112:211—215.

102. Naas J, Gnarpe JA. Demonstration of *Chlamydia pneumo*-*niae* in tissue by immunohistochemistry. APMIS 1999;107: 882—886.

103. Davis KJ, Vogel P, Fritz DL, et al. Bacterial filamentation of *Yersinia pestis* by β-lactam antibiotics in experimentally infected mice. Arch Pathol Lab Med 1997;121:865—868.

104. Davis KJ, Fritz DL, Pitt ML, et al. Pathology of experimental pneumonic plague produced by fraction 1—positive and fraction 1—negative *Yersinia pestis* in African green monkeys *(Cercopithecus aethiops)*. Arch Pathol Lab Med 1996; 120:156—163.

105. Williams ES, Mills K, Kwiatkowski DR, et al. Plague in black-footed ferret *(Mustela nigripes)*. J Wild Dis 1994;30: 581—585.

106. Suffin SC, Kaufmann AF, Whitaker B, et al. *Legionella pneumophila*: Identification in tissue sections by a new immunoenzymatic procedure. Arch Pathol Lab Med 1980; 104:283—286.

107. Maruta K, Miyamoto H, Hamada T, et al. Entry and intracellular growth of *Legionella dumoffii* in alveolar epithelial cells. Am J Respir Crit Care Med 1998;157:1967—1974.

108. Parkash V, Morotti RA, Joshi V, et al. Immunohistochemical detection of *Listeria* antigens in the placenta in perinatal listeriosis. Int J Gynecol Pathol 1998;17:343—350.

109. Chiba M, Fukushima T, Koganei K, et al. *Listeria monocytogenes* in the colon in a case of fulminant ulcerative colitis. Scand J Gastroenterol 1998;33:778—782.

110. Weinstock D, Horton SB, Rowland PH. Rapid diagnosis of *Listeria monocytogenes* by immunohistochemistry in formalin-fixed brain tissue. Vet Pathol 1995;32:193—195.

111. Pospischil A, Wood RL, Anderson TD. Peroxidase-antiperoxidase and immunogold labeling of *Salmonella typhimurium* and *Salmonella cholerasuis* var *kunzendorf* in tissues of experimentally infected swine. Am J Vet Res 1990;51: 619—624.

112. Thygesen P, Martinsen C, Hougen HP, et al. Histologic, cytologic, and bacteriologic examination of experimentally induced *Salmonella typhimurium* infection in Lewis rats. Comp Med 2000;50:124—132.

113. Carabias E, Palenque R, Serrano JM, et al. Evaluation of an immunohistochemical test with polyclonal antibodies raised against mycobacteria used in formalin-fixed tissue compared with mycobacterial-specific culture. APMIS 1998;106:385—388.

114. Kim KM, Lee A, Choi KY, et al. Intestinal tuberculosis: Clinicopathologic analysis and diagnosis by endoscopic biopsy. Am J Gastroenterol 1998;93:606—609.

115. Dumler JS, Walker DH. Diagnostic tests for Rocky Mountain spotted fever and other rickettsial diseases. Dermatol Clin 1994;12:25—36.

116. White WL, Patrick JD, Miller LR, et al. Evaluation of immunoperoxidase techniques to detect *Rickettsia rickettsii* in fixed tissue sections. Am J Clin Pathol 1994;101:747—752.

117. Procop GW, Burchette JL Jr, Howell DN, et al. Immunoperoxidase and immunofluorescent staining of *Rickettsia rickettsii* in skin biopsies. Arch Pathol Lab Med 1997;121: 894—899.

118. Paddock CD, Greer PW, Ferebee TL, et al. Hidden mortality attributable to Rocky Mountain spotted fever: Immunohistochemical detection of fatal, serologically unconfirmed disease. J Infect Dis 1999;179:1469—1476.

119. Ripoll CM, Romondegui CE, Ordonez G, et al. Evidence of rickettsial spotted fever and ehrlichial infections in a subtropical territory of Jujuy Argentina. Am J Trop Med Hyg 1999;61:350—354.

120. Chung KY, Lee MG, Chon CY, et al. Syphilitic gastritis: Demonstration of *Treponema pallidum* with the use of fluorescent treponemal antibody absorption complement and immunoperoxidase stains. J Am Acad Dermatol 1989; 21:183—185.

121. Guarner J, Greer PW, Bartlett J, et al. Congenital syphilis in a newborn: An immunopathologic study. Mod Pathol 1999;12:82—87.

122. Trevejo RT, Rigau-Perez JG, Ashford DA, et al. Epidemic

leptospirosis associated with pulmonary hemorrhage—Nicaragua, 1995. J Infect Dis 1998;178:1457–1463.

123. Lebech A-M, Clemmensen O, Hanse O. Comparison of in vitro culture, immunohistochemical staining, and PCR for detection of *Borrelia burgdorferi* in tissue from experimentally infected animals. J Clin Microbiol 1995;33:2328–2333.

124. Aberer E, Kersten A, Klade H, et al. Heterogeneity of *Borrelia burgdorferi* in the skin. Am J Dermpathol 1996;18:571–579.

125. Schwarz J. The diagnosis of deep mycoses by morphological methods. Hum Pathol 1982;13:519–533.

126. Jensen HE, Schonhyeder H. Immunofluorescent staining of hyphae in the histopathological diagnosis of mycosis in cattle. J Med Vet Mycol 1989;27:33–44.

127. Marques MEA, Coelho KIR, Bacchi CE. Comparison between histochemical and immunohistochemical methods for the diagnosis of sporotrichosis. J Clin Pathol 1992;45:1089–1093.

128. Reed JA, Hemaan BA, Alexander JL, et al. Immunomycology: Rapid and specific immunocytochemical identification of fungi in formalin-fixed, paraffin-embedded material. J Histochem Cytochem 1993;41:1217–1221.

129. Jensen HE, Schonhyeder H, Hotchi M, et al. Diagnosis of systemic mycosis by specific immunohistochemical tests. APMIS 1996;104:241–258.

130. Cooper CR, McGinnis MR. Pathology of *Penicillium marneffei*: an emerging acquired immunodeficiency syndrome–related pathogen. Arch Lab Pathol Med 1997;121:798–804.

131. Kauffman L. Immunohistologic diagnosis of systemic mycosis: An update. Eur J Epidemiol 1992;8:377–382.

132. Verweij PE, Smedts F, Poot T. Immunoperoxidase staining for identification of *Aspergillus* species in routinely processed tissue sections. J Clin Pathol 1996;49:798–801.

133. Breier F, Oesterreicher C, Brugger S, et al. Immunohistochemistry with monoclonal antibody against *Candida albicans* mannan antigen demonstrates cutaneous *Candida* granulomas as evidence of *Candida* sepsis in an immunosuppressed host. Dermatology 1997;194:293–296.

134. Marcilla A, Monteagudo C, Mormeneo S, et al. Monoclonal antibody 3H8: A useful tool in the diagnosis of candidiasis. Microbiology 1999;145:695–701.

135. Fratamico PM, Long WK, Buckley HR. Production and characterization of monoclonal antibodies to a 58-kilodalton antigen of *Aspergillus fumigatus*. Infect Immun 1991;59:316–322.

136. Stryer D, Sarfati J, Goris A, et al. Rat monoclonal antibodies against *Aspergillus* galactomannan. Infect Immun 1992;60:2237–2245.

137. Fenelon LE, Hamilton AJ, Figueroa JI, et al. Production of specific monoclonal antibodies to *Aspergillus* species and their use in immunohistochemical identification of aspergillosis. J Clin Microbiol 1999;37:1221–1223.

138. Wazir JE, Brown I, Martin-Bates E, et al. EB9, a new antibody for the detection of trophozoites of *Pneumocystis carinii* in bronchoalveolar lavage specimens in AIDS. J Clin Pathol 1994;47:1108–1111.

139. Wazir JE, Macrorie SG, Coleman DV. Evaluation of the sensitivity, specificity, and predictive value of monoclonal antibody 3F6 for the detection of *Pneumocystis carinii* pneumonia in bronchoalveolar lavage specimens and induced sputum. Cytopathology 1994;5:82–89.

140. Burke DG, Emancipator SN, Smith MC, et al. Histoplasmosis and kidney disease in patients with AIDS. Clin Infect Dis 1997;25:281–284.

141. Arnold SJ, Kinney MC, McCormick MS, et al. Disseminated toxoplasmosis: Unusual presentations in the immunocompromised host. Arch Pathol Lab Med 1997;121:869–873.

142. Bonnin A, Petrella T, Dubremetz JF, et al. Histopathologic methods for diagnosis of cryptosporidiosis using monoclonal antibodies. Eur J Clin Microbiol Infect Dis 1990;9:664–665.

143. Perez de Suarez E, Perez-Schael I, Perozo-Ruggeri G, et al. Immunocytochemical detection of *Entamoeba histolytica*. Trans R Soc Trop Med Hyg 1987;81:624–626.

144. Azadeh B, Sells PG, Ejeckman GC, et al. Localized *Leishmania* lymphadenitis: Immunohistochemical studies. Am J Clin Pathol 1994;102:11–15.

145. Kenner JR, Aronson NE, Bratthauer GL, et al. Immunohistochemistry to identify *Leishmania* parasites in fixed tissues. J Cutan Pathol 1999;26:130–136.

146. Amato VS, Duarte MIS, Nicodemo AC, et al. An evaluation of clinical, serologic, anatomopathologic and immunohistochemical findings for fifteen patients with mucosal leishmaniasis before and after treatment. Rev Inst Med Trop Sao Paulo 1998;40:23–30.

147. Warnke C, Tuazon CU, Kovacs A, et al. *Toxoplasma* encephalitis in patients with acquired immunodeficiency syndrome: Diagnosis and response to therapy. Am J Trop Med Hyg 1987;36:509.

148. Anez N, Carrasco H, Parada H, et al. Myocardial parasite persistence in chronic chagasic patients. Am J Trop Med Hyg 1999;60:726–732.

149. Reis MM, Higuchi M de L, Benvenuti LA, et al. An in situ quantitative immunohistochemical study of cytokines and IL-2R+ in chronic human chagasic myocarditis: Correlation with the presence of myocardial *Trypanosoma cruzi* antigens. Clin Immun Immunopath 1997;83:165–172.

150. Inglesby TV, O'Toole T, Henderson DA. Preventing the use of biological weapons: Improving response should prevention fail. Clin Infect Dis 2000;30:926–929.

151. Lillibridge SR, Bell AJ, Roman RS. Thoughts for the new millennium: Bioterrorism: Centers for Disease Control and prevention bioterrorism preparedness and response. Am J Infect Control 1999;27:463–464.

152. Franz DR, Zajtchuk R. Biological terrorism: Understanding the threat, preparation, and medical response. Dis Month 2000;46:125–190.

153. Ezzell JW, Abshire TG, Little SF, et al. Identification of *Bacillus anthracis* by using monoclonal antibodies to cell wall galactose-*N*-acetylglucosamine polysaccharide. J Clin Microbiol 1990;28:223–231.

154. van Moll P, Baumgartner W, Eskens U, et al. Immunocytochemical demonstration of *Coxiella burnetii* antigen in the fetal placenta of naturally infected sheep and cattle. J Comp Pathol 1993;109:295–301.

155. Brouqui P, Dumler JS, Raoult D. Immunohistologic demonstration of *Coxiella burnetii* in the valves of patients with Q fever endocarditis. Am J Med 1994;97:451–458.

156. Patterson JS, Maes RK, Mullaney TP, et al. Immunohistochemical diagnosis of eastern equine encephalomyelitis. J Vet Diag Invest 1996;8:156–160.

157. Garen PD, Tsai TF, Powers JM. Human eastern equine encephalitis: Immunohistochemistry and ultrastructure. Mod Pathol 1999;12:646–652.

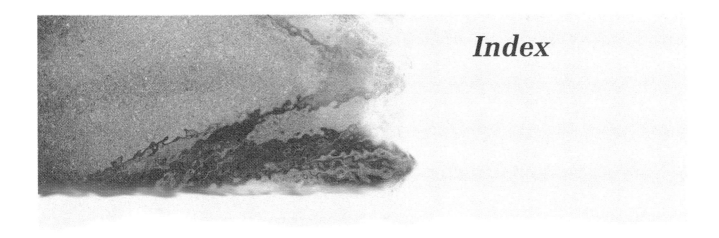

Index

Note: Page numbers followed by the letter f refer to figures and those followed by t refer to tables.